10/98

ESSENTIALS OF
Medical
Microbiology

FIFTH EDITION

ESSENTIALS OF
Medical
Microbiology
FIFTH EDITION

WESLEY A. VOLK, PhD
Professor Emeritus of Microbiology
University of Virginia School of Medicine
Charlottesville, Virginia

BRYAN M. GEBHARDT, PhD
Professor of Ophthalmology and Microbiology
Louisiana State University Eye Center
New Orleans, Louisiana

MARIE-LOUISE HAMMARSKJÖLD, MD, PhD
Associate Director
Myles H. Thaler Center for AIDS and Human Retrovirus Research
University of Virginia Medical Center
Charlottesville, Virginia

ROBERT J. KADNER, PhD
Professor of Microbiology
University of Virginia School of Medicine
Charlottesville, Virginia

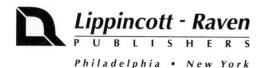
Lippincott - Raven
P U B L I S H E R S
Philadelphia • New York

Acquisitions Editor: Rich Winters
Assistant Editor: Mary Beth Murphy
Project Editor: Bridget H. Meyer
Production Manager: Caren Erlichman
Production Coordinator: David Yurkovich
Senior Design Coordinator: Kathy Kelley-Luedtke
Indexer: Maria Coughlin
Compositor: Bi-Comp, Incorporated
Printer/Binder: Courier Book Company/Kendallville

Library of Congress Cataloging-in-Publication Data

Essentials of medical microbiology / Wesley A. Volk ... [et al.]. —
   5th ed.
       p. cm.
    Includes bibliographical references and index.
    ISBN 0-397-51308-9 (alk. paper)
    1. Medical microbiology.   I. Volk, Wesley A.
    [DNLM: 1. Microbiology.   QW 4 E78 1995]
  QR46.V64   1995
  616'.01—dc20
  DNLM/DLC
  for Library of Congress   95-16385
                                                           CIP

The material contained in this volume was submitted as
previously unpublished material, except in the instances in which
credit has been given to the source from which some of the
illustrative material was derived.

Great care has been taken to maintain the accuracy of the
information contained in the volume. However, neither
Lippincott–Raven Publishers nor the editors can be held responsible
for errors or for any consequences arising from the use of the
information herein.

The authors and publisher have exerted every effort to ensure
that drug selection and dosage set forth in this text are in accord
with current recommendations and practice at the time of
publication. However, in view of ongoing research, changes in
government regulation, and the constant flow of information relating
to drug therapy and drug reactions, the reader is urged to check the
package insert for each drug for any change in indications and
dosage and for added warnings and precautions. This is particularly
important when the recommended agent is a new or infrequently
employed drug.

Materials appearing in this book prepared by individuals as part
of their official duties as U.S. Government employees are not
covered by the above-mentioned copyright.

9 8 7 6 5 4 3 2 1

PREFACE

The overall objectives of this edition remain unchanged from those of the first, namely, to provide a single text that encompasses the fundamentals of basic and medical microbiology as well as a comprehensive coverage of immunology, all of which can be read in a one-semester course.

We would like to stress that this text is neither an outline nor a review, nor is it a collection of isolated examples, leaving important areas of the field untouched. Rather, it is, within the confines of space, a small reference book that should be valuable long after the formal course is completed.

This text does not require a previous knowledge of microbiology, and should be readily understood by any reader who has completed an introduction to biochemistry. It is modeled after the course in microbiology taught to medical students at the University of Virginia, but would also serve as a text for any course whose objectives are to provide a solid understanding of medical microbiology and immunology.

The overall organization of the fifth edition is similar to the previous edition. Users of the previous edition will note, however, that two of the four authors are new to this edition. Bryan M. Gebhardt has revised the unit on immunology and Marie-Louise Hammarskjöld has updated the unit covering virology. All units have undergone extensive revisions including many new or revised illustrations.

The organization of this edition is designed to provide a brief introduction to basic molecular biology before the beginning of the more specialized sections of the text. However, those students who are familiar with microscopy and cell structure, as well as gene structure and function, may choose to omit the first two chapters and begin with the immunology unit in Chapter 3.

Previous users of this text will also note that there has been an extensive rearrangement of Unit 3 and considerable revision of Unit 1. This includes a rearrangement of the order and emphasis of presentation to reflect current advances in basic microbiology. A few of the more notable upgrades include an expanded coverage of the mechanism of antibiotic action and of the prevalence, sources, and transmission of antibiotic resistance. Other revisions include recent advances in the understanding of the molecular mechanisms of bacterial virulence factors, the control of their expression, and some examples of their genetic variability. There is also an expanded discussion of the interplay between bacteria and the immune system.

All of the chapters in Units 4 and 5 have been extensively updated to reflect epidemiology, virulence factors, and mechanisms of immunity for both bacterial and viral diseases. A new section on hantavirus is included as well as an expanded discussion on hepatitis viruses and human retroviruses.

Many thanks are due to David Benjamin for his comments on parts of the revised immunology unit and for his work on earlier editions which provided the basic outline for this unit. We are indebted to J. Thomas Parsons for the earlier virology unit which provided much of the outline used in the present text. We are indebted also to Richard Guerrant and Erik Hewlett for their comments on various chapters in unit 4. And, last, but not least, we wish to extend our warmest appreciation to all of our colleagues who provided help and useful information during the revision of this text.

Wesley A. Volk, PhD
Bryan M. Gebhardt, PhD
Marie-Louise Hammarskjöld, MD, PhD
Robert J. Kadner, PhD

CONTENTS

ESSENTIALS OF
Medical Microbiology
FIFTH EDITION

Introduction to Medical Microbiology

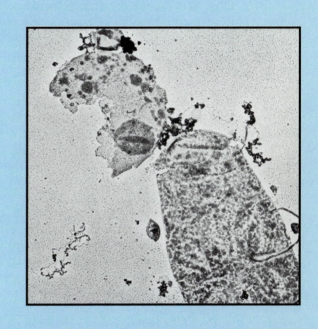

MANY human and animal diseases are caused by microorganisms, and we are learning some molecular details of the mechanisms by which bacteria, viruses, fungi, and protozoa cause diseases and how these diseases can be prevented or treated. Furthermore, we can see the biochemical unity in the living world that allows us to extrapolate our knowledge of bacterial genetics toward a better understanding of the regulation and control of human physiology.

The growth of knowledge in biology during the past half-century is analogous to the advances in physics that have taken us from horsepower to rocket power. This knowledge allows us to question the role of viruses in human cancer, to test the feasibility of genetic engineering to correct heritable defects, and to anticipate an understanding of many hitherto mysterious maladies such as multiple sclerosis, juvenile diabetes, and autoimmune diseases.

Is this what microbiology is all about? In part, yes. Microbiology is that part of biology that primarily involves organisms too small for the naked eye to see. Medical microbiology is the subdivision concerned with the biology of microorganisms that can grow on or in a host organism and produce disease. It also studies the responses of the host to infection.

In this book, we present clues or answers to the following basic questions of medical microbiology: How does the immune system operate to recognize and respond to the presence of an almost infinite variety of infectious agents or foreign objects? How do the various branches of the immune system inactivate or eliminate the different types of infectious agents? How does the overzealous action of the immune system, in its response to the presence of an infectious agent or after its inappropriate targeting of the host's own structures, lead to many of the symptoms of disease? How do successful pathogens evade or subvert the immune system? How do antimicrobial and antiviral agents act, and how is the resistance to these therapeutic agents established and spread? And finally, how are the infectious agents identified, how are they spread, and how do they cause their particular type of disease?

Before we can begin to address these questions, we must first learn what bacteria are, how they grow, and how they can be controlled. Unit One is comprised of two chapters, which briefly compare the structures of eucaryotic and procaryotic cells and introduce the reader to the structure of genes and the expression of genetic information. Knowledge of these subjects is a prerequisite to an understanding of the molecular biology of the immune response, which is discussed in Unit Two, and of the properties of the bacteria, fungi, viruses, and parasites that cause human disease.

Bibliography

BOOKS

Alberts B, Bray D, Lewis J, Raff M, Roberts K, Watson JD. Molecular biology of the cell, ed 3. New York, Garland Publishing, 1994.

Baron EJ, Chang RS, Howard DH, Miller JN, Tanner JA. Medical microbiology. A short course. New York, Wiley-Liss, 1994.

Baron S, ed. Medical microbiology, ed 3. New York, Churchill Livingstone, 1991.

Davis BD, Dulbecco R, Eisen HN, Ginsberg HS. Microbiology, ed 4. Philadelphia, JB Lippincott, 1990.

Gilligan PH, Shapiro DS, Smiley ML. Cases in medical microbiology and infectious diseases. Washington, DC, American Society for Microbiology, 1992.

Jawetz E, Melnick JL, Adelberg EA. Review of medical microbiology, ed 20. Norwalk, CT, Appleton & Lange, 1995.

Joklik WK, Willett HP, Amos BD, Wilfert CM. Zinsser's microbiology, ed 20. Norwalk, CT, Appleton & Lange, 1992.

Mandell GL, Bennett JE, Dolin R, eds. Principles and practices of infectious diseases, ed 4. New York, Churchill Livingstone, 1995.

Pelczar MJ, Chan ECS, Krieg NR. Microbiology, ed 5. New York, McGraw-Hill, 1986.

Ryan KJ, ed. Sherris medical microbiology, ed 3. Norwalk, CT, Appleton & Lange, 1994.

Salyers AA, Whitt DD. Bacterial pathogenesis: a molecular approach. Washington, DC, ASM Press, 1994.

Schaechter M, Medoff G, Schlessinger D. Mechanisms of microbial disease. Baltimore, Williams & Wilkins, 1989.

Essentials of Medical Microbiology, Fifth Edition, edited by Wesley A. Volk,
Bryan M. Gebhardt, Marie-Louise Hammarskjöld, and Robert J. Kadner.
Lippincott-Raven Publishers, Philadelphia © 1996.

Chapter 1

Microbial Cells and Their Function:
A Review of Cell Biology

Medical microbiology involves the study of the activities and interactions of many different types of cells. The bacterial, fungal, and protozoan parasitic cells have structures and products that allow them to cause disease. Viruses infect specific host cells to kill them or alter their growth behavior. The various cells that constitute the immune system respond to the presence of infectious agents to neutralize and eliminate them. In addition, human disorders can result from either excessive or deficient action of any of the cell types of the immune system. Because medical microbiology is concerned with this multiplicity of different cell types and their interactions, a general description of cellular structure and function is presented in this chapter to review the properties of the various types of microorganisms and to emphasize the differences between eucaryotic and procaryotic or bacterial cells.

The Microbial World

In the last century, biologists realized that the simple organisms that constitute the microbial world did not fit into the plant or animal kingdoms. For example, some algae have a plant's characteristic photosynthetic capabilities combined with an animal's motility. Conversely, fungi are immotile but lack other plant-like traits. Thus, in 1886 Haeckel proposed a third kingdom, the Protista, to include the algae, protozoa, fungi, and bacteria. Subsequent advances in microscopy revealed that bacteria possess a very different cellular architecture from that found in the other members of the Protista. The latter have a complex cell structure that is similar to that of plant and animal cells. The algae, fungi, and protozoa, as well as plant and animal cells, are termed *eucaryotic cells.* The bacteria have a much simpler internal organization and are termed *procaryotic cells* to reflect their lack of a true nucleus.

EUCARYOTIC PROTISTS

The eucaryotic protists are comprised of algae, protozoa, fungi (yeasts and molds), and slime molds. Distinctions between these groups are often blurred by the existence of transitional forms. Here we are concerned only with those groups whose members cause disease.

Fungi

The fungi are immotile, nonphotosynthetic protists that usually grow as a mat of branched filaments (hyphae) known as a *mycelium*. The hyphal filaments sometimes are not divided into individual cells by septa, allowing exchange of nuclei and cytoplasm along a considerable length of the growing tip of the hyphae. Mycelial forms, commonly called *molds*, frequently produce both sexual and asexual spores, and the structure, arrangement, and location of the spores are a major taxonomic key to their identification. Most fungi are saprophytic, that is, they degrade organic materials in soil or on vegetation, and they form the mildew that grows on clothes, food, and leather goods in humid conditions. Among the pathogenic fungi, some infect only keratinized layers of skin, whereas others cause serious systemic infections. These are described in Chapter 34.

Some fungi, known as *yeasts*, do not form a mycelium but remain as single cells that generally reproduce by budding. Many yeasts have evolved to grow in high-sugar environments, and those that convert sugar to ethanol and carbon dioxide are widely used for the production of alcoholic beverages (beer, wine, and spirits) or in the baking process because of their ability to produce copious amounts of carbon dioxide in bread dough. Unlike the saprophytic yeasts, many of the systemic fungal pathogens grow as single yeast cells at 37°C but develop a mycelium at 25°C, a condition known as dimorphic growth.

Protozoa

Protozoa are unicellular eucaryotes that have various mechanisms for movement, including ameboid crawling on surfaces and swimming with flagella or cilia. They exhibit a wide variety of shapes and sizes: some are oval or spherical, others are elongated, and some can change shape as they move along a surface. Some species are as small as 5 or 10 μm in diameter, whereas others reach diameters of 1 to 2 mm and are visible to the unaided eye.

Most protozoa reproduce asexually or sexually and, although they do not form spores as do the fungi, many secrete a thick coating around themselves for protection against adverse environments. These organisms are described in Unit Six.

PROCARYOTES

Bacteria are called procaryotic cells because of their much simpler cellular organization than eucaryotic cells and their lack of nuclei and other membrane-bound organelles. Procaryotic cells are divided into two major taxonomic groups, the *eubacteria* and the *archaebacteria* or *archaea;* members of each group are as different from each other as they are from eucaryotic cells. All bacteria of medical importance are in the eubacterial kingdom. Many of the archaebacteria inhabit unusual environmental niches, including extreme thermophiles that thrive in thermal springs and mid-oceanic vents, and extreme halophiles that live in the highly concentrated brine in evaporating salt flats. Other archaebacteria are major inhabitants of rumen flora, marshes, or sewage treatment plants. One major branch of the archaebacteria carry out the unique metabolic reactions of methanogenesis, or the production of methane. One species of methanogenic archaebacteria, *Methanobrevibacter smithii,* is part of the normal human intestinal flora. Some characteristic features of archaebacteria are the presence of isoprenoid ether lipids in place of the fatty acid esters present in eubacteria and eucaryotes, and unique types of cell walls. They carry out several unusual types of metabolic reactions, such as methane synthesis, using enzyme cofactors that are related to, but distinctly different from, the familiar cofactors found in eubacteria or eucaryotes.

Even among the eubacterial procaryotes, there is considerable diversity of cell shape and metabolic capability. The *Cyanobacteria* (formerly called the *blue-green algae*) carry out plant-like photosynthesis with the formation of oxygen. Many other procaryotes are also capable of using light as an energy source, but these bacteria have a simpler photosynthetic system than the photosynthetic eucaryotes or Cyanobacteria and are unable to generate oxygen.

Bacteria inhabit almost every environmental niche on Earth, and some have adapted to survival under extremely harsh conditions, ranging from lakes in Antarctica to boiling hot springs. Most bacteria are unable to grow or even survive in animals or humans and, thus, are only of peripheral interest in medical microbiology. The major groups of bacteria of medical concern are described in Chapter 15 and Unit 4.

VIRUSES

Viruses are infectious particles that can reproduce only when inside a living cell. These obligate intracellular parasites differ from cells in their size, physical and genetic complexity, and pattern of replication. There are viruses specific for almost every organism, but the range of species they can infect usually is restricted. A virus particle consists of a single type of nucleic acid (either RNA or DNA, never both) enclosed in a protein coat, or *capsid*, and, in some cases, surrounded by a membrane. The capsid protects the nucleic acid from attack by enzymes or physical agents and also is responsible for entry of the viral nucleic acid into the cell. Once inside the cell, the viral nucleic acid subverts the host's replication machinery to favor the synthesis of viral nucleic acids and proteins. These new viral subunits are then assembled into progeny virions and released from the cell.

The fate of the virus-infected cell varies for different viruses and ranges from rapid lysis to continued growth of the cell with prolonged release of new virus particles. Some viruses can integrate their nucleic acid into the cell's genome, and thereby remain quiescent within growing cells for long periods before being triggered to reinitiate viral replication and cause lysis of the host cell.

Microscopy

The study of microbes began in 1683 when Antony van Leeuwenhoek (1632 to 1723) described his observations of some of the myriad members of the microbial flora from various environmental sources. His hobby of lens grinding led to the construction of simple but effective microscopes, which allowed him to view the delightful world of "animalcules" of all sizes and shapes. Microscopy still provides a crucial tool for identifying microorganisms and studying their structures and interactions. In this section, some of the types of microscopic techniques used to visualize bacteria and eucaryotic cells are described.

LIGHT MICROSCOPE

van Leeuwenhoek made simple microscopes that contained a single lens capable of 200- to 300-fold magnification (Fig. 1-1). The compound microscopes now in use contain two sets of lenses, the objective lens next to the sample and the ocular lenses next to the observer's eyes. In this arrangement, the magnifications achieved by each set of lenses are multiplied to give the final magnification.

Modern microscopes contain multiple objective lenses mounted on a revolving turret. The low-power (10×) and high-power (44×) objectives are useful for the study of large eucaryotic cells, whereas the oil immersion (97×) objective generally is best for the study of bacteria. Use of the oil immersion lens requires that the sample be covered with a drop of oil, so that the light illuminating the sample passes through the glass slide, the sample, and the oil before entering the objective lens. This greatly reduces the diffraction or bending of light rays that occurs on crossing an interface between media of different refractive indices, such as that between glass and air.

The resolving power of any microscope, namely its ability to discriminate between two adjacent objects, is limited to roughly half the wavelength of the light used. The wavelength of visible light ranges from 400 to 800 nm, so the smallest object that can be observed in a light microscope must be at least 200 nm (0.2 μm). Because the diameters of most bacteria range from 0.3 to 1.0 μm, light microscopes cannot provide information on the internal structure of bacterial cells; therefore, they are used mainly to visualize the general shape of the cell and the reaction to specific staining procedures.

Ultraviolet Microscope

The shorter wavelengths of ultraviolet light (200 to 300 nm) can extend the limit of microscopic resolution to about 0.1 μm. However, ultraviolet light is invisible to the human eye (harmful, in fact), so the image must be

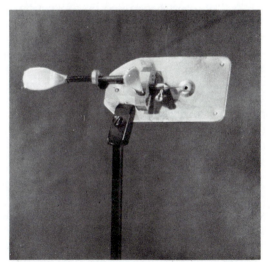
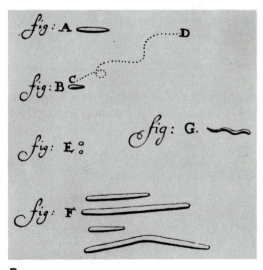

A   **B**

FIGURE 1-1 **A.** Leeuwenhoek used a microscope with a single biconvex lens to view bacteria suspended in a drop of liquid placed on a moveable pin. **B.** Although his microscope was capable of only 200- to 300-fold magnification, Leeuwenhoek was able to achieve these remarkable drawings of different bacterial types, which he submitted to the Royal Society of London.

recorded on a photographic plate or fluorescent screen. Because this light is absorbed by glass, all lenses must be made of quartz; such microscopes are too intricate and expensive for routine use.

Fluorescence Microscope

In fluorescence microscopy, a sample is labeled with a fluorescent dye and illuminated with ultraviolet light. The location of the dye in the specimen is revealed by its fluorescence, or emission of visible light of a longer wavelength. If the dye is selectively taken up by certain cells in a specimen, the presence of those cells can be readily detected. For example, the tubercle bacillus, *Mycobacterium tuberculosis,* will selectively take up the fluorescent dye auramine and appear bright against a dark background, even when small numbers are present in a large population of other types of cells.

Fluorescence microscopy is frequently used to detect microorganisms by coupling a fluorescent dye to a specific antibody that binds only to the target bacterium. The specificity of antigen–antibody reactions is thereby combined with a sensitive and dramatic assay to reveal the presence of a specific organism by its cell-bound fluorescence. This powerful technique can also be used to reveal the presence and cellular location of any antigen. Different antigens within a single preparation can be detected by using specific antibodies labeled with dyes that emit light of different colors.

Dark-Field Microscopy

The dark-field microscope is useful for detecting unstained bacteria in fluids and is particularly valuable for observing thin spirochetes, such as the syphilis organism, *Treponema pallidum.* With a dark-field microscope, a black background is seen against which suspended bacteria appear bright. The dark-field microscope uses a special condenser that illuminates the sample with a hollow cone of light in such a manner that the light is not directed into the objective lens. Only light that is reflected off an object in the sample enters the lens and reveals the shape of that object.

Phase-Contrast Microscopy

Bacterial and animal cells are difficult to see in the light microscope unless the sample has been dried and stained, because of the lack of contrast between the cells and the aqueous medium surrounding them. The phase-contrast microscope enhances the slight differences in refractive index between the cell and the medium, and is used to visualize live bacteria in an unfixed state.

The optics of this instrument are complex; they convert a difference in refractive index at any site in the specimen into a difference in the phase of the light passing through that point. Because of the constructive or destructive interference that occurs with light waves differing in phase, regions of the sample that differ in refractive index are revealed as differences in light intensity. For example, endospores have a low water content and, thus, differ markedly in refractive index from the medium. These structures are much brighter than the surrounding medium or the vegetative cells when viewed in this microscope.

ELECTRON MICROSCOPE

Almost all our understanding of microbial and subcellular ultrastructure comes from use of the electron microscope, a device that uses a beam of electrons rather than light to illuminate the sample. The shorter wavelength of electrons increases the resolving power to about 0.001 μm (1 nm). The image generated by the transmission of electrons through, or their reflection from, the sample is visualized by projection onto a photographic plate or a fluorescent screen. Two types of electron microscopes are used.

Transmission Electron Microscope

The transmission electron microscope yields an image from the electrons that pass through the sample; thus, extremely thin slices (1 μm or less) of the specimen must be used because electrons are readily absorbed by biologic materials. Detection of fine details of cellular structure requires careful techniques for sample fixing, embedding, and sectioning. Freeze drying of samples reduces the distortions caused by conventional dehydration and drying procedures. Examination of serial thin sections permits a detailed reconstruction of organelles or even whole cells in three dimensions. The location of specific proteins within the sectioned samples can be determined by immunoelectron microscopy, in which antibodies that bind to the specific protein are labeled with an electron-dense marker, such as ferritin or colloidal gold. The electron-dense marker is readily detected in the electron micrograph. Alternatively, immunohistochemical methods allow detection of specific enzymes that yield electron-dense reaction products at the site of the enzyme.

Negative staining is a useful technique to complement the examination of sectioned samples. This procedure involves suspension of the sample in solutions of electron-dense heavy metal salts such as phosphotungstate. These salts form deposits on the surface of the particles in the sample and provide a detailed image of surface structures. Shadow casting is another technique used to reveal the surface architecture of an object, especially of viruses. In this case, an electron-dense material

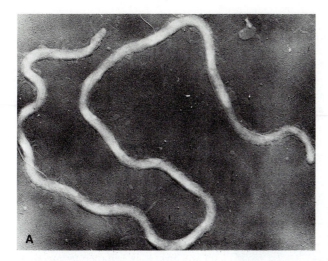

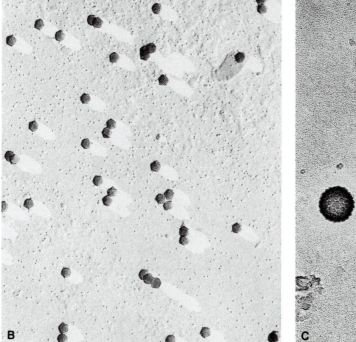

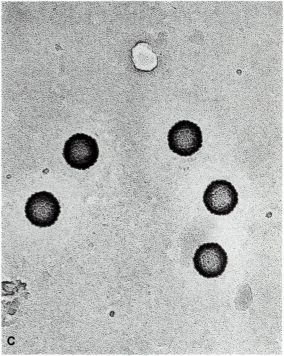

FIGURE 1-2 **A.** Electron micrograph of the spirochete *Spirochaeta stenostrepta* shadowed with platinum. (Original magnification ×12,000.) **B.** Electron micrograph of adenovirus with oblique shadowing. **C.** Electron micrograph of herpesvirus with rotary shadowing.

such as platinum or chromium is deposited at an angle on the sample by placing it in an oblique beam of the metal ions. In this way, an object casts a shadow on the side opposite the direction of the ion beam, resulting in a three-dimensional effect (Fig. 1-2).

Freeze etching is a technique in which the unfixed sample is frozen at very low temperature and then fractured by a sharp blow from a knife. The newly exposed surfaces are replicated by deposition of carbon metal. The fracture planes often extend along cell surfaces, yielding detailed views of surface structures and especially the intramembranous distribution of proteins. Ion bombardment is a technique in which the outer layers of viruses or cells are eroded in an ion beam, to reveal the otherwise inaccessible internal structures.

Scanning Electron Microscope

The scanning electron microscope uses a fine beam or spot of electrons that is focused rapidly back and forth over the specimen. As the electrons strike the surface of particles in the sample, secondary electrons are emitted, which are collected by a detector to provide an image of the specimen's surface. This instrument does not require that the sample be sectioned and provides some spectacular three-dimensional images, as shown in Figure 1-3. In addition, because the energy of the secondary emitted electron is determined by the identity of the scattering atom, the energy spectrum of these electrons provides information about the location and content of the different elements.

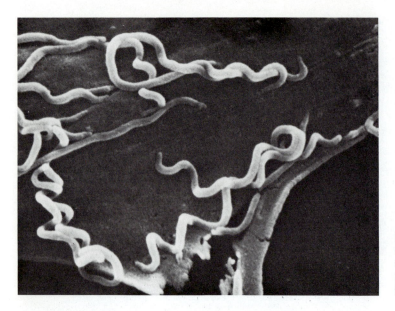

FIGURE 1-3   The three-dimensional qualities of scanning electron microscopy clearly reveal the corkscrew shape of cells of the syphilis-causing spirochete *Treponema pallidum*, attached here to rabbit testicular cells grown in culture. (Original magnification ×8000.)

Eucaryotic Cells: Structure and Function

The following sections briefly summarize the general features of the structure and composition of eucaryotic and procaryotic cells, with emphasis on the differences between these two fundamentally distinct cell types. Eucaryotic cells are larger and more complex than procaryotic cells, and possess intracellular membrane-enclosed organelles, which are invariably absent from procaryotic cells. The following sections describe briefly some of the characteristic structures found in higher eucaryotic cells and their contribution to the life of the cell. The "Closer Look" at the end of the chapter follows the steps involved in the production of an antibody molecule by an antibody-producing cell.

NUCLEUS

The possession of a membrane-enclosed nucleus is the hallmark of any eucaryotic cell. The nucleus contains almost all the cell's deoxyribonucleic acid (DNA), which is carried on chromosomes and represents the cell's genetic information. Diploid organisms contain two versions of each chromosome. In each chromosome, the linear double-stranded DNA is organized into higher order structures and is bound to numerous proteins, the most prevalent of which are the basic and universally conserved histones. The nucleus is the site of DNA replication, in which each chromosome is copied during the synthesis (S) phase of each cell cycle. The mechanism of DNA replication is described in Chapter 2. Chromosomes generally are not visible in the light microscope until they condense into compact units (metaphase chromosomes) long after completion of the S phase and just before cell division, during the mitosis (M) phase of the cell cycle. At that time, the mitotic spindle apparatus forms to pull the two copies of each chromosome into the two progeny

cells. In this process, a cytoskeletal filament, called a microtubule, forms between an attachment site on each chromosome (called the centromere or kinetosome) and the spindle body at one or the other end of the nucleus. The newly replicated chromosomes are pulled apart by their movement along the microtubular strand toward the opposite poles. This system accurately ensures that each progeny cell receives one copy of each chromosome.

The chromosomes are surrounded by the nuclear envelope, which consists of two membrane layers, the outermost of which is contiguous with the endoplasmic reticulum (ER). In some cell types, the nuclear membrane dissolves during the M phase and then forms again around the partitioned chromosomes. The nuclear membrane contains pores through which the mature RNA molecules leave the nucleus en route to the cytoplasm, where they will be translated into protein.

The nucleus is also the site of expression of the genetic information. As described in Chapter 2, the sequence of bases in a particular region of the DNA is copied into an RNA molecule of the same sequence. In eucaryotic cells, the initial RNA copy, or transcript, is modified by the addition of extra nucleotides at both ends and, usually, by the removal of some stretches of sequences within the transcript. These modifications of the RNA transcript are important for its stability and efficient translation and export from the nucleus.

ENDOPLASMIC RETICULUM

The ER is a membranous network that extends throughout the cell. There are two types of ER, termed *rough ER* and *smooth ER,* which have multiple functions, mostly related to the synthesis and processing of proteins. The rough ER is studded with ribosomes that synthesize the proteins destined to become part of other organelles or to be exported from the cell. These proteins are made with a short sequence of amino acids at their end that is removed during the process of export but targets the remainder of the protein for its translation on ribosomes bound to the ER. These ribosomes secrete the new polypeptides across the membrane and into the enclosed lumen of the ER. From there, these new proteins travel in membrane vesicles to the Golgi complex and other sites.

The Golgi complex consists of stacks of smooth ER membranes, and it carries out the further processing (primarily glycosylation) and sorting of proteins that are to be stored, transferred to other organelles, or secreted. Vesicles containing newly synthesized proteins can be observed moving from the rough ER to the Golgi complex and from there to the surface plasma membrane. Because of the complexity of these processes, the secretion of a protein by eucaryotic cells often takes more than an hour to complete.

The smooth ER is also involved in a variety of metabolic functions, including the biosynthesis of hormones and the conversion of some drugs to less toxic or more easily excreted forms.

MITOCHONDRIA

Mitochondria are distinctively shaped organelles that are the primary site of energy generation in the cell. Their membranes contain the respiratory electron transport system and the enzyme responsible for producing adenosine triphosphate (ATP), the primary form of metabolic energy in the cell. Mitochondria accomplish this by a three-step process: (1) Metabolites derived from various nutrients are converted ultimately to acetyl-CoA, which is oxidized to CO_2 by the enzymes of the tricarboxylic acid cycle. (2) The electrons released during this process of oxidation are passed along the proteins of the electron transport chain to oxygen. At several steps of the chain, electron passage results in the expulsion of protons from the interior of the mitochondrion, resulting in the generation of an electrical potential across the membrane. (3) The return of protons back into the mitochondrion through an enzyme complex called the F_1F_0-*proton-translocating adenosine triphosphatase* is coupled to the synthesis of ATP. All these events occur in the innermost of the mitochondrion's two membranes. Mitochondria, like chloroplasts in plant cells, originally were derived from a bacterium and are plastids, capable of self-replication and containing DNA and other machinery that permits the synthesis of a few of their constituent proteins and RNA molecules.

OTHER EUCARYOTIC STRUCTURES

Lysosomes are membrane-bound structures containing numerous hydrolytic enzymes and antimicrobial peptides that digest macromolecules and participate in the killing of ingested microorganisms. Lysosomes fuse with coated membrane vesicles (called *phagosomes*) that have budded in from the surface membrane and enclose portions of the exterior fluid and proteins or particles, including bacteria, that were bound on the cell surface.

Cell shape and numerous functions of the plasma membrane are dependent on the *cytoskeleton*, which is a filamentous scaffold-like structure extending throughout the cytoplasm. There are two basic types of cytoskeletal elements, termed *microtubules* and *microfilaments*. Microtubules are formed by the polymerization of a protein called *tubulin* and are the basic structure of the cytoskeleton. They contribute to chromosome separation during cell division. Microfilaments contain actin and myosin and are necessary for creeping (ameboid) motility. Many eucaryotic cells exhibit ameboid or creeping motion when moving along a surface, but some cell types are motile in liquid with cilia or flagella. These organelles are assembled from microtubules and consist of nine fibrils surrounding two fibers.

The cytoplasm is enclosed by the *plasma membrane,* which contains nutrient transport systems and receptors that are used in intracellular communications. Some nutrients are transported directly across the membrane. Other nutrients are taken up after they bind to receptors on the membrane surface while a segment of the membrane is pinched off and taken into the cell as a membrane vesicle that fuses with lysosomes. This membrane appears to be in constant motion and to be actively recycled from the surface into internal organelles and back. Figure 1-4 shows electron micrographs of two diverse eucaryotic cells, demonstrating many of the organelles found in these cells.

Procaryotic Cell Structure

Procaryotic cells are invariably smaller and simpler than eucaryotic cells. Most bacteria are similar in size to a mitochondrion. Because of their small size and cellular simplicity, many bacteria can divide in less than 30 minutes, in contrast to the 8 to 24 hours needed by many of the higher eucaryotic cells.

Procaryotic cells, examples of which appear in Figure 1-5, possess no separate internal membrane-bound organelles. Any internal membranous structures that do occur are extensions of the cytoplasmic membrane, which is the site of most of the functions carried out by the eucaryotic organelles. There is no nuclear membrane or mitotic apparatus. Instead, a nuclear region is seen, composed of DNA fibrils in direct contact with the cytoplasm. Some bacteria, such as *Escherichia coli,* possess only a single chromosome that, if extended, would be almost a thousand times the length of the cell. Other bacteria contain two chromosomes that have different genetic content. The chromosomes are circular in some bacteria and linear in others. The nucleoid does not condense into a more compact structure during cell division and there is no formation of an obvious mitotic apparatus to pull

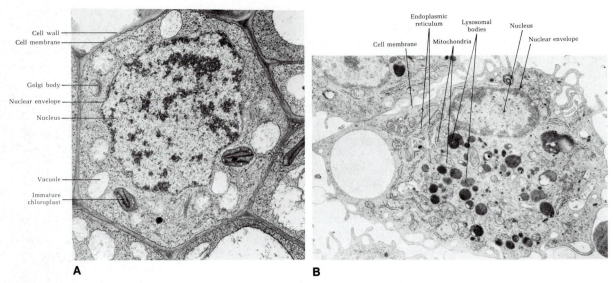

FIGURE 1-4 **A.** Section of a cell from the stem of a young pea plant, *Pisum sativum*. (Original magnification ×9945.) **B.** Section of an animal cell—in this case, a macrophage from a mouse. (Original magnification ×6240.)

the chromosomes apart into the dividing cells, as occurs in eucaryotic cells. Instead, partitioning the chromosomes into the daughter cells appears to be accomplished by attachment of a portion of the DNA to the cytoplasmic membrane or to a cytoskeletal element. Growth of the membrane or movement of the cytoskeleton between the chromosomal attachment sites brings about the segregation of the replicating chromosomes. In bacteria, the cell cycle is not divided into separate S and M phases, and bacterial cell division can occur even while the chromosome is still in the process of replication.

As in mitochondria, energy generation by oxidative phosphorylation in bacteria occurs by formation of a gradient of protons across the cytoplasmic membrane and its utilization for ATP synthesis by the F_1F_0-adenosine triphosphatase. The chlorophyll and other pigments in photosynthetic bacteria are organized into lamellar or tubular extensions of the cytoplasmic membrane, instead of the independent membrane-enclosed chloroplasts.

Bacterial flagella, described in Chapter 17, are much simpler in structure and composition than their eucaryotic counterparts and bring about motility in a fundamentally different manner than do eucaryotic flagella.

Bacteria produce storage granules, but these are never

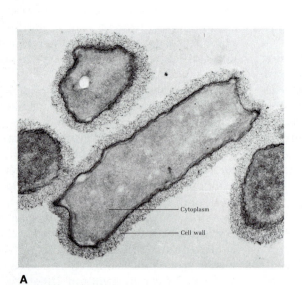

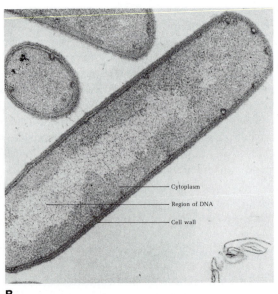

FIGURE 1-5 **A.** Section of bacterium-*Klebsiella aerogenes.* (Original magnification × 20,730.) **B.** Bacterium *Bacillus mucroides* (Original magnification ×26,000.)

TABLE 1-1
Comparison of Eucaryotic and Procaryotic Cells*

Characteristic	Eucaryotes	Procaryotes
Structure		
Organelles	Membrane-bound organelles always present	Never, only ingrowth of plasma membrane
Nucleus	Nuclear membrane and spindle apparatus	DNA in contact with cytoplasm
Cytoskeleton	Prominent	Absent or modest
Flagella and motility	Complex flagella beat in a wave	Simple filament rotates
Multicellular communication	Common	Absent or rare
Composition		
Lipids		
Phosphatidylcholine	Always	Unusual
Complex lipids	Common	Very unusual
Sterols	Always	Only in *Mycoplasma*
Ribosomes	80S = 40S + 60S subunits	70S = 30S + 50S
Cell wall	Absent or made of cellulose	Peptidoglycan with muramic acid
Triglycerides	Common lipid storage form	Rare or never
Genetic Organization		
Chromosomes	Multiple linear	One or two, circular or linear
Ploidy	Often diploid	Haploid
Extrachromosomal DNA	Organellar DNA	Plasmids
Histones and nucleosomes	Present	Absent
Transcription and translation	Separated in time and space, long-lived mRNA	Coupled, often short-lived mRNA
Colinearity of gene and protein	Introns often present	Colinear
mRNA processing	Always: splicing, cap, poly A tail	Never
Gene organization	Single genes; monocistronic mRNA	Operons and polycistronic mRNA
Initiating amino acid	Met	Formyl-Met
Number of RNA polymerases	Three	One
Sexual cycle	Yes, often necessary for reproduction	Absent or not necessary
Genetic exchange	Formation of diploid zygotes	Only part of chromosome

* Many of these designations are invariably observed; others apply to most bacteria of medical importance, but do not apply to all eubacteria and archaebacteria.

enclosed by a membrane. Whereas many eucaryotic cells deposit lipid reserves in the form of triglycerides, many bacteria synthesize a polymeric ester of poly-β-hydroxybutyric acid or related hydroxyacids.

It is particularly noteworthy that procaryotic cells possess smaller ribosomes (70S*) than those in eucaryotic cells (80S). The different ribosomes also exhibit different sensitivities to various inhibitors or antibiotics. Note, however, that the ribosomes in mitochondria and chloroplasts are also 70S and are inhibited by many of the antibiotics that act on bacterial ribosomes.

CHEMICAL COMPOSITION OF PROCARYOTES

Profound differences in structure and chemical composition between eucaryotic and procaryotic cells are also seen in that bacteria usually possess simpler, less evolutionarily advanced constituents than do eucaryotes. Sterols are in-

variably present in eucaryotic cell membranes, but they cannot be synthesized by any bacterium and are incorporated only into the membranes of one group of bacteria, the mycoplasmas. In addition, the lipids of eubacterial membranes are primarily phosphatides, and the complex phospholipids and sphingolipids that are commonly found in eucaryotes are rarely seen in procaryotes. Even such a common lipid as phosphatidylcholine (lecithin) is made by relatively few bacterial species.

Most bacteria make complex lipopolysaccharide-type surface structures that, together with the rigid cell wall, contain unique ingredients. Some of the chemicals peculiar to bacteria include muramic acid in the cell wall, lipid A and dideoxy sugars in the lipopolysaccharide of gramnegative bacteria, and poly-ribitol phosphates in the teichoic acids of gram-positive bacteria. These differences are of considerable importance, both with respect to understanding the structure and classification of bacteria, and because they represent attractive targets for antimicrobial chemotherapy. Table 1-1 summarizes major differences between eucaryotic and procaryotic cells.

* The Svedberg constant (S) is a measure of the rate of sedimentation of a particle during centrifugation and is related to the size of the particle.

A Closer Look

Synthesis, Export, and Processing of Immunoglobulin Molecules

All cells need to make proteins that ultimately arrive at a destination outside the cytoplasm, either in an organelle, on the cell surface, or secreted into the medium. Special mechanisms are necessary to allow proteins to pass across membranes and to be targeted to their proper destination. These topics are under active investigation to define the route for protein translocation and the nature of the signals that allow or prevent movement across a membrane. Some of the targeting signals are well known. The cleavable amino-terminal signal sequences are clearly necessary for the entry of many, perhaps most, proteins into the secretory pathway. However, poorly defined sequences in the mature portion of the polypeptide chain strongly influence or determine the final destination of the protein after it has entered the secretory pathway. There are numerous secreted proteins that lack a cleavable amino-terminal signal sequence, especially in bacteria, where there are multiple specialized protein secretion systems that are highly specific for their client protein.

To provide a closer look at protein secretion, this section follows the passage of an immunoglobulin molecule from the time its mRNA appears in the cytoplasm until the protein is released from the mature B cell or plasma cell. As described later in this book, there is considerable complexity of nuclear events in the gene rearrangements that select from the extensive repertoire of antigen specificities and that determine the particular immunoglobulin isotype to be produced. Alternative splicing of the mRNA into the nucleus controls whether a hydrophobic stretch of amino acids will be present near the carboxyl terminus of the immunoglobulin to serve as a membrane anchor so that the protein remains attached as surface immunoglobulin or is secreted.

As described in detail later in this book, immunoglobulins, or antibodies, are made up of two separate polypeptide chains, termed *light chain* and *heavy chain*. IgG is a heterotetramer, containing two light chains and two heavy chains, with some disulfide bonds connecting different parts within a single polypeptide chain and others connecting separate polypeptide chains together.

SIGNAL SEQUENCE

The ribosomes producing the heavy and light chains are brought to the surface of the rough ER, where a docking complex releases the signal recognition particle and allows protein translation to proceed. Continued translation results in secretion of the polypeptide chain across the membrane into the lumen of the ER. The signal sequence is removed soon after the amino-terminal end of the protein appears in the lumen. Even during their synthesis, the heavy and light chains associate with each other and increase each other's stability and solubility. For IgG, the assembly process involves the formation of a heavy-chain dimer, H_2, onto which the two light chains add sequentially to form H_2L and then H_2L_2. This association is stabilized by the formation of covalent disulfide bonds between and along the polypeptide chains. The process of proper folding of the polypeptide chains into their final structure, and perhaps of associating the separate chains with one another, is facilitated by the presence of a chaperone protein in the ER lumen. Chaperone proteins play a catalytic role in assisting or directing the process of protein folding. In some cases, they retard folding to maintain a protein in an unfolded state that is competent for export and secretion across a membrane (the usual situation for protein export in bacteria) or they help a protein avoid nonproductive but stable folding intermediates. The chaperone involved in immunoglobulin processing is called *BiP*. Also in the ER, mannose oligosaccharides are attached to certain asparagine residues in a process known as *N-linked glycosylation*. N-linked glycosylation occurs at one site on all H chains, termed *region CH_2*. Some immunoglobulin molecules also are glycosylated at other positions. The role of glycosylation includes increasing the solubility of the protein and subtly affecting the protein conformation. In some cases, glycosylation is necessary for release of the protein from the cell.

After completion of synthesis and these covalent modifications, the completed and assembled proteins move to the Golgi complex in membrane vesicles pinched off from the ER. Processing continues in the Golgi complex, where the high-mannose carbohydrates are partially trimmed off and replaced by other sugars in the arrangement typical of the final product. The completed proteins then move in secretory membrane vesicles to the cell surface, where the vesicles fuse with the plasma membrane. In the case of a mature B cell, the mRNA splicing process results in synthesis of the IgG molecule with a carboxyl-terminal hydrophobic segment, and this protein is anchored on the surface when that vesicle fuses with the plasma membrane. The terminally differentiated plasma cells make the secreted form of the same antibody molecule

A Closer Look *continued*

as a result of a different RNA splicing specificity. In this case, fusion of the secretory vesicle with the plasma membrane results in release of the enclosed immunoglobulins into the circulation.

The multimeric IgA and IgM proteins, made up of two or five of the basic four-chain units, are joined together by the 20-kilodalton J chain, which is made only in the cells synthesizing those types of immunoglobulin. In addition, another subunit, known as the *secretory piece* or *secretory component,* is attached to the IgM and IgA molecules that are secreted across mucosal surfaces.

Essentials of Medical Microbiology, Fifth Edition, edited by Wesley A. Volk, Bryan M. Gebhardt, Marie-Louise Hammarskjöld, and Robert J. Kadner. Lippincott-Raven Publishers, Philadelphia © 1996.

Chapter 2

Gene Structure and Function

An unprecedented expansion has occurred in our knowledge of the structure and expression of a cell's genetic information, particularly since the development in the mid-1970s of recombinant DNA techniques that allow the isolation of any gene and the determination of the sequence of bases in its deoxyribonucleic acid (DNA). This chapter describes the basic methods used in nucleic acid analysis and the general picture of gene structure that has resulted from the application of these techniques. A general overview of the mechanism of gene expression and regulation in procaryotic and eucaryotic cells, with emphasis on how the sequence of bases in DNA encodes the sequence of amino acids in individual proteins, is presented.

Nucleic Acid Structure

A cell's genetic information provides the blueprint that determines the amounts and the structure of all the cell's proteins, which in turn determines the amounts of all other cellular constituents. The genetic information in all cells is maintained as the sequence of nucleotide bases in DNA and is expressed by being converted into a corresponding sequence of nucleotide bases in ribonucleic acid (RNA). DNA is made up of the four nucleotide bases, adenine (A), cytidine (C), guanine (G), and thymine (T), which are attached to the sugar 2-deoxyribose and joined together by phosphodiester bonds in a long sugar–phosphate backbone (Fig. 2-1). DNA normally exists as a double-stranded helical molecule, in which two single strands of DNA wrap around one another in the manner first described by Francis Crick and James Watson in

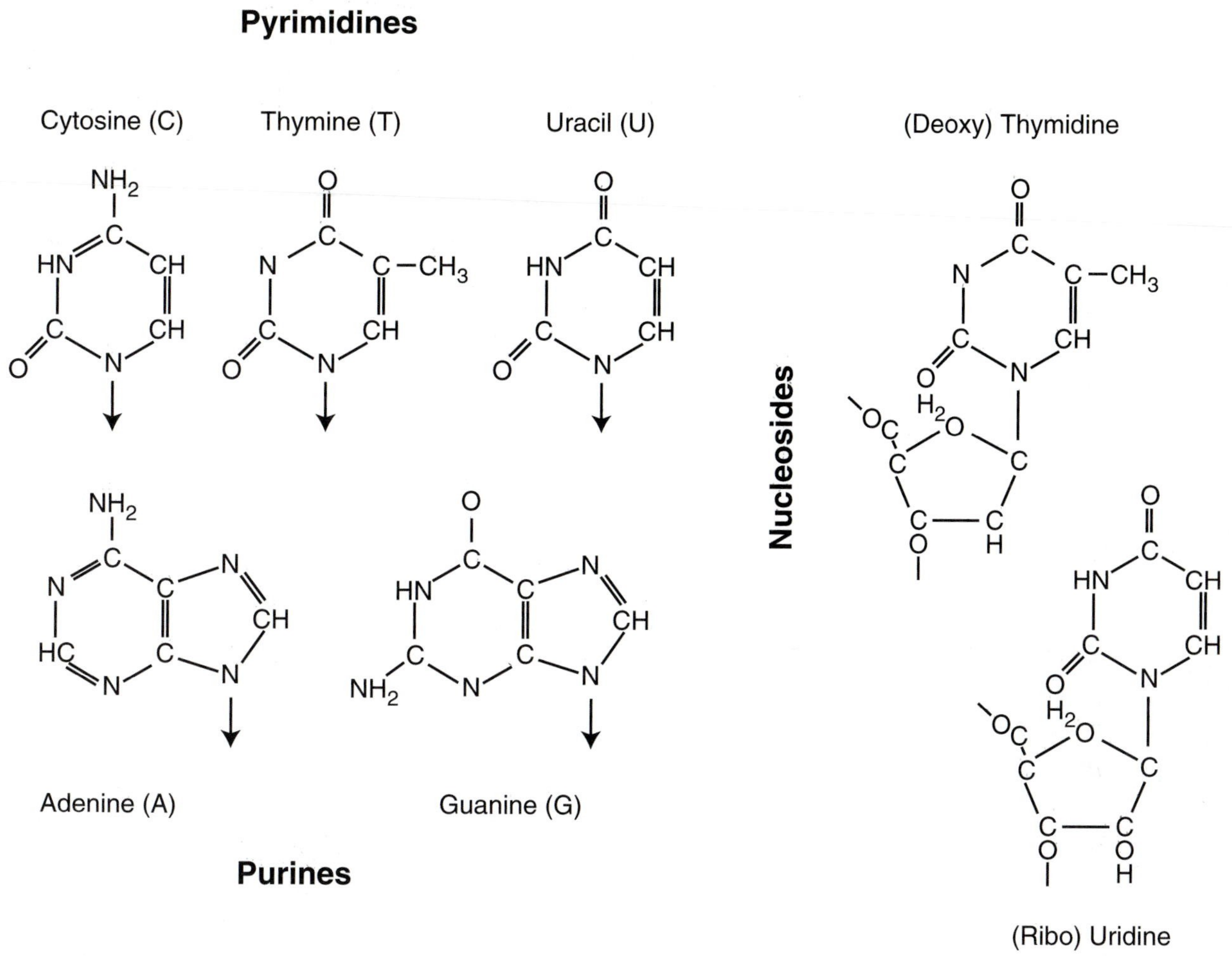

Pyrimidines

Cytosine (C)   Thymine (T)   Uracil (U)

Nucleosides

(Deoxy) Thymidine

Adenine (A)   Guanine (G)

(Ribo) Uridine

Purines

FIGURE 2-1 The purine and pyrimidine bases in nucleic acids. RNA contains uracil in place of thymine. Nucleosides contain a glycosidic bond between the base and the C1 position of deoxyribose in the case of DNA, or ribose in the case of RNA.

1952. The two strands of the double helix are arranged in an antiparallel manner (ie, in an opposite direction when viewed along the phosphodiester backbone). The bases opposite one another at each position along the double helix form base pairs as determined by complementarity rules, such that A forms a base pair with T, and G pairs with C. A and G are purines, with two rings, whereas T and C are pyrimidines, with a single ring. The pairing of A to T and G to C occurs to maximize the energy gained from hydrogen bonding between the nucleotide bases and to keep the helix at a constant diameter along its length (Fig. 2-2). Double-stranded DNA can exist in various forms or conformations, the most prevalent of which is called B-form DNA (Fig. 2-3). In B-form DNA, the helix repeats roughly every 10.5 base pairs or 3.4 nm. RNA differs from DNA in several regards. It contains the base uracil (U) instead of thymine, and the sugar ribose instead of 2-deoxyribose. Although RNA can form a double helix, it usually is copied from DNA as a single strand.

The double strands of DNA melt or separate after heating or exposure to denaturing agents. The temperature at which a DNA melts is a direct function of its G and C content, because the G–C base pair with three hydrogen bonds is more stable than the A–T base pair with two hydrogen bonds. Renaturation of melted DNA strands is a much slower process than melting because it requires that the complementary sequences find each other. Renaturation also requires the presence of salt to reduce the high electrostatic repulsion of the phosphodiester backbone, and it works best at a temperature near the melting temperature to help melt regions of short sequence match.

Several features of DNA make it a good choice as the genetic material. Its high degree of chemical and biologic stability over the range of physiologic pH and salt concentrations enables it to maintain the genetic information relatively intact from one generation to the next. For example, RNA is degraded at an alkaline pH level, but DNA is not. Its long length (some bacterial DNA molecules measure 1 mm) allows it to carry large amounts of information in a small volume. The comple-

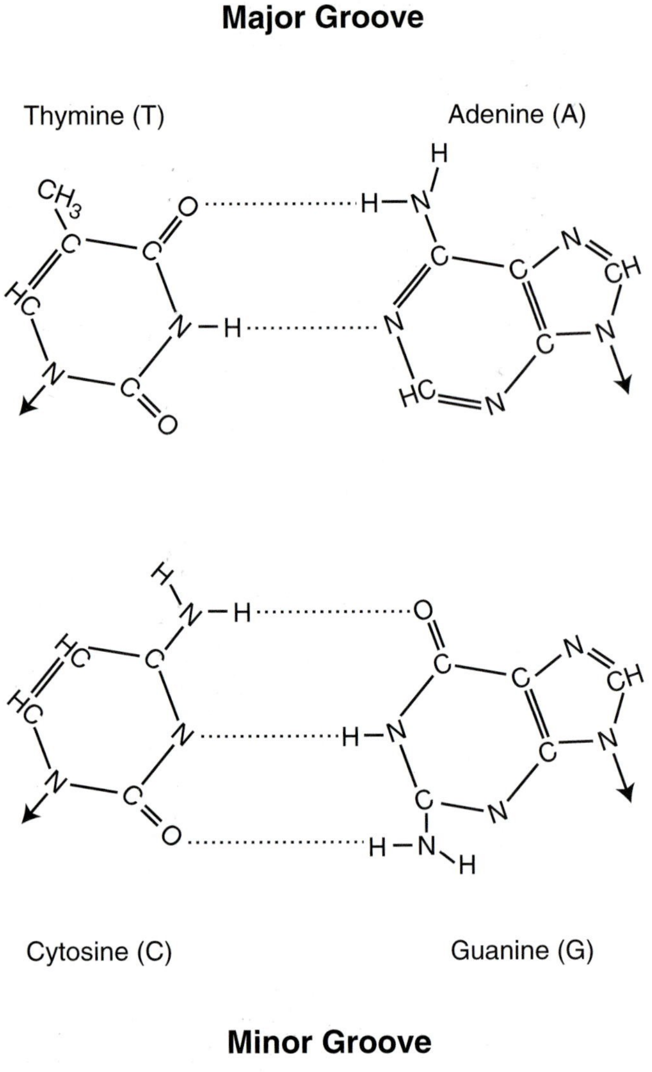

Major Groove

Thymine (T)   Adenine (A)

Cytosine (C)   Guanine (G)

Minor Groove

FIGURE 2-2   Hydrogen-bonding properties of base pairs in the Watson-Crick arrangement. The size of both base pairs is approximately equal. The parts of the molecules exposed in the major groove and minor groove of DNA are indicated.

mentarity rules that determine base-pair specificity provide the mechanism for accurate and rapid replication of each strand so that each progeny cell receives an exact copy of the DNA from its parent. The same process allows accurate and highly regulated copying of the nucleotide sequence of DNA into RNA to encode the proteins that carry out the cell's functions. The double-stranded nature of DNA means that the same information is carried on each strand, providing a degree of redundancy that allows DNA repair processes to remove damaged sequences in one strand using the undamaged strand as template to restore the correct sequence on both strands.

Mutations and the Genetic Code

The term *genetic code* refers to the mechanism by which the genetic information carried in the DNA nucleotide

sequence is decoded into the sequence of amino acids that make up each specific protein. Not all the DNA in an organism codes for a protein; some parts are regulatory regions and other parts play no obvious function. Within the regions that do encode a protein, there is an unambiguous correspondence between the nucleotide and amino acid sequences. This genetic code is said to be a nonoverlapping triplet code, which means that each three bases, or codon, encodes one amino acid. There are 64 possibilities for a triplet of four bases, so multiple codons can specify a single amino acid. For example, there are six codons for arginine, leucine, and serine; four codons for valine, proline, threonine, alanine, and glycine; three codons for isoleucine; one codon for methionine and tryptophan; and two codons for the remaining amino acids. As described further later, three codons specifically signal the end of a coding region and stop synthesis of that protein. The standard genetic code is listed in Table 2-1. This

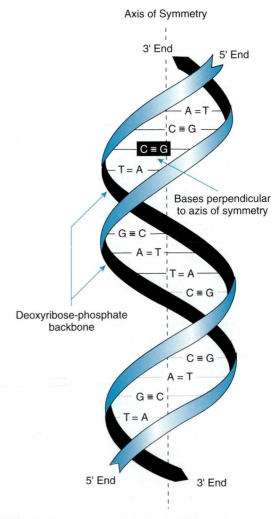

FIGURE 2-3   Structure of B-form DNA. The base pairs are approximately parallel to one another and are perpendicular to the helical axis. Considerable variation of this structure is seen in authentic DNA molecules as a result of changed orientation and nonplanarity of some base pairs.

TABLE 2-1
The Gentic Code: Nucleotide Triplet Codons and the Encoded Amino Acids

First Base	Second Base				Third Base
	U	*C*	*A*	*G*	
U	Phe	Ser	Tyr	Cys	U
	Phe	Ser	Tyr	Cys	C
	Leu	Ser	Ochre*	Opal*	A
	Leu	Ser	Amber*	Trp	G
C	Leu	Pro	His	Arg	U
	Leu	Pro	His	Arg	C
	Leu	Pro	Gln	Arg	A
	Leu	Pro	Gln	Arg	G
A	Ile	Thr	Asn	Ser	U
	Ile	Thr	Asn	Ser	C
	Ile	Thr	Lys	Arg	A
	Met	Thr	Lys	Arg	G
G	Val	Ala	Asp	Gly	U
	Val	Ala	Asp	Gly	C
	Val	Ala	Glu	Gly	A
	Val	Ala	Glu	Gly	G

* Translation termination codons.

characteristic will appear early during the growth of some cultures, later in others, and not at all in other cultures. If each mutant continues to reproduce after its appearance, those cultures in which a mutation appeared early in the growth cycle will contain many mutants, whereas those in which mutation occurred late will contain only a few mutants. In other words, there will be a large fluctuation or variability in the number of variant organisms if they arose as a result of spontaneous mutation. On the other hand, if a proportion of the population adapted to the selective conditions used to identify the mutant types, a fairly constant number of variant organisms would be expected in each of the separate cultures. As shown in Figure 2-4, the large fluctuation in the number of variant

code is not universal and is different for some triplets in some organisms or organelles.

Mutations are genetic changes that result from an alteration in the sequence of nucleotides in DNA. Many mutations have no detectable consequence (phenotype) because they occur in noncoding regions or do not change the amino acid sequence of the encoded protein, owing to the degenerate nature of the genetic code, in which different codons can specify the same amino acid. Even when there is a change in amino acid sequence, many substitutions are not sufficiently detrimental to the protein's function to impair cell behavior. The frequency of mutations at any particular gene in almost any type of cell is typically in the range of 10^{-6} to 10^{-8} per generation. Because most bacterial cultures contain more than 10^8 organisms per milliliter, it is likely that any bacterial culture contains at least one cell with a mutation in any given gene.

Changes in a cell's behavior can result from permanent mutational alterations in the DNA or from programmed regulatory adaptations to changes in the environment. To determine whether the appearance of cells with an altered phenotype is caused by a transient adaptation or by a true mutation, the fluctuation test was designed by Salvador Luria and Max Delbruck. This test is based on the assumption that mutation is a random event but adaptation is not. Thus, in a series of independent cultures, spontaneous mutants altered in some observable

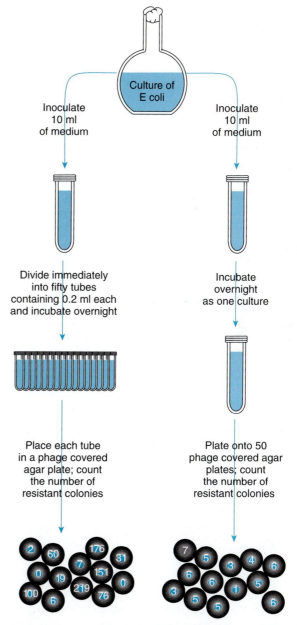

FIGURE 2-4 Fluctuation test. On the left, mutation to phage resistance must have occurred early in the tube that provided 400 resistant organisms and late in the tube with only two resistant organisms. The control plates on the right show little fluctuation.

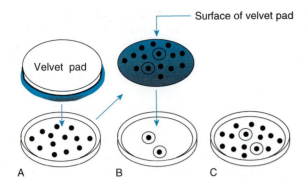

Surface of velvet pad

Velvet pad

A   B   C

FIGURE 2-5 Replica plating. **A.** A sterile velvet pad is pressed lightly on a plate containing microcolonies of staphylococci. **B.** The velvet pad then is pressed lightly on a sterile agar plate containing penicillin. Only two colonies grew in this example. **C.** By noting the position of the colonies that grew, it is possible to go back to the original plate and subculture penicillin-resistant colonies that have never been exposed to penicillin.

organisms in the actual study indicated that they arose as the result of mutation rather than adaptation.

A second method used to show that mutations are spontaneous and not specifically induced by the selection procedure is called *replica plating*. Developed by the Lederbergs, this technique was used to isolate penicillin-resistant staphylococci without ever exposing the bacteria to this antibiotic. A large number of staphylococci were spread on an agar plate and each cell formed a microcolony after several hours. A sterile velvet pad was then pressed onto the surface of the plate so that a few bacteria from each colony adhered to the velvet. When the velvet pad was pressed onto a second agar plate containing penicillin, it produced an exact copy of the original master plate, but only the organisms resistant to penicillin could grow. Based on the location of the penicillin-resistant colonies, it was possible to pick from the original plate the resistant colonies that had never been exposed to the presence of penicillin (Fig. 2-5). Mutations occur constantly in any population and are not induced by the selective conditions used for their identification.

TYPES OF MUTATIONS

Mutations are categorized according to their effect on the DNA sequence or on the phenotype of the organism. *Base-pair substitutions* replace one base for another, which can result in a change of one amino acid in the sequence of the encoded protein. Although some substitutions have no detectable effect on cell function, others can render a protein inactive or thermolabile, or can alter its affinity for a substrate or a feedback inhibitor. Such mutant organisms can exhibit growth only under particular conditions, such as temperature-sensitive growth. Base-substitution or missense mutations are classified as transitions (replacement of a purine for a purine or a pyrimidine for a pyrimidine) or transversions (replacement of a purine for a pyrimidine). *Frame-shift mutations* result from the insertion or loss of one or a few bases, thereby shifting the process of decoding the triplets and resulting in the insertion of amino acids that are unrelated to those in the original protein. *Insertions* or *deletions* are mutations in which larger segments of DNA have been gained or lost. The effect of these changes on the appearance or behavior of the cell depends on the nature and placement of these changes in the coding sequence of each protein.

Nonsense Mutations and Suppressors

Three codons (UAG, UAA, and UGA) are used to signal the end of the coding region for a protein. A mutation that creates one of these termination codons within a gene causes premature termination and synthesis of an incomplete polypeptide. These are called *nonsense mutations,* and they have the trivial names of amber (UAG), ochre (UAA), and opal (UGA) mutations.

A *suppressor mutation* is the general name given to a change in DNA that compensates for the defect caused by the presence of another mutation. Extragenic suppressor mutations occur in a different gene than the original mutation. Nonsense suppressors are mutations that alter the specificity of a transfer RNA (tRNA) so that it inserts an amino acid at the site of a nonsense mutation (protein synthesis and tRNA action are described later). For example, if a mutation occurs in the gene for the tRNA that inserts leucine in response to the codon UUG so that it recognizes the nonsense codon UAG, that suppressor tRNA will insert leucine at the site of any amber mutation and will allow the synthesis of a full-length polypeptide. Thus, amber suppressors can overcome the effect of all amber mutations, although they also can interfere with the termination of polypeptides at the end of normal genes. Nonsense suppressor mutations overcome the premature termination but may not restore complete activity if the amino acid inserted by the nonsense suppressor is incompatible with proper function of the affected protein.

Mutagens

Numerous compounds, known as mutagens, increase the mutation rate of a cell. Some mutagens are base analogues, such as 5-bromouracil (see Fig. 2-2), which can be incorporated into DNA in place of the normal base, in this case, thymine. Mutagenic base analogues have an increased frequency of forming base pairs with an inappropriate base, such as guanine, instead of adenine during chromosome replication.

Other mutagens include alkylating agents, such as nitrogen mustard, ethylene oxide, ethyl methanesulfonate, and *N*-methyl-*N*-nitro-nitrosoguanidine. These agents react with guanine residues in the DNA and cause occasional improper base pairing during chromosome replication or loss of the alkylated base followed by incorporation of any base during repair. The attachment of bulky alkyl groups onto DNA bases can block DNA synthesis, leading to induction of the SOS damage-repair process and the action of an error-prone DNA polymerase. Another potent mutagen is ultraviolet light, which causes the formation of pyrimidine dimers within one DNA strand. Although the presence of a dimer prevents the passage of the DNA replication fork, it is the removal of dimers by the error-prone repair systems that results in the generation of mutations.

Recombinant DNA Techniques

The methods for the generation, isolation, and experimental manipulation of specific fragments of DNA are termed *recombinant DNA techniques* because they involve the construction of hybrid DNA molecules containing portions of DNA from different sources. These techniques are based on several specialized topics of microbiologic research into the processes of plasmid replication, genetic transformation, restriction enzymes, and nucleic acid hybridization.

PLASMIDS

Many bacteria possess plasmids, which are extrachromosomal (usually) circular DNA molecules that are generally dispensable for growth. They range greatly in size, genetic content, and number of copies per cell. Many plasmids confer antibiotic resistance or other traits related to bacterial virulence; some plasmids can mediate their own transfer from one cell to another (see. Chap. 21). With regard to recombinant DNA technology, the key feature of plasmids is that their replication in a bacterial host is controlled by a small portion of the whole plasmid. This region, usually termed *ori*, for origin of DNA replication, contains all the information needed to allow plasmid multiplication by host cell enzyme systems. As long as an *ori* region is present, the rest of the plasmid molecule can be rearranged, eliminated, or replaced by other DNA sequences without affecting the ability of the plasmid to replicate, thereby providing the basis for the construction of plasmids that carry any segment of DNA from any cell source.

TRANSFORMATION

A few bacterial species have the natural capacity to take up fragments of DNA from their medium by a genetic exchange process called *transformation* (see. Chap. 21). However, many types of bacteria can be induced to take up DNA by experimental manipulations, such as exposure to solutions of $CaCl_2$ followed by a brief heat shock. It is common practice to construct or alter a plasmid in a test tube and then return it to a bacterial cell by the process of transformation, thereby permitting the preparation of large amounts of that plasmid DNA (or of the proteins it encodes) and the examination of the effect of that plasmid on its new host cell.

Plasmid DNA also can be introduced into eucaryotic cells by a variety of techniques, including deposition onto the cells of a precipitate of DNA and calcium phosphate, exposure to steep electrical gradients (electroporation), microinjection, and even bombardment with DNA-coated microprojectiles.

RESTRICTION ENZYMES

The experimental manipulation of DNA in plasmids and other vectors was made possible by the discovery of *restriction endonucleases,* which are enzymes that cut DNA molecules at specific base sequences. These enzymes are present in most procaryotic organisms and probably function to eliminate foreign DNA that might enter a cell by transformation or virus infection. A cell's DNA is protected from its own restriction endonucleases by being specifically modified (usually by methylation of bases within the target sequence).

Commonly used restriction enzymes recognize and cut DNA sequences that are 4 to 6 base pairs in length and are palindromic, meaning that the sequence is the same on both strands of the double helix. Some restriction enzymes cleave in the center of the recognition sequence to produce blunt or flush ends. Other enzymes cut off-center to generate complementary or cohesive ("sticky") ends that overlap for two or four bases, as diagrammed in Figure 2-6. Fragments of DNA that were cut with restriction enzymes and have blunt or overhanging complementary ends can be rejoined by action of the enzyme, *DNA ligase.*

As an example of a simple application of this technique, plasmid DNA from the bacterium *Escherichia coli* and chromosomal DNA from another organism can be cleaved with a restriction enzyme, mixed, and resealed with DNA ligase. The resulting complex DNA aggregate is introduced by transformation into *E coli* cells, where the foreign chromosomal DNA can replicate only if it is linked to the plasmid DNA, because only the plasmid has an origin of replication. Plasmid vectors are available that carry genes that confer antibiotic resistance, and selection for this resistance facilitates the isolation of those cells that have acquired plasmids carrying a fragment of foreign DNA. For further manipulation of cloned DNA, fragments generated by cleavage with restriction endonucleases can be purified by electrophoretic separation in an agarose gel and then ligated together with a plasmid or viral vector that has been cut with a restriction enzyme to give complementary ends. The products of ligation reactions are introduced back into bacteria by transforma-

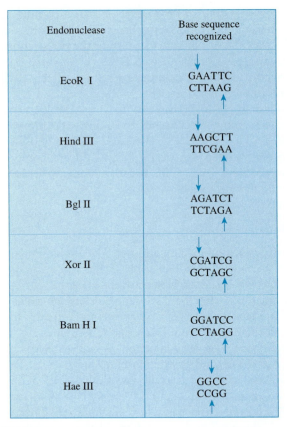

Endonuclease	Base sequence recognized
EcoR I	↓ GAATTC CTTAAG ↑
Hind III	↓ AAGCTT TTCGAA ↑
Bgl II	↓ AGATCT TCTAGA ↑
Xor II	↓ CGATCG GCTAGC ↑
Bam H I	↓ GGATCC CCTAGG ↑
Hae III	↓ GGCC CCGG ↑

FIGURE 2-6   Examples of specific base sequences recognized by restriction endonucleases. Arrows indicate points of cleavage. Note that some enzymes are cut at staggered sites, yielding "sticky ends."

tion. Figure 2-7 illustrates some of the steps involved in recombinant DNA technology.

NUCLEIC ACID HYBRIDIZATION

Nucleic acid hybridization provides a powerful way to identify bacteria transformed with a plasmid carrying a specific DNA fragment or to detect the presence of a particular gene sequence in the genome of other organisms. Hybridization techniques were developed for studies of taxonomy, because the phylogenetic relatedness of bacterial or other species can be estimated from the rate and extent to which DNA from different species forms a double helix (hybridizes, or renatures) after separation of its strands. The more related the species, the more similar are their DNA sequences and the greater are the rate and extent of renaturation. Hybridization can be measured in solution by physical methods that separate renatured from single-stranded DNA, or by treatment with an enzyme that specifically degrades single-stranded nucleic acids (such as the S1 nuclease produced by *Aspergillus oryzae*). For recombinant DNA studies, hybridization is commonly detected by the binding of a radioactively labeled DNA to a solid matrix containing denatured DNA (Fig. 2-8). Typically, DNA fragments are generated by

cleavage with a restriction enzyme, separated by electrophoresis in an agarose gel, and transferred from the gel to a membrane (nitrocellulose or nylon) in the same relative locations as on the agarose gel. The DNA on the membrane then is denatured by alkali and heat, and is bound to the membrane before the membrane is incubated with a radioactively labeled DNA or RNA fragment, called the *probe*. The probe will form a duplex only with DNA fragments that have identical or similar sequences. The filter is washed under conditions that release the probe from sequences with poor match. The labeled probe that remains hybridized to homologous sequences on the filter is detected by autoradiography. This technique is called *Southern hybridization analysis,* after its developer, Edward Southern. Bacterial colonies or phage plaques that carry specific nucleic acid inserts can be detected in a similar manner, after their lysis, transfer to a membrane, and hybridization to a probe. Northern hybridization analysis uses the same procedures for detection of homologous species of cellular RNA.

GENE CLONING

The techniques described for cloning restriction fragments of DNA into plasmid or viral vectors and for detecting specific inserts by hybridization make it possible to isolate specific DNA fragments derived from the chromosome of any organism.

Complementary DNA Cloning

It is often advantageous to clone as DNA a copy of the messenger RNA (mRNA) that encodes a protein of interest from cell lines that produce large amounts of that protein because they have correspondingly amplified levels of its mRNA. This process is called *complementary DNA (cDNA) cloning,* because the first step involves the synthesis of DNA fragments complementary to the mRNA using retroviral enzymes called *RNA-dependent DNA polymerases* (reverse transcriptases; see Chap. 43). The cDNA is then made into a double strand by the action of a DNA polymerase and is ligated into a plasmid or phage vector. The desired clones can be detected within the entire collection of cDNA clones by virtue of their hybridization to a DNA probe that was made from the same gene from another organism, or was a synthetic oligonucleotide whose sequence was deduced from the amino acid sequence of the desired protein. Other cDNA cloning systems have been developed to allow the cloned fragments to be expressed in bacteria as proteins that can be detected with specific antibodies.

Genomic Cloning

A cDNA clone corresponding to a desired gene can be used as a hybridization probe to identify the correspond-

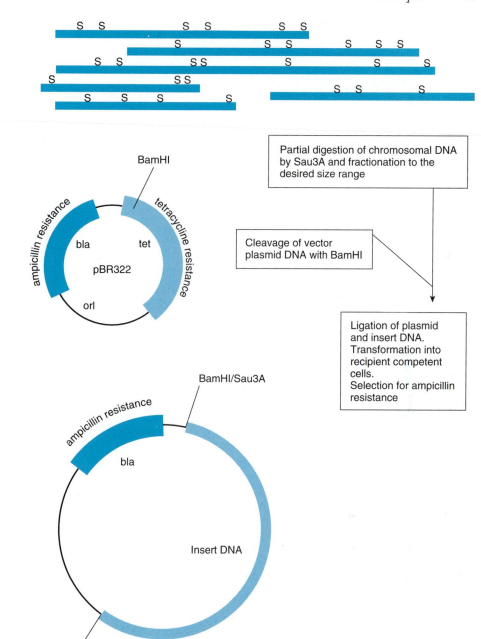

Cloning of foreign DNA into a plasmid vector (pBR322). Plasmid pBR322 DNA is cut with restriction endonuclease *Bam*HI, and the foreign DNA is cut partially with endonuclease *Sau*3A, yielding staggered cuts with the same sticky ends. Reannealing causes some of the foreign DNA to base pair with the sticky ends in pBR322. Because *Bam*HI cuts in pBR322 inside a gene for tetracycline resistance, ligation of the foreign DNA into pBR322 inactivates the *tet*^R gene. Thus, bacteria transformed with pBR322-containing foreign DNA will be ampicillin resistant and tetracycline sensitive, whereas those receiving only religated pBR322 plasmid without an insert will be resistant to both antibiotics.

ing clones in a library of DNA fragments derived directly from the DNA of a cell's genome. Any individual gene represents a small fraction of a genomic library.

When the structure of a cDNA is compared with that of its gene on the eucaryotic chromosome, it is usually found that substantial portions of sequence that were present in and copied from the gene were removed during processing of the mRNA. Isolation of the genomic clone is necessary to reveal which regions were removed during RNA processing and to provide the nucleotide sequences on each side of the gene that may be important for the control of its expression.

DNA Sequencing

An important breakthrough in the analysis of nucleic acids was the development of methods for rapid determination of the nucleotide sequence of cloned DNA. Two different procedures—one chemical, the other enzymatic—have been developed, but the enzymatic method is used most commonly. Briefly, the enzymatic (Sanger) method involves making a copy of the DNA region from a specific DNA primer sequence using a DNA polymerase in the presence of all four of the nucleotide precursors and small amounts of a form of one of the nucleotides that blocks

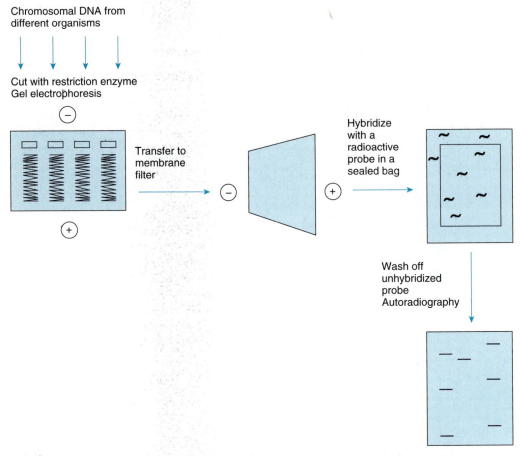

FIGURE 2-8 Schematic diagram of nucleic acid hybridization on a solid support. Cellular RNA or restriction fragments of DNA are separated according to size by electrophoresis through agarose or polyacrylamide gels. The resolved nucleic acid species are transferred either by electrophoresis or by capillary flow to a solid membrane support made of nitrocellulose or nylon. The transferred nucleic acids then are linked tightly to the support. The membrane is exposed to a nucleic acid probe labeled with radioactivity or a chemical marker, and sufficient time is allowed for hybridization of the probe to its homologous sequences immobilized on the filter. The membrane is then washed to remove nonspecifically bound probe. The location of the bound probe then is detected by autoradiography or enzymatic visualization.

further chain growth (2′,3′-dideoxynucleoside triphosphate). Thus, fragments of different lengths are made that correspond to the position of the base in the dideoxynucleotide. Comparison of the fragment lengths with those formed by each of the other three dideoxynucleotides allows direct reading of the DNA sequence. Using these techniques, the sequence of a gene can be determined in perhaps a month, and determining the sequence of an entire human genome is considered feasible.

Polymerase Chain Reaction Techniques

An extremely powerful technique for the isolation of specific DNA sequences has been developed. Called the *polymerase chain reaction*, it involves amplification of the sequences between any two DNA primers by repetitive cycles of primer hybridization to genomic DNA, polymerization of the DNA regions between the two primer-binding sites, and thermal denaturation of the product

from the DNA (schematically diagrammed in Fig. 2-9). This is an exceedingly sensitive technique able to yield large amounts of DNA from a single DNA molecule, giving it considerable promise in forensic medicine and in the detection of the presence and identity of infectious agents.

Gene Structure

Recombinant DNA techniques have allowed detailed knowledge of the structure and sequence of many genes from bacteria and eucaryotic organisms. This revealed substantial differences in the genetic organization of these two life forms.

PROCARYOTIC GENE STRUCTURE

Almost all bacterial genes exhibit an exact *colinearity* between the sequence of nucleotides in the DNA, the se-

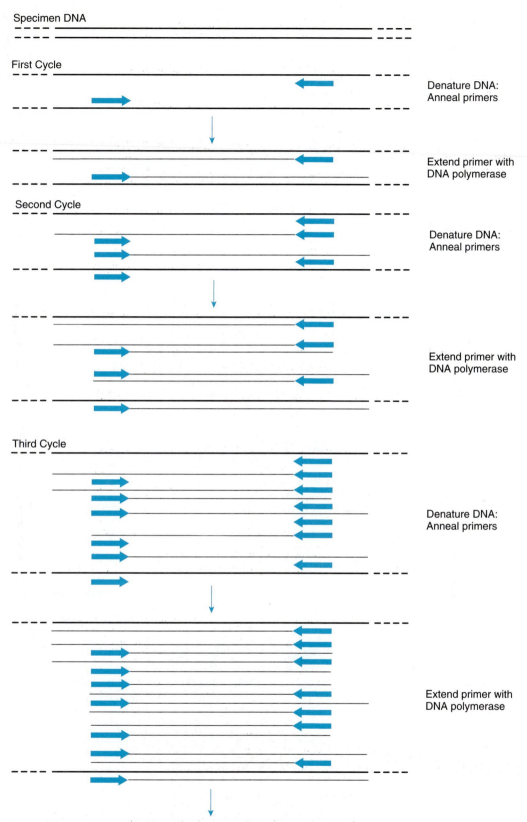

Specimen DNA

First Cycle

Denature DNA:
Anneal primers

Extend primer with
DNA polymerase

Second Cycle

Denature DNA:
Anneal primers

Extend primer with
DNA polymerase

Third Cycle

Denature DNA:
Anneal primers

Extend primer with
DNA polymerase

Repeated cycles of denaturation and primer extension results in exponential
amplification of the DNA sequence between the two primers.

FIGURE 2-9 Polymerase chain reaction (PCR) technique. Any specific DNA sequence can be obtained from a sample of DNA by the repetitive amplification of the sequence lying between the binding site for any two oppositely oriented DNA oligonucleotides serving as primers. This amplification involves repeated cycles of DNA thermal denaturation, annealing of the oligonucleotide primers at a lower temperature, and extension of the primer by template-dependent polymerization. Both primers must bind within about 10 kb of each other for amplification of a distinct product. This technique was made practical by the isolation of very stable DNA polymerases from thermophilic bacteria.

quence of nucleotides in the mRNA copied from the DNA, and the sequence of amino acids in the polypeptide product. Bacterial mRNAs are not modified after their synthesis and are exact copies of the DNA gene. Genes encoding separate steps in a common pathway are often contiguous on the chromosome and are copied into a single multigenic (polycistronic) message. This clustered arrangement of genes is termed an *operon*. The expression of an operon is regulated as a unit from a single control region, which facilitates the regulation of enzyme synthesis and the coordination of the relative amounts of different polypeptides.

EUCARYOTIC GENE STRUCTURE

Most eucaryotic genes differ markedly in structure from bacterial genes. The clearest indication of this difference is the finding that a gene cloned from the chromosome is much larger than the cDNA copy of the RNA derived for that gene. Not all the DNA sequences present in the gene on the chromosome are retained in the final product.

The parts of the gene that are retained in the mRNA are called *exons* (*ex*pressed regi*ons*); some exons make up more than half the coding information for a protein and other exons are as small as the three base pairs that encode a single amino acid (Fig. 2-10).

The exons in the chromosome are interrupted by stretches of DNA called *intervening sequences* or *introns*. During gene expression, an entire region of a chromosome, including exons and introns, is transcribed into a long RNA molecule. The introns are removed from the precursor RNA by an enzyme complex that links the exons together in the same order and orientation as in the chromosome. This process, called *RNA splicing*, requires the recognition of specific base sequences at the beginning and end of each intervening sequence. Eucaryotic RNA usually is modified further at its ends by the addition of a cap structure at the 5′ end and of a tail of 80 to 200 A residues (poly A tail), as described later. After these modifications, the mRNA is released from the nucleus to travel to the ribosomes in the cytoplasm or on the rough endoplasmic reticulum.

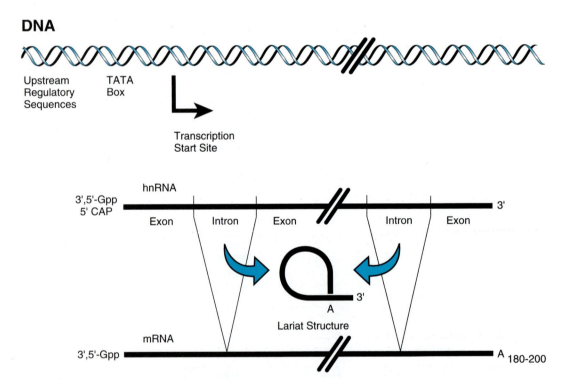

FIGURE 2-10   Diagram of mRNA processing in eucaryotic cells. Sequences in the DNA upstream from the start of RNA synthesis are essential for determining where and how frequently transcription will occur. The TATA box is an AT-rich region that is located a defined distance from the start of synthesis and is present in all promoters. Different upstream regulatory sequences can either increase or decrease transcription. Enhancer elements are DNA sequences that increase transcription and are active in either orientation and in any location with respect to the promoter. A long RNA sequence of heterogeneous length is read from the DNA and then processed by removal of introns through splicing and addition of modifications at the 5′ end (*CAP*) and the 3′ end (*poly A tail*). The CAP structure consists of 7-methylguanosine linked to the 5′ end of the transcript by an unusual 5′-5′-diphosphate bond that is added after synthesis of the mRNA has begun. On the 3′ end is added a poly A tail of about 200 adenosine residues. During removal of the introns in the splicing process, the upstream end of the intron forms a covalent bond to the 2′ hydroxyl group of an adenosine residue within the intron, forming a lariat-like structure.

A gene can contain from 1 to more than 20 introns, which can be much larger than the exons they separate. In some cases, exons correspond to different functional domains or structural motifs of the polypeptide product. This correspondence supports the concept that the apparently inefficient interruptions in eucaryotic genes help to enhance the rate of evolution. Joining of exons from different genes by genetic recombination could allow the assembly of the functional domains of different proteins in novel combinations. In addition, some genes contain alternative splice sites. The choice of one or another splice site results in the formation of different polypeptides that can be identical over most of their length but have different sequences in one region or differ in length because of the presence of additional amino acids at one end. An example is seen in the genes for immunoglobulin molecules, where alternative splicing of the mRNA gives rise to either the soluble form of antibody molecule that is released from the cell or the surface-bound form that has the same binding specificity but with a carboxyl-terminal membrane anchor.

Thus, genes are not static structures but can undergo several forms of reshuffling. In addition to RNA splicing, genome rearrangements have been found that bring distant coding regions into proximity. This process is important for the expression of the genes encoding several components of the immune system.

Chromosome Organization

The DNA of all cells is arranged in superstructures and is associated with various cellular components. Detailed descriptions of chromosome structure can be found in books on cell biology, but a brief review of the major differences between chromosome structure and organization in bacterial and eucaryotic cells is given here.

PROCARYOTIC CHROMOSOME

It is widely stated that bacteria possess a single chromosome, but this assertion is based on examination of a small group of organisms and is not always true. The presence of two chromosomes has been demonstrated in several bacterial types. Bacterial chromosomal DNA is circular in some bacterial types and linear in others. There also are optional, extrachromosomal genetic elements called *plasmids*, which usually are circular DNA molecules that encode various ancillary bacterial functions, such as drug resistance and conjugal genetic transfer (see Chap. 21).

Bacterial DNA is associated with proteins, but no single protein (or family of related proteins) coats or organizes bacterial DNA, as do the histones in the eucaryotic nucleus. A characteristic feature of bacterial DNA (at least in the well-studied *E coli*) is that it is circular and

negatively supercoiled, meaning that it is slightly underwound by about 6 turns per 100 turns of the DNA helix (about 1000 base pairs). Supercoiling makes the DNA helix easier to unwind and is necessary for DNA synthesis, for many recombination processes, and for expression of some genes. Supercoils are put into bacterial DNA by the action of an adenosine triphosphate (ATP)–dependent enzyme called *DNA gyrase.*

Intact bacterial chromosomes can be isolated by gentle lysis of cells. The large nucleoid structures are compact but can be separated from cellular debris and small components by centrifugation. This condensed superstructure appears to be the result of looping of about 50 segments of supercoiled DNA around an RNA core, and it probably is necessary to allow separation of the daughter chromosomes, which otherwise would become hopelessly tangled.

EUCARYOTIC CHROMOSOME

In contrast to the simple single bacterial chromosome, the nuclear DNA of all eucaryotes is carried on multiple chromosomes, which are present in pairs in all diploid organisms. Each chromosome is composed of an extremely long, linear DNA molecule associated with tightly bound basic proteins, called *histones,* as well as a large number of nonhistone proteins. This complex is called *chromatin.*

Viewed through the electron microscope, chromatin has an appearance resembling beads on a string (Fig. 2-11). The beads are called *nucleosomes,* and each nucleosome contains 180 base pairs of DNA wrapped around a complex of eight histone proteins. The DNA between nucleosomes is coated with a different histone than is in the nucleosome. Further coiling of nucleosomes into higher order structures occurs in the interphase chromosome. During mitosis and cell division, the chromosomes condense further to form the compact, discrete, and distinctive mitotic or metaphase structures that are sorted efficiently into the two progeny nuclei.

Chromosome Replication

DNA replication is a semiconservative process in which each strand of the double helix serves as the template directing the synthesis of its complementary strand. Thus, after chromosome replication, each progeny double-stranded DNA molecule contains one newly synthesized strand and one strand from the original double helix. The replication system accurately copies the sequence of nucleotides of the template strand into the sequence in the progeny strand using the complementarity rules that A pairs with T, and G pairs with C.

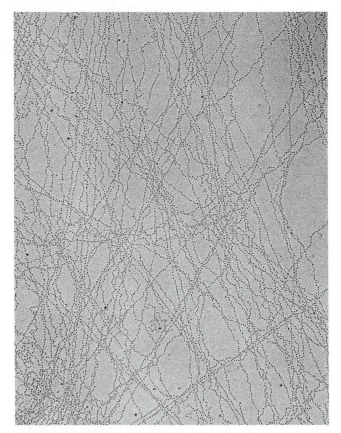

FIGURE 2-11 Electron micrograph of eucaryotic chromatin. Note the beaded appearance of the histone-containing nucleosomes that occur at regular intervals along the strands of DNA. Such structures do not occur on procaryotic DNA. (Original magnification ×410,000.)

PROCARYOTIC CHROMOSOME REPLICATION

Replication of the bacterial chromosome begins at a single, specific site, called the *origin,* and proceeds in both directions around the chromosome, requiring about 40 minutes for completion. The general events that occur as each replication complex proceeds around the chromosome are fairly well understood because of extensive biochemical characterization of the process. The key enzymatic activity is DNA polymerase, which adds deoxyribonucleoside monophosphates onto a growing chain using each DNA strand as the template to specify which of the four deoxyribonucleoside triphosphates will be the next substrate used. The product strand is oriented antiparallel to the template strand.

Of the three DNA polymerases in *E coli,* DNA polymerase III is the one necessary for chromosome replication; the others are involved in the repair of DNA damage and in some processing steps of replication. All DNA polymerases have similar mechanisms and pose two fundamental problems, because they synthesize DNA in only a single direction (5' to 3') and can add new nucleotides only to the 3'-hydroxyl group of an existing chain, or *primer.* During DNA replication, one new strand can

be made in a continuous manner, because its synthesis proceeds in the 5' to 3' direction. Synthesis of the other strand, however, is not so simple and must take place in a discontinuous fashion. This is accomplished by the synthesis in the 5' to 3' direction of short "Okazaki fragments" of DNA, 1000 to 2000 nucleotides in length, beginning as soon as a sufficient stretch of template DNA has become exposed (Fig. 2-12).

The primers required to start the growth of each progeny strand or Okazaki fragment are short RNA molecules (2 to 20 nucleotides) synthesized by a special RNA polymerase, called *DNA primase* or primosome. Once synthesis of each segment has started, the RNA primer is removed and replaced with DNA nucleotides in a process that includes DNA polymerase I. These segments are then joined by the action of DNA ligase. This backward, intermittent replication of the so-called lagging strand allows rapid, faithful, and coordinated copying of the double helix without leaving extensive lengths of single-stranded DNA exposed. Each replication fork adds 750 to 1000 nucleotides per second, meaning that the DNA unwinding machinery operates at 4500 to 6000 rpm.

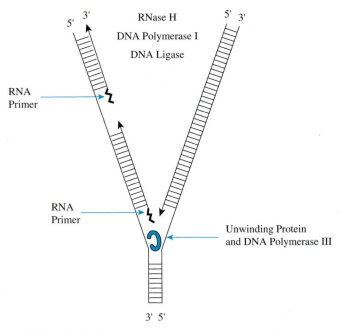

FIGURE 2-12 Highly schematic representation of a replication fork formed during the replication of DNA. An unwinding protein separates the two strands of DNA, and a second protein binds to each strand to keep them apart. Replication can occur only from the 5' end toward the 3' end of each DNA strand. Therefore, on one strand (represented on the right-hand fork), replication is continuous. On the other strand, however, the DNA polymerase must wait until a segment of about a thousand bases becomes unwound and then replicates back toward the newly formed double-stranded DNA in a 5' to 3' direction. Replication is initiated for each discontinuous fragment by a primase that lays down a short chain of RNA, which acts as a primer for the DNA polymerase. As each segment is completed, RNase H removes the RNA primer; DNA polymerase I fills in the gaps with deoxynucleotides; and DNA ligase joins each segment together.

Replication of the bacterial chromosome uses a complex assemblage of enzymes, including the DNA polymerase III holoenzyme, which consists of seven protein subunits, and a primosome complex that contains between three and five proteins. This latter complex is responsible for synthesis of the short RNA primers during replication of the lagging strand.

The controls that govern the time of initiation of chromosome replication are complex and not fully understood. Initiation of replication of many DNA plasmids requires the synthesis of a long RNA molecule to serve as primer. Initiation of chromosome replication depends on the synthesis of specific origin-binding protein, which is coupled to the cell division cycle and is responsive to the nutritional state of the cell. A replication fork can initiate before the previous one has finished. For bacteria dividing more rapidly than every 40 minutes, which is the time required for a pair of bidirectional replication forks to traverse the chromosome, there will be several forks in action at once. Thus, the chromosome that is segregated into the two progeny cells will still be in the process of replication needed for the next cell division.

EUCARYOTIC CHROMOSOME REPLICATION

The enzymes involved in eucaryotic DNA replication have not been characterized as completely as have those in procaryotic cells, but the basic enzymatic mechanisms are similar. There are multiple origins on each chromosome, and replication from each origin proceeds in both directions. DNA synthesis occurs only during the *S phase* of the cell cycle, and many of the enzymes necessary for DNA replication are found in the nucleus only during the S phase. At mitosis, each chromosome that had replicated during the S phase is condensed into compact structures that are pulled apart by the mitotic spindle apparatus to opposite poles of the cell. Another noteworthy feature of each chromosome are its ends, called *telomeres*. Special mechanisms operate to allow their replication, because the ends of any linear molecule cannot be copied by DNA polymerase and eventually would be lost.

Transcription

The genetic information in DNA is expressed by being copied into RNA, a process called *transcription*. RNA is a polynucleotide like DNA, except that RNA contains uracil in place of thymine, and the phosphodiester-linked sugar is ribose instead of deoxyribose. Several classes of RNA are distinguished on the basis of their function and size. mRNAs are heterogeneous in length and carry the information for the synthesis of specific proteins. tRNAs decode the information in the mRNAs to yield the correct sequence of amino acids. Other RNAs play structural roles, and the most abundant of these are the three or four

ribosomal RNAs (rRNAs) that are integral constituents of the ribosome. Another RNA is a component of the protein secretion system, and others participate catalytically in the RNA-splicing reactions. One RNA is the catalytic portion of the enzyme ribonuclease P (RNase P), which helps process tRNAs after their synthesis as a longer fragment.

Transcription is the DNA-dependent polymerization of ribonucleotides in the 5′ to 3′ direction. It occurs after each incoming ribonucleoside triphosphate binds to its complementary base on the DNA template. Generally, only one strand of DNA is copied in any one region, although the other strand is read in other regions. This section describes the mechanism of transcription and the signals that specify where transcription starts (promoters) and stops (terminators).

PROCARYOTIC TRANSCRIPTION

RNA Polymerases

Bacteria possess only one RNA polymerase, which typically contains three polypeptides in the arrangement $\alpha_2\beta\beta'$. The specificity for starting the RNA polymerase at the correct site on the proper strand is provided by the binding of another protein called *sigma (σ) factor*. This protein is involved only in the selection of the promoter, and it dissociates from the polymerase after transcription has started. Any cell contains multiple σ factors that recognize different promoters and allow differential transcription of various families of genes. RNA polymerase that contains σ factor is referred to as the *holoenzyme*, because it faithfully carries out the normal transcription process. The form of the enzyme lacking σ factor, called *core polymerase*, also is able to synthesize RNA, but without regard for proper site or direction of initiation. As in DNA replication, RNA is synthesized in the 5′ to 3′ direction at an average rate of about 30 to 60 nucleotides per second. RNA synthesis does not require a preexisting primer to start chain synthesis.

Promoters

Bacterial promoters are well-defined, short DNA sequences that determine the site where transcription will start. Most promoters in *E coli* consist of short DNA sequences located 35 and 10 base pairs before the start of transcription, and optimal promoter activity occurs with the sequence TTGACA at the −35 region and TATAAT at the −10 region (Fig. 2-13). RNA polymerase holoenzyme binds to the promoter regions in DNA and covers about seven turns of the DNA helix. It opens the DNA double helix to form a stable open–promoter complex. Ribonucleoside triphosphates are polymerized sequentially onto the growing RNA strand as specified by the DNA template. After the RNA chain has reached

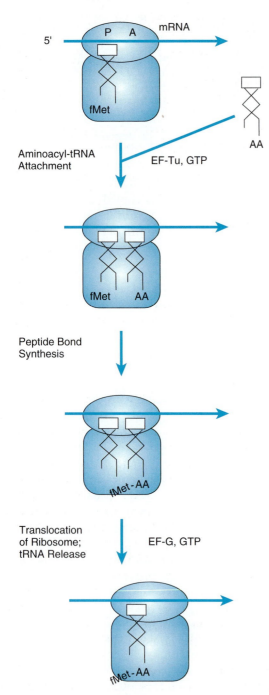

Aminoacyl-tRNA
Attachment

EF-Tu, GTP

Peptide Bond
Synthesis

Translocation
of Ribosome;
tRNA Release

EF-G, GTP

FIGURE 2-13 Summary of transcription and protein synthesis. The structure of a procaryotic promoter determines the site of binding of RNA polymerase and the formation of an open promoter complex. RNA synthesis proceeds in the 5′ to 3′ direction, and the newly formed mRNA can be used immediately to encode synthesis of its polypeptide product. Polypeptide synthesis occurs on the surface of a ribosome as it moves across the mRNA in the 5′ to 3′ direction. Initiation always begins with formyl methionyl tRNA. Peptide bond formation is followed by shifting of the ribosome to the next codon on the mRNA. This liberates the uncharged tRNA and moves the polypeptide-bound tRNA from the A site to the P site on the ribosome, thus exposing a new codon in the A site for the next aminoacyl tRNA.

a length of 4 to 12 nucleotides, the σ factor is released from the complex and the RNA polymerase moves away from the promoter as an elongation complex. During the elongation stage of RNA synthesis, the enzyme opens about 17 base pairs of the DNA to expose the template strand. About 12 nucleotides of the newly synthesized RNA pair with the template strand of DNA before being released with re-formation of the DNA double helix, as the RNA polymerase moves along. The σ factor is replaced by other proteins that allow the enzyme to respond to transcription termination signals. Some terminators, at which RNA synthesis stops and the polymerase dissociates, are characteristic sequences in which a stem and loop structure rich in G and C is followed by a string of U residues; other terminators are less easily recognized sites at which the termination protein *rho* acts to halt transcription.

RNA Processing

Processing of RNA after its synthesis is rare in bacteria. The mRNAs are immediately available for translation, and translation frequently begins while the transcript RNA is still being made. Bacterial mRNAs usually have short lifetimes of less than 2 minutes. The stable rRNAs and tRNAs are synthesized as multiple units from which the proper-sized products are trimmed by the action of specific nucleases. Many of the bases on these RNAs subsequently are modified by the addition of methyl and other groups.

EUCARYOTIC TRANSCRIPTION

RNA Polymerases

Transcription in eucaryotes is a much more complex process than in bacteria. There are three eucaryotic RNA polymerases: one (Pol II) synthesizes mRNA, another (Pol I) makes rRNA, and the third (Pol III) primarily makes tRNA. These enzymes are more complex than the bacterial polymerases, containing more protein subunits and responding to a larger number of activator proteins.

Promoters

The characteristics that determine a transcription start site are complicated and are still being defined. Most promoters possess a TATA site near the start of transcription, but multiple regions, some more than 500 base pairs from the start of a message, are required for proper initiation at some promoters. Sometimes, changes in the DNA far beyond these sites can influence transcription, perhaps by altering the chromatin structure. For some tRNAs and other short genes, the start sites actually are determined by sequences located within the genes themselves rather than by sequences upstream.

In addition to the promoter region, there are important regulatory sequences, called *enhancer* elements, that do not affect the location of the initiation site but greatly increase the frequency with which nearby promoters are read. The orientation of the enhancer elements relative to the promoter does not matter; in fact, enhancers can act even if they are located on the opposite side of the gene from the promoter. Enhancers are important factors in the control of both the immune response (see Chap. 7) and viral replication (see Chap. 41).

RNA Processing

Eucaryotic RNAs are subject to multiple processing events, the most remarkable of which is RNA splicing, or the removal of introns from the initial transcript. Splicing can occur while the transcript is still being made. The process of splicing is carried out by ribonucleoprotein complexes (the "spliceosome") that recognize the two splice sites at each end of each intron and join them together with release of the intron as a so-called lariat structure.

Other modifications of eucaryotic messages are common. To the 5′ end of the mRNA is attached an unusual structure called a *cap*, which is a modified G nucleotide attached to the mRNA at its 5′ end through a diphosphate linkage to yield the surprising situation in which the 5′ end of the mRNA is actually a 3′-end structure. With few exceptions, the cap structure is necessary for the translation of that message into protein. A second modification present in almost all cellular mRNAs is the *poly A tail,* which consists of about 200 A nucleotides added to the 3′ end. These A residues are not encoded in the DNA; instead, a specific sequence in the RNA signals the site where cleavage of the transcript and poly A addition will occur. The poly A tail is necessary for normal stability or translation of the message.

Translation

Translation is the process by which the genetic information contained in the nucleotide sequence of an mRNA is translated into the sequence of amino acids in the product polypeptide. The correspondence between base sequence and amino acid sequence is called the *genetic code,* through which the three contiguous nucleotides in a *codon* code for one amino acid.

TRANSFER RNA

The genetic code is translated by small RNA molecules (70 to 80 nucleotides long) called tRNAs. These form tightly folded, L-shaped structures with several domains essential for their function. At one end of the folded structure (which is actually in the middle of the nucleotide sequence) is the *anticodon loop,* containing three bases complementary and antiparallel to the codons in the mRNA. The recognition of each codon in the mRNA by the anticodon in the tRNA occurs by base pairing and determines the specificity of which amino acid is inserted at each codon. Interestingly, the requirement for specificity in pairing to the third base in the codon is relaxed ("wobble"), so that one tRNA can pair with several codons that differ in the third position.

Each tRNA molecule is recognized by one of the 20 activating enzymes, or aminoacyl-tRNA synthetases. Each synthetase specifically attaches its appropriate amino acid onto the correct tRNAs through the ATP-dependent formation of a covalent bond between the carboxyl group of the amino acid and the 3′-hydroxyl group at the end of the tRNA. Each enzyme can recognize all the tRNAs that should carry that amino acid. The specificity for recognition of the proper tRNA by each synthetase is influenced by specific nucleotides throughout the tRNA molecule, although the sequence of the anticodon loop plays a major role for many of the enzymes.

RIBOSOMES

The process of protein synthesis takes place on particles called *ribosomes*. Ribosomes are composed of rRNAs and ribosomal proteins, and are designated by their sedimentation coefficient (S, or Svedberg unit). An intact procaryotic ribosome, called a *70S particle,* is composed of a 30S and a 50S subparticle, which come apart normally at the end of protein synthesis or when the level of magnesium ions is reduced. The 30S subunit contains one molecule of 16S rRNA (1520 nucleotides) and 32 proteins, all present in a single copy per ribosome. Each 50S subunit contains a molecule of 23S rRNA (3100 nucleotides), a molecule of 5S rRNA (120 nucleotides), and 34 ribosomal proteins, all of which are different from the proteins found in the smaller subunit. The rRNAs play a major role in ribosome function by providing the scaffold for attachment of the ribosomal proteins and by actually carrying out the central steps of peptide bond formation. Ribosomal proteins are relatively small and basic. Ribosomes represent a major component of the cell and can constitute as much as half the weight of the cell.

The overall process of protein synthesis catalyzed by the ribosome is a complex process with three major steps: *initiation,* in which the ribosome assembles at the proper site on the mRNA; *elongation,* in which the tRNA specified by the next codon in the mRNA is selected and bound, the amino acid it carries is coupled onto the growing polypeptide chain, and the ribosome is readied to incorporate the next amino acid; and *termination,* in which the end of the coding region is recognized and the completed polypeptide is released. Figure 2-13 outlines the mechanism of protein synthesis in procaryotic cells.

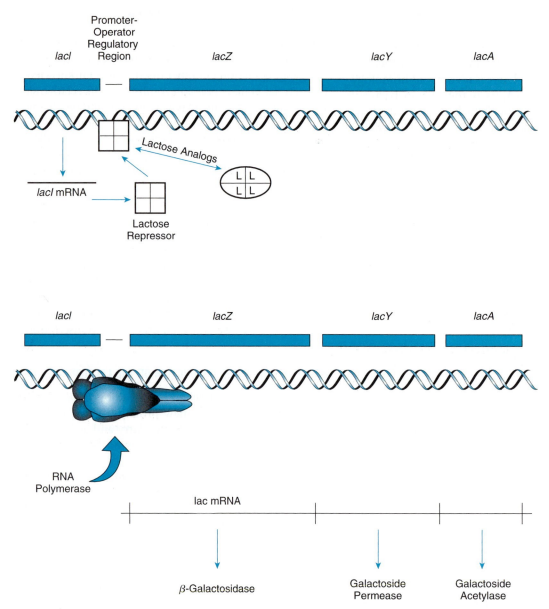

FIGURE 2-14 Model for the regulation of inducible enzyme synthesis in the lac operon. The three structural genes responsible for the transport and breakdown of lactose are arranged as an operon, or series of contiguous genes subject to a common control region. The regulatory gene, *lacI*, encodes a repressor protein which binds to specific sites near the promoter region, and prevents RNA polymerase binding and passage. In the presence of lactose analogs, the repressor protein undergoes a change in shape which reduces its ability to bind to the operator region. Release of the repressor allows RNA polymerase to bind and transcribe the three genes of the operon.

cause a change in the shape of the repressor, reducing its affinity for the operator by a factor of 1000. The RNA polymerase then can attach to the open promoter and copy the operon.

Mutations that destroy the repressor or impair its ability to bind to the operator site result in high-level constitutive expression of the *lac* operon. If a good copy of this gene (*lacI*+) also is present in the cell along with a defective *lacI* gene, the wild-type gene restores inducible behavior (ie, inducibility is dominant in this situation).

Other mutations in *lacI* impair the ability of the repressor to bind allolactose or to change shape in the presence of allolactose. When this type of mutant repressor protein binds to DNA, the *lac* operon is forever silent and cannot be induced by lactose. These mutants are termed I^S, for super-repressed, and cannot be corrected by the presence of *lacI*+ in the same cell.

Mutations can occur in the *lac* operator, which is a symmetric sequence of 18 base pairs, so that the repressor binds with a lower affinity for the altered operator. This results in a higher uninduced level of operon expression, even though the induced level remains normal. Operator-constitutive mutations affect only the operon adjacent to them and not any other *lac* operon in the cell (in a partially diploid cell). This behavior, in which a mutation affects only the gene adjacent to it, is called *cis-dominance*.

The structure of the DNA-binding portion of the *lacI* protein is similar to that of many other bacterial transcription regulators. The part of the protein that specifically recognizes and binds to the DNA forms a structural motif called the helix–turn–helix, in which two helical portions are connected by a short turn. One of the helices binds in the major groove of the DNA and recognizes the specific sequence of 3 to 5 base pairs there. The other helix lies atop the inserted helix and helps stabilize the contact with the DNA. Many regulatory proteins exist as dimers and are arranged so that each helix–turn–helix portion on the two monomers of the complex binds to the same sequence exposed in successive turns of the DNA duplex.

NEGATIVE CONTROL OF REPRESSIBLE PATHWAYS

The same basic mechanism of repressor action operates to control gene expression by *repression*. This type of regulation often is seen with genes for biosynthetic enzymes, in which a surplus of the product of that enzyme's pathway causes decreased production of that enzyme. In this situation, the repressor binds to the operator site only if the low-molecular-weight product of the pathway is present. Depletion of the product and its release from the repressor alters the repressor so that it is released from the operator, resulting in increased transcription of the gene.

POSITIVE CONTROL OF THE ARABINOSE OPERON

In *positive control*, a regulatory protein turns on the expression of the controlled genes, rather than turning them off, as in negative control. In this case, the regulatory gene product is called an *activator*. When the activator is eliminated by mutation or is in an inactive state in the absence of its inducer, it cannot bind to a control region upstream from the controlled gene. The promoter of such genes cannot be recognized by RNA polymerase unless the activator protein is bound nearby. Addition of inducer alters the structure of the activator so that it can bind near the promoter and facilitate the binding of RNA polymerase, possibly by protein–protein interactions.

The best known example of this type of control is the arabinose operon of *E coli*, in which the three catabolic genes of the *araBAD* operon and genes for two transport systems are controlled by the activator produced by the gene *araC* (Fig. 2-15). In the absence of the inducer, L-arabinose, the dimer of the AraC protein forms a loop in DNA by binding to two distant sites. In the presence of

inducer, AraC lets go of the distant site and binds nearer the promoter to stimulate the binding of RNA polymerase. In addition, the *araC* product acts as a repressor to control its own synthesis by binding to its own promoter in competition with the binding of RNA polymerase.

CATABOLITE REPRESSION

Many genes are subject to *global controls*, which respond to features of the general physiologic state of the cell. Various physiologic states or imbalances trigger the production of specific low-molecular-weight compounds, termed *alarmones*, which regulate a variety of cellular processes.

One major global control, called *catabolite repression*, reduces the level of expression of genes for catabolic enzymes when the cells are actively metabolizing a good carbon source, even though their inducing substrate is present. One of the several aspects of this integrative response as used by *E coli* results in decreased production of the alarmone, cyclic-3′,5′-adenosine monophosphate (cAMP), when cells are growing in glucose-containing medium. Glucose inhibits the activity of adenylate cyclase, the enzyme that makes cAMP, indirectly through the phosphotransferase transport system described in Chapter 16. In *E coli*, cAMP stimulates the binding of a transcription-activator protein (called the catabolite gene-activator protein, or CAP) to specific sites on DNA near catabolite-sensitive promoters, which then stimulates the binding of RNA polymerase to increase transcription of those genes. The lower level of cAMP resulting from its lower rate of synthesis in the presence of glucose leads to a decreased transcription of many genes involved in sugar and amino acid transport and degradation pathways, and the synthesis of flagella.

In addition to its effect on gene transcription, glucose inhibits the uptake of many sugars into the cell. This is especially severe if the sugar transport system is at a low level (as it is in uninduced cells before exposure to lactose). This phenomenon of inducer exclusion is another factor that reduces the expression of catabolic genes in the presence of glucose. The net result is that cells of *E coli* exposed to a mixture of glucose and lactose initially use only the glucose; the lactose-degrading enzymes are not produced until all the glucose has been consumed. Although glucose is the preferred nutrient in *E coli*, catabolite repression systems in other bacteria are triggered by other nutrients.

ATTENUATION CONTROL OF THE TRYPTOPHAN OPERON

Many bacterial genes are regulated by *attenuation* controls. This type of control mechanism does not affect the initiation of transcription but regulates the continuation of RNA polymerase into the structural genes (Fig. 2-16). The best studied example of this behavior is the

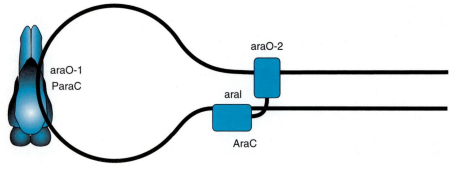

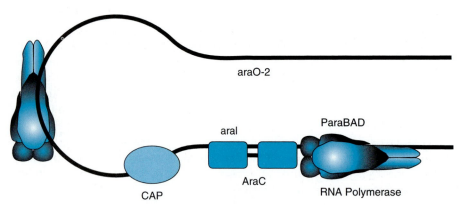

FIGURE 2-15 Schematic diagram of the arabinose operon control region. The *araBAD* operon encodes the three enzymes necessary for the catabolism of arabinose. The *araC* gene encodes a regulatory protein, which is converted in the presence of L-arabinose to a form ($AraC_{II}$) that binds upstream of the *araBAD* operon and stimulates the binding of RNA polymerase (*RNAP*) and the transcription of the operon. Without the binding of the $AraC_{II}$ protein, this operon is not transcribed. The AraC protein also binds to a site upstream of its own gene (araO site). Binding of AraC here prevents the binding of RNA polymerase, thereby regulating the level of AraC protein. The cyclic adenosine monophosphate binding protein (*CAP*) also binds to a specific region and is necessary for efficient expression of the *ara* operon. (Redrawn from Schleif R. The L-arabinose operon. In: Neidhardt FC et al, eds. *Escherichia coli* and *Salmonella typhimurium:* cellular and molecular biology. Washington, DC, American Society for Microbiology, 1987:1473)

trp operon, which contains the five genes responsible for the biosynthesis of tryptophan. In the mRNA transcribed from the *trp* operon, a potential transcription termination structure occurs early in the transcript (after about 140 nucleotides have been made). This termination structure, called the *attenuator,* occurs before the first structural gene is encountered and can halt as many as 95% of the RNA polymerase molecules that have started transcribing the operon. The attenuator region of the RNA has the structure of a stem and loop rich in G and C, followed by a string of U residues, characteristic of rho-independent terminators. The key feature of this system is that the likelihood of forming the secondary structure of the RNA in the attenuator region that results in termination is determined by the tryptophan supply. The RNA in the leader region up to the attenuator can fold into either of two alternative conformations, one of which results in termination, while the other does not. Thus, regulation is a matter of controlling the relative amounts of the two RNA conformations in a process coupled to translation and the site of ribosomal pausing.

Within the leader region in front of the attenuator is a gene for a short (14–amino acid) peptide with two tandem codons for tryptophan. If there is a sufficient supply of Trp-tRNA, this small gene is efficiently translated, the peptide is made, the ribosome stops at the end of the peptide-coding region or falls off, the terminator structure in the mRNA forms, and most of the transcription of the remainder of the *trp* genes is prevented. If the amount of Trp-tRNA is limiting, the ribosome that is translating the peptide stalls at the *trp* codons and covers one of the base-pairing regions that allowed the formation of the terminator structure. As a result, another secondary structure forms in the mRNA that does not cause termination and allows RNA polymerase to proceed all the way through the entire operon. Attenuation control responds to the amount of the amino acid directly able to serve in protein synthesis (ie, the amount charged to its proper tRNA). It is interesting to note that the *trp* operon also is regulated by a repressor whose binding to the promoter–operator region responds to the level of free tryptophan instead of Trp-tRNA.

This type of regulation requires close coupling of transcription and translation, inasmuch as the choice of termination versus continuation must be decided for an RNA polymerase that is in front of the ribosome.

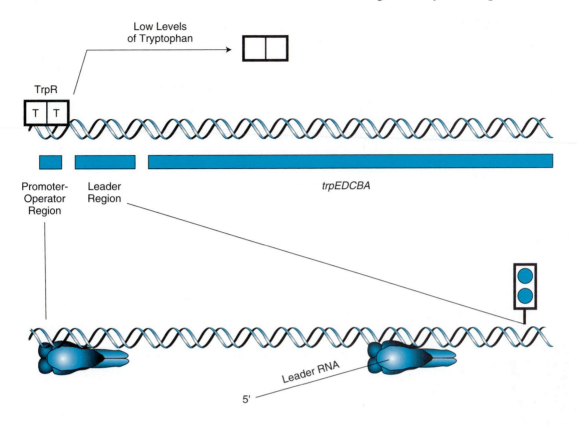

Low Levels
of Tryptophan

TrpR

Promoter-
Operator
Region

Leader
Region

trpEDCBA

Leader RNA

5'

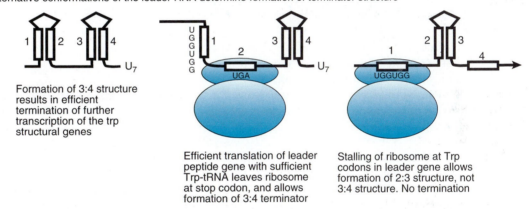

Alternative conformations of the leader RNA determine formation of terminator structure

1   2   3   4 U_7

Formation of 3:4 structure
results in efficient
termination of further
transcription of the trp
structural genes

U
G
G
U
G
G   1   3   4 U_7
          2
        UGA

Efficient translation of leader
peptide gene with sufficient
Trp-tRNA leaves ribosome
at stop codon, and allows
formation of 3:4 terminator

              2   3
              1   4
        UGGUGG

Stalling of ribosome at Trp
codons in leader gene allows
formation of 2:3 structure, not
3:4 structure. No termination

FIGURE 2-16   Model for the dual regulation of the *trp* operon, which contains the five genes involved in tryptophan biosynthesis. The upper part of the diagram shows a schematic representation of the control region. The initiation of transcription is regulated through the competition between the binding of RNA polymerase to the promoter site and the binding of the tryptophan-TrpR repressor at the overlapping operator site. Under conditions of low tryptophan supply, the TrpR aporepressor does not bind to the operator, and transcription is initiated.

The second level of regulation determines whether transcription will continue through the operon or stop at the attenuator site. The center of the diagram shows that the early RNA transcript (leader) has regions that can base pair with other regions. For example, region 2 can pair with either region 1 or region 3. When regions 3 and 4 pair, they form a structure at which termination occurs. The leader also contains a coding region for a small peptide, which contains two tryptophan residues. When Trp-tRNA is plentiful, a ribosome, represented by the large circle in the bottom of the figure, rapidly makes this peptide and then either falls off or stops at the end of the coding region, allowing the base-paired structure 3:4 to form. If Trp-tRNA is scarce, the ribosome stalls in region 1. This allows segment 2 to pair with segment 3, preventing formation of the 3:4 terminator structure and allowing transcription to proceed through the operon.

Similar attenuation controls regulate many other amino acid biosynthetic pathways. In the histidine operon, the leader region in front of the attenuator codes for a peptide that contains seven histidine residues in a row. Genes for some steps of nucleotide biosynthesis or for erythromycin, ampicillin, and chloramphenicol resistance use variations of this attenuation control.

A related form of regulation coordinates the expression of the genes coding for ribosomal proteins to ensure that there is no appreciable pool of free protein subunits. Numerous ribosomal proteins are coded by a single polycistronic mRNA. One of the proteins coded by each mRNA can bind to a site on its mRNA and prevent ribosomes from binding and translating any of the genes. Thus, whenever the level of that ribosomal protein exceeds the amount needed to complex with its rRNA, the free protein prevents its own translation as well as that of several other ribosomal proteins, thereby coupling the production of all the ribosomal proteins with that of the rRNAs.

STRINGENT CONTROL

A global control, called the *stringent response,* occurs in response to the inhibition of protein synthesis. An alarmone, guanosine 3′-diphosphate 5′-diphosphate (ppGpp), is synthesized by a ribosome-associated enzyme when any amino acid is limiting and the ribosome is unable to fill its acceptor site with the appropriate charged tRNA. The resulting elevated levels of ppGpp specifically inhibit the transcription of genes for rRNA, tRNA, and ribosomal proteins while stimulating the transcription of some genes for amino acid biosynthetic enzymes. This alarmone also appears to inhibit key enzymes involved in lipid and cell-wall biosynthesis. In this way, decreases in the rate of protein synthesis can trigger a decrease in the synthesis of other major cellular constituents and prevent gross imbalances in cell composition. In addition, ppGpp might be involved in controlling the rates of rRNA and tRNA synthesis in response to the overall growth rate.

Other global response systems bring about profound changes in gene expression in response to environmental stresses such as heat shock, exposure to peroxide or other toxic oxygen products, shifts in osmolarity or pH of the medium, exposure to alkylating agents, entry into stationary phase, and many others.

Bibliography

JOURNALS

Brock TD. The bacterial nucleus: a history. Microbiol Rev 1988;52:397.

Conaway RC, Conaway JW. General initiation factors for RNA polymerase II. Annu Rev Biochem 1993;62:161.

Gold L. Posttranscriptional regulatory mechanisms in *Escherichia coli.* Annu Rev Biochem 1988;57:199.

Guthrie C, Patterson B. Spliceosomal SNRNAs. Annu Rev Genet 1988;22:387.

Hiraga S. Chromosome and plasmid partitioning in *Escherichia coli.* Annu Rev Biochem 1992;61:283.

Marians KJ. Prokaryotic DNA replication. Annu Rev Biochem 1992;61:673.

Newlon CS. Yeast chromosome replication and segregation. Microbiol Rev 1988;52:568.

Pabo CO, Sauer RT. Transcription factors: structural families and principles of DNA recognition. Annu Rev Biochem 1992;61:1053.

Schleif R. DNA looping. Annu Rev Biochem 1992;61:199.

BOOKS

Neidhardt F, Ingraham JL, Low KB, et al. *Escherichia coli* and *Salmonella typhimurium:* cellular and molecular biology, ed 2. Washington, DC, American Society for Microbiology, 1996

Sambrook J, Fritsch EF, Maniatis T. Molecular cloning: a laboratory manual, ed 2. Cold Spring Harbor, NY, Cold Spring Harbor Laboratory, 1989.

Immunology

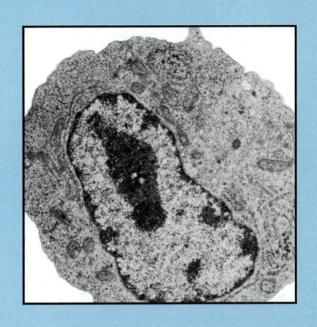

RESISTANCE to infection is called *immunity,* and *immunology* is the study of the cells, molecules, and mechanisms responsible for immunity. The immune response generated by the immune system as the direct result of the presence of an infectious organism leads to the selective removal of that organism. Activation of the immune system not only results in elimination of the offending organism, but also generates memory of this initial exposure to the pathogen. This memory leads to a faster and greater immune response on subsequent exposure to that same pathogen.

The induction of a specific immune response occurs only after recognition of the foreign material by specific receptors on a class of cells called *lymphocytes.* Subsequently, removal of the pathogen requires the release by these lymphocytes of one or more molecules that promote elimination of the organism or neutralization of toxic substances released by the organism.

The practice of medicine requires a knowledge of immunology, because most diseases have an immunologic component in their pathogenesis or treatment. Organ transplantation, infectious diseases, cancer, autoimmune diseases, and allergy are a few examples.

The purpose of this unit is to provide a summary of the immune system and its role in defense against disease.

Bibliography

BOOKS

Abbas A, Lichtman AH, Pober JS. Cellular and molecular immunology, ed 2. Philadelphia, WB Saunders, 1994.

Brostoff J, Scadding GK, Male D, Roitt IM. Clinical immunology. New York, Gower Medical Publishing, 1991.

Gallin JI, Fauci AS, eds. Mucosal immunity: advances in host defense mechanisms, vol 4. New York, Raven Press, 1985.

Golub ES, Green ES. Immunology: a synthesis, ed 2. Sunderland, MA, Sinauer, 1987.

Klein J. Immunology. Boston, Blackwell Scientific, 1990.

Kuby J. Immunology, ed 2. New York, WH Freeman, 1994.

Lichtenstein LM, Fauci AS. Current therapy in allergy and immunology. London, CV Mosby, 1983.

Paul WE, ed. Fundamental immunology, ed 3. New York, Raven Press, 1993.

Roitt I. Essential immunology, ed 7. Oxford, Blackwell Scientific, 1991.

Rose NR, Mackay IR, eds. The autoimmune diseases. New York, Academic Press, 1985.

Stites DP, Perr AI, Parslow TG. Basic and clinical immunology, ed 8. Norwalk, CT, Appleton & Lange, 1994.

Essentials of Medical Microbiology, Fifth Edition, edited by Wesley A. Volk,
Bryan M. Gebhardt, Marie-Louise Hammarskjöld, and Robert J. Kadner.
Lippincott-Raven Publishers, Philadelphia © 1996.

Chapter 3

Immunology: Ancient History and the Modern Era

Ancient History

The recognition that the human body possesses an adaptable immune defense system occurred progressively. Scientists and physicians observed that individuals who survived infection during one of the numerous plagues did not contract the disease again. This awareness was put into practical application as early as the 10th century, when the Turks introduced the practice of inoculating their daughters with extracts of pustules from smallpox victims soon after birth so that they would not contract the disease later, become physically marked (pocked), and thus lose their value on the market as concubines in the harems of the wealthy. Somewhat later, the Lady Mary Wortley Montague, while living with her ambassador husband in Constantinople, following the accepted practice in that part of the world, gave dried powders of smallpox to her newborn child. The result was so successful that she conveyed her joy and the technique to the then Princess of Wales (soon to be Queen of George II), who introduced the practice into Great Britain. This practice, termed *variolation* (variola: smallpox), was not without considerable risk, albeit a chance understandably worth taking, considering the great number of deaths that occurred during a smallpox epidemic, not to mention the disfigurement suffered by many survivors.

Although the practice of smallpox inoculation was disputed, the example set by the Prince and Princess of Wales led to its widespread use. As a result, the great increase in population that began in the middle of the 18th century can be attributed to this practice.

In the English countryside, a new procedure involving the use of material from cowpox pustules was introduced. The first recorded example of this procedure took place in 1774 when an English farmer obtained the material from a neighbor and inoculated his wife. Edward Jenner was the first physician to embark on systematic studies to test the usefulness of cowpox inoculation in preventing smallpox. In 1798, he reported the results of experiments based on the inoculation of James Phipps with cowpox material. Although his evidence appeared conclusive, it initially was met with considerable scorn. The results eventually were accepted, and Jenner was admitted into the learned societies of Europe.

The Modern Era

THE GERM THEORY AND VACCINATION

The science of immunology began with the elegant experiments of the French chemist and bacteriologist Louis Pasteur. During one of his many experiments on the germ theory of disease, he left a culture of the chicken cholera bacterium on the laboratory bench while he was away on holiday. On returning, he found not only that the organisms had lost much of their virulence, but that their inoculation into chickens protected those chickens against infection with fresh organisms. Many subsequent experiments showed that the virulent organism could be *attenuated* by any one of several treatments. Pasteur termed this inoculation with attenuated organisms *vaccination* (*vacca*, "cow") in honor of Edward Jenner.

Subsequently, Pasteur observed that the anthrax bacillus became less virulent for pigs when it was passed through rabbits, but highly virulent when it was passed through pigeons. In 1881, he demonstrated the efficacy of attenuated organisms in preventing anthrax in cattle, sheep, and pigs.

Undoubtedly, Pasteur's most celebrated experiments were those in which he used the rabies virus, which had been attenuated by growth in rabbits, to prevent hydrophobia in humans bitten by rabid animals. Such inoculation was not without problems. We subsequently have learned that injection of attenuated rabies virus, which also contains brain tissue, occasionally is accompanied by the onset of postvaccination rabies encephalitis. Although inoculation with attenuated virus continues today, the virus is grown in human diploid cell line cultures to minimize such side effects.

THE DISCOVERY OF ANTIBODY

In 1888, Emile Roux and Alexandre Yersin demonstrated that supernatants obtained from cultures of the diphtheria organism contained a soluble toxin that could produce all the symptoms of diphtheria. In 1890, von Behring and Kitasato established that injection of animals with the toxin of the diphtheria or tetanus organisms resulted in the production of a serum substance that would prevent disease. In 1892 and 1894, these same individuals demonstrated that injection of serum from such immunized animals into infected children resulted in remarkable cures. This substance was termed *antitoxin,* and subsequently *antibody.* The term *antigen* was applied to the agents responsible for inducing the synthesis of these antibodies.

These early experiments of Pasteur, Roux and Yersin, and von Behring and Kitasato were the foundation for the development of many vaccines used today to prevent diseases such as polio, influenza, and whooping cough. Indeed, the experiments of Jenner led to the highly successful vaccination program that resulted in worldwide eradication of smallpox.

COMPLEMENT

In 1893, Buchner demonstrated that fresh serum killed certain bacteria, but did not do so when heated at 56°C. This thermolabile substance was termed *alexine.* One year later, Bordet showed that the killing activity of serum from animals immunized with cholera organisms was due to two factors, one of which was heat labile and present in normal serum, and the other of which was heat stable and present only in the serum of animals immunized with the organism (ie, it was specific). The heat-labile factor, alexine, is now termed *complement,* and the heat-stable factor is known as *antibody.*

HUMORAL VERSUS CELLULAR IMMUNITY

Antibody and complement, known as humoral factors because they are found in the blood, seemed to account for all that was necessary for protection against disease. However, in 1884, the Russian zoologist Eli Metchnikoff hypothesized a phagocytic basis for immunity. This hypothesis was prompted by two observations. The first was the mobilization of phagocytic cells around rose thorns inserted under the skin of starfish larvae. The second was the direct correlation between the extent of phagocytosis (engulfment) of spores of the fungus *Monospora bicuspidata* and death resulting from infection of the water flea *Daphnia* by this organism.

This hypothesis engendered a lengthy debate among scientists. The debate was not resolved for some time, despite the efforts of the Englishman, Almroth Wright, who demonstrated that specific antibody reinforced or enhanced the killing action of phagocytes, and who coined the term *opsonic* (from the Greek, *opsono-,* meaning "I prepare food for") for this property of blood serum and the term *opsonin* for the serum substance itself.

IMMUNOCHEMISTRY OF ANTIGENS

At this point, it was becoming clear that a hallmark of antibodies is their specificity. This realization led to the use of antibody to distinguish between related and unrelated organisms, to differentiate soluble molecules, and to study the structural basis of antibody specificity. In 1900, Karl Landsteiner, a German chemist, using "natural" antibody, discovered the A, B, and O blood group antigens on human erythrocytes. Shortly thereafter, several reports appeared on the use of antibody to distinguish similar fluids or proteins from different species, as well as to detect similarities (ie, *cross-reactivity*) among antigens from related species. In 1917, Landsteiner initiated a series of experiments on the serologic basis of specificity, which demonstrated that antibody could easily distinguish between closely related antigen molecules, and that large antigens possess multiple sites with which antibody could react. Our knowledge of the structure of antigens and antigenic determinants progressed largely due to the efforts of scientists such as Michael Heidelberger and Elvin Kabat. Research teams headed by David Davies at the National Institutes of Health and Roberto Poljak at the Pasteur Institute have produced detailed crystallographic structures of several antigenic determinants. These studies have paved the way for studies of the structural basis of antigen–antibody interactions.

MULTIVALENCY OF ANTIBODY

At the turn of the century, Bordet and Ehrlich found that antigen and antibody combine in varying proportions, not in fixed ratios. This, in essence, was the first demonstration of the multivalency of antigen and antibody. Beginning in the 1930s, Michael Heidelberger and colleagues developed quantitative immunochemistry using techniques not available to Ehrlich and Bordet. Heidelberger's studies led to the lattice hypothesis, which demonstrated how antigen and antibody can combine in varying proportions, and enabled these investigators to predict the outcome of antigen–antibody interactions. These observations led to other methods for visualizing antigen–antibody interactions, culminating in the development of the double diffusion method by Ouchterlony and of immunoelectrophoresis by Grabar and Williams in 1953.

THE STRUCTURE OF ANTIBODY

In 1938, Arne Tiselius and Elvin Kabat were the first to show that antibodies belong to the class of serum proteins called γ-*globulins*. Subsequently, four different groups of investigators conducted studies that together revealed the basic structure of antibody molecules. In 1959, Porter, using the enzyme papain to cleave the antibody molecule, provided chemical evidence of the multivalency of antibody molecules. In 1960, Edelman and Kunkel demonstrated that antibody was composed of two polypeptide chains, termed *heavy chain* and *light chain*. In 1965, Hilschman and Craig reported the first amino acid sequence of light chain. In 1974, Poljak, using x-ray diffraction, provided the first view of the three-dimensional structure of antibody. In 1966, Bennet and Dryer proposed that the polypeptide chains of antibody are composed of variable and constant regions and, therefore, must each be encoded by two genes. This two-gene–one-polypeptide theory was based on the sequences of only two light chains and, although totally contradictory to the then current one-gene–one-polypeptide dogma, subsequently has been proved to be correct. The experiments of Tonegawa and others have revealed the fine structure of the genes that code for antibodies and the way in which antibody synthesis is regulated.

In 1984, Poljak again provided a breakthrough in our understanding of the molecular basis of the interaction of antigen and antibody when he produced the crystallographic structure of an antigen complexed with its specific antibody. Since then, the detailed structures of other antigen–antibody complexes have been reported, providing a molecular image of the specificity of an immune response.

HYPERSENSITIVITY

In 1890, while attempting to produce a vaccine for tuberculosis, Robert Koch noted that injection of supernatants of the tubercle bacillus into the skin of tuberculous animals resulted in a severe local reaction about 24 hours later. Although he never succeeded in producing a vaccine, he was the first investigator to experimentally produce a *delayed-type hypersensitivity* (DTH) reaction. Koch was incorrect in his interpretation of the cause of this reaction, however, and it was not until the 1930s and thereafter that detailed studies of the mechanisms of DTH were initiated. During the 1930s, Landsteiner and colleagues demonstrated the chemical specificity of DTH reactions and, in 1942, Merrill Chase showed that DTH could be transferred from sensitized to normal animals by lymphoid cells but not by serum. In recent years, it has been shown that DTH reactions are indeed caused by the activation of a specific class of lymphocytes, which mediate DTH through the release of soluble factors.

Charles Richet and Paul Portier were the first investigators to understand that systemic anaphylactic shock could be induced in presensitized animals by relatively bland, nontoxic substances. The reactions noted in sensitized animals were violent, occurring within a few minutes after injection of the challenge dose, and frequently resulted in death. This *immediate hypersensitivity* subsequently was shown to possess the same specificity as other immune responses. The relationship between this type of reaction, asthma, hay fever, and certain local reactions was soon noted, and the term *allergy* was coined. The first demonstration that these allergies might be mediated by antibody was provided by Heinz Kustner and Karl Prausnitz in 1921, when Prausnitz showed that Kustner's sensitivity to fish could be transferred to a normal individual with serum. This was followed somewhat later by the discovery of IgE antibody and its role in immediate hypersensitivity reactions by Kimishige Ishizaka.

Essentials of Medical Microbiology, Fifth Edition, edited by Wesley A. Volk, Bryan M. Gebhardt, Marie-Louise Hammarskjöld, and Robert J. Kadner. Lippincott-Raven Publishers, Philadelphia © 1996.

Chapter 4

Microbial Invasiveness, Nonspecific Host Resistance, and the Inflammatory Response

To understand immunity or, more specifically, the mechanisms by which a host can protect itself from and combat infectious diseases, one must know something about microbial invasiveness. One must also be able to distinguish between infection and disease. All people are "infected" from birth until death—our normal flora are actually an infection, because these organisms obtain their nutrients from our bodies (the host on which they live). Disease occurs when an organism invades an area of the body that is normally sterile, or when a microbe that is not part of the normal flora becomes established in a site where it can cause harm to the host. This difference between infection and disease is important, particularly because an individual can harbor organisms that, although they do not harm that person, can be a source of infection and disease to others. In this chapter, the general properties that enable an organism to cause disease and the nonspecific mechanisms of resistance available to the host to control or eliminate these harmful invaders are discussed.

Microbial Invasion

HOW PATHOGENS ENTER AND LEAVE THE BODY

In general, infective microbes are carried in secretions and excretions from infected areas. In some illnesses (eg, malaria, yellow fever, the viral encephalitides, Rocky Mountain spotted fever, typhus, plague), the body exit site may not be obvious, because the organisms are present in the blood and require a mosquito, tick, flea, or louse for transmission to another host. However, whether it is obvious or not, each disease-producing organism has its own portal or portals of entry as well as a means of escape from the host (Table 4-1).

Microorganisms enter the body at the following sites:

1. *Respiratory tract*—through the nose and mouth. This is the portal of entry for microbes causing respiratory

TABLE 4-1
Portals of Entry of Some Infectious Organisms

Portal of Entry	*Organism*	*Disease*
Skin and mucous membranes	Bacteria:	
	Staphylococcus	Boils and furuncles
	Clostridium tetani	Tetanus
	Francisella tularensis	Tularemia
	Leptospira interrogans	Leptospirosis
Respiratory tract	Viruses:	
	Rhinovirus	Common cold
	Paramyxovirus	Measles (rubeola), mumps
	Bacteria:	
	Streptococcus pneumoniae	Pneumonia
	Mycobacterium tuberculosis	Tuberculosis
Gastrointestinal tract	Viruses:	
	Poliovirus	Poliomyelitis
	Hepatitis B virus	Hepatitis
	Bacteria:	
	Staphylococcus	Food poisoning
	Salmonella typhi	Typhoid fever
	Vibrio cholerae	Cholera
Genitourinary tract	Bacteria:	
	Neisseria gonorrhoeae	Gonorrhea
	Treponema pallidum	Syphilis
	Viruses:	
	Herpes simplex type 2	Cervical cancer
		Primary genital herpes
	Human immunodeficiency virus (HIV)	AIDS
Blood	Viruses:	
	Hepatitis B virus	Hepatitis
	HIV	AIDS
	Bacteria:	
	Rickettsia rickettsii	Rocky Mountain spotted fever
	Sporozoa:	
	Plasmodium	Malaria
	Protozoa:	
	Leishmania	Leishmaniasis

diseases such as the common cold, measles, pneumonia, and tuberculosis.

2. *Gastrointestinal tract*—through the mouth. Examples include agents responsible for typhoid fever, paratyphoid fever, dysentery, cholera, polio, and hepatitis, as well as many food-borne illnesses such as botulism and staphylococcal food poisoning.

3. *Skin and mucous membranes.* Although the skin provides an effective barrier, some organisms appear capable of penetrating the intact skin; in addition, minor breaks such as scratches and punctures frequently occur, allowing the entrance of many organisms. The staphylococcus that causes boils and furuncles frequently enters by this route; however, streptococci also can cause spreading skin infections. Tularemia, leptospirosis, and anthrax are examples of severe systemic diseases usually contracted through the skin from contact with infected animals or animal products.

4. *Genitourinary system.* The mucous membranes of the genital tract are the site of invasion by agents causing sexually transmitted diseases such as gonorrhea and syphilis. In addition, the urinary tract can be infected by microorganisms originating in the blood and infecting the kidney or by the introduction of organisms into the bladder during catheterization.

5. *Blood.* Those organisms that must be introduced directly into the blood to cause disease usually are transmitted from one individual to another by insects that penetrate the skin with their bites. In addition to those mentioned earlier, our advancing civilization has added other ways for direct blood inoculation to occur, such as blood transfusions and organ transplants. Hepatitis has been transmitted by the use of whole blood from individuals who are asymptomatic carriers of the hepatitis virus, and acquired immunodeficiency syndrome has been transmitted by both whole blood and blood

products. Pretesting of blood for the presence of antibodies to these agents has done much to eliminate this type of transmission but has not stopped their spread among intravenous drug users.

The portals of exit for disease agents usually are the same as their portals of entry. Thus, diseases of the respiratory tract are spread through secretions and excretions of the respiratory tract and mouth. Similarly, microorganisms causing enteric infections leave the body by the intestinal tract and are spread through fecal contamination. Skin or wound infections can be spread by drainage from these areas, either directly to another person or through contamination of some inanimate object. Blood infections, which are spread by insects or contaminated needles or syringes, usually leave the individual in a similar manner, through direct contact with a needle or syringe or by ingestion of the microorganisms by a biting insect.

MAJOR PROPERTIES OF PATHOGENIC BACTERIA

Pathogenicity is defined as the ability of a microorganism to cause disease; *virulence* refers to the extent of pathogenicity. Thus, strictly speaking, virulence is a measure of pathogenicity, although many use the two words interchangeably. For an organism to be pathogenic, it must possess certain characteristics or properties not possessed by saprophytic organisms. In many cases, the properties conferring virulence to an organism are either unknown or unclear. However, some bacteria are known to have special structures that protect them from the host's defenses, whereas others may secrete substances that contribute to their virulence. Some of the factors believed to contribute to pathogenicity are described later.

Capsules

Some pathogenic bacteria possess large capsules surrounding their cell walls (Fig. 4-1). The ability of one of these organisms to produce disease depends on the presence of this capsule, and loss of the capsule (as a result of mutation) invariably results in concomitant loss of the ability to produce disease. Possession of a capsule contributes to an organism's disease-producing potential by preventing phagocytosis (engulfment of the encapsulated organisms by the host's phagocytic cells). The exact reason for this antiphagocytic activity is not known, but it seems to be due to surface properties of the capsule that prevent the phagocyte from forming a sufficiently intimate contact with the microorganism to allow phagocytosis to take place. As we shall see later, the binding of antibodies to the capsular antigens provides a coating that can interact with receptors on the phagocyte and permits phagocytosis to occur. For example, immunity to *Streptococcus pneumoniae* depends on antibody to the microor-

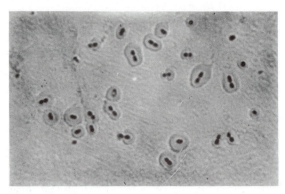

FIGURE 4-1 Encapsulated cells of *Streptococcus pneumoniae*. The capsules around the pairs of cells are swollen by the use of type-specific antibody.

ganism's capsule, and, in the presence of this antibody, the invading organism is rapidly engulfed and destroyed by the host's leukocytes (ie, the antibody is functioning as an opsonin). The chemistry of some of these capsules is discussed in Chapter 16.

Fimbriae

Many non–disease-producing bacteria possess fimbriae, just as many nonpathogenic bacteria possess capsules. This obviously demonstrates that neither capsules nor fimbriae are the sole determinants of the virulence of microorganisms. However, it is known that the possession of fimbriae endows a bacterium with an enhanced ability to adhere to other bacteria and to the membranes of the host's cells and phagocytes. Thus, for some bacteria (eg, *Neisseria gonorrhoeae*, the cause of gonorrhea, and enterotoxigenic *Escherichia coli*, a cause of gastroenteritis), the possession of fimbriae is required for virulence.

Exotoxins

Many pathogenic organisms do not possess antiphagocytic structures, such as capsules or fimbriae, but they have other components that permit them to cause disease. For many microbes, these include the production and secretion of toxic substances. Some of these products, called *exotoxins,* are responsible for the symptoms of such diseases as diphtheria, tetanus, gas gangrene, scarlet fever, the staphylococcal scalded skin syndrome, and toxic shock syndrome. In addition, certain types of food poisoning, such as those caused by *Clostridium botulinum, Clostridium perfringens,* and *Staphylococcus aureus,* also are caused by the presence of exotoxic substances.

There are other pathogenic organisms that neither possess antiphagocytic capsules nor produce exotoxins. With these, it is somewhat more difficult to pinpoint the properties responsible for virulence. However, an array of substances (some of which are enzymes) secreted by some bacteria may play an important role in their ability to cause disease. Many of these substances have not been isolated, purified, or chemically characterized, and they have been given names based on observations of the biologic or chemical activities of crude materials. A few of the more commonly found extracellular products include various hemolysins, which lyse red blood cells; leukocidins, which kill leukocytes; hyaluronidase, which hydrolyzes the hyaluronic acid of connective tissue; collagenase, which hydrolyzes collagen; coagulase, which coagulates plasma to form fibrin clots; and streptokinase, an enzyme that indirectly lyses plasma clots. Still another type of excreted virulence factor is exemplified by siderophores; these are phenolates or hydroxamates that, in some cases, can successfully obtain microbial growth-essential iron from the transferrin or lactoferrin of the host.

Endotoxins

Endotoxins are lipopolysaccharides and components of the cell walls of gram-negative bacteria. They are excreted by the cell in small amounts but, most importantly, they are able to manifest their toxicity while still attached to the bacterial cell wall. The biologic effects of endotoxins are manifold, but the two particularly prominent effects of an infection with gram-negative organisms are fever and shock. Humans are particularly sensitive to minute amounts of endotoxins, and mild gram-negative bacterial infections often cause fever. Larger amounts of endotoxin can cause irreversible shock; this is seen in association with fulminating gram-negative bacteremia.

Despite the toxicity of endotoxins, a microbe's pathogenicity is not entirely explained by its content of endotoxin. Undoubtedly, many of the symptoms of infections by organisms such as *Salmonella typhi* or *Neisseria meningitidis* are a result of endotoxins, but the fact that many nonpathogenic gram-negative bacteria possess equally toxic endotoxins and do not normally produce disease indicates that endotoxin by itself is not the major determinant of virulence by these organisms.

FACTORS IN THE DEVELOPMENT OF DISEASE

Many different factors must come into play for a disease agent to produce an infection. At the outset, the portal of entry must be suitable for the particular pathogen. In many cases, a microorganism is restricted to only one portal of entry—for example, the typhoid fever organism (*S typhi*) must be swallowed and must reach the small intestine in large numbers to cause disease. On the other hand, *S aureus* can use multiple portals of entry; it can cause pneumonia through the respiratory route, boils and furuncles through the skin, internal abscesses through the blood, or food poisoning through the gastrointestinal tract.

The ability to exit from the body and survive also is an important factor in disease development. Some organisms, such as *N meningitidis* and *N gonorrhoeae*, are extremely sensitive to drying and will die after several hours outside the host. Organisms such as the tubercle bacillus, however, can survive in dried sputum or secretions for months and still maintain their pathogenicity.

RELATIONSHIP OF DOSE TO INFECTION

The number of organisms required to cause disease in different settings is an important variable. For example, it may take thousands of staphylococci to cause infection in a clean cut, but a few hundred can infect a suture. On the other hand, some highly virulent organisms, such as *Francisella tularensis,* the organism causing tularemia, can cause severe disease after invasion of the skin by only three or four cells. Thus, the division between pathogens and saprophytes is vague, and it is only at the extremes that clear-cut examples of obligate pathogens (*F tularensis, Treponema pallidum*) or obligate saprophytes (*Bacillus megaterium, Bacillus cereus*) can be seen.

When specific infections are studied, it is evident that some diseases normally are found only in humans (typhoid fever, cholera, syphilis, meningococcal meningitis); thus, humans are necessary for the continued life of the microorganisms involved. It also is apparent that there are many infectious diseases that humans acquire only as accidental hosts. Examples of diseases in this category include yellow fever and malaria (both carried as an endemic infection in jungle monkeys), endemic typhus, Rocky Mountain spotted fever, tularemia, and brucellosis. A third category of infectious organisms, the soil saprophytes, live and grow in the soil, but if introduced through a wound into a susceptible host, can cause serious illness and death. These include such diseases as tetanus, gas gangrene, and the subcutaneous mycoses.

Nonspecific Host Resistance

The complex reactions a host animal undergoes after contact with microorganisms can be grouped under the broadly defined heading of *resistance*. We can categorize such resistance as being of two major types: (1) nonspecific (natural or innate) resistance; and (2) specific resistance (directed against specific microbes).

In the first category, resistance or susceptibility (lack of resistance) to infections can vary from one species of animal to another. For example, mice are extremely susceptible to infection by *S pneumoniae*. Humans, on the other hand, are relatively resistant to *S pneumoniae* infections, as evidenced by the large percentage of persons who carry these organisms in their respiratory tract without symptoms of infection (under some conditions, as many as 50%).

In many cases, it is not known why resistance varies from one species to another or why a disease is mild in one person and severe in another. In some cases, there may be genetic factors that make certain races of people more susceptible to a particular infection than are other races. An example of greater susceptibility to disease is the apparent inordinate vulnerability of Native Americans to tuberculosis. In addition, statistical data indicate that if one identical twin contracts tuberculosis, there is a 75% chance that the other twin also will contract tuberculosis. In contrast, for fraternal twins, there is only a 33% chance that the second twin will contract clinically apparent disease. We do not fully understand the genetic determinants that control this increased susceptibility to infection, although there are a few instances in which genetically determined resistance to a specific disease can be pinpointed. For example, resistance to infection by *Plasmodium vivax* (a causative agent of malaria) is found in almost all African blacks and is attributed to the lack of a specific component on their erythrocyte membrane to which the parasite must bind to invade and multiply within cells.

The age of an individual at the time of infection also is an important factor in determining the severity of the disease. Many diseases, such as mumps, measles, and chickenpox, are mild during childhood but can be exceedingly severe when contracted during adult life.

It is therefore apparent that susceptibility and resistance to infection vary considerably among various species of animals as well as among persons with different genetic backgrounds.

Innate immunity can be divided into three general categories (Table 4-2). Most infectious organisms are faced with external mechanical and chemical barriers that must be surmounted before they can gain entrance to the body. After penetration does occur, they are still faced with a wide variety of chemical and cellular mechanisms that have been finely tuned to prevent further dissemination in the body, which might lead to disease. These mechanical, chemical, and cellular mechanisms of innate immunity are discussed here.

MECHANICAL AND CHEMICAL MECHANISMS OF DEFENSE

Skin and Mucous Membranes

The intact skin and the mucous membranes provide mechanical barriers that prevent the entrance of most microbial species. However, even though the structure of the skin itself undoubtedly gives a great deal of protection, considerably more important are the fatty acids secreted by the sebaceous glands and the propionic acid produced by the normal flora of the skin. Secretions from the sebaceous glands contain both saturated and unsaturated fatty acids that kill many bacteria and fungi. A striking example of this type of resistance to infection is seen in the case

TABLE 4-2
Mechanical, Chemical, and Cellular Mediators of Innate Immunity

Mechanical
   Barriers to penetration—skin as a physical barrier
   Ciliated cells and mucus in respiratory tract
   Washing action of tears, urine

Chemical
   Fatty acids—from normal flora, sebaceous glands
   Propionic acids—from normal flora
   Lysozyme—in tears, blood, sweat, urine
   Acid—stomach, vagina, skin
   Basic polyamines—in plasma
   Complement—in plasma
   Interferons—with antiviral activity
   Acute-phase proteins—C-reactive protein, α_1-antitrypsin, fibrinogen, α_2-macroglobulin

Cellular
   Phagocytic cells such as macrophages and monocytes, polymorphonuclear neutrophils (PMNs), and eosinophils

of the fungi causing ringworm of the scalp (species of *Microsporum* and *Trichophyton*). This infection is difficult to cure in children, but after puberty it disappears without treatment, presumably as a result of a change in the amount and kinds of fatty acids secreted by the sebaceous glands.

Infections caused by organisms that enter through the mucous membranes occur in the conjunctiva, respiratory tract, and genitourinary tract. However, such infections are not commonplace, and it would appear that organisms able to penetrate the mucous membranes must possess special invasive properties. Alternatively, a prior viral infection may result in damage to the mucous membranes, as in influenza, in which destruction of the cilia-bearing epithelial cells allows infection by *S pneumoniae* or *S aureus* to occur more readily. Under normal conditions, the beating action of the cilia on the mucous membranes of the respiratory tract provides for the continuous movement of a fluid layer of mucus. Particles of dust or microorganisms adhere to this mucus and are moved to the exterior, in this way keeping the lungs remarkably free of microorganisms.

Similarly, foreign organisms gaining entry to the genitourinary tract or the eye can be eliminated by the mechanical washing action of urine and tears, respectively.

Chemical Factors

The body produces many antimicrobial substances that are important in preventing infections. Tears are rich in lysozyme, an enzyme that hydrolyzes the peptidoglycan cell wall of many bacteria. Lysozyme also is present in blood and urine, and, as will be seen, it may be an important determinant in the killing of some microorganisms by white blood cells.

Acids of the stomach, vagina, and skin also provide important resistance to infection. For example, if acid in the stomach is neutralized before *S typhi* organisms are ingested, many fewer organisms are needed to cause typhoid fever. Furthermore, although difficult to correlate with specific chemical factors, the microbial antagonism of our normal flora is of great value in preventing the growth of potentially pathogenic organisms. This is readily seen after long-term therapy with broad-spectrum antibiotics—therapy that destroys a large part of the normal flora, allowing yeast, *Candida* organisms, or staphylococci resistant to the antibiotic to proliferate and cause severe infections of the mucous membranes of the mouth or gastrointestinal tract.

Many infectious organisms cause infection by attaching to and multiplying on mucosal surfaces. Subsequent invasion of these tissues or the release of toxic substances by bacteria can lead to local or systemic disease. These bacteria attach by fimbriae on the organism binding to "receptors" on the host cell surfaces. There are numerous defenses against these bacteria, including IgA antibody (see Chap. 5), which specifically binds to the bacterial fimbriae and prevents attachment. Similarly, luminal mucus contains glycoprotein or glycolipid analogues of the host cell receptor that bind to the bacterial fimbriae, also preventing attachment. Not to be outdone, several pathogens produce IgA-specific proteases (*N meningitidis, N gonorrhoeae, S pneumoniae*) or attach directly to cilia, preventing their action (*Bordetella pertussis*).

CELLULAR MECHANISMS OF DEFENSE

In spite of the physical and chemical barriers that normally prevent the entry of microorganisms into our bodies, a day does not pass when bacteria do not enter the bloodstream or connective tissue. This occurs when we cut ourselves, have a difficult bowel movement, brush our teeth, get scratched, step on a sharp object, or even chew gum vigorously. We survive these daily attacks of bacteria primarily because such organisms are quickly removed and killed by phagocytic cells. A brief description of these cells and of their ability to destroy the invading microorganisms is provided later. The differentiation of phagocytes from pluripotential stem cells is discussed in Chapter 7 along with that of the other blood-borne cells.

Polymorphonuclear Neutrophils

Polymorphonuclear neutrophils (also called PMNs, polys, neutrophils, or granulocytes) are the body's major circulating leukocytes. Their function is to remove debris, including bacteria, from the body's tissues by engulfing and destroying the foreign material. This process of engulfing particulate matter is called *phagocytosis.*

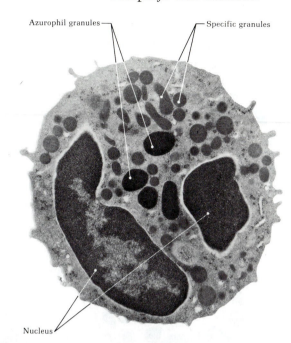

FIGURE 4-2   Electron micrograph of a mature neutrophilic granulocyte (PMN) from rabbit bone marrow, showing two lobes of its dense nucleus and cytoplasmic granules. There are two types of granules: the larger, denser azurophil granules contain peroxidase, lysozyme, and lysosomal enzymes; the smaller, less dense specific granules lack lysosomal enzymes but contain alkaline phosphatase, lysozyme, and lactoferrin. (Original magnification ×25,000.)

A PMN contains a nucleus that is divided into several large segments (hence the name polymorphonuclear) and, as shown in Figure 4-2, contains many granules that stain with neutral dyes (the basis of the name *granulocyte* or *neutrophil*). After many infections, there is a rapid increase in the number of these leukocytes in the blood as a result of an increased rate of release from the bone marrow, a condition known as *leukocytosis.* After some infections, however, particularly those caused by viruses, or severe bacteremia caused by gram-negative organisms, there is a decrease in the number of circulating leukocytes as a result of their sticking to capillary walls. This is referred to as *leukopenia.*

For a PMN to be effective in host defense, it must migrate to the area of the infection, phagocytose the infecting organisms, and finally kill the invader. Each of these steps is described later.

CHEMOTAXIS AND MIGRATION. PMNs are produced in the bone marrow; after differentiation into mature granulocytes, they are released into the bloodstream (Fig. 4-3). From there, they circulate throughout the body and subsequently enter the tissues by squeezing between the cells lining the blood vessels (a process called *diapedesis*). In the event of an infection or inflammation, large numbers of PMNs migrate into the infected area of the body. This directed migration is called *chemotaxis.*

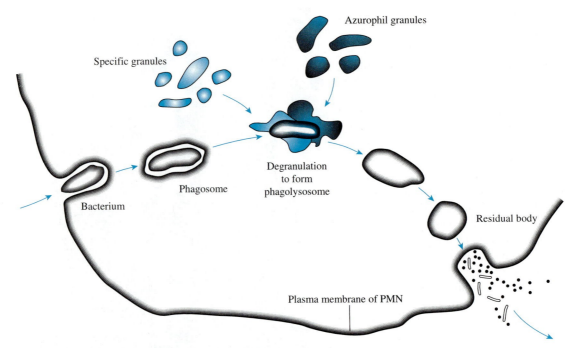

FIGURE 4-5 Phagocytosis and destruction of a bacterium by a PMN. The bacterium is engulfed by the PMN. After engulfment, lysosomal enzymes from azurophil granules along with enzymes in specific granules enter the phagosome by fusion of the granule membranes with the phagosome membrane. The ingested bacterium within the phagolysosome is killed and either digested or retained within a residual body, from which it can be excreted by fusion with the plasma membrane of the PMN.

macrophages also contain numerous low-molecular-weight peptides called *human neutrophil peptides* or *defensins* that kill bacteria. These defensins are basic peptides of 29 to 30 amino acids in length and are rich in cysteine and aromatic amino acids. Although the mechanism by which they kill certain bacteria is not known, defensins probably represent a broad-spectrum antimicrobial system in neutrophils. Certain intracellular pathogens can circumvent killing and degradation by neutrophils. Patricia Fields and her colleagues at the Centers for Disease Control in Atlanta have identified a gene in *Salmonella typhimurium*, an intracellular pathogen, that is necessary for virulence and required for resistance to defensins. Their results are of particular importance, because certain patients with a specific granule deficiency who have frequent and severe infections are almost totally lacking in defensins.

MYELOPEROXIDE–HALIDE–PEROXIDE SYSTEM. The hydrogen peroxide that was produced during the metabolic burst after phagocytosis diffuses from the cytoplasm of the PMN into the phagolysosome. There, in conjunction with MPO and a halide ion from the PMN, it exerts its bactericidal effect. The biochemical mechanism by which the MPO–halide–H_2O_2 system kills the phagocytosed microorganisms is unclear, but the following two proposals have experimental support:

1. The halide involved in this system is the chloride ion, and the microbicidal (killing) effect results from the formation of hypochlorite (a strong oxidizing agent) according to the following equation:

$$H_2O_2 + Cl^- \xrightarrow{\text{MPO}} ClO^- + H_2O$$

2. The halide involved in this system is the iodide ion, and death results from an iodination of microbial proteins catalyzed by MPO in the presence of H_2O_2.

Perhaps both reactions occur. Certainly chloride is present in large amounts, and hypochlorite is an effective microbicidal compound. On the other hand, the addition of iodide to the system suggests that it is much more active than chloride on a molar basis. However, the concentration of iodide in the PMN under physiologic conditions is extremely low, which would argue against iodine as the ion involved in the MPO microbicidal system.

SUPEROXIDE ANION. PMNs form superoxide (O_2^-) during their metabolic burst after phagocytosis. The superoxide ion is extremely toxic (see Chap. 17) and, unless scavenged by the enzyme superoxide dismutase, it can exert a toxic effect on phagocytosed organisms, particularly those anaerobic pathogens that do not possess their own superoxide dismutase. However, another important function of superoxide is to serve as an intermediate in the oxidative production of hydrogen peroxide according to the following equation:

$$O_2^- + O_2^- + 2H^+ \xrightarrow{\text{Superoxide Dismutase}} O_2 + H_2O_2$$

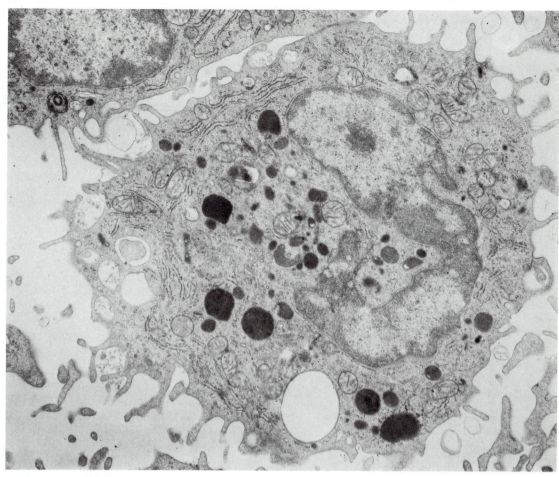

FIGURE 4-6 Electron micrograph of a peritoneal macrophage from a mouse. These cells were obtained from a peritoneal cavity stimulated with a lipid emulsion. Cytoplasmic processes are prominent, some clearly finger-like. Lysosomal dense bodies are numerous, some small and homogeneous, others large and heterogeneous. (Original magnification ×12,000.)

MYELOPEROXIDASE-INDEPENDENT ANTIMICROBIAL SYSTEMS. Additional enzymes are emptied into the phagolysosome during degranulation of the PMN and undoubtedly are involved in the antimicrobial action of this phagocyte. A few of the better understood factors are lysozyme, which hydrolyzes the peptidoglycan cell wall of certain sensitive bacteria; lactoferrin, which can chelate iron present in the phagolysosome and thus prevent growth of the phagocytosed organism; and basic proteins, such as phagocytin and leukin, which have been shown to exert antimicrobial activity. In addition, acid produced by the metabolic activities of the PMN lowers the pH of the phagolysosome to 3 or 4, which alone can cause the death of many microorganisms.

The Monocyte and the Macrophage

A second phagocytic cell, called a *monocyte,* also is produced in the bone marrow and released into the bloodstream. After 1 or 2 days, it migrates through the vessel walls into the surrounding tissues. The monocyte then begins to differentiate into one of several large phagocytic cells called *macrophages* or *mononuclear phagocytes* (Fig. 4-6). These cells are found throughout the body; some are fixed primarily along the blood vessels in the liver, spleen, bone marrow, and lymph nodes, whereas others maintain their motility and are called *wandering* or *tissue macrophages.* Fixed phagocytic macrophages usually are referred to collectively as the *mononuclear phagocyte system.*

The details of macrophage action have been studied less thoroughly than those of PMNs, but the following generalizations can be made:

1. Phagocytosis, including the ability to ingest both foreign particles and antibody-coated bacteria, is analogous to that described for PMNs. Receptors for antibody molecules (Fc portion) and complement (C3b) are present on the membranes of macrophages as they are on PMN membranes.
2. Granules in monocytes, like those in PMNs, contain lysosomal enzymes and, in some species, peroxidase. Macrophages also contain stores of lysosomal enzymes packaged in tiny vesicles. Unlike the situation in

PMNs, lysosomal enzymes are synthesized continuously during the tissue phase of the macrophage, the result being that the mature macrophage possesses many times more lysosomal enzymes than does the monocyte at the time it begins to differentiate into a macrophage.

3. After the formation of the phagosome, lysosomal granules (in monocytes) or stored lysosomal enzymes in vesicles (macrophages) fuse with the phagosome to release their hydrolytic enzymes, forming a phagolysosome.

4. The phagocytosing monocyte or macrophage undergoes a burst of metabolic activity that results in the formation of hydrogen peroxide; however, MPO is not present in these cells in some species. Thus, even though the MPO system seems to be an important microbicidal action of the PMNs, the mononuclear phagocytes make efficient use of killing techniques that have yet to be fully elucidated.

In general, the mononuclear phagocytes are considered to be a second line of defense, because PMNs characteristically are first to arrive at a site of inflammation. Even though both cell types are attracted by bacterial infection, PMNs migrate faster and thus appear first. However, PMNs are short-lived (6 to 8 hours) and, in the event of a chronic infection, are soon replaced by the longer-lived macrophages. In addition, there are certain microorganisms (eg, tubercle bacilli, *Brucella* organisms, and *Toxoplasma* parasites) that preferentially attract macrophages to the site of the infection. Such organisms are phagocytosed by macrophages, but, by an as-yet-unknown mechanism, they are able to inhibit the degranulation of the macrophage. Such organisms, therefore, continue to multiply intracellularly within the macrophage phagosome, usually causing a chronic infection. In some cases, the macrophages (with their intracellular bacteria) pile up into a type of nodule that becomes surrounded by connective tissue. These walled-off nodules are termed *granulomas* or, in the case of tuberculosis, *tubercles*.

Another role played by macrophages appears to be that of one of the mediators of the inflammatory response. It has been shown that, in addition to their phagocytic and intracellular digestive properties, macrophages can secrete various proteases that may be involved in chronic inflammation and delayed-type hypersensitivity reactions (see Chap. 14). The most likely candidate of the various macrophage-secreted enzymes for inducing an inflammatory reaction is a plasminogen activator that converts the humoral proteolytic enzyme, plasminogen, to its active form, plasmin. Interestingly, the administration of steroids (which are antiinflammatory) appears to inhibit the migration of monocytes from the bone marrow, with a resulting inhibition of inflammation and plasminogen-activator secretion. It has been proposed that the normal role of plasminogen activator is to activate plasminogen, which then digests some of the supporting structures of

blood vessels to allow the migration of monocytes into the tissues.

Macrophages play a central role in specific immunity. As effector cells in delayed-type hypersensitivity, they are stimulated by lymphokines secreted by certain lymphocytes. Lymphokine-stimulated macrophages are considerably more active in phagocytosis and killing than are nonstimulated cells; they have been referred to as angry or activated macrophages. As antigen-presenting cells, they are required in the initial stages of the activation of T cells leading to antibody production, cell-mediated lympholysis, and delayed-type hypersensitivity (see Chaps. 13 and 14).

Defects in Intracellular Killing

The role of the phagocyte as a major defense against disease became more obvious with the discovery that some individuals produce leukocytes that are defective in their ability to phagocytose and destroy invading microorganisms. Such persons experience repeated episodes of infection in spite of the presence of high levels of circulating antibodies. Several types of defects are discussed briefly in the following sections.

CHRONIC GRANULOMATOUS DISEASE. Chronic granulomatous disease (CGD) is a frequently fatal genetic disorder characterized by repeated bacterial infections, most commonly with organisms such as *S aureus* or gram-negative rods. Individuals with CGD possess PMNs that phagocytose invading bacteria normally but are unable to kill many of the ingested microorganisms, as indicated in Figure 4-7. There are two forms of this disease. The more

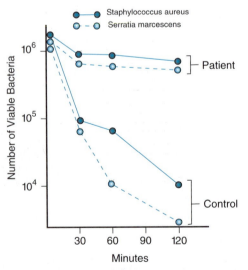

FIGURE 4-7 Impaired killing of bacteria by neutrophils from patients with chronic granulomatous disease (CGD). *Staphylococcus aureus* and *Serratia marcescens* were incubated with PMNs from a patient with CGD and with PMNs from a normal individual. The inability of the patient's PMNs to kill either species of bacterium is readily apparent from the number of viable bacteria.

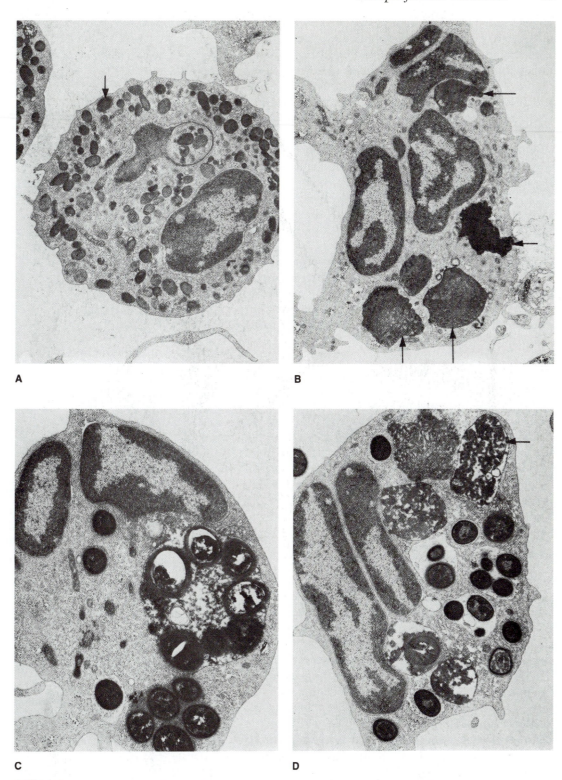

FIGURE 4-8 Electron micrographs of PMNs from normal control subjects and patients with Chediak-Higashi syndrome (CHS). The PMNs have been stained histochemically for peroxidase, causing the azurophil lysosomes to appear dark. **A.** A normal PMN. The arrow points to one of the many small lysosomes. **B.** A PMN from a patient with CHS. The arrows point to the few large lysosomes. **C.** A normal PMN 60 minutes after mixing with staphylococci, showing phagosomal fusion with peroxidase activity in the phagolysosomes and a lack of peroxidase-positive granules in the cytoplasm (compare with **A**). **D.** A PMN from a patient with CHS 60 minutes after mixing with staphylococci. Note the persistence of structurally intact peroxidase-positive giant lysosomes (*arrow*).

frequent, sex-linked form in most cases is associated with the absence of cytochrome *b*, specifically a defect in the 91-kilodalton β subunit. The less frequent autosomal form has normal cytochrome *b* but is characterized by the absence of one or the other of two proteins associated with NADPH oxidase-activating capacity. The PMNs of these patients are unable to produce hydrogen peroxide, although the NADPH oxidase is present in near-normal amounts. Interestingly, organisms that metabolically generate their own H_2O_2, such as streptococci and lactobacilli, are killed normally by CGD PMNs.

CHEDIAK-HIGASHI SYNDROME. Individuals with Chediak-Higashi syndrome have recurrent infections similar to those described for persons with CGD. However, this defect results from the presence of giant lysosomes formed in the promyelocyte, a precursor stem cell to the PMN (Fig. 4-8). These abnormal lysosomes do not fuse readily with a cytoplasmic phagosome. Such cells also have other defects, including a defective chemotactic response to infection.

MYELOPEROXIDASE DEFICIENCY. Individuals whose PMNs completely lack MPO are, for the most part, well and free from recurrent infections, although a case of recurrent candidiasis in an MPO-deficient patient has been reported. It is clear, therefore, that MPO is not the only microbicidal pathway. Phagocytes from MPO-deficient individuals produce H_2O_2 and possess other microbicidal mechanisms that involve superoxide, H_2O_2–ascorbic acid, lysozyme, and the ability to produce an acid pH within the phagolysosome.

Importance of the Phagocytic Cell

The primary importance of the phagocytic cell is well established. The release of phagocytes from the bone marrow and their chemotactic response to infection and inflammation are major defenses in preventing overt disease. Defects in either phagocyte mobilization or the phagocytosis and killing of invading organisms are manifested by frequent infections in spite of the presence of high levels of circulating antibodies. Much that we know concerning the mechanisms of killing invading bacteria has been learned from studies of individuals with defective phagocytes, and it seems probable that additional defects in certain phagocytic cells will be discovered that will add to our knowledge of their microbicidal activities.

The Inflammatory Response

Inflammation is the cellular and vascular response to injury or to the introduction of a foreign particle into the body. Repair of the injury follows the destruction or removal of the foreign object (including bacteria) and the necrotic tissue.

A Closer Look

Our nonspecific resistance mechanisms, sometimes also referred to as innate immunity, form the first line of defense against the disease-causing organisms that we encounter in our daily lives. Humans and animals possess physical barriers to infection, including skin, mucous membranes, and fluids such as tears and mucus, that protect us from the attachment and penetration of infectious organisms. Circulating within our blood and lymph, we have a host of phagocytic cells and an array of accessory molecules, including the complement factors found in the blood and the lysozyme found in tears, which nonspecifically work as enhancing systems for the functions of phagocytic cells, for acquired immune functions, and for the outright killing of invading organisms.

Many microorganisms have evolved ways to resist and evade innate host resistance mechanisms. Similarly, all vertebrates and even the most primitive invertebrates give evidence of having evolved counter-resistance mechanisms to enable them to survive in a threatening environment. The balance between the ability of an infectious organism to circumvent host resistance mechanisms and the ability of host resistance mechanisms to resist or destroy the infectious organism often is tipped in favor of one or the other based on the ability of each to respond to the other. Our cellular mechanisms of defense, bolstered by our chemical and mechanical defense systems, function well under most circumstances. It is only when these systems break down that infection and disease result.

The inflammatory response characterized by an invasion of white blood cells (ie, tissue damage and the formation of pus) is beneficial. Individuals with deficiencies in the number of inflammatory cells and the functions of specific inflammatory cells are susceptible to a multitude of infectious diseases. Soon, it may be possible to reconstitute or correct the cellular defects in such individuals with cell transplants or gene therapy.

Soon after injury, arteriolar dilatation occurs. Increased local blood flow is observed, followed by changes in vascular permeability and subsequent influx of plasma proteins into the site of insult. The changes in vascular permeability result from the release of pharmacologically active agents (ie, prostaglandins) from the damaged cells or from the many cell types that infiltrate the area. The plasma proteins entering the site include components of the complement and coagulation systems (see Chap. 12).

The flow of fluid into the site concentrates red blood cells in the capillaries. This results in decreased blood flow and increased white blood cell migration. Migration of PMNs into the tissue is followed by the migration of monocytes and, eventually, lymphocytes. The degree of influx of cells is influenced by many factors, including the concentration of chemotactic agents such as bacterial products, split products of the complement components, and products of dead or dying cells.

Enzymes released by PMNs and monocytes digest the foreign particles and dead cells. The relative roles of antibody and cell-mediated immune responses, when they do participate, vary depending primarily on the nature of the antigen.

After removal of the foreign object, repair of the wound involves epithelial and endothelial cell proliferation. Proliferation of endothelial cells lining small blood vessels eventually leads to restoration of local microvasculature. Proliferation of epithelial cells results in wound closure. This, combined with infiltration of fibroblasts and subsequent protein (collagen and protein polysaccharides) synthesis, results in scar formation and restoration of connective tissue.

This simplified description of the inflammatory response provides only a brief glimpse of the complex specific and nonspecific mechanisms by which an individual responds to the presence of a foreign particle. It also serves to demonstrate that no single mechanism is sufficient for complete defense against infection. Instead, numerous highly refined defense mechanisms, acting in concert, are responsible for neutralization and removal of the offending substance and repair of the damage incurred as a result of the infection.

Bibliography

BOOKS

Gallin JI, Goldstein IM, Snyderman R. Inflammation: basic principles and clinical correlates, ed 2. New York, Raven Press, 1992.

Lehrer RI, Lichtenstein AK, Ganz T. Defensins: antimicrobial and cytotoxic peptides of mammalian cells. In: Paul WE, Fathman CG, Metzger H, eds. Annual review of immunology, vol 11. Palo Alto, CA, Annual Reviews, 1993:105.

Mims CA. The pathogenesis of infectious disease, ed 3. London, Academic Press, 1987.

Silverstein SC, Steinberg TH. Host defense against bacterial and fungal infections. In: Davis BD, Dulbecco R, Eisen HN, Ginsberg HS, eds. Microbiology, ed 4. Philadelphia, JB Lippincott, 1990.

Essentials of Medical Microbiology, Fifth Edition, edited by Wesley A. Volk,
Bryan M. Gebhardt, Marie-Louise Hammarskjöld, and Robert J. Kadner.
Lippincott-Raven Publishers, Philadelphia © 1996.

Chapter 5

Antibody and Antigen Structure

Antibody Structure

The immune system is able to distinguish between materials that make up the body and those that are foreign. It does not normally react against the body's own cells. However, when it is set into motion by contact with a foreign substance (ie, bacteria, viruses, toxins), a series of complex reactions is activated that aids in eliminating or neutralizing the substance. This ability to recognize "self" as opposed to "nonself" forms the basis for specific acquired immunity.

Foreign materials that gain entrance to the body and induce a specific immune response are called *immunogens,* or *antigens (Ags)*. The resulting specific immune response can be the result of (1) the synthesis and secretion of proteins, called *antibodies (Abs)*, which are found in body fluids such as blood, lymph, tears, and milk (Ab-mediated, or humoral, immunity); (2) the activation of cells that kill other cells, either directly by cell–cell contact or indirectly by activating the intracellular killing mechanisms of phagocytes (cell-mediated immunity); or (3) both.

To understand the mechanisms responsible for self–nonself discrimination, it is necessary to know something about the nature of the foreign substances that can activate the immune system and the nature of the response itself. In Chapters 7, 8, 9, 11, and 13, we describe the cells and organs of the immune system, how they are activated by contact with Ag, and how the immune response is controlled. In this chapter, we describe the chemical and physical properties of Ags and the Abs whose synthesis they induce.

Ab is a glycoprotein (ie, a protein with attached carbohydrate) that is synthesized by cells of the lymphoid lineage in response to exposure to a foreign substance (eg, an infectious organism). This foreign substance can be a small molecule, a large protein or carbohydrate, or an entire microorganism. The small molecule, the protein or carbohydrate, and the molecules of the microorganism are called Ags. The most important property of these Ab molecules is that they specifically bind to the molecule (Ag) that induced their formation.

In the early days of immunology, before the complexity of serum was appreciated, serum proteins were classified according to their solubility as either albumins or globulins. Furthermore, if serum was subjected to electrophoresis, it would separate into albumin and three major globulin components. These globulin components were designated α-, β-, and γ-globulin. Because almost all circulating Abs were found in the γ-globulin fraction (Fig. 5-1), the term *γ-globulin* was used for years as a synonym for circulating Abs. There are exceptions, however, and some Abs with the electrophoretic mobility of α- or β-globulins were found. Therefore, the term *immunoglobulin* (Ig) was coined to refer to Abs and all proteins that show structural similarities to Ab, regardless of their electrophoretic mobility or lack of known Ag-binding specificity.

Studies initiated in the 1950s revealed that most Ab molecules had a molecular weight of about 150,000 daltons and contained 15 to 20 disulfide bonds. Treatment of Ab molecules with sulfhydryl agents to selectively cleave some of these bonds yielded equimolar amounts of two peptide chains. One of the resulting peptides possessed a molecular weight of about 50,000 daltons and was termed *heavy chain;* the other had a molecular weight of about 25,000 daltons and was called *light chain.* The original, intact Ab molecule was shown to have two of the heavy chains (50,000 daltons) and two of the light chains (25,000), which were held together by disulfide bonds.

The British biochemist Rodney Porter demonstrated that digestion of rabbit Ig with the proteolytic enzyme papain cleaved the molecule into two major fragments plus a small amount of short peptides. One fragment (45,000 daltons) still possessed the Ag-binding site and was named *fragment-Ab binding,* or *Fab.* The other fragment (50,000 daltons) could be crystallized and was called *fragment-crystallized,* or *Fc.* Because the Fab fragment contains only one Ag-binding site, the original, divalent Ab molecule was deduced to consist of two Fab fragments and one Fc fragment.

Treatment of Ab molecules with the proteolytic enzyme pepsin generated a single large fragment (100,000 daltons) plus a series of small peptides. The large fragment contained the two Ag-binding sites of the original Ab molecule and was about 10% larger than the two Fab fragments from a papain digestion of Ab; it was named $F(ab')_2$. Mild treatment of $F(ab')_2$ with sulfhydryl reagents cleaved the interchain disulfide bonds, yielding two monovalent pieces termed *Fab'.*

Fab and $F(ab')_2$, possessing Ag-binding sites, were shown to contain both a portion of the heavy chain and the entire light chain, whereas the Fc fragment was found to contain only the remaining parts of the heavy chain.

Therefore, the basic structure of Ab consists of two heavy chains (50,000 daltons each) and two light chains (25,000 daltons each) that are joined by disulfide bonds (Fig. 5-2). Depending on which side of the interchain disulfide bond the heavy chain is cleaved, the reaction with papain or pepsin yields different fragments. Treatment with papain yields two monovalent Fab fragments (45,000 daltons each) and one Fc fragment (50,000 daltons). Treatment with pepsin splits the molecule into one divalent $F(ab')_2$ fragment (100,000 daltons) and some small peptides. It can be seen in Figure 5-2 that the $F(ab')_2$ obtained after pepsin digestion contains a larger portion of heavy chain than does the Fab obtained by papain hydrolysis.

Classes of Immunoglobulins

Most Abs have a molecular weight of 150,000 daltons and are made up of two heavy chains and two light chains. Crude preparations of Ig contain many Abs varying in several structural features, including size (150,000 to 1 million daltons molecular weight), electric charge, and amount of attached carbohydrate. This structural heterogeneity made it difficult to use these Ab populations to determine the relationship between the structure of Ab and its function. However, it was soon recognized that large amounts of single Ig molecules could be obtained from the serum of individuals with a malignancy of the lymphoid system known as *multiple myeloma.* Because this malignancy results from large numbers of daughter cells that have arisen from a single Ab-forming plasma cell (ie, a clone of cells), these cells all synthesize an identical Ig. It also is possible to induce such myelomas

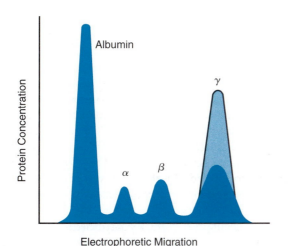

FIGURE 5-1 Electrophoretic separation of serum containing antibodies to a protein antigen. An electric potential was placed across a chamber containing a rabbit serum with antibodies to the protein antigen egg albumin. The proteins in this serum separated into the albumin α-, β-, and γ-globulin fractions as shown. The black pattern shows the size of the protein peaks after absorption of the serum with egg albumin to remove antibody. The shaded γ-globulin peak shows the size of the peak before absorption, demonstrating that the anti-egg albumin antibodies are γ-globulins.

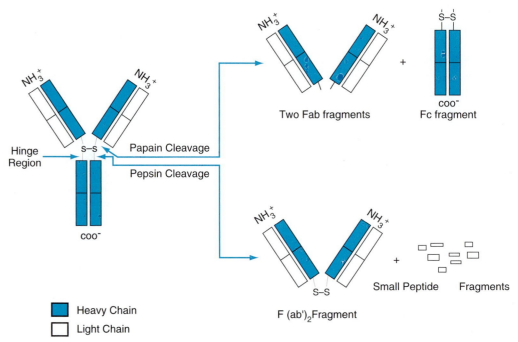

Heavy Chain
Light Chain

FIGURE 5-2 Enzymatic digestion of IgG. The proteins papain and pepsin cleave the antibody molecule in the hinge region. Papain cleavage results in the formation of one Fc fragment and two Fab fragments. Pepsin cleavage yields one F(ab')$_2$ fragment and several small peptides. The hinge region lies between the antigen-binding arms and the carboxy-terminal portion of the molecule and is rich in the amino acids proline and cysteine. This flexible region allows for movement of the antigen-binding arms of the molecule, enabling cross-linking of large antigen molecules.

in mice. The chemical, physical, and biologic properties of many different myeloma proteins have been determined.

Proteins from one species of animal (human or otherwise), when injected into another species, can act as Ags and induce the formation of Abs that specifically bind to the injected protein. Human Igs are foreign to a rabbit. Therefore, rabbits injected with human Ig produce Abs that specifically bind to human Ig. Using this anti-Ig to compare the Igs from a large series of myeloma patients, it was seen that they could be divided into five major classes, and that the antigenic differences among the five classes exist in their heavy chains. These heavy chains have been designated by the Greek letters α, γ, δ, ε, and μ, and the corresponding classes of Ig are named IgA, IgG, IgD, IgE, and IgM. Ig of each class is synthesized by the B lymphocytes of all normal individuals.

Similar studies with human light chains revealed that there are two major types, κ and λ. Both κ and λ light chains are found in association with each class of heavy chain. Thus, the five classes of Ig are distinguished by antigenic differences in their heavy chains. It should be pointed out that any one molecule of Ig will contain only κ or λ light chains, but not both, and only one type of heavy chain. Thus, a single cell normally produces a homogeneous Ig with only a single type of light chain and a single type of heavy chain. Table 5-1 summarizes many of the properties of the various classes and subclasses of Ig discussed in the remainder of this chapter.

IgG

About 70% of the total human Ig is of the IgG class. Its general structure is identical to the prototype Ig described earlier (see Fig. 5-2), that is, a 150,000-dalton glycoprotein consisting of two heavy chains and two light chains. This discussion is confined to human Igs, even though the five major classes of Igs occur in other animals also.

IgG Subclasses

IgG can be subdivided into four subclasses based on antigenic differences (ie, structural differences detected by Abs to human Ig produced in another species) other than those used to divide Ig into classes. These subclasses have been designated IgG1, IgG2, IgG3, and IgG4. The specific antigenic determinants (the sites or structures on the Ag molecule to which the Ab binds) that determine the subclass type of IgG are located in the Fc portion of the Ab molecule. Division into subclasses rather than additional classes of Ig is done because the degree of similarity among the various subclasses of IgG is greater than their overall similarity to the other classes of Ig. For example, members of the IgG subclasses are about 92% identical to each other in heavy-chain constant-region amino acid sequence, yet any one of them is only about 32% identical to the heavy chain of the IgM Ab. Although they are similar in most chemical and physical properties, they can differ in length of the hinge region (described

TABLE 5-1
Properties of Human Immunoglobulins

Ig	Heavy (H)-Chain Designation	Mol. Wt. ($\times 10^{-3}$)	No. of Domains in H-Chain	Mol. Wt. of H-Chain ($\times 10^{-3}$)	Percentage of CHO	Normal Serum Conc. (mg/ml)	Half-life (days)	Fixation of Complement	Attachment to Monocytes
IgG1	γ_1	146	4	51	2–3	9	21 ± 5	+	+
IgG2	γ_2	146	4	51	2–3	3	20 ± 2	±	–
IgG3	γ_3	165	4	60	2–3	1	7 ± 1	+	+
IgG4	γ_4	146	4	51	2–3	0.5	21 ± 2.5	–	–
IgM	μ	970	5	72	9–12	1.5	5	+	–
IgA1	α_1	160	4	52–56	7–11	3	6		–
A₂m(1)									
IgA2	α_2	160	4	55–58	7–11	0.5	6		–
A₂m(2)	α_1 or α_2								
SIgA		380–390	4	52–58	7–11	0–0.05		–	
IgD	δ	172–200	4	60–69	9–11	0.03	3	–	
IgE	ε	188–196	5	72–76	12	0.0003	2.3–4		

CHO, carbohydrate.

61

later), number of interchain disulfide bonds, and, most importantly, biologic effector functions (see Table 5-1).

Using subclass-specific antiserum, it has been shown that IgG1, IgG2, IgG3, and IgG4 constitute about 59%, 30%, 8%, and 3%, respectively, of the total serum IgG. Normal humans possess all four subclasses of IgG, just as they possess all five classes of Ig.

The different classes and subclasses of Ig found in normal individuals are designated as isotypes of Ig. This is in contrast to *allotypes* (discussed later in this chapter), which are determined genetically and vary depending on the gene or genes that the individual inherits.

Electron Microscopy of IgG

Several important features of Ab reactions were observed by Robert Valentine and Michael Green using electron microscopic examination of purified IgG Ab specific for the small organic molecule, dinitrophenol. When dinitrophenol was part of a larger molecule, bis-*N*-dinitrophenyl-octamethylene-diamine (bDOD), which contained a dinitrophenol group at each end (Fig. 5-3*A*), the Ab was able to form dimers, tetramers, and pentamers with this synthetic hapten (depending on the number of bDOD and Ab molecules in a given complex; see Fig. 5-3*B*). These combinations are illustrated schematically in Figure 5-3*C*. The Ag-binding site is located between the light and heavy chains at the N-terminal end of the Fab portion of the molecule. Moreover, careful examination of an electron micrograph of IgG that was treated with pepsin to remove the Fc fragment shows that this treatment had no effect on the ability of the Ab to bind to the hapten and form dimers, trimers, and larger configurations. It also shows pepsin-treated Ab to be missing the external Fc stubs. Finally, the schematic drawing (see Fig. 5-3*C*) clearly shows that the angle between the Fab arms of the molecule must be variable, able to open or close depending on the size of the Ag, or, as in this case, to fit the various multiples of bDOD bound by the Ab.

This region of the Ab molecule is rich in the amino acid proline and has several interchain disulfide bonds between the heavy chains. Because it is believed to be flexible to allow for spreading of the Fab arms, it is called the *hinge* region.

Primary Structure of IgG

Using homogeneous IgG from patients with multiple myeloma, it has been possible to determine the primary structure (ie, the amino acid sequence) of several light and heavy chains. Light chains are particularly easy to obtain, because many of these patients secrete large amounts of pure homogeneous light chains, known as Bence Jones proteins, in their urine.

Determination of the amino acid sequences from many different κ and λ light chains showed that the sequence of the amino-terminal half (about 110 amino acid residues) was extremely variable among different κ chains. However, the sequence of amino acids in the carboxy-terminal half of the light chains was remarkably constant for all κ and λ chains (see allotypes for exceptions). These areas were appropriately named variable-light (V_L) and constant-light (C_L) regions.

Similar analyses of the primary structure of heavy chains from different IgG molecules of the same subclass also showed that about 115 residues at the amino-terminal end were highly variable, whereas the remainder of the heavy chain was constant (exceptions are the allotypic and subclass differences in the constant region). However, because the heavy chain is twice as long as the light chain, the heavy-chain constant region is about three times as long as the light-chain constant region. The IgG molecule contains 12 intrachain disulfide bonds evenly spaced throughout the heavy and light chains, resulting in the formation of several loops in the polypeptide chain. Each loop serves to bring together, in the folded structure, amino acids that are distant from each other in the linear amino acid sequence. Light chains have one disulfide loop in the constant region and one in the variable region. The γ heavy chain of IgG has four disulfide loops: one in the variable region and three in the constant region. Based on such chemical and physical properties, it is easy to see that light chains and heavy chains of IgG are made up of two or more structural domains, each of which is about 110 amino acids in length and contains a single disulfide-bonded loop.

A more detailed model of an IgG molecule showing these variable and constant domains and the intrachain and interchain disulfide bonds is provided in Figure 5-4. The light-chain domains are referred to as V_L and C_L for variable-light and constant-light, whereas the heavy-chain domains are referred to as V_H1, C_H1, C_H2, and C_H3 for the single variable-heavy and three constant-heavy regions. The V_L and V_H domains together form the Ag-binding site of the Ab molecule. The heavy-chain constant domains perform biologic effector functions such as complement fixation, crossing the placenta from mother to fetus, and binding to phagocytes, mast cells, and lymphocytes.

SITE OF ANTIBODY DIVERSITY

The specificity of Ab is a function of the tertiary structure of the variable regions of its light and heavy chains. This, in turn, is a function of the amino acid sequence of the variable regions. If the amino acid sequences from many different Igs are compared, "hot spots" of variability are noted where amino acid substitutions, deletions, or insertions occur within specific areas of the variable regions. Thus, a comparison of the variable regions from Igs of the same family (ie, V_H, V_κ, or V_λ) shows that the major variations and gaps occur at about the same positions in each chain (Fig. 5-5). Human Igs have been shown to possess three such hypervariable regions on their light chains and four on their heavy chains. Mouse Ig and Igs from other species that have been examined have three hypervariable regions on their heavy chains. The amino acids in between the hypervariable regions are called *framework residues,* and the regions within which they reside are called *framework regions.*

These hypervariable regions have been shown to be a part of the Ag-binding site of Ab and are known to form a contact surface that is complementary to the structure on the Ag (the antigenic site, antigenic determinant, or epitope) to which it binds. Therefore, such hypervari-

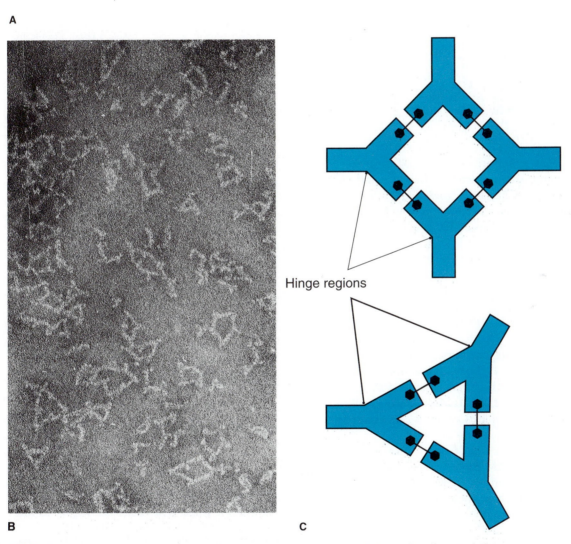

A

B   **C**

FIGURE 5-3 Hapten–antibody interaction. **A.** Structural formula for bis-*N*-dinitrophenyl-octamethylene-diamine, the hapten used to bind IgG to form polymers such as those diagrammed in **C. B.** Electron micrograph of polymers produced by reaction of rabbit anti-DNP IgG with an equivalent amount of the divalent hapten shown in **A**. The antibody molecules are centered at the corners of the polygonal shapes. The Fc fragments project from the corners, and the Fab fragments form the edges of the polygons. Note how the polymers consist of dimers, trimers, tetramers, and pentamers. (Original magnification ×260,000.) **C.** Schematic illustration of a trimer and a tetramer made of IgG antibody as shown in **B**. Note how the arms of the Fab portion must open wider for the tetramer than for the trimer. This demonstrates the flexibility of the hinge region between the Fab and Fc portions of the IgG molecule.

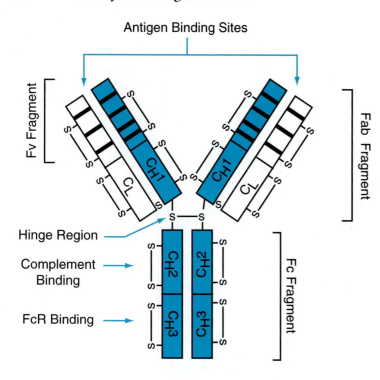

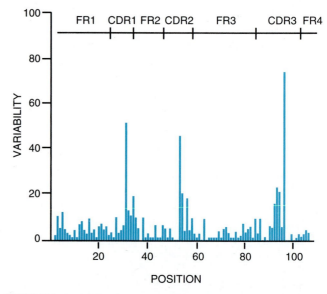

FIGURE 5-4 Diagrammatic representation of the IgG antibody molecule showing its basic structural features. This model illustrates the two-chain structure of the IgG molecule and the position of its Fab and Fc regions. The Fv fragment is another fragment that can be generated by digestion with the proteolytic enzyme trypsin. This fragment contains the variable region domains of the heavy and light chains. Each Fv fragment has a single antigen-combining site. Also shown are (1) the four domains of the heavy chain (V_H, C_H1, C_H2, and C_H3) and the two domains of the light chain (V_L and C_L), each with its intrachain disulfide bond; (2) the four complementarity-determining regions of the heavy chain and the three complementarity-determining regions of the light chain (the dark bands in the Fv portion of each chain); (3) the hinge region; and (4) the heavy-chain domains involved in fixation of complement and binding to Fc receptors on phagocytic cells (monocyte binding).

able regions are called *complementarity-determining regions* (CDRs). Definitive demonstration of the role of the CDRs in Ag binding has been provided by x-ray crystallographic studies on Ag–Ab complexes, such as the one described later in this chapter for the lysozyme–antilysozyme complex.

IgM

IgM was so named because it is a macroglobulin, at least five times larger than IgG. It is a glycoprotein with a molecular weight of about 900,000 daltons. Considerable information concerning its structure has accumulated from the study of IgM isolated from patients with Waldenström's macroglobulinemia. These individuals have a lymphoproliferative disorder that is characterized by the extensive proliferation of a single IgM-producing cell, resulting in the synthesis of copious amounts of a homogeneous IgM.

If the interchain disulfide bonds are broken gently with sulfhydryl agents, the IgM molecule will dissociate into five subunits, each having a molecular weight of about 180,000 daltons. Each of these subunits is made up of two light chains (either κ or λ) and two μ heavy chains. The μ chain is about 20,000 daltons larger than the γ heavy chain of IgG and contains one variable region plus four (rather than three) constant regions. A comparison of the amino acid sequence data with that of IgG indicates that the additional domain is internal. Thus, each IgM molecule actually is made up of five monomeric units, and the general formula for IgM can be written as either $(\mu_2\kappa_2)_5$ or $(\mu_2\lambda_2)_5$. All μ chains within a single IgM molecule are identical.

FIGURE 5-5 Variability in amino acid sequence of immunoglobulin light chains. All light chains have a single amino acid at each position of their linear sequence. However, if the sequences of many light chains are determined and compared, it is seen that certain positions have more possibilities than do others. This figure shows the variability at each position seen within the κ–light-chain variable domain. The variability plotted is equal to the number of different amino acids at a given position divided by the frequency of the most common amino acid at that position. It can be readily seen that there are three regions where the variability is greater. These regions, called the hypervariable regions or the complementarity-determining regions (*CDRs*), are brought together during folding to form part of the antigen-binding site of the antibody molecule. The regions of less variability are called framework regions (*FRs*). The human heavy-chain variable region domain has four regions of high variability (ie, it has four CDR regions), which are brought together during folding to form the remaining portion of the antigen-binding site.

Dissociation of an IgM molecule into its monomeric units also releases a 15,000-dalton peptide that has been designated the J chain. The J chain is synthesized in the same cell as the heavy and light chains of IgM and is covalently linked by means of disulfide bonds to cysteine residues in the carboxy-terminal end of the μ chains. Its function appears to be to join the five monomeric IgMs to form the final secreted molecule, which can be expressed as $(\mu_2\kappa_2)_5$J or $(\mu_2\lambda_2)_5$J.

As described in Chapter 8, Ab-producing cells and their immediate precursors have Igs on their membrane surfaces that act as Ag-specific receptors. IgM and IgD are the most common membrane-bound Igs on the surface of such cells. However, membrane-bound and secreted IgM are not identical. Membrane-bound IgM exists as a monomer that lacks the J chain. The carboxy-terminal 20 amino acids of the heavy chain of secreted IgM, containing the cysteine residue to which the J chain binds, has been replaced by a 41–amino acid section containing primarily hydrophobic amino acids. This section constitutes the transmembrane region of the membrane-bound IgM monomer. (The genetics of Ig synthesis are discussed in Chap. 8.) Figure 5-6 gives a schematic presentation of an IgM molecule (A), as well as models (B) and electron micrographs (C) of the secreted pentameric IgM molecule.

Because IgM contains 10 Fab fragments, and thus 10 Ag-binding sites, one would predict that it could bind 10 Ag molecules. However, it appears that many Ags are so large that, when bound to one binding site on the IgM Ab molecule, they physically prevent the binding of another Ag molecule to an adjacent binding site. Thus, one frequently finds that IgM is capable of binding as few as five molecules of Ag.

IgM usually is the first Ab to appear in the serum after stimulation by an Ag (see Chap. 11). However, IgM synthesis generally is not prolonged, and IgG Abs soon become the most prevalent class. IgM is much more efficient than IgG in its ability to fix complement (see Chap. 12), promoting lysis and death of most gram-negative bacteria. This greater efficiency is due to the proximity of the complement-binding sites on each of the Fc regions of the pentameric secreted IgM. (Membrane-bound IgM does not bind complement.)

IgA

The basic structure of IgA is similar to that of IgG; it contains two identical light chains (either κ or λ) and two identical heavy chains that have been designated α chains. The structural properties of the α chains set IgA apart as a separate class of Ig (see Table 5-1).

In addition to occurring in the serum as a 150,000-dalton monomer, IgA also is found externally in almost all body secretions as a 370,000-dalton dimer. Thus, secretory IgA is present in saliva, tears, seminal fluid, urine,

and colostrum, as well as in the mucus of the lungs and gastrointestinal tract. Secretory IgA is synthesized by plasma cells in the subepithelial tissue and is secreted as a dimer containing four heavy chains, four light chains, and one J chain (identical to the J chain found with pentameric IgM). Another polypeptide chain of 60,000 daltons molecular weight, termed *secretory piece* or *secretory component*, is associated with IgA in secretions. Secretory component is part of a larger cell-surface receptor of epithelial cells called the poly-Ig receptor. This receptor serves to bind the IgA secreted by nearby plasma cells and promotes its intracellular transport through the epithelial cells and into the external secretions at the surface of the secretory organ. Secretory component also seems to protect secretory IgA from degradation by proteolytic enzymes present in secretions. Serum IgA contains neither the J chain nor the secretory component. Schematic models of serum and secretory IgA are shown in Figure 5-7.

Many infectious organisms cause disease by attaching to glycoproteins on the surface of epithelial cells lining mucosal surfaces. If this adhesion is sufficiently strong, the organism will divide, establish a colony, and cause disease by one of several mechanisms (eg, secretion of toxins that cause local and systemic tissue injury). When present in mucus secretions, IgA Ab functions to prevent the attachment of organisms to epithelial cells, thus preventing adhesion, colonization, and infection.

IgA Subclasses

Based on minor antigenic differences in the α chain, IgA is divided into two subclasses, which have been designated IgA1 and IgA2. These subclasses are found in all normal individuals; 80% to 90% of serum IgA is IgA1. Secretory IgA consists of about equal amounts of the two subclasses.

As discussed in the introduction to Unit Four, certain streptococci and pathogenic *Neisseria* secrete proteases that will specifically cleave the heavy chain of IgA1. IgA2 is resistant to such cleavage because it has a shorter hinge region and lacks the proline-rich site cleaved by the proteases.

IgD

The concentration of IgD in the serum is only about 0.2% that of IgG. IgD molecules have a molecular weight of about 180,000 daltons and, like other monomeric Abs, are composed of two light chains and two heavy chains. The heavy chains, designated δ chains, contain about 12% carbohydrate and the antigenic determinants that define this class of Ig.

B lymphocytes (see Chap. 8), which are destined to differentiate into Ab-producing plasma cells, have Igs on their cell surface that serve as Ag-specific receptors. Reaction of Ag with this surface Ig can lead to cell differentia-

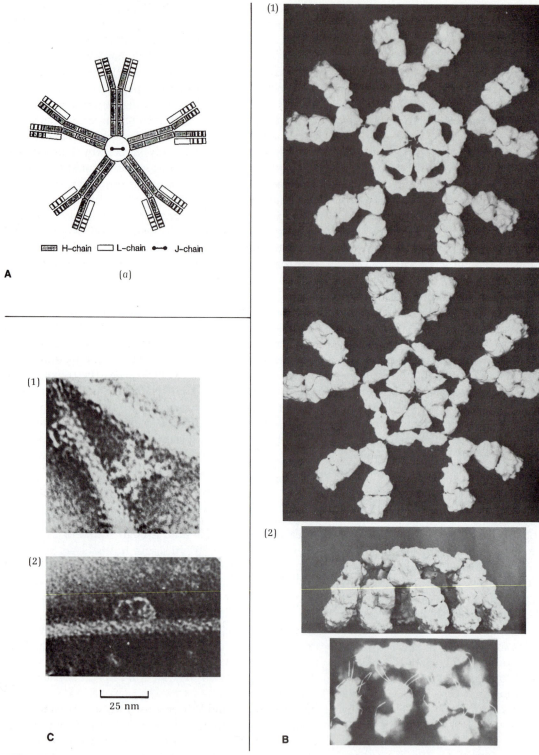

FIGURE 5-6 The structure of IgM. The basic structure of IgM is the same as that of IgG (ie, it has two kinds of polypeptide chains, the μ heavy chain and a light chain [either κ or λ]). **A.** The secretory form of IgM has 5 basic structures, each composed of 2 μ chains and 2 light chains, for a total of 10 μ chains and 10 light chains forming 10 antigen-binding sites. The 5 basic structures are held together by disulfide bonds between the carboxy-terminal regions of the μ heavy chains. It also has a third type of polypeptide chain—the J chain—which is present only on multimeric forms of immunoglobulin. The monomeric form (not shown) of IgM, found only as a receptor on B cells, is composed of a single basic unit with 2 μ chains and 2 light chains; therefore, it has 2 antigen-binding sites. **B.** Part 1 shows case models of pentameric IgM with alternative arrangements of the $C\mu3$ and $C\mu4$ domains. Part 2 shows the "Table" form of IgM corresponding to the "stable" form seen in electron micrographs. **C.** Electron micrographs of IgM antibodies. Part 1 shows IgM cross-linking two bacterial flagella. Part 2 shows IgM in profile bound to a single flagellum.

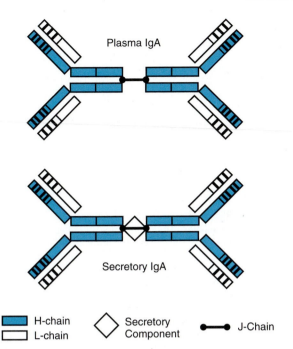

Plasma IgA

Secretory IgA

| ■ H-chain | ◇ Secretory Component | ●━● J-Chain |
| □ L-chain | | |

FIGURE 5-7 The structure of IgA. IgA is found both in the blood and in secretions. In the blood, IgA exists as a monomer, which is composed of two α heavy chains and two light chains (either κ or λ). The dimers and trimers contain the J chain, as do all multimeric forms of immunoglobulin. Secretory IgA is present in various secretions (eg, tears, saliva, mucus, colostrum). Secretory IgA is a dimer of the basic IgA molecule and, in addition to the J chain, contains a fourth polypeptide chain called the *secretory component*. The secretory component is a part of a receptor on the epithelial cells lining the secretory organ. This receptor binds dimeric IgA secreted by plasma cells within the secretory organ and mediates its transfer through the epithelial cell and into the lumen of the secretory organ. On release into the lumen, a portion of the receptor is cleaved and remains with the IgA molecule. As such, this secretory component protects the IgA from digestion by proteolytic enzymes in the lumen.

tion and Ab synthesis. Although IgD occurs in low concentrations in the serum, it is found on the surface of most B lymphocytes as a cell-surface receptor for Ag.

The δ chain of IgD has a molecular weight of 66,000 daltons and contains one variable and three constant domains. The larger size of the δ chain was shown by Frank Putnam and his collaborators to be caused by a long hinge region (about 50 amino acids) between the C_H1 and C_H2 domains. This hinge region is susceptible to cleavage by a variety of proteases, including serum plasmin, and may play a special role in the function of IgD.

IgE

Although IgE is present in serum only in minute concentrations, we have more definitive information concerning its function than we have for serum IgD. IgE is responsible for countless human allergies, including allergies to food, ragweed and other pollens, dust, and almost any other material imaginable (see Chap. 14). The heavy

chains, called ε, are about 20,000 daltons larger than the IgG γ chains and possess an additional domain (see Fig. 5-7). Most of a person's IgE is fixed to the surface of mast cells, and when a specific Ag (such as ragweed pollen) binds with mast cell or basophil membrane-bound IgE, the reaction results in the release of pharmacologically active substances, such as histamine and serotonin, which dilate capillaries, alter vascular permeability, and cause the bronchial constriction characteristic of allergic rhinitis (eg, hay fever). This surface reaction occurs because mast cells and basophils possess receptors specific for the Fc portion of IgE, leaving the Ab-binding site free to react with Ag (allergen).

Although IgE may seem to promote only adverse reactions, it appears to have evolved to provide several protective functions. For example, individuals from tropical areas of the earth can possess 20 times as much IgE as those from northern regions. It also has been noted that IgE levels rise after infection with certain parasites, especially helminths (see Chap. 50). Together, these observations suggest that the normal physiologic function of IgE is to promote the destruction of invading parasites by reacting with Ags on the surface of the parasite while its Fc fragment is bound to a mast cell. Subsequent release of histamine from the mast cell results in increased vascular permeability, an influx of plasma and cells (particularly eosinophils), and destruction of the offending pathogen.

All normal individuals possess IgE, yet certain individuals show a predisposition for multiple allergies to a wide variety of substances. This genetic predisposition to allergy, termed *atopy,* is independent of the ability to produce IgE.

Three-Dimensional Structure of the Antibody-Combining Site

INTERACTION BETWEEN V_H AND V_L DOMAINS

The heavy-chain and light-chain molecules fold and interact in such a way as to bring together amino acids of the CDRs of each chain to form the Ag-binding surface. This Ag-binding surface is discussed in more detail later, but first it is informative to take a closer look at the interface between the V_H and V_L domains. Two structural features are immediately evident. First, each domain interacts with the other through a relatively flat surface made up of several β-pleated sheet structures (Fig. 5-8). Second, about 25% of the amino acids in this interface are from the CDR. These two features may provide a unique way to modify the geometry of the Ag-binding site *without* changing residues within the site itself. For example, changes in the CDR residues at the V_H–V_L interface may cause a change in the position of the V_H and V_L domains relative to each other. This movement then would affect the positions of the heavy- and light-chain CDR residues

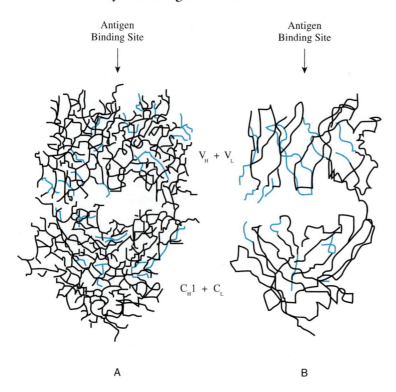

Antigen Binding Site

Antigen Binding Site

$V_H + V_L$

$C_H1 + C_L$

A

B

FIGURE 5-8   Molecular model of the structure of an antibody Fab fragment. **A.** The Fab fragment of a monoclonal antibody to a protein antigen, including all amino acid side chains. **B.** The α-carbon backbone of the same Fab fragment. The heavy- and light-chain variable regions (V_H and V_L, respectively) are loosely associated, forming the domain with the antigen-binding site (*top*), whereas the light-chain constant region (C_L) and the first heavy-chain constant region (C_H1) are shown as a more compact globular domain at the bottom. An entire IgG antibody is about three times the size of this Fab fragment. The black-to-gray shading is indicative of depth, with gray lines representing bonds in the distance and black lines representing amino acids closer to the reader.

within the binding site. Repositioning of potential contact residues within the site undoubtedly would alter the specificity of the Ab.

THE ANTIGEN-BINDING SURFACE

The Ag-binding site of an Ab is a convoluted surface complementary to the surface structure on the Ag molecule to which it binds. (The site on the Ag is discussed later in this chapter.) Figure 5-9 shows two views of the binding site of an Ab molecule. The structure of this site was determined by x-ray diffraction analysis of an Ag–Ab complex. Several features are worthy of attention:

All six CDRs of this Ab contribute to binding of Ag.
A large number of amino acids are involved (13 to 17 residues in the Abs studied so far).
The number of residues each CDR contributes to binding Ag varies from one Ab to the other.

Wherever there is a depression or protrusion on the Ab surface, there is a protrusion or depression, respectively, on the Ag (this will become more evident later). Thus, a close fit between Ag and Ab is achieved, which excludes all solvent molecules; the closer the fit, the stronger the binding.
The surface area involved is 650 to 750 Å, about the same as for other protein–protein interactions. The large number of amino acids involved in the interaction between Ag and Ab (about 13 to 17 on each molecule) explains the high degree of specificity of the interaction.

Allotypes

In contrast to isotypes, allotypes are minor differences in structure that vary from one person to another. For example, the subclass IgG1 from one person can show a

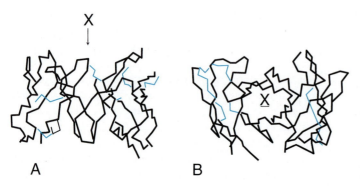

X

A

B

FIGURE 5-9   The antigen-combining site of antibody. Two views of the variable domain of antibody are shown. Both are constructed using only the α-carbon main chain of the V_H and V_L regions of the antibody. **A.** A side view of the variable domain, with the binding site (*X*) at the top. **B.** The same structure rotated 90 degrees toward the reader. The center of the combining site is labeled with an *X* and can include as many as 16 amino acids surrounding this central marker. The light chain is on the left and the heavy chain is on the right. Again, gray shading represents distant amino acids and black shading represents amino acids closer to the reader.

minor structural difference from the IgG1 obtained from another person. These differences are specified by slight differences in coding sequences of the alleles encoding the IgG1 heavy chain. The alleles segregate independently and are inherited as mendelian autosomal genes. There are three general types of allotypes: Gm, Am, and Km.

Gm ALLOTYPES

Gm allotypes occur on the heavy chain (γ) of IgG molecules. About 25 different Gm allotypes have been described (designated by numbers), each representing a different allele that codes for a difference of about two amino acids between one Gm allotype and another. The IgG1 heavy chain can carry two or three different Gm determinants (located at different positions in the heavy chain), whereas the other IgG subclasses carry only a single Gm determinant. Because each of the IgG subclasses is encoded by a different gene (each with two alleles), each IgG subclass has its own Gm markers. Therefore, an individual's Gm allotype could be listed as IgG1, Gm1, Gm3; IgG2, Gm23, IgG3, Gm15; and IgG4, Gm4a. Unlike many genetic loci in which the maternally or paternally acquired gene can be dominant (such as in eye color), the Gm alleles are codominant. Thus, individuals who are heterozygous at a locus express both the paternal and maternal Gm specificity, although any one Ab-synthesizing cell expresses only one of the two allelic genes.

Am ALLOTYPES

The Am allotypes are completely analogous to the Gm allotypes described for IgG, except that they occur on the heavy chain of IgA2. Only two such allotypes have been described: $A_2m(1)$ and $A_2m(2)$.

Km ALLOTYPES

The third allotype, called *Km* (previously termed *InV*), is found only on κ light chains. There appear to be two different amino acid changes at positions 153 and 191 on the κ chain.

Idiotypes

Because of the high degree of variability in the aminoterminal regions of heavy and light chains of an Ab, the Ab-combining site and adjacent variable regions often are unique to that Ab (or at least found infrequently in other Abs). Such V-region–associated structures are called *idiotypes*. It may help to think of idiotypes as being analogous to fingerprint patterns—few of either are the same.

The idiotype on Ab from one individual can be seen as foreign by another individual of the same species who has not, or cannot, form the same structure on his or her own Abs. If it is seen as foreign, this second individual can make an Ab that binds to the idiotype structure on the Ab from the first individual. The Ab made in the second individual is called an anti-idiotype Ab.

Many different amino acid sequence and structural combinations can form an Ab to a single site on an Ag. Each of these combinations results in a unique Ab-binding site, and each unique Ab-binding site can give rise to a unique idiotype. Thus, an Ab response to a single site on an Ag can give rise to many different Abs with many different binding sites and, thus, many different idiotypes. Although Abs can see the same site on an Ag in a variety of ways, there are limits to the variability that will allow the binding to occur. Therefore, among those Abs that do bind, some similarity in binding sites and, as a result, some similarity in idiotypes might be expected. These similar, or shared, idiotypes are called *public idiotypes*.

There also are idiotypes that are unique to a single Ab. These are called *private idiotypes*. For example, an Ab response to site 1 on an Ag molecule contains Abs with 10 different combining sites. Seven of the 10 binding sites, although different, are similar enough that anti-idiotype Ab made to one reacts with all 7. These 7 Abs share a public idiotype. The other 3 Abs also are similar to each other, but are different from the first 7 Abs. These 3 Abs share an idiotype (public idiotype number 2) that is different from the idiotype (public idiotype number 1) shared by the other 7 Abs.

In addition, 1 or more (and perhaps each) of the 10 Abs can have a second V-region–associated structure that is not shared with *any* of the other 9 Abs. This would be a private idiotype.

This lengthy explanation of allotypes and idiotypes is given because both are used as genetic markers in human genetic studies and as markers of variable- and constant-region genes in studies of regulation of immune responses. In addition, an understanding of the nature of idiotypes is required to appreciate how they can complicate efforts to use monoclonal Abs to suppress transplant rejection and to kill malignant lymphoid cells.

Monoclonal Antibodies

Most proteins possess many different antigenic determinants. As a result, serum from an animal or human producing Abs to a protein or cellular constituent contains a complex mixture of Abs. This mixture contains Abs to all determinants as well as Abs that are heterogeneous with respect to heavy-chain isotype, light-chain type, allotype, variable-region sequence, and idiotype. A long-held dream of biomedical scientists was to isolate a single Ab-producing cell and grow it in vitro to provide a source of homogeneous Abs that would bind to only a single antigenic determinant.

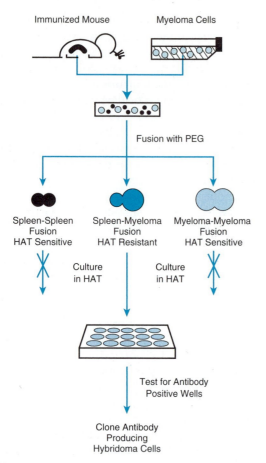

FIGURE 5-10 Production of hybridoma cell lines secreting monoclonal antibodies. The procedure for producing monoclonal antibodies is shown. Activated B cells from an immunized individual (eg, spleen cells from an immunized mouse) are fused with malignant plasma cells isolated from plasmacytomas and adapted to tissue culture. The myeloma cell has a mutant gene that renders it sensitive to the drug aminopterin. The activated B cells, although resistant to aminopterin, have a limited lifetime in culture and die naturally. The B cell–myeloma cell hybrid is resistant to aminopterin because the B cell provides the missing genes. Therefore, the B cell–myeloma cell hybrid (the hybridoma) is the only fusion product that can survive in the hypoxanthine, aminopterin, thymidine (HAT) selective culture medium used. The hybrids are distributed into many culture wells in the multiwell culture plates and are allowed to grow for a short period. The culture supernatant of these wells then is tested for the desired antibody. Those cultures that are positive are cloned, and the hybridoma cell producing the desired antibody is propagated and used as a source of the monoclonal antibody.

Unfortunately, normal Ab-producing cells do not grow indefinitely in tissue culture. In 1975, Georges Köhler and Cesar Milstein overcame this difficulty by fusing normal cells producing the desired Ab from an immunized animal with myeloma cells (malignant lymphocytes that can be propagated easily in vitro) in the presence of a chemical that promotes cell fusion (polyethylene glycol or Sendai virus). This caused the cell membranes of some Ab-producing spleen cells to fuse with the myeloma cells. Such fused cells, called *hybridomas*, have the Ab-producing capability of the normal cell parent

and the in vitro growth properties of the malignant myeloma parent. The normal, nonfused spleen cells cannot survive in culture, whereas the unfused myeloma cells, which can grow in vitro, carry a mutant gene in a critical biosynthetic pathway (ie, a drug marker). The presence of this mutant gene allows the unfused myeloma cell to be killed by adding the appropriate drug in culture. The fused cell is protected from this drug, because the normal spleen cell provides the normal biosynthetic gene. The procedure used to produce hybridoma cell lines secreting monoclonal Abs is shown in Figure 5-10.

Monoclonal Abs are available for thousands of different determinants and are being used widely as research tools to study protein structure and virus and toxin neutralization, and to isolate specific proteins from complex mixtures. Moreover, many commercially available monoclonal Abs are being used in extremely sensitive and specific techniques for the diagnosis of various diseases and, as mentioned earlier, for the experimental treatment of several human diseases.

Antigen Structure: The Chemical Nature of Antigens

Ags can be made up of almost any chemical substance, although most are protein, carbohydrate, lipid, nucleic acid, or a combination of these (eg, glycoproteins, glycolipids, nucleoproteins). Examples of Ags are bacterial capsules, toxins, the cell-wall lipopolysaccharides of gram-negative bacteria, cell-membrane glycoproteins or glycolipids, single- and double-stranded DNA, RNA, ribonucleoproteins, and virtually any viral, fungal, bacterial, or parasitic protein.

THE RELATION OF ANTIGEN TO SELF

Some Ags are more effective in inducing an immune response than are others. First and foremost, an Ag is normally foreign to the host. In general, the greater the difference between the Ag and similar molecules in the host's body, the greater the immune response that is generated. This is directly related to the number of antigenic determinants that are involved and, thus, the number of lymphocytes that are activated. Some proteins, such as diphtheria or tetanus toxoids, are different from self-proteins. Therefore, they are strong Ags and induce a good immune response. Other proteins, such as some cancer cell Ags, are closely related to self-Ags and induce poor, if any, immune responses.

The theory of clonal selection, first proposed by Sir Frank Macfarlane Burnet, postulated that during the prenatal period, the developing lymphoid system learns to distinguish "self" from "nonself." Several mechanisms may be responsible for this self–nonself discrimination (see Chap. 11). As a result, individuals normally develop a long-term tolerance to molecules that are components of their own cells. However, as described in Chapters 11 and 14, immune responses to self-Ags can be generated, resulting in autoimmune disease.

THE ANTIGENIC DETERMINANT

The portion of the Ag that specifically combines with Ab or with the Ag receptor on lymphocytes is called the *antigenic determinant,* or *epitope.* Most Ags are large and possess multiple antigenic determinants. In general, the greater the number of epitopes, the greater the number of lymphocytes that are activated during an immune response.

HAPTENS

Low-molecular-weight organic compounds have been used for many years in studies on the nature of Ags and the interaction between Ag and Ab. These low-molecular-weight molecules, called *haptens,* cannot induce an immune response when injected by themselves (ie, they are not *immunogenic*) but can do so when covalently coupled to a large protein molecule, called the *carrier* molecule, forming a hapten–carrier, or hapten–protein, conjugate (Fig. 5-11). The injection of a hapten–protein conjugate results in an Ab response to the hapten and to epitopes on the carrier protein. The Ab directed to the hapten

reacts with the hapten either on the original carrier, with the hapten conjugated to almost any other macromolecule, or with the "free" hapten itself. Thus, the free hapten cannot induce the formation of Ab, but it can react with the Ab after it is made in response to injection of the hapten–carrier complex. The bDOD molecule discussed earlier (see Fig. 5-3) is a good example of a hapten.

The discovery that free hapten binds to its Ab opened a new area of research concerned with the molecular specificity of Abs. A good example of such research is the series of experiments conducted many years ago by Karl Landsteiner and his colleagues. Slight structural changes were made in the haptens, and the effects of the changes on the reaction with Ab were determined. The specificity of Ab for its inducing antigenic determinant was astonishing. As shown in Table 5-2, merely moving the sulfonic acid group from the *meta* to the *ortho* or *para* positions greatly diminishes their reactivity with Abs induced by the hapten *m*-aminobenzene sulfonic acid conjugated to a carrier protein. Similarly, if the chemical nature of the side group is changed from sulfonic acid to arsenic acid or a carboxyl group, reactivity with Abs to the *m*-aminobenzene sulfonic acid hapten is almost totally lost. Thus, both the chemical nature and the three-dimensional structure of the hapten play major roles in determining the specificity of Ag–Ab interaction.

Abs can distinguish several structural differences between related Ags, such as between the nature (α versus

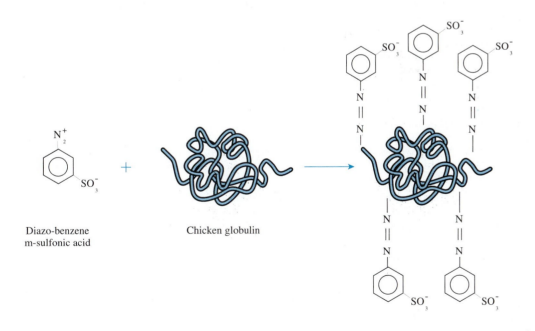

Diazo-benzene
m-sulfonic acid

Chicken globulin

Diazotized hapten coupled
to tyrosine residues of
the chicken globulin

FIGURE 5-11 A hapten–protein antigen conjugate. Schematic diagram illustrating the coupling of an aromatic hapten to a carrier protein. The final protein will induce antibody synthesis to both the carrier protein and the aromatic hapten.

TABLE 5-2
Effect of Moving or Altering Side Groups on Aromatic Haptens

Antigens made from chicken globulin and:	Position of the substituents		
	ortho (NH₂ — R*)	meta (NH₂ — R)	para (NH₂ — R)
Aminobenzene sulfonic acid†	+±‡	+++	±
Aminophenyl arsenic acid	−	+	−
Aminobenzoic acid	−	+	−

* R denotes the group SO_3H, AsO_3H_2, COOH.
† 2 drops of immune serum for *m*-aminobenzene sulfonic acid were added to 0.2 ml of the antigens, diluted 1 : 500.
‡ Readings were taken after standing overnight in the ice box.

β) or position (1 to 3 versus 1 to 4) of glycosidic linkages between sugar residues in a polysaccharide, or between the spatial arrangements of different chemical groups around a single asymmetric carbon atom in the stereoisomers of a given organic molecule. Blood groups constitute another example of the incredible ability of Ab, and thus the immune system, to distinguish small structural differences. In this case, the only difference between type A and type B antigenic determinants on human red blood cells is that the terminal sugar on the type A Ag is *N*-acetyl galactosamine, whereas the terminal sugar on the type B Ag is galactose. Yet, this seemingly minor structural difference can be responsible for a fatal reaction if type A blood is transfused into a type B individual, or vice versa. In addition, as will be seen later, a single amino acid substitution in a large protein also can be discerned by Ab.

There are many clinically important haptens. For example, the antibiotic penicillin is not immunogenic in humans in its free form and does not normally react with the proteins of a patient to form a hapten–carrier conjugate. However, penicillin can be metabolized in the patient, giving rise to several chemically reactive breakdown products, which couple covalently to serum and cellular proteins. Many of these penicillin-derived, hapten–protein conjugates can induce Ab that is reactive with the breakdown product in its free and conjugate forms, and with penicillin itself. In some patients, this Ab response is directly responsible for life-threatening hypersensitivity reactions (see Chap. 14). Other drugs or simple chemical compounds can induce Ab or cell-mediated immune responses responsible for a variety of clinical problems, such as drug-induced hemolytic anemia and contact dermatitis (see Chap. 14).

NATURAL ANTIGENS

Proteins constitute the largest and most diverse group of Ags. Proteins are composed of one or more polypeptide chains, each of which folds into a specific structure in three dimensions. The surface of a protein can be envisioned as an irregular surface made up of the side chains of amino acids and, to a certain extent, those atoms that constitute the backbone chain of the polypeptide. The side chains of the amino acids are in direct contact with the solvent and with each other.

Computer modeling is extremely useful in efforts to more fully understand the molecular basis of immune recognition. It allows direct visualization of the accessible surface of Ags, their individual epitopes, and the way in which the epitopes interact with the Ab-combining sites (Fig. 5-12). In addition, computer modeling can permit examination of the surface of certain viruses for antigenic determinants recognized by neutralizing Abs, and for the position of these epitopes relative to other viral surface structures important in the infectious process.

The three-dimensional structures of most Ags involved in cell–cell interaction during the immune response, or involved in a disease process, are not known. Most studies of antigenicity, therefore, have been conducted on model proteins selected primarily because their three-dimensional structures are known, and because they are readily available in pure form. The validity of using such nonpathogenic models is based on the fact that many apparently innocuous proteins can induce severe, life-threatening immune responses in humans (eg, in immediate hypersensitivity reactions), and on the fact that studies indicate that there is no single structural feature that dictates antigenicity.

FIGURE 5-12 An antigenic determinant of a protein antigen. An antigenic determinant on the protein antigen hen egg white lysozyme is shown in two views. For simplicity, only the α-carbon main chain of the protein is shown except for those residues that make up the antigenic site. In both views, the van der Waals radii are shown for the amino acids within the antigenic site. **A.** A side view of the irregular yet relatively flat surface of the epitope. Two positively charged arginine residues form a slight ridge that projects from the protein surface. These two residues form several salt bridges and hydrogen bonds with three glutamic acid residues in the antibody-combining site. **B.** The same site rotated 90 degrees toward the reader. This view gives an indication of the size of the epitope (12 amino acids), which is about 14% of the entire protein surface.

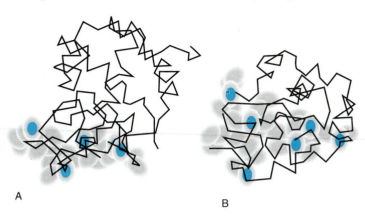

One such protein, chicken egg-white lysozyme (HEL), has been the subject of intensive investigation and is discussed here with regard to the molecular basis of antigenicity. Much of the early work on most of the epitopes on HEL was conducted by Sandra Smith-Gill, Eli Sercarz, and their colleagues. In determining the position of antigenic epitopes, they used two groups of reagents: (1) monoclonal Abs specific for HEL; and (2) a panel of egg-white lysozymes from several species of birds (eg, chicken, turkey, pheasant, and guinea-hen). Each of these lysozymes differs from every other lysozyme by one or more amino acids. By determining the reactivity of the monoclonal Abs with each of the other lysozymes, they were able to correlate reactivity with differences in amino acid sequence. For example, Table 5-3 shows a summary of the data they and others obtained revealing the site of reactivity of two Abs, both of which were made to chicken lysozyme. Ab 2 reacted with both chicken and California quail lysozymes, but not with bobwhite quail lysozyme. The only difference in structure that can explain this reactivity pattern is at position 68, where bobwhite quail lysozyme has a lysine (Lys) residue substituted for the arginine (Arg) that is present in the chicken and California quail lysozymes. In contrast, Ab 1 reacts with chicken and bobwhite quail lysozymes, but not with California

quail lysozyme. The only difference between the lysozymes that can explain this reactivity pattern is at position 121, where those that react have glutamine (Gln) and those that do not, have a different amino acid (eg, histidine [His] in California quail). Thus, the investigators found that the reactivity of one monoclonal Ab with each of the lysozymes correlated exactly with the presence or absence of a given amino acid at one position in the structure. From these data, they inferred that these amino acids are important in the recognition of lysozymes by Ab 1 and Ab 2. Other monoclonal Abs could detect sequence differences elsewhere in the structures of the lysozymes. From these data and knowledge of the three-dimensional structure of HEL, they were able to map epitopes on the surface of the HEL protein molecule.

Studies by Roberto Poljak and colleagues at the Pasteur Institute in Paris, and by Steven Sheriff, Roberto Padlan, and David Davies at the National Institutes of Health in the United States, using x-ray diffraction techniques, have provided the three-dimensional structure of several complexes of three different monoclonal Abs and HEL. The computer-generated models shown in Figure 5-12 are based on their studies. As can be seen, the contact surfaces of the epitope and the Ab-combining site are irregular. Not so obvious is the fact that two amino acids

TABLE 5-3
Antigenically Active Amino Acids of Lysozyme

| Lysozyme† | Amino Acid Position* | | | | | AB1 | AB2 |
	40	55	68	91	121		
HEL	Thr	Ile	Arg	Ser	Gln	+	+
CQEL	Ser	Val	Arg	Thr	His	−	+
BQEL	Ser	Val	Lys	Thr	Gln	+	−

* HEL, chicken egg-white lysozyme; CQEL, California quail egg-white lysozyme; BQEL, Bobwhite quail egg-white lysozyme.
† Position in the linear sequence of amino acids of the polypeptide chain. Lysozyme is 129 amino acids long. Thr, threonine; Ser, serine; Ile, isoleucine; Val, valine; Arg, arginine; Lys, lysine; Gln, glutamine; His, histidine.

that are adjacent to each other on the surface of the protein frequently are distant from each other in the linear amino acid sequence of the polypeptide chain. Understanding this concept of distant amino acids coming together on the surface during folding of the protein is important for a full understanding of antigenicity, because most antigenic determinants recognized by Abs exist only on the surface of the native folded protein, that is, they are topographic. Such antigenic determinants are termed *conformational, topographical assembled,* or *discontinuous epitopes.* This is not a hard and fast rule, however, because some Abs react with linear fragments of protein Ags, so that the antigenic determinants they are recognizing probably are made up of several amino acids that are close to each other both on the surface and in the linear sequence of amino acids of the polypeptide chain. These are termed *sequential, topographical segmented,* or *continuous epitopes.*

The Ab used by Poljak had the reactivity pattern of Ab 1, whereas the Ab used by Steven Sheriff and David Davies had the reactivity of Ab 2 (see Table 5-3). In each case, the crystallographic data confirmed the partial mapping of epitopes accomplished by Smith-Gill using naturally occurring variants of lysozymes. In each case, there are one or two residues in the epitope that protrude slightly from its surface and penetrate into a cleft formed by the Ab-combining site (see Fig. 5-12). In each case, both the Ab and the Ag provide many contact residues (about 15 from Ag and 15 from Ab) from segments of the polypeptide chain distant from each other. Therefore, these epitopes are clearly of the conformational or discontinuous type and exist only on the surface of the lysozyme Ag molecule. Although the contribution of each amino acid to specificity and energy of binding is unknown, it is clear that binding by Ab can be considerably reduced by a single change in the epitope (see Table 5-3).

Many other studies have been conducted on a wide variety of model proteins and have suggested some general rules for understanding antigenicity. First, no single part of a protein Ag is intrinsically more immunogenic than any other part. Second, the entire surface of a protein is potentially immunogenic in that, in one species or another, Abs can be formed, so that the collection of all such Abs would recognize the entire surface. Third, the regions of the surface that are immunogenic in a given responding species or individual, including humans, depend primarily on two factors: (1) the structural differences between the Ag and a similar molecule in the responding individual; and (2) the regulatory mechanisms active in controlling the immune response in that individual. Both these factors are discussed in Chapter 11.

This discussion has been restricted to those antigenic determinants that are recognized by Ab. Similar studies have been carried out with cells specifically activated by Ag during cell-mediated immune responses (T cells; see Chaps. 9 and 11). As discussed in Chapter 11, there appear to be fundamental differences between the determinants recognized by Abs and those recognized by T-cell receptors.

A Closer Look

The complete molecular structure of all the classes of Ab in humans and animals has been determined. Early on, much of this investigation appeared to some to be an exercise in tapestry weaving, but the investigators involved persisted in their pursuit of knowledge, and the results of their work have vindicated this effort. Now that we know the primary amino acid structure of a variety of Ab molecules and have a detailed appreciation of the three-dimensional structure of the Ab-combining site, it is possible to identify the genes that code for Ab-combining sites, isolate these genes, clone them, and use these clones in both basic and clinical investigations. On the research front, we have been able to determine the specificity relations between the amino acids in the Ab-combining site and the amino acids of the Ag to which the Ab-combining site binds. On the clinical side, knowledge of Ab-combining–site genes has afforded us the ability to develop human monoclonal Abs directed against the antigenic epitopes of infectious organisms, cancer cells, and an array of other antigenic structures. These Abs will be useful in defining the protective immune response against infections, cancers, and other disease processes. In addition, it soon should be possible to perform gene therapy and provide patients with genes that will direct the synthesis of protective Abs at specific sites in the body where they are needed. Already, investigators are performing cell and gene therapy experiments in patients who have certain deficiencies or who, for other reasons, are unable to mount a normal immunologic response.

Just as our detailed knowledge of Ab structure and function has allowed us to use these molecules as therapeutic agents, our detailed knowledge of Ags has afforded us the ability to identify those Ags most important for inclusion in vaccines against specific infections and disease processes. It now is possible to create defective viruses for use as vaccines that can protect whole populations against several disease-causing viruses simultaneously. Our ability to generate synthetic vaccines that will simultaneously immunize against two or more pathogens holds great promise.

SYNTHETIC VACCINES

Another approach to the study of Ag structure has been to synthesize peptides with exactly the same sequence as portions of the Ag of interest and to determine whether Ab made to the intact protein will react with these peptides. Similarly, such peptides have been conjugated to a carrier protein (as described earlier for haptens) and used to induce Abs to the peptide. Frequently, these latter Abs have been found to react with the native protein molecule as well.

This has led to attempts to predict which amino acids are involved in the formation of an antigenic determinant. For example, it is known that epitopes recognized by Ab are located on the surface of the Ag molecule. Therefore, if one could predict which segments of the linear sequence exist sequentially on the surface, one could possibly synthesize a peptide with that sequence and use it to induce Ab that would react with the native molecule. Such studies have been conducted, and the results generally bear out the predictions of the amino acids that contribute to the structure of an antigenic determinant. Other algorithms for predicting antigenic structure have been suggested, but no single one is universally applicable. Much of the problem lies in determining which peptides will invoke an immune response that will neutralize a virus or promote removal and destruction of the bacterium causing the disease. Nevertheless, such studies have led to multiple attempts to produce synthetic Ags that could be used to immunize individuals against disease caused by bacteria or viruses. For example, synthetic vaccines have been used experimentally to immunize against diseases such as hepatitis and hoof-and-mouth disease.

The antigenic structure of most Ags of clinical interest has not been determined, either because we do not have the monoclonal Abs necessary or because our knowledge of the three-dimensional structure is limited or lacking. However, recombinant DNA technology has allowed us to infer the amino acid sequence of several viral proteins from their DNA coding sequences. This knowledge of the primary structure of viral proteins, combined with the algorithms for predicting antigenicity, may enable us to produce synthetic vaccines in situations in which the production of safe, effective vaccines by current methods is not yet possible.

The gene encoding the hepatitis B surface Ag (HBsAg) of the hepatitis virus has been cloned and expressed in yeast. This recombinant HBsAg has been approved for use as a vaccine in the United States.

Other methods for producing novel vaccines also have been developed. For example, a recombinant vaccinia virus that contains a gene for the immunogenic glycoprotein of rabies virus has been made. This recombinant virus expresses the rabies glycoprotein on its viral envelope in addition to its own glycoprotein. Immunization of experimental animals with this recombinant virus has led to complete protection against disease following intracerebral injection of rabies virus.

About 1 million new cases of polio are reported annually, most in undeveloped countries. With the use of Ab-resistant mutants of the poliovirus, several amino acids that constitute epitopes on this virus have been identified. Karen Burke and her colleagues in England have used recombinant DNA techniques to construct a hybrid virus containing the epitopes of the three serotypes of poliovirus. Experimental animals immunized with this hybrid vaccine have been shown to produce Ab reactive with all three serotypes. Similar methods can be used to produce improved vaccines against many picornaviruses, including hepatitis A.

More recently, the gene encoding p120, the surface glycoprotein of the human immunodeficiency virus, has been cloned, and the protein has been expressed in insect cells. The use of this recombinant protein as a vaccine for acquired immunodeficiency syndrome is undergoing clinical trials.

Bibliography

JOURNAL

Schumaker VN, Phillips ML, Hanson DC. Dynamic aspects of Ab structure. Mol Immunol 1991;28:1347.

BOOKS

Harriman W, Volk H, Defranoux N, Wabl M. Ig class switch recombination. In: Paul WE, Fathman CG, Metzger H, eds. Annual review of immunology, vol 11. Palo Alto, CA, Annual Reviews, 1993:361.

Schatz DG, Oettinger MA, Schlissel MS. V(D)J recombination: molecular biology and regulation. In: Paul WE, Fathman CG, Metzger H, eds. Annual review of immunology, vol 10. Palo Alto, CA, Annual Reviews, 1992:359.

Staudt LM, Lenardo MJ. Ig gene transcription. In: Paul WE, Fathman CG, Metzger H, eds. Annual review of immunology, vol 9. Palo Alto, CA, Annual Reviews, 1991:378.

Essentials of Medical Microbiology, Fifth Edition, edited by Wesley A. Volk, Bryan M. Gebhardt, Marie-Louise Hammarskjöld, and Robert J. Kadner. Lippincott-Raven Publishers, Philadelphia © 1996.

Chapter 6

Antigen–Antibody Interaction

The study of antigen (Ag)–antibody (Ab) reactions in the laboratory is called *serology,* reflecting the fact that it originally was concerned with the determination of Abs or Ags found in the serum (the amber-colored fluid that exudes from coagulated blood). However, many Abs used in the clinical detection of Ags are derived not from serum, but from the culture fluid of cells producing monoclonal Abs. In addition, the use of standard Ags to detect Abs is carried out with many body fluids other than serum (eg, tears, urine, saliva, and mucus). Nevertheless, using standard tests, a known Ag can be used to assess an individual's serum (or other body fluid) for the presence of a specific Ab, or conversely, a solution containing known Abs can be reacted with organisms isolated from a patient to confirm or to assist in the identification of that organism. Serologic techniques also are used for typing blood in blood banks, for typing organs before transplant operations, for typing immunoglobulins (Igs), for measuring lymphocyte subsets, and for many other clinical tests.

The Nature of the Interaction Between Antigen and Antibody

The interaction between Ag and Ab is fully reversible (equation 1). As for all reversible reactions, it follows the law of mass action, whereby the extent of the reaction is directly proportional to the concentration of the Ag and Ab reactants themselves (equation 2).

$$Ag + Ab \underset{k_b}{\overset{k_f}{\rightleftarrows}} Ag.Ab \tag{1}$$

$$K_A = \frac{[Ag.Ab]}{[Ag][Ab]} \tag{2}$$

The rate of the forward reaction (k_f) is determined largely by the diffusion rates of the reactants, whereas the rate of the backward reaction (k_b) is determined primarily by the strength of the bonds between the Ab-combining site and the antigenic determinant to which it is bound. The forward reaction rates for most Ag–Ab interactions are about equal. Hence, the overall differences in affinity and, therefore, the extent of the reaction at equilibrium of Abs and their respective Ags is determined by the differences in the rates of the backward reactions.

The affinity of Ab reacting with a monovalent Ag (eg, a hapten) can be determined easily by measuring the equilibrium constant of their interaction. However, most Ags are multivalent, that is, they have more than one antigenic determinant on their surface. These determinants can be the same or different, as discussed in Chapter 5. Abs are at least bivalent, with some having more than two Ag-combining sites (eg, IgM and secretory IgA). Therefore, when a complex mixture of Abs, as found in a conventional antiserum, is mixed with a solution of multivalent Ag, the effective affinity can be much greater than the intrinsic affinity for binding at any single site. This is the result of many factors, including alterations in local concentrations of reactants, restrictions on free diffusion of reactants, and multipoint binding of Ab to Ags with more than one determinant of a single type. Determining the affinity of this interaction would be difficult. Therefore, when discussing the interaction of complex Ags and Abs, *avidity* normally is used as a measure of the strength of binding. Regardless, the overall strength of the bonds between Ag and Ab is relatively great, so that the reaction (equation 1) greatly favors the formation of the Ag–Ab complex.

Methods Used to Detect and Measure Antigen and Antibody

Numerous methods can be used to determine the presence or the amount of a specific Ab. The particular method used in each case depends partly on the sensitivity desired, but mostly on the physical state of the Ag—in other words, whether it is on the surface of a cell, a soluble toxin or protein, a virus, or an encapsulated organism. Because most Abs have two or more identical Ag-combining sites, and because most naturally occurring Ags possess multiple, different antigenic determinants, a reaction between Ab and Ag can form a latticework of many Ag and Ab molecules. If the Ag is on the surface of particulate material, such as a bacterium or a red blood cell (RBC), the end result is a clumping of the cells, or *agglutination.* A soluble Ag can form an Ag–Ab lattice that becomes too large to stay in solution, and the result is a *precipitation,* or a precipitin reaction. Other reactions merely measure the gain or loss of a property of the Ag. An example of this is an Ab reaction with a bacterial toxin to neutralize it; the Ab neutralizing the toxin is given the general name *antitoxin.* In still other reactions, Ab neutralizes viruses so that they cannot infect susceptible cells (called *neutralizing Ab*), or Abs, called *opsonins,* can react with bacterial cells to make them more easily phagocytosed by leukocytes.

The multiplicity of names applied to Ab does not indicate different types of Abs for each reaction; it merely denotes the type of reaction being measured. Thus, if sufficient antitoxin is mixed with a soluble toxin, it will produce a precipitin reaction, or, if this soluble toxin is adsorbed to particles such as polystyrene beads, the same specific Ab will agglutinate the beads or enhance their phagocytosis. Therefore, Ab names such as precipitin, agglutinin, antitoxin, and others are used only to indicate the physical state of the Ab or the type of Ag–Ab reaction being measured. With this in mind, several methods used to detect the presence of Ag or Ab in clinical specimens are presented in the following sections.

THE PRECIPITIN REACTION

The precipitin reaction yields a visible precipitate of Ag and Ab. If a solution containing Abs is mixed with a solution of the correct Ag, the mixture will become opalescent within minutes to hours, and a flocculent precipitate will appear in what had been a clear solution. Such reactions usually are carried out by adding a constant amount of Ab (antiserum) to each of a series of 10 or 12 tubes that contain increasing amounts of Ag—in other words, tube 1 contains the least Ag and tube 12 contains the most. During an incubation time of 2 to 24 hours, a reaction occurs between the Ag and its specific Ab, which results in a visible precipitate in those tubes in which the Ab and the Ag are in correct proportion to each other so that they can form an insoluble lattice.

If a quantitative test is desired, it is relatively easy to collect the resulting precipitate and determine the amount of Ag and Ab in each precipitate. Figure 6-1 shows a typical precipitin curve obtained by plotting the amount of Ab in the precipitate against the amount of Ag added to each tube (remember that each tube received an identical amount of Ab). Only a small amount of precipitate is formed in the first few tubes, which contain relatively little Ag, and hence, an excess of Ab. In the tubes containing more Ag, the amount of precipitate increases up to a point, after which it decreases as a result of smaller complexes being formed in the zone of Ag excess. Assays of the supernatant solution will show that those tubes containing too little Ag still contain free Ab. There is no free Ab found in the supernatants of tubes containing high concentrations of Ag, in spite of the fact that little or no precipitation occurred in these tubes. Only in tubes of maximum precipitation are all Ag and all Ab removed from solution.

These zones (see Fig. 6-1) are designated as the zone of Ab excess, the equivalence zone, and the zone of Ag excess. In the zone of Ab excess, all Ag has reacted with Ab and has been precipitated. However, there is free Ab that remains in the supernatant. Conversely, in the zone of Ag excess, all the Ab has reacted with Ag, but complexes of varying sizes are formed. Large complexes precipitate, but many small complexes do not reach the size

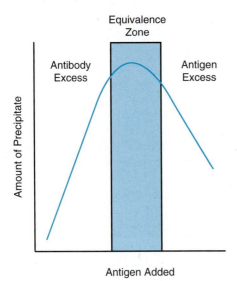

FIGURE 6-1   Precipitin curve. When a complex antigen and antibody to it are mixed, a precipitate is formed. If one begins with a constant amount of antibody and adds increasing amounts of antigen, the amount of precipitate formed increases to a maximum and then decreases. This is a direct function of the valency of the antibody molecule (usually two), the number of antigenic sites on the antigen (usually more than two), and the extent of cross-linking of the antigen molecules by the antibody.

necessary for precipitation to occur, and these remain in solution. Figure 6-2 is a schematic illustration of the type of complexes formed in each zone.

The precipitin curve demonstrates that Ab and Ag must be present in optimal proportions for maximum precipitation to occur, and it also shows that Ab and Ag can react with each other in multiple proportions. Thus, unlike a chemical reaction in which, for example, 1 mol

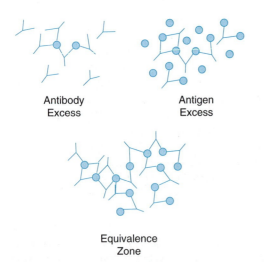

FIGURE 6-2   Complexes formed by antigen and antibody. The complexes depicted here represent those formed in each region of the curve shown in Figure 6-1. In the zone of antibody excess, there is insufficient antigen to precipitate all the antibody. In the zone of antigen excess, there is so much antigen that all the antibody sites are occupied and some soluble complexes are formed. In the equivalence zone, the amount of antigen and antibody are such that *all* antigen and *all* antibody are precipitated.

of Na_2SO_4 reacts with 1 mol of $BaCl_2$ to form 1 mol of $BaSO_4$ and 2 mol of NaCl, Ag–Ab precipitates can contain variable proportions of reactants. One of the advantages of making immune responses that contain Abs of many different specificities is this ability to react in variable proportions, forming large complexes with the Ag that are easily taken up and destroyed by phagocytic cells.

Modifications of the Precipitin Reaction

Several modifications of the classic precipitin reaction have been developed. Such changes are designed either to increase the sensitivity of the reaction or to identify specific Ag–Ab reactions occurring in a system containing multiple Ags and Abs.

DOUBLE DIFFUSION (OUCHTERLONY TECHNIQUE). When soluble Ag and soluble Ab are placed in separate small wells punched into agar that has solidified on a slide or glass plate, the Ag and the Ab will diffuse through the agar. The holes are located only a few millimeters apart, and Ab and Ag will interact to form a line of precipitate in the area in which they are in optimal proportions. Because different Ags diffuse at different rates, and because different Ags can require different concentrations of Ab for optimal precipitation, the position of the precipitin band usually varies for each Ag. In specimens containing several soluble Ags, multiple precipitin lines are observed, each occurring between the wells at a position that depends on the concentration of that particular Ag and its Ab (Fig. 6-3). Thus, this simple diffusion method can be used to detect the presence of one or more Ags or Abs in a clinical specimen. In addition, if set up differently, this gel method can be used to detect similarities or differences in Ags. For example, Figure 6-4 shows the use of various Abs to distinguish between human IgM and IgG, and to detect specific epitopes on human IgG.

RADIAL IMMUNODIFFUSION. Radial immunodiffusion is used to measure the amount of a specific Ag present in a sample and can be used for many Ags. The most widely used diagnostic application of this procedure is to measure the amount of a specific Ig class present in a patient's serum.

The assay is carried out by incorporating monospecific antiserum (antiserum containing only Ab to the Ag being assayed for) into melted agar and allowing the agar to solidify on a glass plate in a thin layer. Holes then are punched into the agar, and different dilutions of the Ag are placed into the various holes. As the Ag diffuses from the hole, a ring of precipitate will form at that position where Ag and Ab are in optimal proportions (Fig. 6-5). The more concentrated the Ag solution, the farther it must diffuse to be in optimal proportion with the constant Ab concentration in the agar gel. Thus, the diameter of the precipitin ring is a quantitative measure of Ag concentration. Using known concentrations of the Ag in question, a standard curve can be prepared by plotting

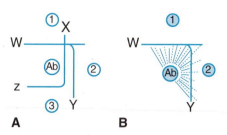

A   **B**

FIGURE 6-3   Double diffusion in agar. The interaction of antigen and antibody in a semisolid medium is illustrated. The test is set up as indicated in the text. **A.** The interaction between an antiserum containing antibodies to the antigens W, X, Y, and Z. It is apparent that only a single antigen was present in the solutions applied to wells 1 and 3, whereas two antigens were present in the solution applied to well 2. Antigen Z from well 3 forms a continuous line with antigen X from well 2. This is a reaction of *identity*, indicating that the two antigens X and Z are the same molecular species. This type of continuous line is not formed by antigen W from well 1 and antigen X from well 2. In fact, the line formed by each of these antigens continues through the line formed by the other, creating *spurs*. This is a reaction of *nonidentity*, indicating that antigens W and X are not related. In contrast, antigen Y does not form a spur over antigen W, although antigen W does form a spur over antigen Y. This is a reaction of *partial identity*, indicating that antigens W and Y are related but that there are some antigenic sites on W that are not on Y. **B.** The formation of the reaction of partial identity. The solid lines radiating out from the antibody well represent the diffusion of antibody that reacts with both antigens. The dashed lines represent antibody that reacts with antigen W but not with antigen Y. The latter antibody does not recognize antigen Y, continues to diffuse through the medium, and reacts with antigen W on the other side, forming the spur.

the diameter of the precipitin ring versus Ag concentration. Once a standard plot is obtained, the diameter of the precipitin ring formed with the unknown Ag can be measured to calculate its concentration.

Radial immunodiffusion is used routinely for the laboratory diagnosis of multiple myeloma or agammaglobulinemia. In either case, Ab to the various classes of Igs (IgG, IgA, IgM, IgD, or IgE) is incorporated into the agar before the agar is allowed to solidify. Aliquots of the patient's serum then are added to the holes punched in the agar. By noting the diameter of the resulting precipitin ring, it is possible to measure the amount of any class of Ig present in the patient's serum.

Nephelometry is supplanting radial immunodiffusion as a method of measuring various Ig classes present in a patient's serum. As discussed earlier, when Abs to various classes of Igs are mixed with serum, Ag–Ab complexes form and create a precipitate in a previously clear solution. Tubes containing known concentrations of Abs to Igs are incubated with different volumes of a patient's serum. The precipitation reaction, seen as a cloudiness, is measured in an instrument called a nephelometer. This instrument interprets the Ag–Ab precipitates as increased light scattering compared to a control tube containing no precipitate. As with the radial immunodiffusion procedure, in nephelometry, standard curves are performed using Ig class standards of known concentrations and Abs to the various Ig classes. Through a certain concentration range,

it is possible to generate a straight line plot when Ig concentration is plotted as a function of the amount of light scattering indicated by the nephelometer. This technique is being used increasingly in hospital laboratories and clinics as a quantitative measure of serum Ig class concentration in patient blood.

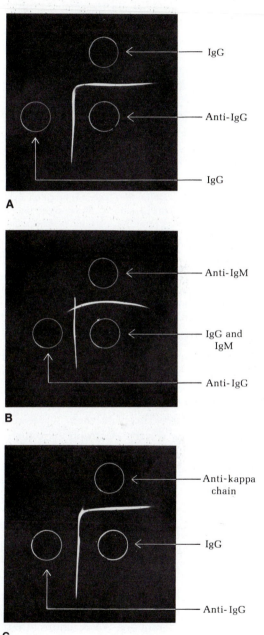

FIGURE 6-4   Examples of double diffusion. **A.** Reaction of identity: human IgG in both antigen wells and anti-human IgG in the antibody wells. Note the absence of spurs. **B.** Reaction of nonidentity: a mixture of human IgG and human IgM in the central antigen well. Anti-human IgM (anti-μ chain) in one antibody well and anti-human IgG (anti-γ chain) in the other antibody well. Note the presence of spurs in both directions. **C.** Reaction of partial identity: human IgG in the central antigen well. Antibody to human κ light chain in one antibody well and antibody to human IgG in the other antibody well. Note the slight spur formed by the anti-IgG over the κ light chain, indicating antigenic sites present on the IgG that are not on the κ light chain. These extra antigenic sites are on the γ heavy chain of the IgG molecule.

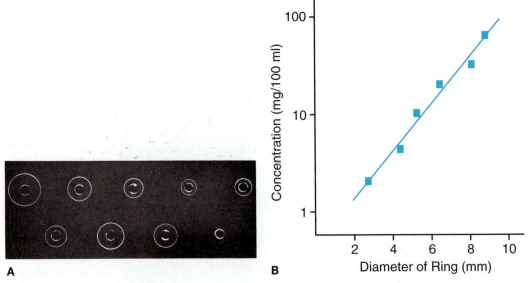

FIGURE 6-5 Radial immunodiffusion. This test is based on a precipitate that is formed as antigen diffuses into a semisolid medium that contains antibody. Because the amount of antibody in the agar bed is constant, the diameter of the precipitin ring formed is a function of the amount of antigen applied. **A.** Anti-IgA is incorporated into the agar and small wells are punched out, into which patient serum or a standard antigen solution is placed. The top row consists of standard amounts of known IgA. The wells in the bottom row receive sera from four different patients. **B.** A curve is drawn by plotting the diameter of the precipitin rings formed by the standard IgA solutions against the logarithm of the concentration of the standard IgA. The concentration of IgA in each patient's serum then is read from this standard curve after measuring the diameter of the ring formed by the patient's serum in the bottom row.

IMMUNOELECTROPHORESIS. Immunoelectrophoresis is a procedure that combines electrophoresis and double diffusion for the separation of Ag–Ab reactions in gels. A small drop of solution containing the Ags (usually proteins) is placed into a small hole punched out of solidified agar on a small glass plate. The plate then is placed in an electric field to allow for the electrophoretic migration of the Ags. Different Ags migrate at different rates or even in different directions, depending on their size and charge, and on the conditions of electrophoresis. After the electrophoresis is completed, a trough is removed from the agar along one or both sides of the plate and the appropriate antiserum is placed in the trough. As before, the Abs and the Ags diffuse toward each other, resulting in the formation of precipitin bands wherever they are in optimal proportions. Because diffusion is a function of the molecular weight and concentration of reactants, gel diffusion alone may not separate precipitin bands formed by different Ag–Ab reactions. Immunoelectrophoresis uses electric charge in addition to diffusion, so it is more likely to separate Ags than is simple diffusion alone. As shown in Figure 6-6, this procedure can be used to separate many Ags, as well as to indicate the potential purity of an Ag.

COUNTERIMMUNOELECTROPHORESIS. Counterimmunoelectrophoresis is another method that takes advantage of the migration of biologic macromolecules in an electric field. However, counterimmunoelectrophoresis can be used only for Ags and Abs that migrate in opposite directions

in the electric field. The test is set up similarly to that for double diffusion in agar (ie, two wells are punched about 1 cm apart in an agar slab on a glass plate). The Ag and Ab solutions are placed in these wells in such a way that when the electric field is applied across the plate, the Ag will migrate toward the Ab, and the Ab will migrate toward the Ag. A precipitin line will form when the Ag and Ab meet in optimal proportions. The advantages of this method over double diffusion in agar are that (1) the electrophoresis focuses the reactants into a small area, allowing the detection of small amounts of Ag or Ab; and (2) it is a much more rapid assay (as little as 30 minutes for some Ags) than is double diffusion in gel. Counterimmunoelectrophoresis is used to detect the presence of anti-DNA Ab in the serum of patients with several autoimmune disorders.

ROCKET ELECTROPHORESIS. Rocket electrophoresis is so named because the precipitin bands resemble rockets. As in radial immunodiffusion, small holes are cut in an agarose gel slab on a glass plate. The agar contains Ab to one or more Ags of interest. The holes are filled with Ag solution, and an electric potential is applied across the plate. The Ags migrate into the gel and precipitate with the Ab in the gel at the appropriate position (Fig. 6-7). The height (distance from the Ag well to the top of the precipitin band) is proportional to the Ag concentration. Thus, this method is primarily a quantitative technique.

TWO-DIMENSIONAL IMMUNOELECTROPHORESIS. The technique of two-dimensional immunoelectrophoresis is a variation of

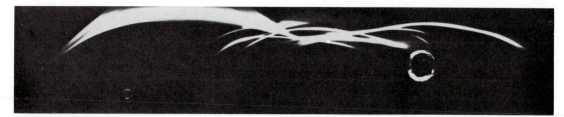

FIGURE 6-6   Immunoelectrophoresis. Human serum is placed in the well (*circle*) and subjected to electrophoresis. After 2 hours, the electric current is turned off and antibody to human serum is placed in a trough along the length of the slide. The precipitin lines are formed where the antibodies and the antigens (separated components of human serum) diffuse together in optimal proportions.

immunoelectrophoresis and rocket electrophoresis. A small trough is cut in an agar gel on a glass plate and filled with the Ag solution. An electric field is placed across the plate, and the Ags migrate into the gel at a rate proportional to their net electric charge. After electrophoresis, the gel slice containing the separated Ags is placed on a second glass plate, and agar containing Ab is poured around the slice. A second electric potential is applied at right angles to the first direction of migration. The preseparated Ags then migrate into the gel containing Ab at a rate proportional to their net charge and precipitate with the Ab in the gel, forming precipitates as for rocket electrophoresis. This method is both qualitative, in that it identifies the Ags that are present, and quantitative, in that it provides an estimate of the amount of each Ag (Fig. 6-8).

AGGLUTINATION REACTIONS

When Ag is present on the surface of a cell or particle, the addition of Ab causes a clumping or *agglutination* of the cells. This reaction is analogous to the precipitin reaction, in that Ab acts as a bridge to form a lattice network of Ab and cells. Because cells are so much larger than a soluble Ag, the result is more visible when the cells aggregate into clumps.

The usual agglutination test actually is only a semi-quantitative measure of Ab because, unlike the precipitin test, the milligrams or moles of Ab that are attached to a clump of bacterial cells usually cannot be determined. Instead, serial dilutions of the Ab solution are made, and a constant amount of cells is added to an exact amount of each Ab dilution. After several hours of incubation at 37°C, clumping is recorded by visual inspection. The titer of the antiserum is given as the reciprocal of the highest dilution that causes clumping. Thus, an antiserum that agglutinated at a dilution of 1:128 (but not at 1:256) would be reported to have a titer of 128. Note that this is not an absolute value, but instead expresses a relative concentration of a specific Ab present in the sample. These agglutination assays normally are carried out in wells of a plastic plate containing multiple wells, as shown in Figure 6-9.

Because a cell has many antigenic determinants on its surface, zones of Ab excess as described for the precipitin

reaction generally are not seen. Occasionally, Abs are formed, however, that will react with the antigenic determinants on a cell but will not cause agglutination (for example, anti-Rh and anti-*Brucella* Ab). Such Abs have been named *blocking Abs,* because they are unable to agglutinate the cells. At one time, blocking Abs were thought to be monovalent (possessing only one Ag-binding site) and, thus, unable to form a lattice. However, this is now known to be untrue, and the best explanation for the inability of these Abs to agglutinate is that there are insufficient antigenic determinants on the RBCs to permit the Ab to overcome the normal electrostatic repulsion that exists among RBCs.

Isoantibodies

Early in the practice of blood transfusion, it was observed that the blood of the recipient had to be compatible with that of the donor if a serious transfusion reaction was to be avoided. It was soon learned that the basis of incompatibility was immunologic in nature, and that some individuals possess Abs in their serum that can lyse other types of RBCs. This led to the discovery of the ABO system of classification for RBCs.

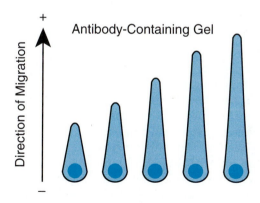

FIGURE 6-7   Rocket electrophoresis. This is another quantitative reaction between antibody and antigen in a semisolid agar medium. Antibody is incorporated into the agar, and a series of wells is punched. Into each of these wells is placed an antigen solution. An electric potential then is applied across the agar slide, and the antigen solution migrates into the agar containing the antibody. As in the passive diffusion of agar methods, a precipitate is formed. The height of the "rocket" formed is proportional to the concentration of antigen applied to the well.

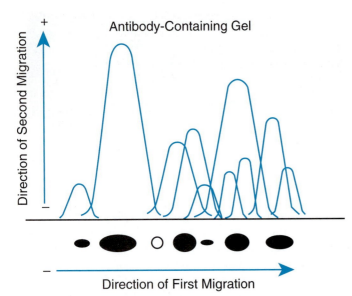

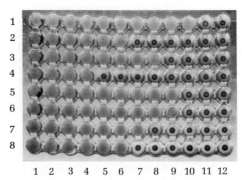

FIGURE 6-9 Hemagglutination is essentially the same as precipitation except that the antigens are molecules present on the surfaces of large objects, such as red blood cells, bacteria, white blood cells, and latex beads. Antibody reacts with these antigens, cross-linking the large objects and leading to agglutination. In this figure, the wells in horizontal rows 1 through 4 contain sheep red blood cells (SRBCs) and antibody to SRBCs. Rows 5 through 8 contain SRBCs that have been coated with human γ-globulin (HGG) and antibody to HGG. A positive reaction is seen as diffuse clumping of the red blood cells (eg, wells 1 through 10 in row 1), whereas a negative reaction appears as a small button of red blood cells that has settled to the bottom of the well (eg, wells 11 and 12 in row 1). Direct reaction of antibody with antigens on cells that are intrinsic to that cell is called *direct agglutination* (as for the SRBC agglutination in rows 1 through 4), whereas reaction of antibody with an antigen that has been placed experimentally on the surface of the cell is called *passive agglutination* (as for the HGG antigen here).

FIGURE 6-8 Two-dimensional immunoelectrophoresis. This method is related to the immunoelectrophoresis procedure shown in Figure 6-6 and to the rocket electrophoresis technique shown in Figure 6-7. An agar slide is prepared and a well is punched out. The antigen solution is placed in this well and subjected to electrophoresis. This separates the antigens in the complex antigen solution based on their net electric charge, as indicated by the dark oval spots at the bottom of the figure. After electrophoresis is completed, the agar containing the separated antigens is placed on the edge of a larger slide, and an agar solution containing antibody is poured over the remainder of the slide (the top two thirds of the figure). An electric potential then is applied perpendicular to the original direction of migration. The previously separated antigens migrate into the antibody-containing agar and form rocket precipitates with the antibody. The number of lines formed depends on the number of antigens recognized by the antibody. The height of the precipitin rockets formed is proportional to the concentration of antigen in the initial solution.

It was observed by pathologist Karl Landsteiner that if serum from several individuals was mixed, in all possible combinations, with RBCs obtained from these persons, the RBCs were agglutinated in some instances. On the basis of these findings, he determined that RBCs could be classified into four major types, which were designated A, B, O, and AB. This classification is based on the presence (or absence) of two Ags, A and B, which can be present together, singly, or not at all on RBCs. These RBC Ags have been termed *isoantigens* (or alloantigens).

Unexpectedly, Landsteiner found that each individual's serum contained isoantibodies (subsequently shown to be of the IgM class) against those A and B isoantigens that were not present on their own RBCs. Thus, as shown in Table 6-1, type A persons possess Ab to type B Ag on RBCs; type B persons possess Ab to type A Ag on RBCs; type O persons have both anti-A and anti-B Abs; and type AB persons have neither of these Abs. The origin of the isoantigens is a heritable trait, but the isoantibodies arise as a result of an Ab response to Ags of intestinal microorganisms that are structurally similar to the A and B isoantigens. The occurrence of structurally similar Ags from widely diverse sources is not unusual; one such Ag,

named *Forssman Ag*, stimulates the formation of Abs capable of lysing RBCs of sheep (in the presence of complement) and is found in many animals and bacteria. Abs to Forssman Ag are referred to as *heterophile Abs*, and their presence in humans is used as a diagnostic aid for infectious mononucleosis.

A sometimes fatal transfusion reaction with fever, prostration, and renal insufficiency can occur if a patient receives blood from a donor with a different blood type; this results from the hemolysis of the transfused cells by the patient's own isoantibodies and serum complement. Careful agglutination assays must be carried out to ensure compatibility between donor and recipient. One test uses standard Abs to blood-group Ags to determine the blood group of both the recipient and the donor. In another test, serum from the recipient is added to donor cells as a final test of compatibility of the recipient for cells of the chosen donor before transfusion.

TABLE 6-1

Isoantigens and Isoantibodies Associated With the ABO Classification of Red Blood Cells (RBC)

Blood Type	Isoantigen on RBC	Isoantibody in Serum
A	A	B
B	B	A
AB	AB	None
O	None	AB

Rh Factor

The Rh factor (so-called because it also occurs on the RBCs of rhesus monkeys) is an Ag that is found on RBCs of about 85% of the human population but is not related to the A and B Ags. Unlike in the ABO system, isoantibodies to Rh Ag do not occur. If, however, an Rh-negative individual receives Rh-positive RBCs, that person will respond by making Ab to the Rh Ag.

This is particularly dangerous when a mother is Rh negative and the father is Rh positive because, if the fetus is genetically Rh positive, any fetal blood that enters the mother's circulation can induce the formation of IgG Abs to the Rh Ag on the fetal RBCs. Once formed, these IgG anti-Rh Abs will cross the placenta, react with the RBCs of the fetus, and cause a severe hemolytic disease known as *erythroblastosis fetalis*.

During a normal pregnancy of an Rh-negative woman, the number of Rh-positive fetal RBCs that cross the placenta to the mother is insufficient to induce a *primary* immune response (see Chap. 11). Therefore, during the first pregnancy, the child is not in danger. However, during delivery of the first child, a relatively large dose of fetal RBCs is transferred to the mother and, in most cases, this delivery dose is sufficient to induce a primary immune response. Then, during a second similar pregnancy, the small number of Rh-positive fetal RBCs that cross the placenta are sufficient to induce a *secondary* or *booster* response in the mother. The IgG anti-Rh Abs formed will cross the placenta and react with the Rh-positive fetal RBCs, causing a severe hemolytic reaction. Note that the normally occurring isoantibodies to the ABO blood group Ags do not present the same problem, because they are of the IgM isotype and do not cross the placenta—a nice evolutionary solution to a potentially great problem.

To prevent this problem, an excess of Ab to the Rh-positive RBCs is injected into an Rh-negative mother bearing an Rh-positive fetus immediately after each delivery. This injected Ab reacts with and destroys the fetal RBCs transferred at delivery *before they can induce a pri-* *mary response*. Fortunately, even though there are 27 known Rh specificities, only one Ag (ie, Rh-D) appears to be sufficiently strong to stimulate the synthesis of destructive, hemolytic Abs; hence, anti-D Abs (Rhogam) are used in these cases.

COOMBS ANTIGLOBULIN TEST. Anti-Rh Abs are of the IgG type, but they normally will not agglutinate Rh-positive RBCs. The best explanation for this observation is that there are insufficient Rh-factor sites to permit IgG anti-Rh Ab to overcome the normal electrostatic repulsive force between RBCs. The British immunologist, R.R.A. Coombs, reasoned that if RBCs were coated with anti-Rh Abs, the addition of Abs to the Rh Abs would cause the erythrocytes to agglutinate. The antiglobulin test for Rh Abs that he originally devised is still used today. There are two such tests. The most direct, and least used, test involves the addition of antihuman Ig to RBCs thought to have anti-Rh Ab on their surface (eg, RBCs from an individual undergoing a transfusion reaction after matching for the ABO and other blood groups). Agglutination indicates the presence of human Ab on the surface of these cells. The second Coombs test, the indirect Coombs test, is accomplished by first reacting standard Rh-positive RBCs with the serum to be tested or reacting RBCs of an unknown Rh type with a standard anti-Rh Ab, and then, after a short incubation, adding antihuman Ig. If the serum contains Rh Abs or the RBCs are Rh-positive, agglutination will occur, as shown schematically in Figure 6-10.

Passive Agglutination Reactions

Because the difference between a precipitin reaction and an agglutination reaction is based on whether the Ag is soluble or particulate, the same Ags and Abs used in a precipitin reaction can be measured as an agglutination reaction, if the soluble Ag is artificially bound to the surface of a cell or particle. (Synthetic particles such as latex beads can be used; because RBCs can be made to readily adsorb many soluble Ags, however, they are often used for this purpose.)

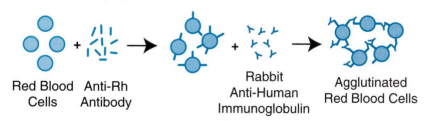

Red Blood Cells Anti-Rh Antibody Rabbit Anti-Human Immunoglobulin Agglutinated Red Blood Cells

FIGURE 6-10 Coombs antiglobulin test. Often, antibodies fail to agglutinate red blood cells, even though the antigens they recognize are on the surface of the cells and the antibodies react with them. Although this originally was thought to be due to antibodies that were incomplete (ie, had only a single binding site), it is now known to occur for other reasons. This absence of agglutination in the presence of reaction with antigen can be overcome by cross-linking the antibody that has reacted with the antigen by adding antibody to the original antibody molecule. For example, human antibody to the rhesus antigen (Rh antigen on Rh+ human red blood cells) will react but will not cross-link the Rh+ red blood cells. To detect this anti-Rh antibody, a rabbit anti-human immunoglobulin is added. This rabbit antibody then reacts with the "coated" red blood cells and causes agglutination. This is the basis of the blood test for Rh antigen in humans.

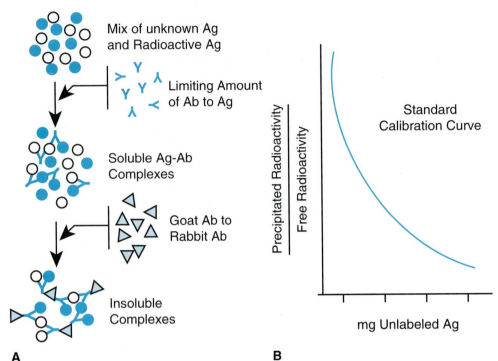

A   B

FIGURE 6-11 The radioimmunoassay is used to detect and measure trace amounts of antigen, such as insulin and human growth hormone. **A.** The ratio of precipitated radioactivity to free radioactivity is measured after the reaction. **B.** The amount of unlabeled antigen present then can be determined from a calibration curve. The standard calibration curve is prepared in a similar manner, using a constant amount of radioactively labeled antigen with varying, but known, amounts of unlabeled antigen.

Most polysaccharides or lipopolysaccharides, but not proteins, spontaneously adsorb to the surfaces of RBCs. Therefore, some form of chemical reagent must be used to conjugate the protein to the RBC surface. Agglutination of these protein-coated RBCs with Ab is referred to as *passive agglutination*. Using such artificial conjugation methods, the agglutination reaction can be used to detect and semiquantitate Abs to virtually any soluble protein Ag.

ASSAYS USING "TAGGED" ANTIGENS OR ANTIBODIES

The most versatile and sensitive immunologic methods involve the use of known Ags or Abs that have been "tagged" with a molecule that is detected easily in small amounts. The tags normally used are radioisotopes, enzymes, and fluorescent compounds. Several of the most widely used methods are discussed in this section.

Radioimmunoassay

Several different versions of the radioimmunoassay (RIA) are available. The one most commonly employed is used for the detection and measurement of trace amounts of haptens or Ags. The entire procedure is based on competition for the reactive sites on the specific Ab between a known amount of a highly radioactive Ag and an unknown amount of the same, but nonradioactive, Ag (Fig. 6-11). If no unlabeled Ag is present, the Ag–Ab complex will be highly radioactive (see Fig. 6-11A). If equimolar amounts of radioactive and nonradioactive Ag are present, the complexes will contain only half as much radioactivity, and if there is a huge excess of unlabeled Ag (see Fig. 6-11B), the complexes will contain little radioactivity.

Thus, a standard curve can be prepared for a specific system by adding increasing *known* amounts of nonradioactive Ag and measuring the decrease in radioactivity occurring in the Ag–Ab complexes. This curve will allow the measurement of Ag present by merely counting the radioactivity present in the test Ag–Ab precipitated complexes.

RIAs usually are carried out in Ag excess, and the concentrations of Ab and Ag used are so small that precipitation does not occur. Therefore, the soluble Ag–Ab complexes must be separated from any residual soluble radioactive Ag before counting. This can be accomplished by several techniques. For example, using albumin as an Ag, R.S. Farr showed in 1958 that soluble Ag–Ab complexes could be precipitated by adding ammonium sulfate to a final concentration of 40% saturation. The Farr technique is now used to precipitate the radioactive Ag–Ab complexes formed during the RIA, but it is of value only if free Ag remains soluble in 40% ammonium sulfate.

Another procedure for precipitating Ag–Ab complexes out of solution is the double Ab technique. This method (see Fig. 6-11) is based on the fact that Abs are antigenic if injected into a foreign host. Thus, the injection of human Ig into a rabbit induces rabbit Abs that react with and precipitate human Abs. Therefore, if the RIA uses human Abs, rabbit antiserum containing antihuman Igs can be added to the solution containing the Ag–Ab complexes. This will form even larger complexes, resulting in the precipitation of the soluble Ag–Ab complexes formed during the RIA. The precipitate then can be counted for incorporated radioactivity.

Because of its extreme sensitivity (measuring picograms of Ag per milliliter), the RIA is used to measure the concentration of certain hormones, such as insulin, testosterone, growth hormone, and glucagon. It also is used to determine the presence of the hepatitis B Ag, which can be present in the serum of asymptomatic blood donors.

Solid-phase modifications of the RIA take advantage of the fact that most proteins strongly adsorb to polystyrene wells, forming a monomolecular film. Therefore, Ab can be adsorbed to the wells and known amounts of radioactive Ag and unknown amounts of Ag to be measured can be added to the adsorbed Ab. After allowing several hours for the reaction to occur, the wells are thoroughly washed, and the amount of radioactivity bound to the Ab is determined.

Protein Ag also can be adsorbed to polystyrene wells, and such wells then can be used for the sensitive detection of Abs to that protein. In such cases, however, a second radioactively labeled Ab directed against the first Ab would have to be added in the final step to determine whether Ab had bound to the adsorbed protein.

Enzyme-Linked Immunosorbent Assay

The radioactive tag used in RIA techniques can be replaced with an enzyme. When this enzyme is linked to an Ab and used to detect and measure other Abs or Ags, the assay is called the *enzyme-linked immunosorbent assay (ELISA)*. All ELISAs depend on the ability to covalently attach an active enzyme (such as alkaline phosphatase or horseradish peroxidase) to an Ab molecule. Such enzymes catalyze reactions that are extremely sensitive but easy to measure. The assay is carried out in a manner identical to that described for solid-phase RIA, except that after all unreacted material is washed away, the substrate for the enzyme is added (usually one that will yield a colored product, such as p-nitrophenol phosphate for alkaline phosphatase), and the conversion of the substrate from colorless to color is a measure of Ag–Ab interaction. The ELISA method is not as sensitive as RIA, but it has gained wide acceptance because the use of radioactive materials is avoided.

IMMUNOBLOT. Also called the Western blot, the immunoblot uses enzyme-linked Ab to detect Ags in complex mixtures of proteins. This method involves the separation of Ags in the complex mixture by electrophoresis in a semisolid medium such as agarose gel or polyacrylamide gels. After electrophoretic separation, the Ags are transferred (*blotted*) to a piece of nitrocellulose filter paper, reproducing the banding pattern found in the original gel. The protein of interest is detected by adding either radioactive Ab or enzyme-linked Ab. The Ag–Ab reaction is detected by exposing the paper to photographic film or incubating it in the enzyme's substrate, respectively. In addition to being semiquantitative, this method can provide other information (eg, molecular weight and number of polypeptide chains of the Ag). An example of

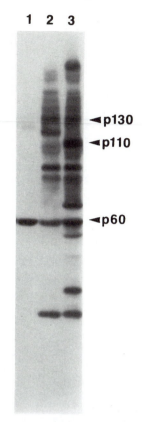

FIGURE 6-12 Immunoblot. Labeled antibodies can be used to detect proteins in complex antigenic mixtures. One such method is the immunoblot or Western blot, shown here. Complex or purified protein populations are separated according to size by electrophoresis on polyacrylamide gels. The separated proteins are transferred ("blotted") onto nitrocellulose or a similar matrix, which strongly binds the proteins and can be subjected to washing and staining techniques. The transferred "blot" then is incubated with the antibody of choice. In this case, three protein solutions underwent electrophoresis: lane 1 contained a purified preparation of the oncogene pp60$_{src}$, and lanes 2 and 3 contained extracts of two different cell types. The labeled antibody was a monoclonal antibody to the hapten phosphotyrosine. Thus, this antibody detects proteins that have been phosphorylated on a tyrosine residue. The p130, p110, and p60 phosphotyrosine proteins are indicated.

the radioactive version of this assay is shown in Figure 6-12.

Fluorescent Antibody Methods

Certain small-molecular-weight chemicals absorb light (energy) of one wavelength and emit (fluoresce) light of another wavelength. Such fluorescent compounds can be coupled to Ab molecules and the fluorophor–Ab conjugate can be used to detect Ags on cells, in tissue sections, on solid surfaces, and in solution. For example, if cells carrying a given Ag are treated with a fluorescent Ab, the entire complex becomes visible when viewed with a special fluorescence microscope. Similarly, an assay essentially identical to the solid-phase RIA or ELISA methods described earlier can be performed with fluorescent Ab; the difference is the method used to detect the tagged Ab at the end of the assay.

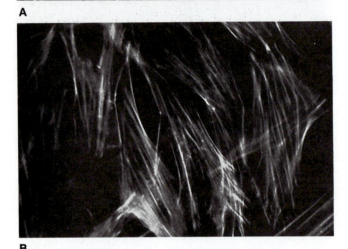

A

B

FIGURE 6-13 Fluorescence microscopy. Fluorescent antibody can be used to stain cells for the presence of specific antigens before viewing by microscopy. **A.** In the example given here, fibroblasts are viewed using Nomarski optics. Note the position of the nuclei, cytoplasm, and cellular processes. **B.** These same cells are viewed by fluorescence microscopy after staining with a fluorescent antibody specific for the protein actin, a component of the cell's cytoskeleton. Note the typical long filaments that underlie the plasma membrane.

As an example of the use of fluorescent Ab in diagnostic bacteriology, antihuman Ig can be conjugated with a fluorescent compound. These Abs then can be used to detect, in a patient's serum, Abs to any organism, such as the one that causes typhoid fever, *Salmonella typhi*. A dilution of the patient's serum is mixed with the *S typhi* organisms and, after a few minutes, the excess serum is washed off. If the patient's serum contained Ab to *S typhi*, these Abs would have reacted with the Ags on the surface of the bacterial cells. The fluorescent antihuman Ig subsequently added then would react with the human Ig (ie, the patient's Ab) on the *S typhi*, causing the bacterial cells to fluoresce. If the patient's serum did not contain specific Abs to *S typhi*, no human Ig would react with the bacterial cells, and the subsequent addition of the fluorescent antihuman Ig would not result in the presence of fluorescent cells. The same technique is used for many different types of Ab reactions, because the fluorescent antihuman Ig

will react with all human Abs. This method is frequently referred to as the *indirect* fluorescent method (or the fluorescent sandwich method), because the second Ab carries the fluorescent compound.

An Ab specific for the Ag (eg, bacteria, cell) can be prepared, conjugated with the fluorescent compound, and used in a *direct* fluorescent assay without a second Ab. For example, the same fluorescent antihuman Ig used to detect patient Ab to *S typhi* can be used in a direct assay to detect and count the number of B cells (see Chaps. 7 and 8), by reacting with the B cell's Ig receptors in complex mixtures of cells.

An example of the use of fluorescent Ab to demonstrate the intracellular position of the cytoskeletal protein, actin, is shown in Figure 6-13.

FLUORESCENCE-ACTIVATED CELL SORTING. A powerful application of fluorescent Ab technology has gained wide acceptance in both research and clinical medicine in recent years. This method, termed fluorescence-activated cell sorting (FACS), or cytofluorography, combines the use of fluorescent Abs and an instrument capable of detecting single cells (by light scatter or fluorescence). A complex mixture of cells (eg, peripheral blood mononuclear cells) is mixed with a fluorescent Ab (eg, the monoclonal anti-CD4 Abs that detect the inducer T-cell subset; see Chap. 9), incubated, and then washed to remove all excess Ab. These cells then are placed in the FACS instrument. The instrument dilutes the mixture of cells so that any given drop will contain no more than one cell, and analyzes individual drops for the presence of fluorescent or non-fluorescent cells (at the rate of thousands of cells per second). Cell number, size, and fluorescence intensity can be determined simultaneously to a degree of accuracy previously impossible. This technique is used to determine absolute and relative cell numbers in a wide variety of clinical disorders. For example, FACS analysis is used to demonstrate the preferential loss of the CD4-positive, inducer T-cell subset in patients with acquired immunodeficiency syndrome. An example of the ability of FACS analysis to measure human CD4-positive cells in peripheral blood is shown in Figure 6-14.

SPECIAL IMMUNOLOGIC TESTS

Other serologic tests are available that are highly specialized and sometimes difficult to process. One example of these is the *Treponema pallidum* immobilization test for syphilis. This test is based on the fact that live organisms become immobilized if mixed with serum containing specific antisyphilitic Abs. Complement fixation is another specialized technique for the determination of specific Abs and is discussed in Chapter 12.

The hemagglutination inhibition test (RBC agglutination inhibition) is used to identify certain viruses that, by themselves, routinely cause the agglutination of RBCs. However, if specific Abs to the virus are added, agglutina-

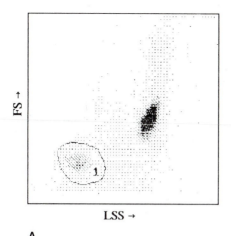 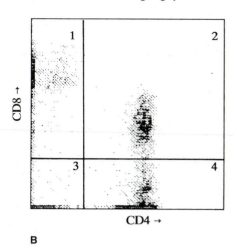

A   **B**

FIGURE 6-14. Cytofluorographic analysis of human peripheral blood lymphocytes. Analysis of peripheral mononuclear cells from a patient with intermittent bilateral symmetric parotid swelling as the only clinical symptom. This individual had a normal white blood cell count and a slightly elevated lymphocyte count. **A.** The peripheral mononuclear cells were isolated and separated into lymphocytes (*circled area*), monocytes, and granulocytes based on their light-scattering properties (FS, forward scatter; LSS, logside scatter). **B.** The cells then were stained with fluorescent antibodies to the CD4 and CD8 cell-surface markers characteristic of thymocytes and peripheral T cells. The lymphocytes were distributed into four quadrants based on their reactivity with these two antisera. Quadrant 1 contains CD4⁻ CD8⁺ cells characteristic of normal class I–restricted T cells of the cytotoxic T-cell subset; quadrant 4 contains CD4⁺CD8⁻ cells characteristic of normal class II–restricted T cells of the helper T-cell subset; quadrant 3 contains double-negative CD4⁻CD8⁻ cells, primarily B cells; and quadrant 2 contains cells not normally found in peripheral blood that have the unusual CD4⁺CD8⁺ phenotype. The CD4⁺CD8⁺ cells are also T cell receptor positive (TCR⁺) and thus more characteristic of thymocytes. Unlike most normal thymocytes, however, these cells also are CD1⁺. (Courtesy of David Normanfell and Michael Williams, University of Virginia)

A Closer Look

The history of immunology contains a wealth of spin-off techniques that have benefited scientists in widely divergent fields. Clinically, it is now routine to be able to detect and measure small amounts of Ags and Abs in the blood, tissues, and other bodily fluids of human beings. Some incredibly sensitive methods are available for measuring Ab concentrations in extremely small volumes of body fluids. The availability of such methods has strengthened the clinician's ability to diagnose and treat a variety of diseases.

On the research front, a vast array of techniques and methods is used routinely not only by immunologists, but by microbiologists, biochemists, molecular biologists, physiologists, anatomists, and more. The ability of Abs to bind Ag with high avidity and to act as probes for the identification of minor components in a complex mixture forms the basis and bulwark of much of the research conducted by investigators around the world. Many systems for studying Ag–Ab interaction have been automated in both clinical and research laboratories.

tion is inhibited. Thus, using known antisera, an unknown virus can be identified or a known virus can be measured. Ab also can be labeled with ferritin (a protein that contains a high concentration of iron) and used as an electron-dense probe for Ag when viewed in an electron microscope.

The described examples represent only a small fraction of the methods used to detect and measure Ag or Ab. The method of choice is dictated primarily by the source of the reactants and the expected sensitivity required.

Bibliography

JOURNAL

Richards FF, Konigsberg WH, Rosenstein RW, Varga JM. On the specificity of Abs. Science 1975;187:130.

BOOKS

Feldman H, Rodbard D. Mathematical theory of radioimmunoassay. In: Odell WD, Daughaday WH, eds. Principles of competitive protein-binding assay. Philadelphia, JB Lippincott, 1971:158.

Shokat KM, Schultz PG. Catalytic antibodies. In: Paul WE, Fathman CG, Metzger H, eds. Annual review of immunology, vol 8. Palo Alto, CA, Annual Reviews, 1990:335.

Voller A, Bidwell D, Bartless A. Enzyme-linked immunosorbent assay. In: Rose NR, Friedman H, eds. Manual of clinical immunology, ed 2. Washington, DC, American Society of Microbiology, 1980:359.

Essentials of Medical Microbiology, Fifth Edition, edited by Wesley A. Volk, Bryan M. Gebhardt, Marie-Louise Hammarskjöld, and Robert J. Kadner. Lippincott-Raven Publishers, Philadelphia © 1996.

Chapter 7

Hemopoiesis and Lymphoid Organs

Hemopoiesis

Blood-borne cells have finite life-spans and, therefore, must be constantly renewed. This renewal process is called *hemopoiesis* (from the Greek, *hemo,* meaning blood, and *poiein,* meaning to make). The cells responsible for both innate and acquired immunity are blood-borne elements and are all derived from a common, self-renewing, pluripotential stem cell (Fig. 7-1).

STEM CELLS

All circulating blood cells (red blood cells, white blood cells, and platelets) arise from the differentiation of a single, self-renewing, pluripotential stem cell. Early in embryonic development, these stem cells originate in the yolk sac. Later, during fetal life, they are found in the liver, and at birth, they reside in the bone marrow, where they remain throughout life. Evidence for their yolk sac origin was obtained by M.A.S. Moore and D. Metcalf, who demonstrated that the livers of 7-day-old mouse embryos cultured with yolk sac contain stem cells, whereas those cultured in the absence of yolk sac are devoid of stem cells. The fact that stem cells are transported in the blood has been deduced from several observations involving natural or experimentally created parabiosis. For example, dizygotic cattle twins, which are genetically dissimilar yet share the same placental circulation in utero, possess circulating blood cells of their twin's phenotype in addition to cells of their own. This could occur only if each calf's stem cells entered the common placental circulation and were subsequently seeded in the other calf. These animals continue to produce cells of both genotypes throughout their lives and have been termed *chimeras* (after a legendary monster who was represented as having a lion's head, a goat's body, and a serpent's tail).

Stem cells emigrate from the yolk sac to the liver and subsequently to the bone marrow, from which they continue to replicate and provide precursors to all blood

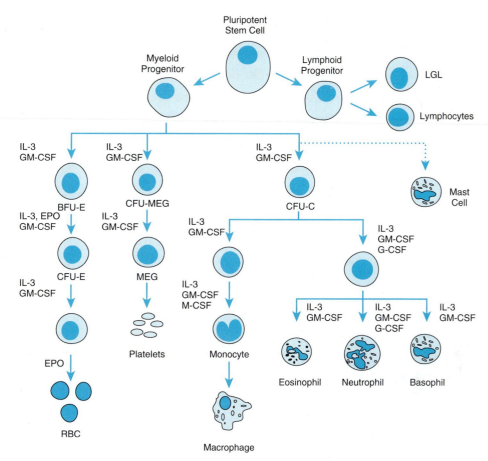

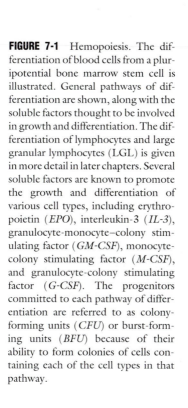

FIGURE 7-1 Hemopoiesis. The differentiation of blood cells from a pluripotential bone marrow stem cell is illustrated. General pathways of differentiation are shown, along with the soluble factors thought to be involved in growth and differentiation. The differentiation of lymphocytes and large granular lymphocytes (LGL) is given in more detail in later chapters. Several soluble factors are known to promote the growth and differentiation of various cell types, including erythropoietin (*EPO*), interleukin-3 (*IL-3*), granulocyte-monocyte–colony stimulating factor (*GM-CSF*), monocyte-colony stimulating factor (*M-CSF*), and granulocyte-colony stimulating factor (*G-CSF*). The progenitors committed to each pathway of differentiation are referred to as colony-forming units (*CFU*) or burst-forming units (*BFU*) because of their ability to form colonies of cells containing each of the cell types in that pathway.

cell types. Transplantation of bone marrow into individuals lacking hemopoietic stem cells (either naturally or experimentally, such as after lethal irradiation) restores all normal circulating cells, whereas transplantation of cells from other organs (eg, spleen, lymph nodes, thymus, or blood) restores only certain cell types.

The pluripotential stem cell, until fairly recently, has been a theoretical concept invoked to explain many natural phenomena involving the formation of blood-borne elements. Evidence that many cell types originate from a common stem cell was provided by J.E. Till and E.A. McCulloch. They injected syngeneic (genetically identical) bone marrow into lethally irradiated mice; before injection, however, the bone marrow cells were lightly irradiated to make a few recognizable chromosomal breaks. Nodules (or colonies) developed in the recipient animal's spleen, and some nodules contained representatives of the four major types of circulating blood cells (ie, granulocytes, lymphocytes, erythrocytes, and megakaryocytes). Because most of these various cell types were found to have identical chromosomal aberrations (induced by the irradiation of the bone marrow cells before transfer), the cells in each nodule were determined to be derived from a single stem cell. Figure 7-1 illustrates the formation of mature cells from a single pluripotential stem cell.

Irving Weissman and his colleagues at Stanford University accomplished a goal long sought by biomedical scientists. They isolated a pure population of pluripotential stem cells from bone marrow of mice and are attempting to do the same in humans. These isolated pluripotential stem cells have been shown to proliferate and differentiate into myelomonocytic cells, B cells, and T cells. Only 30 of these cells are required to save 50% of lethally irradiated mice and to reconstitute *all* blood cell types in the survivors. If this feat can be accomplished in humans, the potential for treating and studying diseases involving the immune system (eg, aplastic anemia and certain leukemias) cannot be overstated.

As differentiation from the pluripotential stem cell proceeds, some choices must be made. For example, the pluripotential stem cell must decide whether to divide and reproduce itself or to differentiate. If it decides to differentiate, it will enter either the lymphoid or the nonlymphoid pathway. As differentiation proceeds, several "decision" points along the pathway are reached, such as differentiation into the erythroid, monocytic, or granulocytic lineages. The mechanisms by which these critical decisions are made are not well known but are influenced at least partially by a group of protein mediators (Table 7-1), which are discussed in more detail later.

TABLE 7-1
Soluble Mediators of Hemopoiesis

Factor	Molecular Weight	Source
Interleukin-3	15–30 kd (15)*	T cells
Erythropoietin (EPO)	46 kd	Kidney
GM-CSF	15–30 kd (15)*	T cells
		Fibroblasts
G-CSF	20 kd	Monocytes
		Fibroblasts
M-CSF	70–90 kd (26)†	Monocytes
		Fibroblasts
	40–50 kd (16)†	Monocytes
		Fibroblasts

G-CSF, granulocyte-colony stimulating factor; GM-CSF, granulocyte-mono-cyte–colony stimulating factor; M-CSF, monocyte-colony stimulating factor; kd, kilodalton.

* Molecular weight varies because of varying degrees of glycosylation. The number in parentheses is the molecular weight based on primary amino acid sequence inferred from the sequence of the cloned DNA.

† The two forms of M-CSF are encoded by the same gene. Each is a disulfide-bonded homodimer. The molecular weight ranges indicate varying degrees of glycosylation. The numbers in parentheses represent the molecular weight of the nonglycosylated monomer peptides inferred from DNA sequences.

It is beyond the scope of this book to present hemopoiesis in the detail it deserves. The differentiation of the lymphoid lineage responsible for acquired immunity is described briefly here and is discussed in more detail in Chapters 8 and 9. The differentiation of the nonlymphoid lineages involved in innate immunity is described here.

LYMPHOID DIFFERENTIATION

Specific immune responses are mediated by two distinct cell types: lymphocytes and accessory cells. The lymphocytes are made up of two general sets, termed *B lymphocytes* (B cells) and *T lymphocytes* (T cells). If the pluripotential stem cell is to enter the lymphoid lineage and differentiate into a lymphoid stem cell, there are only two subsequent major possibilities. If it is to become a T cell, it leaves the bone marrow and emigrates to the thymus, where it differentiates further under the influence of the thymic microenvironment and soluble factors produced by the thymic epithelium. The resulting T cells are responsible for specific cell-mediated immunity and for regulation of specific, acquired immune responses. This pathway to the thymus most probably requires at least one differentiating step from the lymphoid stem cell to a T-cell progenitor.

However, if the lymphoid stem cell is destined to become a B cell, it remains in the bone marrow (in birds, it emigrates to a specialized organ called the bursa of Fabricius), where it undergoes several more differentiating steps before it gains the ability to produce and secrete

antibody in response to the presence of infectious organisms.

In either case, once differentiation into a T cell or a B cell has occurred, these cells leave their primary site of differentiation and emigrate to the peripheral lymphoid organs (the spleen and lymph nodes), where they await encounter with infectious organisms that have escaped the innate defense system. The differentiating pathways leading to the formation of B cells and T cells are discussed in more detail in Chapters 8 and 9.

NONLYMPHOID DIFFERENTIATION

Differentiation along the nonlymphoid lineage offers more choices, and most such cells perform a wide variety of functions in defense against disease (see Fig. 7-1). It could be said that, indirectly, all but the erythrocyte might play such a role. For example, platelets are the main source of histamine, which is involved in promoting vascular permeability and smooth muscle contraction during elimination of certain infectious organisms (eg, helminths). Most cells of the granulocytic and monocytic lineages are professional phagocytes whose function is to ingest and destroy infectious organisms. Natural killer cells are capable of killing a wide variety of tumor cells and, thus, probably play a major surveillance role in controlling the appearance of malignant cells. Monocytes and their tissue-resident descendants, macrophages, play a central nonspecific role in the activation of acquired immune responses and as nonspecific effector cells in delayed-type hypersensitivity responses.

SOLUBLE FACTORS IN HEMOPOIESIS

Many soluble factors, synthesized and secreted by blood-borne white blood cells, have been shown to influence hemopoiesis. The genes, or cDNA, encoding some of these factors have been cloned and expressed, producing recombinant factors. These factors influence both the proliferation and the differentiation of a variety of cells in the nonlymphoid and lymphoid lineages (see Table 7-1).

Interleukin-3

Although the role of interleukin-3 (from *inter,* meaning between, and *leukin,* meaning leukocytes) in hemopoiesis is not clearly defined, this 28,000-dalton glycoprotein stimulates the growth and differentiation of most blood-borne cells. It may function in concert with one or more specific differentiation factors to promote rapid proliferation of differentiating cells.

Erythropoietin

Erythropoietin is a 46,000-dalton glycoprotein produced by the kidney in response to changing red blood cell concentrations in the circulation. It appears to promote red blood cell formation by acting on several red blood cell precursors. Its effect on each precursor depends on the concentration of erythropoietin in the blood.

Colony-Stimulating Factors

Colony-stimulating factors are a group of glycoproteins, so called because they promote the formation of colonies of differentiated cells from single multipotential stem cells (see Table 7-1). All colony-stimulating factors induce both proliferation and differentiation, although their differentiation-inducing activity is more restricted than their ability to promote proliferation.

GRANULOCYTE-COLONY STIMULATING FACTOR. Granulocyte-colony stimulating factor (G-CSF) has two main biologic activities. First, it promotes the growth and differentiation of neutrophilic granulocytes from progenitor cells. Second, it has a significant effect on the activity of mature neutrophils, such that it can enhance the ability of neutrophils to produce superoxide anions in response to external stimuli and to phagocytize foreign particles. In vivo studies using human G-CSF produced by recombinant DNA techniques showed that G-CSF is capable of inducing a significant elevation in the white blood cell count in both normal and cyclophosphamide-treated monkeys (an experimental treatment used to induce bone marrow aplasia and pancytopenia). The new cells were found to be primarily neutrophils.

MONOCYTE-COLONY STIMULATING FACTOR. Monocyte-colony stimulating factor (M-CSF) occurs in two forms. Neither is overwhelmingly potent in stimulating the growth of macrophage colonies from human progenitors, but both have major effects on murine progenitor cells. However, this may be caused by a greater difficulty in growing the human cells in vitro. Although in vivo studies with M-CSF have not been conducted, both forms are active as stimulators of mature macrophage function in vitro.

GRANULOCYTE-MONOCYTE–COLONY STIMULATING FACTOR. Granulocyte-monocyte–colony stimulating factor (GM-CSF) appears to act at an earlier stage than does either G-CSF or M-CSF. It may be responsible for stimulating the growth and differentiation of early progenitor cells, giving rise to those on which G-CSF and M-CSF act. GM-CSF also is capable of enhancing the activity of many mature cell types (eg, neutrophils, macrophages, and eosinophils), in contrast to G-CSF and M-CSF, which are essentially cell specific. Human GM-CSF dramatically increases white blood cell counts when given intravenously to monkeys. More recently, Steven Clark and Robert Kamen reported the successful use of recombinant human GM-CSF to correct neutropenia in certain patients with the acquired immunodeficiency syndrome. In addition, Steven Clark and his associates showed that human GM-CSF and human interleukin-3 can act synergistically to stimulate hemopoiesis in monkeys. Their results were consistent with the idea that interleukin-3 expands an early cell population that is then acted on by GM-CSF to complete its development.

As with the isolation of the pluripotential stem cell discussed earlier, the cloning and production of these factors, which affect hemopoiesis, should greatly benefit treatment of a variety of diseases in humans.

Primary Lymphoid Organs

The duality of the immune system was suggested when it was discovered that sensitivity to some bacteria and fungi could not be transferred from one animal to another with antiserum but could be transferred using living white blood cells. It therefore appeared that the body possessed two immune systems: one mediated by antibody and the other mediated only by intact living white blood cells.

Our current knowledge of the origins of these two immune systems arose from experiments with birds and mice. Experiments in chickens demonstrated the existence of two distinct organs necessary for the development of immune responses: the bursa of Fabricius as the site of development of antibody-producing potential, and the thymus as the site of development of cell-mediated immune responses. Similar experiments in mice and other mammals defined a similar role in cell-mediated immunity for the mammalian thymus but failed to reveal an organ with a function equivalent to that of the bursa. It is now known that the mammalian bone marrow fulfills that role.

Thus, these two organ types are referred to as primary lymphoid organs, because they are the sites of *initial* differentiation of precursors into the various functional cell types, that is, T cells and B cells.

BURSA OF FABRICIUS

The bursa of Fabricius is the organ in avian species that provides the microenvironment for the differentiation of those lymphocytes that ultimately differentiate into the cell that produces and secretes antibody. Such cells are termed *B cells* to designate their origin in the bursa. The bursa begins as a sac-like invagination of the avian intestinal wall leading to the formation of follicles. Several days before hatching, differentiated B cells begin to enter the circulation. Removal of the bursa (either surgically or chemically) from newly hatched chickens destroys their ability to produce circulating antibodies but does not affect their ability to mount cell-mediated immune responses.

BONE MARROW

The mammalian bone marrow is the site not only of hemopoiesis, but also of initial differentiation of stem cells to B cells. This is demonstrated most clearly by the in vitro generation of functional B lymphocytes in cultures of bone marrow cells. This suggests either that a specific microenvironment in the bone marrow is not necessary for initial B-cell differentiation or that it can be readily duplicated in cultures of dissociated bone marrow cells.

THYMUS

The thymus is essentially fully developed at birth, existing as two lateral lobes above the pericardium and extending into the neck on the front and sides of the trachea. The embryonic thymus consists of a mass of connected epithelial cells surrounded by a thin capsule. In utero, precursor cells (prothymocytes) differentiate from lymphoid stem cells and emigrate from the bone marrow and infiltrate the thymus, wedging between the epithelial cells to form a meshwork of branched epithelial cells and lymphocytes. This infiltration of the thymus by precursor cells does not seem to occur continuously, but in discrete bursts dictated by the thymic environment itself rather than by the bone marrow. The outermost epithelium, called the *cortex,* becomes heavily populated with the resulting thymocytes, whereas the central area, termed the *medulla,* contains far fewer lymphocytes, at least some of which are derived from the cortical thymocytes (Fig. 7-2).

Histologically, the thymus is divided into a series of lobules extending from the periphery to the central area, including both the cortex and the medulla. The newly arrived prothymocytes enter the cortex from the bone marrow and begin dividing rapidly (generation time, 6 to 9 hours); surprisingly, though, most of these thymocytes die within 3 to 5 days without ever leaving the cortex.

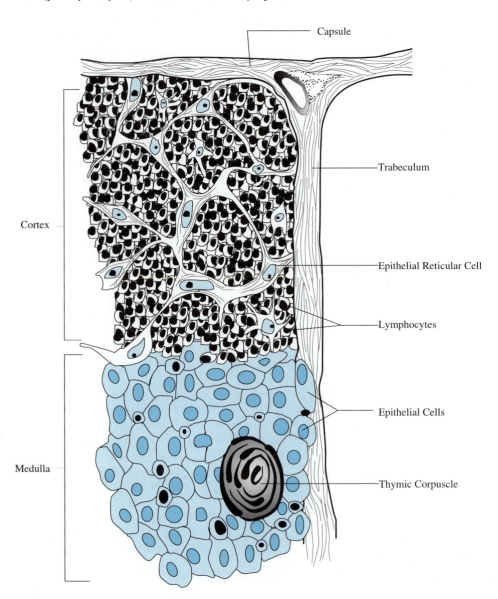

FIGURE 7-2 Structure of the thymus. Portion of a thymic lobe. The capsule and trabecula are mainly connective tissue containing blood vessels and some lymphocytes, granulocytes, and plasma cells. The cortex contains large numbers of lymphocytes. As a result, the epithelial cells are stellate yet remain attached to one another. The medulla is mainly epithelial but contains a significant proportion of lymphocytes. Some epithelial cells are arranged concentrically and form a thymic corpuscle.

During differentiation from prothymocyte to thymocyte to T cell, the cell synthesizes several cell-surface molecules, which characterize the phenotype of the cell. Several of these cell-surface molecules are markers of distinct functional subsets of T cells (see Chap. 9), and several are directly involved in the initial recognition events leading to T-cell activation (see Chap. 11).

Differentiation of a small proportion of thymocytes to T cells (thymus-derived lymphocytes) is followed immediately by emigration of these T cells to the peripheral lymphoid organs as mature cells that are already committed to particular functions and antigen specificity.

The control of differentiation within the thymus is not clearly understood but involves cells bearing certain molecules encoded by genes within the major histocompatibility locus (MHC; see Chap. 10), one or more hormones, and growth and differentiation factors secreted by thymic epithelial cells. The MHC-encoded molecules are involved in T cells learning to distinguish self from nonself, whereas the hormones and cytokines are involved in proliferation and in the differentiating process itself.

Several such hormones (eg, thymosin and thymopoietin) have been isolated from the thymus of various species and have been used in many clinical trials involving individuals who are wholly or partially deficient in thymic, or T-cell, function; for example, they have been used in children with the DiGeorge syndrome who have a congenital thymic deficiency.

Soon after puberty, the thymus begins to atrophy without any apparent immediate effect on the peripheral T-cell numbers or on T-cell function. This is probably because T cells are long-lived and can circulate in the resting state for long periods.

The role of the thymus in the development of cell-mediated immunity has been clearly demonstrated by experiments in which removal of the thymus results in the absence of all cell-mediated immune responses and partially inhibited antibody formation. Cellular immune deficiency also is seen in individuals in whom differentiation of the thymus fails or does not proceed normally.

Secondary Lymphoid Organs

After differentiation in the primary lymphoid organs, B cells and T cells enter the circulation and migrate to the secondary lymphoid organs, namely the spleen, lymph nodes, Peyer's patches, appendix, and tonsils, where they continue to mature. It is in these organs that B and T lymphocytes are stimulated by antigen.

LYMPH NODES

Lymph nodes are small, complex organs that serve as junction points between blood and lymph vessels. Two major areas can be distinguished within a lymph node: a central medulla containing primarily T lymphocytes and a peripheral cortex containing follicles of B lymphocytes (Fig. 7-3). A large number of lymphocytes, mainly T cells, continuously enter the bloodstream and circulate back again to the lymph nodes. Each lymph node has several lymph channels (called *afferent lymph channels*) that drain into it and a single large lymph vessel (called the *efferent lymph channel*) that carries the lymph fluid and lymphocytes to the thoracic duct, which empties into a large vein in the neck.

Lymph nodes serve as very efficient filters. Antigens entering a lymph node are trapped by phagocytic cells (primarily macrophages), which process the antigen and present it to the lymphocytes. This trapping, processing, and presentation of antigen to lymphocytes is the initial step in the induction of specific immune responses (see later and Chap. 11) and results in the antigen-specific activation of both B cells and T cells. B-cell activation occurs in the follicular areas of the lymph node. These B cells respond to antigen, with the help of nonspecific accessory cells and antigen-specific T cells, by dividing and differentiating into antibody-producing plasma cells. The areas that contain large numbers of dividing B cells within the secondary follicles thus formed are called *germinal centers*. About 1 week after antigen stimulation, the germinal centers and interfollicular areas become filled with antibody-producing plasma cells. Memory B cells and T cells also are formed and are disseminated throughout the body through the efferent lymph and blood circulatory system. This circulation of primed cells ensures an adequate subsequent response to a second contact with the antigen, no matter where in the body the secondary contact occurs.

Thus, antigen (eg, bacteria) in the connective tissue will enter the lymph and flow into the lymph node through the afferent lymph channels. After it is within the lymph node, the antigen encounters all elements of the specific immune system (ie, macrophages, B cells, T cells) and many elements of the nonspecific immune system as well.

SPLEEN

The spleen is a secondary lymphoid organ, within which antibody synthesis to most blood-borne antigens occurs. The major areas discernible within the spleen are the white pulp, consisting primarily of lymphocytes and macrophages, and the red pulp, consisting of erythrocyte-rich blood (Fig. 7-4). Arteries entering the spleen are surrounded by a sheath of T cells and macrophages (the periarteriolar sheath). Isolated within this sheath are primary follicles of B cells similar to those occurring in lymph nodes. Blood-borne antigens entering the spleen are phagocytized and processed by macrophages and fixed phagocytic mononuclear cells. Presentation of antigens on the surface of such accessory cells to the splenic lym-

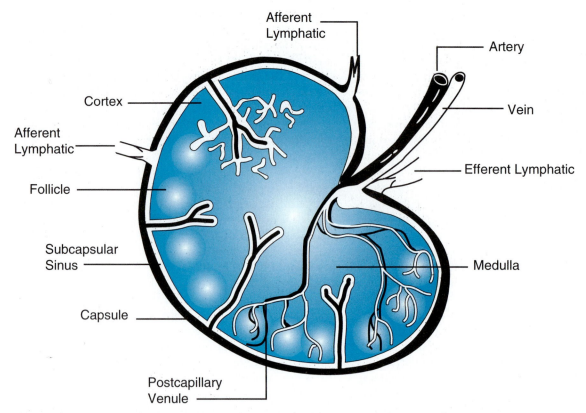

FIGURE 7-3 Lymph node. Lymph containing lymphocytes enters through the afferent lymphatics and exits through the efferent lymphatic. The cortex contains densely packed lymphocytes and its development is thymic dependent, whereas the development of the medulla (especially the medullary cords) is B-cell dependent. Follicles can be of two types: (1) primary follicles, which are collections of small lymphocytes lying in webs of dendritic cells; or (2) secondary follicles, which form as the result of antigen stimulation and are made up of two parts, with the mantle being the same as the primary follicle and the germinal center being responsible for the production of antibody-synthesizing cells (ie, plasma cells).

phocytes results in the formation of secondary follicles containing germinal centers of dividing and differentiating B cells.

PEYER'S PATCHES

Another type of peripheral lymphoid organ exists in the intestinal tissue of mammals. This gut-associated lymphoid tissue (Fig. 7-5) is composed primarily of Peyer's patches and the appendix. Peyer's patches are small patches of organized lymphoid tissue along the intestine containing B cells (in germinal centers) and T cells. It is believed that these gut-associated lymphoid organs play a primary role in defense against infectious organisms entering through the digestive tract.

LYMPHOCYTE CIRCULATION AND HOMING

Most lymphocytes circulate between the various secondary lymphoid organs through the lymph and blood vessels (Fig. 7-6). T cells appear to circulate more frequently

than do B cells, and activated lymphocytes may circulate more often than do cells that have yet to encounter antigen. This recirculation provides a mechanism by which lymphocytes of all specificities and states of activation can reach all regions of the body.

Lymphocytes appear to be preferentially retained in one or the other lymphoid organ as a result of a specific interaction between receptors on the surface of the lymphocyte and molecules on the epithelial cells of high endothelial venules (HEV) that exist within the lymphoid organ. Several types of receptor–HEV interactions can occur, resulting in the "homing" of some lymphocytes to lymph nodes, others to Peyer's patches, and so on. Lymphocytes taken from Peyer's patches and injected intravenously into an irradiated recipient preferentially localize in the recipient's Peyer's patches. It has been shown by John Cebra and colleagues that such selective homing of lymphocytes also reflects on the immunoglobulin class specificity of these cells. IgA-producing B cells home to the Peyer's patches and IgM- and IgG-producing B cells localize in the spleen and lymph nodes.

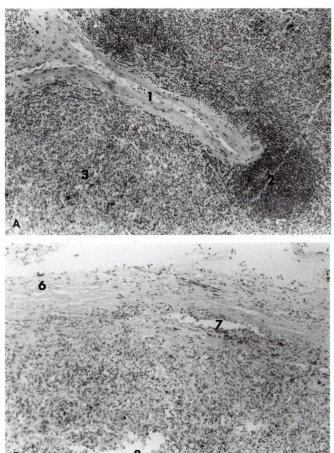

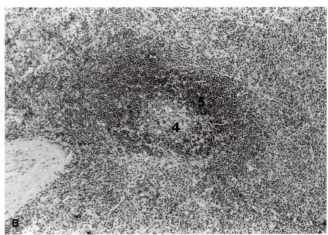

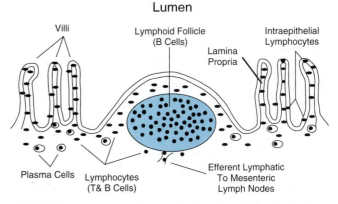

FIGURE 7-4 Microanatomy of the spleen. **A.** A central artery (1) surrounded by a sheath of T lymphocytes (2). The splenic red pulp (3) consists of erythrocytes, macrophages, and other leukocytes. **B.** A splenic germinal center (4) consisting of proliferating B cells surrounded by a cuff of small dense B cells **C.** (5). The splenic covering (6) consists of a connective tissue capsule within which lymphatic vessels (7) are found. Splenic sinuses (8) are open areas in the red pulp in which filtration of the blood occurs in this organ.

Irving Weissman and colleagues have produced a monoclonal antibody to an 80,000-dalton lymph-node–specific HEV receptor present on some lymphocytes. Binding of this antibody to a mixture of lymphocytes prevents localization in the lymph nodes but not in other lymphoid organs. Weissman also used this antibody to detect cells possessing this receptor in the thymus of adult mice. Cells with this marker were found to reside almost entirely in the cortical region of the thymus and represented a small proportion (about 1%) of the total cortical thymocytes. Using this antibody, Weissman was able to isolate this small subset of thymocytes and to obtain data indicating that they may be the immediate precursors of the peripheral T lymphocytes.

Even more recently, Weissman and colleagues have cloned the cDNA for the molecule responsible for homing to lymph nodes in mice. It is a transmembrane protein with an unusual mosaic structure. It has a terminal lectin-like domain, another domain similar to epidermal growth factor, and a repeat structure similar to that found in several other regulatory proteins. A detailed analysis of the structure–function relationships of this molecule in mice and humans should permit a better understanding of the mechanisms controlling the recirculation of lymphocytes and their homing to specific lymphoid organs.

FIGURE 7-5 Gut-associated lymphoid tissue. Several lymphoid tissues are associated with the gastrointestinal tract (eg, the appendix, tonsils, and Peyer's patches). Shown here is a diagram of a Peyer's patch in the small intestine. The basic design of this lymphoid organ is similar to that of the lymph node. There are B-cell– and T-cell–dependent areas. After antigen stimulation, the primary follicles develop germinal centers, which are areas of intense B-cell activation and differentiation. Plasma cells underlying the epithelial cells of the gut secrete IgA antibody molecules that interact with receptors on the epithelial cells. This secretory IgA is transported through the epithelial cell and released into the lumen of the gut. Also found are T cells with several types of antigen-specific receptors. Of particular interest are those T cells with the γ/δ T-cell receptors. Gut-associated lymphoid tissue is primarily responsible for defense against intestinal pathogens and other antigens that enter through the gastrointestinal tract.

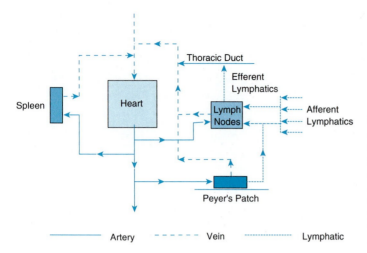

Spleen

Heart

Thoracic Duct

Efferent
Lymphatics

Lymph
Nodes

Afferent
Lymphatics

Peyer's Patch

——— Artery   - - - - - Vein   ········· Lymphatic

FIGURE 7-6   Lymphocyte recirculation. Both T cells and B cells are constantly recirculating throughout the body. As a result, antigenic stimulation (ie, infection) can provide systemic protection from reinfection regardless of where the second site of infection might occur. Shown here is a schematic illustration of the circulatory pathway, including both blood and lymph systems. Although lymphocytes do recirculate, many have cell-surface receptors that promote "homing" to one or the other lymphoid tissue (eg, some T cells preferentially home to Peyer's patches, whereas others home to other lymph nodes).

A Closer Look

The organization of the primary and secondary lymphoid organs has evolved to facilitate the maturation of the adaptive immune system's function. Embryonic stem cells differentiate early and populate the primary lymphoid organs, including the bone marrow and thymus of vertebrates. Animals or humans who experience genetic defects in the differentiation of the primary hematopoietic stem cells, or in whom the embryogenesis of the primary lymphoid organs fails to occur normally, are destined to be born with a variety of immunologic deficiency diseases.

Failure of bone marrow stem cells to develop into the B-lymphocyte lineage can result in an infant being born with congenital immunoglobulin deficiency disease. All infants are protected early in life by maternal antibodies that cross the placenta in utero. Once these maternal antibodies decline with age and the infant fails to replace them with its own antibodies, the immunologic deficiency becomes apparent. Such infants are susceptible to a variety of bacterial infections and can die if their deficiency is not recognized and treated properly.

It is possible to treat humans who have total or isolated immunoglobulin deficiencies with preparations of human immune globulin. Many patients have been given years of infection-free life by virtue of periodic injections with the immunoglobulin fraction obtained from the blood of normal donors. A goal of modern clinical immunologic research is to develop a means of correcting B-lymphocyte deficiency through cell and gene therapy. Such therapies may be developed soon, certainly by the turn of the century.

Thymic deficiencies resulting from abnormal development of the thymus gland or genetic defects in thymic precursor cells are rare, but have been recorded in humans. Infants born with thymic aplasia or thymic hypoplasia are subject to a variety of fungal and viral infections. In many instances, little or nothing can be done to protect these infants from infection, and they die before reaching maturity. For years, investigators have made heroic attempts to save these infants using thymus transplantation, reconstitution of thymus cell function with thymus cell transplants, and reconstitution of T-lymphocyte function with a variety of factors derived from the thymus gland. To date, no one therapeutic approach has enabled us to correct the major thymic deficiencies that are life-threatening in infants born without a normal thymus gland. Perhaps when we are able to recognize the presence of a thymic abnormality in utero, it will be possible to perform thymic reconstitution before birth using cell or gene therapy. Other efforts are being directed toward correcting thymic T-lymphocyte deficiencies and abnormalities that occur in adults as a result of infections, such as those associated with the acquired immunodeficiency syndrome and those that occur after debilitating, iatrogenically induced T-lymphocyte deficiency disease.

Accessory Cells

The vital role of phagocytic cells in immunity became evident from the studies of Eli Metchnikoff in the last century (see Chap. 3). It was not until the mid-1960s, however, that the role of at least one type of phagocytic cell in the induction of immune responses was demonstrated. In 1967, Donald Mosier clearly showed that a glass-adherent cell was required for the in vitro generation of antibody responses. Histologic studies showed that these cells were macrophages. Subsequent investigations in many laboratories have demonstrated that such accessory cells function in the induction of all T-cell–dependent immune responses.

Many different cell types can perform these accessory cell functions, including mononuclear phagocytes, tissue-fixed macrophages, Langerhans cells, dendritic cells, and B cells. Macrophages, Langerhans cells, and B cells express Fc receptors, complement receptors, and class II antigens on their surfaces, whereas dendritic cells express only class II antigens. All these cell types express a variety of other surface markers.

These accessory cells function to ingest and process an antigen, and to present that processed antigen to the T lymphocytes. For most antigens, this ingestion and processing is an obligatory step for antigen-specific activation of helper T cells and delayed-type hypersensitivity T cells (see Chap. 11). Because helper T cells are required for the induction of cytotoxic T-cell responses, the accessory cell plays a major role in the initiation of that form of cell-mediated immunity as well.

Although all accessory cells can ingest and process antigen, only those that express cell-surface class II molecules can function as antigen-presenting cells for helper T cells. As discussed in Chapter 11, these MHC-encoded molecules play a vital role in the initiation of immune responses.

Bibliography

JOURNALS

Clark SC, Kamen R. The human hematopoietic colony-stimulating factors. Science 1987;236:1229.

Osmond DG. B cell development in the bone marrow. Semin Immunol 1990;2:173.

Paige CJ, Cumano A, Wu GE. B cell commitment. Semin Immunol 1991;3:173.

Phillips RA. Hematopoietic stem cells: concepts, assays, and controversies. Semin Immunol 1991;3:337.

Weill JC, Redynaud CA. Early B-cell development in chicken, sheep and rabbits. Curr Opin Immunol 1992;4:177.

BOOKS

Ikuta K, Uchida N, Friedman J, Weissman IL. Lymphocyte development from stem cells. In: Paul WE, Fathman CG, Metzger H, eds. Annual review of immunology, vol 10. Palo Alto, CA, Annual Reviews, 1992:759.

Kantor AB, Herzenberg LA. Origin of murine B cell lineages. In: Paul WE, Fathman CG, Metzger H, eds. Annual review of immunology, vol 11. Palo Alto, CA, Annual Reviews, 1993:501.

MacLennan ICM. Germinal centers. In: Paul WE, Fathman CG, Metzger H, eds. Annual review of immunology, vol 12. Palo Alto, CA, Annual Reviews, 1994:117.

Essentials of Medical Microbiology, Fifth Edition, edited by Wesley A. Volk,
Bryan M. Gebhardt, Marie-Louise Hammarskjöld, and Robert J. Kadner.
Lippincott-Raven Publishers, Philadelphia © 1996.

Chapter 8

B-Cell Development, Receptors, and Genes

B-Cell Development

The mammalian B cell arises from a stem cell in the bone marrow (see Chap. 7). On reaching a functionally mature stage in its differentiation, it leaves the bone marrow and emigrates to the peripheral lymphoid organs where, on contact with antigen, it can differentiate into an antibody-producing plasma cell. This differentiation occurs in a stepwise fashion and is accompanied by the appearance of new surface and cytoplasmic markers at each step of differentiation. The following sections describe the more important surface markers found on cells of the B-cell lineage and outline the antigen-independent and antigen-dependent differentiating steps leading from the stem cell to the antibody-producing plasma cell.

B-CELL MARKERS

Surface Immunoglobulin

All B cells possess antigen-specific surface immunoglobulin (sIg). This sIg serves as a specific surface receptor, recognizing and interacting with only a single antigenic determinant on the antigen. Interaction of antigen with this receptor, in the proper environment, activates the B cell, leading to proliferation and differentiation. Each B cell possesses about 10^5 sIg molecules, primarily of the IgM and IgD classes. After activation, the class of this sIg receptor can change (see later). Thus, within a large population of B cells, cells can be found with any one or more of the immunoglobulin (Ig) classes as the antigen-specific receptor.

    The antigen specificity of the sIg receptor on a B cell is predetermined, and the sole effect of antigen is to select out a cell with the appropriate specificity and induce it to expand clonally and differentiate into a cell that will produce the antibody it has been predetermined to make.

Class II (Ia) Molecules

Class II molecules (previously called Ia antigens; see Chap. 10) are surface proteins present primarily on B cells and macrophages, although certain activated T cells and other cell types also can express these markers. These proteins are encoded by genes within the major histocompatibility locus (MHC) and are involved in the cell–cell interactions between certain T cells and antigen-presenting cells (see Chaps. 11 and 13).

Fc Receptors

Receptors for the Fc portion of Ig are found on all B cells, macrophages, and certain subsets of T cells. These receptors bind antigen–antibody complexes and are thought to be directly involved in regulating immune responses (see Chap. 11).

Complement Receptors

Complement is a part of the nonspecific immune system (see Chap. 12). It is made up of a group of at least 20 serum proteins that interact in a defined manner to promote the elimination of infectious organisms. Receptors for one of these complement proteins (ie, the third component or certain of its fragments) are found on most B cells. Again, this receptor is thought to play a role in the regulation of the B-cell response to antigen.

Other B-Cell Markers

The resting mature B cell has receptors for interferon and interleukin-4 (also called B-cell stimulatory factor-1). After activation, it acquires receptors for transferrin, interleukin-2 (also known as T-cell growth factor), interleukin-5 (also known as B-cell growth factor-II) and interleukin-6 (also called B-cell stimulatory factor-2). Interferon and the interleukins are growth and differentiation factors released by activated T cells (see Chaps. 9 and 11).

ANTIGEN-INDEPENDENT B-CELL DIFFERENTIATION

During ontogeny, the first recognizable B cell possesses only surface IgM. As embryonic development proceeds, these sIg-bearing B cells acquire Fc receptors, surface IgD, class II molecules (Ia antigens), and complement receptors, in essentially that order. Thus, most B cells in mature individuals have the following cell-surface phenotype: $IgM^+IgD^+FcR^+Ia^+CR^+$. Plasma cells, which are descendants of B cells, lack all these markers.

The bone marrow is the site not only of hemopoiesis, as discussed in Chapter 7, but also of the initial differentiation of stem cells to B cells. The strongest evidence for this conclusion is the observation that the in vitro culture of bone marrow cells that have been depleted of B cells by one or more techniques results in the generation of new B cells. The rate at which these cells are regenerated precludes the possibility that the depletion was incomplete and that the newly arising B cells were derived, not from stem cells, but from the few B cells that were not eliminated.

Stem Cell to Pre–B Cell

The first recognizable cell of the B-cell lineage is the pre–B cell (Fig. 8-1). This cell differentiates in the bone marrow from the pluripotential stem cell in one or more steps through a lymphoid stem cell. The pre–B cell is characterized by the presence of the μ heavy chain of IgM in its cytoplasm. At the molecular level, this involves the rearrangement of DNA to form a mature heavy-chain gene (see later). No light chain, either κ or λ, is expressed; thus, no sIg is found. Because no sIg is present, this cell cannot be activated by antigen.

Some pre–B cells possess surface Fc receptors, but the fact that not all pre–B cells possess Fc receptors suggests that the expression of this cell-surface marker occurs after μ-chain expression but before the next differentiating step.

Pre–B Cell to Immature B Cell

Expression of a light-chain gene, either κ or λ but not both, is the next step in B-cell differentiation. This involves the rearrangement of DNA to form a mature light-chain gene (see later). Synthesis of light chain and its association with the already present μ heavy chain results in the insertion of complete *monomeric* IgM into the cell membrane. Interaction between antigen and the newly acquired IgM antigen-specific receptor on this immature B cell can lead to either activation or inactivation, depending on the conditions in which interaction occurs. All immature B cells possess Fc receptors.

Immature B Cell to Mature B Cell

The $sIgM^+FcR^+$ immature B cell leaves the bone marrow and migrates to the peripheral lymphoid organs (ie, the spleen, lymph nodes, and Peyer's patches). Soon after arriving in its new home, the cell begins to express the δ heavy chain of IgD in addition to the μ chain already present. This chain combines with the already expressed light chain and is inserted as IgD into the cell membrane as a second antigen-specific receptor. The antigen specificity of the IgM and IgD surface molecules is identical. The reason for two different Igs with identical specificity is unknown, but must be related to the activation or inactivation of specific B cells by antigen. Some B cells appear to mature yet do not express δ chain, suggesting that expression of IgD is not a necessary differentiating event leading to antibody synthesis.

As the B cell is expressing IgD receptors, it also is beginning to express the cell-surface class II molecules. Soon thereafter, most mature B cells acquire receptors

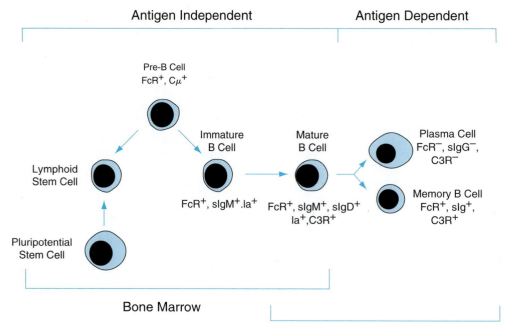

FIGURE 8-1 B-lymphocyte differentiation. B-cell differentiation occurs in two stages. The first stage is entirely independent of the presence of antigen and results in the formation of B cells expressing immunoglobulin receptors specific for a given antigen. This stage begins with differentiation of a progenitor committed to forming lymphocytes. The evidence for the existence of this lymphoid stem cell is entirely circumstantial. Differentiation then proceeds through stages, each defined by the presence or absence of several cell-surface molecules. The end result is the formation of a B cell, expressing both IgM and IgD, which can be activated by antigen. The second stage of B-cell differentiation occurs in the peripheral lymphoid organs and depends on the presence of a specific antigen (eg, an infection) and its interaction with specific receptors on B cells and T cells. This stage begins with a B cell expressing surface immunoglobulin and results in the proliferation of that B cell and the differentiation of its daughter cells both to plasma cells secreting antibody and to memory B cells (an expanded population of B cells usually expressing immunoglobulin receptors of a different isotype but of the same antigen specificity).

for the third component of complement. Thus, the cell-surface phenotype of most mature B cells is IgM^+IgD^+ $FcR^+Ia^+CR^-$ or $IgM^+IgD^+FcR^+Ia^+CR^+$. Most resting B cells in the peripheral lymphoid compartments are of this phenotype.

All the antibody specificities present in an individual's lymphoid system arise from antigen-independent differentiating events. The subsequent activation of B cells, therefore, results solely from antigen interaction with these specific receptors on B cells that have been preprogrammed for both specificity and function.

ANTIGEN-DEPENDENT B-CELL DIFFERENTIATION

Antigen, under certain defined conditions, stimulates the mature B cell to undergo both proliferation and differentiation. Depending on the conditions involved, this activation results in either terminal differentiation to an antibody-producing plasma cell or production of both plasma cells and memory B cells. Barring somatic mutation, a plasma cell secretes antibody with a specificity identical

to that of the receptor on the B cell from which it was derived. The first antibody secreted is IgM. Expression of other Ig isotypes depends to a large degree on a subsequent T-cell–mediated switch in the heavy-chain constant-region synthesis (see later).

The differentiation and proliferation of B cells, specific for most antigens, to antibody-secreting plasma cells and memory B cells requires the interaction of both macrophages and certain subsets of T cells with antigen, and the interaction of the B cells with the resulting activated T cells (see Chap. 11). Memory B cells resemble virgin resting B lymphocytes in most aspects, except that memory B cells turn over less rapidly and, in most cases, have undergone a switch in heavy-chain gene expression.

IMMUNOGLOBULIN IN THE NEWBORN

All antibody present in humans at birth was acquired in utero from the maternal circulation by transplacental transfer. Because IgG is the only Ig isotype capable of crossing the placenta, it is the only Ig present in the newborn at birth. Newborn humans begin to synthesize their own antibody soon after birth, and adult levels are reached by 1 year of age for IgM, about 5 to 7 years of age for IgG, and about 10 to 12 years of age for IgA. The absence of overt Ig synthesis in utero is not due to the absence of the appropriate B cells, but to negative control mechanisms existing during the late prenatal and early neonatal periods. Antibody responsiveness to different antigens is acquired at different times after birth. For example, antibody responses to most protein antigens can be induced in newborns, whereas the ability to respond to certain polysaccharide antigens appears much later. This must be taken into account when considering the timing of immunization with protein or polysaccharide vaccines, and may account for the newborn's susceptibility to certain infections.

Antibody and B-Cell Receptor Genes

Antigen activates both T cells and B cells by interacting with specific receptors on their surface. The nature of B-cell receptors for antigen was relatively easy to demonstrate. B-cell receptors are membrane-bound immunoglobulins (mIgs) that possess the same specificity as the Igs that will be secreted by the B-cell–derived plasma cell. The nature of the T-cell receptor, however, was much more difficult to ascertain and has been described only recently. The difficulty in describing the T-cell receptor

arose from the fact that the T cell only recognizes antigen presented by MHC molecules occurring on the surface of other cells (ie, macrophages, Langerhans cells, dendritic cells, and B cells; see Chaps. 9, 10, 11, and 13). These molecules are encoded by genes within the MHC.

It is now known that antibody, the B-cell and T-cell antigen receptors, and the MHC-encoded cell-surface molecules belong to a structurally related group of molecules called the Ig superfamily. Figure 8-2 is a diagram of the structure of representatives of each of these molecules. They have been drawn so that the structural similarities are maximized. Not shown are the similarities in primary structure or other members of the superfamily.

Thus, most of the molecules involved in antigen recognition and in cell–cell interaction in the immune response are closely related. The structure of antibody is discussed in Chapter 5. The structure of the MHC-encoded molecules and the genes that encode them are discussed in Chapter 10. The structure of the T-cell receptor and the genes that encode it are discussed in Chapter 9. The structure of the genes that encode antibody and the B-cell receptor and the mechanisms by which these genes are manipulated to give rise to antibody or receptor diversity are the topics discussed here.

MOLECULAR BIOLOGY OF ANTIBODY SYNTHESIS

Three gene clusters encode the heavy chain and each of the light chains of Ig. Each cluster segregates indepen-

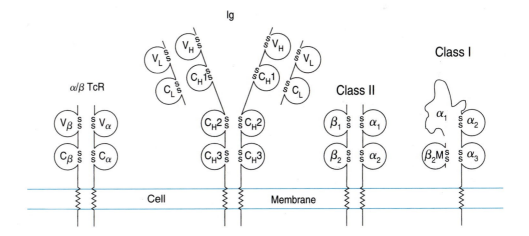

FIGURE 8-2 The immunoglobulin superfamily. Antibodies (and thus B-cell receptors) belong to a group of cell-surface molecules that are involved in recognition of antigen and cell–cell interaction. This family of molecules was so named because its members bear structural similarity to immunoglobulin. Shown here are four of the many molecules of the immunoglobulin superfamily: immunoglobulin itself portrayed as a surface receptor, the α/β T-cell receptor, and the class I and class II major histocompatibility complex molecules. These four molecules are of particular importance in both B-cell and T-cell activation by antigen. The structural similarities are depicted by the disulfide-bonded loops within structural domains. Amino acid sequences and functional similarities, which are not shown here, are discussed in the text.

dently and, therefore, resides on a different chromosome. The variable and constant regions for κ chain form one cluster, those for λ chain make up another cluster, and those for all the different heavy chains form a third cluster. Within each cluster, the variable-region (V-region) genes are clearly separated from the constant-region (C-region) genes, indicating that some rearrangement of genetic material must occur to produce an mRNA within which the variable and constant regions are contiguous. The constant-region genes for each of the heavy-chain isotypes are closely linked on the same chromosome, and all share a common V_H pool. Considerable rearrangement of genetic material occurs to enable a given V_H region to be expressed with any of the heavy-chain isotypes.

Recombinant DNA technology has made it possible to study Ig gene structure, both in embryonic germline cells and in cells of the B-cell lineage. These studies have revealed a complex mechanism for antibody and B-cell receptor synthesis and for the generation of the diversity occurring within the antibody-combining site. The following discussion is based on many studies using multiple systems, including the human system. With few minor exceptions, Ig gene rearrangement is identical in all mammalian systems studied.

Light-Chain Gene Rearrangement

Using Southern blot analysis, it has been shown that the V_L-region (either κ or λ) genes are considerably more distant from the C_L-region gene in lymphoid stem cell DNA than they are in DNA obtained from mature B cells or myeloma cells. In other words, there is a rearrangement of these genes in the Ig-producing cells that bring the V_L-gene segment much closer to the C_L-gene segment.

In subsequent studies, the V_L and C_L genes were cloned individually. When the virgin genes from embryonic cells were sequenced, they were found to encode only the first 97 amino acids of the V_L chain. The nucleotide sequences coding for the remaining 12 amino acids of the V_L region were subsequently located near the C_L-region gene. However, when genomic DNA from myeloma cells was examined, the sequences encoding the first 97 amino acids were contiguous with the small genomic sequence encoding the carboxy-terminal 12 amino acids of V_L. These latter nucleotide sequences have been termed the *J segment,* because rearrangement results in a *joining* of the major part of the V_L to this region of the chromosome. (Note that this J is a gene region and has nothing to do with the J chain found in secretory IgM and IgA.) Thus, the codons for the first two complementarity-determining regions (CDRs; see Chap. 5) of light chain are contained in the V_L gene, and the codons for the third CDR are within the J_L gene.

The mouse κ–light-chain genes have been studied more extensively than any other light-chain cluster. There are about 50 different groups of V_κ-chain genes. Each group contains 5 to 10 closely linked genes, each of which is separated from the others by noncoding sequences (ie, introns; Fig. 8-3). All V_κ genes within a given group are more closely related to each other in sequence than they are to the genes occurring in other groups. This suggests that members of each group arose relatively recently in evolution from a single ancestral gene by gene duplication.

The DNA sequence that encodes the final 12 amino acids on the carboxy-terminal end of the V_κ chain is located near the C_L gene. There are five J genes separated from each other by about 300 bases and from the C_L gene by about 2.5 to 4.0 kilobases.

During differentiation from a pre–B cell to an immature B cell, rearrangement of the light-chain DNA occurs so that a V_L gene is brought into juxtaposition randomly with one of the J genes (see Fig. 8-3). Because each J gene codes for different amino acids, and because the J region of the light chain contributes to the third CDR, multiple J segments contribute to the diversity of the antibody molecule.

The choice of which V_L gene and which J segments rearrange appears to be a random event, but once it occurs, that cell is forever committed to synthesize the rearranged V_L and the J segment adjacent to it. The process of rearrangement results in a deletion of the DNA between the rearranged V_L gene and the J segment that it joins, and, as shown in Figure 8-3, the final active gene still contains the other V_L genes 5′ to the chosen V_L gene and the remaining J genes on the 3′ side of the selected J gene.

In all species studied, there is a single C_κ gene. The λ-chain gene cluster is more complex, and in humans there are six C_λ genes, each with its own pool of V_λ genes. Although not known in detail, it is presumed that the choice between λ-chain groups and between the V-region genes within a group is also random in a manner similar to that described for κ-gene rearrangements.

Transcription of the Light-Chain Gene

The rearranged form of the light-chain gene contains one intron between the leader coding sequences and the C_L gene, one intron between each residual J gene, and one intron between the 3′-most J gene and the C_L gene. This entire rearranged gene (including introns and exons) is transcribed into a long precursor mRNA. This precursor RNA is subsequently processed by removal of the introns and splicing together of the exons to yield functional mRNA with all the coding sequences contiguous with one another. The exact mechanism by which splicing occurs is not fully understood, but it is known that each intron begins with the nucleotides GT and ends with AG. It is thought that these short sequences provide a recognition site for the mRNA-processing enzymes.

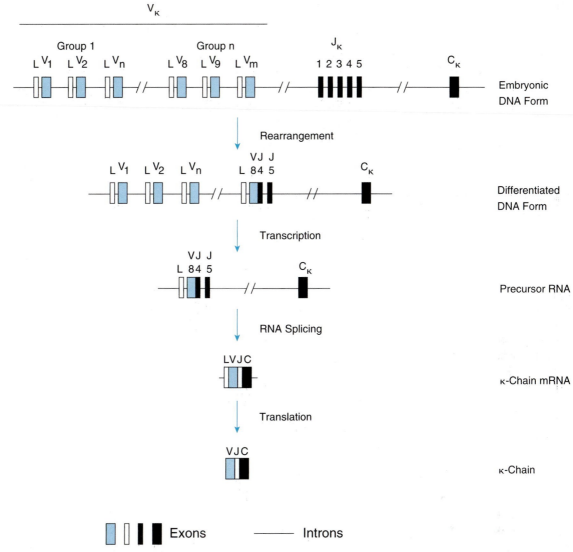

FIGURE 8-3 κ–light-chain gene rearrangement during B-cell differentiation. The sequence of genetic events leading to the production of κ light chain is shown. In the germline genome, the exons encoding the variable region of light chain are well separated. During antigen-independent differentiation, a rearrangement of DNA occurs to bring a V-region exon into juxtaposition with a J-region exon, forming the differentiated gene encoding the κ light chain. This gene is transcribed into a precursor RNA, which is processed (spliced), resulting in the removal of all noncoding sequences and the production of a mature mRNA with all coding sequences contiguous. After translation of this mRNA and subsequent removal of the signal sequence, a mature κ light chain is produced.

Heavy-Chain Gene Rearrangements

Like the light-chain genes, heavy-chain variable-region genes (V_H) occur in groups. Again, members within a group are more closely related to each other than to the members of another group. Each V_H gene is separated by a short intron from an exon (L), which encodes a leader sequence, and each L–V_H gene complex is separated from other L–V_H gene complexes within the group by noncoding sequences.

Comparison of DNA sequences from germline embryonic cells and mature antibody-producing cells demonstrates that V_H-gene segments also undergo a rearrangement during differentiation. However, V_H-gene rearrangement is more complex than that of the V_L genes. It has been reported that germline V_H segments contain the coding sequences for amino acids 1 through 101, and that the J genes encode for amino acids 107 through 123. The missing six amino acids were found to be encoded in a third gene segment, designated D (for diversity), lying between the V_H and J_H genes (Fig. 8-4). There are several such D genes. The length of these D genes varies, giving rise to the known differences in length of the fourth CDR of the human heavy-chain variable region.

During differentiation from a stem cell to the pre–B cell, the first joining event is between a D and a J_H segment (see Fig. 8-4). As with light-chain gene rearrangement,

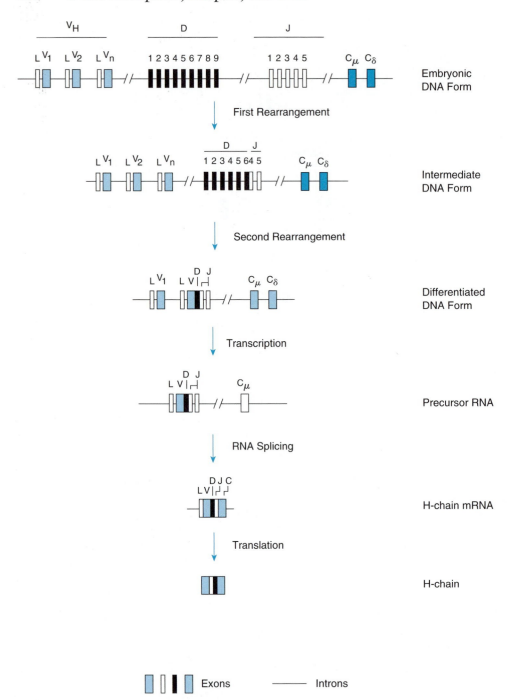

FIGURE 8-4 Heavy-chain gene rearrangement during B-cell differentiation. The sequence of events leading to the production of a mature H-chain gene is similar to that described for κ light chain in Figure 8-3. However, there is a third exon involved in coding for the mature variable region of the heavy-chain polypeptide. This exon is the D-region exon and encodes for most of the four complementarity-determining regions of heavy chain. During antigen-independent differentiation, a rearrangement of DNA occurs that joins a D-region exon with a J-region exon. A subsequent rearrangement brings the chosen V-region exon into juxtaposition with the already rearranged DJ exons. Once these rearrangements are successfully concluded and a mature differentiated H-chain gene is formed, the entire gene is transcribed and the precursor mRNA is processed, giving rise to a mature mRNA with all coding sequences contiguous. This mature mRNA then is translated into a completed heavy chain. The first heavy chain synthesized is the μ chain of the IgM antibody.

Constant-Region Genes

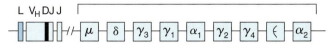

FIGURE 8-5 The human heavy-chain gene locus. The mature, differentiated heavy-chain locus has rearranged variable-region genes as described in Figure 8-4. The exons encoding the constant regions of each of the classes and subclasses of heavy chain are located downstream from the rearranged V-region genes. The order of these constant-region genes is shown here. Note: genes encoding subclasses of a given isotype are not necessarily adjacent to one another.

this results in the deletion of the DNA between the chosen D and J genes. This preliminary joining event can result in the production of DJ_HC_H transcripts from a conserved promoter 5′ to the D segment but 3′ to the V_H genes. The function of these truncated transcripts is not known, although there is some evidence that they are translated.

The next step in the formation of an active heavy-chain gene is the joining of a V_H gene to the already joined DJ_H segment. Again, rearrangement results in the deletion of DNA between the chosen V_H and the chosen D genes (see Fig. 8-4). However, it is not known whether the DNA is lost (by some deletional mechanism) or just relocated (by unequal sister chromatid exchange).

As stated earlier, the heavy-chain constant-region genes (which together encode all the heavy-chain isotypes) all share a common V_H-gene pool. Sequence analysis of cloned DNA has shown that the human C_H-gene segments are encoded by closely linked genes, each of which is separated from the others by a 5- to 30-kilobase intron (Fig. 8-5). These C_H-gene segments are on the 3′ side of the rearranged LV_HDJ_H segment and, in humans, occur in the following order: $5'\text{-}C_\mu$, C_δ, $C_\gamma3$, $C_\gamma1$, $C_\alpha1$, $C_\gamma2$, $C_\gamma4$, C_ε, $C_\alpha2\text{-}3'$. Initiation of Ig synthesis involves the transcription of the LV_HDJ_H segment with the C_μ gene. The result is that the first antibody produced during an immune response is IgM.

As will be discussed later, subsequent gene rearrangements result in a "switch," permitting the synthesis of the same LV_HDJ_H with a different C_H gene (ie, a different isotype or subclass of antibody bearing the same variable region).

Transcription of the Heavy-Chain Gene

Figure 8-6 is a schematic illustration of the rearranged μ-chain gene showing that introns exist between the DNA sequences encoding each domain of μ chain. These introns are spliced out of the precursor RNA to form a functional mRNA. A similar constant-region gene structure and mRNA-splicing mechanism occurs for each of the other isotype genes.

Figure 8-7 illustrates the rearranged heavy-chain locus, showing two additional exons, designated M_μ, which are separated from the $C_\mu4$ exon by an intervening sequence. The first M_μ exon encodes for a hydrophobic 41–amino acid peptide used to anchor membrane-bound IgM to the membrane. This sequence is highly conserved between genes for all the Ig isotypes. The second M_μ exon encodes for a short cytoplasmic tail. There are two polyadenylation sites: one located close to the $C_\mu4$ domain and the other located immediately after the two M_μ exons. Use of the first polyadenylation site results in the production of mRNA for the secreted form of μ chain, whereas use of the second site results in the production of mRNA for the membrane form of μ chain. The controlling elements for the preferential synthesis of one or the other form of mRNA are not known but may involve specific splicing enzymes or specific control of polyadenylation site usage. Regardless of which precursor RNA is made, subsequent splicing removes all the introns (between L and V_H, between V_HDJ_H and C_H, between the domain exons of C_H, between the C_{sec} and C_{mem} exons, and between the C_{mem} exons themselves), providing a

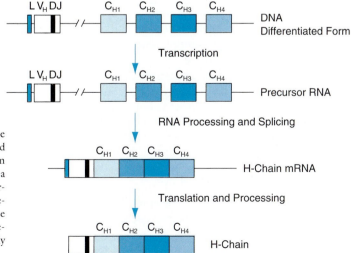

FIGURE 8-6 Structure and expression of a heavy-chain gene. The structure of a model heavy-chain gene is shown, with a rearranged V-region gene with the V, D, and J exons contiguous. The diagram also shows that each of the constant-region domains is encoded by a separate exon. Transcription of both introns and exons gives a precursor mRNA. Subsequent processing removes all introns—those between the V-region and the constant-region genes, as well as those between each of the exons encoding the C-region domains. Subsequent translation leads to the mature H-chain protein. Note: only IgM and IgE have four C-region domains.

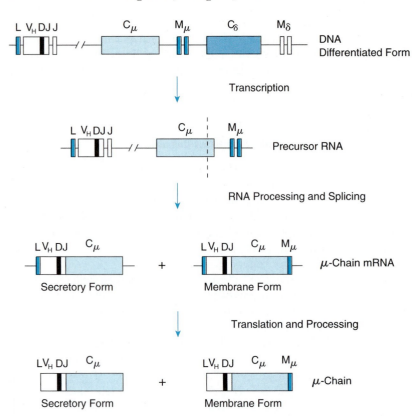

FIGURE 8-7 Formation and translation of mRNA for secretory and membrane-bound IgM. IgM can exist in two forms: as the antigen-specific monomeric receptor on B cells or as a secreted pentameric antibody. Transcription of the mature H-chain gene results in the production of a single large precursor mRNA, which contains all the information for the production of mRNA encoding both forms of μ chain. Subsequent splicing of this large precursor mRNA gives rise to one or both mature mRNA species. Production of the membrane form of μ chain results from splicing the precursor RNA at a site within the exon for the $C_\mu 4$ domain (*dotted line*) and fusing it to the exons (the M_μ sequences) encoding the transmembrane and cytoplasmic portions of the membrane form. Splicing at a site on the 3′ end of the $C_\mu 4$ exon results in an mRNA encoding the secretory form of μ chain.

functional mRNA, with all expressed sequences contiguous to each other.

As discussed earlier, all B cells have mIg, and, although most B cells have IgM and IgD, B cells with mIg of other isotypes arise after stimulation with antigen. Each heavy-chain isotype gene has exons (similar to the M_μ exons) 3′ to the constant-region genes encoding transmembrane and cytoplasmic segments of membrane-bound heavy chain. In all B cells, the production of mIg or secreted Ig of each isotype appears to be regulated in a manner essentially identical to that described earlier for the μ chain.

Thus, mIg functions as the antigen-specific receptor. Antigen binding to this receptor Ig will induce, under the proper conditions, proliferation or differentiation of the B cell to antibody-forming plasma cells and memory B cells. After activation, there is no change in the light-chain or the $V_H DJ_H$ gene being transcribed and translated. The only changes that do occur are in the constant region of the heavy chain. Thus, the secreted antibody has the same specificity as did the Ig receptor on the original B cell.

Regulation of Gene Rearrangement

This complex system of gene rearrangement is thought to be catalyzed by enzymes called *recombinases*. Sequence analysis of cloned germline (nonrearranged) Ig genes shows that all gene segments possess specific flanking base

sequences that are, most probably, the recognition sites for these recombinases. The highly conserved arrangement of these sequences determines which rearrangements can occur. For example, on the 3′ side of all V_L-gene segments, there is a conserved seven-nucleotide sequence (CACAGTC) and a conserved nine-nucleotide sequence (ACAAAAACC or ACATAAACC; Fig. 8-8). These sequences are separated by 23 nucleotides of essentially random sequence (ie, a spacer sequence). Similarly, on the 5′ side of each J_L segment are the same seven-nucleotide and nine-nucleotide sequences. However, those 5′ to J_L are separated by a 12-nucleotide spacer. During rearrangement, it has been suggested that base pairing occurs between the heptamers and between the nonamers, forming a structure that is recognized by the recombinase. This structure results from the fact that the length of the spacers is such that the 12-base spacer represents a single turn of the DNA helix, whereas the 23-base spacer represents two turns. This arrangement allows the heptamers and nonamers from each participating gene to be located on the same side of the DNA helix. Cleavage and ligation of DNA at this juncture would result in a DNA segment with contiguous V and J sequences. If this rearrangement is such that the V- and J-region sequences are in frame (ie, it does not give premature transcriptional or translational termination), a functional variable-region gene is formed.

Similar sequences are found in the germline heavy-chain gene. However, significant variations are seen in

Ig Genes

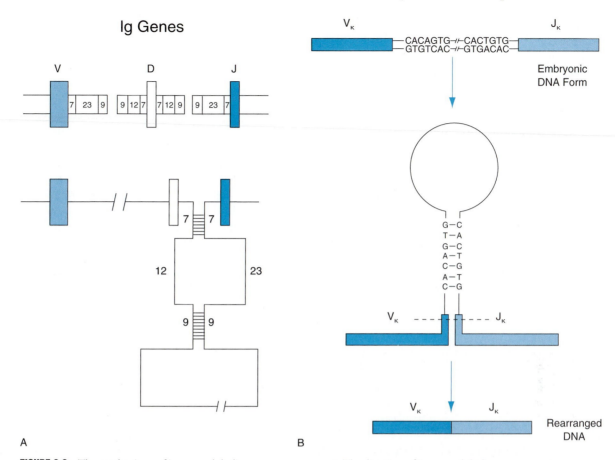

FIGURE 8-8 The mechanisms of immunoglobulin gene rearrangement. The direction of immunoglobulin gene rearrangement during differentiation is controlled by nucleotide sequences within the introns 5′ and 3′ to the V-, D-, and J-region exons. Specific base pairing between heptanucleotide sequences and between nonanucleotide sequences adjacent to V-region exons brings these exons into juxtaposition, enabling subsequent recombinational events to bring the appropriate coding sequences together. Furthermore, the separation of the heptanucleotide and nonanucleotide sequences adjacent to any one exon determines which exons can be joined. **A.** The arrangement around the V, D, and J exons encoding an H-chain V region is one example. The V exon has 3′ heptanucleotide and nonanucleotide sequences separated by a 23-base spacer. A similar arrangement is seen 5′ to the J exon. However, the D exon has 5′ and 3′ heptanucleotide and nonanucleotide sequences separated by a 12-base spacer. The 12/23 rule for immunoglobulin gene rearrangement states that an exon with a 3′ 23-base spacer can rearrange only with an exon with a 5′ 12-base spacer. This requirement makes sense if one realizes that 12 bases is equivalent to one turn of the DNA helix, whereas 23 bases is equivalent to two turns of the helix. This requirement results in the same strand of DNA being brought together and presented to the recombinase enzyme responsible for joining of the DNA segments. Thus, for H chain, the V exon can join only to the D exon and not to the J exon, and so forth. **B.** A similar situation is illustrated for the κ–light-chain gene, showing that the heptanucleotide and nonanucleotide sequences are inverted repeats. For simplicity, the nonanucleotide inverted repeat is omitted. Cleavage and ligation would occur at the dotted line, eliminating the intervening sequences.

the 12- and 23-spacer sequences. In contrast to the V_L gene discussed above, on the 3′ side of each V_H gene, the heptamer and nonamer conserved sequences are separated by a 23-nucleotide spacer. On the 5′ side of each J_H gene, the conserved sequences also are separated by a 23-nucleotide spacer. However, on *both* sides of the D gene, these conserved sequences are separated by a 12-nucleotide spacer. If the 12/23 rule discussed earlier is invoked for the heavy-chain locus, it is obvious that the V_H gene can recombine with the D gene but not with

the J gene, and that the D gene can recombine with both the V_H gene and a J_H gene (see Fig. 8-8).

Humans and mice with severe combined immunodeficiency disease (SCID) are unable to produce appreciable numbers of functional B cells or T cells. The defect in SCID mice that leads to this disease appears to be related to extremely low recombinase activity, which is responsible for the rearrangement of the Ig heavy- and light-chain genes and for similar rearrangements in the formation of functional antigen-specific receptors on T cells (see Chap.

9). The basis for the defect in human SCID is unknown, but most probably also is due to a lack of the recombinase.

Regulation of Heavy-Chain and Light-Chain Gene Transcription

Heavy- and light-chain gene transcription is under the control of promoter sequences 5' to each V-region coding sequence. In addition, this transcription is under the control of positive regulatory elements, termed *enhancers.* These enhancer elements are specific DNA sequences located in the intron between the J gene and the C gene for each Ig chain (Fig. 8-9; see Figs. 8-3 and 8-4). These enhancer sequences act in a *cis,* distance-independent manner (at least up to several kilobases), in conjunction with a soluble factor essential for their activity, to promote transcription from a V_H or V_L promoter.

Each unjoined V gene (embryonic form) possesses its own promoter, yet it is not transcribed at detectable levels in B cells. After rearrangement during B-cell maturation, the V-gene promoter is thought to be brought sufficiently close to the enhancer to allow activation.

Evidence indicates that one or more soluble factors that bind to enhancer sequences may be required for activation of transcription. These transcription factors appear to be tissue-specific in that soluble factors from lymphoid cells, but not from fibroblasts, enhance transcription of mature Ig genes.

Thus, differentiation from a stem cell to a B cell involves the rearrangement of Ig variable-region genes so that each is brought into proximity to an enhancer element 3' to the J segment and 5' to the constant-region gene (see Figs. 8-3 and 8-4). Production of tissue-specific factors that bind to the enhancer sequence promotes subsequent transcription of the mature Ig gene.

Heavy-Chain Class Switch

It is well established that after gene rearrangement of the variable regions of either light or heavy chains has occurred, a particular cell is committed to synthesize that specific V region. This is not true for the constant region of the heavy chains, however, because it has been shown that a cell can switch from the synthesis of IgM to that of another class. This switch involves an additional gene rearrangement in which the V_HDJ_H-gene segment is rearranged and transcribed with a different class of constant heavy-chain gene. This switch allows each of the various biologic effector functions associated with the different Ig isotypes to be expressed with the same antigen-binding specificity.

The details of such a switch are not completely known, but data indicate that after antigen activation, an IgM^+IgD^+ B cell can differentiate and begin to express another heavy-chain isotype. This class switch occurs by recombination between switch regions (see Fig. 8-9) that are 5' to each C_H gene (except for the δ-chain gene) and 3' to the enhancer sequences discussed earlier. Each switch region is made up of repeating (15 or so) short (50 to 80 bases) nucleotide sequences. All recombinations studied thus far involving a heavy-chain switch have occurred within one of these repeating sequences. The switch site for each heavy-chain gene differs in sequence

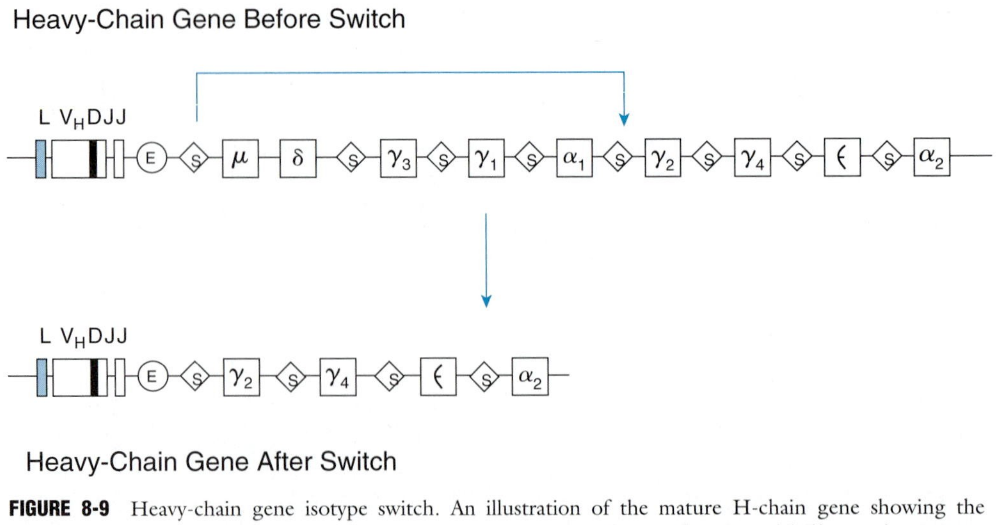

Heavy-Chain Gene Before Switch

Heavy-Chain Gene After Switch

FIGURE 8-9 Heavy-chain gene isotype switch. An illustration of the mature H-chain gene showing the rearranged V, D, and J exons; the H-chain constant-region genes; the switch regions (*S*) 5' to each constant-region gene; and the enhancer sequences (*E*) located 5' to the constant region gene and 3' to the rearranged V-region genes. The H-chain switch results in the enhancer sequences being placed 5' to the switch site of any one of the other constant-region genes. The switch can occur either by deletion of DNA between the two switch sites or by sister chromatid exchange. Note: the δ-chain gene is the only H-chain gene without a 5' switch region.

and size of the repeat, with the μ-chain switch site being the shortest and simplest. Within each of the other switch sites are sequences homologous to the μ-chain switch sequence. The role these μ-like sequences play in the isotype switch is not fully understood.

It has been shown that the DNA between the switch site 5' to C_μ and the switch site 5' to the newly expressed heavy chain is missing, but whether this occurs by a deletional mechanism or by unequal sister chromatid exchange is not fully established.

One seeming paradox of the deletion of heavy-chain genes during switching is evident in the sIgs of B cells, in which both IgM and IgD (and in some instances, other isotypes) are synthesized simultaneously as surface receptors. To explain these observations, it has been postulated that extremely long precursor RNA molecules are produced that contain the coding sequences for δ chain (or other isotype) in addition to those for μ chain. Subsequent splicing would yield mRNA encoding for each of the heavy-chain isotypes.

Because the switch involves DNA sequences 3' to the enhancer elements and the V_HDJ_H gene, the new heavy-chain gene is under the same transcriptional control as was the μ gene in the parental B cell.

ALLELIC EXCLUSION

Because each individual inherits one chromosome of each pair from each parent, each antibody-producing cell contains a paternal chromosome specifying one allotype and a maternal chromosome encoding a different allotype. Analysis of Igs produced by a heterozygous individual shows that about half carry the maternal allotype and the other half carry the paternal allotype. It is clear that both allelic forms of the Ig gene are being transcribed. However, in any one cell, only one allele is expressed. Thus, expression of the maternal allele is *excluded* in some cells and expression of the paternal allele is *excluded* in others. This *allelic exclusion* occurs within each of the light- and heavy-chain loci.

At the molecular level, this could occur if only one chromosome undergoes gene rearrangement, or if the second chromosome undergoes a faulty rearrangement that causes it to be nonfunctional. DNA sequencing of myeloma genes indicates that both processes can occur. It has been estimated that a large fraction of the heavy-chain gene rearrangements are nonfunctional on both chromosomes; thus, the probability of a functional rearrangement occurring on both chromosomes within a single cell is small. Cells with this double faulty rearrangement at the heavy-chain locus are thought to be deleted.

In many cases, however, light-chain rearrangements have occurred on only a single chromosome, perhaps reflecting the fewer number of rearrangements necessary to form a functional gene. The exception are λ-light-chain–expressing B cells in which both κ-chain genes are aberrantly rearranged.

GENERATION OF DIVERSITY

The immune system of a single individual has the ability to synthesize antibody to any one of a large number (perhaps tens of millions) of antigenic determinants. There are several possible mechanisms that, if acting in concert, could generate the necessary diversity.

Combinatorial Association

There are about 100 to 300 V_H genes, 10 D genes, and 4 J_H genes. All possible combinations of these would give 4000 (using the conservative number of 100 V_H genes) different possible heavy-chain variable-region genes. Similar calculations for 100 to 300 V_κ and 4 J_κ genes give a possible 400 κ-chain genes. Taking into account the fact that there are 6 λ-chain constant-region genes in humans, each with its own V_λ-gene pool, about 2400 (6 × 400) λ-chain genes can be estimated. Assuming the random association of any light chain with any heavy chain, 1,600,000 (400 × 4000) antibody molecules with κ light chain and 9,600,000 (2400 × 4000) antibody molecules with λ light chain would be predicted, providing a number that is already in the tens of millions.

Flexible Recombination

During rearrangement of V_L to J_L, D to J_H, and V_H to DJ_H, the exact point of recombination is flexible within a few nucleotides. This results in the formation of different codons that can cause amino acid changes in the third CDR of either light chain or in the fourth CDR of the heavy chain. This recombinational flexibility has been observed at the DNA and at the protein level. The increase in diversity to be expected from such a mechanism is at least 4-fold for each light chain and 16-fold for heavy chain (4-fold for D-to-J_H joining and 4-fold for V-to-DJ_H joining). This would increase the number of κ light chains from 400 to 1600, the number of λ light chains from 2400 to 9600, and the number of heavy chains from 4000 to 64,000. The resulting number of antibodies would be about 10^9 molecules. It can quickly be seen that even if a small fraction (eg, 1%) of these molecules were possible, the number would readily exceed that necessary to respond to a very large number of antigens.

N-Region Addition

It has been shown that a few additional base pairs can be added during the rearrangement process. In the heavy-chain gene, these additions are found in the rearranged

VDJ gene on each side of the D-gene sequences; in the light-chain genes, the additions are found in the rearranged gene between the V and J sequences. Thus, during rearrangement, and probably soon after recombinase cleavage of the DNA (see earlier), extra nucleotides are added to the exposed free ends of the DNA by a mechanism proposed to involve the enzyme terminal deoxynucleotide transferase. The number (although few) and type of nucleotides added appear to be random.

Somatic Mutation

Random mutation within the sequences encoding the V region of light or heavy chain would be expected to generate further antigen-binding specificities. Such mutations have been observed and seem to occur more frequently, but not exclusively, in B cells that have undergone the heavy-chain isotype switch. Furthermore, most of the mutations seem to occur in the variable region, not the constant region, of the heavy-chain gene. The mechanism responsible for this "switch-related" somatic mutation is not known.

GENE REARRANGEMENT AND B-CELL DIFFERENTIATION

The molecular events discussed earlier are given in sufficient detail to enable the reader to appreciate the complex series of events leading to the formation of B cells with functional antigen-specific receptors and the changes in these receptors observed after interaction with antigen. The summary given here is designed to place these molecular events in the proper context of the differentiating steps discussed at the beginning of the chapter.

The differentiation of a lymphoid stem cell to a pre–B cell is the first recognizable step leading to cells of the B-cell lineage. During this differentiating step, the heavy-chain gene rearranges, leading to expression of the μ chain, which remains in the cytoplasm.

The next differentiating step is the formation of an immature B cell with IgM monomers on its surface. During the differentiating step from the pre–B cell to the immature B cell, the light-chain genes rearrange. The κ-chain genes are the first to rearrange. If successful, all rearrangements stop and κ light chain is produced. If unsuccessful, rearrangement at the λ-chain locus is initiated, and λ light chain is produced. Whichever light chain is produced, it associates with the membrane form of μ chain, and monomer IgM is inserted into the plasma membrane as the antigen-specific receptor. It is at this stage that the cells emigrate from the bone marrow to the peripheral lymphoid organs. Soon after arrival in the peripheral lymphoid organs, mature B cells are formed from immature B cells. This is accompanied by the expression of δ chain *in addition to the μ chain*, and both IgM and IgD are inserted into the membrane as antigen-

specific receptors. The same rearranged VDJ gene is used to form the light chain. Only one light chain is expressed, and it is associated with both μ and δ chains. Therefore, the IgD and IgM receptors on a given mature B cell have identical antigen-binding sites.

All these differentiating steps occur in the absence of specific antigen. Thus, B-cell maturation, including selection of the specificity of its antigen receptors, is a preprogrammed series of events. The role of antigen is merely to interact with B cells expressing the appropriate

A Closer Look

The detailed molecular structure of Ig genes and the molecular rearrangements that occur during B-lymphocyte development are now reasonably well understood. This knowledge has enabled us to understand antibody diversity and has resulted in the more precise diagnosis of various B-lymphocyte malignancies, including leukemias and lymphomas.

Complete understanding of B-cell and T-cell development and expression of the antibody repertoire by B cells and of the T-cell–receptor repertoire by T cells will enable us to customize the immune system and reconstitute specific immune deficiencies in patients who require correction as a result of inborn errors or acquired deficiencies.

Our accumulated knowledge regarding the differentiation of B lymphocytes before and after encounter with antigen has greatly facilitated investigations of the normal functioning of these cells, as well as permitted us to understand the defects and deficiencies that can occur in them. Severe combined immunodeficiency (SCID) can be caused by the inability of lymphocyte–stem cells to differentiate and by enzyme deficiencies such as adenosine deaminase (ADA) deficiency. One of the main thrusts of somatic cell gene therapy is to treat SCID in humans by using cells carrying the functional gene, the gene for ADA in this example, to repair the gene defect in a patient. The first clinical trials using this approach were performed in 1990 with promising results. Arising from these studies will be not only a better understanding of B-lymphocyte maturation, but also a coordinated effort and ability to correct defects and errors when they occur. Perhaps, in the future, we will be able to direct B-lymphocyte development and differentiation along specific lines so as to vaccinate essentially everyone against specific infectious agents before these agents are encountered naturally.

receptor and to cause them to expand clonally and further differentiate into antibody-secreting plasma cells and memory B cells.

After antigen stimulation, B cells can switch from expressing Ig of one isotype and begin expressing that of another. This antigen-driven differentiating event involves further rearrangement of heavy-chain DNA. However, in this case, the rearrangement merely results in moving the intact rearranged VDJ gene to a position in front of one of the genes encoding the constant regions of another isotype. This differentiating step is accompanied by a fairly high rate of somatic mutation of the DNA encoding the variable region of the resulting heavy chain. Although not exclusive to cells undergoing the isotype switch, this somatic mutation appears to have occurred more frequently in those cells that have switched.

Bibliography

BOOKS

Ikuta K, Uchida N, Friedman J, Weissman IL. Lymphocyte development from stem cells. In: Paul WE, Fathman CG, Metzger H, eds. Annual review of immunology, vol 10. Palo Alto, CA, Annual Reviews, 1992:759.

Kantor AB, Herzenberg LA. Origin of murine B cell lineages. In: Paul WE, Fathman CG, Metzger H, eds. Annual review of immunology, vol 11. Palo Alto, CA, Annual Reviews, 1993:501.

Ravetch JV, Kinet J-P. Fc receptors. In: Paul WE, Fathman CG, Metzger H, eds. Annual review of immunology, vol 9. Palo Alto, CA, Annual Reviews, 1991:457.

Reth M. Antigen receptors on B lymphocytes. In: Paul WE, Fathman CG, Metzger H, eds. Annual review of immunology, vol 10. Palo Alto, CA, Annual Reviews, 1992:97.

Staudt LM, Lenardo MJ. Immunoglobulin gene transcription. In: Paul WE, Fathman CG, Metzger H, eds. Annual review of immunology, vol 9. Palo Alto, CA, Annual Reviews, 1991:378.

Essentials of Medical Microbiology, Fifth Edition, edited by Wesley A. Volk, Bryan M. Gebhardt, Marie-Louise Hammarskjöld, and Robert J. Kadner. Lippincott-Raven Publishers, Philadelphia © 1996.

Chapter 9

T-Cell Development, Receptors, and Genes

T cells are those cells whose differentiation is dependent on the microenvironment present in the thymus. As discussed briefly in Chapter 7, T cells are antigen-specific cells that are involved both in cell-mediated immune responses and in the generation of antibody responses.

Our knowledge of T cells and the mechanisms by which they interact with other cell types is derived from many different kinds of studies. Antibodies have been produced that recognize human T-cell differentiation molecules. These antibodies have been used to study the expression of cell-surface markers during the differentiation of T cells in the thymus. They also have been used to aid in the isolation of some of these cell-surface molecules for structural analysis. Recombinant DNA technology has been used to study the expression of several genes that are important in T-cell differentiation and in the antigen-activation of mature T cells. What has emerged from these studies is a molecular model of the T-cell recognition complex made up of several polypeptides, each playing a separate, yet coordinated, role in T-cell recognition of antigen and transduction of the recognition signal to the interior of the cell. In addition, numerous studies have provided a clearer understanding of the mechanisms by which T cells, after activation, perform their various functions. They have shown that T cells function primarily by secretion of protein molecules that interact with a wide variety of other cell types. The end result is the regulation of immune responses to most foreign organisms and direct participation in the elimination of cells harboring certain infectious organisms.

The role of T cells in the control of immune responses and the elimination of foreign organisms is discussed in later chapters. In this chapter, we discuss the developmental pathway leading to the formation of T cells. We describe the T-cell recognition complex present on mature T cells. This includes a detailed discussion of the genes that encode the antigen-specific component (the *T-cell receptor* or *TCR*) of the T-cell recognition complex and the way in which the diversity required for responding to a variety of infectious organisms is derived. Finally, TCR expression during ontogeny is discussed, along with

TABLE 9-1
Properties of Components of the T-cell Recognition Complex

Component	Polypeptide* Chain	Molecular† Weight (daltons)	Glycosylated
TCR (Ti)	α	49,000–54,000	+
	β	43,000	+
CD3	γ	25,000	+
	δ	20,000	+
	ε	20,000	–
	ζ	20,000	–
CD4		55,000–60,000	+
CD8		32,000–35,000	+

* The TCR is composed of two polypeptide chains. The CD3 molecule has six polypeptide chains, one each of the γ-, δ- and ε-chains and three ζ-chains. Both the CD4 and CD8 polypeptide chains are monomeric.
† Molecular weights are given for the glycosylated forms and may vary, depending on the extent of glycosylation. Therefore, the ranges most frequently observed are given here.

the selective processes occurring in the thymus that lead to the repertoire of antigen-specific T cells in the mature organism.

T-Cell Development

Many cell-surface molecules on thymocytes and thymus-derived lymphocytes (T cells) are differentiation markers (ie, they are present only at certain stages of the differentiating pathway). The term *CD,* for *c*luster of *d*ifferentiation, and a number are assigned to each marker as it is discovered and shown to be unique (eg, CD2, CD3, CD4). Many CD markers have been defined, and Table

9-1 lists those that apply to this discussion of T-cell differentiation. It also lists some properties of these markers.

ANTIGEN-INDEPENDENT T-CELL DIFFERENTIATION

The overall T-cell differentiation scheme is shown in Figure 9-1. CD3 is a cell-surface molecule present on most thymocytes and all peripheral T cells. It is closely associated with the antigen-specific receptor on T cells and is an integral part of the TCR.

The CD4 and CD8 molecules are useful in defining thymocyte subpopulations and functional T-cell subsets. Each of these molecules also is an integral part of the T-cell antigen-specific recognition complex. Using these markers, thymic lymphocytes can be divided into five major subpopulations as follows:

1. Cortical stem CD3⁻4⁻8⁻ cells, which constitute about 5% of the total thymocyte population.
2. CD3⁺4⁻8⁻ double-negative cortical thymocytes, which are a minor population (10%) and express the γ/δ TCR (see later).
3. CD3⁺4⁺8⁺ (double-positive) cells, which constitute most of the cortical thymocytes (70%) and express the α/β TCR.
4. α/β⁺CD4⁺8⁻ medullary cells (10%).
5. α/β⁺CD4⁻8⁺ medullary cells (5%).

A few other subpopulations, each representing a small fraction of the total thymocytes, also are found. In the mouse, one such subpopulation in the cortex bears markers of mature T cells, yet represents only about 1% to 3% of the total thymocytes. This subpopulation also bears a cell-surface receptor that recognizes a ligand on epithelial cells of high endothelial venules in lymph nodes and Peyer's patches and is responsible for lymphocyte homing to specific lymphoid organs. As discussed in Chapter 7, Weissman and colleagues have shown that these cortical

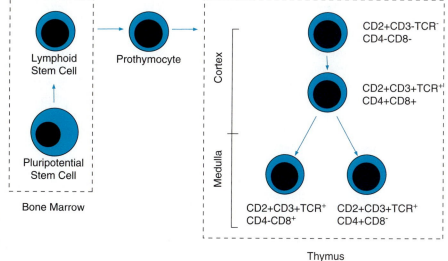

FIGURE 9-1 T-cell development pathway. T-lymphocyte development begins in the bone marrow with a pluripotential stem cell, as it does for all blood cells. A prothymocyte, committed to the T-cell pathway, emigrates from the bone marrow to the thymus, where it undergoes a series of differentiating steps leading to all varieties of mature T lymphocytes. Thymic differentiation begins in the cortex and proceeds to the medulla. It is accompanied by the acquisition or loss of cell-surface molecules. Each of the cell-surface molecules indicated in this figure plays a role in differentiation to mature thymocytes and, later, in activation of the mature T cell by foreign antigen.

thymocytes may be the precursors of the peripheral T cells.

T-Cell Subsets

There are two possible pathways of T-cell differentiation (see Fig. 9-1).

The hypothesis that the medullary thymocytes are the direct precursors of peripheral T cells is based solely on the observation that the two medullary subpopulations are functionally mature. The suggestion that cortical thymocytes are the precursors of mature T cells is supported by experimental observations, some of which were discussed earlier.

The end result of the thymocyte differentiation is the production of two distinct functional subsets of T cells:

1. Helper T cells (Th cells), which regulate antigen-specific activation of B cells and effector T cells.
2. Cytotoxic T cells (Tc cells), which also are involved in cell-mediated immune responses and lyse target cells by direct cell–cell contact.

Subpopulations of Th cells and cytotoxic T cells may yet be defined. There is considerable evidence for the existence of Th1 and Th2 subpopulations of Th cells. Th1 cells produce interleukin-2 and γ-interferon; Th2 cells produce interleukin-4 and interleukin-5. Within the cytotoxic T-cell subset, there may be a subpopulation of regulatory cells that dampen immune responses (ie, suppressor T cells).

In humans, these two functional subsets belong to two phenotypic groups of T lymphocytes. The Th cells have the $CD3^+4^+8^-$ phenotype. The cytotoxic T cells have the $CD3^+4^-8^+$ phenotype.

ANTIGEN-DEPENDENT T-CELL DIFFERENTIATION

The formation of these subsets of T cells is a normal differentiating event and is entirely independent of the presence of antigen. Moreover, as with B cells, the effect of antigen is merely to react with those T cells bearing receptors for that antigen and to activate the selected T cells to perform a preprogrammed function. Here we see that a major prediction of the clonal selection theory of Burnet and Fenner (see Chap. 3) has proved to be accurate.

Antigen activation leads to both the production of effector T cells and the generation of memory T cells. There are memory T cells for each functional subset and, in some cases, they can be distinguished from unstimulated virgin cells. For example, activated human Th cells, but not virgin Th cells, express class II (Ia; see Chap. 10) antigen on their surface. Expression of Th cell function by virgin Th cells requires DNA, RNA, and protein synthesis,

but memory Th cells do not require DNA synthesis to provide help to Tc or B cells. However, DNA synthesis always is required to generate memory cells.

Antigen-specific activation of the T-cell subsets is discussed in greater detail in later chapters.

T-Cell Receptors and Genes

THE T-CELL RECOGNITION COMPLEX

The nature of the antigen-specific TCR was far more difficult to characterize than that of the B-cell receptor. T cells, in general, do not bind free antigen as do B cells; instead, they recognize a foreign antigen in association with cell-surface molecules encoded by genes in the major histocompatibility complex (MHC; see Chap. 10). This property, termed *MHC restriction*, is common to recognition of antigen by most T cells. Therefore, the use of antigen as a probe for the receptor proved unsuccessful, and numerous attempts to use antisera that are specific for the variable or constant regions of immunoglobulin (Ig) as probes for the TCR gave ambiguous results. These latter experiments were based on the assumption that because both B cells and T cells are antigen specific, they probably use receptors that are structurally and, therefore, antigenically related. Significant insight into the real nature of the TCR was gained with the production of antisera that are specific for individual T-cell clones.

Normal T cells can be propagated in vitro and, after cloning, can be used to immunize mice for the production of monoclonal antibodies (Mabs). In 1982 and 1983, Ellis Reinherz and colleagues cloned human T cells and prepared Mabs that were specific for each clone. These Mabs then were used to immunoprecipitate radioactively labeled molecules from the surface of the T-cell clones. In each case, the Mab reacted with a glycoprotein having a molecular weight of about 90,000 daltons. This glycoprotein was found to be a heterodimer made up of two glycosylated polypeptides with molecular weights of about 50,000 (α chain) and 43,000 (β chain) daltons, which were cross-linked by a disulfide bond to give the 90,000-dalton α/β-heterodimeric molecule recognized by the Mab.

Other studies, using a variety of Mabs, revealed that the CD3, CD4, and CD8 molecules also are involved in the antigen-recognition and T-cell activation process. Antibodies to the CD3, CD4, or CD8 molecules either enhance or inhibit T-cell activation, but these molecules are not clonally specific and are not involved in antigen recognition per se. All three of these CD molecules, however, were found to be physically associated with the 90,000-dalton clonally specific TCR glycoprotein on the surface of the T cell.

The α/β, clonally specific, heterodimeric TCR is present on most peripheral T cells in association with the

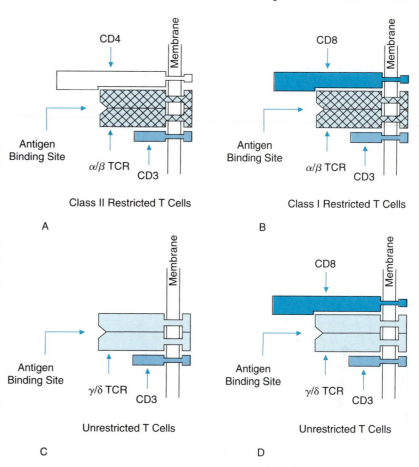

FIGURE 9-2 The T-cell recognition complex. T cells with different cell-surface antigen recognition structures have been demonstrated. The minimal recognition complex is composed of a heterodimeric, antigen-specific receptor (TCR) and an invariant CD3 molecule. T cells with the α/β TCR (**A** and **B**) also have either the invariant CD4 or CD8 molecule as part of their recognition complex. Whether a T cell has the CD4 or the CD8 molecule depends on whether the TCR recognizes antigen complexed with class II or class I major histocompatibility complex (MHC) molecules, respectively. T cells with γ/δ TCRs (**C** and **D**) also have been described. These cells also have the invariant CD3 molecule as part of their recognition complex, and some have the CD8 molecule as well, although the γ/δ TCR does not appear to recognize antigen complexed with either class I or class II MHC molecules. Other cell-surface adhesion molecules, such as lymphocyte functional antigen-1, also play a nonspecific role in T-cell interaction with other cells. The α/β cells represent 90% to 95% of the circulating T-cell pool. The γ/δ cells, although they make up only 5% to 10% of the circulating T-cell pool, represent the major population in the skin and in the intraepithelial spaces between cells lining the intestine.

CD3 and either the CD4 or the CD8, but not both, cell-surface molecules. Thus, most peripheral T cells are either of the $TCR^+CD3^+4^+8^-$ or the $TCR^+CD3^+4^-8^+$ phenotype. These complexes constitute the minimum T-cell, antigen-specific recognition complex (Fig. 9-2*A* and *B*, respectively). The properties of the polypeptides that make up each of these cell surface molecules are given in Table 9-1.

T cells with a different recognition complex also have been described (see Fig. 9-2*C* and *D*). These cells express an antigen-specific, heterodimeric receptor (TcR) made up of two polypeptide chains (γ and δ) that are structurally related to the heterodimeric α and β chains discussed earlier. These γ/δ cells are of either the $CD3^-4^-8^-$ or the $CD3^+4^-8^+$ phenotype and constitute only 0.5% to 10% of the peripheral T-cell pool.

Thus, there are two general types of T cells with recognition complexes that see antigen differently. Most T cells are α/β^+ (they also express CD3 and either CD4 or CD8) and recognize antigen in the context of MHC-gene products. The γ/δ^+ minor population of T cells (that also express CD3 and occasionally CD8) is not MHC-restricted in their recognition of antigen. Whether these latter T cells see antigen in association with another cell-surface molecule is not known.

The Heterodimeric Antigen-Specific Receptor (TCR)

The α, β, γ, and δ chains of the TCRs are cell-surface glycoproteins structurally related to the Ig heavy and light chains (ie, they are members of the Ig superfamily; Fig. 9-3). Each polypeptide chain contains four domains: two extracellular domains, one transmembrane domain, and one cytoplasmic domain. The α and β chains of the α/β TCR are disulfide bonded to each other on the cell surface, as are the γ and δ chains of the γ/δ TCR. The β chain appears to have seven hypervariable (complementarity-determining) regions (or at least a high level of variability), as opposed to three for human Ig light chain and four for human Ig heavy chain. The structure of the genes encoding each of these polypeptide chains is shown in Figure 9-4. The mechanisms by which these genes rearrange to provide the wide diversity required for recognition of the vast array of antigens are described later.

THE β-CHAIN GENE. Cloning of the β-chain gene was described independently by Mark Davis and colleagues at Stanford University and by Tak Mak and collaborators at Toronto. Structural analyses of the β-chain genes from several different human and mouse T-cell clones revealed the structure shown in Figure 9-4*A*. Like the heavy-chain

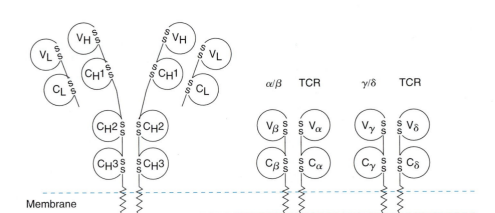

FIGURE 9-3 The TCR polypeptide chains are members of the immunoglobulin superfamily. Each TCR is made up of two distinct polypeptide chains (either α and β or γ and δ), both of which are structurally similar to the H- and L-chain genes of immunoglobulin and several other cell–cell interaction molecules. Each TCR polypeptide chain has four functional domains: the variable, constant, and transmembrane regions, and the cytoplasmic tail.

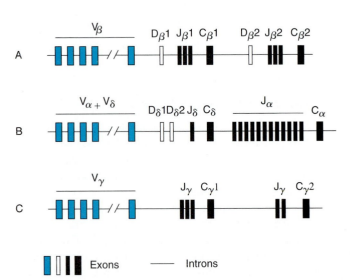

FIGURE 9-4 Structure of the genes encoding the TCR polypeptide chains. Each TCR locus is made up of multiple coding sequences (exons) separated by noncoding regions (introns), similar to that described in Chapter 8 for immunoglobulin H and L chains. The α-chain locus (**B**) has multiple V and J genes, along with a single C-region gene. The γ-chain locus (**C**) also has multiple V genes but has two C-region genes, each with its own set of J_α genes. The $J_\alpha C_\alpha$ sets share the same V-region gene pool. The β-chain locus (**A**) has a structure similar to that of the γ locus in that there are two C-region genes, each with its own set of J_β genes. In addition, each C_β gene has its own D-region gene. The $D_\beta J_\beta C_\beta$ sets share the same V_β gene pool. The δ-chain locus has an unusual location: it resides entirely within the α-chain locus (**B**). It has a single C-region gene, two D-region genes, and one J gene. The V_δ genes are interspersed with the V_α genes. Because of the unusual structure of the α and δ loci, rearrangement of the α-chain genes results in excision of the D_δ, J_δ, and C_δ genes, precluding subsequent expression of the δ-chain locus in α/β^+ T cells.

gene of Ig, the β-chain gene is made up of multiple V-, D-, and J-region genes; unlike the Ig heavy-chain gene, however, it has two essentially identical constant-region genes (that are not isotypes). Each constant-region gene has its own set of D- and J-segment genes. Both sets of DJ-segment genes share a pool of about 70 V-region genes.

β-CHAIN GENE REARRANGEMENT. The rearrangement of the β-chain gene during differentiation is similar to that of the heavy-chain gene of Ig (see Chap. 8). The same 12/23 rule governs the order and direction of rearrangement, and the recombinases used are thought to be the same as those that mediate Ig-gene rearrangement. These recombinases presumably recognize specific sequences 5' and 3' to the appropriate V_β, D_β, and J_β genes. The main difference between Ig heavy-chain gene rearrangement and TCR β-chain gene rearrangement is that a given V_β-region gene can be joined to the D_β gene of either C_β set, effectively doubling the number of possible VDJ mature TCR genes.

THE α-CHAIN GENE. The structure of the α-chain gene is shown in Figure 9-4B. This gene has about 50 V-region genes, 50 J-region genes, and a single C-region gene. No D-region gene has been found for this locus. During differentiation, rearrangement occurs only after successful rearrangement of the β-chain gene and gives rise to a $V_\alpha J_\alpha$ gene—a structure analogous to that of the Ig light-chain gene.

α-Chain DNA clones from Th cells and cytotoxic T cells have been shown to contain the same C-region coding sequence, although the V regions are different. This seems to eliminate the possibility that the constant region of the TCR determines a T cell's function.

THE γ-CHAIN GENE. The γ-chain gene encodes a glycoprotein with a molecular weight of 55,000 daltons. The γ locus is made up of four C-region genes, each with a single J-region gene and 1 to 3 V-region genes (see Fig. 9-4C). It is not known whether all four C_γ genes are active.

Rearrangement of genes within this locus obeys the same 12/23 rule as does rearrangement of genes within the α-chain and β-chain loci. Because of the small number of V-region and J-region genes, the germline diversity is limited. Therefore, the other mechanisms of generating diversity (see later) are of greater importance.

THE δ-CHAIN GENE. The δ-chain gene has been described only recently (see Fig. 9-4B). It has limited germline diversity in that there are only 10 V-region genes, with their usage split between fetal and adult life. There are two D_δ-genes, one J_δ-gene, and one C_δ-gene. The position of the δ locus on the human chromosome is unusual in that it is located entirely within the TCR α-chain locus. The D_δ, J_δ, and C_δ genes are located between the V_α and the J_α genes and are deleted during rearrangement of the α-chain genes, thus precluding coexpression of the α-chain and δ-chain genes. To complicate events further, V_δ genes are either intermixed with the V_α genes or are a subset of the V_α genes.

Generation of Diversity in the T-Cell Receptor

Germline diversity in the α and β chains is large. In addition, recombinational error during VDJ or VJ joining and N-region addition of extra nucleotides at the junctional sites does occur. These mechanisms, together with combinatorial association of the α and β chains, give rise to a large T-cell repertoire that is at least equivalent to that seen for the Igs (see Chap. 8).

In contrast, the limitation in the number of germline γ and δ V-region genes would appear to limit the diversity that could be obtained in the γ/δ TCR. However, the δ-chain gene has a unique property that would permit generation of great diversity. The arrangement of the recombinase recognition sequences (ie, the nonamer, heptamer, and 12- or 23-base spacer nucleotides) 3′ and 5′ to the V_δ, D_δ, and J_δ genes is different (Fig. 9-5) from that found in the TCR α-, β-, and γ-chain genes or in the Ig heavy- and light-chain genes. Application of the 12/23 rule (see Chap. 8) to this locus allows VJ, VDJ, or VDDJ joining events to occur, giving rise to zero, one, or two D_δ-gene segments in the functionally mature variable-region gene encoding the δ chain. Furthermore, there is evidence for *extensive* N-region addition. Thus, the potential repertoire for the γ/δ TCR is extremely large.

In contrast to Ig genes, there is no evidence for somatic mutation occurring in the TCR genes, at least not at frequencies greater than those seen for random mutation in any gene of the human chromosome. Thus, somatic mutation does not play a role in generating the T-cell repertoire.

Transcription and Translation

Transcription of mature antigen-specific receptor genes in T cells occurs in a manner similar to that for Ig genes in B cells (see Chap. 8). After rearrangement to form functional VDJ (or VJ) genes, the entire DNA sequence from 5′ to the V gene through the C-region gene (including all introns) is transcribed into precursor mRNA. Subsequent splicing and polyadenylation results in a functional mRNA with all coding sequences contiguous. These mRNAs then are translated to give the polypeptide chains of the TCR.

Allelic Exclusion

Only one of the two alleles for each of the α, β, γ, and δ genes is expressed in any given cell. Once successful rearrangement to form a VDJ or VJ gene occurs, subsequent rearrangement at that locus ceases. This allelic exclusion allows for maximum precision of the T-cell system and focuses on the minimum number of cells necessary to respond to foreign antigen.

The CD3, CD4, and CD8 Coreceptors

The CD3 cell-surface marker is a part of the antigen-recognition system of T cells. The CD3 molecule is a glycoprotein made up of six invariant polypeptide chains (γ, δ, ε, and ζ [there are three copies of ζ]), with the properties shown in Table 9-1. The γ chain of CD3 is not to be confused with the γ chain described earlier as part of an antigen-specific receptor on a small population of T cells. There is no structural homology between any of the CD3 polypeptide chains and any member of the Ig superfamily.

Incubation of T cells with antibody to CD3 induces proliferation and increased calcium flux in these cells. Based on the effect of anti-CD3 antibody, it is concluded that the CD3 molecule plays a role in signal transduction, possibly as a Ca^{2+} channel structure. Thus, CD3 is a *coreceptor* in association with the TCR.

Antibodies to the CD4 and CD8 cell-surface molecules block antigen-mediated activation of the CD4$^+$8$^-$ and CD4$^-$8$^+$ T-cell subsets, respectively. Thus, each of these molecules is a component of the T-cell recognition complex. The CD4 molecule is a glycoprotein with a molecular weight of 55,000 daltons that is expressed primarily on T cells of the helper/inducer subset. The CD8 34,000-dalton glycoprotein is expressed by the cytotoxic T-cell subset. Both molecules exhibit significant structural homology with Ig; thus, they are members of the Ig superfamily of cell-surface proteins.

Although it is not totally clear what role the CD8 and CD4 molecules might play in T-cell activation, there

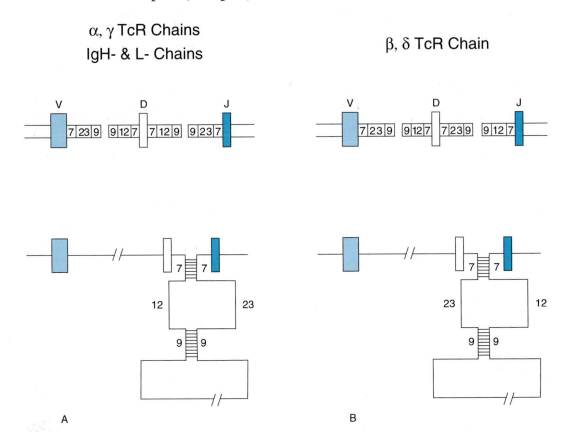

FIGURE 9-5 Mechanisms of T-cell gene rearrangement. T-cell receptor and immunoglobulin gene rearrangement to form functional genes is mediated by specific nonamer (*9*) and heptamer (*7*) base sequences flanking each V, D, and J exon. These nonamer and heptamer sequences are separated by either 12 or 23 base pairs, which represent one and two turns of the DNA helix, respectively. The arrangement of the 12– and 23–base-pair segments around the V, D, and J genes determines which rearrangements can occur. Genes with a 3' 23-base segment can rearrange only with genes that have a 5' 12-base segment. **A.** One example is the general structure of the immunoglobulin H-chain locus. For this locus, the V gene can rearrange with the D gene, but not with the J gene. Similarly, the D gene can rearrange with both the V gene and the J gene, but only in a single orientation. Thus, functional rearrangement of the H-chain locus gives rise only to VDJ genes. The TCR α and γ loci and the immunoglobulin L-chain locus do not have D-region genes, and the order of bases 5' to the J gene is 9-12-7-J. Therefore, only VJ gene rearrangements can occur for these three loci. The 12- and 23-base separator segments allow the same strand of DNA from distant regions to be presented on the face of the DNA molecule, which interacts with the recombinase enzyme that catalyzes the joining event.

B. The structures of the TCR β and δ loci are different. For these loci, the V gene can rearrange with either the D gene or the J gene, giving rise to VJ and VDJ rearranged genes. Additional D-region genes in the δ-chain locus have the same order of segments, allowing for D-to-D joining as well. Thus, for the δ-chain locus, VJ, VDJ, and VDDJ functional rearrangements have been observed. Although the β-chain locus can undergo VJ or VDJ joining, the VJ option rarely is seen. This multitude of possible rearrangements within the δ chain locus can give rise to a large degree of diversity, with few V, D, and J genes.

is good evidence that they interact with class I and class II molecules, respectively. There is mounting evidence that each member of the Ig superfamily interacts with another, yet different, member of the family on another cell (ie, the TCR—with either class I or class II—together with antigen; CD8 with class I; and CD4 with class II). These interactions would tend to direct the CD8⁺ subset to class I–positive target cells (eg, virally infected cells) and the CD4⁺ subset to class II–positive cells (eg, macrophages and B cells).

T-Cell Receptor Gene Expression During Ontogeny

As discussed earlier, gene rearrangements, giving rise to mature TCR genes occur in the thymus. As in heavy-chain gene rearrangement in B cells, the first step appears to involve D-to-J joining, because DJC transcripts are abundant in thymocytes but not in T cells. Rearrangement of the β-chain and γ-chain genes occurs early, followed by rearrangement of the α-chain or δ-chain genes. (Remember that rearrangement of the α-

A Closer Look

The differentiation and maturation of T lymphocytes in the thymus gland is a coordinated process during which T cells express differentiation markers and antigen-specific receptors, and undergo a process of selection whereby self-reactive cells are eliminated and cells capable of recognizing foreign antigens are permitted to survive and proliferate. The processes whereby T lymphocytes mature and, as a population, express an incredible diversity of antigen-specific TCRs is truly one of the remarkable feats of nature.

The germline diversity of the TCR α and β chains is large. Additional diversity beyond that available in the germline comes about as a result of recombinational diversity, which occurs during VDJ and VJ joining, and as a result of end-region additions and deletions of nucleotides in the VDJ segments. Thus, the diversity and extent of the T-cell repertoire are at least equivalent to the diversity of antigen specificities of antibodies.

In a truly remarkable display of adaptation, T lymphocytes learn to discriminate self from nonself during differentiation in the thymus gland. This process whereby self-reactive cells are eliminated and cells capable of recognizing foreign antigens are positively selected for is thought to be an intrathymic occurrence. Some immunologists believe that there may be a postthymic mechanism for the induction of self-tolerance and the elimination of self-reactive cells. However, the evidence for this postthymic system and the mechanism whereby self-reactive cells in the periphery can be deleted or rendered anergic is not understood. It is a tribute to molecular immunologists that they have identified the T-lymphocyte antigen receptor, mapped its detailed structure, and demonstrated its role in T-cell recognition of antigens in association with self-MHC molecules. Armed with this knowledge, we are on the brink of being able to engineer immunologic specificity at the cellular level; we soon will be able to reconstitute specific immunologic defects in patients who have T-cell immune deficiency diseases. Enzyme deficiencies such as purine nucleoside phosphorylase (PNP) and adenosine deaminase deficiencies (ADA), which cause life-threatening immune deficiency disease, have been treated with the technique of somatic cell gene therapy. A patient's T lymphocytes are transfected in vitro with a vector carrying the functional gene and then infused back into the blood. Initial results in terms of numbers of T cells and T cell functional activity are encouraging.

chain gene results in deletion of most of the δ-chain gene.) These rearrangements occur before expression of the CD3/TCR complex on the cell surface. Tonegawa and colleagues have shown that mRNAs that encode the β chain and the γ chain are relatively abundant, and those that encode the α chain and the δ chain are relatively scarce in immature thymocytes. During further development, the level of the α- and δ-chain mRNAs increases, but in different cells. Both V_γ and V_δ are rearranged and expressed in abundance in fetal, but not adult, thymocytes, indicating coordinate control of γ- and δ-gene expression during different stages of differentiation. In $CD3^+4^+8^+$ thymocytes, the β-chain mRNA remains constant, although the α-chain mRNA increases, resulting in expression of the α/β TCR. These latter cells then give rise to the mature $\alpha/\beta CD3^+4^+8^-$ and $\alpha/\beta CD3^+4^-8^+$ cell-surface phenotypes. In a small population of maturing $CD3^+4^-8^-$ thymocytes expressing the γ-chain gene, the δ-chain gene is rearranged, rather than the α-chain gene, resulting in expression of the γ/δ TCR.

SELF–NONSELF DISCRIMINATION IN THE THYMUS

Thymocyte maturation depends primarily on interaction with thymic epithelial cells. Whether T-cell maturation also requires contact with other cells or whether soluble, secreted growth and differentiation factors alone are adequate is still being investigated.

As stated earlier, the TCR does not recognize antigens in solution, as does the B-cell Ig receptor. Rather, it recognizes a complex consisting of antigen bound to either the class I or the class II MHC molecule on the surface of a cell. Thus, each T cell is MHC restricted. During development of T cells in the thymus, both a positive and a negative selection occurs, which limits the spectrum of specificities of the T cells leaving the thymus. This selection determines the ability of mature T cells to discriminate between *self* and *nonself* throughout life.

The positive-selection step expands those cells that are capable of recognizing antigen plus self-MHC (class I or class II). In the negative-selection step, those cells that recognize either self-antigen plus self-MHC or self-MHC alone are eliminated. It is not known which step occurs first, but the overall result is the expansion of T-cell clones that recognize foreign antigen and the elimination of T-cell clones that recognize self-antigens.

Bibliography

JOURNALS

Kroemer G, Martinez A-C. Clonal deletion and anergy: from models to reality. Res Immunol 1992;143:267.
Robey EA, Fowlkes BJ, Pardoll DM. Molecular mechanisms for lineage commitment in T cell development. Semin Immunol 1990;2:25.
Sprent J. The thymus and T cell tolerance. Today's Life Sci 1991;3:14.

BOOKS

Cohen JJ, Duke RC, Fadok VA, Sellins KS. Apoptosis and programmed cell death in immunity. In: Paul WE, Fathman CG, Metzger H, eds. Annual review of immunology, vol 10. Palo Alto, CA, Annual Reviews, 1992:267.

Janeway CA Jr. The T cell receptor as a multicomponent signalling machine: CD4/CD8 coreceptors and CD45 in T cell activation. In: Paul WE, Fathman CG, Metzger H, eds. Annual review of immunology, vol 10. Palo Alto, CA, Annual Reviews, 1992: 645.

Leiden JM. Transcriptional regulation of T cell receptor genes. In: Paul WE, Fathman CG, Metzger H, eds. Annual review of immunology, vol 11. Palo Alto, CA, Annual Reviews, 1993:539.

Matis LA. The molecular basis of T-cell specificity. In: Paul WE, Fathman CG, Metzger H, eds. Annual review of immunology, vol 8. Palo Alto, CA, Annual Reviews, 1990:65

Moss PAH, Rosenberg WMC, Bell JI. The human T-cell receptor in health and disease. In: Paul WE, Fathman CG, Metzger H, eds. Annual review of immunology, vol 10. Palo Alto, CA, Annual Reviews, 1992:71.

Robey E, Fowlkes BJ. Selective events in T-cell development. In: Paul WE, Fathman CG, Metzger H, eds. Annual review of immunology, vol 12. Palo Alto, CA, Annual Reviews, 1994:675.

Essentials of Medical Microbiology, Fifth Edition, edited by Wesley A. Volk,
Bryan M. Gebhardt, Marie-Louise Hammarskjöld, and Robert J. Kadner.
Lippincott-Raven Publishers, Philadelphia © 1996.

Chapter 10

The Major Histocompatibility Complex and Transplantation

Transplantation of tissue from one individual to another invariably leads to rejection of the transplant by the immune system of the recipient. This rejection is specific for cell-surface antigens on the transplanted tissue. These antigens are called *alloantigens* and are encoded by any one of numerous genetic loci within the genome. In mammals, one set of closely linked genes is of primary importance in determining the outcome of transplantation. These genes also play a central role in controlling immune responses to essentially all antigens.

In this chapter, these genes, their products, and their role in transplantation are discussed. The role these genes play in controlling various types of immune responses is discussed in Chapters 11 and 13, and their specific disease associations are presented in Chapter 14.

Transplantable Tumors

Human organ transplantation has had a long and, until relatively recently, unsuccessful history. The discovery of the genetic basis for graft rejection and the development of effective immunosuppressive drugs have made it possible to prolong life by transplanting tissues and organs from one individual to another. Although much is known about the mechanisms of graft rejection, we are still far from achieving a 100% success rate. This is primarily because of the adaptability of the immune system and the extreme polymorphism of the cell-surface antigens responsible for rejection.

The early studies in transplantation biology were concerned more with the transplantability of spontaneously arising tumors from one mouse to another than with the replacement of failed organs in humans. Nevertheless, these studies were of immense value, because they provided an understanding of the genetic and structural basis of graft rejection.

Using outbred strains of mice, George Snell and colleagues showed that a tumor arising spontaneously in one mouse typically was rejected when transplanted to another

TABLE 10-3
Properties Associated With the Major
Histocompatibility Complex

Immune response (Ir) genes (control of immune responses)

Restriction of antigen recognition by T cells (control of immune responses)

Structural genes for major transplantation antigens (graft rejection)

Alloantigen stimulation of cytotoxic T cells (graft rejection)

Stimulation of the mixed lymphocyte reaction (MLC, MLR) (graft rejection)

Graft-versus-host reactions (GVH)

By definition, the cell-surface antigens encoded by genes in each of the H loci are capable of eliciting an immune response and, thus, graft rejection. Because of the large number of H loci, one can appreciate the difficulty that is faced in preventing graft rejection in an outbred species, such as humans, and can marvel at the success that has been achieved.

Unlike studies in mice, which have used inbred and recombinant inbred strains, research into the human MHC has relied almost entirely on population and family studies and, more recently, on recombinant DNA techniques. The MHC in humans is referred to as the human leukocyte antigen (HLA) complex and that in the mouse is referred to as the H-2 complex.

Functions Associated With the Major Histocompatibility Complex

Many immunologic properties have been attributed to genes residing within the MHC (Table 10-3). Graft rejec-

tion already has been mentioned; the others are discussed in the remainder of the immunology section of this book.

The Human Leukocyte Antigen Complex

The structure of the MHC in humans is shown in Figure 10-2. There are three classes of genes with which we must be concerned: *class I, class II,* and *class III* genes. The products of these classes of genes and their role in transplantation and immune responses are discussed later.

CLASS I LOCI

The genes encoding the major transplantation antigens are the *HLA-A, HLA-B,* and *HLA-C* loci in humans. The products of these loci are similar in structure and are referred to as the *class I antigens* (see Fig. 10-2).

In humans, the alloantisera used to detect class I antigens are obtained from multiparous women (ie, women who have had multiple pregnancies), from individuals who have received multiple transfusions, from individuals who have received and rejected grafts, and from volunteers who have been immunized with cells from another individual with a different HLA haplotype (ie, a different combination of genes within the HLA complex).

Class I antigens are expressed on essentially all nucleated cells and, in some species (ie, mice, but not humans), on red blood cells as well (Table 10-4).

Structure of Class I Antigens

Class I antigens are made up of two polypeptide chains (Fig. 10-3). The smaller of these two chains, called β_2-

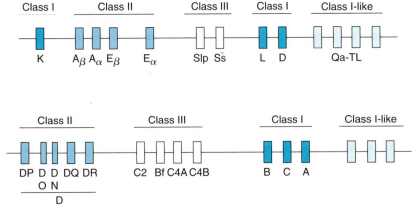

FIGURE 10-2 Genetic map of the mouse and human major histocompatibility complexes (MHCs). MHCs encode proteins involved in graft rejection and in regulation of immune responses. These proteins are grouped into three classes. Class I genes encode a family of structurally related proteins that are the targets for graft rejection and are involved in the regulation of immune responses to endogenously produced antigens such as viral and tumor antigens (see Chaps. 11 and 13). Class II genes encode another group of structurally related antigens that also are involved in graft rejection and in the regulation of immune responses to exogenously produced but processed soluble antigens (see Chap. 11). Class III genes encode several proteins that are members of the complement cascade (see Chap. 12). This illustration incorporates the new human leukocyte antigen nomenclature adopted by the Nomenclature Committee on Leukocyte Antigens in 1987.

TABLE 10-4
Properties of Some Products of the Major Histocompatibility Complex (MHC)

	HLA-A	HLA-B	HLA-C	HLA-D
PRESENT ON				
Macrophages	+	+	+	+
T cells	+	+	+	±
B cells	+	+	+	+
All other nucleated cells*	+	+	+	−
CHARACTERISTICS				
Molecular weight of polypeptide chains†	44,000	44,000	44,000	33,000
	12,000	12,000	12,000	25,000
Immune response (Ir) genes‡	+	+	+	+
Class of antigen	I	I	I	II

* Class II gene products (Ia antigens, HLA-D region products) are found on macrophages, on some activated T cells, and on some other nucleated cells such as epithelial cells and B lymphocytes. Their presence on these other cell types does not necessarily mean that these cells can present antigen in the initiation of immmune responses.
† The 12,000-dalton peptide associated with the HLA-A, HLA-B, and HLA-C molecules is β_2-microglobulin and is encoded by a gene outside the MHC.
‡ Both class I and class II gene products control immune responses by similar mechanisms.

microglobulin (β_2-M), is encoded by a gene located outside the MHC. It has a molecular weight of 12,000 daltons and is the amino acid sequence that is constant for each species. β_2-M is noncovalently associated with all class I antigens on the surface of cells, regardless of which class I locus encodes them.

Structurally, β_2-M is related to immunoglobulin (Ig). Its amino acid sequence is similar to that of antibody heavy chains. It is the same length as an Ig domain (ie, about 110 amino acids long) and possesses an intrachain disulfide bond, as does each domain of antibody heavy and light chains. Thus, β_2-M is a member of the *Ig superfamily* (see Chap. 5).

The larger polypeptide chain of the class I antigen is encoded by the HLA-A, HLA-B, or HLA-C locus. It has a molecular weight of 44,000 daltons and, like β_2-M, bears structural homology to Ig (see Fig. 10-3). Thus, it too is a member of the Ig superfamily. This larger chain has five structural domains. One domain is hydrophobic and is inserted into the plasma membrane of the cell. Another domain is highly charged, is on the cytoplasmic side of the membrane, and presumably serves as an anchor to keep the molecule in the membrane or as a functional link to the interior of the cell. The external portion of this class I polypeptide is divided into three domains: α_1, α_2, and α_3 (see Fig. 10-3).

FIGURE 10-3 Both the class I and the class II MHC-encoded proteins are structurally related to immunoglobulin and are involved in cell–cell interaction in the generation and regulation of immune responses. Therefore, they are members of the larger group of proteins called the immunoglobulin superfamily. Shown here are some of the basic structural properties of these proteins, emphasizing their similarity to immunoglobulin. Both polypeptides of the class II molecule are encoded by genes within the MHC, as is the larger polypeptide chain of the class I molecule. The smaller peptide (β_2-microglobulin [β_2-M]) of the class I molecule is invariant within a species, is associated with *all* class I molecules on the surface of a cell, and is encoded by a gene outside the MHC.

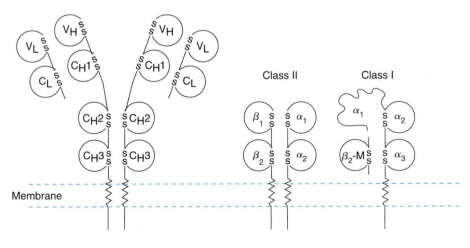

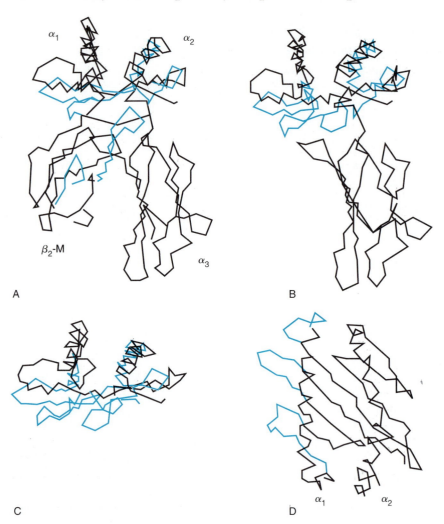

FIGURE 10-4 Graphic representation of the three-dimensional structure of a class I molecule. The structures shown here were generated with the Molecular Modeling System developed at the University of California, San Diego, using atomic coordinates for the HLA-A2 class I molecule, kindly provided by Dr. Pamela Bjorkman of Stanford University. Only the α-carbon backbone of the polypeptides is shown. **A.** The extracellular portions of the class I molecule are shown (the transmembrane and cytoplasmic tail of the larger polypeptide chain is missing). Each of the domains is labeled, as is the β_2-microglobulin (β_2-M) protein. The peptide–antigen-binding site is located at the top of the molecule and is formed by the α_1 and α_2 domains. Both these domains have highly variable polymorphic regions that form much of the binding site. These polymorphic residues also are those residues that form the antigenic regions responsible for graft rejection. **B.** The same molecule is shown without the β_2-M peptide. **C.** The α_3 domain has been removed, leaving only the peptide–antigen-binding domains of the HLA-A2 molecule. The α-helical "sides" of the peptide-binding site are particularly evident in this representation. **D.** The molecule from **C** has been rotated 90 degrees. The reader is now looking down to the peptide-binding groove. Two α helices, one from each of the α_1 and α_2 domains, form the walls of the groove, whereas β-sheet structures, also from each domain, form the floor of the binding site. The structure of the class II MHC molecules is thought to be similar.

The three-dimensional structure of a class I molecule has been determined and is shown in Figure 10-4. The α_1 and α_2 domains combine to form a deep pocket at the most external face of the molecule. The floor of the pocket is made up of antiparallel β-sheet structures and the walls are formed by α helices. The α_1 and α_2 domains each contribute one half of the floor and one wall to the structure. There is evidence that this pocket is the binding site for antigen-derived peptides (see Chaps. 11 and 13). Polymorphic residues (ie, amino acids that differ from individual to individual, see later) in the class I molecule are located along the floor and walls of this pocket.

The roles of the polymorphic residues and the antigen-derived peptide, as well as other details of this structure, are discussed in Chapters 11 and 13 with regard to presentation of antigen to T cells.

Gene Structure

As described in Chapter 8 for antibody and in Chapter 9 for the T-cell receptor, the domains of the class I antigens correspond well to the exons at the DNA level (Fig. 10-5). However, unlike the genes that encode antibody and the T-cell receptor, there is no rearrangement of DNA to form the mature functional genes encoding the class I polypeptide chain. Transcription of the gene and removal of intervening sequences at the RNA level produce a mature mRNA molecule with all coding sequences contiguous to one another.

Polymorphism

Many different *alleles* can be present at each of the HLA-A, HLA-B, and HLA-C loci (Table 10-5), although each individual possesses a maximum of two at each locus (one on each chromosome). This polymorphism is detectable by graft rejection and serologically by antibody. In structural terms, polymorphism represents differences in amino acid sequence and, thus, in the overall surface structure of the large 44,000-dalton polypeptide chain encoded by each of these loci. If a comparison of the amino acid sequences of proteins encoded by the HLA-A, HLA-B, and HLA-C loci obtained from numerous individuals is carried out, the following results are seen:

TABLE 10-5
Listing of Recognized Human Leukocyte Antigen (HLA) Specificities*

HLA-A	HLA-B	HLA-B	HLA-C	HLA-D	HLA-DR	HLA-DQ	HLA-DP
A1	B5	Bw50(21)	Cw1	Dw1	DR1	DQw1	DPw1
A2	B7	B51(5)	Cw2	Dw2	DR2	DQw2	DPw2
A3	B8	Bw52(5)	Cw3	Dw3	DR3	DQw4	DPw4
A9	B12	Bw53	Cw4	Dw4	DR4	DQw5	DPw5
A10	B13	Bw54(w22)	Cw5	Dw5	DR5	DQw5(w1)	DPw6
A11	B14	Bw55(w22)	Cw6	Dw6	DRw6	DQw6(w1)	
Aw19	B15	Bw56(w22)	Cw7	Dw7	DR7	DQw7(3)	
A23(9)	B16	Bw57(17)	Cw8	Dw8	DRw8	DQw8(w3)	
A24(9)	B17	Bw58(17)	Cw9(w3)	Dw9	DR9	DQw9(w3)	
A25(10)	B18	Bw59	Cw10(w3)	Dw10	DRw10		
A26(10)	B21	Bw60(40)	Cw11	Dw11(w7)	DRw11(5)		
A28	Bw22	Bw61(40)		Dw12	DRw12(5)		
A29(w19)	B27	Bw62(15)		Dw13	DRw13(w6)		
A30(w19)	B35	Bw63(15)		Dw14	DRw14(w6)		
A31(w19)	B37	Bw64(14)		Dw15	DRw15(2)		
A32(w19)	B38(16)	Bw65(14)		Dw16	DRw16(2)		
Aw33(w19)	B39(16)	Bw67		Dw17(w7)	DRw17(3)		
Aw34(10)	B40	Bw70		Dw18(w6)	DRw18(3)		
Aw36	Bw41	Bw71(w70)		Dw19(w6)	DRw52		
Aw43	Bw42	Bw72(w70)		Dw20	DRw53		
Aw66(10)	B44(12)	Bw73		Dw21			
Aw68(28)	B45(12)	Bw75(15)		Dw22			
Aw69(28)	Bw46	Bw76(15)		Dw23			
Aw74(w19)	Bw47	Bw77(15)		Dw24			
	Bw48	Bw4		Dw25			
	B49(21)	Bw6		Dw26			

* The above are the recognized HLA specificities. The listing is based on the 1987 report of the Nomenclature Committee on Leukocyte Antigens, dated November 21–23, 1987, as published in Human Immunology 1989;26:3–14. The "w" in the listing (as in Aw19) represents a workshop-designated specificity. Numbers in parentheses after some specificities represent split specificities (eg, A23(9) and A24(9) are HLA-A specificities that have recently been separated from the A9 specificity).

1. All proteins encoded by the HLA-A locus are similar to each other and to those proteins encoded by the HLA-B and HLA-C loci. Based on its sequence alone, the class I locus that encoded a protein cannot be predicted. Thus, all the class I genes have evolved by gene duplication from a single ancestral gene.
2. Most of the amino acid sequence of class I proteins is fairly constant—a situation somewhat similar to the framework sequences in the variable region of Ig (see Chap. 5).
3. Most of the sequence differences among class I antigens fall into just a few regions, that is, within certain segments of the α_1 and α_2 extracellular domains (see Fig. 10-3).

Thus, the antigenic differences that give rise to allograft rejection between different individuals are the result of the structural differences in α_1 and α_2 extracellular domains. Again, this is similar to the Ig situation, in which the residues in the antigen-binding site all map to the complementarity-determining regions (see Chap. 5). As discussed in Chapter 13, these structural differences are responsible in part for differences in the recognition of foreign antigens by cytotoxic T cells.

Serologic and recombinant DNA analyses of the mouse and human MHCs have revealed many class I genes other than the HLA-A, HLA-B, and HLA-C loci, such as the Qa and TLa loci in mice and the Qa/TLa-like genes in humans. Some of these genes are pseu-

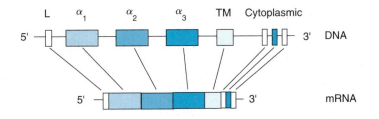

FIGURE 10-5 Structure of a gene encoding a class I molecule. The class I molecules are encoded by a series of exons corresponding to the functional domains of the molecule. After transcription and splicing of the precursor RNA, the mature mRNA has all the coding sequences contiguous to one another. Subsequent translation and processing lead to the mature polypeptide shown in Figure 10-4. L, signal peptide; α_1, α_2, and α_3 exons, external domains; TM, transmembrane.

dogenes, that is, they do not encode functional proteins. Compared to the HLA-A, HLA-B, and HLA-C genes, there is little or no polymorphism in the products of these other class I genes, and their role, if any, in allograft rejection or in the regulation of immune responses is not known.

The class I genes are codominant, meaning that both alleles at any given locus are expressed in the same cell. Therefore, in an individual who is homozygous at each locus (ie, has the same allele on each chromosome), any given cell has only one type of gene product from each locus. However, in an individual who is heterozygous at each locus (ie, has different alleles on each of the two chromosomes), any given cell has two different types of gene products for each locus. The implications of the codominant expression of class I alleles on allograft rejection and immune responses are discussed later.

CLASS II LOCI

A distinct class of alloantigens encoded by genes within the MHC, which are different from those encoded by the class I genes, originally was detected in mixed lymphocyte culture. It was noted that if lymphocytes from two unrelated animals of the same species or from two unrelated human beings were mixed together in tissue culture, the cells would recognize the class II antigen differences between them and respond by dividing. This response by lymphocytes in mixed lymphocyte culture is called the mixed lymphocyte reaction and can be used to detect class II antigen differences between donors and recipients of allografts. The products of some of the class II genes now can be detected by serology, and the genes have been mapped to the HLA-D region of the human MHC and to the H-2A and H-2E regions of the mouse MHC.

In the mouse, these H-2 regions originally were defined as that portion of the mouse MHC that contained genes regulating immune responses. These genes were called *Ir genes* (for *i*mmune-*r*esponse genes), and the products they encoded were subsequently called *Ia antigens* (for *I*-region–*a*ssociated products).

Although the data defining Ir genes in humans are far less precise than they are in mice, it was found that several loci within the HLA-D region of the MHC encode for proteins similar in structure to the Ia-antigen products of the Ir genes in mice. These loci in the human MHC are called the HLA-DP, HLA-DQ, and HLA-DR regions. It is inferred that the Ia antigens encoded by these three loci function to regulate immune responses in humans, as do their structural counterparts in mice (see Chaps. 11 and 13).

The products of the DP, DQ, and DR loci are termed *class II* antigens. They are detected by either serologic or mixed lymphocyte culture techniques. Because they are similar in structure, they all are referred to as class II antigens, regardless of the method used to detect them.

The class II antigens have a more limited cellular distribution than do the class I antigens (see Table 10-4). They are found on a few cell types, most of which are involved in the initiation or control of immune responses. These include some macrophages, some dendritic cells, most B cells, some activated T cells (but not virgin T cells), and certain epithelial cells.

Structure of Class II Antigens

Class II molecules are made up of two polypeptide chains, termed α and β (see Fig. 10-3). Both polypeptide chains are encoded by genes within the MHC (see Fig. 10-2). These chains have molecular weights of 33,000 and 25,000 daltons, respectively, and both are glycoproteins.

The class II molecule exists on the cell surface as a heterodimer of one α chain and one β chain. Both chains show structural similarities to Ig, to the T-cell receptor, and to the class I antigens. Thus, class II antigens also belong to the Ig superfamily of cell-surface receptors.

Each chain of the class II molecule consists of two extracellular domains (α_1 and α_2 or β_1 and β_2), one hydrophobic transmembrane region, and one cytoplasmic, highly charged domain (see Fig. 10-3).

Because of the overall similarity in primary structure of classes I and II, and because of their similar function in immune responses (see Chaps. 11 and 13), the three-dimensional structure of the class II molecule is thought to resemble that of class I molecules. However, in the case of the class II molecule, the peptide-binding pocket is believed to be formed by the α_1 domain of the α chain and the β_1 domain of the β chain. Similarly, it is thought that the polymorphic residues in these two chains are found in the floor and walls of the pocket. The role that this pocket and the polymorphic residues play in antigen presentation and T-cell activation is discussed in Chapter 11.

Gene Structure

The use of recombinant DNA technology has revealed that within each of the DP, DQ, and DR loci, there are several genes encoding α chains and several genes encoding β chains (Fig. 10-6). For example, within the DP locus, there are two genes encoding α chains ($DP_\alpha I$ and $DP_\alpha II$) and two genes encoding β chains ($DP_\beta I$ and $DP_\beta II$). It is unclear whether all these genes are functional genes or whether the α chains and β chains from a given locus can associate in any combination of α chains and β chains. If a random association of the α and β chains that are encoded within a given locus is permitted, the number of possible combinations increases significantly. For example, with two DP_α chains and two DP_β chains, random association would lead to four possible DP heter-

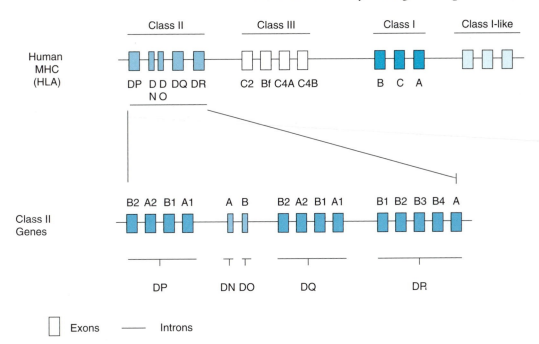

FIGURE 10-6 Fine structure of the HLA-D (class II) region of the human major histocompatibility complex (*MHC*). The DR, DQ, and DP regions each have genes encoding α- and β-polypeptide chains. Only single genes have been demonstrated within the DO and DN regions. The A genes and B genes within each locus encode α chains and β chains, respectively. The DR-B2, DP-A2, and DP-B2 genes are pseudogenes. It is not known whether the DQ-A2 and DQ-B2 genes are expressed. The DR-B1 gene encodes the β chain, which determines the specificities DR1, DR3, DR4, DR5, and so forth. The DR-B3 gene encodes the β chain, which determines the DRw52, DRw24, DRw25, and DRw26 specificities. The DR-B4 gene encodes the β chain, which determines the DRw53 specificity. Association of the DR α-polypeptide chain with more than one DR β chain can result in more than one functional HLA-DR molecule on the cell surface. Similar associations are possible at the other loci, although it is not known whether all such combinations are possible.

odimers (αIβI, αIβII, αIIβII, and αIIβI) in a homozygous individual, and to 16 possible DP heterodimers in a heterozygous individual. The functional implications of a random association of these polypeptide chains are discussed in Chapters 11 and 13.

As with other members of the Ig superfamily, the structural domains of the α and β polypeptide chains correspond well to the exons at the DNA level. After transcription and splicing of precursor RNA, the mature mRNA has all the coding segments contiguous with one another.

Polymorphism

Like the class I antigens, the class II antigens are polymorphic (see Table 10-5 for a listing of the known alleles). This polymorphism is detected structurally and immunologically. On a structural basis, the polymorphism, and thus the antigenic and functional differences between allelic products, are restricted primarily to the α_1 and β_1 domains of the two polypeptide chains. However, most of the variability occurs in the β chain of the class II molecule.

The alleles of a given class II locus are codominant, meaning that all alleles at a given locus are expressed on a single cell at the same time. However, there is variable expression of the DP, DQ, and DR genes. The DR-gene products are found on all B cells, most macrophages and dendritic cells, and some activated T cells. The DP- and DQ-gene products, however, appear to be expressed at lower levels and possibly by fewer cells. The functional significance of the variable expression of the class II genes has yet to be determined.

OTHER HUMAN LEUKOCYTE ANTIGEN LOCI

Several other loci within the MHC are of interest but are not discussed in detail here:

1. The genes that encode the C2, C4, and factor B proteins of the complement system. These genes have been termed class III genes (see Fig. 10-2), and their products are discussed in detail in Chapter 12.
2. The genes that control the expression of certain red blood cell antigens (eg, Chido and Rogers). Whether these loci encode the antigen itself or some other regulatory molecule is not known.

SUMMARY

The MHC is a cluster of genes that encode several structurally and antigenically distinct classes of cell-surface molecules. The class I antigens are encoded by several different loci (eg, HLA-A, HLA-B, and HLA-C), for which there are multiple alleles in the population. These antigens are detected by serology and by transplantation. They are made up of two polypeptide chains: an invariant chain with a molecular weight of 12,000 daltons called β_2-M that is found associated with all class I molecules, and is encoded by a gene outside the MHC and a larger chain with a molecular weight of 44,000 daltons that can vary in sequence between different allelic forms of the same locus and between loci. These antigens are found on all nucleated cells and are the targets of cytotoxic T cells that are responsible for graft rejection. They also are involved in the regulation of immune responses to viruses (a topic discussed elsewhere in this text).

The class II antigens (also called *Ia antigens*) are encoded by the HLA-DP, HLA-DQ, and HLA-DR loci (all of which reside within the HLA-D region of the HLA complex), for which there are multiple alleles in the population. These antigens are detected by serology, by mixed lymphocyte culture, and by transplantation. They are made up of two polypeptide chains with molecular weights of 33,000 and 25,000 daltons, both of which are encoded by genes within the MHC. Both chains vary in amino acid sequence, giving rise to antigenic differences between allelic forms. These class II antigens are found only on certain cell types and are involved in the regulation of immune responses to most antigens.

Transplantation

Transplantation antigens are, by definition, those antigens that affect the survival of tissue or organ allografts. There are three classes of transplantation antigens: (1) the ABO blood group antigens (ABO incompatibility is a major barrier to transplantation, and matching of donor and recipient for these antigens is of utmost importance); (2) MHC antigens (both class I and class II antigens are of major importance; the effect of mismatching at these loci is discussed later); and (3) minor histocompatibility antigens (these are any other, ill-defined differences that can affect transplant outcome). There are many minor H loci, making attempts at matching donor and recipient difficult. Fortunately, immunosuppressive drug treatment is effective in cases of rejection caused by minor H loci incompatibilities. Although the minor, or weak, H loci cannot be ignored, the *major barrier to allograft survival is antigens coded for by the MHC*.

CLASS I LOCI

Although MHC antigens are immunogenic, there is some variability in the intensity or strength of the immune response elicited against the different MHC antigens. A factor of major concern in transplantation is the *donor–recipient match*. Rejection is controlled more easily when there are no or few MHC antigen differences between the donor and the recipient. When several MHC antigen mismatches are present, a vigorous allograft rejection response occurs. For example, Figure 10-7 shows the HLA-A and HLA-B pedigree of a family. The haplotypes of the father (ie, the alleles on each chromosome) are $A_{11}B_5$ on one chromosome and A_2B_{37} on the other chromosome. The haplotypes of the mother are A_9B_6 and $A_{23}B_{10}$. The genotype (ie, the alleles on both chromosomes) for the father is $A_{11}B_5/A_2B_{37}$, and that for the mother is $A_9B_6/A_{23}B_{10}$.

Each child's genotype is determined by the parental genotypes. Each child normally inherits an intact haplotype from each parent. (This is because the genes are

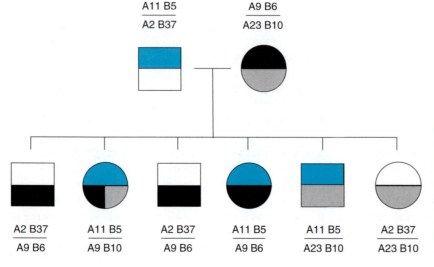

FIGURE 10-7 Inheritance pattern of HLA-A and HLA-B genes within a family. In general, each child receives one complete gene complex (a haplotype) from each parent. However, occasionally, a recombinational event occurs leading to the formation of a new haplotype within the family (eg, A9,B10 for child 2). The effect of this inheritance pattern and the recombinational event on the outcome of transplantation between members of the family is discussed in the text.

linked closely on the chromosome, and the chance of a recombination occurring in a single generation is small.) For example, the first child inherited the A_2B_{37} haplotype from his father and the A_9B_6 haplotype from his mother. Thus, his genotype is distinct from that of either parent; this is true for the other children as well.

Two of the children (numbers 1 and 3) have the same genotype. A particular phenotype has an equal likelihood of occurring in each of the children. The other four children possess unique genotypes, that is, each has a genotype that is different from that of each sibling and from that of each parent. The genotype of the second child is an entirely new haplotype and could have resulted only from recombination between the HLA-A and HLA-B loci of the mother.

Therefore, what are the chances of a successful transplant between any two members of this family?

1. All children differ from their parents by two of the four alleles.
2. Children 1 and 3 share all alleles but differ from the other children by one of four, two of four, or all four alleles.
3. Children 4, 5, and 6 differ from each other and from the parents by two or more alleles. Child 4 shares no alleles at all with child 6. Thus, they are no better matched to each other than they are to their parents.
4. Child 2 shares one of four alleles with children 1, 3, and 6; two of four alleles with his parents; and three of four alleles with children 4 and 5.

The match, therefore, ranges from a complete match (0/4 mismatch; child 1 and child 3, in whom all four alleles match) to a complete mismatch (4/4 mismatch; children 4 and 6 in whom no alleles match) within this family. Because the success of a transplant exchanged between two members of a family depends on the degree of matching, it is critical to identify the two individuals who have the most HLA antigens in common.

In the case of transplanting a kidney from one family member to another, the typing (usually using serologic methods) and the matching for HLA antigens can be done precisely. Because the MHC usually is inherited as a unit, typing for HLA-A and HLA-B alone allows the class I genotype of the family to be determined. However, this is not true for unrelated donors and recipients, because the identity of any locus for which typing is not done cannot be predicted. This is of major concern, because cadaveric donors are a major source of kidneys for renal transplantation.

The results of a study conducted by Festenstein and his colleagues in London serve to demonstrate the success of renal transplantation efforts (Fig. 10-8). The graft survival rate (regardless of the number of mismatches between donor and recipient) 5 years after transplantation was about 60% for patients receiving their first transplant and about 40% for those receiving their second transplant.

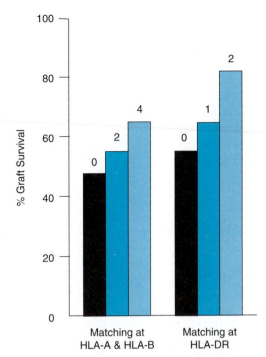

FIGURE 10-8 Effect of major histocompatibility complex (MHC) gene matching on graft survival. Two-year cadaveric kidney allograft survival rates are shown. The left panel indicates matching at the class I HLA-A and HLA-B loci with no consideration for match at the class II loci. The right panel indicates matching at the class II HLA-DR locus with no consideration for match at the class I loci. The numbers above each column indicate the number of matches at the indicated loci. For example, on the left, the data represent 0/4, 2/4, and 4/4 matches at the four class I alleles (two at HLA-A and two at HLA-B). Numerous studies suggest the importance of matching donor and recipient for class II MHC antigens.

The survival rate of allografts ranged from 54% for a 3/4 or 4/4 HLA-A and HLA-B match to 32% for a 0/4 or 1/4 HLA-A and HLA-B match. Thus, matching at the two class I loci has a significant effect on allograft survival.

CLASS II LOCI

The mixed lymphocyte reaction, which is used to identify class II antigens and differences between donor and recipient, can be applied only to those cases in which both the donor and the recipient are living. Improvements in serologic typing of the HLA-DR–encoded antigens have revealed that matching at the HLA-DR locus may be more important than matching at the class I loci. This is probably because recognition of the class II antigens is the primary event responsible for induction of the immune response to the grafted allogeneic tissue (see Chap. 13).

Figure 10-8 shows the effect of matching at the class II HLA-DR locus without regard to matching at the class I loci. Although these data cover only a 2-year follow-up period, they make clear that matching at the class II HLA-DR locus has a significant effect on graft survival (there is a 15% to 20% difference between no match and a complete match at this locus). Furthermore, a complete match at the HLA-DR locus (regardless of class I genotype) is considerably better than a complete match at the class I loci (regardless of class II phenotype), with graft survival rates of 75% for a complete match at class II versus 60% for a complete match at class I.

There is extensive polymorphism in the HLA-DR, DQ, and DP genes, although the relative role of each of the class II antigens coded for by these genes in allograft rejection is unclear. It is apparent that typing and matching for class II antigens may be of greater prognostic value in transplantation than is typing and matching of class I antigens.

ALLOGRAFT REJECTION

The immune response of the recipient to antigens on the donor allograft is the major cause of failure of organ transplants. Because of our inability to regulate totally the recipient's immune response, 10% to 30% of all cadaveric renal allografts are lost due to irreversible rejection within the first 3 months after transplantation.

In this discussion, allograft rejection is classified as hyperacute, acute, or chronic. There are other classification schemes that may be more precise, but this one best suits the purposes of this chapter.

Hyperacute Rejection

If, at the time of transplantation, the patient's serum antibodies are reactive with the alloantigens on the graft, rejection will begin within minutes or hours. This type of rejection is antibody mediated and unresponsive to immunosuppressive therapy. The presence of these antibodies in the recipient's serum is an indication that the allograft should not be performed.

Acute Rejection

Acute rejection is the typical first-set rejection (a primary response) previously discussed. The recipient is not immune to the antigens of the donor. The first evidence of acute rejection is a mild swelling of the kidney occurring 1 to 3 weeks after transplantation. This is followed by decreased renal function and urine output. Biopsies performed at this time often show mononuclear cell (macrophages and lymphocytes) infiltration. Immunosuppressive drug therapy usually is effective in stopping this form of rejection if it is initiated soon enough. Acute rejection appears to be caused by $CD4^-8^+$ cytotoxic T cells specific for class I antigens on the transplanted organ, or by $CD4^+8^-$ cells that induce macrophage-mediated damage

of the transplant (see Chap. 13). Acute rejection is totally independent of antibody.

Chronic Rejection

Chronic rejection of allografts usually begins months after transplantation and proceeds gradually over a period of months or years. The reasons for the slow progression of chronic rejection are not known, although it is clear that both T cells and antibody are involved. Reversal of chronic rejection by immunosuppressive drugs often fails.

Occasionally, an episode of acute rejection is initiated several months after engraftment. In these cases, the acute rejection seems to have been triggered by some other event (eg, a blood transfusion or viral infection) that in some unknown way alters or stimulates the recipient's immune system so that an immune attack on the graft is initiated.

IMMUNOSUPPRESSION

Allograft rejection is prevented with immunosuppressive drug therapy. The basis for such therapy is suppression of the immune response of the recipient. Each immunosuppressive agent has advantages and disadvantages, but *none specifically suppresses* the immune response to the graft. Therefore, immunity to all antigens, including infectious organisms, is suppressed as well. Specific suppression of the immune response to graft alloantigens has been accomplished in experimental situations using inbred animals but is not yet achievable in humans. Suppression of the immune response to prevent allograft rejection also significantly reduces the patient's ability to ward off infection by many microorganisms. The possibility of overwhelming bacterial infection remains one of the more significant hazards of immunosuppressive therapy after transplantation.

Numerous immunosuppressive agents are used, and several are discussed briefly here.

Corticosteroids

Prednisolone and prednisone are the corticosteroids used most often. These drugs are antiinflammatory agents given before transplantation, starting in relatively high dosages and tapering gradually to maintenance dosages. Infection, hypertension, and peptic ulceration are some of the possible side effects. Corticosteroids reduce the expression of class II molecules and inhibit the release of interleukin-1, interleukin-2, and γ-interferon, all of which are involved in the activation of T cells (see Chaps. 11 and 13). These agents also inhibit the production of new T cells in the thymus.

Azathioprine

The induction of immune responses requires the proliferation of lymphocytes. Azathioprine is a purine analogue and inhibits DNA synthesis. Methotrexate inhibits nucleotide precursor biosynthesis. These agents work only on dividing cells. Although both these agents prevent lymphocyte proliferation during alloantigenic stimulation, they also prevent proliferation of bone marrow cells. Thus, the margin between effective and toxic doses of such agents is small. Cyclophosphamide (Cytoxan) and chlorambucil can damage DNA directly and, thus, can affect both dividing and nondividing cells.

Antilymphocyte Serum

Antisera to human lymphocytes can be prepared in animals. If prepared correctly, the major reactivity of such antilymphocyte serum is against T cells. However, its usefulness in human transplantation is controversial. Although it seems to affect T-cell function, it does not prolong graft survival beyond that obtained with corticosteroids or other drugs alone, with which it usually is given.

Monoclonal Anti–T-Cell Antibodies

A monoclonal antibody to the CD3 pan-T-cell–surface marker (see Chap. 9) has been used successfully to reverse acute renal rejection episodes. T cells are cleared immediately (15 to 45 minutes) from the circulation and reappear within 48 hours. Therefore, the effectiveness of this antibody is limited to control of acute rejection.

Ideally, one would like to develop a panel of monoclonal reagents that could selectively affect the various T-cell subsets. Use of this cocktail of monoclonal antibodies might make it possible to manipulate the immune system to the patient's benefit.

Cyclosporin A

Cyclosporin A, or cyclosporine, is a neutral, hydrophobic, cyclic peptide made up of 11 amino acids that originally was isolated from a fungus. It is being used experimentally to study the immune response and clinically to suppress allograft rejection. Cyclosporin A is also being tested as a therapy for certain autoimmune diseases (eg, posterior uveitis, type I diabetes mellitus).

Early studies suggested that this compound differentially suppresses T-cell–mediated immune reactions. Although our understanding of its mechanism of action and its specificity has undergone some fine tuning, cyclosporin A appears to be a potent immunosuppressive agent, apparently preventing lymphocyte activation rather than effector function. Thus, the drug seems to be most effective when administration is begun before or at the time of allograft transplantation; in general, treatment with cyclosporin A or other immunosuppressive drugs must be continued indefinitely.

Cyclosporin A has some side effects and is toxic to the kidney. Whether lower-dose protocols will reduce the incidence of this serious adverse effect remains to be seen.

Blood Transfusions

In 1974, Opelz and Terasaki reported that patients who received blood transfusions before renal transplantation had better graft survival rates than those who did not receive transfusions. Since that time, clinical transplantation groups have shown that blood transfusion just before, or at the time of, renal transplantation significantly improves organ survival. The mechanism for this effect remains obscure, although it has been speculated that immunologic unresponsiveness can be induced by the transfused blood cells.

OTHER ORGANS AND TISSUES

Technically, it is possible to transplant a variety of organs, including lung, liver, heart, and pancreas, although the success rate for these organs is lower when compared with that of renal allografts. The basic principles, types of therapy, and mechanisms of rejection briefly discussed earlier also apply in these cases. The major obstacle to widespread transplantation of organs and tissues is not the technical limitations, but immunologic rejection of the grafts.

Bone Marrow Transplantation

Bone marrow transplantation deserves special consideration, not only because of the many types of diseases to which it applies, but also because of the special problems that arise as a result of the transplantation of bone marrow cells, which include some immunologically competent lymphocytes.

Some of the diseases treated by bone marrow transplantation include certain leukemias, breast cancer, various immunodeficiency diseases (eg, severe combined immunodeficiency; see Chap. 14), and aplastic anemia. In each case, there is the possibility that the host's immune system may reject the graft. However, it also is possible that the grafted tissue may react to and reject the recipient. This *graft-versus-host (GVH)* reaction is mediated by donor lymphocytes in the grafted bone marrow, which recognize and respond to the HLA antigens of the recipient.

In bone marrow transplantation, the recipient's immune system often is impaired by the primary disease or by the therapy given for it (eg, irradiation or chemotherapy). Ideally, the recipient could be rendered immunologically tolerant (see Chap. 11) to the alloantigens of the donor,

TABLE 11-1
Monokines and Lymphokines Involved in Regulation of Immune Responses

Factor	Other Name(s)	Source	Properties	Effect on Human Cells
IL-1	LAF	Macrophages T cells B cells Epithelial cells	15–17 kd	Promotes early B-cell differentiation
IL-2	TCGF	Activated T cells	15 kd	Promotes proliferation of B and T cells
IL-3	Multi-CSF	Activated T cells	34 kd	Induces growth of hemopoietic cells
IL-4	BCGF-1 BCDF-ε BCDF-γ BSF-I	Activated T cells	20 kd	Promotes IgE production, induces increased FcεR on B cells and mast cells
IL-5	BCGF-II	Activated T cells	30–60 kd	Promotes IgM and IgA production, promotes eosinophil differentiation
IL-6	BSF-II HGF	Monocytes Fibroblasts T cells	20 kd	Promotes growth of plasma cells, promotes Ig secretion
IFN-γ		T cells NK cells	20–25 kd	Induces class II expression on cells, promotes antimicrobial activity of macrophages, promotes NK cell activity, induces FcγR expression on monocytic cells, with IL-4 promotes IgG production
IL-10	CSIF	T cells B cells Macrophages Keratinocytes	17–21 kd	Inhibits cytokine production by Th1 cells, NK cells, and macrophages; stimulates B-cell proliferation and differentiation

BCDF, B-cell differentiation factor; BCGF, B-cell growth factor; CSF, colony-stimulating factor; CSIF, cytokine synthesis inhibitory factor; HGF, hepatocyte growth factor; IFN-γ, interferon gamma; IL, interleukin; LAF, leukocyte activating factor; NK, natural killer; TCGF, T-cell growth factor.

by antigen in the presence of a positive regulatory cell, the Th cell. Each activated effector cell then performs its preprogrammed function, for example, antibody synthesis or killing of virally infected cells. Down-regulation of these immune responses is provided by a negative regulatory effect brought about by cytokines such as interleukin (IL)-10, produced by the Th subset called Th$_2$. The lymphocytes are thought to exert positive regulatory actions mediated by IL-2 and interferon gamma (IFN-γ).

The induction and control of antibody responses to foreign and self-antigens are the topics of the remainder of this chapter. The induction and control of cell-mediated immune responses (eg, those mediated by Tc cells and Th cells) are discussed in Chapter 13.

SIGNAL TRANSDUCTION AND SECOND MESSENGER PATHWAYS IN LYMPHOCYTES

The literature dealing with signal transduction and second messenger pathways is replete with details regarding the events that take place after receptor–ligand interaction at the surface of a cell. Lymphocytes have served as models for the study of transmembrane signaling and the investigation of second messenger pathways in part because of the convenience in obtaining large numbers of these cells in relatively pure form and because they can be maintained in tissue culture in synchronous growth using a variety of growth factors and mitogens. From the overview of signal transduction and second-messenger regulation of lymphocyte activation, it is apparent that considerable similarity exists in the transduction and messenger pathways in T and B lymphocytes.

To begin with, B-lymphocyte membrane immunoglobulin, the T-cell antigen receptor/CD3 complex, the CD4 and CD8 coreceptor molecules, and the IL-2 receptor (IL-2R) function in their respective lymphocyte subtypes to transduce signals from the cell membrane to the interior of the cell. It is well known that protein tyrosine kinases (PTKs) are activated upon cell membrane interaction of receptors with ligands in both T and B lymphocytes. There is still much to learn regarding how these common pathways in lymphocytes from distinctly different lineages, which have different functions, can selectively activate and repress different transcriptional events in these separate cell types.

T CELLS. The α/β and γ/δ chains of the T-cell receptor (TCR) complex designated Ti are involved in recognition of antigen presented by antigen-presenting cells (APCs). The TCR chains have short cytoplasmic tails and do not function as signal transduction systems for intracellular activation events. Other molecules of the TCR—the CD3 complex known as the γ, δ, and ε chains—actually serve to couple the α and β chains of the TCR to the intracellular signal transduction pathways. In addition to the γ, δ, and ε chains, a fourth chain exists known as ζ which is noncovalently associated with the CD3 complex of the TCR. The ζ chain has a short extracellular domain and a long intracellular domain. A homologue of the ζ chain on T-cell membranes is on the IgG–Fc receptor (IgG-FcR) of natural killer cells. The molecules of the CD3 complex—γ, δ, ε, and ζ—couple the TCR to the intracellular compartment, and the IgG-FcRs perform a similar function on natural killer cells. They activate protein tyrosine phosphorylation of tyrosine residues after interaction of the TCR with antigen on an APC. At least 10 repeating cytoplasmic components, or motifs, allow one TCR to interact with, and activate, many copies of the same signal transduction system. This amplification increases the sensitivity of the TCR interaction with antigen. After transduction of the signal from the plasma membrane to the intracellular compartment, several members of the Src

family of PTKs are involved in further regulation of cellular activation. Thus, the FynPTK, LckPTK, LynPTK, and ZAP-70 SrcPTKs have been shown to be involved in T-cell activation. One of the major consequences of TCR-mediated PTK activation is activation of the phosphatidyl inositol second messenger pathway within the cell. The activation of the kinases ultimately results in transduction of signals into the nucleus of the cell where gene activation, DNA synthesis, transcription, and cell division are initiated (Fig. 11-2). As indicated earlier, considerable redundancy exists in the pathways used in transmembrane signaling and second messenger signal transfer to the nucleus in T lymphocytes and B lymphocytes (compare Fig. 11-2 and Fig. 11-3). Thus, it is not clear how common pathways in different cell types lead to expression of different cellular functions.

B CELLS. As previously indicated, B-cell membrane immunoglobulin receptors interact with antigens and signals are transduced across the plasma membrane, activating

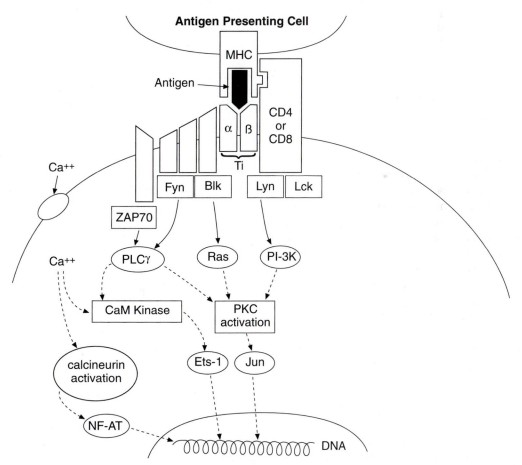

FIGURE 11-2 T-lymphocyte activation. The recognition of an antigen on an antigen-presenting cell by the T-cell receptor results in signal transduction across the plasma membrane of the lymphocyte. A series of kinases are activated, which phosphorylate second messengers in the cytoplasm. A consequence of protein tyrosine kinase activation is a stimulation of phosphatidylinositol second messenger systems, leading to calcium mobilization and activation of transcription regulatory proteins, which interact with specific segments of DNA, including lymphokine genes such as interleukin-2, interleukin-4, and interferon gamma. These activation mechanisms also result in entry of the cell into the cell cycle and culminate in mitosis.

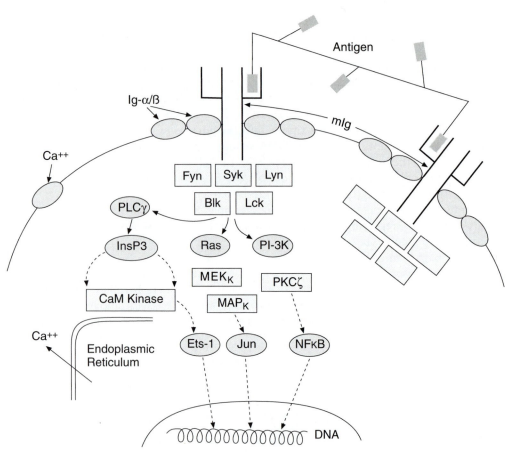

FIGURE 11-3   B-lymphocyte activation. Antigen cross-linking of B-lymphocyte immunoglobulin activates a series of the Src family of tyrosine kinases, including Fyn, Syk, Lyn, and others. These kinases act as signal transducers, resulting in protein tyrosine kinase phosphorylation events. Ultimately, calcium mobilization and phospholipid cleavage take place, and inositol 4,5-triphosphate and diacylglycerol are generated. These and other phospholipid products activate additional kinases, which phosphorylate DNA-binding proteins, including Ets-1, Jun, and NFkB. These activation events stimulate B-lymphocyte synthesis of cellular RNA and protein and cause the cell to enter the cell cycle.

intracellular PTKs in much the same way as occurs in T lymphocytes. It is known that the membrane immunoglobulin protein complex of B cells is homologous to the CD3 complex, which is associated with the TCR on T lymphocytes. On B cells adjacent to the immunoglobulin receptor, there is a disulfide-bridged heterodimeric complex referred to as Ig α/β which contains amino acid sequences that bind to cytoplasmic effector systems, including members of the Src family of tyrosine kinases, such as are activated after T-cell recognition of antigen. Activation of a number of PTKs within the cell occurs shortly after cross-linking of B-cell immunoglobulin receptors by antigen. These kinases include Fyn, Lyn, Blk, and others. Whether these tyrosine kinases are activated in parallel or as a cascade is not clear. Nevertheless, these and other kinases serve as a transduction system ultimately resulting in nuclear activation of specific genes in the B lymphocytes. The biochemical cascade that occurs intracellularly after tyrosine kinase activation involves protein tyrosine phosphorylation. These activation events include the phosphorylation of phosphatidylinositol 4,5-diphos-

phate–specific phospholipase C, PLC-γ. This, in turn, results in the hydrolytic cleavage of phospholipids producing inositol 1,4,5-triphosphate (InsP$_3$) and diacylglycerol (DAG). InsP$_3$ mediates Ca^{2+} changes, which activate calcium calmodulin kinase II (CaM kinase II), which phosphorylates the Ets-1 DNA binding protein. The regulatory action of Ets-1 on gene transcription is altered by phosphorylation, thus completing the cascade from the cell membrane to the gene.

A second biochemical pathway activated intracellularly in B cells after antigen binding involves a G protein known as p21ras. Ras is activated within minutes of immunoglobulin–antigen interaction and regulates the sequential activation of serine/threonine phosphorylation of the microtubule-associated protein kinases, ERK2 kinase, MEK, and subsequently microtubule-associated protein kinase 2 (MAPk). MAPk may indirectly regulate gene expression; this kinase is known to catalyze the phosphorylation of c-Jun, which regulates gene activity in B lymphocytes.

A third event occurring intracellularly in B cells after

stimulation by antigen involves the activation of phosphatidylinositol 3 kinase. This enzyme phosphorylates inositol phospholipids, and these phospholipids are important in stimulating proliferation, possibly by activating protein kinase C (PKC) ζ, which activates NFkB, a mediator of gene transcription and cell division.

Ultimately, signal transduction from the B-lymphocyte membrane immunoglobulin receptor involves the activation of PTKs, which diverge intracellularly, activating several enzymatic processes that stimulate serine/threonine kinases. These kinases may, in turn, regulate gene transcription in the B cells, resulting in a differentiated cellular response (see Fig. 11-3). As indicated previously, such signal transduction events and second messenger pathways are recognized as a common pattern in receptor-mediated signaling from the cell surface to the interior of the cell. Much is yet to be learned regarding the specificity of these various second-messenger pathways, and it is still undetermined how genes are differentially activated and inactivated in T cells and B cells so as to permit these cells to maintain their unique functional properties.

HELPER T-CELL ACTIVATION

An essential step in the induction of immune responses to most antigens is the activation of the Th cell. (The cell-surface phenotype of the Th cell in humans is $CD3^+4^+8^-$.) This activation occurs in several steps:

1. Antigen is taken up and processed by the antigen presenting cell (APC) (eg, a macrophage, a dendritic cell, or a B lymphocyte). This involves antigen interaction with the APC cell surface, endocytosis of the antigen, partial or incomplete digestion of the antigen, and the expression of the antigen fragment in the groove or cleft of a major histocompatibility complex (MHC) molecule on the APC cell surface (Fig. 11-4). Processing of antigen within the cell occurs in acidic compartments such as endosomes or the phagolysosomes. Drugs, such as chloroquine, that increase the pH in these compartments inhibit antigen presentation, although they do not prevent endocytosis of the antigen by the cell. Similarly, processing of protein antigens is blocked by the addition of protease inhibitors (eg, leupeptin). Indeed, preprocessed protein antigen (ie, peptides derived from an in vitro digestion of the antigen) can substitute for whole antigen, even if fixed APCs are used that are unable to internalize and process antigen. Thus, in most situations, processing of most protein antigens is a prerequisite for T-cell recognition of antigen on the APC cell surface.
2. It is well established that Th cells recognize antigen on the surface of APCs in the context of class II MHC molecules (see Chap. 10). This *dual recognition* of an

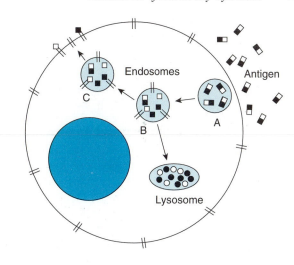

|| Class II Molecule   ●&○ Fully Degraded Antigen   □&■ Antigen-Derived Peptides

FIGURE 11-4 Antigen processing by the antigen-presenting cell (APC). The activation of helper T (Th) cells depends on the uptake and processing of soluble foreign antigen molecules by nonspecific APCs. The antigen undergoes endocytosis by the cell and is degraded in acidic intracellular compartments (thought to be the light endosomes). Fragments of the antigen are taken up by class II molecules and presented as peptide–class II complexes on the surface of the APC. The association between the peptide antigen and the class II molecule is thought to first occur in the intracellular compartment before appearance of the complex on the cell surface. Class II–restricted T cells specifically recognize and interact with this complex. A number of cell types can perform this antigen-presentation function.

antigen and a class II molecule is responsible for the *MHC restriction* discussed in Chapters 9 and 10. Specific binding of peptides, derived from protein antigen, to isolated class II molecules has been directly demonstrated. Therefore, the Th cell recognizes a *complex* of peptide antigen and a class II molecule, and only cells that express class II molecules can function as APCs in the activation of Th cells. The class II molecule exhibits a relatively broad specificity (compared with the highly specific B-cell receptors and TCRs) in that a given class II molecule can bind peptides derived from a broad range of proteins that have no apparent structural similarity with one another. Because of the importance of this binding of peptides derived from protein antigens by class II molecules (and, is seen later, by class I molecules as well) to the initiation of immune responses and to the development of synthetic vaccines, the nature and specificity of this binding are areas of intense investigation.

3. The APC subsequently releases a soluble factor called *IL-1* (see Table 11-1). Incidentally, macrophage-derived factors are collectively referred to as *monokines*. The recognition of the class II–antigen peptide complex by the Th on the APC surface, combined with the binding of IL-1 to IL-1 receptors on the T-cell

membrane, provides the first signal which drives the Th from the resting G_0 state into G_1 of the cell cycle (Fig. 11-5).

4. As the Th cell progresses into the cell cycle, it begins to express cell-surface receptors for another soluble factor, *IL-2* (or T-cell growth factor; see Table 11-1). Subsequent interaction of these IL-2R–positive Th cells with IL-2 drives the cells through the remainder of the cell cycle (see Fig. 11-5). This interaction is the second signal required for Th activation. The rate and extent of proliferation induced are directly proportional to the amount of IL-1 released, the density of cell-surface IL-2R, and the concentration of IL-2.

5. The overall result of this APC–antigen–Th cell interaction is the clonal proliferation of the Th cell *and* the production, by the Th cell, of a variety of soluble factors collectively referred to as *lymphokines*. These lymphokines include B-cell and T-cell growth and differentiation factors including IL-2 (see Table 11-1). IL-2 is a product of the Th cell as well as a growth factor for Th cells and is a good example of an autocrine growth factor (ie, it is required by the cell that produces it).

6. The early biochemical events underlying transition from the resting cell stage to the proliferating cell stage seem to be similar, if not identical, to the triggering of activation pathways observed in a number of cell types (Fig. 11-6). Interaction of antigen (with or without other signals) with its membrane receptor activates membrane phospholipase C, releasing inositol triphosphate and DAG by the hydrolysis of membrane phosphatidyl inositol biphosphate. Activation of PKC by DAG indirectly affects ion pumps and intracellular ion concentrations. Ion concentrations, in turn, affect the activity of certain protein kinases. Inositol triphosphate induces the release of Ca^{2+} from intracellular stores, activating other protein kinases and thus protein phosphorylation, which precedes DNA synthesis.

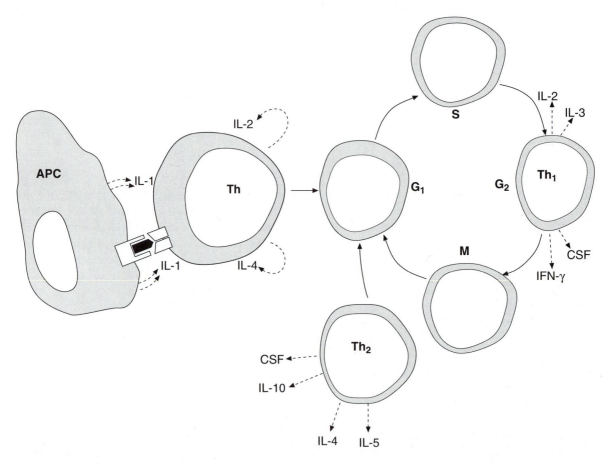

FIGURE 11-5   Antigen-specific activation of helper T (Th) cells. Th cells are activated after the recognition of a peptide antigen-class II major histocompatibility complex (MHC) by the T-cell receptor. Interleukin-1 (IL-1) is involved in this initial event, which causes the G_0-to-G_1 transition in the cell cycle and the acquisition of receptors for the growth factors IL-2 and IL-4. Interaction of IL-2 and IL-4 with these newly acquired receptors causes the T cells to continue through the remainder of the cell cycle. In addition, expression of other genes is induced, leading to the secretion of a number of lymphokines by the Th cells. Th1 cells secrete IL-1, IL-3, interferon gamma (IFN-γ), and various colony-stimulating factors (CSF). Th2 cells secrete IL-4, IL-5, and IL-10, as well as CSFs. The types of T- and B-cell responses regulated by each of the helper T cell subsets (Th1 and Th2) depend on the cytokines that each secretes.

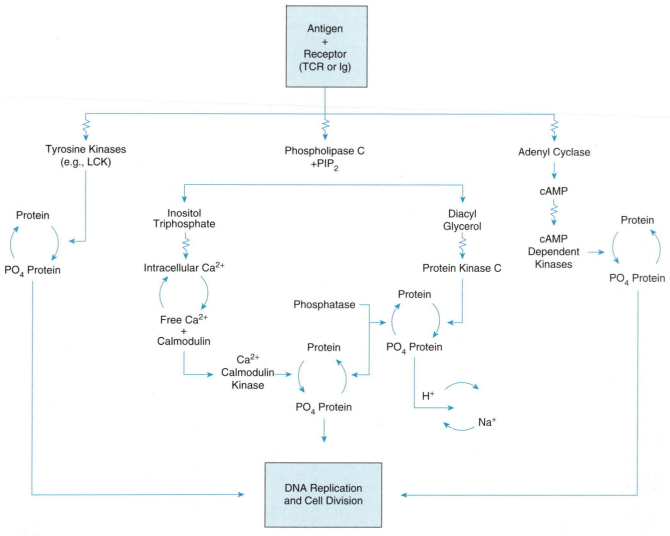

FIGURE 11-6   Early biochemical events in T-cell and B-cell activation. Antigen interaction with specific receptors on T cells and B cells initiates a series of biochemical events leading to DNA replication and cell division which are similar to those seen upon activation of many cell types. (1) Activation of tyrosine kinases: for example, a tyrosine kinase termed *lymphocyte cell kinase* (LCK) has been shown to be associated with the CD4 and CD8 polypeptides of the T-cell receptor complex. Evidence suggests that on activation of the T cell, the CD4-associated (or CD8-associated) LCK phosphorylates one of the chains of the CD3 component of the receptor complex. (2) Antigen-receptor interaction is also known to activate phospholipase C, which leads to production of inositol triphosphate and diacylglycerol from phosphatidyl inositol biphosphate (PIP_2). Inositol triphosphate releases Ca^{2+} from intracellular stores, whereas diacylglycerol activates protein kinase C (PKC). This increase in Ca^{2+} and PKC activity results in protein phosphorylation, which affects a number of activities, including membrane ion pumps. (3) Antigen-receptor interaction also results in activation of adenyl cyclase, leading to activation of the cAMP-dependent protein kinases.

The proliferation of the Th cell yields an expanded pool of antigen-specific Th cells. Subsequent activation of this enlarged pool of Th cells by second contact with antigen produces a more rapid and heightened response, that is, a secondary response.

Co-Stimulatory Signals Required for T-Cell Activation

The interaction of the TCR complex with a peptide antigen in the groove of a self-MHC molecule is the primary signal that a T lymphocyte must receive to become activated and participate in an immune response. The TCR, in conjunction with either the CD4 or CD8 molecules on helper and cytotoxic T cells, respectively, provides the primary stimulus to T cells to enter into an antigen-specific immune response.

Several years ago, Kevin Lafferty and others recognized that antigen-specific T-lymphocyte responses require more than antigen recognition by the T cell. It soon became clear that second or co-stimulatory signals are required for lymphocyte activation and entry into specific immune responses. Because it is known that antigen presentation to T lymphocytes is performed by so-called professional APCs, it is clear that, in addition to the recognition of antigen on self-MHC molecules, the T cells have to form a second or co-stimulatory receptor–ligand relationship with the APC. Many investigators have contributed to the discovery and molecular characterization of various receptors and ligands on APCs and T cells. For example, the molecular characterization of the CD28 molecule on T cells and the B7 molecule on APCs preceded the functional characterization of these molecules.

Within the last few years, Peter Linsley and coworkers and Jeffrey Bluestone and colleagues elucidated the function of the CD28 receptor and its B7 ligand in T-cell co-stimulation. These investigators showed that after the interaction of the TCR with a self-MHC–peptide complex, the CD28 and B7 interaction must take place for the T cell to undergo activation, functional differentiation, and participation in an antigen-specific immune response (Fig. 11-7). There are other examples of T-cell APC co-stimulatory interactions; the CD28-B7 interaction will be used here as the prototype to define the functional significance of the co-stimulatory signaling in T-cell activation.

CD28 is a 44-kilodalton glycoprotein that is present on the surface of all CD4$^+$ and approximately 50% of CD8$^+$ human T lymphocytes; all mouse T cells express this glycoprotein. Perturbation of the CD28 molecule with anti-CD28 antibodies mimics the co-stimulatory CD28-B7 signal to the T cell, causing the T cell to pro-

duce lymphokines and enter the cell cycle. Both similarities and differences exist between the signal transduction events that take pace after the TCR interacts with the self-MHC–peptide complex and CD28 interacts with the B7 molecule. The TCR transduction pathway is sensitive to the immunosuppressive drug, cyclosporin A, and inhibitors of PKC, whereas CD28-B7 transduction is not affected by these mediators. Interestingly, both CD28-B7 and TCR signal transduction are sensitive to tyrosine kinase inhibitors. Thus, there are some common elements and some differences in both receptor–ligand interactions.

Gordon Freeman and Richard Hodes have discovered a variant of the B7 molecule on APCs. Thus, the original B7 molecule is one of a family of at least two B7 subtypes designated B7-1 and B7-2. In the latest modeling of the expression of B7 molecules by APCs, it seems that the B7-2 molecule may be constitutively expressed; mRNA transcripts for the B7-2 molecule are present in APCs before they are actively involved in antigen presentation. The B7-1 molecule, on the other hand, is expressed by APCs after some delay. B7-1 appears on the APC membrane 24 to 48 hours after the APC has provided the antigenic stimulus to T cells through the interaction of self-MHC–peptide complex with the TCR.

The significance of the observations regarding the necessity of co-stimulatory signals for antigen-specific T-cell activation lies in the potential to manipulate this interaction to modulate and even prevent antigen-specific immune responses both experimentally and clinically. Evidence suggests that if a T cell receives an antigenic stimu-

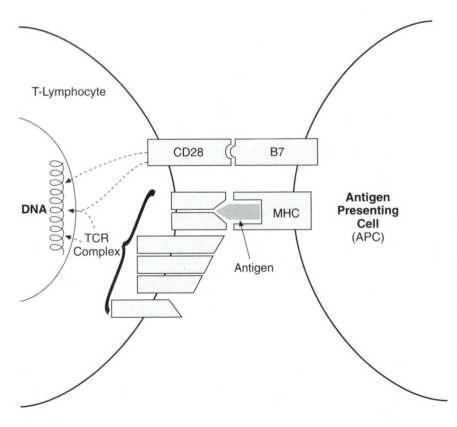

FIGURE 11-7 T-lymphocyte co-stimulatory signaling. The primary signal that a T lymphocyte receives is through the binding of the T-cell receptor (TCR) to the antigen presented on a self-MHC antigen molecule. An example of a second or co-stimulatory signal, which T lymphocytes must receive, is the interaction of the CD28 molecule on the T lymphocyte with the B7 ligand on an antigen-presenting cell. This second, or co-stimulatory, interaction must take place for the T cell to respond to the antigen.

lus by the TCR interacting with antigen on self-MHC but fails to receive the co-stimulatory signal provided by the CD28-B7 interaction, the T cells are rendered impotent or anergic. Some investigators have speculated that blocking the co-stimulatory interaction may be one route to the induction of antigen-specific T-cell tolerance. The results of several studies reveal that if the CD28-B7 interaction is blocked, an antigen-specific T-cell response is prevented from developing.

The discovery of a CD28 homologue on activated T cells called CTLA4, which has a higher affinity for B7 than CD28, has been used to block T-lymphocyte co-stimulation (Fig. 11-8). The creation of a soluble version of the CTLA4 molecule called CTLA4-Ig has been used in the laboratories of Linsley and Ledbetter and of Jeffrey Bluestone to modulate antigen-specific T-cell responses in mice. Remarkably, it was shown that human pancreatic acinar cells survived for 100 days or more under the kidney capsule of mouse hosts. The survival of human cells in mice for this period of time suggests that useful clinical opportunities lie ahead; it should be possible to engineer molecules such as CTLA4-Ig, which can be used to safely and effectively suppress unwanted T-lymphocyte responses.

B-CELL ACTIVATION

Antigens can be divided into two categories based on their apparent need for Th cells for the induction of antibody synthesis: (1) those that require Th cells, referred to as T-dependent antigens (TD-antigens); and (2) those that do not require Th cells, called T-independent antigens (TI-antigens).

The first step in the induction of antibody responses to TD-antigens is the activation of Th cells. This has been discussed earlier. B cells can take up antigen either specifically, via their immunoglobulin receptors, or by nonspecific endocytosis. Specific uptake is a far more efficient process, requiring at least 1000-fold less antigen for stimulation than does nonspecific endocytosis. Therefore, in normal situations where antigen is in low concentrations (eg, early in infection), the immunoglobulin receptor serves to *focus* the antigen on the important B cells. This focusing of antigen results in a specific antibody response rather than in generalized immunoglobulin biosynthesis.

This immunoglobulin receptor–mediated endocytosis results in the internalization and processing of the antigen by B cells in a manner essentially identical to that described earlier for the APC in Th activation (see Fig. 11-4). Processed antigen (ie, peptide) then is repositioned on the B-cell surface in association with the B cell's class II molecules (Fig. 11-9).

The B cell, therefore, is also an APC. The role of IL-1 in the interaction between B cells and Th cells is uncertain. Apparently, B cells do not secrete this monokine, but several reports suggest that IL-1 is present in a membrane-bound form on B cells. In addition, although B cells can function as APCs for activating Th cells during induction of antibody responses, it is not clear that they can present antigen to virgin Th cells.

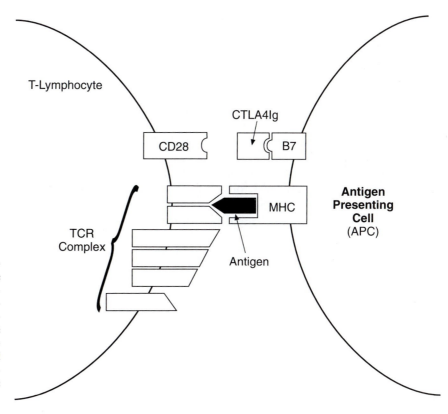

FIGURE 11-8 Blocking T-lymphocyte co-stimulation. The production of a high-affinity soluble ligand termed *CTLA4-Ig* has been used to prevent the co-stimulatory signaling of T lymphocytes upon antigen recognition on an antigen-presenting cell (APC). CTLA4-Ig binds to the B7 coreceptor molecule on the APC and prevents the T cell from receiving the second signal through the CD28 receptor. The failure to receive the second signal renders the T lymphocyte unresponsive or anergic.

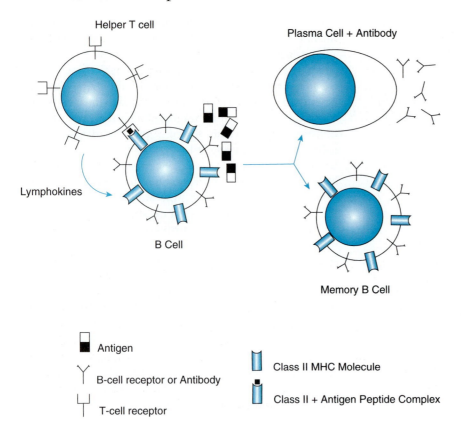

Helper T cell

Plasma Cell + Antibody

Lymphokines

B Cell

Memory B Cell

☐ Antigen

Y B-cell receptor or Antibody

⊔ T-cell receptor

▯ Class II MHC Molecule

▮ Class II + Antigen Peptide Complex

FIGURE 11-9 Induction of an antibody response to a T-dependent antigen. Antigen is recognized and bound by the B-cell immunoglobulin antigen-specific receptor. Receptor-mediated endocytosis of the antigen (and the immunoglobulin receptor itself) leads to processing of the antigen, as described for APCs in Figure 11-2. A fragment of the antigen is bound by a class II molecule and is presented on the B-cell surface as a peptide–class II complex. A helper T (Th) cell, which has been preactivated by interaction with an identical peptide–class II complex on an APC, interacts with this complex on the B cell. This Th cell is then activated and delivers both proliferative and differentiative signals (many in the form of secreted lymphokines) to the B cell, causing the formation of memory B cells and plasma cells, which synthesize and secrete antibody. On subsequent contact with antigen and Th cells, the memory B cell gives rise to more memory B cells and to more plasma cells secreting antibody.

The activated Th cell then interacts with this peptide–class II complex, resulting in the release of lymphokines by the Th cell *at the B-cell surface*. These factors provide signals of growth and differentiation that, together with signals derived from its interaction with antigen, drive the B cell to proliferate and to differentiate into antibody-producing plasma cells and memory B cells (Fig. 11-10; see Fig. 11-9).

The peptide bound by the class II molecule for presentation to the Th cell can be any part of the protein that makes up a complex antigen recognized by the B-cell receptor. The induction of antibody responses to viruses is an important example. Virus are complex structures composed of several proteins, DNA or RNA and, in certain cases, lipids from the host cell in which the virus replicated. A given B cell will recognize only a single epitope on one of the viral *surface* proteins. Uptake of the viral particle via immunoglobulin receptor-mediated endocytosis and the subsequent degradation of the viral proteins may result in many antigenic peptides, one or more from *each* viral protein. Thus, B cells that recognize epitopes on viral surfaces can be helped by Th cells, which are specific for peptides derived from any protein of that virus, whether on the surface (viral glycoprotein) or not (eg, nucleocapsid or matrix proteins). Therefore, the epitope recognized by the Th cell need not be on the same molecule as the epitope recognized by the B cell, but it must be on the same antigenic complex that was recognized and processed by that B cell. The chief requirement

is that the antigenic epitope recognized by the Th cell must be part of whatever the B cell specifically recognizes, internalizes, and processes, whether it be a complex, multiprotein antigen such as a virus, or a simple soluble protein antigen such as tetanus toxin.

This Th cell–B cell interaction can cause the B cell to switch from producing IgM to producing antibody of another isotype. As discussed in Chapter 8, this switch involves a translocation of the heavy-chain VDJ gene from a position adjacent to the μ-chain constant-region gene to another constant-region gene. Because of this switch, some plasma cells will be producing antibody of one isotype, and the memory B cells will begin to express receptors of a different isotype.

This Th cell-driven switch in heavy-chain constant-region expression is also accompanied by a dramatic increase in somatic mutation in the VDJ gene, presumably giving rise to some of the amino acid sequence diversity and the maturation in affinity of the antibody.

HELPER T-CELL FACTORS (LYMPHOKINES)

As discussed earlier, the Th cell is responsible for a number of the growth and differentiation signals given to the B cell during immune responses. Evidence suggests that the Th cell controls B-cell proliferation and differentiation by secreting soluble factors, generally referred to as cytokines or lymphokines which interact with the B cell (and, as is seen later, other T cells).

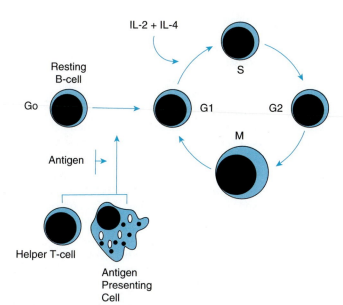

FIGURE 11-10 B-cell activation. Activation of a resting B cell requires several discrete signals. Signal 1 is delivered by cell–cell interaction with a preactivated helper T (Th) cell. This signal involves direct contact between the two cell types (Th cell recognition of antigen–class II complex on the B-cell surface) and most probably interaction of the B cell with the lymphokine, IL-1. Signal 1 drives the resting B cell from G_0 to G_1 of the cell cycle and induces the production of receptors for other lymphokines (eg, IL-2 and IL-4). Interaction of these receptors with the Th cell–produced lymphokines drives the B cell through the remainder of the cell cycle. These early events result in the expansion of the pool of B cells recognizing a given antigen.

The first step in B-cell activation requires cell–cell contact with the Th cell, resulting in progression of the resting B cell from G_0 to G_1 of the cell cycle. During this progression, the B cell begins to express receptors for IL-2 and a number of other Th-derived lymphokines. Subsequent interaction of the B cell with IL-2 drives the B cell through the remainder of the cell cycle (see Fig. 11-10), resulting in clonal expansion of the antigen-specific B cell.

Further differentiation into memory B cells and antibody-producing plasma cells appears to require other Th-derived lymphokines. A number of these lymphokines have been isolated, and their effect on B-cell growth and differentiation is the subject of intense study (see Table 11-1). The possibility that the role of IL-1 in B-cell activation is the same as it is in Th activation (ie, induction of expression of receptors for IL-2) has already been discussed. During or after clonal expansion, interaction of other lymphokines (IL-4, IL-5, IL-6, and IFN-γ) with their specific receptors on the B cell will induce a variety of effects, such as differentiation into plasma cells and memory cells (Fig. 11-11), increased expression of class II molecules, increased antibody secretion, expression of Fc receptors (FcRs), and preferential expression of antibody of a given isotype (see Fig. 11-11).

HETEROGENEITY OF HELPER T CELLS

Multiple examples exist in humans and in experimental animals of antibody responses in which a single immunoglobulin class, allotype, or idiotype is dominant. There is

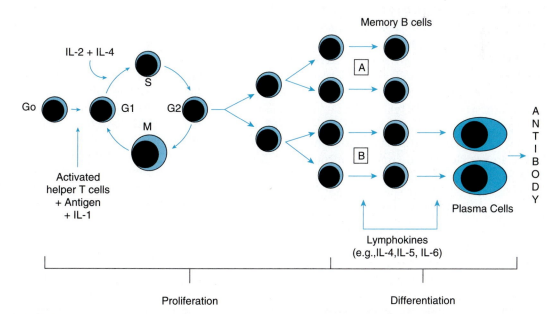

FIGURE 11-11 Role of lymphokines in B-cell proliferation and differentiation. A number of factors are released by macrophages and other antigen-presenting cells (monokines) and by T cells (lymphokines). These factors act at specific points in the proliferative and differentiative pathway leading to memory B cells (**A**) and antibody-secreting plasma cells (**B**). Some factors act early, some act later, and others (eg, IL-4) exert effects at several points in this pathway.

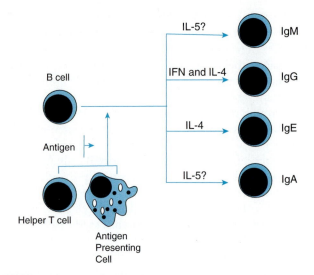

FIGURE 11-12   Role of helper T (Th) cells in the preferential expression of immunoglobulin isotypes. Certain Th cell clones can have a preferential effect on the expression of one or the other antibody isotypes. This effect is probably mediated by the type and concentration of lymphokine secreted by the Th cell clone. For example, it has been shown that secretion of IL-4 results in elevated production of IgE antibody. Secretion of interferon gamma and IL-4 increases IgG antibody production, and it is thought that secretion of IL-5 promotes IgM or IgA production. It is not known whether these factors influence production of a given isotype by promoting expansion of B cells already producing that isotype or by inducing an isotype switch in antibody-producing cells.

evidence that selective secretion of certain lymphokines is responsible for this phenomenon (Fig. 11-12). For example, it has been shown that two classes of Th cells, Th1 and Th2, exist. Th1 cells secrete IL-2 and IFN-γ, whereas Th2 cells secrete IL-4 and IL-5. Both subsets of Th cells activate B lymphocytes; Th1 cells induce B cells to switch from IgM to IgG, and Th2 cells induce B-cell switching from IgM to IgG or IgE. The subsets promote IgG synthesis, although it is unclear whether both promote synthesis of all four IgG subclasses. The conditions that result in preferential activation of one type of Th or preferential secretion of certain lymphokines by a single Th cell are not clear. Furthermore, evidence suggests that preferential expression of certain allotypes or idiotypes by B cells occurs, but this property has not yet been linked to any known lymphokine. It is not known whether these lymphokines can directly induce the isotype switch in B cells or whether they selectively expand B cells that have already undergone the switch as the result of other signals. Either way, the control of isotype expression permits the immune system to be focused on the synthesis of the antibody with the required biologic activity (eg, IgE and IgG in response to parasitic infections, IgA in response to infections on mucosal surfaces, and IgM and IgG to infections by organisms sensitive to complement).

T-INDEPENDENT ANTIGENS

As mentioned earlier, certain antigens do not require Th to induce antibody responses. These are called T independent or TI-antigens. They are normally large molecules that are poorly catabolized, possess repeating antigenic determinants, and often possess properties that render them mitogenic for lymphocytes when present at high concentrations. TI-antigens are present on the surface of infectious organisms. An example is the lipopolysaccharide of gram-negative organisms such as *Escherichia coli* or *Salmonella typhi* or the pneumococcal polysaccharide of the various species of *S pneumoniae*. Induction of antibody responses by these antigens may involve binding to both immunoglobulin receptors and mitogen receptors on B cells. Binding of a TI-antigen to a B cell results in extensive cross-linking of the immunoglobulin receptors. This cross-linking combined with the mitogenic activity of other structures on the antigen suffices to provide proliferative signals and certain signals of differentiation to the B cell. It is not known why these antigens are T-cell independent. Perhaps it is because they are poorly catabolized, or perhaps class II antigens do not bind these antigens or smaller oligomers derived from them. Either way, Th cells, which require corecognition of antigen and class II, are not stimulated.

KINETICS OF ANTIBODY FORMATION

As one might expect, the rate and extent of antibody formation are influenced by several different factors. These include the nature and concentration of the antigen, the frequency of Th and B cells specific for the antigen, and the efficiency of antigen processing by the APC. An adjuvant is a substance that is used to enhance the immunogenicity of soluble antigens. The exact mechanisms by which adjuvants exert their effect on immunogenicity is not clear, but it is interesting that many adjuvants contain substances that are mitogenic for lymphocytes. Examples of adjuvants are alum-precipitated toxoids, which have been used extensively in human immunizations, and water and oil emulsions of antigen-containing killed tubercle bacilli, which have been used widely in animal immunizations. This latter mixture, called *Freund's complete adjuvant,* causes a fairly intense inflammatory response at the site of injection.

Primary Response

The appearance of antibodies in the blood after an initial exposure to antigen is known as the *primary antibody response*. The rate and the extent of the primary response are dependent on the nature of the antigen, the size of the dose administered, the route of administration, and the frequency of the antigen-specific Th and B cells. Figure 11-13 shows the kinetics of an antibody response

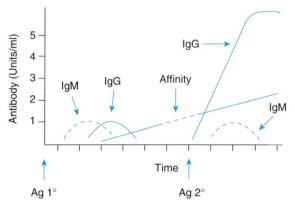

FIGURE 11-13 Kinetics of the antibody response. The kinetics of the appearance of antibody in blood plasma are shown after first and subsequent contacts with antigen. After a primary response (1°), there is a latent period before appearance of antibody. IgM antibody is the first to appear, followed by IgG and other isotypes. After a short period, the concentration of circulating antibody declines. On subsequent contact (2°) with antigen, memory B cells are stimulated and immediately respond by differentiating to plasma cells secreting antibody. The shortened latent period in the secondary response is primarily because of the expanded pool of B cells after primary stimulation (ie, there are more B cells and, thus, antibody is detected earlier). The secondary response is also of a much greater magnitude, again reflecting the greatly expanded pool of B cells after primary stimulation. In addition, the relative amount of IgG antibody in the secondary response is much greater than that of IgM (which is approximately the same as in the 1° response). This enhanced IgG response reflects the fact that many of the memory B cells have already undergone an isotype switch from μ- to γ-heavy chain expression. The affinity of antibody for its antigen also increases with time after antigen contact. This increasing affinity for antigen reflects an in vivo selection for B cells with high-affinity receptors while the antigen concentration decreases.

after an initial (primary) and subsequent (secondary) exposure to a theoretical antigen. Measurable antibody begins to appear about 5 days after the initial exposure to an antigen and reaches a peak in 2 to 3 weeks. The duration of antibody in the serum is dependent on continued stimulation of antibody production and on the normal catabolic turnover rate of immunoglobulin, which is different for each class of immunoglobulin. (The half-life of human IgG is about 23 days.)

Notice that IgM is the first antibody produced in the primary response and that the affinity of the antibody for the antigen increases with time. The fact that the first antibody produced is IgM should not be surprising, because after DNA rearrangement during differentiation from a stem cell to a B cell, the VDJ gene is directly upstream from the μ-chain constant-region gene. Thus, B cells with the VDJ μ-chain constant-region arrangement are present in a high frequency.

The increase in affinity during the primary response probably results from two factors. First, as discussed earlier and in Chapter 8, the heavy-chain switch is accompanied by somatic mutation in the VDJ genes. These somatic mutations may yield antibody molecules with a

greater affinity for antigen. Second, as antibody is produced, the concentration of antigen capable of stimulating B cells decreases. Residual antigen binds preferentially to B cells bearing immunoglobulin receptors with high affinity. Thus, as antigen concentration decreases, stimulation of B cells with high-affinity receptors occurs.

As B cells undergo the heavy-chain switch, antibody of the IgG and other classes begins to appear. The nature of the antibody produced depends on a number of factors, not the least of which is the nature of the immunoglobulin-specific Th cell that is activated (see earlier). In most cases in which one examines antibody in the blood, the IgG isotype is predominant. However, IgA is the predominant isotype in the secretions (eg, tears and colostrum).

As antigen is removed, fewer and fewer cells are stimulated. Serum antibody concentrations begin to decline as the terminally differentiated plasma cells cease to produce antibody and die.

Secondary Response

As is shown in Figure 11-13, a second exposure to antigen, months or even years later, produces an almost immediate appearance of antibodies (within 1 to 3 days), reaching concentrations that may be 10 to 15 times greater than that which occurred during the primary response. This may happen even if there was no measurable antibody at the time of the second exposure to antigen. This heightened response is caused almost entirely by the activation of relatively large numbers of memory Th and memory B cells that resulted from the clonal proliferation after primary stimulation. Because most of these memory cells have already undergone the switch, IgG antibody is synthesized almost immediately.

The affinity of the antibody produced during a secondary response begins at about the level that was present at the end of the primary response. Again, this should not be surprising, because the majority of the memory cells activated are those that were generated near the end of the primary response.

The response to TI-antigens is different. First, the isotype of the antibody produced is largely IgM, regardless of the number of times antigen is encountered. Second, because memory Th cells, to a large extent, are responsible for the heightened response after second exposure to antigen and because TI-antigens do not activate Th cells, the response to most TI-antigens will be of about the same magnitude on second and subsequent contacts as it is on first contact.

MHC Restriction and Dual Recognition

As mentioned earlier, activation of the Th cell requires that the Th cell interact with both antigen and a class II

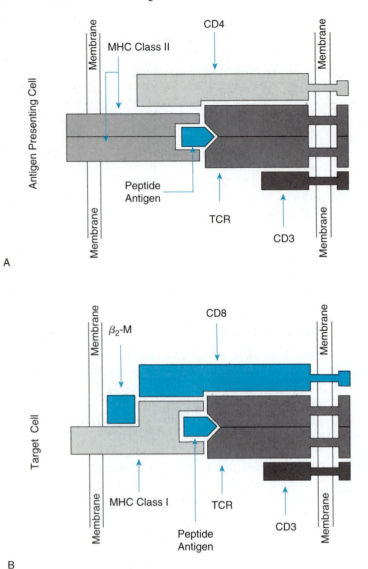

FIGURE 11-14   Model for MHC-restricted antigen recognition by T cells. The antigen-specific T-cell receptor (TCR) recognizes antigen complexed with either class II (**A**) or class I (**B**) MHC-encoded proteins on the surface of an antigen-presenting cell, a B cell, or a target cell. Class II–restricted T cells are CD4$^+$, whereas class I–restricted T cells are CD8$^+$. Evidence strongly suggests that the CD4 and CD8 invariant molecules interact with nonpolymorphic portions of the class II or class I MHC molecules, respectively. This restricted recognition is thought to result in phosphorylation of a ζ-chain of the CD3 part of this recognition complex, leading to increased Ca^{2+} flux and signal transduction. Although most class II–restricted T cells are helper cells, some cytotoxic T cells are class II restricted. Conversely, evidence suggests that some helper cells can be class I restricted.

molecule on the APC surface. This phenomenon is referred to as *dual recognition*. Moreover, such dual recognition is restricted in that the Th cell can respond only to an antigen that is complexed with class II molecules of its own genotype. This is referred to as *MHC restriction*.

Dual recognition and MHC restriction are general phenomena that are common to Th cells and cytotoxic T cells. Th cells are *restricted to recognizing antigen plus class II molecules*, whereas cytotoxic T cells are *restricted to recognizing antigen plus class I molecules*.

The T-Cell Recognition Complex

As discussed briefly in Chapter 9, the minimal T-cell recognition complex includes the heterodimeric antigen-specific TCR (termed *Ti*), the CD3 molecule, and either the CD4 or CD8 molecule, depending on whether the T cell is CD4$^+$8$^-$ or CD4$^-$8$^+$, respectively. A diagrammatic representation of this recognition complex is shown in Figure 11-14.

The CD3, CD4, and CD8 molecules from different individuals and different T-cell clones are invariant in structure. Antibody to the CD4 or CD8 molecules blocks activation of T cells, regardless of their antigen specificity. The CD3 and TcR molecules are physically associated with each other on the T-cell surface, and antibody to either can activate the T cell. However, antibody to CD3 activates T cells, regardless of the antigen specificity of the T cell, whereas antibody to TcR activates only the T-cell clone used to produce the anti-TcR antibody (ie, anti-TcR antibody is clonally specific).

The CD4 molecule appears to react with a nonvariable (monomorphic) portion of the class II molecule, whereas the CD8 molecule appears to react with a monomorphic portion of the class I molecule. Thus, the CD4 molecule on a CD4$^+$ T cell may serve to direct that cell to a target cell bearing the class II MHC products (eg,

CD4$^+$ Th cells would be directed to class II$^+$ macrophages and B cells). Similarly, the CD8 molecule on a CD8$^+$ T cell may serve to direct that cell to a target bearing the class I MHC products. For example, a CD8$^+$ Tc cell (see Chap. 13) would be directed to class I$^+$ virally infected target cells.

The model shown in Figure 11-14 is a minimal model and, at first glance, one might question the need for such complexity. However, the complexity is explicable if the recognition complex is viewed as having an antigen-specific receptor (the TCR molecule) linked to a signal transducer (the CD3 molecule) whose interaction with specific cell types is directed and stabilized by an anchor (the CD4 or CD8 molecule).

Figure 11-14 shows the interaction of a CD4$^+$8$^-$ Th cell with an APC that has processed the antigen for which the Th cell is specific. The complementarity-determining regions (CDRs) of the TCR polypeptide chains have formed a binding site that interacts with the peptide–class II complex. (The structure of class I and class II molecules is discussed in Chap. 10.) Some polymorphic residues of the class II molecule are involved in binding the peptide and others in binding to the TCR. The CD4 molecule binds to monomorphic (invariant) residues on the Class II molecule. This specific interaction leads to signal transduction via the CD3 molecule.

Other invariant, cell-surface adhesions are involved in this cell–cell interaction: for example, lymphocyte function antigen-1 on the T-cell surface and intracellular adhesion molecule-1 on the APC or target-cell surface. However, their role is to nonspecifically stabilize the complex formed by the more specific interactions described earlier.

Because the binding pocket of each class II (and class I) molecule has a specific composition and stereochemical configuration, it will bind only certain peptide fragments of antigen. The differences in peptide specificity of different class II molecules are determined by polymorphic residues in this pocket. Thus, during processing in the cell, individual allelic class II products can bind only certain of the peptides produced from a given protein. Some class II molecules may not bind to any peptide derived from a given protein. If this occurs for all class II molecules in an individual, no immune response against that protein will be made. Thus, an individual who has a limited number of class II alleles (eg, individuals homozygous at the class II loci) may be more susceptible to infection by a particular organism. Conversely, heterozygous individuals (with different alleles at the class II loci) will have more different class II products and thus a greater chance of binding and presenting antigens from a variety of infectious organisms.

Control of Immune Responses

A number of mechanisms control immune responses. Each of the mechanisms, briefly discussed here, has been shown to function in experimental situations. In most cases, it has been difficult to demonstrate their effects in systems not amenable to manipulation, for example, in humans, but it is assumed that they do function in our species as well.

COMPLEMENT AND Fc RECEPTORS

B cells possess receptors for certain components of complement and for the Fc portion of immunoglobulin (FcR). There are numerous reports that the reaction of these receptors with antigen–antibody complexes, with or without attached complement, respectively, can affect B-cell activation. For example, the complex serves to cross-link the FcR (via the antibody portion of the complex) and the immunoglobulin receptor (via the antigen portion of the complex), leading to down-regulation of antibody production by that B cell.

Similarly, certain T cells are known to have receptors for the Fc portion of immunoglobulin and to interact with antibody in the form of antigen–antibody complexes. The relevance of this interaction is not yet evident.

ANTIIDIOTYPE NETWORKS

The ability of an individual to produce an antiidiotypic antibody to his own antibody suggests that such an antiidiotype can act as a feedback control mechanism. Indeed, Niels Jerne has postulated that the antiidiotypic response is one of several components of a finely balanced control network affecting immune responses. He has proposed that the continued production of antibody results in the production of antiidiotypic antibody. This antiidiotype antibody would tend to suppress the response of B cells bearing immunoglobulin receptors of the same idiotype as the antibody produced originally.

SUPPRESSOR T CELLS

The notion of a distinct subset of T lymphocytes that specifically suppress immune responses evolved from experiments in which lymphocytes were transferred from one animal to another and the transferred cells seemed to prevent or suppress the development of an immune response in the recipient. Ultimately, antigen-specific and -nonspecific suppressor factors were identified as soluble mediators of T-cell–mediated suppression. But, because a distinct subset of T cells that mediate only inhibitory or suppressive activity has not been identified and because a wealth of data supports the positive and negative regulatory actions of cytokines and cell–cell interactions on immune responses, it is more reasonable to reinterpret the observations regarding T-suppressor cells in light of this new information. Essentially, all the actions and effects attributed to T-suppressor cells, that is, immunologic tolerance, suppression of antibody production, and suppression of cell-mediated immune responses, can be explained and understood in light of the knowledge regarding cell–cell interactions, pleiotropic effects of cytokines, and inactivation of antigen-specific lymphocytes by these mechanisms.

Tolerance

Immunologic tolerance is defined as the absence of a specific immune response resulting from a previous exposure to the inducing antigen. The most notable example is immunologic tolerance to self. Obviously, this lack of response is not mediated through no defect in the inherent antigenicity of self, because such self-molecules readily stimulate an immune response if introduced into another individual. Recall that this recognition of self versus nonself was proposed by Burnet to occur during fetal life by a mechanism in which those cells capable of making antibody to self were destroyed. Dizygotic cattle twins share the same placental circulation and exchange blood stem cells in utero. This natural occurrence is reminiscent of successful bone marrow transplantation in humans. The exchanged stem cells induce tolerance and survive in the cattle twins. As adults, each twin fails to respond to the histocompatibility antigens on cells from its twin. This failure to respond is because of the induction of specific immunologic tolerance during fetal life. In another example of tolerance, certain strains of mice that are genetically deficient in the C5-complement component (see Chap. 12) make vigorous antibody responses when immunized with pure C5 taken from normal animals. Neither normal mice nor the offspring of normal and C5-deficient mice respond to similar immunizations. This clearly demonstrates the immunologic tolerance to endogenous C5 in the normal and F1 hybrid mice and the absence of tolerance in the C5-deficient mice.

Experimentally, immunologic tolerance has been amply demonstrated with both living and nonliving antigens. In both cases, the immunologically mature individual is unable to react to the tolerogen (the antigen used to induce tolerance) when it is subsequently given in immunogenic form.

PARAMETERS THAT AFFECT THE INDUCTION OF TOLERANCE

A number of parameters have an effect on the ease with which immunologic tolerance can be induced. These include age, dose of antigen, route of tolerogen administration, physical nature of the antigen, and various treatments that reduce activation of positive regulatory cells of the immune response.

Age

The younger the recipient, the easier it is to induce tolerance, and, of course, it is easiest in utero. This undoubt-edly reflects both the number and immunologic maturity of the lymphocytes that constitute the immune system. Immature B cells (see Chap. 8) are far more sensitive to tolerance induction than are mature B cells. This may account, in part, for the increased ease of tolerance induction during fetal and neonatal life.

It has long been known that allograft tolerance can be easily induced in neonatal mice injected with suspensions of allogeneic spleen cells. However, neonatal mice given IL-2 at the same time as allogeneic spleen cells do not develop tolerance. This suggests that neonatal T cells have a reduced capacity to produce the IL-2 that is necessary for clonal expansion of T cells and B cells during activation by antigen, and that, in the absence of antigen-driven clonal expansion, tolerance is induced. That this may be true is suggested by the following observations:

- Administration of IL-2 prevents induction of tolerance in adult animals.
- Neonatal T cells produce little IL-2 on stimulation with agents known to induce it.
- Treatments known to reduce the numbers of IL-2–producing T cells facilitate the induction of tolerance in adult animals (eg, total lymphoid irradiation and injections of anti–T-cell antibodies such as anti-lymphocyte serum [ALS], anti-CD3, and anti-CD4).
- Drugs (eg, cyclosporin A) that inhibit IL-2 production prevent tolerance induction in adult animals.

This is not meant to imply that IL-2 production is the only factor involved, because even in the absence of overt IL-2 production, it is still much more difficult to induce tolerance in mature lymphoid cells.

Nature of Tolerogen

It has been demonstrated experimentally that it is easier to induce tolerance to a soluble macromolecule than to an aggregated antigen. A plausible explanation for this phenomenon is that aggregated antigens are readily phagocytized by macrophages, where they can be presented to Th cells, which, in turn, would provide help to B cell-antibody synthesis. On the contrary, soluble antigens are not so easily processed. The route of tolerogen contact is also important, probably for the same reasons, that is, intravenously administered antigens make faster contact with more cells at higher concentrations, compared with antigens administered subcutaneously or intraperitoneally.

Genetic Background

Extensive studies in experimental animals have made it clear that the genetic background of the individual plays a major role in determining whether tolerance will or will not be induced. It may be that such factors as homozygosity versus heterozygosity at the class I and class II loci, the presence or absence of T cells with TCRs capable of recognizing antigen in an MHC-restricted manner, the ability to process a given antigen in a manner that results in antigenically active peptides, and the capacity of the tolerogen to induce negative cytokine regulatory production are all important.

T-CELL VERSUS B-CELL TOLERANCE

Tolerance can be induced in both T cells and B cells. Jacques Chiller, Gail Habicht, and William Weigle conducted a classic experiment that provided considerable insight into the conditions necessary to induce experimental tolerance in these two cell types. They injected various doses of a monomeric antigen into a number of mice to induce tolerance. After varying periods of time, the mice were killed; their bone marrow or thymus cells were mixed with normal thymus cells or bone marrow, respectively, and injected into irradiated mice to assess which cell type was responsible for tolerance to the antigen, how quickly tolerance arose, and how long it lasted. Figure 11-15 shows that, under conditions in which high doses of tolerogen were injected, T-cell tolerance was almost immediate and total and was still at the 50% level after 23 weeks. On the other hand, B cells did not become tolerant for about a week, and the tolerance was completely lost after 6 to 7 weeks. In an identical experiment in which considerably less tolerogen was given, T-cell tolerance was essentially identical to that in the first experiment, but B-cell tolerance did not develop. Thus, contact with a high dose of tolerogen induced both T-cell and B-cell tolerance, even though B-cell tolerance was of much

shorter duration than that induced in T cells, whereas a low dose of tolerogen induced only T-cell tolerance. Notice that these studies were conducted with adult mice, suggesting that the high dose of tolerogen required for the development of B-cell tolerance probably reflects the concentration needed to eliminate (or inactivate) mature B cells, because neonatal tolerance involving immature B cells is much easier to induce.

MECHANISMS OF TOLERANCE

A number of theories explain the natural and experimental tolerance systems that have been observed, but they can be grouped into two categories: clonal deletion and clonal anergy.

Clonal Deletion

The discussions in this chapter have shown that several cell types are required for antibody production, and as is seen in Chapter 13, they are also required for the induction of cell-mediated immune responses. Thus, it follows that if any one or more of the required cell types (eg, B or T cells) can be removed or permanently inactivated, a person would be unable to respond immunologically to that antigen (specific tolerance) while maintaining an ability to respond to all other nonrelated antigens. All theories of clonal deletion-type tolerance involve the specific removal or inactivation of B or T cells after contact with antigen at the right time, in the correct dosage, and by way of the correct route.

A special form of clonal deletion is that proposed in 1975 by Sir Gustav Nossal called *clonal abortion*. This theory proposes that during development in utero or during development from bone marrow stem cells in adults, specific lymphocytes pass through a stage of differentiation in which they are exquisitely sensitive to clonal elimination by contact with antigen. Such a mechanism could account for the continuous elimination of clones directed toward self that constantly arise from stem cells throughout life. The fact that immature B cells (surface IgM$^+$IgD$^-$) are up to 1000-fold more susceptible to tolerance induction than are mature B cells provides support for this concept.

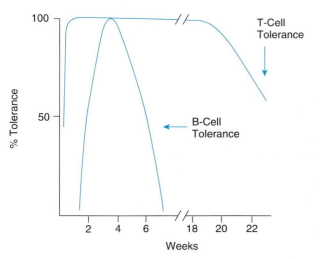

FIGURE 11-15 Kinetics of tolerance in T cells and B cells. The kinetics of tolerance in mouse T cells and B cells after a single contact with the soluble antigen, human gamma globulin (HGG) are shown. It is clear that tolerance is induced much earlier and lasts much longer in T cells than in B cells. In addition, tolerance in T cells can be induced with much lower concentrations of antigen.

Clonal Anergy

It has already been shown that negative-control mechanisms can affect all types of immune responses. Therefore, it seems reasonable to propose that if antigen were to preferentially activate a negative-control cytokine response, a person could not mount an immune response to that antigen, even though such a person possessed all the genetic potential for producing the response.

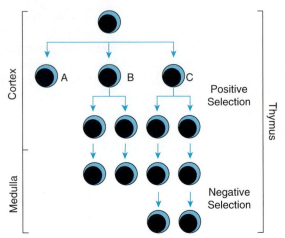

FIGURE 11-16   Positive and negative selection during T-cell differentiation in the thymus. Both positive and negative selection of T cells occurs during T-cell differentiation in the thymus. This selection is mediated by class II+ and class I+ cells resident in the thymus. The target cells appear to be the CD3+4+−8+TCR+ thymocytes. This process results first in selection for self-MHC–restricted T cells and then selection against T cells recognizing self-antigen in the context of self-MHC. The positive selection provides a pool of T cells that are capable of seeing any antigen (self and otherwise) in the context of self-MHC. The negative selection results in the elimination of the cells (arising from the positive selection) that see self-antigen complexed with self–class I or self–class II MHC. This induction of tolerance to self-antigen + self-MHC prevents subsequent development of autoimmune disorders.

A SPECIAL ROLE FOR THE THYMUS IN INDUCTION OF SELF-TOLERANCE

Chapter 9 discussed the role of the thymus in T-cell differentiation and in the development of the T-cell repertoire. It was also mentioned that the thymus is the site for initial self–nonself discrimination and that both positive and negative selection for or against certain antigenic specificities is known to occur. During T-cell differentiation, there is the possibility of developing TCRs that recognize self-MHC molecules (both class I and class II) with high affinity and of developing TCRs that recognize a complex of self-peptide and self-MHC with high affinity. Self-peptides would be any peptides derived from any self-protein produced by the developing individual. If this development of a high-affinity anti-self repertoire were permitted, the organism (human or animal) would not survive. Therefore, the positive- and negative-selection steps occurring in the thymus during T-cell differentiation have evolved to eliminate any possible anti-self–T-cell clones (Fig. 11-16). The positive-selection step would select (clonally expand) those T-cell clones with TCRs having low affinity for self-MHC alone (in essence selecting against those with high affinity for self-MHC alone). The negative-selection step would select against (clonal elimination) those developing T-cell clones with TCRs that recognize self-MHC plus self-peptide with high affinity. Both types of selection are known to occur and experimentally have been demonstrated to function in vivo.

This selection mechanism in the thymus would continue for as long as the thymus functions in T-cell differentiation. Such a mechanism may also explain why most autoimmune phenomena (see Chap. 14) involve tissue-specific antigens. These antigens, other than those specific to the thymus, would not be present in the thymus during T-cell differentiation. Thus, T cells specific for these antigens would not be eliminated during the selection process.

Related to such a mechanism is the effect of a failure of costimulation in T cells. Clearly, once the TCR binds to an antigen–MHC complex, the T cell must receive a second signal such as the interaction of a ligand called B7 with the C28 receptor on the T cell. If this second, co-stimulatory signal is not received, the T cell is rendered anergic or unresponsive. Clonal anergy is reversible, an observation that helps to explain the reversible nature of immunologic tolerance.

A Closer Look

The mechanisms of regulation of the immune response have long been a mystery to immunologists and an area of intense investigation. The activation of T and B cells during the antigen-specific immune response has been found to require cell–cell interaction between APCs, T cells, and B cells. In addition, a variety of cytokines, products of macrophages in the case of monokines and lymphocytes in the case of cytokines, are critical to the maturation of an antigen-specific immune response. T-cell and B-cell growth factors, activating factors, and co-stimulatory molecules must be present in a coordinated way for the development of an immune response. Of course, the entire response is dependent on the interaction of antigen-specific receptors on T cells with self-MHC molecules, which present the antigen.

The nature of modulation or suppression of immune responses has captured the interest of immunologists from all branches of this science. Over the years, a variety of regulatory mechanisms have been discov-

A Closer Look *continued*

ered, including idiotype and antiidiotype networks, antibody feedback on antigen-specific antibody responses, and various forms of immunologic deviation, immunologic tolerance, and immunologic suppression.

One of the most controversial areas in the investigation of the regulation of immune responses is the existence and role of suppressor T lymphocytes in the regulatory process. In the 1970s, T-suppressor lymphocytes were discovered and elevated to the status of a central immunoregulatory cell in virtually all forms and varieties of immune responses. In the late 1980s, because of a failure to definitively identify, clone, and propagate a distinct T-suppressor lymphocyte subset, coupled with the fact that no single lymphocyte membrane marker has ever been consistently associated with a cell having the suppressor cell phenotype, the existence of this category of cells came into question. In the 1990s, there has been a resurgence of interest in T-lymphocyte–mediated suppression of specific immune responses. As has happened in the past, extremes of enthusiasm, pro and con, regarding T-lymphocyte–mediated suppression may have led investigators astray. It seems likely that immunologists will define interacting networks of cells (eg, T and B lymphocytes, macrophages, and others) that communicate and regulate each other by exchange of soluble mediators. The existence of a unifunctional T suppressor lymphocyte subpopulation is deemed unlikely. The role of cytokine networks and cellular interaction in the positive and negative regulation of antigen-specific immune responses is coming to be appreciated. Much of the activation and regulation of immune responses believed to be mediated by T-suppressor cells can be explained through the interactions of the various subsets of T lymphocytes. Clearly, co-stimulatory signals are necessary for the activation of T cells, and some cytokines, such as the interleukins and IFN-γ, may play a modulatory or even suppressive role during the generation of an immune response.

An area of investigation that has not yielded definitive answers is immunologic tolerance. Various parameters of antigen-specific unresponsiveness (tolerance) and mechanisms for the induction of tolerance have been defined. Both B and T lymphocytes become immunologically tolerant, but whether the tolerance mechanisms are different for these two cell types and whether one represents a form of anergy and the other a form of deletion is still not apparent. The development of protocols for the induction of antigen-specific immunologic tolerance that will be useful clinically to prevent unwanted immune responses in patients is a central goal of such investigations.

Bibliography

JOURNALS

Greenspan NS, Bona CA. Idiotypes: structure and immunogenicity. FASEB J 1992;7:437.

Noelle RJ, Snow EC. T helper cell-dependent B cell activation. FASEB J 1991;5:2770.

BOOKS

Cambier JC, Pleiman CM, Clark MR. Signal transduction by the B-cell antigen receptor and its coreceptors. In: Paul WE, Fathman CG, Metzger H, eds. Annual review of immunology, vol 12. Palo Alto, Annual Reviews, 1994:457.

Chan AC, Desai DM, Weis A. The role of protein tyrosine kinases and protein tyrosine phosphatases in T-cell antigen receptor signal transduction. In: Paul WE, Fathman CG, Metzger H, eds. Annual review of immunology, vol 12. Palo Alto, Annual Reviews, 1994:555.

Fitch FW, McKisic MD, Lancki DW, Gajewski TF. Differential regulation of murine T lymphocyte subsets. In: Paul WE, Fathman CG, Metzger H, eds. Annual review of immunology, vol 11. Palo Alto, Annual Reviews, 1993:29.

Janeway CA Jr. In: Greene MI, Nisonoff A, eds. Biology of Idiotypes. New York, Plenum, 1984:349.

Jorgensen JL, Reay PA, Ehrich EW, Davis MM. Molecular components of T-cell recognition. In: Paul, WE, Fathman CG, Metzger H, eds. Annual review of immunology, vol 10. Palo Alto, Annual Reviews, 1992:835.

Linsley PS, Ledbetter JA. The role of CD28 receptor during T cell responses to antigen. In: Paul WE, Fathman CG, Metzger H, eds. Annual review of immunology, vol 11. Palo Alto, Annual Reviews, 1993:191.

Matzinger P. Tolerance, danger, and the extended family. In: Paul WE, Fathman CG, Metzger H, eds. Annual review of immunology, vol 12. Palo Alto, Annual Reviews, 1994:991.

Miller JFAP, Morahan G. Peripheral T cell tolerance. In: Paul WE, Fathman CG, Metzger H, eds. Annual review of immunology, vol 10. Palo Alto, Annual Reviews, 1992:52.

Parker DC. T cell-dependent B cell activation. In: Paul WE, Fathman CG, Metzger H, eds. Annual review of immunology, vol 11. Palo Alto, Annual Reviews, 1993:331.

Rothbard JB, Gefter ML. Interactions between immunogenic peptides and MHC proteins. In: Paul WE, Fathman CG, Metzger H, eds. Annual review of immunology, vol 9. Palo Alto, Annual Reviews, 1991:527.

Essentials of Medical Microbiology, Fifth Edition, edited by Wesley A. Volk, Bryan M. Gebhardt, Marie-Louise Hammarskjöld, and Robert J. Kadner. Lippincott-Raven Publishers, Philadelphia © 1996.

Chapter 12

Complement

Nearly 100 years ago, it was observed that antiserum could exert two entirely different effects on gram-negative bacteria or red blood cells (RBCs). In one case, when fresh antiserum was used, such cells were lysed. On the other hand, if the antiserum was heated to 56°C for 30 minutes or aged about 1 week, it could no longer cause lysis but instead would agglutinate the bacteria or RBCs. However, when fresh normal serum, such as guinea pig serum, was added to the heated or aged antiserum, the ability to cause cell lysis was regained. The lytic effect, therefore, requires two factors: (1) specific antibody, and (2) a labile component present in normal serum. This latter substance has been given the name *complement*. Subsequent research has revealed that complement is a multicomponent system composed of many different proteins.

The activation of the complement proteins proceeds by two triggered enzyme systems, wherein a series of inactive proteolytic enzymes (zymogens) are converted into biologically active proteases, each possessing an extremely fine specificity for its substrate. There are two pathways for the activation of the system, each initiated by a different sequence of events. The classic pathway of complement activation is set in motion by antigen–antibody complexes, whereas the alternate pathway, which is phylogenetically much older, is entirely independent of antigen–antibody reactions. Instead, certain components are activated by the presence of a series of foreign substances, not the least of which are infecting bacteria and viruses. The two pathways, however, have much in common, particularly the fact that their final membrane-attack components are identical.

Biologic Function of the Complement System

Before the details of the classic pathway of complement activation are outlined, the biologic function of this system should be considered. This function can best be appreciated by noticing that after antibody has reacted with its antigen, it can do little more. In other words, antibody might precipitate an antigen or, if the antigen is cellular, might cause agglutination but, with the exception of the neutralization of toxins or of virus infectivity, antibody alone is an ineffective means of protection against infection. Thus, for practical purposes, the major function of an antibody is to recognize a foreign antigen and bind to it. By doing so, it provides a site for phagocyte interaction and for the initiation of the reactions of the complement system. It is the activation of this system that (1) leads to the lysis of foreign cells, (2) further enhances phagocytosis of invading microorganisms, and (3) causes local inflammation, stimulating the chemotactic activity of the host's leukocytes.

In addition, after activation of the system, interaction of one or more complement components with specific receptors on cell surfaces can result in (1) enhancement of antibody-dependent cellular cytotoxicity (ADCC) (see Chap. 13); (2) increased oxidative metabolism; (3) secretion of vasoactive amines and leukotrienes (see Chap. 14); (4) secretion of monokines (see Chap. 13); (5) stimulation of prostaglandin and thromboxane pathways; (6) modulation of lymphocyte activation and antibody responses; and (7) mobilization of leukocytes from the bone marrow. The following sections are concerned with a step-by-step dissection of the component parts and reactions of this system and the role that it plays in the destruction of foreign cells.

Classic Pathway of Complement Activation

The operation of the complement system consists of a number of reactions, each of which activates the next reaction in the series. A primary event must occur, however, to initiate the reactions that eventually involve the many components of the complement system (Table 12-1). In the case of the classic pathway, the initiating event occurs when the first component of complement reacts with antigen–antibody complexes in which the antibody is either IgM or IgG. IgA, IgD, and IgE are not effective in activating complement.

Once initiated, the activation of the complement system may have various effects, depending on the type of foreign cell involved in the antigen–antibody reaction. In the case of a gram-negative bacterium, the integrity of the cell membrane is destroyed, permitting the lysozyme-mediated lysis and death of the cell. Gram-positive organisms are not lysed, but the activation of complement by a gram-positive cell and antibody results in the release of fragments of complement components that aid in phagocytosis by binding to the antigen, providing a receptor for the host leukocyte. In addition, many eukaryotic cells, such as RBCs or virus-infected cells, are lysed by complement. The complex reactions that produce all these effects can be divided into three series of reactions involving the

TABLE 12-1
Components of the Human Complement System

Protein	Serum Concentration ($\mu g/mL$)	Molecular Weight (daltons)	Number of Chains
Classic Pathway			
C1q	180	410,000	18
C1r	50	83,000	1
C1s	40	83,000	1
C2	25	117,000	1
C3	1600	185,000	2
C4	640	206,000	3
C5	70	191,000	2
C6	64	120,000	1
C7	56	110,000	1
C8	55	151,000	3
C9	59	71,000	1
Alternate Pathway			
Factor B (B)	200	93,000	—
Factor D (D)	1	24,000	—
Factor H (H)	500	150,000	—
Factor I (I)	34	88,000	—
Properdin	20	224,000	—

complement system: (1) the activation of the recognition unit, (2) the assembly of the activation unit, and (3) the assembly of the attack unit. Figure 12-1 summarizes the reactions of complement leading to the formation of the attack complex, and Figure 12-2 shows a schematic model of this series of reactions.

THE RECOGNITION UNIT

Of the nine known components of the classic pathway, only the first component, C1, is involved in the recognition unit. This component, as indicated in Table 12-1, is composed of three different proteins—C1q, C1r, and C1s—which interact with each other on an antigen–antibody complex. It appears that antigen–antibody reactions bring numerous antibody molecules into aggregates that can be cross-linked by C1q. This clustering of antibody molecules can be mimicked by mild heating or chemically cross-linking antibodies to form an aggregate in the absence of antigen. Such artificial aggregates easily react with C1q, leading to complement activation.

The reaction begins when C1q, the recognition subunit of C1, binds to the constant region of the antibody complexes. The binding site for C1q is located in the fourth domain (C_H4) of IgM and in the second domain (C_H2) of IgG. Some variability exists in the capacity of the IgG subclasses to activate complement. The reason for this is unknown.

ACTIVATION OF RECOGNITION UNIT:

C1 + Ab → Ab-C1 (Ab-C1q-C1r-C1s) → *C1s*

ASSEMBLY OF ACTIVATION UNIT:

C1s
↓
C4 → C4a + C4b

C1s
↓
C2 → C2a + C2b
C4b + C2a → *C4b2a* C3 Convertase

C4b2a
↓
C3 → C3a + C3b
C4b2a + C3a → *C4b2a3b* C5 Convertase

ASSEMBLY OF MEMBRANE ATTACK COMPLEX:

C4b2a3b
↓
C5 → C5a + C5b
C5b + C6 + C7 → C5b67
C5b67 + C8 + C9 → C5b6789$_n$

FIGURE 12-1   The classic pathway of complement activation. All activated enzymes are in color. Ab, antibody.

C1q is an unusual protein made of three subunits occurring as dimers, each possessing three chains (designated A, B, and C) about 200 amino acids long. The A and B chains are linked to the C chain; therefore, each molecule of assembled C1q has 18 chains that can be designated as $(A_6B_6C_6)$. The most unusual feature of these chains, however, is that the major part of the amino-terminal half of each chain consists of a repeating triplet of glycine–X–Y, where X is often proline and Y is frequently 4-hydroxyproline or hydroxylysine. Such a structure is similar to the helical part of collagen, and, as in collagen, these sequences impart a stable helical structure to the amino-terminal half of C1q. The carboxy terminal half of C1q consists of globular regions, or "heads," that contain the binding sites for the Fc region of antibody. C1q has six such heads and consequently can potentially bind six antibody molecules. For complement to be activated, simultaneous binding of antibody by two or more C1q heads must occur. The requirement for cross-linking is exemplified by the fact that a single molecule of IgM on the surface of an RBC is sufficient to cause complement-mediated lysis, whereas it has been calculated that a RBC must bind an average of 700 molecules of IgG to ensure

MEMBRANE

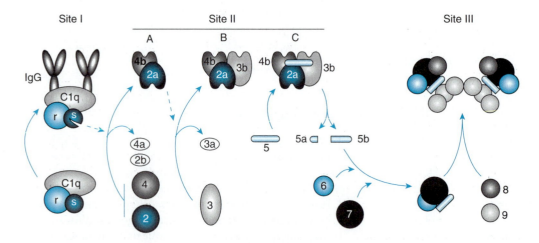

FLUID PHASE

FIGURE 12-2   The three-site model of antibody-dependent complement activation at a cell surface. The C1 complex reversibly interacts with antibody molecules that have bound to cell-surface antigen molecules. Through an internal reaction, the C1s subunit of C1 is activated. This activated C1s protease cleaves first the C4 and then the C2 complement components. The C4b cleavage product binds to appropriate sites on the membrane (*Site II*) as shown in *A*. The C2a cleavage product binds to the membrane-bound C4b, resulting in a new proteolytic enzyme called *C3 convertase*. The C3 convertase hydrolyzes the third component of complement (C3), producing C3a and C3b. The C3b portion then associates with the C4bC2a enzyme (*B* in *Site II*), resulting in an enzyme, *C5 convertase*, with a new substrate specificity. The fifth component of complement, C5, binds to the C4b and C3b portions of the C5 convertase, is cleaved, and is released into the fluid phase. The C5b product then associates with C6 and C7, forming a complex that is stabilized by interaction with the membrane at *Site III*. Components C8 and C9 then associate with the C5b67 complex on the membrane, leading to membrane destabilization and lysis.

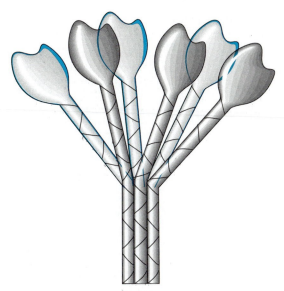

FIGURE 12-3 Model of the human C1q complement component. C1q has six helical stalks, each with a collagen-like structure and each topped with a globular head. The heads contain the sites which bind to the Fc portion of antibody.

statistically that two molecules are close enough to be cross-linked by C1q. Figure 12-3 illustrates a schematic molecule of C1q.

C1r and C1s are both present in the C1 complex as inactive proteases. Limited amino acid sequence studies have shown considerable homology between these two components, as well as some homology with other serine proteases. In the presence of Ca^{2+}, they are bound to the collagen portion of C1q as a tetrameric complex consisting of two molecules each of C1r and C1s [(C1r$_2$C1s$_2$)C1q]. In solution, C1q, C1r, and C1s exist in an easily dissociable complex, but after C1q cross-links antibody, this association becomes much more stable, presumably because of a conformational change in C1q. The actual binding to C1q appears to occur through C1r, because isolated C1r will bind to antibody–C1q, whereas C1s will not.

After binding to antibody–C1q, a conformational change occurs in C1r, which exposes an enzymatic site that catalyses its own hydrolysis, converting it into an active serine protease ($\overline{C1r}$) whose only known substrate is C1s. (Complement components that have been modified to become enzymatically active are written with a bar over the complement designation, as in $\overline{C1r}$.) Once activated, $\overline{C1r}$ splits off a peptide from C1s, converting C1s also into a serine protease, $\overline{C1s}$, which initiates the assembly of the activation unit.

ASSEMBLY OF THE ACTIVATION UNIT

The first step in the assembly of the activation unit occurs when $\overline{C1s}$ splits off a 77–amino acid vasoactive polypeptide (C4a) from the N-terminal chain of C4 to generate

C4b. This exposes an intrachain thioester bond within C4b, which is the reactive site responsible for attachment to the cell membrane or to the cross-linked antibody molecules bound to C1q or to those immediately adjacent. Unbound molecules of C4b are rapidly inactivated. $\overline{C1s}$ also cleaves C2 into two components: C2a (a 70,000-dalton fragment) and C2b (a 30,000-dalton polypeptide).

At this point, C2a remains bound to the antibody-bound or membrane-bound C4b to form a new active protease, $\overline{C4b2a}$, which is called C3 convertase. The catalytic site of C3 convertase exists in the C2a fragment, and the role of C4b appears to be one of binding C2a, thus stabilizing the C3 convertase. The newly formed C3 convertase, $\overline{C4b2a}$, cleaves C3 into two fragments, C3a and C3b, again exposing a highly reactive thioester bond in C3b. The C3b molecule reacts with residues on the cell surface, on the antigen–antibody complex, or on the C3 convertase itself, forming a new enzymatically active complex, $\overline{C4b2a3b}$, called C5 convertase. Those C3b molecules that do not immediately react with sites nearby are inactivated by hydrolysis of this thioester bond. This $\overline{C4b2a3b}$ is the activation unit of the classic pathway, and its function is to split C5 into C5a and C5b, which initiates the formation of the membrane-attack complex. Interestingly, both C3 convertase and C5 convertase use the same catalytic site in the bound C2a. In the C5 convertase molecule, C3b acts as a binding site for the C5 substrate. It seems probable, however, that the C5 convertase continues to split C3 into C3a and C3b. Figure 12-4 illustrates the structure of C3 and shows how it is converted into an active subunit.

ASSEMBLY OF THE MEMBRANE-ATTACK COMPLEX

The splitting of C5 by C5 convertase is the last enzymatic reaction involved in the classic pathway of complement activation; the subsequent assembly of the remaining components of the attack complex are nonenzymatic, occurring spontaneously as follows:

1. C5b reacts with one molecule of C6, forming a relatively stable complex of C5b6. C5b alone is very unstable in serum, with a half-life measured in milliseconds; however, C5b is stabilized by reacting with C6 while still bound to the C3b of the C5 convertase.
2. In the fluid phase, C7 is added to C5b6 to create C5b67, the first component of the attack complex that has membrane-binding properties. C5b67 has a half-life of about 100 milliseconds in the fluid phase, but it is stabilized by binding directly to the membrane, independent of C3b.
3. C5b67 now expresses a C8-binding site, and when C8 binds to the complex, it is inserted into the lipid bilayer. At this point, the complex is capable of slow lysis of susceptible cells, which becomes more rapid with the addition of C9 in the next step. However, animals

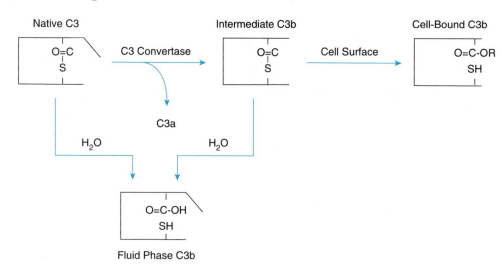

FIGURE 12-4 C3 activation. C3 is cleaved by the proteolytic enzyme C3 convertase. This cleavage results in the exposure of an internal thioester bond. This C3b may be stabilized by reaction of the highly reactive thioester bond with sites on the cell surface, permitting it to function as a component of other enzymes in the complement pathway or as an opsonin that promotes phagocytosis. However, if the highly reactive thioester bond reacts with water, the C3b is inactivated and further degraded by serum proteases.

deficient in the C9 component are able to deal with most infections normally.

4. Aggregation of C5b–8 within the membrane then occurs, resulting in formation of a C9-binding site. Interaction of C9 with this site causes a conformational change in C9, exposing hydrophobic regions and facilitating its insertion into the membrane and its polymerization into a poly–C9 complex. See Table 12-1 for a summary of the components of the entire activation pathway.

OTHER MECHANISMS OF ACTIVATING THE CLASSIC PATHWAY

The classic pathway of complement activation is normally thought of as one initiated by antigen–antibody complexes but, actually, it involves C1, C2, and C4 to form the C3 convertase, because the alternate pathway of activation uses a different C3 convertase. With this definition, several other elements can be added that activate the classic pathway, namely, viral membranes, the lipid A portion of endotoxin, mitochondrial membranes, and miscellaneous polycations and polyanions such as heparin, protamine, and nucleic acids. The mechanism whereby these compounds initiate C1 activation is unknown, but it can be assumed that any substance possessing binding sites for C1q might initiate this pathway.

Interestingly, nonprimate retroviruses activate primate C1 directly. This activation is dependent on the C1s portion of C1. This may be the primary mode of defense against these viruses, because it is known that primates do not produce antibody to these nonprimate retroviruses. It may be that the viruses are cleared from the body by activating the classic pathway before antibody synthesis is induced.

Alternate Pathway of Complement Activation

The alternate pathway of complement activation (the *properdin pathway*) does not require the presence of antibodies for initiation and, as a result, provides a mechanism of nonspecific resistance to infection. Moreover, this pathway does not use C1, C4, or C2, which are the early reactants in the classic pathway of complement activation. Remember, however, that the overall result of this pathway is the same as that of the classic pathway: C3 is split into C3a and C3b, and C5 is cleaved to form C5a and C5b, thus permitting the spontaneous formation of the C5b–9 membrane-attack complex. The enzymes catalyzing these conversions are different from the C3 and C5 convertases described for the classic pathway of complement activation.

RECOGNITION AND ASSEMBLY

This pathway bypasses both the recognition unit and the assembly of the activation unit as described for the classic pathway. Instead, there are at least three normal serum proteins that, when activated together with C3, form a functional C3 convertase and a C5 convertase. These are factor B, factor D, and properdin (P). Table 12-1 lists the major properties of these proteins. To fully comprehend this pathway, the reader should keep the following facts in mind:

1. These are normal serum proteins, and the alternate pathway routinely undergoes activation in the absence of any stimulus.
2. In the absence of initiators (which is discussed later), the initial complexes of the alternate pathway are rapidly destroyed.
3. In the presence of these initiators, such complexes are stabilized, and complement is activated to form the identical membrane-attack complexes described for the classic pathway.

Reaction Sequence

The pathway appears to be initiated in the following steps:

1. The C3 molecule has an internal intrachain thioester bond formed by the reaction of the side chains of two amino acids: cysteine and glutamic acid (see Fig.

12-4). In the blood, this thioester bond reacts with a molecule of H_2O to form the unstable C3–H_2O complex. This unstable, yet active, complex then binds to serum factor B to form another unstable complex, C3B. The factor B portion of the C3B complex is split by factor D (a normal serine protease) into two fragments, Ba and Bb. Ba is a 33,000-dalton peptide that is released during the reaction, and Bb is a 60,000-dalton peptide that remains bound to C3 to form a C$\overline{3Bb}$ complex. The C$\overline{3Bb}$ acts, probably in the fluid phase, as an initial C3 convertase to split C3 into C3a and C3b.

2. C3b binds factor B, forming the transient intermediate C3bB, which is then subject to cleavage by factor D, to form C$\overline{3bBb}$. This is the active C3 convertase of the alternate pathway.

   Notice that there have been two C3 convertases formed to this point (ie, C$\overline{3Bb}$ and C$\overline{3bBb}$) that differ in the form of the C3 portion but that have the same enzymatic specificity. The C$\overline{3bBb}$ enzyme, however, is capable of reacting with surfaces (eg, the cell membrane) and thus can be stabilized.

3. As more C3b is generated by C$\overline{3bBb}$, it continues to attach to the membrane. When an additional molecule of C3b becomes bound to the C$\overline{3bBb}$, the specificity of the convertase is shifted to a C5 convertase (designated C$\overline{3bBb3b}$).

4. Properdin enters the reaction sequence and binds to both the C3 and C5 convertase to protect the complex from the action of factor I (a normal component of serum that is capable of inactivating C3b). Properdin interaction, therefore, is the terminal event in the assembly of the activation unit for this pathway.

5. Once the C5 convertase is formed, C5 is cleaved to form C5a and C5b, and the spontaneous formation of the attack complex (C5b–9) quickly follows. The formation of this attack complex proceeds in the same manner as it does in the classic pathway discussed above.

The Amplification Loop

As is illustrated in Figure 12-5, once C3b is formed and reacts with factor B, there is a rapid formation of a membrane-bound C3 convertase, which initiates an amplification loop to form more C3 convertase by cleaving more C3 into C3a and C3b, which, in turn, reacts with factor B to form more C3 convertase and C5 convertase. It should be pointed out that C3b generated by the classic pathway may also initiate the amplification loop, producing additional convertases. Thus, it can be seen that these two pathways of complement activation have much in common, differing only in the initial events leading to the formation of C3b and C5b.

The Lytic Event

It is now well established that membrane-bound C5b–8 can cause slow lysis of a susceptible cell and that the addition of C9 greatly accelerates the cell lysis. However, no real consensus exists concerning exactly how lysis occurs. Aggregation of the C5b–8 complex in the membrane clearly forms a binding site for C9. Interaction of C9 with this site induces large conformational changes in C9, exposing hydrophobic regions responsible for insertion of C9 in the membrane and the formation of poly–C9. Poly–C9 is composed of 12 to 18 molecules of C9 and is the ring-like structure seen in electron micrographs of cells treated with antibody and complement (Fig. 12-6). The poly–C9 structure forms at high concentrations and is not required for efficient lysis. Lysis of the cell to which the membrane-attack complex is bound occurs primarily by extensive disruption of the lipid bilayer, an increase in membrane permeability, and marked changes in membrane potential, pH, and cytosoliccation concentrations, leading to complete loss of electrochemical gradients and rupture of the plasmamembrane.

FIGURE 12-5 The alternate pathway of complement activation. Soluble C3 spontaneously interacts with factor B in solution. This complex is converted to a C3 convertase enzyme by factor D. Fluid-phase C3 is cleaved by this C3 convertase, leading to the production of C3b, which, in turn, can form a second C3 convertase on the membrane by interaction with factor B and factor D. The membrane-bound C3 convertase can be converted into C5 convertase by interaction with other C3b peptides or can continue to produce more C3b by cleaving more C3. This latter amplification loop can continue to produce more C3b and, thus, more C3 convertase and more C5 convertase, thereby amplifying the effect of the single initial reaction. The C5 convertase cleaves C5, and the resulting C5b initiates formation of the attack complex in the same way as described for the classic pathway in Figure 12-1. Notice that the amplification loop, shown by the heavy line, operates whenever C3b is formed, whether by the alternate or the classic pathway of activation.

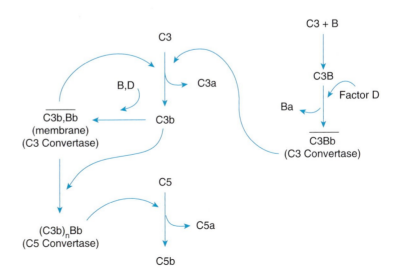

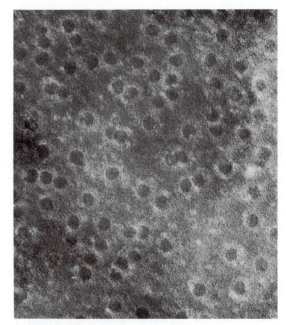

FIGURE 12-6 Antibody- and complement-treated sheep red blood cell membranes. Sheep red blood cells were treated with antibody to red-cell antigens and with human serum as a source of complement. The membranes of the treated red cells were then examined by electron microscopy. This photograph shows the typical lesions formed by such treatment. The round lesions result from aggregation of the C9 component of complement in the red-cell membrane. This poly-C9 is a result of assembly of the attack complex after initial complement activation by antibody complexed with red-cell surface antigen. Lysis of the cell is a result of membrane destabilization after assembly of this complex.

Control of the Complement System

If no controls for the complement system existed, the first molecule of C3b formed would initiate the amplification loop, resulting in a depletion of C3, formation of the attack complex, and damage to host cell membranes. Moreover, as is discussed later in this chapter, a number of the split products of complement components do not enter into the formation of the attack complex and can exert a deleterious effect on nearby cells. Thus, careful regulation of this system is a necessity. The following sections describe these controls and how they interact in each of the activation pathways. Table 12-2 lists the control proteins.

C1 INHIBITOR

Normal serum contains a glycoprotein called *C1 inhibitor,* which rapidly binds to C$\overline{1}$s and plasmin, forming an unusually stable complex. The reaction is nonenzymatic inasmuch as neither C$\overline{1}$s nor plasmin is cleaved, but the catalytic site for both enzymes is blocked by the C1 inhibitor. Interestingly, C1 inhibitor also inhibits enzymes of the kinin-forming, fibrinolytic, and coagulation systems such as kallikrein, Hageman factor, and plasmin. Individuals with deficiencies in C1 inactivator experience fluid accumulation that, particularly if localized in the larynx, can be fatal. This syndrome, called *hereditary angioedema,* appears to result from a kinin-like C2 fragment generated by excess C$\overline{1}$s. Other examples of the interaction of the complement system with the kinin, fibrinolytic, and coagulation systems are given later in this chapter.

FACTOR I

Control of C3b is necessary for the regulation of both the classic and the alternate pathways. Normal serum contains an endopeptidase, called *factor I,* that cleaves the chain of C3b, destroying both the hemolytic and immune adherence properties catalyzed by C3b. Subsequent action by serum plasmin cleaves the inactivated C3b into smaller peptides known as C3c and C3d.

C4b is also cleaved and inactivated by an endopeptidase that is believed to be identical to factor I.

FACTOR H

Factor H is a nonenzymatic protein that exists as a tetramer in normal serum. It has a strong affinity for C3b,

TABLE 12-2
Control Proteins in the Complement System

Control Protein	Activity
C1 inhibitor	Blocks active site of C1s and plasmin
Factor I	Cleaves C3b and possibly C4b
Factor H	Binds C3b and prevents binding of factor B, removes Bb from alternate pathway C3 convertase, enhances factor I action on C3b
C4 binding protein	Enhances C4b degradation
Decay-accelerating factor (DAF)	Membrane protein; inhibits C3 convertases
Vitronectin	Binds fluid phase C5b67 complex and prevents its deposition on membranes
Homologous restriction factor	Membrane protein; inhibits C9 binding to C5b678 complex on membrane
Complement receptor-1 (CR-1)	Membrane protein on human RBCs and platelets; binds C3b and prevents amplification loop

and, after binding C3b, it exerts its control in three ways: (1) it prevents factor B from binding to C3b; (2) it removes factor Bb from active C3 convertase of the alternate system; and (3) it enhances the binding of factor I to membrane-bound C3b by at least 30-fold, thereby greatly increasing the rate of C3b inactivation.

C4-BINDING PROTEIN

C4-binding protein is a normal human serum protein that binds tightly to activated C4, apparently accelerating the rate of enzymatic inactivation. Such a reaction is analogous to the effect of factor H on the activity of factor I on C3b.

DECAY-ACCELERATING FACTOR

Decay-accelerating factor (DAF) is a normal membrane protein present on erythrocytes, granulocytes, monocytes, and platelets. DAF inhibits the activity of the C3 convertases (eg, C3bBb) that are critical for the amplification loop and for the formation of the C5 convertase in both pathways of complement activation. Patients with paroxysmal nocturnal hemoglobinuria have an intermittent hemolytic anemia and may also have pancytopenia, thrombotic episodes, and nonlymphocytic leukemia. Cells from these patients have been shown to be deficient in, or totally lacking, DAF.

This protein presumably prevents the further activity of C3 convertases deposited on host cell surfaces as the result of complement activation (perhaps in response to infection).

VITRONECTIN

Vitronectin, also known as the *S protein* of the complement system, is a plasma protein that binds to fluid-phase C5b67 and prevents diffusion to adjacent bystander cell membranes. The resulting SC5b67 complexes are lytically inactive and circulate in the plasma until cleared. The presence of SC5b67 complexes in the plasma may prove to be a specific diagnostic indicator of intravascular complement activation leading to C5b–9 formation.

HOMOLOGOUS RESTRICTION FACTOR

Also known as C9-binding protein, homologous restriction factor seems to block C9 binding by the C5b–8 membrane-bound complex. This phosphoinositol-linked protein is present on all blood cells and vascular surfaces and is species specific. This protein (like DAF discussed earlier) is missing from membranes of the hemolytically sensitive cells in patients with paroxysmal nocturnal hemoglobinuria.

COMPLEMENT RECEPTOR-1

A complement receptor (CR-1) for C3b is present on human RBCs and on platelets. This receptor binds C3b

and functions (as does factor H) to prevent the initiation of the amplification loop. Thus, the activation of complement on autologous surfaces is inhibited by both DAF and CR-1, preventing bystander self-lysis. CR-1 also serves as an immune adherence receptor, promoting removal of C3b-containing complexes.

ACTIVATOR SURFACES FOR THE ALTERNATE PATHWAY

It has previously been stated that the alternate pathway is continually being activated by factor D through splitting of C3B to C3Bb, the initial C3 convertase of this system. Also, it has been discussed how this complex is quickly destroyed by normal serum components to prevent a runaway activation of the entire system. But, obviously, if the alternative system is to be of value to the host, there must be ways of stabilizing the initial components to provide an active C5 convertase to initiate the formation of the membrane attack complex.

Stabilization and, hence, effective activation of the alternate pathway are mediated by a host of polysaccharides, such as those in bacterial membranes (lipopolysaccharide, LPS), yeast cell walls (zymosan), inulin (polyfructose), some animal RBCs (such as rabbit), and neuraminic acid-poor or neuraminidase-treated membranes in general. The various activating agents seem to have little in common, except to provide an activator surface for the binding of C3bBb, which protects it from inactivation by factor H and factor I. Interestingly, surfaces rich in neuraminic acid (sialic acid) do not serve as activator surfaces, and the C3bBb is quickly destroyed. If, however, the neuraminic acid is enzymatically removed from a nonactivating RBC, this same RBC becomes a potent activator of the alternate pathway.

Mechanism of Alternate Pathway Activation

A hypothesis to explain how an activator surface differs from a nonactivator surface is illustrated in Figure 12-7. This hypothesis states that when C3b interacts with an activator surface, its factor H binding site is blocked or changed, preventing inactivation by factor I and permitting the formation of C3bBb. A nonactivator site, however, such as a neuraminic acid–rich RBC, retains the C3b binding site for factor H, resulting in a rapid inactivation of C3b or C3bBb.

Biologic Activity of Intermediates Formed During Complement Activation

Notice that the activation of one recognition unit (C1s) may eventually cleave many molecules of C3 and C5 and that the amount of both of these components is further amplified by the presence of C3b. Thus, many molecules of C3a, C3b, C5a, and C5b are formed, and

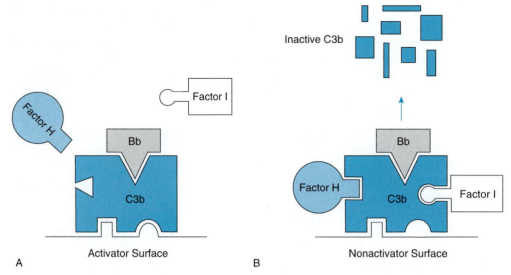

FIGURE 12-7 Activator and nonactivator cell surfaces. Not all cell surfaces are capable of stabilizing C3b after complement activation. The diagram shows a model explaining the mechanisms responsible for this difference. C3b is inactivated by a proteolytic enzyme called *C3b inactivator* or *factor I*. The activity of this enzyme is promoted by interaction of another protein, factor H, with the C3b molecule. Binding of C3b to an "activator" surface **A** is thought to result in a conformational change in the C3b molecule that prevents binding of factor H which, in turn, fails to promote cleavage by factor I. However, as shown in **B**, binding of C3b to a nonactivator surface fails to induce this conformational change. Thus, factor H can still bind to C3b and promote inactivation of C3b by factor I.

some of them are involved in events other than the lysis of the target cell.

ANAPHYLATOXINS

Early studies revealed that the injection of complement-activated serum into a normal guinea pig results in rapid shock and death, similar to that seen in the classic antigen–antibody anaphylaxis (see Chap. 14). The biologic mediators of complement-induced anaphylaxis were consequently named *anaphylatoxins*. This activity is known to reside in the C3a and C5a generated by both pathways of complement activation.

Both C3a and C5a bind to the membranes of mast cells and basophils, causing the release of pharmacologically active mediators such as histamine and serotonin. The role of these mediators in immediate-type hypersensitivity is discussed in Chapter 14, but their major effects are to increase capillary permeability and to cause the constriction of smooth muscle. Large concentrations of C3a and C5a result in fatal shock, but the release of small amounts of histamine may be beneficial by increasing capillary permeability at the site of inflammation. These split products also cause degranulation of polymorphonuclear neutrophils (PMNs), resulting in the release of lysosomal enzymes that further contribute to local inflammation.

Although small amounts of histamine at the site of inflammation may be beneficial, large amounts are disastrous. Fortunately, serum contains an inactivator that rapidly destroys C3a and C5a. This inactivator is a carboxypeptidase B that cleaves the carboxy terminal arginine from each of these anaphylatoxins, resulting in their inactivation.

CHEMOTAXIS

Any substance that attracts leukocytes to an area of inflammation is a chemotactic agent. Factors Ba (the split product from the alternate pathway) and C5a are both chemotactic for PMNs and macrophages, thus contributing to local inflammation. C5b67, the partially formed attack complex, also has been implicated as a chemotactic agent. Interestingly, although the removal of the terminal arginine from C5a by carboxypeptidase B completely eliminates all anaphylatoxic activity, its removal does not affect the chemotactic activity of C5a.

IMMUNE ADHERENCE

C3b is an effective opsonin, stimulating the phagocytosis of antigen–antibody aggregates, cells, and viruses. Its opsonic effectiveness stems from the presence of specific C3b receptors on PMNs, monocytes, macrophages, and mast cells. C3b also binds to antigen–antibody aggregates and to antibody-sensitized cells and viruses. Thus, C3b can act as a bridge to bring antibody-coated material into intimate contact with phagocytic cells, inducing their phagocytosis and destruction.

Complement Deficiencies

Some animals and humans have been found to possess genetic defects that result either in a deficiency in a complement component or in a deficient regulatory system for the control of the activated components of complement. In some deficiencies, such as C2 deficiency, few problems appear, probably because the alternate pathway of complement activation can still be used. Deficiencies in C1r and C4 are noticed in systemic lupus erythematosus (SLE)–like disease. The genes encoding C2, C4, and factor B are examples of class III genes, and they reside within the major histocompatibility complex (see Chap. 10), as do a number of other genes involved in the regulation of immune responses. Notice that about 40% of individuals deficient in these complement components have SLE, suggesting an involvement of genes within the major histocompatibility complex in the pathogenesis of SLE. Other deficiencies, such as a lack of C3 or of the regulators of the activated components, invariably lead to recurrent bacterial infections.

Defects at the C3 level have been observed both in individuals who are unable to synthesize C3 and in those who lack factor I, which functions to destroy the C3b component. Persons with this latter condition, therefore, are subject to C3b amplification (as described for the alternate pathway), with the result that essentially all of the normal C3 will be split into C3a and C3b. This causes abnormally low serum levels of C3. Those persons who are unable to synthesize C3 or who lack factor I are subject to recurrent infections, apparently because they cannot form the attack complex, mount an effective chemotactic response, or stimulate phagocytosis.

A regulatory deficiency has been described in which the inhibitor that inactivates C1s is lacking. Obviously, unless there is some way to turn off the recognition unit, the cascade of reactions involving the complement series may result in considerable damage to the host. Normal serum contains a glycoprotein that rapidly inactivates C1s. Individuals lacking this inactivator experience occasional local accumulations of fluid. Table 12-3 summarizes the complement deficiencies.

Complement Fixation

As described earlier in this chapter, complement reacts with antigen–antibody complexes involving IgM and IgG. As a result, complement undergoes a series of complex reactions and is depleted, or *fixed*. The measurement of complement fixation in vitro thus provides a sensitive technique for the determination of antigen–antibody reactions. A complement fixation test can be used to determine the presence or absence of an antigen–antibody reaction in the following manner.

First, serum from an individual is heated to 56°C for 30 minutes to inactivate any complement present. Then, to assess the level of antibody in the serum, a series of twofold dilutions of the serum is made, after which known amounts of complement (usually in the form of fresh guinea pig serum) and antigen are added to each tube of diluted antiserum. The assay is incubated overnight to allow complement to fix and any resultant lytically effective molecules to decay. Because these assays contain small amounts of antibody and antigen, no visible reaction occurs, and the only way to ascertain whether a reaction has occurred is to determine whether the added complement was fixed, that is, used up. To do this, an indicator system must be added to the reaction tubes.

The indicator system consists of sheep RBCs and antibody to sheep RBCs, which cause lysis only in the presence of complement. If no complement is present, no lysis occurs. Therefore, looking at the test system, it is seen that if antibodies are present in the individual's serum, complement will have been fixed, and the subsequently added indicator system does not undergo lysis. On the other hand, if the person's serum does not contain the antibodies for which the test is being done, complement will still be available for the lysis of the indicator system and lysis of indicator RBCs will be measured as hemolysis. The amount of RBC lysis that occurs can be determined by centrifuging unlysed RBCs and measuring the amount of hemoglobin that has been released into the supernatant solution with a spectrophotometer. The percentage of RBCs lysed can be plotted against the dilution of antibody present in the test system, but, in actual practice, the antibody titer is usually reported as the reciprocal of the serum dilution that resulted in the lysis of half of the added RBCs. Notice that because of the complexity of the complement system, any complement fixation test must include controls to ascertain that neither the antigen nor the antiserum alone could inactivate complement and that, in the absence of both antigen and antiserum, the added complement was effective for the lysis of the RBCs.

TABLE 12-3
Human Genetic Deficiencies of Complement Components

Deficiency	Observed Abnormality
C1r	Systemic lupus erythematosus–like disease, frequently fatal from overwhelming infection
C2	Many appear healthy, but may be associated with connective-tissue disease
C3	Recurrent bacterial infections
C4	Systemic lupus erythematosus–like disease; subject to immune-complex disease
C5	Recurrent infections—lupus-like disease
C6, C7, C8	Recurrent infections—disseminated gonorrhea
C1qINA	Hereditary angioneurotic edema
Factor I	Low C3 levels with recurrent bacterial infections

TABLE 12-4
Cross-Talk Between Complement and Other Protein Systems

Enzyme	Substrate	Result
Kallikrein	C1	Cleaving of C1s
	C5	Chemotaxin activity
	Factor B	Loss of factor B activity
Thrombin	C3	Anaphylatoxin activity
	C5	Chemotaxin activity
	Factor B	Loss of factor B activity
Plasmin	C1	Activation of C1s
	C3	Anaphylatoxin activity
	C5	Chemotaxin activity
	Factor B	Loss of factor B activity
	C1 Inhibitor	Blocking of plasmin activity

Complement fixation tests can be used as an aid for the diagnosis of syphilis (the Wassermann test), pertussis, gonorrhea, histoplasmosis, and a number of other diseases.

Interactions Between Complement and Other Protein Systems

As might be expected, a system as seemingly complex as the complement system does not operate in a void. Proteins of the complement system do interact with proteins of other complex systems, that is, the coagulation, fibrinolytic, and kinin systems. The effects of various enzymes from these other systems on various components of the complement system are given in Table 12-4. Although the activity of any one of these enzymes on complement in solution may be less than expected for a biologically important reaction, it is becoming increasingly clear that cell surfaces and cofactors do exert significant effects on these enzymes, so that their biologic effectiveness between systems becomes much more meaningful.

Examples of the interaction between components of the various systems are many. Plasmin has been shown to cleave C3 to give C3b- and C3a-like fragments, which possess chemotactic and anaphylatoxic activities. Protein S of the coagulation system circulates as a complex with C4-binding protein, although the biologic significance of this interaction is unknown. Kallikrein has been shown to cleave C5 with the release of a fragment that is chemotactic for PMNs.

Human platelets react directly with antigen–antibody complexes through cell-surface Fc receptors. Experimental results suggest that activation of platelets to release vasoactive, granule-associated amines occurs by mechanisms requiring complement. This may occur because of platelet lysis via the classic pathway of complement activation or by nonlytic mechanisms that also involve complement.

A Closer Look

Complement is a biologic effector mechanism that enhances the potency and action of a variety of soluble molecular and cellular mediators of immunity. Complement is a complex system of serum proteins that act in a coordinated way to mediate and enhance the phagocytosis of foreign particles, facilitate the destruction and lysis of certain bacteria and virus-infected cells, and participate in enhancing inflammatory reactions and certain aspects of allergic phenomena.

The alternate and classic pathways of complement activation are two versions of a series of interacting events leading to the same endpoint. The alternate pathway often is believed to be the more primitive of these two pathways because this pathway can be initiated by certain bacterial cell wall components, enzymes, and other nonspecific initiators. Both the classic and alternate pathways, once activated, result in the generation of a series of enzymes, anaphylatoxins, and chemotactic factors that mediate cell lysis, enhance vascular permeability and cause smooth muscle contraction, and attract polymorphonuclear leukocytes to a site of infection and tissue damage. The complement system is a tightly regulated, but ever-ready effector system that we have in our blood. Patients who have isolated complement deficiencies, such as C1, C2, C3, or C4 deficiencies, typically are prone to pyogenic infections, and commonly these patients have associated diseases, particularly systemic lupus erythematosus or glomerular nephritis. Also, a variety of abnormalities of regulatory complement proteins result in altered susceptibility to pyogenic infections and other nonspecific disease syndromes. The complement system plays a key role as an accessory system for enhancing the actions of antibody and cellular immune defense mechanisms.

Bibliography

JOURNALS

Bhakdi S, Tranum-Jensen J. Complement lysis: a hole is a hole. Immunol Today 1991;12:318.

Colten HR, Rosen FS. Complement deficiencies. In: Paul WE, Fathman CG, Metzger H, eds. Annual review of immunology, vol 10. Palo Alto, Annual Reviews, 1992:809.

Esser AF. Big MAC attack: complement proteins cause leaky patches. Immunol Today 1991;12:316.

Farries TC, Atkinson JP. Evolution of the complement system. Immunol Today 1991;12:295.

Liszewski MK, Atkinson JP. Complement system and immune complex diseases. In: Stein JH, ed. Internal medicine. Boston, Little, Brown, & Co, 1990.

Podak ER. Perforin: structure, function, and regulation. Curr Top Microbiol Immunol 1992;178:175.

Essentials of Medical Microbiology, Fifth Edition, edited by Wesley A. Volk,
Bryan M. Gebhardt, Marie-Louise Hammarskjöld, and Robert J. Kadner.
Lippincott-Raven Publishers, Philadelphia © 1996.

Chapter 13

Cell-Mediated Immunity

The immune system of vertebrate animals can be divided into two parts based on the function of each: the humoral immune system, which involves antibody-mediated functions; and the cellular immune system, which involves T-lymphocyte–mediated functions. The two parts or systems are separate entities, but they are not mutually exclusive. Thus, the same antigen frequently induces both antibody synthesis and a cellular immune response.

Antigen-specific cell-mediated immunity is mediated by T lymphocytes. A second, smaller population of cells (which have the morphologic features of lymphocytes but lack T- or B-cell markers, mediate cellular cytotoxicity, and are not antigen specific) includes natural killer (NK) and killer (K) cells. The T-cell group is composed of (1) helper T (Th) cells, which, on recognition of foreign antigens presented on the surface of antigen-presenting cells (APCs), perform their function by secreting biologically active factors that stimulate other cell types that are involved in cellular immune reactions; and (2) T cytotoxic cells (Tc cells), which kill target cells (tumor cells, virus-infected cells, or allograft cells) by release of lysins after recognition of foreign antigens on the target cell membrane. The NK group kills target cells by mechanisms similar to those that the Tc cell uses. The NK cells kill some tumor cells but lack antigen-specific receptors. K cells recognize antibody-coated target cells by means of a cell–surface Fc receptor on the K cell.

Delayed-Type Hypersensitivity

Delayed-type hypersensitivity (DTH), in contrast to immediate hypersensitivity discussed in Chapter 14, derives its name from an immune reaction that develops hours after injection of the antigen. Like immediate hypersensitivity, this reaction can be elicited by many seemingly innocuous substances and can result in considerable damage in the responding individual. Unlike immediate hypersensitivity, however, the beneficial aspects of this type of response are more apparent, in that DTH is the prime mode of defense against intracellular bacteria and most fungi. In fact, it was in patients with chronic infectious diseases that DTH was first observed.

The classic example of DTH is the response to the proteins of the tubercle bacillus (*Mycobacterium tuberculosis*) in individuals infected with this organism. In the late 19th century, Koch and von Pirquet were attempting to produce a vaccine for tuberculosis; they took the filtrate from a culture of *M tuberculosis* and injected it into the skin of a number of individuals. Twelve to 18 hours later, they noticed the appearance of erythema (redness) at the injection site. An indurated bump (swelling) slowly appeared. Both the erythema and swelling progressed, reaching maximum intensity at about 24 to 48 hours (a delayed reaction, and thus the name delayed-type hypersensitivity). The extent and severity of the reaction varied, and indeed, in some individuals, severe necrosis and ulceration resulted. This was the first example of what is the routinely used tuberculin skin test.

The preparation of the antigen solution used in such skin tests has evolved from a crude filtrate of the tubercle bacillus containing bacterial proteins (called *old tuberculin*) to a purified protein derivative from these filtrates called PPD. A similar relationship exists between an antigen-specific DTH reaction and the protein antigens of many other microbial agents in a variety of chronic diseases caused by bacteria, viruses, fungi, and protozoa (Table 13-1).

HISTOLOGY OF THE DTH RESPONSE

The DTH response described above is independent of antibody and is mediated by Th cells and macrophages. The histologic features of the DTH reaction are considerably different from those of an antibody-mediated hypersensitivity such as the Arthus reaction (see Chap. 14).

TABLE 13-1
Some Microbial Products Used to Elicit Delayed-Type Skin Reactions in Sensitive Individuals

Factor	Activity
Tuberculosis	Tuberculin (purified protein derivative prepared from culture filtrate)
Brucellosis	Brucellergin (purified preparation from culture filtrate)
Leprosy	Lepromin (prepared from culture filtrate)
Histoplasmosis	Histoplasmin (concentrated culture filtrate)
Blastomycosis	Blastomycin (concentrated culture filtrate)
Coccidiodomycosis	Coccidiodin (concentrated culture filtrate)
Mumps	Killed mumps virus
Contact dermatitis	Patch test with simple chemicals

Soon after contact with antigen (2 to 3 hours), there is an initial infiltration of polymorphonuclear neutrophils (PMNs). This is followed by an influx of lymphocytes and macrophages in the perivascular area; this influx of mononuclear cells becomes increasingly larger as the PMNs disperse. With time, as the swelling and erythema disappear, the lymphocytes and macrophages also disperse. Continuing antigenic stimulation (eg, chronic infection) can lead to granuloma formation while macrophages, having ingested large amounts of cellular debris, form epithelioid cells and giant cells.

CELLS MEDIATING DELAYED-TYPE HYPERSENSITIVITY

The DTH response is dependent on both antigen-specific Th cells and macrophages. Indeed, the macrophages play a role in the activation of the Th cells and also are, in turn, activated by the lymphocytes to become the terminal effector cells of DTH.

The Th Cell

The Th cell has the cell–surface phenotype α/β TCR$^+$CD3$^+$4$^+$8$^-$. The activation of the Th cell occurs in the manner described in Chapter 11. The antigen is processed by the macrophage (the APC) and is presented to the Th cell in association with a class II major histocompatibility complex (MHC) molecule on the macrophage cell membrane. Thus, the activation of Th cells requires *dual recognition* and is *MHC restricted*. Appropriate interaction between the macrophage and the antigen-specific Th cell results in the production of interleukin-1 (IL-1) by the macrophage. Th cells that have received the appropriate two signals (IL-1 and antigen–class II complex) enter into the cell cycle where, on reaction with interleukin-2 (IL-2; produced by other antigen-specific Th cells), they proliferate and differentiate into activated Th cells and memory Th cells.

The Macrophage

Many bacteria (eg, tubercle bacilli) survive after having been ingested by macrophages. However, macrophages from infected individuals can acquire an augmented ability to kill these intracellular parasites as well as any other unrelated organisms that happen to be around.

Compared with normal macrophages, activated macrophages are larger, have more lysosomes and lysosomal enzymes, and secrete enzymes involved in the inflammatory response, that is, complement components, collagenase, and plasminogen activator. They are also metabolically different from resting macrophages; for example, they have increased glucose transport and increased glucose oxidation to CO_2 and form superoxide anion O_2^-

TABLE 13-2
Soluble Factors Mediating Delayed-Type Hypersensitivity

Factor	Activity*
Migration inhibition factor (MIF)	Inhibits random migration of macrophages
Chemotactic factors	Attract PMNs and macrophages to the site of infection
Macrophage arming factor (MAF)	Activates macrophages
Mitogenic factors	Induce lymphocyte proliferation (and, in some cases, differentiation)
Lymphotoxin	Cell destruction
Interferon-γ	Activates macrophages, upregulates class II MHC molecule expression, and facilitates monocyte egress from capillaries

MHC, major histocompatibility complex; PMNs, polymorphonuclear leukocytes.
* In vitro activities. In vivo activity is inferred.

and H_2O_2, both of which are probably responsible for the destruction of intracellular pathogens.

Thus, after presentation of antigen to activate the Th cell, the macrophage is, in turn, activated by the soluble factors released by the lymphocyte to become an effector cell that is directly involved in the elimination of the offending organism.

SOLUBLE FACTORS MEDIATING DELAYED-TYPE HYPERSENSITIVITY

On activation, the Th cells release a variety of mediators collectively called *lymphokines* (or cytokines), which are responsible for the many manifestations of the DTH reaction (Table 13-2). All of these factors, except possibly transfer factor, are nonspecific in their action. Therefore, the *specificity* of the DTH reaction resides in the antigen-specific activation of the Th cells.

The lymphokines listed in Table 13-2 are only a few of the factors released by lymphocytes. Each has been characterized using in vitro assays; the in vivo functions of the lymphokines are presumed to be identical to their actions in vitro. Thus, the in vitro activities listed in Table 13-2 can account for much of what is known to occur in vivo. For example, contact with antigen causes the Th cell to release factors that are chemotactic for macrophages, resulting in the accumulation of macrophages at the site of infection. The presence of migration inhibition factor prevents the subsequent dispersal of macrophages but not PMNs, making the macrophage the predominant phagocytic cell. Secretion of macrophage arming factor by the Th cell causes these macrophages to become much more metabolically active, increasing their ability to inactivate the offending organisms. Liberation of mitogenic

factors results in a rapid local proliferation of lymphocytes, accounting for the buildup of lymphocytes at the site of infection. Release of lymphotoxin by these lymphocytes will then cause dissolution of the offending organisms.

ALLERGIC CONTACT DERMATITIS

Allergic contact dermatitis (contact hypersensitivity) is the most familiar form of DTH. The inducing agents (antigens) are usually low–molecular-weight substances such as metals (nickel, chromate), plant products (poison ivy catechols), cosmetics (hair dye, preservatives, perfumes), and medications (topical antibiotics). The most common route of contact is the skin. Only substances that can combine *covalently* with host proteins are successful in eliciting contact dermatitis, that is, they are true haptens. They must also possess solubility and diffusion properties, which allow them to pass through unbroken skin. Many are found to be fat soluble (hydrophobic), indicating that they enter via the sebaceous glands. However, if the skin is broken, many other materials may sensitize a susceptible individual. These chemically reactive products (haptens) combine with carrier proteins in the skin or blood. The hapten–carrier complexes, in turn, undergo endocytosis, are processed by the APC, and are presented to Th cells as a complex consisting of the class II–MHC molecule and the hapten–carrier-derived peptide.

The histologic features of the reaction are the same as those described for the tuberculin reaction. As for all DTH reactions, once sensitization (immunization) occurs, contact dermatitis resulting from a subsequent exposure to the same antigen is not limited to the area in which initial contact was made. This is because the specific cells responsible, that is, the Th cells, circulate throughout the body.

CUTANEOUS BASOPHILIC HYPERSENSITIVITY

Mast cells and basophils may also play a role in DTH reactions in the skin and elsewhere. Humans develop a form of *cutaneous basophilic hypersensitivity* (CBH) that peaks at 24 to 48 hours, during which time basophils are prominent. CBH differs from classic DTH in that it occurs primarily in the upper dermis with little deposition of fibrin. CBH reactions are mainly erythematous, with little induration, and are seen most frequently when sensitization (first exposure) occurred relatively recently. Such responses have been seen with a wide variety of antigens.

CONTROL OF DTH RESPONSES

Control of DTH reactions is essentially the same as for other T-cell responses. As shown in Chapter 11, Th cells mediate negative control on immune responses by producing cytokines that suppress Th cell function.

Cytotoxic Cells

The existence of cytotoxic cells was first suspected when it was reported that thoracic duct lymphocytes obtained from dogs that had rejected kidney allografts were able to destroy donor kidney cells in vitro. This type of experiment was repeated using mice that were injected with allogeneic spleen cells or that had received allogeneic skin grafts. After 5 days, the spleens from the recipient animals were removed and assayed for the presence of alloantibody-producing cells and for cells that were cytotoxic for the donor's cells. Cytotoxicity was demonstrated in the absence of antibody-forming cells, and this cytotoxicity was completely eliminated by removing T cells. The effector cells responsible for this specific killing are called *cytotoxic T lymphocytes* (CTL or Tc cells; Fig. 13-1). Most Tc cells are of the CD3$^+$4$^-$8$^+$ phenotype, have a T-cell receptor (TCR) composed of the α/β heterodimer, and kill target cells in an MHC-restricted manner (see Chaps. 9 through and 11).

It was soon noticed that lymphocytes from normal, nonimmune individuals could nonspecifically kill a variety of tumor cells under certain conditions. These cells are referred to as *natural killer* (NK) *cells*. It was also observed that a population of lymphocyte-like cells could kill antibody-coated target cells. This antibody-dependent cellular cytotoxicity (ADCC) is mediated by cytolytic cells called *killer* (K) *cells*. Both these cells belong to a subpopulation of lymphocytes called *large granular lymphocytes* (LGLs) because of their size and the presence of large azurophilic granules in their cytoplasm.

Tc cells with TCRs composed of the γ/δ heterodimer have been demonstrated in the intestine. These cells have a CD3$^+$4$^-$8$^+$ cell-surface phenotype but are not restricted by MHC molecules in their killing of target cells, and their antigen specificity is unknown.

A summary of the properties of these four cytolytic cells is given in Table 13-3. A more detailed description of each cell type and the mechanisms by which they kill their target cells is given below.

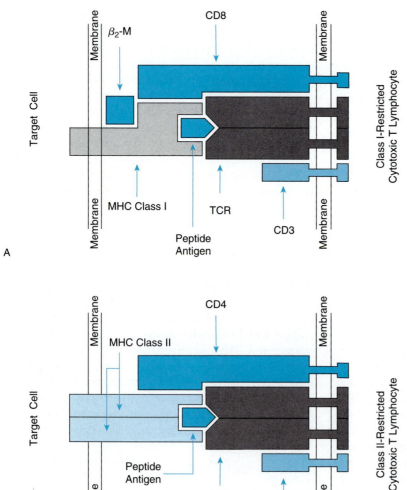

FIGURE 13-1 Antigen recognition by class I– and class II–restricted cytotoxic T (Tc) cells. Cytotoxic T lymphocytes may recognize antigen complexed with either class I **A** or class II **B** MHC molecules on target cell surfaces. Class I–restricted Tc cells are CD8$^+$ and represent the majority of Tc cells. Class II–restricted Tc cells are CD4$^+$. Thus, it is the type of MHC molecule on the target cell that presents antigen, and not the function of the T cell, that determines the nature of the MHC restriction of Tc cells.

TABLE 13-3
Properties of Cytotoxic Cells

Cytotoxic Cell	Receptor	MHC Restriction	Cell Surface CD Phenotype	Target
Tc-I*	α/β	Class I	CD3$^+$4$^-$8$^+$	Class I plus peptide
Tc-II	α/β	Class II	CD3$^+$4$^+$8$^-$	Class II plus peptide
Tc-III	γ/δ	Unknown†	CD3$^+$4$^-$8$^-$	Bacteria(?)
			CD3$^+$4$^-$8$^+$	
NK	Unknown	No	CD16$^+$3$^-$4$^-$8$^-$	Various tumor cells
K	FcγR	No	CD16$^+$3$^-$4$^-$8$^-$	Antibody-coated cells

Tc, cytotoxic T lymphocyte; K, killer; MHC, major histocompatibility complex; NK, natural killer.

* The I, II, and III categories are not an official designation but are used merely to distinguish between the three types of Tc cells.

† There have been some reports that these Tc cells may be restricted by class I–like molecules.

CYTOTOXIC T LYMPHOCYTES (Tc CELLS)

Most cytotoxic T lymphocytes (Tc cells) bear the α/β heterodimeric TCR (the α/β TCR; see Chap. 9). They are involved in elimination of virus-infected cells and tumor cells and in the rejection of allogeneic and xenogeneic transplants.

Tc Cells With the α/β T-Cell Receptors

All of these Tc cells recognize antigen in association with either a class I or a class II MHC molecule (ie, they are MHC restricted). Those α/β TCR$^+$ Tc cells that are class I restricted have the CD3$^+$4$^-$8$^+$ phenotype, whereas those that are restricted by class II molecules are CD3$^+$4$^+$8$^-$ (see Table 13-3). The Class I–restricted Tc cells are by far the most numerous cytolytic cells in the peripheral lymphoid organs.

Tc Cells With the γ/δ T-Cell Receptors

Most γ/δ TCR–expressing cells are of the CD3$^+$4$^-$8$^-$ phenotype and are found in small numbers in the thymus and peripheral lymphoid organs (see Chap. 9). T lymphocytes have been demonstrated residing between the columnar epithelial cells of the villi of the small intestine. These *intraepithelial lymphocytes* (IEL) express the γ/δ TCR but are CD4$^-$8$^+$ or CD4$^-$8$^-$. The cytotoxic activity of γ/δ TCR–expressing cells appears not to be MHC restricted, and until recently there were few clues as to which antigens these cells recognize. However, Lefrancois and Goodman found that IELs taken from mice born and raised in a germ-free environment showed little or no cytolytic activity, whereas IELs taken from mice raised in a conventional (or natural) environment were constitutively cytolytically active (as measured by indirect methods). This result suggests that IELs in normal mice have been activated by environmental pathogens in the intestine. Lefrancois and Goodman also reasoned, as have others, that the γ/δ TCR may have evolved before the α/β TCR, because the primordial immune system would develop a protective mechanism against infection of the digestive tract before requiring one monitoring the internal milieu.

Tc-Cell Activation

The following discussion of Tc-cell activation and the mechanisms by which Tc cells recognize and kill target cells has been shown to be true for the α/β TCR–expressing Tc cells. The mechanisms by which the γ/δ TCR–expressing Tc cells recognize antigen, are activated, and kill target cells are unknown. However, because both cell types have similar antigen-specific receptors, one might assume that except for the difference in MHC restriction during antigen recognition, they operate by similar methods.

The kinetics of a primary and secondary Tc-cell response are much the same as those seen in an antibody response (see Chap. 11). A measurable Tc-cell response to initial contact with antigen (a primary response) can be detected in about 10 days to 2 weeks. On subsequent contact with the same antigen (eg, 1 or 2 months later, during which time cytolytic activity has waned), memory Tc cells undergo rapid clonal proliferation and activation into cytolytically active Tc cells. The lag period between contact with the antigen and the detectable appearance of Tc cells, in both the primary and the secondary response, depends on the nature of the antigen (viral antigen, or minor or major transplantation antigen) and the number of precursor Tc cells with TCRs specific for the antigen in question.

The activation of Tc cells occurs in several steps, as shown in Figure 13-2. The first step is the activation of Th cells, as described in Chapter 11. Antigen is ingested, processed, and presented in association with a class II

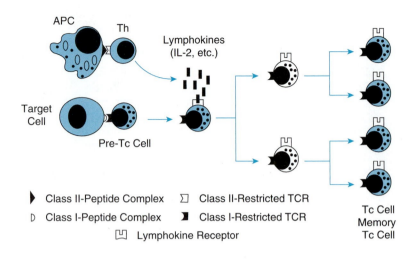

Class II-Peptide Complex   ⊠ Class II-Restricted TCR

Class I-Peptide Complex   ▮ Class I-Restricted TCR

ᕼ Lymphokine Receptor

FIGURE 13-2   Activation of cytotoxic T (Tc) lymphocytes. Tc cell activation requires recognition of peptide antigen (eg, a virus-encoded antigen or an alloantigen on an organ transplant) complexed with MHC molecules. This recognition leads to production of receptors for lymphokines, such as interleukin-2 (IL-2). IL-2 is produced by helper T (Th) cells (see Chap. 11) that have been activated after recognition of processed antigen in association with class II MHC molecules on antigen-presenting cells. Interaction of IL-2 with the IL-2 receptors on the activated Tc cell leads to proliferation and further differentiation to effector Tc cells and memory Tc cells. It is not known whether memory and effector Tc cells differ substantially from each other.

molecule to the Th cell by an APC. This activated Th cell synthesizes and secretes IL-2. The antigen may be a viral glycoprotein or an alloantigen released from an allograft, that is, a major or minor histocompatibility (transplantation) antigen.

At the same time, the Tc cell interacts with antigen, either on the surface of an APC, a virus-infected cell, a tumor cell, or cells expressing foreign major or minor histocompatibility antigens. This interaction induces the Tc cell to express a receptor for IL-2. Other poorly understood differentiative events occur as well. The IL-2 secreted by the Th cell reacts with the newly acquired IL-2 receptor on the Tc cell and induces proliferation and further differentiation. In contrast to what occurs in induction of antibody responses, direct cell–cell contact between the Th cells and Tc cells is not required, and the Th cell requirement in Tc cell activation can be replaced, at least in vitro, by IL-2. Therefore, the primary role of the Th cell in Tc-cell activation may be the synthesis and secretion of this lymphokine.

The activated, or effector, Tc cells recognize and bind to the antigen on the surface of the target cell. A series of subsequent events, which are described later, leads to lysis of the target cell.

These interactions between the Th cell and the APC, and between the Tc cell and the stimulator cell bearing the antigen, result in the generation of functional Tc cells as well as memory Tc cells and memory Th cells. It is not known how memory Tc cells and effector Tc cells differ; they may be the same cell in different stages of the life cycle or in different stages of activation.

Dual Recognition and MHC Restriction by Tc Cells

Although Tc cells were discovered after studies of allograft rejection in dogs, these cells did not evolve thousands of years ago on the chance that surgeons would one day appear on the evolutionary scene with the desire to transfer tissue from one individual to another. Tc cells more

likely evolved as a mechanism of defense against a class of pathogens that are capable of infecting almost any cell type. Viruses are the main example of this type of pathogen.

α/β TCR–expressing Tc cells recognize antigen in association with class I or class II MHC-encoded molecules. It was thought that Tc cells recognized two distinct entities on the surface of target cells. For example, it was believed that after virus infection, a viral antigen is synthesized and inserted into the membrane, where it is recognized as an intact viral protein along with the MHC molecule. However, clearly the Tc cell recognizes antigen-derived peptides bound to the MHC molecule (see Fig. 13-1). Townsend and colleagues demonstrated the existence of influenza virus nucleoprotein (NP)–specific Tc cells. Since NP is a DNA-binding protein and is not expressed on the surface of infected cells as an intact protein, the Tc cells must recognize another form of the NP. Using peptides derived from NPs and a series of mutant NP molecules with deletions in selected regions of the protein, Townsend was able to demonstrate that the NP-specific Tc cell indeed recognizes peptides from selected regions of the NP molecules. Thus, both Th cells and Tc cells apparently recognize processed antigen that is bound by class II or class I MHC molecules respectively.

Another series of experiments demonstrated that two distinct pathways exist for processing and presentation of antigen to α/β TCR$^+$ Tc cells. One pathway is sensitive to treatment with chloroquine or protease inhibitors and does not require protein synthesis. This pathway is responsible for presentation of antigen to class II–restricted CD4$^+$8$^-$ Tc cells. This pathway is presumably the same as that required for processing and presentation of soluble antigens to CD4$^+$8$^-$ Th cells (see Chap. 11). Thus, a common pathway involving endocytosis and processing of exogenous antigen in an acidic, intracellular compartment is responsible for presentation of antigen-derived peptides to both class II–restricted Th cells and to class II–restricted Tc cells (Fig. 13-3B). The second pathway

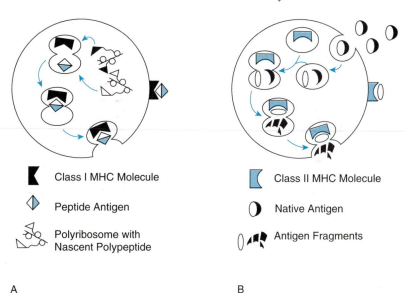

A　　　　　　　　　　　　　　　　　　　B

FIGURE 13-3 Class I and class II MHC-restricted presentation of antigen. Antigen is processed differently for presentation by class I or class II molecules to T cells. Class I–restricted T cells (including cytotoxic T [Tc] lymphocytes) recognize antigen that has been produced within the cell on which it is presented. For example, **A** shows the production of class I MHC molecules on membrane-bound polyribosomes and the production of a viral protein on soluble polyribosomes. Some of this endogenously produced viral antigen is then processed into peptides and combines with the class I MHC molecule. The complex is transferred to the cell membrane where it is recognized by class I–restricted, CD8+ T cells. Most Tc cells recognize antigens processed by this pathway, leading to lysis of cells actively producing the foreign antigen, be it viral, tumoral, or otherwise. This pathway does not require endocytosis, nor does it occur in acidic intracellular compartments. **B** shows the uptake of exogenous antigen (by either nonspecific or receptor-mediated endocytosis), degradation, and presentation of antigen fragments complexed to class II MHC molecules. This complex is recognized by class II–restricted, CD4+ T cells. The pathway shown in **B** requires endocytosis and occurs in acidic intracellular compartments such as light endosomes. In addition, a large portion of the class II molecules used in this pathway seem to recycle from the cell surface to the light endosomes and back to the cell surface. Most Th cells recognize antigen processed by this pathway and thus promote responses to circulating foreign antigens such as bacteria, toxins, certain viruses, and so forth. A small proportion of Tc cells seem to recognize antigen processed by this second pathway and, therefore, presumably, can kill cells that have engulfed antigen through endocytosis (eg, viruses), perhaps preventing initiation of viral replication in cells that have ingested intact virus.

is not sensitive to chloroquine and protease inhibitors but does require protein synthesis. This pathway is responsible for presentation of peptides derived from endogenous antigen to class I–restricted Tc cells (see Fig. 13-3*A*).

ALLOREACTIVITY. In the case of most allografts, the foreign antigen is a class I molecule on the surface of cells of the allograft. Tc cell clones specific for human HLA class I molecules have been isolated that recognize the class I molecule when expressed on human cells but not when expressed on murine cells after transfection of the murine cells with the gene encoding the class I molecule. The human class I molecule expressed by the murine cell appears to be normal in all other aspects. Thus, these allo-specific Tc cell clones seem to be recognizing the alloantigen plus some other entity that is present on human cells

but not murine cells. The other entity is thought to be a peptide derived from proteins endogenous to cells of the allograft. Therefore, Tc-cell responses to allografts probably are most specific for polymorphic residues on the class I molecule of the grafted cells *plus* a peptide derived from molecules endogenous to the allograft cell itself. Tc cells of this type would not have been eliminated during selection of the T-cell repertoire in the thymus of the graft recipient, because the class I molecule involved in thymic selection is different from that expressed on the grafted cells (see Chap. 9 for a discussion of thymic selection in developing the T-cell repertoire).

Tc cells are specific for a complex composed of two components: the MHC molecule and an antigen-derived peptide. If either component is missing, recognition and activation of that T cell will not occur. In the allograft

Image legends:

Class I MHC Molecule

Peptide Antigen

Polyribosome with Nascent Polypeptide

Class II MHC Molecule

Native Antigen

Antigen Fragments

example given above, the antigen from which the peptide is derived may be identical to the same molecule made by the recipient's own cells. One might wonder, therefore, why Tc cells induced by the allograft do not react with the recipient's own tissues. The answer is that the second component of the complex (ie, the MHC molecule) is different, and because recognition of both components must occur, the Tc cells that are specific for the allograft cannot react with self-tissue even if the peptide is present.

Heterozygosity at the MHC Loci

Different clones of Tc cells are specific for different antigenic determinants on a viral antigen in conjunction with each of the HLA-A, -B, and -C gene products. For example, for an individual who is homozygous at each of the class I loci, three types of virus-specific Tc cells may exist: one for virus plus HLA-A, one for virus plus HLA-B, and one for virus plus HLA-C. In an individual heterozygous at each allele, six types of Tc cells would theoretically be present, one for virus plus each of the two alleles of each of the three loci. Being heterozygous at each of the MHC loci, therefore, confers a selective advantage. For example, if Tc cells recognizing virus plus one allelic product are somehow lost, Tc cells recognizing the same virus in association with another allelic product confer protection. Similar arguments apply to class II–restricted Tc cells or Th cells.

Mechanism of Lysis

The events occurring during Tc cell-mediated lysis have been divided into several steps, as shown in Figure 13-4 and as discussed later.

RECOGNITION AND ADHESION. After activation, the Tc cell interacts with the target cell by means of its recognition complex (see Fig. 13-1). Conjugate formation proceeds by a Mg^{2+}-dependent step involving interdigitation of cellular processes of the target and Tc effector cells, maximizing surface area contact. Adhesion may also involve other cell-surface molecules, such as lymphocyte function antigen (LFA)-1 on the Tc cell interacting with intercellular adhesion molecule (ICAM)-1 on the target cell. This LFA-1–ICAM-1 interaction does not seem to be actively involved in cell recognition but is involved in stabilizing the cell–cell interaction initiated by the specific T-cell recognition complex. The recognition complex is not actively involved in the lytic process because it can be replaced by artificially cross-linking the Tc cells and any target cell, regardless of specificity.

This recognition and adhesion is an active process. It can be inhibited by decreasing temperature or by the addition of energy poisons such as azide. It can also be

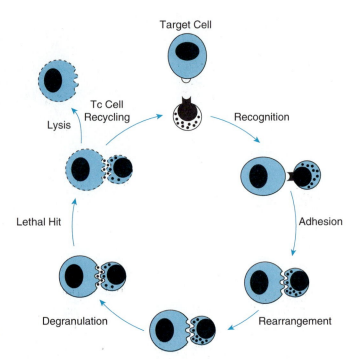

FIGURE 13-4   The cytotoxic T (Tc) lymphocyte lytic process. The process leading to lysis of target cells by Tc cells begins by specific recognition of the antigen–MHC complex on the target cell by the T-cell receptor. Other molecules on the T-cell surface then promote adhesion of the T cell to the target cell. Soon thereafter, cytoplasmic granules containing a number of active molecules, including perforin, begin to move from the distal portion of the Tc cell and accumulate at the interface between the Tc cell and the target cell. Degranulation at the interface results in release of perforin and other active components. Although the process is not completely understood, perforin clearly aggregates on the surface of the target cell, forming complexes similar to those seen with antibody and complement (see Chap. 12). Assembly of this polyperforin then presumably leads to destabilization of the membrane, rapid ion exchange, and lysis. The Tc cell is not affected by this process and survives to kill other target cells.

inhibited by addition of cytochalasin B, suggesting a role for microfilaments and microtubules.

PROGRAMMING FOR LYSIS. Programming for lysis is a general term used to describe a series of metabolic events that lead to irreversible damage to the target cell.

EFFECTOR-CELL REARRANGEMENT. The Tc effector cell possesses a number of cytoplasmic granules that contain lysosomal enzymes and an extremely potent membrane-active cytolytic agent. While the Tc effector cell contacts the target cell, these granules are located distal to the target cell (Fig. 13-5). Soon after target cell–effector Tc cell contact, a Ca^{2+} and energy-dependent rearrangement process occurs. There is evidence for cytoskeletal rearrangement as well as movement of the cytoplasmic granules to a position underlying the point of adhesion between the Tc effector cell and the target cell. The details of the mechanisms by which these rearrangements occur

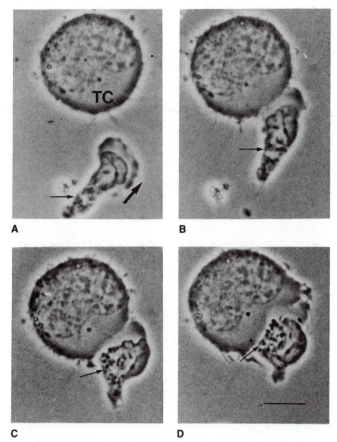

FIGURE 13-5 Reorientation of granules after cytotoxic T (Tc) lymphocyte interaction with a target cell. Shown here are phase contrast micrographs of a Tc cell approaching and interacting with a target cell (TC), which it can kill. The *small arrows* indicate granule position within the Tc cell. The *large arrow* indicates direction of Tc cell movement before contact. **A.** The Tc cell has a granule-free leading edge, a nucleus, and a granule-filled uropod in the rear. **B.** The Tc cell has made contact with the target cell. **C.** Two minutes after contact, the Tc cell has begun to round up and initiate granule movement. **D.** Ten minutes after contact, the Tc-cell granules occupy a position in the zone of Tc cell–target cell contact.

have yet to be determined. However, the overall result of the rearrangement is to locate the granules containing the lytic agents in a position appropriate for subsequent lysis of the target cell (ie, beneath the Tc-cell plasma membrane at the region of contact with the target cell).

EFFECTOR GRANULE EXOCYTOSIS. The mechanism by which Tc cells cause lysis of target cells has long evaded immunologists. However, T cells can be cloned and maintained in culture for long periods of time as fully functional cells. Studies with cloned Tc cells (and NK cells; see below) have shed light on the lytic mechanism.

Lysis appears to occur after exocytosis of the granules, as discussed above, and release of their contents at the interface between the cytotoxic cell and the target cell. The contents of the spaces between the cells have the staining properties of the granules. Deposition of granule contents on the target-cell membrane has been demon-

strated to include acid phosphatase and aryl sulfatase as well as several cylindrical structures that are known to appear in the granules immediately after recognition and adhesion. The formation and release of these cylindrical structures are Ca^{2+} dependent. Furthermore, the granules have been isolated, and their contents have been shown to possess Ca^{2+}-dependent lytic properties.

This secretory process is unusual in that it occurs in a rapidly developing polarized process; that is, secretion occurs only in the area of contact between the target cell and the Tc effector cell. A similar polarized secretory process occurs in mast cells (see Chap. 14) and phagocytic cells when they are given a surface stimulus.

LETHAL HIT. Target cells can be lysed by treatment with isolated granules, and antibody to the granule contents can block this lysis. Furthermore, Fab fragments of antibody to granular contents will block lysis by whole cells. Because the antibody cannot get into the Tc cell, it must block by reacting with released materials. There are a number of different components within the granules. In addition to several lysosomal enzymes, such as acid phosphatase, β-glucuronidase, and aryl sulfatase, a protein called *perforin* has been isolated. This protein, on interaction with membranes, is capable of self-aggregation, forming a cylindrical complex called *polyperforin,* forming "holes" in the membrane similar to those seen in cells treated with complement (see Chap. 12). Indeed, perforin is structurally related to the C9 component of complement and polyperforin may be similar in function to poly-C9. Although it is not known whether other proteins are involved in the membrane attack complex formed by perforin (as in the C5b–8 complex in complement-mediated lysis), it is possible that the mechanisms of lysis are similar.

The complex series of events outlined above, which takes approximately 6 to 10 minutes, results in a change in membrane permeability and in osmotic swelling. Subsequent lysis of the target cell, that is, membrane disruption and loss of cytoplasmic contents, does not require continued contact with the Tc effector cell and may take several hours.

The lytic cycle described above proceeds in one direction and has no effect on the Tc cell itself. This "immunity" from lysis by its own granule contents is probably temporary and is induced during the programming for lysis stage. The lack of permanent resistance to lysis is evidenced by the fact that cytotoxic T cells from one strain of mouse can serve as target cells for MHC-specific Tc effector cells from another strain of mouse.

Control of Tc-Cell Development and Function

Negative control of the induction of Tc cells is mediated by Th cells. These Th cells are activated by antigen and function by preventing release of soluble factors (including IL-2) necessary for the proliferation and differentiation of Tc cells and memory Tc cells.

LARGE GRANULAR LYMPHOCYTES

There are several other cell types that contribute to cell-mediated immunity in all vertebrate species thus far studied. These are collectively referred to as LGLs and include the NK cells and the K cells responsible for ADCC. Although some individual LGLs express either NK or K cell activity, most LGLs can kill by either mechanism, suggesting that NK and K cells are the same cell or different cells in the same differentiative pathway.

Immune surveillance is a term used to describe a putative naturally occurring system for monitoring and controlling the appearance of malignant cells. Although the evidence for such a surveillance system is meager, the discovery of NK and K cells has provided clues to a potential cellular mechanism for such a surveillance system.

Natural Killer Cells

Natural killer cells were so named because they were originally found in the lymphoid tissues of normal mice and were shown to be able to kill a wide variety of tumor cells in the absence of any antigenic stimulation. NK cells appear to be lymphocytes, but they lack most of the cell–surface markers characteristic of B cells and T cells (see Chaps. 8 and 9); their lineage is uncertain. They are classified as lymphocytes because they have the morphologic features of lymphocytes; also, they are bone marrow derived, their distribution is restricted to lymphoid tissue, and, at least in mice, they possess several cell–surface markers that are restricted to lymphocytes.

NK cells differ from Tc cells in other properties as well: they are not inducible by antigen, they lack the classic antigen-specificity of T cells and B cells, and they are not restricted by MHC-encoded proteins. Indeed, freshly isolated NK cells show germline arrangement for the genes encoding the TCR polypeptides. Therefore, whatever their recognition system is, it does not include any of the known TCR polypeptides.

NK activity can be enhanced by lymphokines, specifically interferon-γ. Indeed, the rationale for using interferon as antitumor therapy in clinical trials is based largely on the enhancement of NK antitumor activity by this cytokine.

The mechanism by which NK cells kill tumor cells is similar, if not identical, to that described for Tc effector cells. Although there is no specific recognition (in the same sense as with Tc cells) of the target cells, the adhesion, programming for lysis, and lethal hit events are strikingly similar (see Fig. 13-4). Much of the evidence for the granule exocytosis model of lysis comes from studies of NK cells.

Killer Cells

Killer cells have Fc receptors on their surfaces by which they recognize and exert a cytotoxic activity toward antibody-coated target cells. This activity is referred to as antibody-dependent cellular cytotoxicity (ADCC). Although macrophages and polymorphonuclear leukocytes can, at times, mediate such effects, the K cell, which is a mononuclear cell with non-T, non-B cell characteristics, is of particular interest. These cells are LGLs containing azurophilic granules and are either identical to or closely related to NK cells. As discussed above, most LGLs have both NK- and K-cell activity. However, the recognition mechanism by which each activity is initiated is different in that the ADCC activity, but not the NK activity, of these double-function cells can be blocked by antibody to the Fc receptor.

The mechanism by which K cells mediate their cytotoxic effect is probably the same as that of the NK cell and Tc cell. Drugs that inhibit energy metabolism, but not those that block DNA synthesis, block K-cell lytic activity. K cells have not been cloned, as have Tc cells and NK cells. However, their activity, and thus their apparent specificity, is entirely dependent on the presence of IgG antibody.

SUMMARY OF CELL–CELL INTERACTIONS IN SPECIFIC IMMUNE RESPONSES

The last two chapters have described how immune responses are induced and regulated. Figure 13-6 gives an overall scheme of this induction and regulation, showing the many features common to all responses.

1. There are three specific defense mechanisms:
   a. Those mediated by antibody, such as the inactivation of toxins, opsonization of bacteria, neutralization of viral infectivity, antibody-mediated complement-dependent lysis, and ADCC;
   b. Those mediated by Tc cells, such as the elimination of virus-infected cells or tumor cells; and
   c. Those mediated by Th cells, such as the elimination of intracellular parasites.
2. There are four requirements for the induction of each of these mechanisms:
   a. Antigen;
   b. APCs (macrophages, dendritic cells);
   c. Th cells; and
   d. A resting B cell, Tc cell, or Th cell.
3. In all cases, the B or T cell is precommitted to antigen specificity and function.
4. MHC-restricted activation of Th cells enables these cells to deliver proliferative and differentiative signals to the effector cells or memory cells.
5. This same dual recognition involving antigen and MHC-encoded class II molecules occurs in the activation of virgin Th cells and of memory Th cells.

Differentiation   **Proliferation**   **Effector Function, memory**

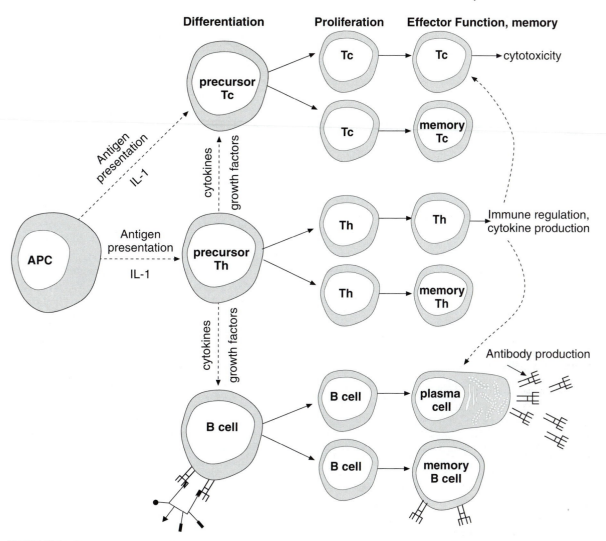

FIGURE 13-6 A summary of the induction and regulation of immune responses. The generation of an immune response is arbitrarily divided into three phases: (1) *Differentiation*, during which precursor T cells recognize antigens presented to them by antigen-presenting cells (APC) and B cells recognize antigens using immunoglobulin receptors. (2) *Proliferation*, during which antigen-specific T and B cells increase in numbers to expand the immune response. This is often referred to as clonal expansion. (3) *Effector function and memory*, during which T-cytotoxic (Tc) cells kill antigen-expressing cells and T-helper (Th) cells produce immunoregulatory cytokines, which modulate the activities of T-cytotoxic cells and B cells and the production and secretion of antibodies by plasma cells. Each of the lymphocyte subpopulations also differentiates into memory cells, which can respond in future immune responses to the same antigen.

6. In each case, activation of the resting B cell, Tc cell, or Th cell (or memory cell) requires recognition of antigen (and for T cells, recognition of MHC-encoded products) in addition to the signals received from the Th cells.

7. The MHC-gene product (class I or class II) seen by the virgin, memory, or effector T cell in association with antigen depends on the cell involved (ie, class I or class II for Tc cells and class II for Th cells).

8. Differentiation of the virgin T cell results in the generation of effector cells and memory cells.

9. Activation of memory cells results in the generation of effector cells and more memory cells.

10. In the case of antibody formation, the Th cell also

delivers a differentiative signal to the B cell, which results in the immunoglobulin isotype produced. This can result in expression of all of the biologic functions of antibody in the response to a given antigen.

11. In antibody responses, a Th cell also secretes lymphokines that enhance expression of a given isotype, allotype, or idiotype of immunoglobulin.

12. The negative control by the Th cell is mediated by regulatory cytokines. This prevents further induction and the amplification of immune responses.

13. In antibody formation, Th cells can specifically modify expression of a given isotype, allotype, or idiotype.

A Closer Look

The phrase *cell-mediated immunity* is generally synonymous with antigen-specific immunity mediated by T lymphocytes. Subcategories of cell-mediated immune reactions include the delayed-type hypersensitivity reaction, cell-mediated cytotoxicity mediated by cytotoxic T lymphocytes, and certain other forms of T-lymphocyte–mediated immune regulation.

Delayed-type hypersensitivity, discovered nearly a century ago, has become the prototypic measure of cellular immune function in humans and is widely used to determine if a patient has been infected by certain microorganisms such as *Mycobacterium tuberculosis.* Beyond its usefulness as a measure of an individual's exposure to an infectious agent when measured in the skin, the delayed-type hypersensitivity reaction is an essential cellular defense mechanism that enables the body to resist and suppress the spread of certain infectious agents.

Cellular cytotoxicity mediated by antigen-specific lymphocytes is a key factor in eliminating virus-infected cells expressing cell membrane antigens dictated by the virus. The role of T-cytotoxic lymphocytes in the destruction of syngeneic tumors is less clear. Evidently, all forms of antigen-specific cell-mediated immune reactions are dependent on the expression of antigen-specific receptors on T-cell membrane and the interaction of these receptors with a self–major histocompatibility complex molecule presenting a foreign peptide on the membrane of an antigen-presenting cell.

There are some forms of non–antigen-specific cellular immunity, which include natural killer (NK) and killer (K) cells. NK cells and K cells have the morphologic features of lymphocytes but do not express typical T- or B-lymphocyte surface membrane markers. These cells, which kill certain kinds of tumor cells and other target cells, are not antigen-specific, do not proliferate in response to antigen, and are not known to be involved in antigen-specific recognition, such as occurs with T and B cells. NK cells may be an important arm of a primordial immune surveillance system that evolved to eliminate effete cells, tumor cells, and certain parasites. K cells acquire specificity by virtue of their cell membrane Fc receptors for immunoglobulin.

Patients who have defects in cellular immune function may have congenital thymic deficiencies. Regardless of the origin of the T-lymphocyte deficiency, such patients are highly susceptible to viral and fungal infections. Therapies designed to reverse such deficiencies have not met with much success, although cellular and gene therapy may offer some hope.

Bibliography

JOURNALS

Dinarello CA. Role of interleukin-1 in infectious diseases. Immunol Rev 1992;127:119.

Goldstein P, Ojcius DM, Young JD-E. Cell death mechanisms and the immune system. Immunol Rev 1991;121:29.

Kaplan G, Cohn ZA. Leprosy and cell-mediated immunity. Curr Opin Immunol 1991;3:91.

Moretta L, Ciccione E, Moretta A, Hoglund P, Ohlen C, Karre K. Allorecognition by NK cells: nonself or no self? Immunol Today 1992;12:300.

Yagita H, Nakata M, Kawasaki A, Shinkai Y, Okumura K. Role of perforin in lymphocyte-mediated cytolysis. Adv Immunol 1992;51:215.

BOOKS

Romagnani S. Lymphokine production by human T cells in disease states. In: Paul WE, Fathman CG, Metzger, eds. Annual review of immunology, vol 12. Palo Alto, Annual Reviews, 1994: 227.

Sher A, Coffman RL. Regulation of immunity to parasites by T cells and T cell-derived cytokines. In: Paul WE, Fathman CG, Metzger H, eds. Annual review of immunology, vol 10. Palo Alto, Annual Reviews, 1992:385.

Essentials of Medical Microbiology, Fifth Edition, edited by Wesley A. Volk, Bryan M. Gebhardt, Marie-Louise Hammarskjöld, and Robert J. Kadner. Lippincott-Raven Publishers, Philadelphia © 1996.

Chapter 14

Immunopathology

Hypersensitivity

Immune responses to foreign antigens are, for the most part, beneficial to the responding individual. Nevertheless, at times the response to a seemingly innocuous antigen can result in tissue damage and even death. The term *allergy* (from the Greek word meaning altered reaction) was coined by von Pirquet merely to indicate an *altered reactivity* on second contact with an antigen. In time, however, the term allergy has become synonymous with hypersensitivity, which means an altered reactivity to an antigen that can result in damage to the individual.

Early studies of hypersensitivity reactions revealed that some occur within minutes after a second exposure to an antigen, whereas others may require 24 to 48 hours to attain a maximum reaction. The former is referred to as *immediate hypersensitivity* and the latter as *delayed hypersensitivity*. Based on the mechanisms of these reactions, Gell and Coombs divided hypersensitivities into four types (Table 14-1). Although the four types are distinct, notice that hypersensitivity to any given antigen

Classification	Manifestations	Effector Components
I	Anaphylaxis (anaphylactic shock, asthma, hives, drug allergies)	IgE, mast cells
II	Cytotoxic antibody (hemolytic anemia, Rh incompatibility, transfusion reactions)	IgM, IgG, complement
III	Antigen–antibody complexes (serum sickness, Arthus reaction, glomerulo-nephritis)	IgG, antigen, complement
IV	Cell-mediated (DTH) (tuberculosis, contact dermatitis)	T cells, macrophages

DTH, delayed-type hypersensitivity.

may occur because of any one or more of these four mechanisms. Delayed-type hypersensitivity (type IV) is discussed in Chapter 13. Types I, II, and III are discussed in this chapter.

IMMEDIATE HYPERSENSITIVITY (TYPE I)

Immediate hypersensitivity is a reaction that occurs within minutes, or at the most hours, after a second contact with an antigen (allergen). Depending to a great extent on the route by which the antigen enters the body of the sensitized individual, an immediate hypersensitivity reaction may vary from a severe and frequently fatal systemic reaction to a local manifestation such as food allergy, hay fever, asthma, or cutaneous anaphylaxis. On contact with an antigen, immediate hypersensitivity reactions result from the release of pharmacologically active substances from mediator cells, such as mast cells and basophils. These pharmacologically active substances react with vascular endothelial and smooth muscle cells, resulting in increased vascular permeability and the contraction of smooth muscle.

Early studies of allergies were hampered by the lack of an in vitro assay for antibodies to specific allergens. In fact, it was originally believed that the antibodies causing such immediate allergic reactions were monovalent, although it is now known that the inability to detect them was a function of their extremely low serum concentration (about 0.1 to 0.5 µg/mL, depending on the age of the individual) and the insensitivity of the then-available in vitro serologic tests. Fortunately, an in vivo technique for their detection became available when it was shown that such allergic responses could be transferred to a nonallergic individual. This was first demonstrated in 1921 by Carl Prausnitz in the following manner. He injected serum from an associate named Heinz Küstner (who was highly allergic to fish) into his own skin, and 1 day later, a minute amount of fish extract was injected into the same site. Within minutes, a pale, elevated area arose, which was surrounded by an area of redness (*erythema*).

This same reaction, designated as a *wheal and flare reaction*, also occurs in an allergic individual when small amounts of the specific allergen are injected into the skin. The skin-sensitizing antibodies responsible for this reaction have been referred to as *reagins*. A test for allergy that is based on the injection of serum from an allergic individual into the skin of a normal volunteer, followed by the injection of minute amounts of the allergen, is referred to as the Prausnitz-Küstner (P-K) test.

The subsequent discovery of two patients with multiple myeloma who produced large amounts of a hitherto undescribed class of immunoglobulin made it possible to produce specific antibodies to these myeloma proteins. This antibody did not react with heavy chains of known immunoglobulins but did react with reagins. Thus, reagins constituted a new class of immunoglobulin, designated as IgE. The structure and properties of IgE antibody are discussed in Chapter 5.

IgE as a Homocytotropic Antibody

If reaginic antibody is injected into the skin, it remains localized for a long period of time. This IgE antibody is found primarily bound to mast cells, which concentrate in the mucosal surfaces of the intestine, respiratory tract, and skin, and on blood leukocytes known as basophils. Immunoglobulins that bind to cells are called *cytotropic* antibodies. Those that bind only to cells obtained from the same species as the antibody are called *homocytotropic*, whereas those that bind to cells of other species (but not to their own cells) are referred to as *heterocytotropic*. Notice that IgE antibody binds to the mast cell or basophil by its Fc portion, thus leaving its Fab portions free to interact with antigen.

Although all normal individuals produce some IgE antibodies, certain individuals seem to be predisposed to allergies. This predisposition is called *atopy*, and atopic individuals frequently show allergies to a variety of apparently unrelated allergenic molecules.

Measurement of IgE

Formerly, measurement of reaginic antibody could be done only by an in vivo assay, such as the P-K test, or by injecting small amounts of allergen into the skin of an allergic individual and looking for a wheal and flare reaction. The availability of myeloma IgE has made it possible to produce highly specific monoclonal antibodies to IgE; using this antibody, a radioimmunoassay has been developed that detects as little as 0.1 ng to 1 ng of IgE (Fig. 14-1*A*). An in vitro assay for IgE antibody specific for a given allergen is also available. The radioallergosorbent test (RAST) uses allergen adsorbed to small beads of a complex carbohydrate, which are then mixed with the serum to be tested. After an appropriate incubation period, the particles are washed and allowed to react with radioactively labeled anti-IgE. The amount of radioactivity binding to the beads is a measure of the IgE antibody that has bound to the specific allergen (see Fig. 14-1*B*).

Antigens That Induce Immediate Hypersensitivity

Many of the compounds that induce immediate hypersensitivity are present in the environment. However, a number of other compounds, with which humans come in contact because of the nature of customs and society, also can be highly allergenic. Examples of different types of agents that can induce immediate hypersensitivity are listed in Table 14-2. The list is long and includes antigens of all types. The most familiar of these are the pollens, venoms, and foods. However, of particular interest and concern is that many antibiotics, diagnostic agents, drugs, and anesthetics can be allergens for some individuals.

Anaphylaxis

Anaphylactic reactions occur as a result of pharmacologically active mediators, that are released when an antigen binds to cytotropic antibody on the surface of a mast cell or basophil. The availability of antigen influences the rate of release of the mediators and, hence, the type and severity of the anaphylactic symptoms. Because antigen availability usually depends on the route by which antigen enters the body, this criterion can be used to divide anaphylaxis into various subtypes.

SYSTEMIC ANAPHYLAXIS. This extremely severe reaction frequently results in death within minutes after contact with an allergen. Before the availability of antibiotics, most

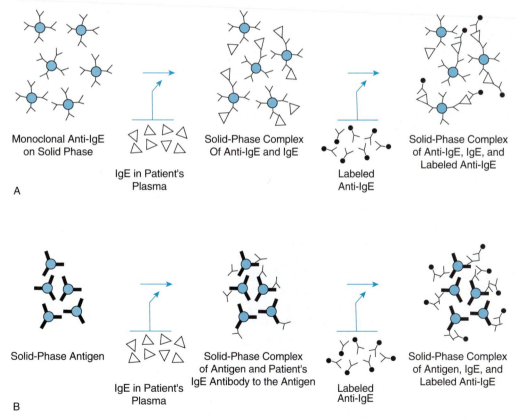

FIGURE 14-1 Determination of IgE concentration in human body fluids. Radioimmunoassays for determining the concentration of total **A** and antigen-specific **B** IgE antibody are shown. Both are indirect assays requiring capturing of IgE in patient plasma or secretions by solid-phase monoclonal anti-IgE **A** or solid-phase antigen **B**. In both cases the bound IgE is then detected with a radioactively labeled anti-IgE antibody, for example, rabbit anti-human IgE.

TABLE 14-2
Some Common Allergens

House dust mite fecal protein
Cockroach protein
Animal serum proteins (in therapeutic antisera)
Animal danders
Eggs
Antibiotics (penicillin)
Seminal fluid
Pollens
Venoms (bees, fire ants)
Seafood
Hormones (insulin)
Molds (*Aspergillus*)

cases of human anaphylaxis were caused by the injection of heterologous (foreign) antiserum into a highly sensitive individual. However, antibiotic therapy has greatly reduced the use of animal-derived antisera for the treatment of disease. Unfortunately, antibiotic therapy itself has become an important cause of human systemic anaphylaxis. For example, although penicillin is chemically innocuous to the body, some persons become remarkably hypersensitive to this antibiotic. This occurs because the metabolic breakdown of injected penicillin can result in the formation of chemically reactive haptens. These haptens can then bind to self-proteins and initiate immune responses. In some individuals, an IgE response is induced. After a subsequent injection of penicillin, the antibiotic reacts with penicillin-specific IgE antibody on the surface of mast cells. This causes a rapid release of histamine and other vasoactive amines into the circulation. The most common cause of systemic anaphylaxis in humans is insect stings (eg, in individuals who are highly sensitive to bee or wasp stings).

Fatal systemic anaphylaxis in humans involves hypotensive shock, respiratory arrest, cardiac failure, and suffocation from blockage of the upper airway caused by edema.

LOCAL ANAPHYLAXIS. Local anaphylactic reactions, sometimes called atopic allergies, occur spontaneously in about 35 million Americans (about 15% of the population). The antigens involved are common environmental allergens such as pollens, dander, house dust, and various foods. Interestingly, studies have shown that up to 90% of asthmatics allergic to house dust develop a wheal and flare reaction when injected with extracts of mites, and that the specific allergen in such cases is a glycoprotein occurring in the mite feces. Symptoms depend on the route of entry of the allergen. For example, pollens and dander that are usually inhaled cause asthma or hay fever, while ingested allergens in foods produce symptoms of gastrointestinal upset, hives, or atopic dermatitis.

Effect of Cytotropic IgE–Antigen Reactions

The mechanism by which antigen–IgE interaction results in immediate hypersensitivity is shown in Figure 14-2 and can be summarized as follows:

1. After an initial contact with an antigen, the individual produces IgE antibodies, which bind to the surface of mast cells and basophils. On second contact with the same antigen, several IgE antibodies on the cell surface are cross-linked by a single antigen molecule or an aggregate of antigen molecules. This cross-linking of

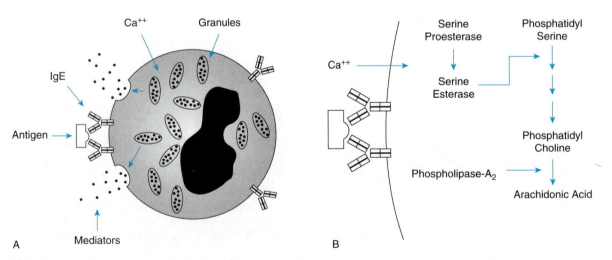

FIGURE 14-2   Antigen-induced mediator release from mast cells. IgE antibody bound to mast cells by IgE Fc receptors is cross-linked by specific antigen **A**, resulting in an influx of Ca^{2+} followed by a rise in intracellular cyclic AMP. This induces degranulation and mediator (eg, histamine) release. **B**. It also results in activation of phospholipase-A_2, which, in turn, catalyzes production of arachidonic acid from membrane phospholipids. Arachidonic acid then is processed into prostaglandins and thromboxanes by cyclooxygenase and into leukotrienes by lipoxygenase (see Table 14-3).

IgE antibody on mast cell surfaces is an absolute requirement.

2. Bridging of two IgE molecules at the mast cell surface initiates a series of events that are incompletely understood. The activation of a membrane serine protease initiates a series of reactions converting phosphatidylserine to phosphatidylcholine. As a result, the structure of the local membrane is modified, permitting an influx of Ca^{2+} ions.

3. The Ca^{2+} influx activates phospholipase-A_2, which converts the phosphatidylcholine to lysophosphatidylcholine and arachidonic acid. Arachidonic acid is the precursor of two classes of potent pharmacologically active agents, the prostaglandins and the leukotrienes.

4. The Ca^{2+} influx also initiates the assembly of a microtubule–microfilament network, along which cytoplasmic granules move on their way to the cell surface. Fusion of the granule membrane with the plasma membrane leads to the release of a number of components (degranulation), each of which has a specific effect on one or more cell types. The release of these mediators begins soon after initial contact with antigen. Fusion of the plasma membrane with the granule membrane involves only those granules in the vicinity of the stimulus (ie, the IgE–antigen interaction). Thus, degranulation is a polarized phenomenon similar to the degranulation of cytotoxic T (Tc) cells and natural killer (NK) cells (see Chap. 13). Continued release of mediators requires constant stimulation; thus, the release of antigen from the cell surface results in decreased mediator secretion.

There are two phases of anaphylactic reaction. The early phase occurs during the first 10 to 15 minutes, as described earlier, and involves mediator release. The response generated is caused primarily by histamine release from mast cells or basophils. The second, or late phase response, occurs 3 to 11 hours later and occasionally is more profound than is the early phase. The pharmacologically active agents responsible for this late-phase response include histamine, but this phase is caused mostly by release of inflammatory agents, such as the leukotrienes (but not the prostaglandins), chemoattractants for eosinophils, such as platelet-activating factor (PAF) released by the mast cell or basophil, and interleukin-5 released by activated T cells (see Chap. 11). Histologic examination of the skin lesion or a pulmonary lavage in asthmatics shows a multicellular picture, including eosinophils and neutrophils.

Pharmacologically Active Mediators

The process described above initiates the release of a number of pharmacologically active agents (Table 14-3). These include histamine, serotonin, bradykinin, PAF, prostaglandins, and the leukotrienes (formerly known as slow-reacting substances of anaphylaxis, SRS-A). Also included are other agents whose structures are unknown but whose activities have been described.

Evidence that some of these compounds are involved in immediate hypersensitivity reactions comes from their ability to induce hypersensitivity reactions, from their presence in antigen-induced hypersensitivity reactions, and from the ability of specific antagonists to partially prevent certain manifestations of the immediate hypersensitivity reaction.

HISTAMINE. Histamine is derived from the amino acid histidine and is localized in the granules of mast cells and basophils and in the platelets of some species. There are two types of histamine receptors on cell surfaces. Interaction of histamine with the H1 receptor results in contraction of smooth muscle and an increase in vascular permeability. Interaction of histamine with the H2 receptor leads to increased gastric secretion and to decreased mediator release from mast cells and basophils by a feedback mechanism. Antihistamines are classified as anti-H1 and anti-H2, depending on the target receptor. Histamine is rapidly degraded in the blood by histaminases.

SEROTONIN. The role of serotonin in human immediate hypersensitivity is not known. It is present in the platelets of most species, but only in rats and mice is it found in mast cells and basophils. Its precursor is the amino acid tryptophan, and it induces contraction of smooth muscle, increased vascular permeability, and capillary dilatation.

BRADYKININ. Although the role of bradykinin in immediate hypersensitivity has yet to be proved, it seems that it may act synergistically with prostaglandins to produce contraction of smooth muscle, increased vascular permeability, and a decrease in blood pressure. It also produces pain. Bradykinin is a nonapeptide produced by the action of kallikrein on plasma proteins called kininogens. It is rapidly degraded by specific plasma kininases.

PROTEASES. Mast cell and basophil granules are found to contain a number of proteolytic enzymes. The principal proteases found are *tryptase* and *chymase,* with specificities similar to those of trypsin and chymotrypsin, respectively. These enzymes most probably are involved in the digestion of blood vessel basement membranes, resulting in increased permeability to a variety of cell types.

HEPARIN PROTEOGLYCAN AND CHONDROITIN SULFATE. Heparin proteoglycan and chondroitin sulfate are highly negatively charged and are responsible for packaging of the protease molecules in the mast cell and basophil granules. In addition, they remain associated with the proteases after release, perhaps stabilizing the enzymes and preventing their inactivation.

TABLE 14-3
The Structure and Function of Some Pharmacologically Active Mediators of Immediate Hypersensitivity

Mediator	Precursor	Structure	Effects
Histamine	Histidine	NH_2-CH_2-CH_2— (imidazole ring)	Contracts smooth muscle, increases vascular permeability
Serotonin	Tryptophan	NH_2-CH_2-CH_2— (indole ring with OH)	Increases vascular permeability, contracts smooth muscle
Bradykinin	Plasma proteins		Produces pain, swelling, and edema; contracts smooth muscle; increases vascular permeability; induces capillary dilation
Heparin proteoglycan			Initiates formation of complexes with proteases
Proteolytic enzymes			Degrades basement membranes
Eosinophil chemotactic factor of anaphylaxis (ECF-A)			Attracts eosinophils
Prostaglandin D_2	Arachidonic acid	(structure)	Induces airway muscle contraction, augments histamine release
Leukotrienes	Arachidonic acid	Gln-Cys-Gly (structure) Leukotriene C4	Contracts smooth muscle, increases vascular permeability, causes bronchoconstriction
Platelet-activating factor		H_2C-O-$(CH_2)_2$-CH_3 H_2C-C-O-CH H_2C-O-P-O-Choline	Induces histamine release from platelets

CHEMOTACTIC FACTORS. Several chemotactic factors are also released during IgE-mediated degranulation. Eosinophil chemotactic factor of anaphylaxis and neutrophil chemotactic factor probably are responsible for the multicellular infiltration during the late phase of the IgE-mediated hypersensitivity response.

PLATELET-ACTIVATING FACTOR. Platelet-activating factor (PAF) stimulates platelets to release a variety of vasoactive amines, especially histamine. It is a low–molecular-weight lipid, which induces a rapid wheal and flare reaction when injected into human skin. It is lethal in small amounts when injected into a number of species and produces the symptoms of IgE-mediated systemic anaphylaxis when injected into rabbits. PAF is also known to be a potent chemoattractant for eosinophils and plays a major role in the multicellular late-phase response.

LEUKOTRIENES. The major effect of the synthesis and release of leukotrienes is bronchoconstriction of the smaller airways. Leukotrienes have stronger and longer-lasting effects than does histamine (eg, they induce slow contractions of smooth muscle). Leukotrienes C_4, D_4, and E_4 are produced in a stepwise fashion from arachidonic acid (see Table 14-3). The role of these compounds may vary, depending on the allergen involved and the site of the allergic response. Leukotrienes have been shown to be released from lung tissue of asthmatics exposed to specific allergens, and they may be responsible for the inability of antihistamines to completely alleviate the asthmatic reaction.

PROSTAGLANDINS. Prostaglandins, which also are products of arachidonic acid metabolism, are formed and released after antigen–IgE interaction at the mast cell surface.

Prostaglandin D_2 appears to be the only prostaglandin with significant activity in immediate hypersensitivity. In the skin, prostaglandin D_2 causes increased vascular permeability and vasodilation accompanied by neutrophil infiltration, and in the respiratory tract, it causes bronchoconstriction.

Pharmacologic Control of Mediator Release and Action

Control of immediate hypersensitivity reactions usually occurs at one of two levels (or both), that is, during or after degranulation.

1. Antigen activation of the mast cell is modulated by cAMP. Agents that cause an increase in cAMP (eg, epinephrine or the methylxanthines; it is not known whether these agents affect cAMP levels in vivo) inhibit this activation. Both epinephrine and methylxanthines are direct bronchodilators, and epinephrine is the agent of choice for treatment of systemic anaphylaxis. It is rapidly absorbed after intramuscular or subcutaneous injection because of the vasodilation caused by degranulation. It acts to prevent degranulation and prevents many of the end-organ effects of the mediators by constricting blood vessels and increasing the heart rate. The use of epinephrine is potentially hazardous, however, because the injection of high doses (usually 1 mg or more) can cause serious or fatal ventricular arrhythmias.
2. Increased Ca^{2+} flux results in activation of phospholipase-A_2, leading to the synthesis of arachidonic acid and the assembly of the microtubule–microfilament network required for degranulation. Sodium chromoglycate seems to stabilize the mast cell membrane, preventing this influx of Ca^{2+}.
3. After degranulation occurs, one must rely on the capacity of compounds to block the effects of the mediators on their target tissues or to counteract their actions. Antihistamines are routinely used, and, when necessary, corticosteroids, epinephrine, and other agents may be helpful, as described earlier. Corticosteroids prevent the late-phase cellular infiltration and are, therefore, the agent of choice for this response.

Other Anaphylatoxins

A number of other agents are known to induce mast cell degranulation. All do so by bypassing the IgE receptor and interacting with other receptors on the mast cell membrane. These include neutrophilic basic protein and the split products from complement activation, C3a and C5a.

After activation of complement, the interaction of either C3a or C5a with mast cell membranes induces localized permeability changes, causing an increase in the flow of plasma into the site of infection. These two ana-phylatoxins are inactivated by the plasma enzyme carboxypeptidase-B, which removes a carboxy terminal arginine residue.

Neutrophilic basic protein is a substance released by neutrophils after their interaction with immune complexes. Its effect is identical to that described earlier for the complement split products (ie, it induces a localized permeability change with subsequent increased plasma flow to the site of the antigen–antibody complexes).

Immunotherapy

Another method of potentially preventing anaphylactic responses is to inject the individual with increasingly larger doses of pure allergen over a long period of time. The exact mechanism by which these injections work is not known, and such procedures are not always effective. Explanations for the beneficial effect of immunotherapy include the fact that such injections result in the synthesis of large amounts of IgG antibody specific for the allergen. This excess of IgG could compete with the IgE antibody for the allergen and effectively prevent it from reacting with mast cell–bound IgE. The production of large amounts of IgG antibody, however, cannot be the sole mechanism, because immunotherapy has been successful in the absence of demonstrable synthesis of allergen-specific IgG antibody. Other studies have attempted to determine the ability of IgG subclasses to block basophil mediator release induced by allergen. No single IgG subclass seemed to be a particularly good inhibitor.

Another possible mechanism whereby immunotherapy works is that the injections of allergen may induce a state of "tolerance" or nonreactivity. Therefore, the individual would no longer be able to produce antibody, IgE or otherwise, to the allergen. The mechanism by which this tolerant state might be induced or maintained is unknown. Some investigators believe that immunotherapy works by altering the Th1 and Th2 cell profiles so that the cytokines produced by the T-cell subsets act to suppress IgE production.

Clearly, however, most patients who do respond to immunotherapy have basophils that do not respond well to allergen, nor do they respond well to nonspecific stimuli. This suggests a change in the basophils and mast cells themselves, resulting from immunotherapy.

TYPES II AND III HYPERSENSITIVITIES

Types II and III hypersensitivities in a sense are related, because both involve the formation of antigen–antibody complexes, whether they occur on a cell surface, in solution in the blood, or in tissues. In most cases, the activation of complement—with its anaphylatoxic, chemotactic, and lytic properties—is probably responsible for the deleterious effects. Three examples of such hypersensitivities are hemolytic anemia induced by certain drugs, the Arthus reaction, and immune complex disease.

Drug-Induced Hemolytic Anemia

A type II hypersensitivity reaction involving hemolytic anemia may be induced by administration of certain drugs. The drug acts as a hapten, covalently binding to the surface of red blood cells (RBCs). The hypersensitivity reaction results from the production of a complement-fixing antibody to the drug. Reaction of this antibody with the RBC-bound drug activates the complement system, resulting in RBC lysis and anemia. Treatment involves cessation of drug therapy. An example of drug-induced hemolytic anemia is the response of some patients to the drug alpha-methyldopa during treatment for hypertension.

The Arthus Reaction

The Arthus reaction is a type III hypersensitivity reaction. It is an inflammatory response initiated by the combination of exogenously administered antigen, usually intramuscularly, with preexisting IgG antibody, which is localized in the walls of blood vessels in various tissues. The Arthus reaction is characterized by sequential accumulation of neutrophils and mononuclear phagocytes, increased vascular permeability, edema, hemorrhage, fibrin deposition, and, finally, tissue destruction. Much of this reaction results from the chemotactic and anaphylatoxic properties of the split products of complement. Indeed, in animals, the removal of complement before the injection of antigen prevents the damaging effects, even though antigen–antibody complexes are found in the vessel walls. In humans, such a response may occur after the injection of tetanus toxoid into an individual who already has circulating antibody to this antigen.

Immune Complex Disease

Immune complex disease (serum sickness) is another example of type III hypersensitivity that results from the formation of circulating complexes of antigen and antibody. Complexes formed in the presence of a slight excess of antigen are particularly effective in inducing this reaction. Deposition of these complexes in vessel walls can induce a complement-mediated vasculitis. In addition, prolonged immune complex circulation may cause tissue injury to the kidneys (complex nephritis) by deposition of the complexes in the glomeruli, which may result in complement activation and inflammation. This reaction is manifested clinically by an increase in protein in the urine (proteinuria). If a chronic state is induced by continued exposure to antigen, the subsequent nephritis invariably results in severe disease and sometimes death. For example, in patients with systemic lupus erythematosus (SLE), the chronic presence of DNA–anti-DNA complexes can result in renal failure and death.

Extensive studies of serum sickness in several animal models have given rise to a fairly accurate description of the mechanisms responsible for immune complex disease. The mechanism involves the deposition of immune complexes along vascular membranes (including the glomerular basement membrane), causing the activation of complement. The formation of the complement-derived chemotactic and anaphylatoxic factors leads to extensive vascular permeability changes and the infiltration of neutrophils. Tissue injury results from the subsequent release of their lysosomal enzymes.

Group A streptococcal infections have long been known to cause acute glomerulonephritis. The specific nature of the streptococcal antigen involved in this immune complex disease is not known, but several laboratories have demonstrated the presence of IgG, complement, and streptococcal antigens in the granular deposits along the glomerular capillary walls.

Chronic glomerulonephritis has been reported to be associated also with malaria and hepatitis B infections. In both cases, it seems likely that the immune system is presented with large amounts of antigen over an extended period of time, causing immune complex disease.

Tumor Immunology

IMMUNOLOGIC SURVEILLANCE

The concept of immunologic surveillance was proposed to account for the relative paucity of tumors in the young and the increased frequency of cancer in proportion to age. This theory states that the immune system maintains surveillance, destroying malignant cells as they arise.

Although the concept appears logical and the theory is widely invoked, it is not proved. Much effort has been expended to test this theory in vitro and in vivo, in mice and humans, with the same results. Often small doses of tumor cells are not rejected, leading to the formation of tumors. Moreover, spontaneous tumors do not arise at a greater frequency in congenitally immune-deficient animals compared with normal animals. However, there is a higher-than-normal frequency of certain tumors in immunosuppressed mice and humans.

The original concept of immunologic surveillance as a function of the immune system in which T lymphocytes recognize and destroy tumor cells expressing tumor specific antigens no longer seems tenable.

TUMOR ANTIGENS

Immunologic surveillance and tumor immunology were predicated on the assumption that differences exist in the cell surfaces of normal and malignant cells, and that these differences could be detected by the immune system. The general terms *tumor-associated antigens* and *tumor-specific antigens* were coined to enable categorization of cell membrane molecules on tumor cells.

Chemically Induced Tumor Antigens

The antigens induced by chemical carcinogens seem to be incredibly diverse, even within a group of different tumors induced by the same carcinogen. For example, different tumors taken from different mice, or indeed, from different sites on the same mouse, but all induced by exposure to the same carcinogen (eg, methylcholanthrene), seem to be antigenically different from each other. In mice, these tumor antigens are detected by transplantation rejection methods; if a mouse is injected with small numbers of tumor cells, it makes an immune response and may reject a subsequent larger tumorigenic dose of cells from the same tumor. Thus, these antigens are referred to as *tumor-specific transplantation antigens* (TSTAs).

Attempts to demonstrate an antibody response to TSTAs have been generally unsuccessful. Therefore, it was concluded that cell-mediated mechanisms (see Chap. 13) are responsible for immunity to chemically induced tumors. Some investigators believe that TSTAs are intracellular proteins, and that stimulation of an immune response in these experimental systems is the result of T-cell recognition of a tumor-derived peptide presented on a class I or class II major histocompatibility complex (MHC) molecule on the membrane of the tumor cell. The peptide, of course, would be a degradation product of the putative intracellular TSTA. Extensive studies are being performed to isolate cytotoxic T-lymphocyte (Tc) clones specific for TSTAs. If successful, use of such T-cell clones as probes for TSTAs might permit the isolation and characterization of these antigens. The knowledge that immune responses to these tumors are primarily cell-mediated may help to guide us in the development of vaccines and other therapies directed against tumors.

The existence of tumor-specific antigens (TSAs) has not been conclusively demonstrated. It may be that some proteins produced by human tumor cells are mutated and, therefore, are altered versions of the same proteins expressed by normal noncancerous cells. It is also possible that the products of some oncogenes serve as tumor antigens on human cells. Clearly, there is much to learn in this regard; the future of tumor antigen–specific immunotherapy in humans is not close at hand.

Virus-Encoded Tumor Antigens

Tumors induced by viruses are well documented in animals. Injection of such oncogenic viruses into immunologically naive animals (neonatal, thymectomized, or congenitally athymic) usually elicits progressively growing, fatal tumors. Frequently, injection of a tumor virus into mature animals results in tumors that grow and then regress, producing an immunity specific for tumors induced by that virus.

All tumors induced by a given oncogenic virus possess similar antigens, as opposed to the diverse antigens induced by chemical carcinogens. Some of these antigens are encoded by the viral genome and are found on the viral envelope as well as on the tumor cell. Again, evidence for such antigens in human cancer is scant; few human tumors have been shown to be of viral origin. Burkitt's lymphoma may be an exception. These tumors arise from cells that apparently have been transformed after infection with the Epstein-Barr virus. This virus encodes an antigen that is found on such transformed cells.

Considering the fact that Tc cells may recognize peptides derived from any foreign protein, whether expressed inside or on the surface of the tumor cell, it is possible that any virus-encoded product could serve as a TSA. Examples are oncogene products, polymerases, and nucleoproteins. The reality is that none of these molecules has become useful clinically as a target for immunotherapy in humans.

Cellular Oncogenes

Clearly normal cells have genes that are the normal cellular homologue of viral oncogenes. These protooncogenes in normal cells are involved in a number of normal metabolic events, such as control of cell proliferation and differentiation. Point mutations in these protooncogenes have been observed and, in several cases, are thought to be responsible for tumorigenesis. Although it has not been demonstrated so far, it is possible that peptides derived from these mutant proteins are sufficiently different from normal to be recognized by T cells in conjunction with MHC class I or class II molecules. If so, then specific immunotherapy against such tumors would require definition of the structural difference between the mutant and normal protooncogenes—a process that may be prohibitively time-consuming and expensive.

Oncofetal Antigens

Some years ago an antiserum was prepared in rabbits by injecting extracts of human colon cancer. The antiserum was absorbed with noncancerous tissue obtained from the same individual. The resultant antibodies that were not absorbed were found to react with colon cancer cells and normal embryonic colon cells but not with normal adult colon cells. This antigen was termed carcinoembryonic antigen (CEA), and it was shown that patients with various gastrointestinal cancers had significantly elevated levels of CEA in their blood. It was subsequently shown, however, that this antigen was also present in normal human serum at low levels and in patients with certain other inflammatory disorders. It has, therefore, been suggested that its use in screening for cancer be discontinued, because it lacks the specificity needed to discriminate between certain malignant and benign disorders. A test for prostate cancer, based on the presence of a so-called prostate specific antigen (PSA) in the blood of patients, has been developed and has recently come into widespread use, although the accuracy and clinical utility are still controversial.

Idiotypes

Some cell-surface determinants other than TSTAs are tumor specific and could act as targets for immunotherapy using a xenogeneic antiserum (ie, an antiserum produced in another species). For example, a B-cell lymphoma is a clone of cells derived from a single parent B cell within which the oncogenic event occurred. Antibodies to the variable region of the immunoglobulin receptor on these B-cell lymphomas can be produced. The antigenic determinant in the variable region is called an *idiotype* and the antibody an *antiidiotype* (see Chap. 5). Antiidiotype made to one clone of B cells reacts only with members of that clone and with no others. Therefore, treatment of a B-cell lymphoma with the antiidiotype could be used to eliminate the malignant cells without affecting other normal B cells. Such an immunotherapeutic approach has been used in humans with limited success. The antiidiotype is of animal origin and can be immunogenic in the patient. Consequently, the immune response of the patient may limit the effectiveness of such therapy. In addition, use of this antiidiotype therapy allows clonal expansion of lymphoma cells that have mutated their surface receptor so that it is no longer recognized by the antiidiotype antibody used in the therapy. Thus, combination therapy using the antiidiotype immunotherapy to eliminate most of the tumor cells together with chemotherapy to prevent outgrowth of mutant cells may be required.

CELLS INVOLVED IN TUMOR IMMUNITY

Studies in animals and in vitro have implicated five cell types in antitumor defenses. They are the B cell, the T cell, the macrophage, the natural killer (NK) cell, and the killer (K) cell (or antibody-dependent cellular cytotoxicity [ADCC]).

B Cells

Antibody (the product of B cells) seems to be somewhat effective, in the presence of complement, against tumors of the hemopoietic system (eg, leukemia), for example, the antiidiotype discussed earlier.

T Cells

Cell-mediated immunity was to be the magic bullet to eliminate solid tumors. It was thought that helper T (Th) cells act as effector cells, activating macrophages to kill

tumor cells, and that cytotoxic T (Tc) cells recognize tumor antigens and kill tumor cells. However, demonstration of effective antigen-specific cell-mediated immunity in human cancer has not been accomplished.

If T cells are important, one might predict that T-cell–deficient animals and humans would have a high incidence of spontaneous cancer. Mice that have been thymectomized at birth and thus lack mature T cells show a much greater incidence of tumors when exposed to Maloney sarcoma virus or to polyoma virus. This seems to support a role for T cells. However, such thymectomized mice do not have a higher frequency of spontaneous tumors. This seems to argue against immunologic surveillance and a role for T cells. These mice, however, have a strikingly increased level of NK cells that are active.

In humans, about 10% of immunodeficient children (see later) develop cancer, supporting the concept of immune surveillance. However, most of these tumors are of lymphoid origin, and it is uncertain whether the increased frequency is because of decreased surveillance or some other mechanism associated with the lymphoid system imbalance. An increased incidence of tumors occurs in patients with adult-onset immunodeficiencies, and in patients treated with immunosuppressive drugs after kidney transplantation, there is an 80% increase in the risk of developing cancer. Sixty percent of these tumors are of epithelial origin and about 40% are of lymphoid origin. Therefore, one must question if these tumors reflect the immunodeficient state, the drug, or a pathologic lymphoid disorder.

Patients with acquired immunodeficiency syndrome have a much greater than normal frequency of Kaposi's sarcoma. It is not known whether this is because of the emergence of tumor cells that were held in check by immunologic surveillance or because of the emergence of agents (viruses?) that induce the tumor.

Macrophages

Macrophages are activated by T-cell–derived lymphokines (see Chap. 13), and such macrophages can kill tumor cells in vitro. In vivo, they have been shown to infiltrate tumors, but, as the tumor progresses, the macrophages are less active and do not respond well to lymphokines. Much of the tumoricidal activity of macrophages is probably caused by the secretion of *tumor necrosis factor* (TNF) by these cells. Human TNF is a protein of 157 amino acids and is closely related to lymphotoxin, a protein secreted by activated Th cells. TNF is a pleotropic polypeptide that has a number of biologic activities. It is crucial in inflammatory processes and in immunity and stimulates other cells to produce a variety of other proteins. TNF acts synergistically with interferon to kill tumor cells, exerting its lethal effect by an unknown mechanism that probably involves a variety of cell types.

Natural Killer Cells

Natural killer cells are discussed in Chapter 13. They can kill certain virus-infected cells, tumor cells, and some embryonic cells. They are found naturally in blood and tissue. Their numbers are not increased by exposure to antigen, and they may be present in increased numbers in athymic individuals. Thus, these cells may be responsible for the fact that athymic individuals do not experience more spontaneous tumors than do normal persons.

NK cells recognize tumor cells without restriction by MHC-encoded molecules, and there is no memory, as seen with T cells. They are not antigen specific because they can kill a variety of different tumor cells. In mice, transfer of large numbers of NK cells can protect recipient mice against certain tumors. Also, some evidence in humans links tumor load to NK cell numbers.

NK cells are regulated by interferon, which increases their number and activity. Prostaglandins inhibit NK cell activity.

Killer Cells

The activity of K cells resides in their receptors for the Fc portion of antibody. Thus, these cells kill after binding to antibody on antibody-coated tumor cells. The role of K cells in antitumor defense is speculative.

MECHANISMS OF ESCAPE FROM SURVEILLANCE

If surveillance by either NK or K cells does exist, it is not foolproof because tumors do arise. Each of the five cell types mentioned earlier relies, to a certain extent, on specific lymphocytes for its function. Macrophage antitumor activity depends on activation by lymphokines, and lymphokines are products of T cells. NK cells are increased in number and activity by interferon-γ, and this cytokine is the product of lymphocytes. The K cell requires antibody to function. Thus, any mechanism affecting lymphocyte (B- and T-cell) function may have some effect on surveillance, regardless of the effector cell.

MODULATION. Removal of antigens from the surface of tumor cells by antibody may occur and results in the inability of specific cells (Tc) or other antibody to kill tumor cells.

IMMUNOSELECTION. Activation of responses to cell-surface molecules can result in the selection of the variant (mutated) tumor cells that lack the recognized molecule. Thus, a tumor antigen–specific defense mechanism may select for variant tumors by killing the antigen-expressing cells and allowing the nonexpressing cells to live and grow.

ENHANCEMENT. The binding of specific antibody to a tumor cell, if not effective in removing that cell, may block other defense mechanisms by physically preventing effector cells from reaching the tumor cell. This results in enhanced growth, compared with growth in the absence of antibody. In experimental animals, this mechanism seems to occur even in the presence of K cells for undetermined reasons.

TREATMENT OF TUMORS

There are four general classes of treatment for cancer: surgical removal of the tumor, treatment with ionizing radiation, chemotherapy, and immunotherapy. The first three are relatively self-explanatory and are not dealt with here. The last, immunotherapy, deserves some comment.

Other than the use of antiidiotype, as mentioned earlier, there are several approaches that are being studied in experimental systems and tested in limited clinical trials in humans.

Macrophage-Activating Systems

The injection of nonspecific agents, such as an avirulent mycobacterium (bacille Calmette-Guérin) and certain polynucleotides, is known to stimulate macrophages, to increase whatever tumoricidal activity these cells might have, and to increase the number of NK cells. Such treatment has been used to treat a variety of human cancers, and there is some limited beneficial effect (ie, prolonged survival but no cures) for only two types of cancer: acute myelogenous leukemia and stage I lung cancer.

Interferon

The rationale for the use of this protein is based on its demonstrated antiviral effects and on the observation that it stimulates NK-cell activity. The results of attempts to treat cancer in humans with interferon have been disappointing.

Site-Specific Delivery Mechanisms

A number of experimental studies using toxin or radioactive compounds coupled to antitumor antibody have yielded moderately encouraging results. After injection of these conjugates, the antibody specifically (or preferentially) reacts with the antigen on the surface of the tumor cell. The tumor cell is then killed by radiation (in the case of the isotope–antibody conjugate) or by the toxin (in the case of the toxin–antibody conjugate). Thus, the antibody serves as a site-specific agent, which delivers the killing agent to the tumor cell. Although complete removal of solid tumors has yet to be accomplished by the use of such conjugates, there have been reports of dramatic decreases in tumor loads. Perhaps a combination of therapies might prove more effective, for example, a combination of surgical removal, chemotherapy, and administration of antibody–toxin conjugates.

LAK- and TIL-Cell Therapy

Steven Rosenberg at the National Institutes of Health has devised another approach to tumor therapy. This approach is based on the theory that most patients have lymphocytes (T cells, NK or K cells) capable of killing the specific tumor cells in question. The first attempts by Rosenberg used peripheral blood of the patient as the source of white cells. After in vitro stimulation with interleukin-2 (IL-2) to expand the population of antitumor cells, these lymphokine-activated killer (LAK) cells were reinjected into the patient along with additional IL-2 to promote further expansion in vivo. This LAK cell therapy worked well in experimental animals, showing major effects on established liver or pulmonary metastases. To achieve these dramatic results, combination therapy of LAK cells and IL-2 was necessary. Successful treatment of sarcomas, melanomas, and colon adenocarcinomas has been demonstrated.

In humans with certain types of tumors, LAK-cell therapy also showed promise, with significant regression of metastatic cancer in some patients with colon cancer, melanoma, renal cell cancer, and primary lung adenocarcinoma. Significant reduction of metastases in the lung, liver, and subcutaneous tissues has been observed. However, the quantity of IL-2 necessary to achieve optimal effects caused major side effects and prohibited its use in many patients. These side-effects include fever, chills, headache, malaise, nausea, diarrhea, and fluid retention.

To avoid these side-effects, Rosenberg proposed that a population of tumor-specific lymphocytes could be isolated from the tumor itself. If true, then a greater response with fewer cells and much less IL-2 might be achieved. He then began to isolate tumor-infiltrating lymphocytes (*TIL* cells) from various tumors induced experimentally in mice. After IL-2–mediated expansion of these TIL cells in vitro, significant tumor regression in vivo was observed using fewer cells than were required for the LAK-cell therapy discussed earlier. This TIL-cell therapy is undergoing clinical trials in humans.

LAK cells in humans are CD3⁻ and kill target tumor cells in an MHC-*unrestricted* manner. These cells are, therefore, probably NK or K cells. LAK cells are unable to kill freshly isolated normal cells. However, if the surfaces of these normal cells are slightly perturbed by a variety of treatments, they are converted to LAK-sensitive target cells. The cell-surface phenotype of TIL cells has not yet been definitively established.

Immunodeficiency Diseases

A number of disorders involve defects in antibody production or cell-mediated immunity, or both. Many of these are heritable defects, and some are acquired. Regardless of the functional deficiency observed, there are few instances in which the individuals affected are totally deficient in B or T cells. These disorders seem to be rare; the most common have reported frequencies between 0.03% and 0.97%.

B-CELL DEFICIENCIES

Selective IgA Deficiency

A severe paucity in both serum and secretory IgA is the most common immunodeficiency disorder known. These patients have less than 5% of normal serum IgA levels, even though they have normal serum levels of IgG and IgM. Such persons do not seem to have overt diseases, but they do experience frequent respiratory infections and, surprisingly, are more subject than normal to IgE-mediated hypersensitivities and autoimmune disorders.

Forty percent of patients with a selective IgA deficiency have circulating anti-IgA antibody. Transfusion of such patients with whole blood, plasma, or certain other blood products can result in fatal anaphylactic reactions.

The mechanism of selective IgA deficiency is obscure, but because normal levels of B cells possessing surface IgA are present, it is assumed that such cells are incapable of being stimulated by antigen, or that the IgA antibody produced is rapidly being removed from circulation.

Sex-Linked Agammaglobulinemia

Sex-linked agammaglobulinemia, also known as Bruton's disease, is characterized by a severe deficiency in mature B cells possessing surface immunoglobulin. This disorder is restricted to males and is characterized by recurrent infections with pyogenic bacteria beginning at 6 to 8 months of age (about the time maternally received IgG antibodies disappear). Such children frequently have a family history of brothers or maternal uncles with recurring infections. Because their T-cell–mediated responses are normal, individuals with Bruton's agammaglobulinemia can usually handle viral, fungal, and some bacterial diseases. This disease is treated by routine injections of normal immune globulin.

The molecular basis of this disorder is unknown, but the fact that these patients possess normal pre-B cells containing cytoplasmic μ-chain suggests that the block in differentiation occurs after the B cell has undergone immunoglobulin heavy-chain rearrangement but before light-chain rearrangement (in some cases) and before light-chain expression (in all cases).

Variable Immune Deficiencies

Any defects in regulatory or structural genes of immunoglobulin families could likely result in nonfunctional pre-B cells or their B-cell progeny. Such deficiencies are rare or minor and are identified only because of recurrent infections. One such case involved a young boy who was completely unable to make κ-chains. Because κ-chains contain a large repertoire of variable-region genes, it is not surprising that such an individual might be deficient in response to certain antigenic stimuli.

A number of individuals with varied immunodeficiencies possess normal mature B cells, but, as in IgA deficiency, such cells are unable to differentiate into plasma cells. The mechanism for this is unclear. In at least one case, the defect in maturation of an immunocompetent B cell resulted from an inheritable deficiency in a transport protein for vitamin B_{12}. Treatment with large amounts of B_{12} corrected this abnormality.

In some cases of hypogammaglobulinemia (low levels of immunoglobulin), it was shown that B cells from such individuals could be stimulated to synthesize IgG, but they could not secrete it because they lacked one or more enzymes necessary to glycosylate the synthesized immunoglobulin. Such nonglycosylated immunoglobulin is unable to cross the plasma membrane.

T-CELL DEFICIENCIES

Defects in Thymus Development

The failure to develop a functional thymus (thymic aplasia) leads to a class of T-cell immunodeficiency diseases characterized by a failure of T-cell maturation. One such malady, termed the Di George syndrome, follows a failure of the development of organs from the third and fourth pharyngeal pouches with a resulting deficiency in thymus and parathyroid gland functions. Two other types of thymic aplasia, called ataxia telangiectasia and Nezelof's syndrome, are inherited as autosomal-recessive diseases.

Such persons usually possess normal, or slightly increased, numbers of B cells and a significant number of plasma cells, but lack normal numbers of T cells. These individuals have recurrent infections with opportunistic agents such as viruses and fungi, are susceptible to graft-versus-host disease after transfusion or transplantation with allogeneic bone marrow cells, and frequently die after vaccination with live virus (eg, vaccinia virus).

Intestinal Lymphangiectasia

Intestinal lymphangiectasia occurs in individuals who make perfectly normal B and T cells, but in whom, because of a lymphatic channel abnormality, almost all long-lived T cells are emptied into the intestinal tract from which they are excreted. Such persons are usually unable to mount a positive delayed-type hypersensitivity skin response, and, in the several cases reported, could accept skin grafts from unrelated donors.

Humoral immunity appears normal, because B cells do not circulate at the same rate as do T cells, but, as

a result of abnormal cell-mediated immune responses, afflicted individuals have an increased incidence of fungal infections, tuberculosis, and reticuloendothelial malignancies.

SEVERE COMBINED IMMUNODEFICIENCY DISEASE

The leading clinical sign of severe combined immunodeficiency disease (SCID) is recurring infections starting early in infancy and involving all surfaces of the body. Moreover, these infections are caused by both pyogenic and saprophytic bacteria, as well as viruses, protozoa, and fungi. Most such persons die young. By definition, SCID refers to that disorder in which an individual lacks both T cells and B cells. There are, however, several causes of this disorder.

Swiss-Type Agammaglobulinemia

Although the pathogenesis is undefined, the majority of Swiss-type agammaglobulinemia disorders are inherited either through a sex-linked pattern or as an autosomal-recessive trait. Such persons are born with stem-cell defects and lack both antibody and cell-mediated immunity.

Adenosine Deaminase Deficiency

Adenosine deaminase deficiency was the first immunodeficiency disease demonstrated to be related to the absence of a specific enzyme. Adenosine deaminase converts adenosine and deoxyadenosine to inosine and deoxyinosine, respectively. In its absence, deoxyadenosine is secreted in the urine, and there is a buildup of dATP, ATP, and cAMP in RBCs and lymphocytes. The mechanism by which this deficiency causes SCID is not clear, but several theories have been proposed. One suggests that the resulting increase in dATP inhibits ribonucleotide reductase, leading to a suppression of deoxynucleotides and, hence, of DNA synthesis. Evidence also has been presented that dATP inhibits protein synthesis.

The disease may be acquired as a sex-linked disorder, and this defect accounts for between one third and one half of all autosomal SCID.

Miscellaneous Combined Immunodeficiency Diseases

Reticular dysgenesis is probably the most severe type of SCID. It is characterized by a deficiency in a primitive hematopoietic cell; persons with this disease are deficient in all blood leukocytes and usually die within a few days of birth.

Acquired SCID usually is seen in adolescence or in young adult life. Nothing concerning its etiology is known, because such persons generally have no previous history of recurrent infections.

THERAPY OF IMMUNODEFICIENCY DISEASES

Therapy of immunodeficiency disease relies either on replacing missing soluble factors or on implanting immunologically functional tissues. For example, periodic injections of immunoglobulin are used to treat Bruton's agammaglobulinemia. Adenosine deaminase deficiencies are treated by the periodic injection of previously frozen and irradiated RBCs; such cells permit purine entrance and allow residual enzymes to catalyze the missing degradative step. Soon, perhaps, somatic cell gene therapy may be used to correct this defect. Hormone injections (thymosin) have shown some success as therapy for selective T-cell deficiencies.

Transplantation of immunologically competent tissues, such as bone marrow cells, has been successful for a number of patients with SCID. Normally the donors for such transplants are siblings or other members of the family who possess identical HLA loci. As discussed in Chapter 10, matching at HLA loci is necessary to prevent fatal graft-versus-host disease. Fetal thymus transplants have proved successful in a few cases of Di George syndrome, but thymic transplants for SCID have been disappointing. Greater success has been achieved with combined thymus and fetal liver cell transplants, the latter obtained from fetuses of less than 12 weeks' gestational age. Cultured thymic epithelium containing no host lymphocytes also has been used to treat thymic aplasia.

Autoimmune Diseases

Our discussion of the immune system has described a mechanism for the generation of diversity among B cells and T cells that provides them with an almost limitless potential to bind to a large array of different molecules. Yet with all this vast potential for reactivity, a functional immune system must be able to discriminate between self and nonself. Unfortunately, this discrimination does not always occur, and the resultant destruction is termed autoimmune disease. Susceptibility to most diseases that are thought to involve immune responses to self-antigens is often associated with a particular haplotype at one or more genetic loci within the MHC.

Most studies linking the MHC and disease in animals were conducted with inbred strains of mice or rats. Obviously, a different approach had to be used in studies with humans. Two general methods have been used, and each has been effective. In one approach, a search is conducted in human populations for an association between a disease or immunologic characteristic and the presence of a given HLA antigen. The suitability of this approach was demonstrated by the observation of a close association between the HLA-B27 antigen and ankylosing spondylitis (inflammatory arthritis of the spine). In the second method, genetic linkage studies are carried out in families or in closed populations (eg, the Amish in western Pennsylvania) and in relatively inbred populations (eg, the Tuareg tribe in northern Africa).

Studies using recombinant DNA techniques and direct sequencing of the suspected HLA genes have revealed some interesting associations between disease susceptibility and specific amino acids in the polypeptide chains of a class II product of an HLA-D region gene.

Some of these diseases and their associated MHC haplotypes are shown in Table 14-4. Several are discussed here.

SYSTEMIC LUPUS ERYTHEMATOSUS

Systemic lupus erythematosus is a multisystem disorder characterized by the presence of a variety of autoantibodies that are responsible for immunologically mediated tissue injury. It is considered the prototype of all autoimmune diseases. One of the early signs of SLE is a rash, occurring over the nose and cheeks, giving rise to the original name *lupus erythematosus*, meaning "red wolf." This rash is exacerbated by sunlight. Multiple organs are involved, including the kidneys, nervous system, cardiovascular system, lung, gastrointestinal tract, skin, and lymph nodes.

Pathologic features include acute or chronic inflammation with deposition of fibrinoid material in connective tissue and blood vessel walls, mononuclear infiltration, and proliferation of fibroblasts. Renal involvement is seen in about 50% of the patients. These patients may have severely reduced renal function. Examination of kidney biopsy specimens from these patients shows extensive deposits of immunoglobulins and complement components in the submembranous tissue of the glomerular capillary loops. Skin biopsy specimens show deposition of IgG, IgA, IgM, C3, and C1q in the form of a linear or finely granular deposit at the dermal–epidermal junction. Similar deposits are seen in other connective tissue diseases.

Pathology involving the nervous system, cardiovascular system, lung, and gastrointestinal tract is observed in greater than 20% of the patients (20% to 90%, depending on the organ involved). Although the etiology of SLE is unknown, some evidence suggests that certain of the autoantibodies found can induce tissue injury. For example, DNA–anti-DNA complexes have been eluted from the kidneys, and it is likely that complement-mediated tissue injury is initiated by immune complexes deposited in the kidney and other sites.

Patients with SLE exhibit altered immune responsiveness. Evidence shows decreased T-cell numbers and increased antibody production (primarily to self-antigens). Furthermore, there is evidence of a strong genetic predisposition to develop SLE along with an association between the frequency of the disease and certain HLA haplotypes. Overall, these clinical observations suggest a combination of factors resulting in defective immune

TABLE 14-4
Autoimmune Diseases and MHC Association

Disease	Tissue Affected	Immune Response		Relative Risk*
		Antibodies	HLA Type	
AUTOIMMUNE DISORDERS				
Sjögren's syndrome	Salivary and lacrimal glands	Antinuclear	Dw3	5
Rheumatoid arthritis	Joints	Anti-Ig, antinuclear	Dw3, Dw4	3
Systemic lupus erythematosus	Kidneys, lung, skin, brain	Antinuclear, primarily anti-DNA	DR2	3
Polymyositis	Muscle	Antinuclear	—	—
Scleroderma	Skin, lungs, kidneys, GI tract	Antinucleolar	—	—
Graves' disease	Thyroid	Anti-TSH receptor	Dw3	4
Hashimoto's disease	Thyroid	Antimembrane, antithyroglobulin	—	—
Myasthenia gravis	Muscle	Antiacetylcholine receptor	B8, Dw3	4
Pernicious anemia	Gastric mucosa	Antiparietal cells Anti-intrinsic factor	DR5	3
Primary biliary cirrhosis	Liver	Antimitochondria	—	—
Autoimmune hemolytic anemia	Red blood cells	Antimembrane	—	—
Addison's disease	Adrenal glands	Several to gland	DR3	3
Multiple sclerosis	Muscle	—	DR2	4
Type I diabetes mellitus	β cell of pancreas	Anti-insulin	Dw2	0
		β-Cell specific Tc cell (?)	Dw3†	3
			Dw4	4
SELECTED HLA-ASSOCIATED DISEASES (NOT OBVIOUS AUTOIMMUNE DISORDERS)				
Ankylosing spondylitis	Joints (sacroiliac)	—	B27	> 100
Reiter's disease	Joints, eyes, mucous membranes	—	B27	40
Celiac disease	Small intestine	—	B8, Dw3	10
Psoriasis	Skin, joints	—	B13	5
Anterior uveitis	Eye	—	B27	15

Tc cell, cytotoxic T lymphocyte; GI, gastrointestinal; MHC, major histocompatibility complex; TSH, thyroid-stimulating hormone.

* Relative risk describes frequency associations between HLA types and diseases. Thus a relative risk of 1 means that an HLA type is expressed at the same frequency in a diseased and control population. Values above 1 reveal an association between an HLA type and a disease.

† Using molecular probes and DNA sequencing, a high correlation has been demonstrated between Type I diabetes mellitus and the type of amino acid at position 57 of the DQβ polypeptide chain. The mechanism responsible for this association is not known.

regulation, leading to increased autoantibody production and disease.

TYPE I (INSULIN-DEPENDENT) DIABETES MELLITUS

Type I diabetes (insulin-dependent diabetes mellitus [IDDM]) is characterized by little or no endogenous insulin secretory capacity and usually develops in juveniles. It is an HLA-associated autoimmune disease, and although the specific antigen on the β cells of the pancreas to which the autoimmune response is directed has not been identified, it is clear that this disease results, at least in part, from an activation of the cell-mediated immune system. Development of IDDM is a slow process, occurring over a period of years. At some time in genetically susceptible individuals, an unknown triggering event occurs, leading to an autoimmune reaction against the pancreatic β cells. For a period thereafter, there is a progressive decline in insulin production in the presence of normal blood glucose levels and in the absence of other overt clinical symptoms. This decline is followed by clinical diabetes resulting from complete destruction of the β cells.

Some evidence suggests that IDDM is mediated by autoimmune T cells. Spontaneous diabetes in the BB rat closely parallels the human disease. In both humans and rats, the disease is characterized by mononuclear infiltration of the pancreas prior to complete destruction of the insulin-producing β cells. In humans and rats, onset of disease is preceded by an increase in circulating T cells expressing class II MHC molecules (a marker for activated T cells; see Chaps. 9 and 11). The disease may be transferred to normal rats with lymphocytes (but not serum) from newly diagnosed diabetic BB rats. Moreover, immunologic intervention, such as transfer of normal T cells or bone marrow to the prediabetic animal, can prevent onset of the disease in the diabetes-prone BB rat. Lastly, β cells taken from normal rats are destroyed when transplanted into a diabetic BB rat. In humans, D. E. Sutherland has shown that when pancreatic tissue is transplanted from normal individuals to their identical diabetic twins, mononuclear infiltration and β-cell destruction occur within several weeks. Anti–islet cell antibodies are found in both prediabetic BB rats and genetically susceptible humans. These anti–islet cell antibodies are not directed to β-cell antigens and thus are probably not involved in β-cell destruction.

At least two genes are involved in the genetic susceptibility of individuals to IDDM. One of these genes maps within the MHC locus (see Chap. 10). Early studies demonstrated a close association between onset of IDDM and the HLA-DR3 and DR4 haplotypes and a negative association with the HLA-DR2 haplotype. Second, it was found that heterozygous individuals possessing the DR3 *and* the DR4 haplotypes are at a much greater risk than those homozygous at the DR locus (see Table 14-4). This clearly suggests a multi–MHC-gene effect on susceptibility to disease. The disease in the BB rat is also closely associated with a particular MHC haplotype, and in the nonobese diabetic mouse (another animal model for spontaneous diabetes), the disease is associated with the I-A class II locus, which is analogous to the HLA-DQ locus in humans.

Using recombinant DNA technology, a number of investigators have shown that susceptibility to IDDM is more closely associated with the HLA-DQ genes than it is with the HLA-DR genes (see Chap. 10). John Todd and colleagues at Stanford University determined the DNA sequences of genes encoding the DR_β, DQ_α, and DQ_β class II polypeptide chains from diabetic and nondiabetic individuals. Their results showed that, although there were no sequences unique to diabetic individuals, there was a striking correlation between susceptibility and an amino acid at the polymorphic position 57 of the DQ_β-chain. Type I diabetes susceptibility is positively correlated with the neutral residues alanine, valine, and serine and negatively correlated with the amino acid aspartic acid at this position.

These data clearly implicate residue 57 in disease susceptibility. However, the mechanism by which residue 57 influences disease is unknown. One explanation might be that specific residues create an HLA-DQ site that is capable of binding and presenting a β-cell–derived self-peptide to responding T cells. Alternatively, as suggested by Todd and associates, DQ molecules possessing these residues may fail to bind a self-peptide and, thus, may be unable to delete self-reactive T cells during their differentiation in the thymus (see Chaps. 9 and 11). Each of the above possible mechanisms may result directly from the participation of residue 57 in binding of self-peptide or indirectly by influencing the conformation of the peptide-binding site of the DQ molecule.

This correlation with position 57 of the DQ_β-chain does not explain all of the HLA associations with IDDM. However, it is entirely possible that differences in other residues in or near the binding pocket could either promote or prohibit binding of the same or different β-cell–specific self-peptides.

The low concordance rate for IDDM in HLA-identical siblings and in identical monozygotic twins indicates that other genes play a major role. One other set of genes that may be responsible are the genes encoding the antigen-specific T-cell receptor (see Chap. 9). Indeed, even identical monozygotic twins may not be identical in the repertoire of specificities expressed on their T and B cells. During differentiation of these lymphocytes, rearrangement of the genes encoding the polypeptide chains of their antigen-specific receptors is thought to involve *random* selection of V, D, and J genes. Thus, even identical twins may have significantly different repertoires that lead to different immune response capabilities and to different susceptibilities to disease.

Other studies, using the same sequencing methods, have shown similar correlations between specific amino acid residues and susceptibility to rheumatoid arthritis and pemphigus vulgaris.

ANTIRECEPTOR AUTOIMMUNE DISEASES

Several autoimmune diseases are associated with circulating antibody specific for cell-surface receptors. Of these, Graves' disease and myasthenia gravis are of particular interest and are the best understood. Each is briefly discussed here.

Graves' Disease

Graves' disease accounts for about 85% of all hyperthyroidism. It occurs most frequently in young women, although it can occur in either sex at any age. Susceptibility is certainly multigenic but has been associated with the HLA-DR3 haplotype in the MHC locus. It is generally characterized by hyperthyroidism and diffuse thyroid enlargement and by the presence of circulating antibodies directed against the thyroid-stimulating hormone (TSH) receptor on the membrane of the thyroid gland.

Three types of antibodies may be found:

1. Stimulatory antibody, which on reaction with the TSH receptor, mimics TSH itself and stimulates the gland, inducing iodide uptake, iodination of thyroglobulin, and secretion of the T3 and T4 thyroid hormones. Secretion of the hormones results in suppression of TSH release by the pituitary without affecting the levels of circulating antibody to the TSH receptor. Thus, chronic stimulation results in hyperthyroidism. This antibody can be demonstrated in almost all patients.

2. Inhibitory antibody, present in about 25% of patients with Graves' disease, has the opposite effect, resulting in hypothyroidism.
3. A third, less well-characterized antibody, induces goiter formation without hormone release. The TSH receptor is known to be composed of a transmembrane glycoprotein and a ganglioside unit. There is some experimental evidence that the stimulatory antibodies are directed to the ganglioside moiety and the inhibitory antibodies are directed toward the glycoprotein. The clinical picture probably reflects the relative proportions of the three antibodies.

Myasthenia Gravis

Myasthenia gravis is a progressive disease that is characterized by increasing muscle weakness and fatigue, ending with loss of breathing control by the diaphragm and trunk muscles. Thymus involvement is suggested by the occurrence of thymomas in 10% of the patients and the presence of germinal centers in the thymus of 60% of affected individuals. Genetic susceptibility to this disease is associated with the HLA-DR3 MHC haplotype. This disease is associated with antibodies specific for the acetylcholine receptor (AchR) at the neuromuscular junction. Interaction of this antibody with the AchR inhibits receipt of a signal for muscular contraction at the postsynaptic surface, although the signal is transmitted across the synaptic cleft. In addition, these antibodies can cause modulation and depletion of AchRs from the cell surface.

OTHER MHC-ASSOCIATED DISEASES

There are a number of other diseases for which individuals with a particular HLA haplotype are at increased risk. Table 14-4 lists a number of diseases having a more or less strong association with various HLA haplotypes. Two examples are briefly discussed here to illustrate several points.

Idiopathic Hemochromatosis

Idiopathic hemochromatosis is associated with the HLA-A3 haplotype but not with any class II molecule. Discovery of the pathogenesis of this disease demonstrated that it results from a defect in iron metabolism mediated by a gene closely linked to the HLA-A locus. The fact that this disease does not result from an immunologic mechanism shows that caution must be exercised in interpreting an apparent association between disease and any given HLA haplotype.

Ankylosing Spondylitis

The discovery of the close association between HLA-B27 and ankylosing spondylitis (AS) first demonstrated the validity of population studies. The reason for this high association is unknown. However, it has been shown that rabbit antibody to *Klebsiella* is cytotoxic for lymphocytes of B27⁺ patients with AS but not for B27⁺ individuals without AS or for cells of B27⁻ individuals. Cells from healthy B27⁺ individuals can be rendered susceptible to the rabbit anti-*Klebsiella* antibody by preincubation with extracts of the microorganism. A possible explanation is that *Klebsiella* (and possibly other bacterial products) is more likely to associate with the B27 molecule than with any other HLA molecule and renders the cells susceptible to the antibody.

MECHANISMS OF AUTOIMMUNE DISEASES AND HLA ASSOCIATION WITH DISEASE

It is well established that both positive and negative control of immune responses is mediated by genes mapping within the MHC. Indeed, evidence suggests a direct role for the products of these genes in certain autoimmune disorders. A number of immunologic and nonimmunologic mechanisms have been proposed to account for the association between a given HLA haplotype and a given disease. A few of the more plausible suggestions are presented here.

1. The relevant gene does not encode a class I or a class II product but resides within the MHC and is in linkage disequilibrium (see Chap. 10) with a given HLA gene. Idiopathic hemochromatosis is an example of this mechanism. Another excellent example is the gene responsible for 21-hydroxylase deficiency in chronic adrenal hyperplasia. This deficiency is associated with HLA-B5, but family studies have shown that the HLA-B gene itself is not responsible.
2. The HLA gene product may be a viral receptor, and, thus, the host range of the virus depends on the HLA haplotype. Some evidence exists for this mechanism in mice.
3. It is possible that the HLA gene product and the antigens of an infectious organism are similar (molecular mimicry). Tolerance to self would lead to tolerance to the microorganism, infection, and disease. In contrast, an immune response generated to an infectious organism could cross-react with self-antigens. Cross-reactivity between streptococcal antigens and heart tissue may be partially responsible for rheumatic fever. Amino acid sequence similarities have been found for a number of infectious organisms and human proteins, for example, between measles virus P3 protein and human corticotropin, between measles virus P3 and myelin basic protein, between human immunodeficiency virus p24 and human IgG constant region, and between *Klebsiella* antigen and HLA-B27, as discussed earlier for ankylosing spondylitis.
4. Any event leading to alteration of a self-molecule, and, thus, loss of tolerance, would map to the MHC. The

altered molecule may activate helper cells or bypass self-specific suppression, leading to immune responses that subsequently react with self.

5. Clearly the selection processes occurring in the thymus and those responsible for B-cell tolerance are not fool-proof. Therefore, autoreactive clones do emerge as mature functional B or T cells. These cells, specific for any given self-antigen, would be of low frequency and normally would be held in check. However, their presence clearly signals a potential hazard.

6. As suggested for susceptibility to IDDM, any change in the HLA gene leading to altered binding and presentation of self-peptide to either Tc or Th cells may result in an autoimmune response. Similarly, any change in the TCR genes leading to recognition of self-peptide

in association with class I or class II molecules would have a similar effect.

7. Any shift in the idiotype–antiidiotype regulatory network could result in antiidiotypic antibodies that mimic self-antigen and thus mimic the normal physiologic function of the self-molecule in question. This mechanism could explain the stimulatory and inhibitory actions of antireceptor antibodies seen in Graves' disease and myasthenia gravis.

In summary, in most cases, the etiologic agent initiating the autoimmune response is unknown. Therefore, although many of these mechanisms have been experimentally demonstrated, there is as yet little evidence that any one (or more) is as yet involved in the pathogenesis of any given autoimmune disorder in the human population.

A Closer Look

Immediate hypersensitivity reactions mediated by immunoglobulin E (IgE) antibodies have plagued human beings in the form of allergy, asthma, and a variety of other atopic conditions. Much has been learned about the initiation of allergic reactions and the mediators that are produced, and some knowledge has been gained regarding how to treat and suppress these often-debilitating reactions. It has also become clear that the immediate hypersensitivity response plays an important role in the killing and expulsion of parasites in certain parasitic infestations.

In the 1970s, war was declared on cancer. An important division in this battle against cancer was to be represented by tumor immunology. The great hope was that we would be able to identify tumor-specific antigens (TSAs) and thus would be able to direct the tumor-bearing host's immune system against cells expressing such TSAs. The destruction of these tumor cells would represent a focused antitumor immune response that would eliminate the cancer. In spite of all that has been learned, little has come of the potential for using the immune system to destroy cancer cells. TSAs have been elusive and the ability to potentiate antitumor immunity in clinical settings has not borne fruit. Nevertheless, protocols are still being tested that are designed to potentiate nonspecific antitumor mechanisms mediated by lymphokine-activated killer cells and tumor-infiltrating lymphocytes. Clearly, there is much to learn and a long way to go in developing effective antitumor therapies mediated through our own immune systems.

A host of immunologic deficiency diseases exists; fortunately, they are rare. This chapter categorizes and defines a variety of B- and T-cell deficiencies, as well as a number of severe combined immune deficiency conditions. B-cell deficiencies are somewhat less life threatening than T-cell deficiencies and can often be treated with periodic gamma globulin injections. T-lymphocyte deficiencies are often severe, debilitating diseases that cannot be corrected and ultimately lead to death. Especially troublesome and serious are the combined immune deficiency diseases. Heroic efforts have been made to try to perform cell and tissue transplants into patients who have T-cell or combined immune deficiency diseases, or both, with little success. Nevertheless, it seems that investigators are on the threshold of developing new ways of correcting immune deficiency diseases, perhaps through the use of gene therapy and cell transplants.

Autoimmune diseases are some of the most insidious, chronic, and difficult to treat conditions in human beings. Conditions such as systemic lupus erythematosus, insulin-dependent diabetes, and myasthenia gravis are chronic conditions affecting a small percentage of humans. Often these diseases occur in one sex or the other and show up in particular age groups. The cause and origin of any of these autoimmune diseases are still unknown. There is much to learn in this regard. Furthermore, the effective treatment and reversal of these chronic autoimmune diseases are still largely experimental. The association of certain autoimmune diseases with major histocompatibility complex genotypes has spurred much research into the origin of these diseases and, as well, has stirred great interest in new approaches to the prevention, cure, and treatment of these conditions.

Bibliography

JOURNALS

Altmann DM, Sansom D, Marsh SGE. What is the basis for HLA-DQ associations with autoimmune disease? Immunol Today 1991; 12:267.

Atkinson MA, Maclaren NK. What causes diabetes? Sci Am 1990; 263:62.

Bousquet J, Hejjaoui A, Michel FB. Specific immunotherapy in asthma. J Allergy Clin Immunol 1990;96:292.

Creticos PS. Immunotherapy with allergens. JAMA 1992;268:2834.

Klein G. Immunological surveillance against neoplasia. Harvey Lect 1975;69:71.

McFadden ER Jr, Gilbert IA. Asthma. N Engl J Med 1992;327:1928.

Old LJ. Cancer immunology: the search for specificity. G.H.A. Clows Memorial Lecture. Cancer Res 1981;41:361.

Stiehm RE. New and old immunodeficiencies. Pediatr Res 1993;33:S2.

Todd JA. Genetic control of autoimmunity in type-1 diabetes. Immunol Today 1990;11:122.

Wall JR, Salvi M, Bernard NF, Boucher A, Haegert D. Thyroid-associated ophthalmopathy: a model for the association of organ-specific autoimmune disorders. Immunol Today 1991;12:150.

WHO Scientific Group. Primary immunodeficiency diseases. Immunodefic Rev 1992;3:195.

BOOKS

Cooper MD, Burrows PD, Kubagawa H. Ontogeny of B cells and their abnormal development in immunodeficiency disease. In: Aiuti F, Cooper MD, Good RA, Rosen R, eds. Recent advances in immunodeficiencies. New York, Raven Press, 1986:19.

Marsh DG, Bias WB. The genetics of atopic allergy. In: Samter M, Talmage DW, Frank MM, Austen KF, Claman HN, eds. Immunologic diseases, ed 4. Boston, Little, Brown, & Co, 1988:981.

Rosenberg SA. Adoptive cellular therapy: clinical applications. In: DeVita VT, Hellman S, Rosenberg SA, eds. Biologic therapy of cancer. Philadelphia, JB Lippincott, 1991:214.

Rossini AA, Mordes JP, Like AA. Immunology of insulin-dependent diabetes mellitus. In: Paul WE, Fathman CG, Metzger H, eds. Annual review of immunology, vol 3. Palo Alto, Annual Reviews, 1985:289.

Thomas L. In: Lawrence HS, ed. Discussion of cellular and humoral aspects of the hypersensitivity states. New York, Hoeber-Harper, 1959:529.

Yunginger JW. Clinical significance of IgE. In: Middleton E Jr, Reed CE, Ellis EF, Adkinson NF Jr, Yunginger JW, eds. Allergy: principles and practice, ed 3. St. Louis, CV Mosby, 1988:849.

Bacterial Physiology and Genetics

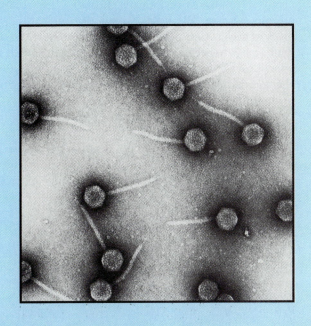

ABOUT 300 years have passed since van Leeuwenhoek first observed his little animalcules and reported his findings to the Royal Society of London. At that time it was beyond anyone's imagination that these tiny creatures could be more than a curiosity.

The last century, however, has witnessed a virtual explosion in the knowledge of biology, and much of it has centered about these same tiny cells. We know that microorganisms are essential to life on earth through their photosynthetic capacity and their ability to recycle many organic and inorganic compounds, especially carbon and nitrogen sources. We also know that some microorganisms are injurious to humans through their ability to produce disease. We have learned that we can control many of their activities for beneficial purposes or to reduce their ability to cause harm, but we have also learned that infectious agents like bacteria can continually adapt to changes in their environment and thereby can elude many of the human efforts to control them.

This ability to control microorganisms stems from our knowledge of what they are and what they can do. In other words, we have learned much about their molecular biology and have been able to exploit this knowledge for our own benefit. Furthermore, our knowledge of bacteria has shed light and provided models for understanding how similar processes occur in higher organisms.

Unit Three acquaints the reader with the knowledge of what bacteria can do and how we can use this information to our advantage. To this end, the discussions center around the structural and metabolic attributes of bacteria, the effects of various antibiotics on bacteria, and the genetic transfer mechanisms occurring in bacteria.

Bibliography

BOOKS

Moat AG, Foster JW. Microbial physiology, ed 3. New York, Wiley Interscience, 1995.

Neidhardt FC, Ingraham JL, Low KB, Magasanik B, Schaechter M, Umbarger HE. *Escherichia coli* and *Salmonella typhimurium*: cellular and molecular biology, ed 2. Washington DC, American Society for Microbiology, 1996.

Roth JA, ed. Virulence mechanisms of bacterial pathogens. Washington DC, American Society for Microbiology, 1988.

Salyers AA, Whitt DD. Bacterial pathogenesis: a molecular approach. Washington, ASM Press, 1994.

Starr MP, Stolp H, Trueper HG, Balows A, Schlegel HG, eds. The prokaryotes. Berlin, Springer-Verlag, 1981.

Essentials of Medical Microbiology, Fifth Edition, edited by Wesley A. Volk, Bryan M. Gebhardt, Marie-Louise Hammarskjöld, and Robert J. Kadner. Lippincott-Raven Publishers, Philadelphia © 1996.

Chapter 15

Bacterial Morphology and Taxonomy

This chapter presents the general characteristics of bacteria and describes how they are identified and classified using the techniques of morphology, biochemistry, immunology, and genetics. Insights into the relatedness among various bacteria are summarized, and a brief description of the major groups and types of bacteria that are important in medical microbiology is included.

Characteristics of Bacteria

The structural and genetic characteristics that distinguish bacteria from eucaryotic organisms were introduced in Chapters 1 and 2. Bacteria comprise an extremely diverse and widespread group of organisms, capable of inhabiting almost every environmental niche on earth and possessing broad metabolic capabilities. Only a small fraction of bacteria cause disease in humans or animals. Bacteria are unicellular organisms with relatively few examples of obvious cooperation among cells, other than some metabolic synergies. The primary characteristic of procaryotic or bacterial cells is the simplicity of their structure and genetic organization, which helps foster their rapid rates of growth. Examples of this structural simplicity include the small size and relatively simple shapes of bacterial cells, which enables rapid multiplication and growth of the cells and efficient diffusion of nutrients and signals throughout the cell. The absence of intracellular membrane-enclosed organelles also simplifies the process of cell division, but requires that the cytoplasmic membrane be able to carry out all of the complex functions normally performed by all of the eucaryotic organelles. The most striking feature of the chemical composition of bacteria is in their lipid content, where considerable simplicity in terms of the absence of sterols and of complex phospholipids is the usual case. The absence of sterols reflects the fact that most bacteria possess a rigid cell wall and do not require the membrane rigidity conferred by sterols. The simple lipid composition is probably related to the lack of intercellular communication and the existence of different types of signaling systems that do not depend on inositol lipids or arachidonic acid derivatives. Bacterial phospholipids need only provide a suitable membrane barrier against hydrophilic compounds and a matrix for the activity of membrane enzymes.

All bacteria have a simple genetic style. Their genome is much smaller than that of eucaryotic cells, but the amount of coding capacity is not proportionately decreased relative to the genome size. Bacterial chromosomes contain little noncoding regions, which are common in the eucaryotic genome with extensive repetitive DNA regions and introns. Although all bacteria probably can transfer genetic information, this transfer never involves formation of diploid zygotes, as in eucaryotic organisms, but occurs by exchange of relatively small portions of each organism's genome. This discussion does not suggest that bacteria are somehow rudimentary or primitive, but rather that they have forsaken features of cellular communication and cooperation for the sake of rapid growth and response to environmental changes. As will be discussed later, bacteria are efficient at responding to novel environmental challenges, such as the development of a new antibiotic.

Classification of Bacteria

Like other organisms, bacteria are given a binomial name indicating their genus, species, and, if appropriate, subspecies or serotypes. These names are printed in italics; examples include organisms such as *Escherichia coli* and *Bacteroides fragilis* subsp *fragilis*. A comprehensive system for the classification of bacteria is presented in *Bergey's Manual of Determinative Bacteriology,* which was first published in 1923. This system intended to aid in the identification of bacterial isolates and, while avoiding implications of actual phylogenetic relationships, divided all bacteria into various parts (or hierarchies), based on their prominent morphologic and metabolic characteristics. In this classification system, bacterial genera are subdivided into groupings, namely, families (names ending in -aceae), orders (-ales), classes (-aceae), and divisions (-es). These groupings provide no implications about the actual evolutionary or phylogenetic relationships among different bacteria, and no fossil records exist to provide a history of the line of descent of the various genera. Another impediment to the establishment of phylogenetic relationships among bacteria results from their rapid evolutionary change and exchange of DNA among distant genera, which causes a blurring of many features that are used for a classification. Whereas the classifications and groupings of bacteria based only on prominent morphologic and biochemical features are useful for routine identification, recent development of identification methods and of convincing phylogenetic relationships among different bacterial genera have arisen through analysis of DNA sequences.

MORPHOLOGIC CLASSIFICATIONS

Morphologic features provide major criteria for classification of bacteria, namely, the size and shape of the cells and their formation of characteristic cellular aggregates. Morphologic characteristics are routinely determined after the bacteria are stained by procedures that allow the visualization of the general shape of the cells and, in many cases, reveal additional features of cellular content or structure that are useful for identification.

Techniques for Microscopic Study of Bacteria

VISUALIZING LIVING BACTERIA. Living bacteria are difficult to see using the light microscope because individual cells appear almost colorless, even though the culture as a whole may be highly colored. Use of the phase-contrast microscope enhances the ability to examine unstained cells. A routine test that requires observation of living bacteria is the determination of motility. In these observations, remember that for a bacterium to be considered motile, it must swim in a definite direction, in contrast to the Brownian motion shown by nonmotile bacteria that bounce back and forth because of bombardment from water molecules. Wet mounts of bacteria can be prepared by placing a drop of a liquid culture onto a glass slide and covering it with a cover slip. The edges of the cover slip can be sealed with petroleum jelly to reduce evaporation of liquid and convection currents.

GENERAL STAINING PROCEDURES. Bacteria are usually observed in stained smears using staining procedures that permit detection of the size, shape, and arrangement of cells and can reveal the presence of certain cellular structures, such as endospores and flagella or the character of the cell wall. To prepare bacteria for staining, a small amount of culture is dispersed in a drop of water on a glass slide. After the smear is allowed to dry at room temperature, a faint haze should be visible, indicating that the cell density is not too great to allow detection of the normal cell aggregates. The bacteria are fixed to the glass by gentle heating in a flame.

Most stains are salts of a colored ion. In basic dyes, the cation (positive ion) is colored, whereas in acidic dyes, the color is carried by the anion (negative ion). Bacteria have a high affinity for basic dyes because of the high content of negatively charged macromolecules in the cell wall, nucleic acids, and ribosomes. Commonly used basic dyes are crystal violet, safranin, and methylene blue. Covering a smear with one of these dyes for 30 to 60 seconds, followed by rinsing with water, is sufficient to stain many types of bacteria and reveal the size and shape of the cell. When some basic dyes bind to highly negatively charged cellular constituents, they undergo a change in color, the metachromatic shift. Blue dyes, such as methylene blue, appear red when bound to nucleic acid or polyphosphate granules.

Acidic dyes are repelled by the negative charge of the bacterial cell, and dyes such as Congo red or nigrosin can be used for negative staining, where the background is colored, and the colorless cell bodies are apparent. This technique is valuable for examination of smaller cells.

Another form of negative staining is used for detection of the capsules around cells, which are not stained by the common dyes. Cells are suspended in India ink, which provides a black background in which the clear cells are visible. Because the ink particles are too large to penetrate into the capsule, encapsulated cells show a large, clear area surrounding the cell body.

GRAM STAIN. An extremely important staining reaction was developed in 1884 by a Danish physician, Christian Gram. The procedure has four steps: (1) the heat-fixed smear is covered with a solution of gentian or crystal violet; (2) after 60 seconds the dye is washed off, and the smear is flooded with an iodine solution; (3) after 60 seconds the iodine solution is washed off with water, and the slide is rinsed with 95% alcohol for 15 to 30 seconds; and (4) the slide is counterstained for 30 seconds with safranin (a red dye) or Bismarck brown.

The violet basic dye and the iodine form a large, complex aggregate within the heat-fixed cell. This complex can be readily washed out of some types of bacteria with alcohol; these are called gram-negative organisms. These appear red in the final slide, because they are stained only with the safranin dye. Other bacteria retain the dye complex during the alcohol wash; these are called gram-positive organisms. They appear blue or bluish purple, because the red counterstain is not detectable on cells that have retained the intensely colored blue complex.

As is described in Chapter 17, the gram-staining reaction of a cell is a reflection of the nature of its cell wall. The walls of gram-positive bacteria are much thicker and more cross-linked than in gram-negative cells, and it is this cell-wall meshwork that traps the large dye complex. Gram-negative bacteria have much thinner, lipid-containing walls, which are partly dissolved by alcohol, allowing the dye complex to be washed out of the cell body.

ACID-FAST STAIN. The acid-fast stain (Ziehl-Neelsen stain or modifications) is used primarily for the detection of bacteria in the genus *Mycobacterium,* which includes the agents of tuberculosis and leprosy. Mycobacteria have a hydrophobic surface that resists entry of dyes by the usual staining procedures. To get dyes into these cells, methods such as heating the organisms in the stain or including detergents in the stain are necessary. Once these cells are stained by carbolfuchsin (a mixture of phenol and the dye fuchsin), they retain the stain even when washed with 95% alcohol containing 3% HCl—hence, the term *acid fast.* All other bacteria are decolorized by this procedure. This stain allows the detection of small numbers of acid-fast bacteria, even when they are present with large numbers of other cells, as in the sputum from a patient with tuberculosis.

Shapes of Bacterial Cells

Medically important bacteria are classified in the following general shapes: (1) cocci, or spherical cells; (2) bacilli, or cylindrical rod-shaped cells; and (3) spiral and curved forms. A few bacteria exhibit filamentous morphologic features consisting of branched tubes, and some bacteria lack a constant shape and characteristically have a variable (pleomorphic) morphologic type. Figure 15-1 illustrates the major morphologic groups of bacteria.

COCCI. Cocci (singular, coccus; from the Greek word for berry) are generally spherical, although often elongated in one dimension. Cocci often adhere to one another in groups that are characteristic of a species. For example, most streptococci form long chains of cells, because all progeny cells divide in the same plane and do not easily separate. *Streptococcus pneumoniae* may also occur in short chains, but occur mainly in pairs. Cocci that divide sequentially in two perpendicular planes form tetrads of cells and belong to the genus *Gaffkya,* and cocci in the genus *Sarcina* divide sequentially in three planes to form cubical packets. Cells that divide in random planes form irregular clusters of cells and include the genera *Staphylococcus* and *Micrococcus.*

BACILLI. Bacilli (singular, bacillus; meaning "little staff") are rod shaped. The ends of some bacilli are rounded, whereas those of others (ie, fusiform bacteria) are more tapered. Some bacilli are so short that they are called *coccobacilli.* All bacilli divide across the narrow axis and some form long chains. However, unlike the cocci, the length of the chains of bacilli is not an identifying characteristic.

SPIRAL FORMS. The spiral bacteria can be divided into three groups. *Vibrios* are curved rods, resembling commas. *Spirilla* are S-shaped but do not extend for more than one sine wave, whereas *spirochetes* are helical and flexible (to varying degrees), spiral-shaped organisms that are always longer than one wave.

Colony Morphology

Occasionally features of bacterial colonies provide some taxonomic information, such as their size (indicative of the growth rate), appearance (eg, fried-egg shape of *Mycoplasma* colonies), or color (eg, the golden pigmentation on certain media gave *S. aureus* its name). The production of smooth, glistening, wet-looking colonies is frequently associated with virulent organisms that produce copious antiphagocytic capsules or long surface polysaccharide

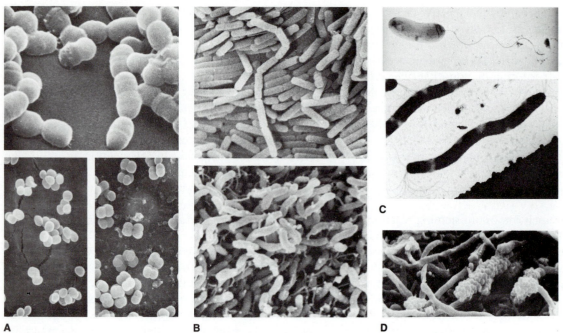

FIGURE 15-1   Forms of bacteria. **A.** Cocci. (*Top*) *Streptococcus mutans*, demonstrating pairs and short chains. (Original magnification ×9400). (*Bottom left*) Single cells and small clusters of *Staphylococcus epidermidis*. (Original magnification ×3000.) (*Bottom right*) Pairs, tetrads, and regular clusters of *Micrococcus luteus*. (Original magnification ×3000.) **B.** Bacilli. (*Top*) Single cells and short chains of *Bacillus cereus*. (Original magnification ×1700.) (*Bottom*) Flagellated bacilli (unnamed) associated with peridontitis. (Original magnification ×3700.) **C.** (*Top*) A cell of *Vibrio cholerae:* notice curved cell and single flagellum. (Original magnification ×8470.) (*Bottom*) The spirillum *Aquaspirillum bengal:* notice polar tufts of flagella. (Original magnification ×2870.) **D.** Variety of organisms in dental plaque after 3 days without brushing. (Original magnification ×1360.)

chains. Certain bacteria growing on media containing red blood cells display hemolysis, or apparent lysis of the red blood cells surrounding the colonies. The type of hemolytic reactions is a primary feature for identification of many bacteria. As described later, specialized media have been developed to distinguish various types of bacteria on the basis of colony color.

BIOCHEMICAL CLASSIFICATIONS

In addition to the appearance of individual cells and colonies, taxonomic classifications make use of the biochemical properties of an organism. Each type of bacterium possesses a characteristic complement of enzymes and metabolic pathways. The presence of these pathways determines the ability of that organism to grow in various environments or on particular media. For example, the response of bacteria to oxygen and their ability to grow in its presence or absence is an easily measured and extremely useful feature in bacterial classification. The response to oxygen is determined in part by the presence of enzymes that detoxify reactive oxygen species. For example, the enzyme catalase, which eliminates hydrogen peroxide, can be detected by the evolution of bubbles of oxygen gas when a solution of hydrogen peroxide is dropped on a bacterial colony; the possession of catalase provides an

easy way to distinguish between *Staphylococcus* and *Streptococcus* (catalase-negative) organisms. Many bacteria, including some medically important species, are rapidly killed on exposure to oxygen, and special precautions are needed for their detection.

Other taxonomically useful criteria include the ability to use specific nutrients for growth or the presence of enzymes that metabolize specific chemicals. To use a specific nutrient, for example, a sugar or amino acid, the bacterium must possess a transport system able to bring that compound into the cell as well as the enzymes to convert the compound into a metabolite that can enter one of the central metabolic pathways. The ability to use specific sugars is a primary basis for assignment of a bacterium to a particular species within many genera. The measurement of growth using one sugar as sole carbon source is impractical for bacteria having complex nutritional requirements, and it is common to test for the production of acid by such cells growing on a rich medium containing that sugar, as described in Chapter 16. For example, *E coli* metabolize the disaccharide lactose, salmonellae do not, and shigella do so slowly or not at all. Simple methods are available to test for the production of characteristic metabolic products, such as gas or hydrogen sulfide. The presence of diagnostic enzymes that differentiate among various species or genera often can be detected by colorimetric assays linked to pH changes or the production of a reactive product. For example, the production of high levels of urease by *Proteus* organisms, but not most other enteric bacteria, is easily detected with a pH-indicator dye as a result of the increase in pH that occurs when urea is broken down to ammonia. Bacteria that possess cytochrome *c* can be identified colorimetrically by the dichlorophenol–indophenol oxidase reaction. Colonies of bacteria that produce H_2S can be detected by its reaction with ferrous salts to produce a black ferrous sulfide precipitate.

Relatedness among different bacterial isolates can be estimated by a numerical analysis, in which 100 to 300 biochemical characteristics are compared for each strain. A similarity index is calculated for each pair of organisms, using the formula $S = NS/(NS + ND)$, where S is the similarity index, NS is the number of characters shared by both organisms, and ND is the number of characters that are different. The higher the value of S, the more related are the pair of strains. Examination of a large number of biochemical parameters reduces the bias inherent in less extensive classification schemes that are based on the presence or absence of only a few key enzymes.

Serologic classifications are used routinely to distinguish among species, subspecies, or serotypes within a genus. These tests employ antibodies as sensitive and specific probes for the presence of various chemicals and antigenic conformations present on the bacterial surface. The use of monoclonal antibodies has greatly increased the specificity for many such probes. Typing by sensitivity of an isolate of *S. aureus* to a panel of bacteriophages frequently was used for epidemiologic tracing of those isolates.

GENETIC CLASSIFICATIONS

Whereas taxonomic classification systems are useful for the identification of bacterial isolates and for the separation of species within a genus, they were impractical for indicating phylogenetic or evolutionary relationships among different genera and for formulating higher groupings of bacteria. Phylogenetic relationships basically define the length of time since two current organisms diverged from a common progenitor. This timing process can be measured from the number of base changes that have occurred in related segments of the DNA of the two organisms, with the assumption that there is a reasonably constant probability at which base changes occur. The difficulty of relying on morphologic or biochemical characteristics as an index of the evolution of bacteria can be exemplified as follows. A single base change could render a bacterium unable to metabolize glucitol, for example, and this organism would seem to be closely related to its progenitor except for the difference in the utilization of the unusual sugar glucitol. On the other hand, another single base change could eliminate the ability to form

spores or to produce catalase (and hence, to grow well aerobically), and this organism would seem to be distinct from its progenitor, despite the fact that it also has only a single base change. Prominent features of a bacterium can be lost as readily as can minor traits, but the former changes would receive far more weight in the usual taxonomic schemes.

The phylogenetic relationships among different bacteria are estimated by determining the degrees of similarity between their nucleic acid sequences.

DNA Homology

One of the earlier tests of the genetic relatedness between two organisms is the measurement of DNA homology by nucleic acid hybridization techniques. The DNA from one organism is made radioactive and mixed with an excess of small DNA fragments from the test organism. These mixed samples are heated to separate the strands of DNA and are then slowly cooled to allow the reformation of double-stranded regions by the pairing of homologous portions of the two DNAs. The DNA homology between the two organisms is revealed by the rate and extent to which the test DNA forms stable double-stranded duplexes with that from the reference organism. The amount of radioactivity present in the double-stranded DNA species can be determined by chromatographic procedures that separate single-stranded DNA from double-stranded species, or by the degradation of nonhybridized single-stranded DNA by the action of the S1 nuclease. This technique is useful only for closely related organisms, because changes in DNA sequence can prevent specific solution hybridization, even though substantial homology is still present.

HYBRIDIZATION TECHNIQUES. Hybridization techniques, in which one of the nucleic acids is immobilized on a solid support, are being increasingly used in the clinical laboratory for more immediate problems than the genealogy of bacteria. Using cloning techniques, it is possible to obtain portions of a genome that are uniquely present in a given genus, species, or subspecies. Such cloned DNA fragments provide the basis for simple and rapid tests for the presence of that type of organism in a clinical specimen. The ease, specificity, and sensitivity of hybridization techniques to detect homologous sequences promise to make this type of approach practical for routine use. It is also possible to use the DNA from a drug-resistance determinant to test for the presence of that determinant in a clinical sample, thereby allowing the investigator to identify an organism and determine its drug-resistance properties without having to wait for the organism to grow. The development of polymerase chain reaction (PCR) techniques to amplify the portion of DNA that lies between two specific sequences provides an even more sensitive and simple procedure for identification of the

TABLE 15-1
Some Bacteria of Medical Importance

Family Genus and Species	Disease	Features
GRAM-POSITIVE COCCI		
Staphyloccoccus (Gram-positive spheres in irregular clusters; facultative anaerobe; catalase positive; no spores)		
S. aureus	Abscesses, toxic shock	Coagulase positive
S. epidermidis	Nosocomial infections	Coagulase negative, skin flora
S. saprophyticus	Urinary tract infections in young women	
Streptococcus (Gram-positive spheres in pairs or chains; homofermentative aerotolerant; catalase negative)		
S. pyogenes	Pharyngitis, skin infections, rheumatic fever, glomerulonephritis	β-Hemolytic
S. agalactiae	Neonatal meningitis	
S. pneumoniae	Lobar pneumonia, meningitis	α-Hemolytic; lancet shaped, bile soluble
Enterococcus faecalis	Secondary infection, SBE	Grows in 6.5% salt
GRAM-POSITIVE RODS, SPORE FORMING		
Bacillus (Rod shaped; aerobe or facultative anaerobe)		
B. anthracis	Anthrax	
Clostridium (rod shaped; anaerobic; spores are larger than cell)		
C. botulinum	Botulism	Multiple neurotoxins
C. difficile	Pseudomembranous colitis	Two exotoxins
C. perfringens	Gas gangrene	
C. tetani	Tetanus	Single neurotoxin
GRAM-POSITIVE RODS, NOT SPORE-FORMING		
Listeria (Short rod; facultative anaerobe; catalase-positive)		
L. monocytogenes	Meningitis	Food-borne; intracellular growth
Corynebacterium (Rod or club shaped cells, irregular staining and cell clusters; facultative anaerobe)		
C. diphtheriae	Diphtheria	Exotoxin blocks protein synthesis
Actinomyces (nonmotile, not acid-fast, form filaments, facultative anaerobe, catalase-negative)		
A. israelii	Actinomycosis	
MYCOBACTERIA (Acid-fast rods, gram-positive, aerobes, catalase-positive, nonmotile; high content of lipids in cell wall)		
Mycobacterium tuberculosis	Tuberculosis	Very slow growth
M. avium - M. intracellulare	Chronic pulmonary infection; disseminated in immunocompromised host	
M. leprae	Leprosy	
MYCOPLASMAS (Small cells; lack cell wall; sterol-containing membrane; small genome size; pleomorphic shape)		
Mycoplasma pneumoniae	Primary atypical pneumonia	Intracellular growth
Ureaplasma urealyticum	Nongonococcal urethreitis	
NOCARDIA (Gram-positive aerobic, often acid fast; irregular shapes with long filaments and fragments; produce mycolic acids)		
Nocardia asteroides	Pulmonary nocardiosis	
GRAM-NEGATIVE AEROBIC RODS AND COCCI		
Bordetella (Minute, nonmotile coccobacilli)		
B. pertussis	Whooping cough	
Brucella (Coccobacilli, nonmotile, facultative intracellular growth, catalase positive)		
B. abortus	Brucellosis	
B. melitensis		
Francisella (Minute pleomorphic; requires cysteine in blood agar)		
F. tularensis	Tularemia	
Legionella (Motile, catalase positive, requires cysteine)		
L. pneumophila	Legionnaire's pneumonia	

TABLE 15-1 *(Continued)*

Family Genus and Species	Disease	Features

Neisseria (Nonmotile diplococci, catalase and oxidase positive)
  1 *N. gonorrhoeae* — Gonorrhoeae
  2 *N. meningitidis* — Epidemic meningitis
Pseudomonas (Straight or curved rods, motile, catalase and oxidase positive, respiratory metabolism)
  1 *P. aeruginosa* — Wound, burn, urinary tract infections, pneumonia in cystic fibrosis

GRAM-NEGATIVE FACULTATIVE ANAEROBIC RODS

Enterobacteria (Small rods, intestinal inhabitants, catalase positive; ferment glucose)

Family Genus and Species	Disease	Features
Enterobacter aerogenes	Opportunistic, UTI	Motile, butanediol, lactose fermenter
Escherichia coli	Diarrhea, UTI, meningitis, septicemia	Motile, lactose fermenter to acid and gas
Klebsiella pneumoniae	Pneumonia, UTI	Nonmotile, capsulated
Proteus mirabilis	UTI	Urease
Salmonella typhi	Typhoid fever	Only human
Salmonella sp.	Food poisoning	Acid and gas
Shigella dysenteriae	Bacillary dysentery	Nonmotile, no gas
Yersinia pestis	Bubonic plague	Lactose negative
Yersinia enterocolitica	Gastroenteritis	

Vibrio (Curved rods, polar flagella, catalase and oxidase positive)

V. cholerae	Cholera	
V. parahaemolyticus	Gastroenteritis	Seafood contaminant

Pasteurellae (Nonmotile rods, catalase and oxidase positive, require organic nitrogen source)

Pasteurella multocida	Cat bite	
Haemophilus influenzae	Meningitis, pediatric disease	Require NAD and hemin

GRAM-NEGATIVE, AEROBIC/MICROAEROPHILIC

Campylobacter fetus	Septicemia	Slender curved rod
C. jejuni	Enteritis	
Helicobacter pylori	Ulcers	

GRAM-NEGATIVE, ANAEROBIC RODS

Bacteroides (Rod with curved ends, major intestinal flora)

B. fragilis	Anaerobic or multistrain abscesses	
Fusobacterium sp.	Abscesses, dental infections	

GRAM-NEGATIVE, OBLIGATE INTRACELLULAR PARASITES

Rickettsia (Small rods, associated with arthropods)

R. prowazekii	Epidemic typhus	Growth in vacuole
R. rickettsii	Rocky Mountain Spotted Fever	Growth in cytoplasm and nucleus
Coxiella burnetii	Q fever	Growth in vacuoles, airborne spread

Chlamydia (Cocci, developmental cycle in cytoplasm)

C. trachomatis	Trachoma, Lymphogranuloma venereum	
C. psittaci	Psittacosis	

SPIROCHETES: GRAM-NEGATIVE HELICAL BACTERIA

Borrelia burgdorferi	Lyme disease	Irregular coils
B. hermsii	Tick-borne relapsing fever	
Treponema pallidum	Syphilis	Tightly coiled, microaerophilic, not growable in media
Leptospira interrogans	Leptospirosis	Flexible, tightly coiled

SBE, subacute bacterial endocarditis

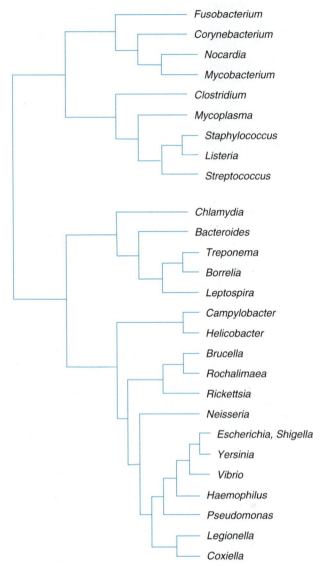

FIGURE 15-2   Relatedness among some bacteria of medical importance as revealed by comparison of the nucleotide sequences of their 16S ribosomal RNAs. Lengths of the horizontal lines are not drawn to scale with respect to the degree of relatedness.

presence of an specific DNA sequence, and these developments are sure to be widely used in clinical microbiology.

DNA SEQUENCES OF RIBOSOMAL RNA. The principle underlying the use of hybridization techniques for taxonomic studies is that the extent of hybridization between nucleic acids from more distantly related organisms decreases as a result of the base changes that have occurred since the two organisms diverged from their common progenitor. It is routine to count the number of base changes directly by determination of the DNA sequence of particular genes, rather than indirectly by hybridization. The most widely used test genes for this purpose are the ribosomal RNAs (rRNA). All bacteria possess rRNAs (16S, 23S, 5S) whose

structures and functions are strongly conserved. The rRNAs exhibit considerable base-pairing between different parts of the same molecule, and many portions of the rRNAs are sites for the specific binding of ribosomal proteins. Because of the need to maintain these secondary structures and RNA–protein interactions, the sequence of rRNA can only change slowly. Most base substitutions affecting the gene for an rRNA must be balanced by a compensatory change elsewhere in the rRNA molecule or in the gene for a ribosomal protein. Thus, rRNAs represent useful evolutionary clocks in which different parts of the molecule appear to undergo base changes at different rates. Rapid techniques for the determination of DNA sequence allow comparisons of the entire rRNA sequence. The nucleotide sequences of rRNAs from many bacteria have been determined, and they provide a quantitative measurement of the genetic relatedness of various bacteria and other organisms.

GENETIC TAXONOMY. Measurement of the number of base differences in the rRNAs allows construction of phylogenetic trees showing the evolutionary distances between organisms, as exemplified in Figure 15-2. Interpretation of these data led to some startling and provocative conclusions about the origins of species. Three major phylogenetic kingdoms (Eubacterium, Archaea, and Eucaryotae) are proposed, each being roughly equally distant from the others, although the exact route of descent is a controversial topic, which is not of immediate relevance for this book.

Some intriguing findings came from analysis of the nucleotide sequence relationships among the eubacteria. The gram-positive bacteria comprise a single phylogenetic grouping, whereas the gram-negative bacteria are much more diverse, falling into as many as 10 distinct groups. Perhaps the gram-negative cell-wall architecture is the original version present in the first successful eubacteria. Whereas cell-wall architecture is a major taxonomic criterion, the absence of a wall does not seem to represent a separate evolutionary track, because the wall-less mycoplasmas are most closely related to organisms from the genus *Clostridium*, a major group of gram-positive anaerobic bacteria. Similarly, photosynthetic organisms are found in most phylogenetic units, interspersed with nonphotosynthetic forms. It is unlikely that the complex photosynthetic system arose several times, suggesting that photosynthetic capability was present in the earliest eubacteria. One implication of this finding is that the earliest successful cells were able to generate energy from light rather than from the degradation of organic materials. The analysis of nucleotide sequences has thus provided new views of the origin of life and of the development of species.

Although the use of nucleic acid sequences as a tool for bacterial taxonomy is a recent development, it provides a coherent and quantitative approach for the grouping of

A Closer Look

Nucleic Acid Probes: Clinical Impact of DNA Sequences and Family Trees

The development of recombinant DNA techniques in the 1970s has revolutionized the study and understanding of gene structure and expression. Many of these techniques are also seeing increased uses in the clinical microbiology laboratory by providing a means for the rapid, sensitive, and very specific detection and identification of infectious agents in human samples, and for tracing the source and spread of a particular organism associated with a local bacterial or viral epidemic. Listed here are some of the types of DNA hybridization and amplification tests that are being used in clinical microbiology.

The purpose of these tests is to provide a more rapid and specific way to detect the presence of an infectious agent in a clinical sample. Traditional microbiological testing required the isolation and growth of the causative bacterium or virus from the clinical sample. This type of testing requires substantial time before the growth of the entity is apparent, and is limited by the difficulties of eliminating the background represented by the presence of the normal bacterial flora, and by the fact that some bacteria and viruses grow very slowly or require special media and conditions, if they can be grown at all. Hence, there seems to be a tremendous advantage to the application of diagnostic techniques that identify bacteria by detecting the presence of genus-specific or species-specific DNA sequences. These techniques are being continuously developed, and this topic is changing at a rapid pace.

Some diagnostic tests are based on DNA hybridization, which is based on the fact that there exist some segments of DNA that are shared by all members of a particular bacterial genus or species, or type of virus, but which are not present in members of other genera or species. Such specific sequences are found on a fortuitous basis, and the coding properties of these specific sequences are unimportant. The availability of a specific sequence, or probe, allows detection of that bacterial type in any clinical sample, even in the presence of substantial amounts of DNA from the human host and other bacterial types. When the DNA in the clinical sample is denatured to separate the two strands and then mixed with the specific probe, the probe will hybridize only to its complementary DNA sequence, if it happens to be present. Hybridization can be detected on a solid support or in solution after the unbound probe has been removed by washing the support under conditions to reduce or eliminate nonspecific binding to related but nonidentical DNA sequences. Detection of the hybridization of the probe DNA to its specific complement can be determined by radioactive labeling of the probe with ^{32}P-labeled nucleotides followed by detection of bound radioactivity by exposure to x-ray film, as is the routine procedure in the research laboratory. For work in the clinical laboratory, it is greatly desirable to avoid reliance of radioactive materials, owing to the short lifetime of radioactive probes, the expense and risk of their use, disposal and monitoring, and the need for specialized training. Hence, numerous nonradioactive methods have been developed. For example, it is possible to prepare the probe DNA so that it contains a modified nucleotide base that contains the vitamin biotin. The incorporation of the biotinylated nucleotide does not interfere with the hybridization efficiency or specificity. The biotinylated DNA probe that is hybridized to DNA from the clinical specimen can be detected by taking advantage of the very tight and specific binding to biotin of the protein streptavidin. To detect the bound biotin, streptavidin that has been covalently linked to an enzyme, such as alkaline phosphatase or peroxidase, that gives a colored product when a substrate is added, is used. Another nonradioactive label is the steroid digoxigenin, which can be detected with a specific antibody.

These DNA hybridization tests can also be used in the same approach to detect not the particular species of bacterium, but the presence of a particular virulence or drug-resistance determinant. In these cases, the DNA probe is obtained from the gene for the determinant of interest.

Another very valuable tool for detection of specific DNA sequences makes use of the amplification possible in the polymerase chain reaction (PCR). This technique amplified the DNA sequence that is located between the sites for binding of two DNA primers, which are chosen to hybridize some distance apart on opposite strands of the DNA. Specificity of this process is very high, because if the sequences to which either primer binds is missing, or is too far away, or is on the wrong DNA strand, there will be no amplification and no product of the expected size will be produced. The amplification provided by the PCR technique results from the repetition of the cycles of extension of the added primers used the DNA in the clinical sample as template, followed by denaturation of the extended product and re-hybridization to the added primers. This technique became practicable only with the isolation of very heat-stable forms of DNA polymerase iso-

which can respond differently to changes in the growth medium and can influence the growth of other bacteria in the population. Pure cultures usually are isolated by spreading a sample of cells over the surface of a suitable medium. Growth media have been developed for the isolation or identification of many specific types of bacteria; some media are selective, meaning that they contain ingredients that inhibit the growth of certain other bacteria. For example, bile salts and basic dyes often are included in media used for the isolation of enteric bacteria, because these reagents prevent the growth of most gram-positive bacteria. Other media are termed differential, meaning that they permit the differentiation of organisms on the basis of some biochemical property. For example, media used for the isolation of enteric bacteria incorporate lactose and an acid-base indicator into a peptone-containing medium. Colonies formed by bacteria able to produce acid from lactose are readily distinguished by their color from colonies of lactose-nonfermenting bacteria, which grow on the peptone present in the medium but produce an alkaline reaction owing to their metabolism of the amino acids and peptides.

Almost all media used for the purification of bacteria are solidified by the addition of agar, a complex polysaccharide isolated from seaweed. Solutions containing agar melt when heated to about 95°C, but must be cooled to about 45°C before they will form a solid gel. These solutions can be kept molten at temperatures above 50°C and, if desired, can be mixed with heat-labile ingredients before being poured into Petri plates or tubes and allowed to harden. Fortunately, few bacteria degrade agar.

Bacteria will grow when distributed on an agar surface of a suitable medium by pouring or by spreading with a wire loop (Fig. 16-1). Wherever a single cell has been deposited, a visible colony can arise containing 10^6 to 10^9 bacteria, all of which are the progeny of the original cell. An isolated colony thereby provides the pure culture needed for subsequent studies of the growth and drug-resistance properties of the bacterial isolate. It is good practice to restreak each single colony on a similar medium to ensure the absence of any contaminating bacteria.

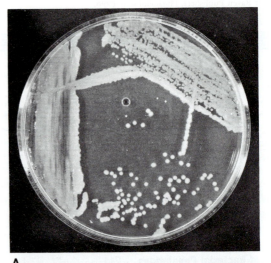

A

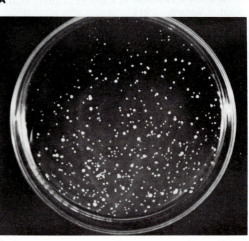

B

FIGURE 16-1   A. The streak-plate technique is used to isolate bacterial colonies for pure cultures. Each individual colony contains the progeny of a single cell. Notice how the number of cells decreases as one goes from the heavy part of the streak to an area of isolated single colonies. **B.** Pour plate prepared from dilution of a bacterial culture. Plates are prepared by inoculating tubes of cooled, but still molten, nutrient agar with various dilutions of bacterial culture. The inoculated agar tubes then are poured into Petri dishes and allowed to solidify. As with the streak plate, each colony represents the progeny of a single bacterial cell.

Determination of Bacterial Mass

To measure the growth parameters and the effect of antibiotics on a particular bacterial strain, the change of cell mass and number of living cells should be determined. Some antibiotics cause a decrease in viability but no change in cell mass, others only inhibit growth, and others cause cell lysis. No single method allows both measurements. Cell mass can be determined from the dry weight, although this requires large samples and considerable time. Rapid colorimetric assays are available for measurement of the amount of cell protein, and a sensitive assay can be used to determine the amount of ATP. The simplest and most frequently employed technique is the mea-

surement of the optical density or turbidity of a liquid culture. This assay is based on the fact that light scattering by particles, such as bacterial cells, is related to their number, size, and mass. The determination of certain metabolic activities, such as dye reduction by the electron transport components or the release of radioactive CO_2 from a labeled substrate, are far more sensitive than those based on turbidity but more involved for routine analyses.

Determination of Cell Number

The total number of cells, both living and dead, can be determined microscopically by using a special glass slide, called a Petroff-Hauser chamber, which has a graduated

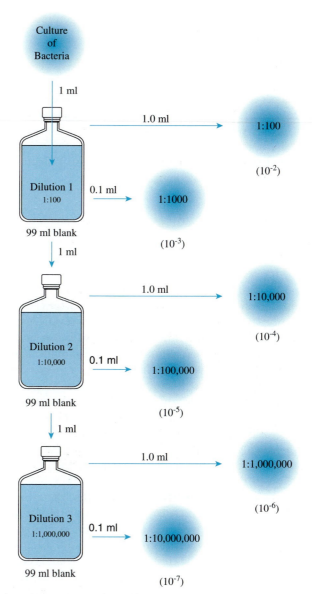

FIGURE 16-2 Serial dilutions for counting bacteria. Circles represent platings, and all dilutions are expressed as the dilution per milliliter of the original culture. Thus, when 0.1 ml of a 10^{-2} dilution is plated, this is expressed as a 10^{-3} dilution, because it represents one tenth as many cells as would be used by plating 1 ml of the 10^{-2} dilution.

section of known volume. An electronic particle counter, known as a Coulter counter, provides rapid and quantitative measurements of the number of cells and their volumes.

The number of living cells in a sample can be determined by plating dilutions of the original culture onto the surface of an agar medium or by mixing the diluted sample with the melted agar medium before pouring it into a Petri dish to harden. The number of colonies that arise after 1 or 2 days' incubation is counted and multiplied by the dilution factor to yield the number of viable cells per milliliter in the original sample. Figure 16-2 illustrates such a dilution scheme, in which the sam-

ple was diluted by a factor of 10^{-6}, and 0.1 mL was plated onto the surface of the plate. In this case, if 90 colonies were found on the plate after incubation, one calculates that there were 90×10^6 cells per 0.1 mL, or 9×10^8 viable cells per milliliter of the original sample. Clinical samples expected to have few cells, such as urine or clear water, can be concentrated by centrifugation or filtration rather than diluted before plating.

PHASES OF GROWTH

The size of a population of bacteria in a favorable growth medium increases exponentially. The generation time or doubling time is a measure of the time required for the population to double and is influenced by numerous growth conditions. The optimal generation time varies for different organisms, ranging from as short as 8 to 10 minutes for *Clostridium perfringens* and some *Vibrio* species to as long as 15 to 20 hours for *Mycobacterium tuberculosis.* Because many bacteria have generation times in the range of 30 to 120 minutes, bacterial populations can quickly become large. For example, one *Escherichia coli* cell with a 30-minute doubling time will grow overnight into more than one billion (10^9) cells. If cell division could continue at the same rate, it would require only an additional 37 hours for the progeny of that single cell to cover the United States to a depth of 1 meter. This example stresses the rapidity of logarithmic bacterial growth and suggests the necessity for quickly diluting and plating samples when determining the cell numbers.

To portray the growth curve of a bacterial culture, the number or mass of cells usually is plotted on a logarithmic scale as a function of time (Fig. 16-3). A typical growth curve contains four major phases.

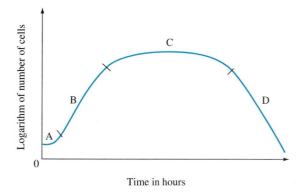

FIGURE 16-3 Typical growth curve illustrating the phases of growth occurring when bacteria are inoculated into a culture medium. **A.** Lag phase: cells begin to synthesize inducible enzymes and use stored food reserves. **B.** Logarithmic growth phase: the rate of multiplication is constant. **C.** Stationary phase: death rate is equal to rate of increase. **D.** Death phase: cells begin to die at a more rapid rate than they reproduce. The slope of this phase varies from one genus to another and may last from less than 1 day to several months.

LAG PHASE. When bacteria are inoculated into fresh medium, reproduction does not usually begin immediately. During the lag phase, the synthesis of enzymes and other macromolecules needed for growth in the new medium occurs and cell mass and size begin to increase before cell division initiates. The length of the lag phase depends on the kind of bacteria, the age and size of the inoculum, the nature of the medium from which they were taken, and the nutrients present in the new medium.

LOG OR EXPONENTIAL GROWTH PHASE. During the exponential growth phase, cell mass and numbers increase in a logarithmic manner with a constant generation time. This is a period of balanced growth, during which all cellular constituents are manufactured in constant proportion. The rate of cell division is, of course, dependent on the type of organism, the nature of the medium, the temperature, and, for aerobic organisms, the rate of aeration.

Both cell number and mass increase in a coordinate manner during log phase, and measurements of either parameter can be used to determine the generation time. Because each cell generation results in a doubling of the population, the following equation applies:

$$B_t = B_0 \times 2^n$$

where B_t and B_0 are the number of bacteria or their mass at time t and initial time 0, respectively, and n is the number of generations that have occurred between time 0 and time t. Taking the logarithm (to the base 10) of both sides the equation yields:

$$\log B_t = \log B_0 + n \log 2$$

Because $n = t/g$ where t is the time and g is the generation time in minutes per doubling, the equation above can be rearranged to yield:

$$\log B_t - \log B_0 = \log 2 \times t/g.$$

This equation can be rearranged to solve for any unknown when given three of the four parameters ($\log 2 = 0.301$). A frequently employed function is called the *specific growth rate*, which is given the symbol, μ, and is in units of doublings per hour:

$$\mu = \ln 2/g = (\ln B_t - \ln B_0)/t.$$

STATIONARY PHASE. Logarithmic growth eventually slows because of accumulation of waste products, exhaustion of nutrients, change in pH, or a decrease in oxygen tension. The population then enters the stationary phase in which the number of viable cells remains about constant. Usually, a steady state occurs in which some cells die and others continue to divide. Notice that entry into the stationary phase or even starvation for a required nutrient need not result in the killing of most bacteria. Many cells entering stationary phase display a substantial change in their pattern of gene expression leading to changes in cell shape and increased resistance to many types of environ-

mental stresses, such as ultraviolet light, oxygen radicals, and many mutagens.

DEATH PHASE. Eventually the rate of death exceeds the rate of reproduction, and the number of viable cells declines. The length of time before all cells have died differs markedly for various organisms. Some species have a very short death phase, whereas others may take weeks before all the cells in the culture have died. During this phase, cells often assume unusual shapes, making it difficult to recognize bacteria in old cultures.

EFFECT OF GROWTH RATE ON CELL SIZE AND COMPOSITION

Using specialized growth techniques that maintain cells in a constant environment and, thus, at a constant rate of growth, as well as batch cultures in media of different composition, it has been possible to define the effect of growth rate on the size and composition of bacterial cells. Faster growing cells are larger, contain more DNA per cell, and more RNA per unit of DNA. To grow faster, cells must contain more ribosomes and other components for macromolecular synthesis. In *E. coli* the rate of ribosome synthesis increases roughly in proportion to the square of the growth rate constant, μ, so that the number of ribosomes per cell increases from about 7000 in slow-growing cells ($\mu = 0.6$ doublings per hour) to 70,000 in fast-growing cells ($\mu = 2.5$ doublings per hour). In these cells, the proportion of ribosomal RNA increases from 35% of the total RNA to about 73%.

As the cells grow faster in richer media, the rate of DNA replication must increase proportionally. However, the rate of movement of the replication fork is relatively constant in all but very slowly growing cells, and there is a maximal rate at which the chromosome can be replicated, which, in the case of *E coli*, is 42 minutes. Thus, cells that are growing faster than every 42 minutes possess multiple copies of their chromosome and initiate a new round of chromosome replication before the previous round has finished. As a result, fast-growing cells partition into each progeny cell several chromosomal copies that are still in the process of replication. For this reason, the control of cell division is responsive not to the start of DNA replication, but to the completion of a chromosome.

Bacterial Nutrition

In this section, the nutrients that must be provided to obtain bacterial growth are considered. Bacteria can be classified on the basis of the nature of their sources of energy and of the carbon used for construction of their cell materials. Organisms that gain energy from light are called *phototrophs,* whereas those that obtain energy from alterations of chemicals are called *chemotrophs.* Organisms that use carbon dioxide as their sole source of carbon are called *autotrophs,* whereas those that require organic carbon are called *heterotrophs.* These terms can be combined to reflect the various possible sources of energy and carbon. All of the bacteria of medical importance are classified as *chemoheterotrophs,* meaning that they use organic compounds as both carbon and energy sources.

CARBON SOURCE

For bacteria of medical importance, an organic source of carbon must be provided. This usually serves as both the source of carbon for biosynthetic processes and the material whose metabolism provides the energy required for cell growth. The mechanisms by which bacteria acquire energy from sugars are described later. Few carbon-containing compounds cannot be used by some bacteria as a carbon source. Bacteria are known that degrade wood, methanol, phenols, or hydrocarbons, such as asphalt or gasoline. Most pathogens, however, are limited to metabolism of simple carbohydrates, amino acids, or lipids.

NITROGEN SOURCE

Proteins, nucleic acids and many other cell constituents contain nitrogen, and, thus, substantial amounts of nitrogen must be provided for cell growth. A few free-living organisms can convert the dinitrogen gas in the atmosphere into ammonia, which is then incorporated into cellular constituents. Many other bacteria can use inorganic sources of nitrogen, such as ammonium ions or nitrate. Other less-versatile bacteria, including many pathogens, require organic nitrogen in the form of glutamine or glutamate, asparagine, arginine, or peptide digests.

INORGANIC IONS

All organisms require phosphate as a component of lipids and nucleic acids and for the storage of energy and the metabolism of carbohydrates. Sulfur, usually in the form of sulfate, can supply the sulfur in the amino acids cysteine and methionine. Most organisms possess the enzymes that reduce sulfate to the oxidation state (S^{2-}) present in biologic materials. Other ions are cofactors for numerous enzymes. Any growth medium must contain sufficient amounts of Mg^{2+}, and, occasionally, Na^+ and Ca^{2+}. Many other ions are needed but in such minute amounts that the contaminating amounts present in water and the other ingredients provide sufficient levels of these trace elements. These include Mn, Zn, B, Se, Mo, Ni, Co, and Cu.

Acquisition of Iron

One inorganic ion that deserves special consideration is iron. Iron is a constituent of catalase, cytochromes, non-heme iron-containing proteins, and a number of enzymes involved in intermediary metabolism. Hence, iron is required by almost all organisms. However, under aerobic conditions, iron is present primarily as the ferric (Fe^{3+}) ion, which in neutral or alkaline solutions forms large, insoluble complexes, leaving a remarkably small amount of iron free in solution (as low as 10^{-17} M). Consequently, all aerobic organisms have developed mechanisms to solubilize iron from these insoluble complexes and to transport it into the cell. Bacteria and some fungi accomplish this by excreting low–molecular-weight iron chelators, called siderophores, which bind iron with high affinity and extract it from the insoluble complexes. The iron-binding groupings in most siderophores are either catechols (such as 2,3-dihydroxybenzoate) or secondary hydroxamates. The soluble ferric-siderophores then are taken up into the bacterial cell by high-affinity transport systems, after which the iron is released from the siderophore and reduced to the ferrous state. Many bacteria can acquire iron complexed to their own siderophore as well as siderophores produced by other bacteria or fungi.

In animals, essentially all of the iron is bound to proteins, such as transferrin in serum, lactoferrin in milk, ferritin in liver, or conalbumin in eggs. Thus, the growth of an infecting bacterium within a host depends on its ability to produce sufficient siderophores to be able to compete with and remove the iron from the host's iron-binding proteins. Bacterial mutants that are defective in the production or accumulation of a siderophore usually are avirulent for systemic infection. The virulence of bacteria that do not grow in serum but remain, for example, in the intestinal tract, such as *V. cholerae,* does not seem to be dependent on the operation of siderophore-mediated iron uptake. Perhaps the anaerobic, iron-rich conditions in the intestine allow maintenance of growth-sufficient levels of soluble ferrous ion. Some systemic pathogens do not appear to produce a siderophore, but acquire iron directly from heme (eg, *Haemophilus*) or host proteins, such as transferrin or hemoglobin (e.g., *Neisseria*).

Conditions that increase the amount of free iron in serum are associated with an increased risk of systemic bacterial infection. Hemolytic anemia and malnutrition increase the degree of saturation of transferrin by increasing the amount of serum iron or by decreasing the concentration of serum proteins, respectively. The parenteral injection of iron has the same effect of increasing the serum iron load and the risk of septicemia. The major site of regulation of the host's serum iron level is at the stage of intestinal adsorption, and this is circumvented by iron injection.

Laboratory experiments demonstrate that the growth of many bacteria is inhibited by serum, even after inactivation of complement. This growth inhibition is often overcome by adding excess iron or by increasing the size of the inoculum (thereby increasing the concentration of siderophore in the medium). Thus, the growth of invading pathogens in serum or tissues is impaired by the extremely low level of available iron. The host can take advantage of the bacterium's obligate requirement for iron and lowers the level of iron in the serum by decreasing the intestinal adsorption of iron and increasing its sequestration in the liver in ferritin in response to many bacterial infections.

The ability of a bacterium to compete successfully with the host for iron is an important virulence determinant. In some strains of *E coli*, virulence is associated with the presence of a transmissible plasmid (pColV), which encodes the ability to produce and accumulate a new siderophore, called aerobactin. This siderophore normally is not produced by *E coli* but is produced by other bacteria, such as *Shigella*.

The accumulation by gram-negative bacteria of the ferric-siderophore complexes makes use of specific transport proteins in the outer membrane, several of which are responsible for the uptake of siderophores synthesized by other organisms.

ESSENTIAL METABOLITES

To reproduce, all bacteria must synthesize their own macromolecules. However, bacteria differ considerably in their ability to make their biosynthetic precursors and intermediates, such as amino acids, vitamins, purines, and pyrimidines. Many of the enteric bacteria and pseudomonads are able to grow in a synthetic medium containing only a simple carbon source and inorganic ions, demonstrating that these species are capable of synthesizing all of their biosynthetic intermediates from the carbon source in the medium. Many other bacteria have lost the ability to synthesize one or more essential metabolites and, therefore, require their addition to the growth medium. The nature of such requirements varies, ranging from only a few amino acids for *Bacillus* species to a long list of amino acids, bases, and vitamins for the streptococci. Some organisms (*Haemophilus*) require lysed red blood cells as a source of hemin and nicotinamide-adenine dinucleotide (NAD), and the obligate intracellular parasites can reproduce only within a living eucaryotic host cell.

Effect of Environment on Bacterial Growth

A number of conditions other than adequate nutrition strongly influence the rate of growth. Major variables include temperature, pH, and oxygen supply.

TEMPERATURE

Each bacterial species has an optimal temperature for growth and a temperature range above and below which growth is blocked. Bacteria are placed into one of three groups according to the temperature range allowing optimal growth. The largest group of bacteria, which includes all of the pathogenic forms, are the mesophiles, in which

growth occurs between 10°C and 45°C, with optimal growth between 20°C and 40°C. Psychrophiles are cold-loving organisms that grow between −5°C and 30°C and have an optimal range between 10°C and 20°C; these organisms can grow effectively in solutions kept in a refrigerator. Thermophiles have a growth range from 25°C to 100°C, and most have an optimal temperature range between 50°C and 60°C. Members of this group can be found growing in hot springs and oceanic thermal vents at temperatures near boiling; others are found in compost piles that have generated considerable heat as a result of bacterial metabolism.

The basis for the response of an organism to temperature is not clear. Metabolic reactions occur more rapidly with increasing temperature up to the point at which the enzyme is denatured. Protein stability is a major factor in setting the upper range of growth temperatures. At the lower temperatures conducive to bacterial growth, it is often the assembly of proteins into complexes, such as ribosomes, that becomes limiting.

pH

The pH of the culture medium affects the growth rate; usually there is an optimal value for growth and a wide range over which growth will occur. Although some bacteria can grow at a pH as low as 1 or 2, and others flourish at a pH around 10, most organisms grow best at a neutral or slightly alkaline pH (7.0 to 7.4). *V cholerae* is the only pathogen that grows well above pH 8, whereas most other bacteria grow in a pH range of 6 to 7.5, and numerous fungi grow well at pH 4 or 5.

The pH is one of the major factors that limits the growth of bacterial cultures, and organisms that ferment sugars to produce acids may lower the pH of the medium down to the point at which growth is prevented. Many bacteria keep a constant internal pH of 7.4, and this internal pH becomes too difficult to maintain when the pH gradient becomes greater than 2 or 3 units. In addition, the organic acids produced by fermentation reactions accumulate within the interior of the cell and inhibit metabolic reactions.

Osmolarity

The osmolarity of the medium influences the rate of growth, and bacteria must be able to adapt to changes from one osmolarity to another. Thus, a transfer to media of higher osmolarity often is followed by increased accumulation of ions (mainly K^+) to increase the internal osmolarity. Growth in medium of higher osmolarity (>0.5 M NaCl) requires the production of osmoprotectants, such as glycine betaine, proline, the disaccharide trehalose, and the peptide N-acetyl-glutaminyl-glutamine amide. Osmoprotectants are compounds that allow retention of protein structure and function even at the high intracellular concentrations needed to balance the osmotic stress of high external salt concentrations.

OXYGEN AND REDOX POTENTIAL

A major classification key for bacteria is their response to the presence of oxygen. Several factors are involved in this response. Some bacteria are able to use oxygen as electron acceptor in the energetically efficient process of aerobic respiration, whereas others lack respiration and rely on oxygen-independent fermentative metabolism. In addition, the presence of oxygen gives rise to toxic metabolic products that are lethal for bacteria that lack the means to destroy them. Oxygen readily acquires electrons from other chemicals, especially the quinones, flavoproteins and iron-sulfur proteins of electron transport systems. The transfer to oxygen of two or one electrons results in the formation of hydrogen peroxide (H_2O_2) or the reactive superoxide radical (O_2^-), respectively. Peroxide and superoxide react with water in the presence of iron to form the highly reactive hydroxyl radical ($OH\cdot$). Each of these three reactive oxygen species is toxic for cells through their reactions with lipids, nucleic acids, and proteins.

The ability of cells to grow in the presence of oxygen is largely determined by their ability to eliminate the toxic oxygen by-products; three enzymes play prominent roles. Catalase is a heme-containing enzyme that is found in aerobes and facultative anaerobes and destroys hydrogen peroxide:

$$2\ H_2O_2 \rightarrow 2\ H_2O + O_2.$$

Superoxide dismutase is found in all oxygen-tolerant bacteria and generally occurs in two forms: one containing iron and the other containing manganese. Some bacteria have only one form and others produce a Cu,Zn-containing form. These enzymes inactivate the superoxide radical:

$$O_2^- + O_2^- + 2\ H^+ \rightarrow H_2O_2 + O_2.$$

A third group of enzymes are the peroxidases, which catalyze the destruction of H_2O_2 with the simultaneous oxidation of an organic acceptor.

The presence of these three types of enzymes and of metabolic pathways that require particular oxidation-reduction potentials are major determinants of the response of bacteria to oxygen. Based on these responses, four groups are described.

1. *Obligate aerobes* (such as mycobacteria, pseudomonads, and some bacilli) generally require oxygen for growth, because their only energy-yielding metabolic reactions are electron transfers to oxygen or nitrate. They are unable to generate a net increase in ATP in the absence of this type of electron transfer. These organisms possess both catalase and superoxide dismutase to allow them to tolerate the presence of oxygen.

2. *Facultative anaerobes* (including the enteric bacteria and *Staphylococcus*) are capable of growth in the presence or absence of oxygen and actually change their metabolic machinery in response. When they grow in the absence of oxygen, the heme proteins of the normal respiratory chain are not produced. These organisms possess both catalase and superoxide dismutase, and the amount of these enzymes is influenced by the oxygen level of the medium, becoming low in the complete absence of oxygen.

3. *Microaerophilic organisms* (most lactic acid bacteria and streptococci) grow in the presence of oxygen but cannot use it as a final electron acceptor. Such organisms derive their energy solely from fermentative reactions that occur in the absence of oxygen, because they lack a cytochrome system that can transfer electrons to oxygen. These organisms grow best at low oxygen tensions. Their reduced growth at atmospheric oxygen levels may reflect their lack of catalase and the presence of superoxide dismutase. Their preference for the presence of low levels of oxygen probably is associated with the involvement of oxygen in certain steps of intermediary metabolism, such as the biosynthesis of pyrimidines and unsaturated fatty acids.

4. *Obligate anaerobes* grow only in the absence of oxygen but vary considerably in their sensitivity to it. None use oxygen in their metabolism or possesses the enzyme catalase. All have metabolic systems that function only at low oxidation-reduction potentials. Some, the aerotolerant anaerobes, can survive limited exposure to air because of their possession of sufficient levels of superoxide dismutase. Many obligate anaerobes are extremely sensitive to the presence of oxygen and are rapidly killed by exposure to air. As a result, special precautions must be taken for their isolation and study. These organisms generally lack superoxide dismutase.

Bacterial Metabolism

The term *metabolism* refers to all the chemical processes that occur within a cell, including those involved in interconversions of small molecules, the synthesis of the precursors of macromolecules, and the reactions that generate a cell's energy supply. The reactions of *anabolism* are involved in the synthesis of cellular constituents and require energy; the reactions of *catabolism* carry out the oxidation of a substrate accompanied by the liberation and storage of metabolic energy and the formation of degradation products. Anabolic reactions generally are similar for all types of cells, because the pathways for biosynthesis of the precursors of proteins, nucleic acids, lipids, and polysaccharides do not differ much among all living organisms. Catabolic reactions in bacteria are exceedingly diverse, where energy sources range from inorganic compounds such as sulfide, ferrous ion, or hydrogen to the organic materials such as carbohydrates, amino acids, or lipids.

The major catabolic and anabolic reactions used in bacterial metabolism are briefly described later in this chapter to illustrate some mechanisms of energy generation and storage and to show how these reactions help in the identification of bacterial types based on their characteristic nutritional requirements, carbon source utilization, and metabolic end products.

ENERGY LIBERATION AND STORAGE

When chemical oxidations are carried out in a test tube, the energy liberated is lost as heat. Living cells trap some of the energy released by metabolic oxidations and store it for use in other reactions.

The oxidation of glucose to carbon dioxide and water:

$$C_6H_{12}O_6 + 6\ O_2 \rightarrow 6\ CO_2 + 6\ H_2O$$

releases 686,000 cal/mol. In the biologic oxidation of glucose, this reaction occurs not in a single step but involves 20 to 30 individual reactions. Several of these reactions are designed to couple the release of energy during substrate oxidation to another process that leads to the formation of ATP.

The coupling process for trapping metabolic energy occurs by either of two basic mechanisms:

1. In *substrate-level phosphorylation*, an energy-rich phosphate bond is formed during catabolism of the substrate and is transferred directly to the formation of ATP. This process is exemplified by two reactions of glycolysis (the conversion of glucose to two molecules of lactic acid). A molecule of glyceraldehyde-3-phosphate is oxidized in the presence of inorganic phosphate to form 1,3-diphosphoglyceric acid, which contains an energy-rich acyl-phosphate bond. The acyl-phosphate formed in the first reaction is transferred to ADP to form ATP in the second reaction.
2. ATP formation also occurs by the process called *oxidative phosphorylation*, in which electrons released by substrate oxidation are passed through an electron transport chain. Operation of the electron transport chain results in the generation of a proton-motive force that can be used for many energy-requiring processes, including synthesis of ATP.

The catabolism of any organic energy source (carbohydrate, amino acid, lipid) involves its oxidation, or the transfer of electrons from the energy source to an electron acceptor. The electrons released during substrate oxidation are usually transferred to NAD to form the reduced derivative NADH. The NADH must be oxidized back to NAD to allow continued operation of the catabolic pathway. One mechanism for NADH oxidation is through transfer of electrons to the electron transport chain and ultimately to an inorganic electron acceptor,

such as oxygen or nitrate in the process called *respiration*. This process is coupled with oxidative phosphorylation and can yield up to three ATP molecules per NADH oxidized.

In the absence of an inorganic electron acceptor, the NADH formed during catabolism must be reoxidized by transfer of electrons to some organic compound during *fermentation*. Lower yields of energy are available from this process than from respiration, because the span in redox potential and, hence, the maximum amount of energy available from the overall reaction, is substantially smaller when organic compounds serve as electron acceptors.

CARBOHYDRATE METABOLISM

Although many bacteria are unable to metabolize sugars, the ability to do so is widespread and provides a major taxonomic key. Simple tests to determine whether a particular bacterium is able to ferment a specific sugar are based on the fact that many of the products of sugar fermentation pathways are acids. An acid-base indicator dye can be added to a medium (either liquid or solidified with agar) containing the specific sugar and a source of amino acids to support bacterial growth. Production of acid as a result of sugar fermentation is indicated by a color change in the medium surrounding each colony. Bacteria that metabolize sugars solely by respiratory pathways produce CO_2, but no acid, and would not be revealed by this test. Because the specific acids formed during fermentations often are characteristic for each genus, separation and identification of fermentation end products by gas chromatography is a useful tool for the rapid identification of anaerobes.

Catabolism of sugars can be visualized as several blocks of reactions. The first step is the conversion of the carbohydrate into a form that enters one of the central catabolic pathways. For example, the catabolism of lactose in *E coli* occurs by its cleavage to glucose and galactose and the conversion of galactose by three enzymatic reactions into glucose-1-phosphate. After its phosphorylation, the glucose molecules are processed by the enzymes of glycolysis or other metabolic pathways. The ability of a bacterial species to use a particular sugar is thus dependent on the ability to synthesize the enzymes that convert that sugar into glucose or another central metabolite.

Formation of Pyruvic Acid

The second major set of reactions of sugar catabolism are those that convert glucose or other hexoses into the three-carbon compound pyruvate. There are several distinct reaction pathways by which this can occur; the most familiar of these is the widely distributed Embden-Meyerhof pathway of glycolysis (Fig. 16-4). The glycolytic pathway comprises nine enzymatic reactions and begins with the sequential phosphorylation and isomerization of glucose

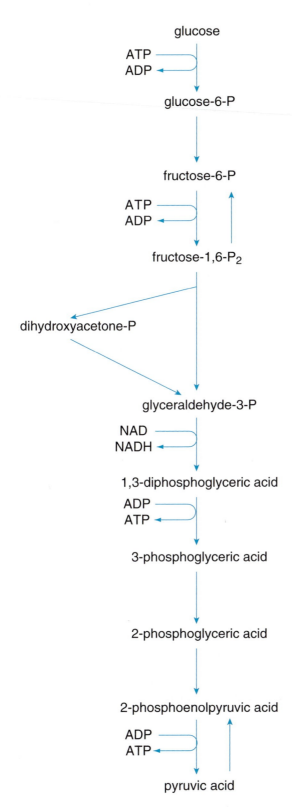

FIGURE 16-4 Embden-Meyerhof pathway for the dissimilation of glucose. Notice that one molecule of fructose 1,6-bisphosphate is split into two three-carbon compounds that are in equilibrium with each other. Thus, as the glyceraldehyde 3-phosphate is oxidized, the dihydroxyacetone phosphate is converted to more glyceraldehyde 3-phosphate. Each molecule of the six-carbon glucose gives rise to two of each of the three-carbon intermediates. Two molecules of ATP are required to initiate the pathway, but four molecules of ATP are formed by the glycolytic conversion of one molecule of glucose to pyruvic acid.

to yield fructose-1,6-bisphosphate at the expense of two molecules of ATP. This six-carbon compound is then cleaved into two three-carbon compounds, which are each oxidized and converted to pyruvic acid with the formation of two molecules of ATP, yielding a net gain of two ATPs per glucose metabolized. Two molecules of NADH are formed and must be reoxidized to NAD.

Other pathways can be used by bacteria for the catabolism of glucose. These pathways begin with the oxidation of glucose-6-phosphate to 6-phosphogluconolactone, which is converted to 6-phosphogluconic acid. Some pathways use a form of the pentose phosphate pathway (Fig. 16-5), in which the 6-phosphogluconic acid is oxidized, with the loss of a molecule of CO_2, to yield a pentose phosphate. This five-carbon compound is converted by the action of the transaldolase and transketolase enzymes to either hexose phosphate or glyceraldehyde-3-phosphate, which is converted to pyruvic acid by enzymes of the Embden-Meyerhof pathway. A few bacteria carry out a heterolactic acid fermentation in which a pentose phosphate is split to yield acetylphosphate and glyceraldehyde-3-phosphate.

In the Entner-Doudoroff pathway (see Fig. 16-5), the 6-phosphogluconic acid is converted to 2-keto-3-deoxy-6-phosphogluconic acid. This intermediate is then cleaved in one step to form pyruvic acid and glyceraldehyde-3-phosphate, which is converted to pyruvic acid by the same reactions as operate in glycolysis. This pathway requires fewer enzymes and reaction steps than the glycolytic scheme, but results in the net formation of only one molecule of ATP during conversion of one molecule of glucose to pyruvic acid.

Formation of Fermentation Products

Bacteria can employ many different metabolic pathways for the conversion of pyruvic acid to characteristic fermentation end products. All of these pathways must bring about the reoxidation of the NADH generated during the conversion of glucose to pyruvate. In addition, some of these pathways extract additional energy through the synthesis of ATP or allow further bacterial growth by releasing less toxic end products. Just a few of these pathways are described here and in Figure 16-6.

HOMOLACTIC ACID FERMENTATION. The direct reduction of pyruvic acid to lactic acid by the enzyme lactate dehydrogenase occurs in some streptococci and lactobacilli, as well as in mammalian skeletal muscle. Release of the product lactic acid makes the medium acidic and inhibits further bacterial growth, which is a useful reaction in many types of food preservation.

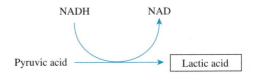

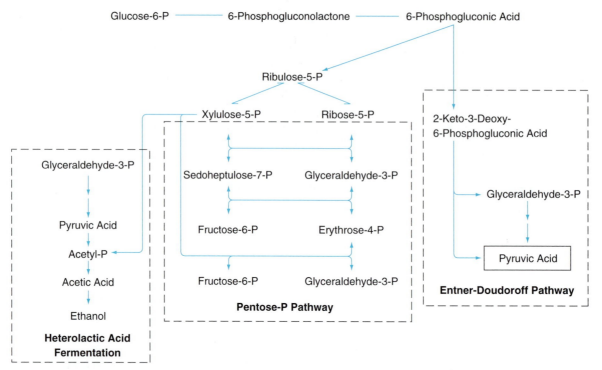

FIGURE 16-5 Other pathways of glucose catabolism. Glucose-6-phosphate can be metabolized through oxidative pathways that branch from the formation of 6-phosphogluconic acid. The pentose phosphate pathway makes use of the enzymes transketolase and transaldolase for the conversion of pentoses to hexoses and trioses. Notice that the erythrose 4-phosphate can accept a two-carbon intermediate from a molecule of sedoheptulose 7-phosphate to form fructose 6-phosphate and ribulose 5-phosphate. The complete oxidation of one molecule of glucose requires six revolutions of the cycle, with each revolution liberating one molecule of CO_2 and forming two molecules of NADPH. This pathway thus provides a pathway for the formation of ribose 5-phosphate for nucleic acid biosynthesis, a source of NADPH for many biosynthetic reactions, and a second pathway for the aerobic oxidation of glucose to CO_2 and H_2O. Heterolactic acid fermentation is carried out by members of the genus *Leuconostoc* and some species of *Lactobacillus*. The Entner-Doudoroff fermentation is used by some enterics and members of the genera *Zymomonas* and *Acinetobacter*. Both pathways use a single step to cleave a pentose or hexose, respectively, to small products.

ETHANOLIC FERMENTATION. The enzyme pyruvate decarboxylase releases carbon dioxide from pyruvic acid, with the formation of acetaldehyde, which is reduced by alcohol dehydrogenase to ethanol. These reactions occur in yeast and are crucial for the baking and brewing industries. Although the end products are neutral and the pH of the medium does not change much, ethanol is toxic and its accumulation limits further growth.

MIXED-ACID FERMENTATION. This complicated scheme occurs in the enteric bacteria and is named because of its production of multiple acidic products. The key reaction is the phosphoroclastic cleavage (pyruvate:formate-lyase), which converts pyruvic acid to formic acid and acetyl-CoA. Many enteric bacteria contain the enzyme formate:hydrogen-lyase, which splits the formic acid to form the gases hydrogen and carbon dioxide. Members of the

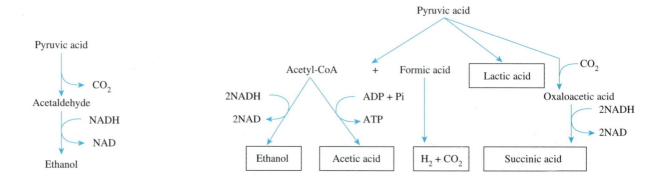

genus *Shigella* and some species of *Salmonella* lack this enzyme and thus do not produce gas during sugar fermentation. Gas production is an important taxonomic feature for the enteric bacteria. The acetyl-CoA has two metabolic fates. It is converted to acetyl-phosphate, from which the phosphate group is transferred to ADP, forming ATP and acetic acid. This formation of acetic acid from acetyl-CoA generates energy but does not reoxidize NADH. Thus, for every molecule of acetyl-CoA that is released as acetic acid, another acetyl-CoA must be reduced by two NADH molecules via acetaldehyde to ethanol. Lactic acid and succinic acid are also released during mixed-acid fermentation.

BUTYLENE-GLYCOL FERMENTATION. Members of the genus *Enterobacter* carry out mixed-acid fermentation but have an additional pathway to form 2,3-butylene glycol from pyruvate. Because 2,3-butylene glycol is relatively nontoxic compared with the acids and ethanol produced in the other pathways, its production allows cells to reach higher population densities before their growth is inhibited by the accumulation of toxic products. The decreased acid production and the presence of *acetoin,* an intermediate in 2,3-butylene glycol synthesis, helps to differentiate the lactose-fermenting species of *Enterobacter* from *Escherichia* in tests of environmental water supplies. The free-living *Enterobacter* species are likely to be found in water sources, but the presence of *Escherichia,* an inhabitant of intestinal tracts, is an indication of recent fecal contamination. Butylene-glycol fermentation, without the other parts of mixed-acid fermentation, is carried out by members of the genus *Bacillus.*

$$2\ CH_3COCOOH$$
Pyruvic acid

$$CH_3COHCOOH + CO_2$$
$$|$$
$$C=O$$
$$|$$
$$CH_3$$
Acetolactic acid

$$CO_2$$

$$CH_3CHOHCOCH_3$$
Acetoin

NADH

NAD

$$CH_3CHOHCHOHCH_3$$
2,3 Butylene glycol

OTHER FERMENTATION PATHWAYS. Members of the genera *Propionibacterium* and *Veillonella* convert pyruvate, through succinate and methylmalonyl-CoA, into propionic acid. Members of *Clostridium* produce a variety of organic compounds, including acetone, isopropanol, butanol, and butyric acid.

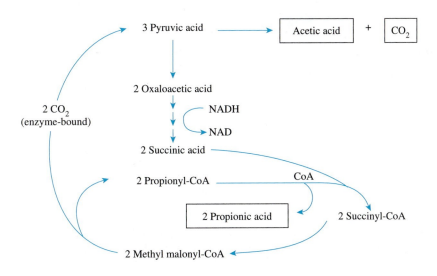

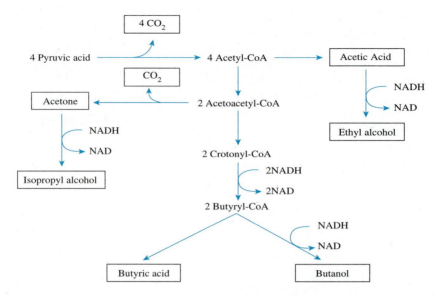

Products of Respiration

Respiration occurs when an inorganic compound is the final electron acceptor. During aerobic respiration, the acceptor is oxygen, but anaerobic respiration occurs with nitrate, nitrite, sulfate, or carbon dioxide in place of oxygen. Oxygen is the preferred electron acceptor and provides the maximum energy yield whereas nitrate is the

preferred electron acceptor for anaerobic respiration. The end products of respiratory metabolism are very different from the products of fermentation because respiration provides an effective route for disposal of electrons and reoxidation of the NADH formed during glycolysis to pyruvate.

The operation of the electron transport chain yields much more energy, in the form of ATP, than does glycoly-

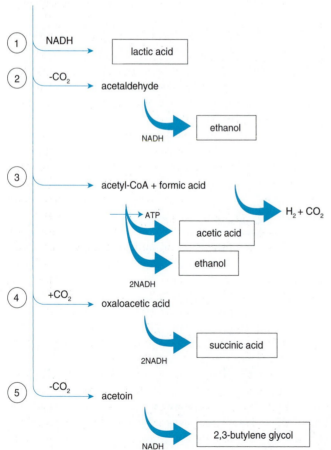

FIGURE 16-6 A few bacterial fermentation pathways. Branch 1 is the production of lactic acid by a D- or L-lactate dehydrogenase during homolactic fermentation. Branch 2 is the ethanolic fermentation pathway of yeast. The several steps of mixed acid fermentation add branch 3 to the reactions of branches 1, 2, and 4. Branch 5 is the pathway of 2,3-butylene glycol synthesis.

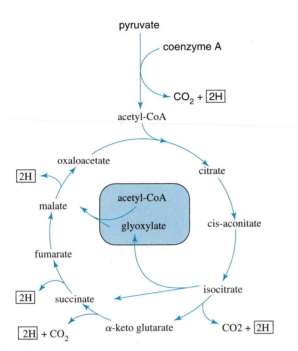

pyruvate

coenzyme A

CO_2 + 2H

acetyl-CoA

oxaloacetate

citrate

2H

malate

acetyl-CoA

glyoxylate

cis-aconitate

fumarate

2H

succinate

isocitrate

2H + CO_2

α-keto glutarate

CO2 + 2H

FIGURE 16-7 Tricarboxylic acid (TCA) cycle. Notice that each turn of the cycle liberates eight protons, which drive ATP formation via oxidative phosphorylation. The shaded area illustrates the glyoxylate cycle, which bypasses the decarboxylation steps of the TCA cycle and allows formation of additional four-carbon intermediates to replenish those lost to biosynthetic reactions.

sis. Cells exhibit a much lower rate of sugar consumption when they are able to respire, because the same amount of cellular ATP can be formed from the metabolism of fewer substrate molecules. In addition, pyruvate can be fully oxidized by means of the Krebs tricarboxylic acid cycle (Fig. 16-7) to carbon dioxide and water, resulting in greatly reduced release of acidic material during respiration than during fermentation. Both the NADH formed during glycolysis and the electrons released during the oxidation steps of the tricarboxylic acid cycle are transferred through the electron transport chain to oxygen and generate considerable additional energy.

BIOENERGETICS

Bioenergetics refers to those processes that generate cellular energy or use it for the physical and chemical tasks a cell must perform. Findings over the last decade have established the uniformity of bioenergetic processes throughout biology and have emphasized the central role of ion gradients in energy storage.

Respiratory Chains

The key feature of respiratory metabolism is the operation of an energy-conserving electron transport system that carries out the transfer of electrons from NADH and other electron donors to oxygen or other acceptors. Bacterial

electron transport chains are similar in principle to the mitochondrial pathway, although they are substantially different in detail. These differences reflect the much broader range of metabolic capabilities of bacteria and their different environmental niches. A simplified representation of the *E coli* electron transport system is given in Figure 16-8. Electrons pass along a series of electron carriers of increasingly higher redox potential. These carriers are all arranged in the cytoplasmic membrane and include flavoproteins, quinones, nonheme iron proteins, and cytochromes. Electrons from donors of different redox potential, such as NADH, succinyl-CoA or glycerol-3-phosphate, enter the electron transport chain through soluble or membrane-bound dehydrogenases. The reducing equivalents are transferred to membrane pool of quinones, which serve as mobile electron carriers to couple the dehydrogenases to the terminal reductases. These enzymes transfer electrons to the terminal electron acceptors, which are oxygen in aerobic respiration and nitrate, nitrite fumarate, sulfate, or CO_2 during anaerobic respiration.

Oxidative Phosphorylation

A model for the chemiosmotic operation of the electron transport system was developed by Peter Mitchell and provides the most satisfying general description of the capture of the energy released at different steps of electron transport. The concepts underlying this hypothesis account for a wide variety of bioenergetic phenomena occurring in bacteria, mitochondria, chloroplasts, and other cells. This model recognizes the importance of the vectorial distribution of the electron transport chain within the cytoplasmic membrane and the fact that energy capture occurs only when the transport chain is contained in a sealed membrane structure.

Electron transport results in the movement of protons across the cytoplasmic membrane, that is, from inside to outside the bacterial cell (see Fig. 16-8B). Some electron carriers, such as flavins and quinones, acquire hydrogens when they are reduced and thus can carry both electrons and protons across the cytoplasmic membrane. Other electron carriers, like cytochromes, carry only electrons. In some of the electron transport steps, a flavoprotein or quinone can pick up one or two electrons and protons on the cytoplasmic side of the membrane and then diffuse across the membrane to react with the next electron carrier on the other side of the membrane. If the next carrier can accept only electrons, the protons will be released into the medium outside the cell, resulting in the net movement of protons across the membrane and separation of charge. Other mechanisms also can result in the movement of protons across the membrane. The exact number of protons that are translocated per electron is difficult to determine and differs depending on the electron donor and acceptor. Thus, unlike sub-

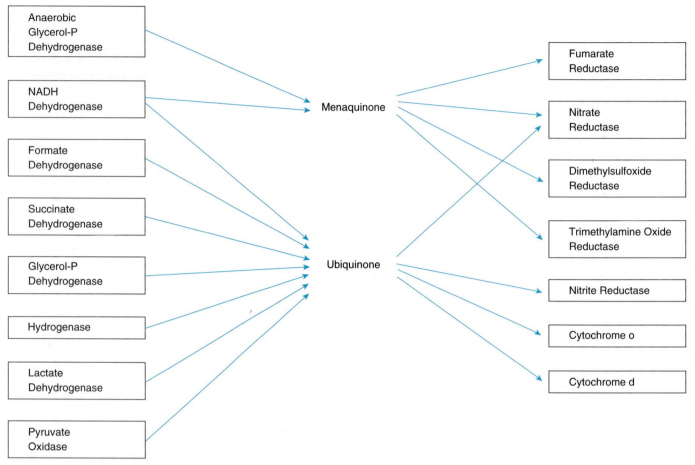

FIGURE 16-8 Schematic diagram of the coupling of electron flow to proton translocation and the generation of a proton-motive force. Quinones can carry both protons and electrons across the membrane as a hydride, whereas the cytochromes can only carry electrons. Protons liberated from the oxidation of NADH are passed through the membrane to the exterior. The accompanying electron is passed by a nonheme iron carrier to quinone. As shown, the electrons terminate in the cytochrome system where they are eventually accepted by oxygen to form water. Q, ubiquinone; MQ, anaerobically produced menaquinone.

strate-level phosphorylation, the energy from electron transport is trapped not by the synthesis of an energy-rich chemical intermediate, but in the transmembrane gradient of protons.

The separation of charge that results from the movement of protons generates an electrical potential across the membrane (interior negatively charged) in the range of 100 to 200 mV. Under certain conditions, continued proton extrusion can generate a substantial difference in the chemical concentration of protons, or a pH gradient, across the membrane. Many cells maintain an internal pH of 7.5, and, thus, a pH gradient occurs only if the external pH is less than 7.5. The membrane potential and the pH gradient together make up the electrochemical potential across the membrane, commonly called the *proton-motive force*. This force attracts protons back into the cell and is coupled with the performance of a wide variety of metabolic and mechanical work.

Oxidative phosphorylation uses the proton-motive force to drive the synthesis of ATP (Fig. 16-9). This is accomplished by an enzyme complex that is highly conserved among bacteria, mitochondria, and chloroplasts and is called the F_1F_0–proton-translocating ATPase, or *ATP synthase*. The bacterial enzyme complex possesses eight different protein subunits, most of which occur in multiple copies. The F_0 portion of this complex is embedded in and spans the cytoplasmic membrane, and the F_1 portion extends into the cytoplasm. The enzyme couples the downhill passage of protons across the membrane back into the cell to the synthesis of ATP. This enzyme can operate in the reverse direction to allow bacteria lacking an electron transport system to generate a proton-motive force by using the energy from the hydrolysis of ATP generated during fermentation.

Chemical agents known as uncouplers block ATP synthesis without affecting electron transport or the activity of the ATPase. They are hydrophobic compounds with an ionizable group, such as 2,4-dinitrophenol, and they can cross the membrane in either the ionized or neutral form. Uncouplers act as protonophores and allow protons

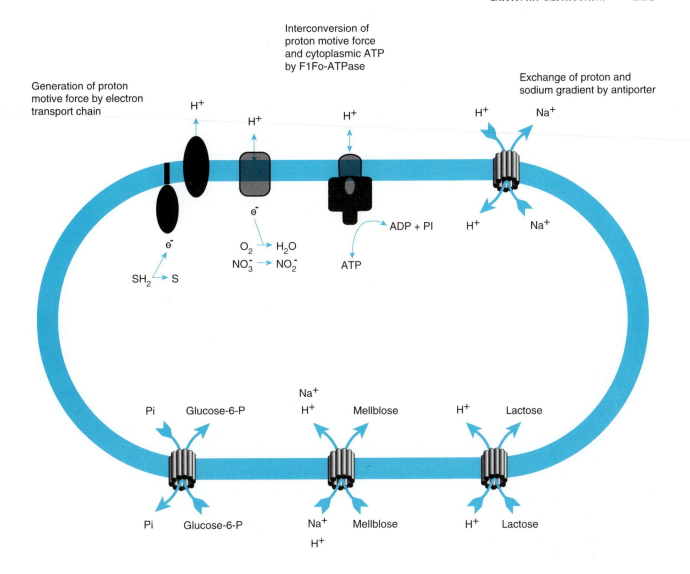

Generation of proton motive force by electron transport chain

Interconversion of proton motive force and cytoplasmic ATP by F1Fo-ATPase

Exchange of proton and sodium gradient by antiporter

Use of ion gradients to transport nutrients

FIGURE 16-9 Ion gradients as driving forces in bacteria. The proton-motive force generated by proton extrusion by the electron transport system results in creation of an electrical potential (interior negative) and a chemical gradient (interior alkaline). The return of protons to the cytoplasm is coupled by transport proteins to drive the accumulation of other substrates or is used by the F_1F_0–proton-translocation ATPase for synthesis of ATP. Fermentative cells can use the ATPase in reverse direction to generate a proton-motive force from ATP.

to enter the cell without being coupled to any of the work-generating systems, thereby dissipating the proton-motive force. Carriers of other ions also can dissipate the electrical potential or pH gradient.

Nutrient Transport

Most nutrients for bacteria are hydrophilic substances and hence require the operation of specific transport systems for their passage across the cytoplasmic membrane into the cell. Bacterial transport systems usually allow the accumulation of a substrate to a much higher concentration inside the cell than in the external environment. They

also have fairly high affinities for their substrates, which help bacteria compete with surrounding cells for the limited nutrients in the environment. Transport systems are divided into several groups on the basis of their mechanism of action and the form of metabolic energy used to bring about the accumulation of the substrate.

ACTIVE TRANSPORT. Active transport systems use metabolic energy directly to drive the movement of their substrates against a concentration gradient. In some systems, solute accumulation is driven by coupling to the electrical potential or the gradients of protons or sodium ions across the cytoplasmic membrane. In these systems, a substrate molecule binds with high affinity (Km of 0.1 to 100 $\mu M/L$) to a specific site on the transport protein (also called a *permease*). The binding of one or more protons to the carrier can either increase the affinity of the carrier for the substrate or increase the rate at which the carrier moves its substrate across the membrane. Because the proton-motive force results in a more negative charge on the interior of the cell relative to the exterior, the ability of a proton to bind to the carrier is higher on the exterior side than on the inner side of the membrane, and thus transport out of the cell occurs at a lower rate than does entry. The accumulation of substrate is thereby coupled with the movement of protons in response to their electrochemical gradient.

Accumulation of positively charged nutrients, such as lysine or K^+, does not require the simultaneous transport of a proton (symport) but occurs in response to the electrical potential, which draws the substrate into the negatively charged interior. In some cases, positively charged ions such as Na^+ and Ca^{2+} are pumped out of the cell; their carriers act as an antiport to exchange incoming protons for outgoing Na^+ ions.

Most transport systems that are driven by the proton-motive force use only membrane-bound proteins and can function in cytoplasmic membrane vesicles free of cytoplasmic constituents.

Another mechanism of energy coupling makes use of substrate-binding proteins that are present in the periplasmic space between the cytoplasmic and outer membranes of gram-negative bacteria. These proteins are readily released from cells by osmotic shock treatments or by disruption of the outer membrane. These transport systems are driven by ATP hydrolysis rather than the proton-motive force. This type of ATP-driven transport system can be found in gram-positive bacteria which lack a periplasmic space. In these cases, the sugar-binding proteins are anchored to the cell membrane by a lipoprotein anchor.

A few transport systems (such as ones that mediate uptake of Mg^{2+} or K^+) are related in structure and sequence to the ion-translocating P-type ATPases of eucaryotic cells and use ATP hydrolysis as the driving force for ion uptake.

GROUP TRANSLOCATION. The process of group translocation brings about the simultaneous transport of a substrate into the cell and its modification. The product of the reaction usually is a poor substrate for the transport system and is thereby trapped inside the cell. The best characterized group translocation process is the phosphoenolpyruvate-sugar phosphotransferase system (PTS), which catalyzes the simultaneous transport and phosphorylation of a number of sugars and sugar alcohols.

A complex series of reactions participate in the phosphotransferase reaction, as shown later. The energy source is phosphoenolpyruvate, whose phosphate group is transferred first to a soluble enzyme called *enzyme I* and then to a histidine residue on a small, heat-stable protein called *HPr*. The phosphate on HPr is then sequentially transferred to two sugar-specific proteins or protein domains, which can be cytoplasmic or membrane bound. The last protein in the process is the transmembrane transport protein, which transfers the phosphate to a sugar while the sugar is being transported into the cell.

The PTS system does not phosphorylate internal sugars, which must be acted on by cytoplasmic kinases. In addition, the PTS system is not used for the uptake of all sugars, and different bacterial species can accumulate a particular sugar by different transport mechanisms. For example, *E coli* transports glucose by the PTS and lactose by proton symport, whereas *S aureus* transports lactose by the PTS. PTS systems are present in both gram-positive and gram-negative bacteria, but not all bacteria possess PTS transport activity.

Purines and pyrimidines also may enter the cell by a form of group translocation in which the base is converted to the nucleoside during transport.

Facilitated diffusion systems, in which a substrate simply reaches an equal concentration on both sides of the cytoplasmic membrane, may not be present in bacteria, at least in *E coli*. Passive diffusion is, by definition, not associated with any specific membrane protein. Only a few compounds, such as water, oxygen, dinitrogen, fatty acids, and other lipid-soluble compounds, enter a cell by passive diffusion.

UTILIZATION OF NONCARBOHYDRATE SUBSTRATES

Bacteria are extremely versatile in the range of compounds that they can degrade; in fact, probably few organic compounds exist that cannot be degraded by bacteria. Many pathways for the metabolism of various exotic compounds have been elucidated, but the organisms of interest in medical microbiology use a rather limited range of nutrients.

Protein Utilization

The entry of intact proteins into a bacterial cell is extremely rare. However, many bacteria secrete a variety of proteases that hydrolyze proteins into peptides and amino acids, which can be taken up by means of active transport systems in any bacterium. Transported amino acids may be incorporated into bacterial proteins or degraded by catabolic pathways. Catabolism usually is initiated by the action of deaminases or decarboxylases, followed by further degradation to yield metabolites that can be used as an energy source or for biosynthesis of cellular constituents.

Fat Utilization

Fats and other lipids are broken down by the action of enzymes known as *lipases,* which hydrolyze the fatty acids or the polar head groups from triglycerides or glycerol phospholipids. The liberated glycerol can be phosphorylated, oxidized to glyceraldehyde-3-phosphate, and metabolized by the enzymes of the Embden-Meyerhof glycolytic pathway. The fatty acids are degraded by the β-oxidation pathway similar to that found in mitochondria.

Many of the proteases and lipases secreted by bacterial cells have detrimental effects on eucaryotic cells, including their lysis. For this reason, many of the enzymes that bacteria use to provide nutrients are classified by the microbiologist as toxins.

BIOSYNTHESIS OF MICROBIAL INTERMEDIATES

Bacteria differ in their number of growth requirements. Some bacteria can grow with only a single carbohydrate or amino acid as their sole carbon and energy source; others require a number of preformed compounds such as amino acids, purines, pyrimidines, and vitamins. Obviously, bacteria that can synthesize most of their biosynthetic intermediates will be able to grow in a simpler medium.

All of the cell's biosynthetic intermediates are synthesized from some component of the central catabolic pathways of glycolysis, the pentose phosphate pathway or the tricarboxylic acid cycle, as summarized in Figure 16-10. The biosynthesis of all 20 amino acids can be assigned

(text continues on page 230)

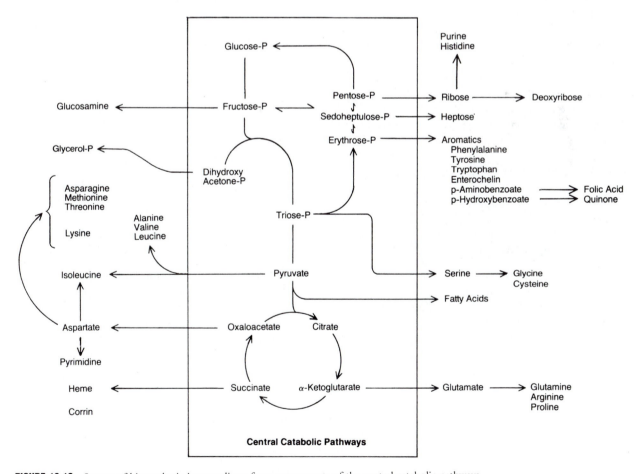

FIGURE 16-10 Source of biosynthetic intermediates from components of the central catabolic pathways.

A Closer Look
Iron and Air

To help organize the bewildering numbers of types of bacteria of medical importance, bacteria are split into major groupings based on certain obvious differences, such as their reaction in the gram stain, the shape of the cell, and their ability to grow in the absence or presence of air. As recognized in the preceding chapter, many of these seemingly fundamental differences may not be as profound as the conservation of DNA sequences for building a family tree of the evolutionary development of bacteria. They nonetheless represent very useful tools for the identification of bacteria and may also provide clues about the sites and nature of the infection and about the response of the bacterium to different types of antibiotics.

This section takes a look at the way bacteria respond to the presence or absence of oxygen and iron. These are two of the major nutrients, and their availability influences strongly the ability of cells to grow optimally and cause disease. It is striking how closely these two very different nutrients are intertwined.

The distinction between the four types of growth behavior to aerobic or anoxic conditions is based on the rather complex responses that different cells make to the metabolic opportunities and difficulties posed by the presence of oxygen. The strong electron-accepting activity of dioxygen (O_2) makes aerobic respiration so efficient by allowing the maximal possible energy yield to be obtained from the breakdown of a cell's energy source, such as glucose. This high redox potential of O_2 has several other, less desirable consequences. As described in this chapter, O_2 can react with various components of the electron transport system to give rise to toxic and reactive oxygen species, particularly hydrogen peroxide and the superoxide radical. Production of toxic levels of superoxide in phagocytic vacuoles is also a major aspect of the antibacterial action of neutrophils. Superoxide radical rapidly inactivates several proteins that contain susceptible structural components called iron-sulfur centers. Some of these highly superoxide-labile enzymes play key roles in glucose metabolism or amino acid synthesis. The existence of such sensitive targets helps explain why superoxide, which is not a potent oxidizing agent, can inhibit bacterial growth without causing general cellular damage or actual killing. In addition, peroxide and superoxide react together to form the very reactive hydroxyl radical, which kills bacteria by causing DNA strand breakage. Other highly reactive products are nitric oxide (NO) and peroxynitrile (ONOO).

Formation of these highly reactive and lethal molecules by aerobic organisms is reduced or prevented by the action of enzymes, such as catalase and peroxidases, which reduce hydrogen peroxide, and superoxide dismutases, which convert superoxide to peroxide and water. By reducing the levels of peroxide and superoxide, these enzymes reduce formation of the more reactive products. As described earlier, the levels of these enzymes in bacteria is roughly related to the ability of that bacterium to grow in the presence of atmospheric oxygen. Some types of superoxide dismutases exist in the periplasmic space, where they are well suited to inactivate externally generated superoxide. This localization probably contributes to survival of those bacteria in phagocytic cells producing superoxide.

There are multiple interesting levels of interaction between oxygen and iron supplies. Cellular levels of iron affect the rate of formation of oxygen products. Ferrous iron catalyzes the formation of hydroxyl radicals in the presence of peroxide, by the process called the Fenton reaction. On the other hand, iron also helps to protect cells against the toxic effects of oxygen. Some species of bacteria possess two types of superoxide dismutases, one of which carries iron as a prosthetic group, the other which carries manganese. Catalase, which rids the cell of peroxide, is a heme protein and hence contains iron.

Oxygen affects the ability of cells to acquire iron. Iron is needed for the growth and metabolism of almost all types of cells, and is involved in a wide variety of metabolic pathways. It is an essential component of the heme group present in cytochromes, which are important components of electron transport chains, and in catalase. Many other proteins that carry out electron transport or other oxidation-reduction processes contain noncovalently bound iron-sulfur clusters; some enzymes contain iron as a bound cofactor. Thus, a wide variety of metabolic pathways require a sufficient cellular supply of iron. Most organisms require a dietary supply of iron, and only a few lactobacilli have been reported to be able to grow in the absence of added iron. It would seem that iron should be readily available in the environment, since it is a major component of the earth's surface crust. Iron exists in solution in two oxidation states: ferrous (Fe[II]) and ferric (Fe[III]). In the reduced or ferrous form, iron is fairly soluble and is readily available for cells. However, in the presence of air, ferrous iron is oxidized to the ferric form, which forms ferric hydroxide complexes of remarkably low solubility; the concentration of soluble

A Closer Look *continued*

ferric ion is around 10^{-18} M at pH 8 (corresponding to about 600 molecules per mL). Hence, all cells living in an aerobic environment must possess some mechanism to acquire iron, and not just the soluble molecules, which are too scarce to allow appreciable growth. There must be a mechanism to obtain iron from the insoluble hydroxide complexes (rust) and to keep it soluble until each cell can acquire sufficient iron.

Bacteria have developed several mechanisms for this task. Many free-living or pathogenic bacteria synthesize and secrete small high-affinity iron chelators, called siderophores. These generally comprise two chemical classes, catechols and hydroxamates. Catechol-type siderophores contain one to three moieties of 2,3-dihydroxybenzoate. For example, enterobactin, the siderophore produced by *E. coli* and *S. typhimurium*, is a cyclic trimer of N-2,3-dihydroxybenzoyl-serines linked together by ester bonds. Enterobactin binds ferric iron with very high affinity and effectively brings iron into solution from its insoluble precipitates. Possible drawbacks to the dependence on enterobactin are that it is not as stable a chemical as are most hydroxamates, that owing to its highly aromatic nature it adsorbs to many surfaces and to serum proteins, and that it binds iron so tightly that it actually has to be broken down by the action of an esterase to allow it to release iron once inside the cell. Hydroxamate-type siderophores generally have a lower affinity for iron than catechol-types like enterobactin, but they are more stable chemicals and are less readily adsorbed nonspecifically. Other types of chemicals can be used as siderophores, including organic acids, such as citrate.

The essential step for iron acquisition involves the action of a specific transport system that recognizes the iron-siderophore complex in the environment and transports it into the cell with high affinity. *E. coli* possess one transport system for iron-enterobactin, and another one which seems to take up iron bound to some breakdown products of enterobactin. In addition to the secretion and reacquisition of their own siderophores, most microorganisms can acquire iron bound to other siderophores produced by other organisms. Thus, *E. coli* normally produces transport systems for several different hydroxamate-type siderophores produced by various fungi.

An interesting example of the role of an extended range of siderophore utilization is provided by the finding that the presence of a plasmid, called pCoIV, was associated with increased virulence of strains of *E. coli* that cause porcine diarrhea. This plasmid was named for its ability to encode synthesis of the toxic peptide, colicin V. However, the basis for the increased virulence was not related to colicin production but occurred because the plasmid also encoded genes for the synthesis and transport of a hydroxamate-type siderophore, called aerobactin. This siderophore is not normally produced by *E. coli*, but is made by numerous related bacterial types. It seems paradoxical that production and transport of a siderophore that is less efficient at binding iron that is enterobactin would prove beneficial to cells that produce enterobactin.

The transport systems for siderophores in the gram-negative bacteria have several unusual features. The outer membranes of gram-negative bacteria are, in general, poorly penetrated by hydrophobic compounds. Hydrophilic compounds pass through the outer membrane by diffusing through the aqueous channels formed by the porin proteins. Ferric-siderophores appear to be too large to pass efficiently through the porin channels, at least at the concentrations that are normally encountered. Hence, gram-negative bacteria produce outer membrane proteins that bind their siderophore substrate with high affinity and participate in their energy-dependent uptake into the cell by a complex process. Bacteria produce several iron transporters, and they are usually recognized by the fact that their synthesis is repressed when the cells are grown with excess iron and are increased when the cells are grown under iron-limiting conditions. A related protein is used in some organisms for the uptake of vitamin B_{12}, which is also too large and scarce to enter efficiently through the porin channels. In humans, iron is taken up from dietary sources relatively inefficiently—only about 2% is taken up normally. Iron is transported through serum in complex with the serum protein, transferrin. Lactoferrin is an iron-binding protein in milk and other body fluids. In normal individuals, serum transferrin is only about 30% saturated with iron, which means that there is such an extensive reserve capacity that the concentration of free iron in serum is probably nil. Hence, bacteria must be able to acquire iron from transferrin in order to grow in serum. Siderophores with a high affinity for iron, such as enterobactin, are able to extract iron from transferrin, thereby providing any bacterium able to transport that siderophore with a rich source of iron from the human host's own supply. Serum that has been heated at 56°C to inactivate complement still inhibits growth of bacteria because of its ability to sequester iron. This inhibition is overcome by providing additional iron to overwhelm the buffering capacity of the transferrin, or by using a larger inoculum of bacteria which produce

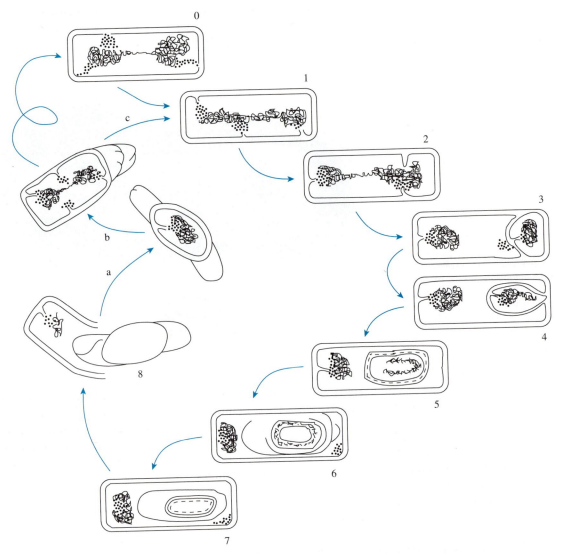

FIGURE 17-2   Diagrammatic summary of sporulation in a species of *Bacillus.* Stages 1 through 4 represent steps in forespore development. At stage 5, cortex development commences (*dotted line*) and continues through stage 6, when the coat protein is deposited. Stage 7 is characterized by the dehydration of the spore protoplast and the accumulation of dipicolinic acid and calcium in the spore. At stage 8, the spore is completely refractile and a lytic enzyme acts to release the spore. Also shown are germination (*a*) and outgrowth to a primary cell (*b*) from which the cell may, under special conditions, enter sporulation (*c*) by shortcut (the *microcycle*); normally, however, the cell undergoes logarithmic growth (*spiral arrow*).

can, called the cortex, is laid down between the two membranes. While the cortex is being synthesized by enzymes in the inner spore membrane, an external spore coat composed of a tough keratin-like protein is made on the outer spore membrane. The spores of some species are enclosed within an additional layer called the exosporium. The mature spore is eventually released on lysis of the remainder of the bacterium (Fig. 17-3).

The most striking characteristic of spores is their extreme resistance to chemical or physical agents. Most chemicals do not cross the spore surface, and spores are poorly stained unless first treated at high temperature or in the presence of strong detergents. Some spores can remain viable for many years under normal soil conditions, and many spores will even survive in boiling water for surprisingly long periods. They are extremely resistant to drying and to most disinfectants, including ultraviolet light. Certain killing of spores requires exposure to moist heat under pressure (for example, in an autoclave, which uses high-pressure steam to attain temperatures of 121°C for 15 minutes) or to dry heat (150°C for at least 1 hour).

The basis for the extraordinary resistance of spores is complex and not fully understood. Contributory factors include the presence of the impervious and impermeable surface layers and the extremely low water content within the spore. Spores of many species contain large amounts

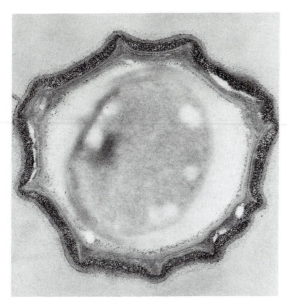

FIGURE 17-3 Spore of *Bacillus fastidiosus.* (Original magnification ×53,590.)

of calcium, most of which is in a complex with dipicolinic acid, which is not found in the vegetative cell before onset of sporulation. However, the role of this compound is unclear, inasmuch as mutants of *B subtilis* devoid of calcium dipicolinate produce spores with normal heat resistance.

Although endospores can remain dormant for long periods of time, they germinate in response to a specific trigger. The nature of the trigger differs for each species and can be a particular amino acid, pyrimidine, or sugar in a suitable aqueous environment. Within a short period of time, the spore loses its refractility and heat resistance; it then swells and absorbs water, after which the spore coat ruptures, and a new vegetative cell grows out.

Most spore-forming bacteria are inhabitants of soil, but bacterial spores are found almost everywhere. Many of the spore-forming bacteria produce potent toxins. For example, the anaerobe *C botulinum* is a serious cause of food poisoning as a consequence of its growth in nonacidic foods that were incompletely heated during canning. Spores can germinate, grow, and elaborate a toxin in the anaerobic environment of the canned food. Botulism toxin is extremely potent, but it is inactivated by heating and has a relatively slow onset of action. The need to kill all spores is the reason such lengthy heating regimens are employed in canneries and other food-processing operations.

Cytoplasmic Membrane

The cytoplasm of all bacterial cells is surrounded by the cytoplasmic membrane, which is the interface between the cell and its environment. This membrane carries out a wide variety of important functions, including most of the activities performed by the organelles of eucaryotic cells. These functions include the following:

Respiratory electron transport for the generation of a transmembrane proton gradient and oxidative phosphorylation to use that proton gradient for the formation of ATP.

Synthesis and export of the precursors of peptidoglycan, teichoic acids, and outer membrane components.

Secretion of extracellular and periplasmic enzymes and toxins.

Segregation of chromosomal and plasmid DNA into daughter cells.

Operation of numerous high-affinity nutrient transport systems able to concentrate their substrates inside the cell at concentrations as much as 1000 times higher than their external level.

The cytoplasmic membrane of most bacteria is composed of about 50% to 70% protein and 30% to 50% phospholipid by weight and contains small amounts of carbohydrate. The phospholipids form a typical bilayer into which the constituent proteins are embedded (Fig. 17-4). The major phospholipids are phosphatidyl glycerol, phosphatidyl ethanolamine, and diphosphatidyl glycerol (cardiolipin). Phosphatidyl choline (lecithin) and sphingolipids are present in only some bacterial species, and, although no procaryotic cell can synthesize sterols, the mycoplasmas incorporate them from the growth medium into their cell membrane. The predominant fatty acids contain 16 or 18 carbons and exist in both saturated and monounsaturated forms. Cyclopropane and branched fatty acids are often encountered, although usually in minor amounts.

Mesosomes and other invaginations of the cytoplasmic membrane are frequently observed in some or-

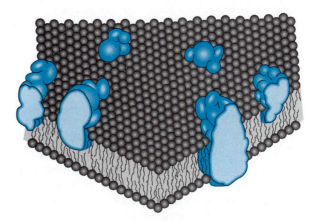

FIGURE 17-4 Fluid-mosaic model for membrane structure. In this representation of the Singer-Nicolson model, the solid bodies represent the globular integral proteins, which at long range are randomly distributed in the plane of the membrane. The small circles represent the hydrophilic ends of the membrane phospholipids, and the wavy lines represent the component fatty acids of the phospholipids.

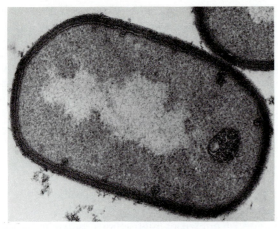

FIGURE 17-5   A number of mesosomes have invaginated from the cytoplasmic membrane in this section of a *Bacillus fastidiosus* cell. A larger mesosome, not continuous with the membrane in the plane of this section, is located to the right.

ganisms (Fig. 17-5). They provide increased membrane surface for enzymes such as the photosynthetic system or electron transport, among others. It has been proposed that mesosomes near the septum of gram-positive cells are involved in chromosome separation. Mesosomes that form elsewhere along the wall may be involved in secretion of extracellular proteins or in the metabolism of hydrocarbons.

Cell Envelope

The cell envelope, or cell wall, lies outside the cytoplasmic membrane. Its structure determines the shape of the cell and provides the rigidity and strength necessary to allow the cell to withstand the turgor pressure generated by the high intracellular concentrations of ions, metabolites, and macromolecules. Because the cell envelope makes contact with the environment, its constituents are the major antigenic determinants of the cell, and some of them contribute directly to the virulence of the organism. Cell envelopes also contain unique chemical moieties, which provide effective targets for the action of antibacterial agents.

Most bacteria of medical importance can be divided into two groups on the basis of their reaction in the gram-staining procedure. The gram-staining reaction of an organism is determined by its possession of one of two distinct types of cell-wall architecture. When observed by electron microscopic examination, the wall of a gram-positive bacterium is seen to be thick and homogeneous, sometimes having distinctive structures or dense layers at the inner and outer surfaces. The inner surface is always in contact with the cytoplasmic membrane. In striking contrast, the envelope of the gram-negative cell is marked by the presence of an outer membrane that surrounds a thin, rigid layer. This envelope is only rarely attached to the cytoplasmic membrane. The one component com-

mon to both types of wall is a large polymer called peptidoglycan or murein.

PEPTIDOGLYCAN

Peptidoglycan, a structure unique to bacteria, is responsible for the shape and structural rigidity of the cell. It is present in all eubacterial cells except the mycoplasmas; a related structure is present in the walls of some archaebacteria. Peptidoglycan is an enormous polymer composed of long polysaccharide chains cross-linked by peptide bridges. Each polysaccharide chain consists of repeating disaccharides of *N*-acetylglucosamine and *N*-acetylmuramic acid (Fig. 17-6*A*). The latter amino sugar is derived from *N*-acetylglucosamine by attachment of a lactyl group to the hydroxyl group on C3. The carboxyl group of *N*-acetylmuramic acid is linked a peptide, which is synthesized as a pentapeptide, but is normally found in the completed peptidoglycan as a tetrapeptide. These tetrapeptides can be cross-linked to one another to connect adjacent glycan chains into a strong, rigid structure. The peptidoglycan envelope can be isolated free of other cellular components and retains the size and shape of the intact cell.

The composition and linkages of the peptide chain vary substantially among different organisms, but there are several common features found in most bacteria. The peptide consists of alternating L- and D-amino acids. The amino acid at the amino end linked to *N*-acetylmuramic acid is L-alanine linked to D-glutamic acid, which is often joined through its γ-carboxyl in an isopeptide bond to the third amino acid. The third amino acid contains two amino groups: in gram-positive bacteria, it is lysine or ornithine; in gram-negative bacteria, this diamino acid is most commonly diaminopimelic acid. The fourth amino acid is always D-alanine.

This peptide is initially synthesized as a pentapeptide with an additional D-alanine residue that is removed when one peptide chain is cross-linked to another (see Fig. 17-6*B*). The linkage between peptide chains joins the carboxyl group of the remaining terminal D-alanine on one glycan chain to the free amino group of the diamino acid on an adjacent chain. In gram-negative bacteria and in some gram-positive ones (*Mycobacterium, Nocardia, Bacillus,* and *Corynebacterium*), the peptide bond is formed directly between the D-alanine and the diamino acid. In other gram-positive bacteria, these amino acids are linked together by an additional peptide bridge (see Fig. 17-6*C*), thereby allowing distant glycan chains to be joined together. The composition of these cross-bridges is variable; some examples are shown in Table 17-1.

Further modifications of the peptide portion of peptidoglycan are common. Usually one, and occasionally both, terminal D-alanines are removed from peptide chains that are not involved in a cross-link. The entire peptide unit is missing from about 30% of the sites in *E coli* and at least 50% of the sites in *Micrococcus luteus,* and

Linkage hydrolyzed
by lysozyme

CH₂OH   CH₂OH

        β(1-4)   β(1-4)

OH

NHCOCH₃   NHCOCH₃

N-acetylglucosamine   *N*-acetylmuramic acid

HC—CH₃

C=O

L-alanine

D-isoglutamamide

L-lysine

A   D-alanine

FIGURE 17-6   A. Structure of the repeating unit of cell-wall peptidoglycan in *Staphylococcus aureus*. **B.** Peptidoglycan structure showing cross-linking of linear polymers of *N*-acetylglucosamine (G) and *N*-acetylmuramic acid (M) as it exists in most gram-negative bacteria. Notice the D-alanine of one tetrapeptide is linked directly to the diamino acid of a second tetrapeptide. **C.** Peptidoglycan structure as seen in staphylococci, in which an added peptide bridge (ie, pentaglycine) joins the two linear polymers.

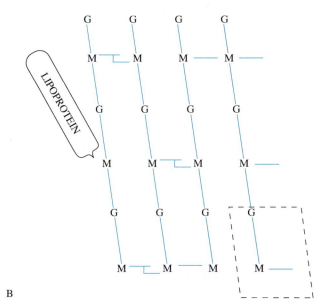

B

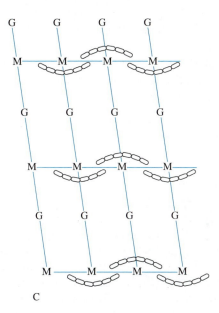

C

the extent of cross-linking of the glycan chains in these organisms is correspondingly reduced. In contrast, the glycan chains of *Staphylococcus aureus* retain all peptide chains, and all are fully involved in cross-linking. In some organisms, additional amino acids are attached to the D-glutamic acid residue, and carbohydrates or proteins may be covalently attached to peptidoglycan.

Lytic Enzymes

A number of enzymes cleave peptidoglycan and cause bacterial lysis. These enzymes fall into three general types:

1. Endo-*N*-acetyl hexosaminidases, known as lysozymes, cleave the glycan chains by hydrolyzing the glycosidic bond between *N*-acetylmuramic acid and *N*-acetylglucosamine. Lysozymes are present in serum, tears, white blood cells, and egg white.

2. Endopeptidases cleave the peptide cross-links at D-alanine or at various interchain peptide bridges. For example, lysostaphin splits the glycine peptide bridge in *S aureus*.

3. Amidases cleave the entire peptide chain from the glycan chain by splitting the bond between muramic acid and the first L-alanine.

Because of the high osmolarity of bacterial cytoplasm, disruption of the peptidoglycan layer by the inhibition of its synthesis or cross-linking or by the action of lytic enzymes results in the bulging of the cell membrane

TABLE 17-1
Representative Compositions of Peptidoglycan Peptide Bridges

Organism	Peptide Bridge
Staphylococcus epidermis	Gly$_{2-4}$ → L-Ser → Gly
Streptococcus sp	L-Ala → Gly → L-Ala
S salivarius	Gly → L-Thr
Lactobacillus viridescens	L-Ser → L-Ala
L cremoris	L-Ala → L-Ser
Arthrobacter citreus	L-Ala$_2$ → L-Thr
Micrococcus roseus	L-Ala$_3$ → L-Thr

through weakened areas of the wall and the eventual lysis of the cell. Lysis can be prevented if the cells are kept in a medium of high osmolarity. Cells lacking their walls round up into spheres and, although stable in the presence of high concentrations of salts or sucrose, lyse upon dilution of the osmoprotectant. The wall-less forms of gram-positive bacteria are called *protoplasts*. In the case of the gram-negative organisms, the external envelope components are not fully removed, and the osmotically sensitive forms are called *spheroplasts*.

GRAM-POSITIVE CELL WALLS

The cell walls of gram-positive bacteria are thick (20 to 80 nm) and relatively homogeneous (Fig. 17-7*A*). They consist largely of peptidoglycan (40% to 80% of the total weight of the wall) that is extensively cross-linked in three dimensions to form a thick polymeric mesh. Most of the remainder of the wall are cell-wall polysaccharides, including teichoic acids and related polymers, as well as nonteichoic acids and acidic and neutral polysaccharides. Proteins can be present in the wall and may have considerable biologic importance but rarely form an organized structure.

The peptide cross-links in the peptidoglycan of gram-positive bacteria are more extensive and are frequently longer than those occurring in the cell walls of gram-negative bacteria, resulting in a strong three-dimensional network. Peptidoglycan of gram-positive cells is accessible to lysozymes and other lytic enzymes in the medium, but some bacteria are resistant to their action as a result of the modification of their glycan chains by acetylation of a hydroxyl group on the muramic acid or by removal of the *N*-acetyl group from glucosamine.

Teichoic Acids

Teichoic acids (from the Greek word for wall) are acidic polymers in the walls of gram-positive bacteria. There are two major types of teichoic acid—ribitol teichoic acid and glycerol teichoic acid—which are long polymers of ribitol (a five-carbon sugar alcohol) or glycerol, linked through phosphodiester bridges (Fig. 17-8). The free hydroxyl groups of both types of teichoic acids are substituted with various amino acids, amines, amino sugars, or mono-, di-, or trisaccharides. Some organisms possess teichoic acid polymers in which every other glycerol or ribitol is replaced by *N*-acetylglucosamine or some other sugar. When bacteria are grown under conditions of phosphate limitation, they can produce teichuronic acids in

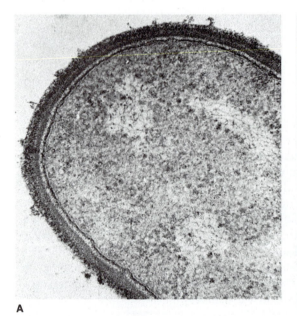
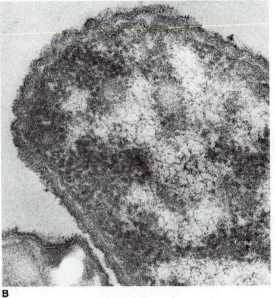

A   **B**

FIGURE 17-7   A. A portion of the gram-positive bacterium *Bacillus fastidiosus;* notice the cell wall's thick peptidoglycan layer immediately surrounding the cytoplasmic membrane. **B.** The gram-negative bacterium *Enterobacter aerogenes;* both the cytoplasmic membrane and the outer membrane are visible along some sections of the cell wall.

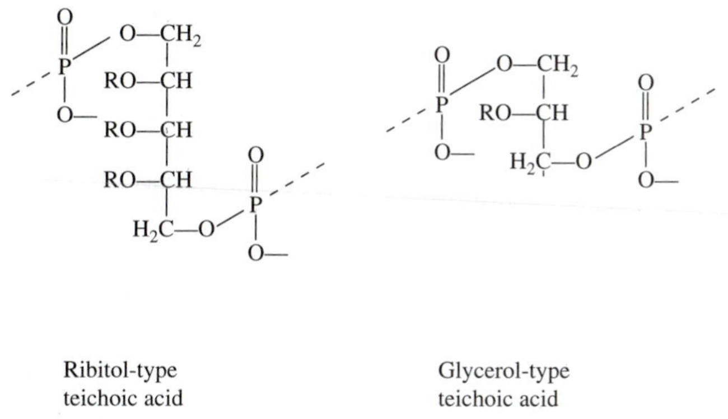

Ribitol-type
teichoic acid

Glycerol-type
teichoic acid

FIGURE 17-8 Teichoic acids are usually long chains of glycerol or ribitol joined together with phosphodiester bridges. The R group for glycerol teichoic acid is frequently D-alanine, whereas for the ribitol-type teichoic acid it may be glucose, succinate, N-acetylglucosamine, D-alanine, or short oligosaccharides. Substitutions vary considerably, even within a species.

which the glycerol or ribitol groups are joined by acidic monosaccharides, such as glucuronic acid, instead of phosphate. The substituted teichoic acids are major antigenic determinants and are the basis for the serologic identification of many species of gram-positive bacteria. The ability of antibodies to react with teichoic acids in whole cells shows that these polymers can extend through the wall into the medium.

Ribitol teichoic acids are usually linked to the 6-hydroxyl group of N-acetylmuramic acid in peptidoglycan and are termed *wall teichoic acids*, whereas glycerol teichoic acid is linked to a glycolipid in the cytoplasmic membrane and is, hence, termed *membrane or lipoteichoic acid.*

Membrane teichoic acids are present in all gram-positive bacteria, but their function is not well defined. Mutants have been isolated that lack these teichoic acids, and most of them are defective in cell septation and peptidoglycan biosynthesis. In *Streptococcus pneumoniae,* replacement of the choline normally present on the teichoic acid–like C polysaccharide with ethanolamine prevents separation of daughter cells, resulting in formation of long filaments instead of the usual diplococci. This suggests that the teichoic acids might regulate the autolytic reactions necessary for cell growth and septation. This substitution for choline also blocks the ability of cells to take up free DNA and affects the cell's response to antibiotic inhibitors of cell-wall assembly.

Other Components

Although the basic structure of the gram-positive cell wall is a thick mesh of peptidoglycan interlaced with teichoic acids, other components may be present and confer important antigenic or medical properties, as described in the sections on specific pathogens. Examples are the branched, group-specific rhamnose polymers present in

many streptococci and the M and F adhesin proteins of the group A streptococci.

Envelope of Acid-Fast Bacteria

Lipids are not present in the walls of most gram-positive bacteria, but they can comprise up to one third of the weight of the walls of the acid-fast bacteria. These organisms, discussed in Chapter 31, have the basic gram-positive wall structure, but their cell walls contain about equal amounts of peptidoglycan, lipid, and an arabinogalactan polysaccharide. About half of the lipids are *mycolic acids,* which are large (C_{32} to C_{90}) α-substituted, β-hydroxy fatty acids. The mycolic acids are esterified to cell-wall polysaccharides, and, when attached to the arabinogalactan, they form a large, water-insoluble complex known as wax D. Mycolic acids also are esterified to extractable glycolipids and to trehalose (a disaccharide of glucose). The lipid chains appear to be organized into a structure related to that of a membrane, which restricts the passage of chemical to the cell surface. There is a porin-like protein that forms a channel for passage of nutrients through the cell wall, which is reminiscent of the situation with gram-negative cells. The large amount of lipid on the cell surface is thought to be responsible for the peculiar staining properties of these organisms as well as their general stickiness and hydrophobic nature.

GRAM-NEGATIVE CELL WALLS

The cell envelope of gram-negative bacteria is considerably more complex than the wall of gram-positive bacteria. It is a multilayered structure composed of an outer membrane lying atop a thin peptidoglycan layer, which is separated from the cytoplasmic membrane by the periplasmic space (see Fig. 17-7B). The envelope contains four major constituents: peptidoglycan in the rigid layer, and, in the outer membrane, phospholipids, proteins, and a unique glycolipid called lipopolysaccharide (LPS). The following sections describe each of these components, their arrangement in the intact gram-negative envelope, and the mechanism whereby the unusual structure of the envelope confers many of the properties characteristic of gram-negative bacteria.

Peptidoglycan (Murein) and Murein Lipoprotein

The peptidoglycan, or murein, layer of gram-negative bacteria differs in some respects from that of gram-positive cells. The peptidoglycan of the gram-negative wall is probably only one molecule thick and, thus, is cross-linked in only two dimensions, in contrast to the thick, three-dimensional peptidoglycan matrix in the gram-positive wall. The gram-negative wall is, therefore, more flexible and porous, although sufficiently strong to protect the cell against osmotic lysis. Cross-links between peptide chains extend directly from the carboxyl group of the terminal D-alanine on one chain to the free amino group of a diaminopimelic acid on an adjacent chain. Only about 50% of the potential cross-links are formed, and, in the remainder, there is either a free tetrapeptide or no peptide at all. In rod-shaped cells of *E coli,* the glycan chains are oriented perpendicular to the long axis of the cell, in the nature of a belt.

Roughly 10% of the tetrapeptide units are covalently linked to an unusual lipoprotein by a bond from the amino group of a diaminopimelic acid to the carboxyl-terminal lysine of the protein. This murein lipoprotein is small (7500 daltons) and strongly lipophilic, owing, in part, to the attachment of three fatty acids, one in amide linkage to the terminal amino group and two esterified to S-glyceryl-cysteine, the *N*-terminal amino acid. The remainder of the protein is folded in an extremely stable α-helical structure and is embedded in the outer membrane. For every molecule of the lipoprotein that is covalently attached to the peptidoglycan, there are about two unattached or free molecules, with a total of about 10^5 molecules of this protein per cell. Murein lipoprotein helps to anchor the outer membrane to the peptidoglycan and to maintain the structure and organization of the outer membrane.

Lipopolysaccharide Structure

Lipopolysaccharide is a complex and unique glycolipid that is present in all gram-negative bacteria. It consists of three distinct, covalently linked regions: lipid A, core polysaccharide, and O-specific polysaccharide side chains. The lipid A portion is embedded in the outer leaflet of the outer membrane, and the carbohydrate chains extend into the medium. Remarkable variability exists in the composition and arrangement of the O-specific polysaccharide side chains. The following section describes the structure of LPS in *Escherichia* and *Salmonella;* the basic features are present in many other gram-negative bacteria, but there are also many differences in detail.

The lipid A portion of LPS (Fig. 17-9*A*) consists of a disaccharide of β-1,6-linked glucosamines, which is esterified at two hydroxyl and two amino groups with the unusual C_{14} fatty acid, 3-hydroxy myristic acid. As shown in Figure 17-9, other fatty acids can be joined in ester linkage to the hydroxyl group of some of the 3-hydroxy myristic acid residues at certain positions. The lengths of the fatty acids and the residues that are esterified on the 3-hydroxy fatty acid differ among different genera, but are fairly constant within a species. Phosphate groups are attached to positions 1 and 4' at the ends of the glucosamines, and in *Salmonella,* the unusual sugar, 4-aminoarabinose, is attached to the 4'-phosphate. Other enteric bacteria have different sugars linked to this phosphate, and many organisms have ethanolamine phosphate esterified to the 1 position. Lipid A is somewhat analogous

to a glycerol-based phospholipid, but is much larger and more rigid, owing to the presence of about six saturated fatty acyl chains.

Attached to the hydroxyl group at position C6' on lipid A is the long polysaccharide chain (see Fig. 17-9*B*). Its inner portion, called the *core polysaccharide,* is similar within a genus and contains two unusual sugars, the 8-carbon 2-keto-3-deoxyoctulosonic acid (KDO) and a 7-carbon heptose. The other sugars in the core are glucose, galactose, and *N*-acetylglucosamine. The heptoses usually are modified by the addition of phosphate, pyrophosphate, or ethanolamine phosphate.

Attached to the terminal sugar of the core is the outer portion of the polysaccharide chain, termed the O-specific side chain. This portion consists of variable numbers (0 to 50) of repeating oligosaccharide units of three to five sugars each. The side chains often contain unusual sugars, such as 6-deoxyhexoses, 3,6-dideoxyhexoses, 6-deoxyaminohexoses, 3-aminohexoses, and aminohexuronic acids. This portion of the LPS, with its unusual sugars, is the major serologic determinant of many gram-negative bacteria. For example, over 1000 different serologic combinations are found in *Salmonella,* most of which are the result of variations in the composition of the O-specific side chain.

Mutant organisms that are unable to add any one of the core sugars or to attach the O-specific side chain are called rough or R mutants, because their colonies are rougher and drier in appearance than colonies with full-length LPS. Addition of the core sugars and attachment of the O-side chain is a sequential process, and, thus, any mutant unable to add any one sugar generally will be unable to add any subsequent sugars. Rough mutants arise frequently when bacteria are cultured in the laboratory. Although rough strains are better suited for growth on agar medium, they invariably have decreased virulence or survival in an animal host. Deep-rough mutant strains that are unable to add the heptose groups to KDO usually exhibit a severe deficiency in the function and protein content of the outer membrane. Mutants that cannot synthesize the KDO portion are unable to grow, and the minimal structure compatible with bacterial viability is lipid A with two KDO groups. The lipid A of some strains, including the pathogens *Neisseria* and *Chlamydia,* have short or no saccharide chains, respectively, beyond the KDO.

BIOLOGIC EFFECTS OF LIPOPOLYSACCHARIDE. The LPS from most gram-negative bacteria is toxic to mammals, and many of the symptoms of systemic gram-negative infection can be reproduced with purified LPS. Because LPS is an integral part of the cell wall, it is often called *endotoxin,* in contrast to the exotoxins, which are products normally released from cells. The toxicity of LPS resides in the lipid A portion, although the polysaccharide portion enhances toxicity by keeping the hydrophobic lipid portion water

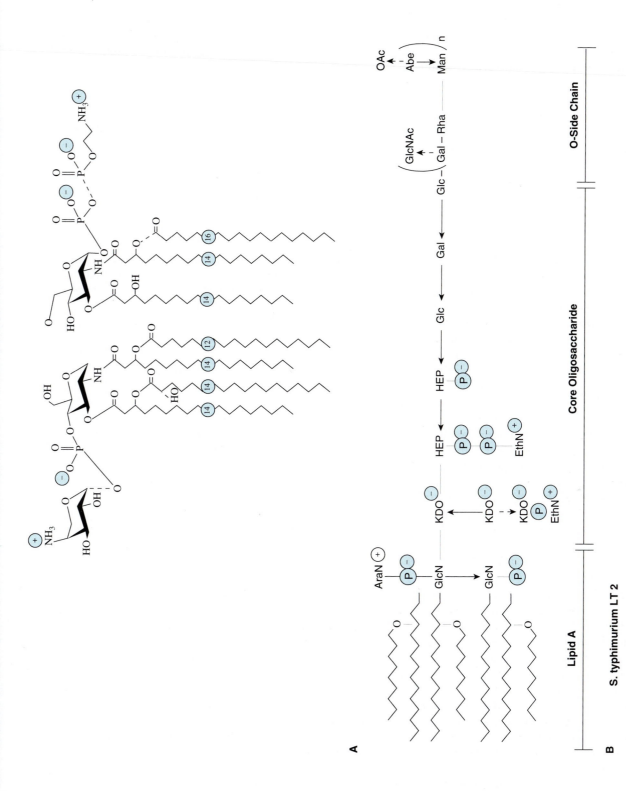

A

B   **S. typhimurium LT 2**

FIGURE 17-9 **A.** Structure of lipid A as it exists in *Salmonella minnesota.* Dotted lines indicate incomplete substitution. KDO is linked to the primary hydroxyl group in position 6′. Numbers in circles indicate the number of carbon atoms in the acyl chains. **B.** Schematic diagram of lipopolysaccharide in *Salmonella typhimurium.* The three distinct segments are lipid A, the core oligosaccharide, and the repeating O-specific side chain. GlcN, glucosamine; KDO, 2-keto-3-deoxyoctulosonic acid; HEP, *manno*-heptose; Glc, glucose; Gal, galactose; GlcNAc, *N*-acetylglucosamine; Rha, rhamnose; Man, mannose; Abe, abequose.

soluble. LPS from many gram-negative bacteria, including avirulent rough strains, exhibits comparable toxicities. The LPS from some bacteria, such as the photosynthetic *Rhodobacter* species, are not toxic and even antagonize the toxic effect of LPS from enteric bacteria; these may provide a therapeutic tool.

Investigations of the effect of LPS in mammalian systems, as well as clinical observations, have shown that the injection of LPS or the presence of an overwhelming gram-negative infection results in severe, frequently fatal shock, often accompanied by severe diarrhea. Sublethal doses of LPS produce a wide range of pathologic effects, the most characteristic of which is fever. Endotoxin stimulates leukocytes and monocytes to release an *endogenous pyrogen,* which acts on the hypothalamus to trigger fever. Other effects of LPS include leukopenia (decreased blood leukocytes) and hyperglycemia (increase in blood sugar). Endotoxin can also activate the complement cascade, leading to local tissue damage, and the clotting system, leading to disseminated intravascular coagulation. Circulatory abnormalities include initial arteriolar and venous constriction (chills) followed by peripheral vascular dilation, increased vascular permeability and shock, impaired blood circulation, organ damage, and acidosis. LPS also affects the immune system by activating macrophages, stimulating division of B cells, and acting as a general adjuvant.

Because gram-negative bacteria continuously shed small amounts of their outer membrane into their medium (5% per generation), any solution in which these bacteria have grown, even though sterile, will have a pyrogenic effect. Distillation or reverse osmosis through semipermeable membranes is necessary to remove LPS from solution, and it is necessary to test that all solutions to be injected into humans are free of pyrogens. This was formerly determined by measuring fever production in rabbits, but the presence of nanogram amounts of endotoxin can be detected by the clotting of hemolymph (blood) from the horseshoe crab (*Limulus*).

The multiple toxic reactions in response to LPS seem to result from the production of several powerful physiologic mediators by host cells exposed to LPS. Interleukin-1 (IL-1) is a prominent cytokine produced by monocytes, macrophages, vascular endothelial cells, various lymphocytes, and epithelial cells. Properties exhibited by IL-1 include its action on hypothalamic neurons as an endogenous pyrogen, stimulation of prostaglandin-E_2 synthesis, induction of sleep through increased synthesis of neuropeptides (including endorphins, ACTH, and somatostatin), decreased plasma levels of zinc and iron, and decreased activity of lipoprotein lipase (leading to anorexia and tissue wasting). Another cytokine produced by macrophages is tumor necrosis factor (also called cachectin), which causes many of the same manifestations of endotoxic shock as IL-1. These two proteins act in a synergistic manner, and the synthesis of both is stimulated at the level of translation by exposure to LPS. The ability of LPS to affect levels of multiple cytokines with overlapping physiologic effects is one reason for the difficulty of efforts to interfere with endotoxic shock by blocking cytokine production, circulation or binding to cellular receptors. Nonetheless, interference with LPS synthesis and action is a promising area for development of new antimicrobial and therapeutic agents.

Proteins and Phospholipids

Besides LPS, the other major components of the outer membrane are proteins and phospholipids. The phospholipids are similar to those in the cytoplasmic membrane, being primarily phosphatidyl ethanolamine and phosphatidyl glycerol. The remainder of the outer membrane is comprised of relatively few different types of proteins. About five polypeptides are present in major amounts, including murein lipoprotein and the porins, which are trimeric molecules that form aqueous channels through the outer membrane to allow passage of hydrophilic molecules. Some other major proteins, such as OmpA protein of *E coli*, perhaps play a structural role because its loss through mutation confers no obvious transport defect. An additional 10 to 30 minor proteins are involved in nutrient transport or the maintenance of the structure or composition of the outer membrane.

In addition, the outer membrane of all Enterobacteriaceae contains another cell-surface glycolipid, called the enterobacterial common antigen. It is a linear polysaccharide of *N*-acetylglucosamine-*N*-acetylmannosaminuronic acid-*N*-acetylfucosamine, linked to a membrane phospholipid.

Organization of the Outer Membrane

The organization of the components of the outer membrane gives rise to a membrane of unusual, highly ordered structure and atypical functional properties. Like all membranes, the outer membrane consists of two lipid leaflets with opposing hydrophobic regions. LPS is located exclusively in the outer leaflet and is essentially the only lipid in that layer; phospholipid is present almost entirely in the inner leaflet. LPS is much less fluid than are phospholipids, partly because the diglucosamine backbone is relatively large and the fatty acids are more highly saturated than in the phospholipids, and partly because the LPS chains are cross-linked to one another through Ca^{2+}, or polyamine salt bridges between the phosphate groups in the core sugar region. Moreover, the major outer membrane proteins are complexed through salt bridges and direct protein contacts to each other, to the LPS, and to the murein lipoprotein, resulting in a stable structure. All of these properties make the outer membrane unusually rigid, and the movement of proteins or LPS molecules along the plane of this membrane is remarkably slow. A schematic diagram of the outer membrane is shown in Figure 17-10.

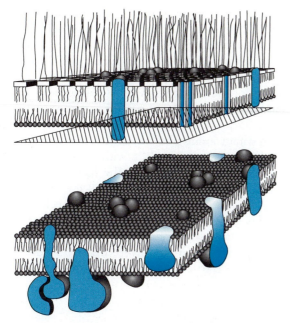

FIGURE 17-10 Schematic representation of the gram-negative cell envelope. The lower structure portrays the cytoplasmic membrane, a phospholipid bilayer in which various proteins, many of which span the membrane, are embedded. Overlying this membrane is the peptidoglycan layer to which the outer membrane is bound through the helical murein lipoprotein. Spanning the outer membrane are a number of proteins, including the trimeric porins that allow entry of nutrients. The outer membrane is shown with an inner leaflet of glycerol phosphatides and an outer leaflet of lipopolysaccharide from which the polysaccharide chains extend into the medium.

Properties of the Outer Membrane

The structure of the outer membrane imparts two unusual properties to most gram-negative bacteria. Because the membrane is so rigid, and because regions of phospholipid–phospholipid bilayer are rare, the membrane is not readily penetrated by hydrophobic compounds and is, therefore, resistant to dissolution by detergents. This property enables many gram-negative bacteria to grow in the presence of detergents that are lethal for gram-positive cells. Treatment of gram-negative cells with metal chelators disrupts the salt bridges between outer membrane components and results in loss of about half of the cell's LPS and a decrease in its barrier function against nonpolar compounds like antibiotics and detergents. Similarly, mutations that delete certain major outer membrane proteins or that affect synthesis of the inner core sugars or phosphate groups on LPS decrease this barrier function. Presumably, in these cases, the outer surface is not as tightly cross-linked, or the absence of large amounts of protein is compensated by the appearance of phospholipids in the outer layer, providing a route for entry of hydrophobic molecules.

In contrast to the poor passage of hydrophobic compounds, the outer membrane is unusually permeable to many hydrophilic compounds. Nutrients diffuse through pores formed by the porin proteins, which associate in the outer membrane as trimers. The diameter of the resulting channel imposes a size limitation on the nutrients that a cell can employ. For example, the porins of enteric bacteria only allow passage of molecules with molecular weights below 600 Da, about the size of a trisaccharide or a tetrapeptide. The porin channels exhibit little steric specificity and most appear to be negatively charged, because anions enter more slowly than cations. An anion-preferring porin is induced by conditions of phosphate limitation. Some of the minor proteins in the outer membrane provide specific transport systems for nutrients whose diffusion through the porin would be too slow to satisfy nutritional requirements. Several minor proteins serve as porin-like diffusion channels for specific classes of molecules, such as oligosaccharides or nucleosides. Others carry out high-affinity active transport of iron-siderophore complexes or of vitamin B_{12}. The importance of the possession of efficient systems for acquisition of iron complexed to siderophores or host proteins has been established as a virulence factor for some bacteria.

Basis for Gram Reaction

The response of an organism in the gram stain is a consequence of its cell-wall structure and not the presence of any particular chemical. Treatment with crystal violet and Gram's iodine results in formation of large, insoluble blue-dye complexes inside the cell. During the ethanol-washing step, cell membranes are dissolved. However, the blue-dye complex is retained in gram-positive cells by the thick peptidoglycan mesh, whereas it is readily washed out through the thin peptidoglycan layer remaining in gram-negative cells after both membranes have been dissolved. Gram-positive cells from old cultures may stain gram-negative because their peptidoglycan layer is thinner or partly disrupted.

CONSEQUENCES OF CELL-WALL STRUCTURE

Some general characteristics shared by most gram-positive or gram-negative bacteria are direct consequences of their cell-wall structure. The thick mesh of peptidoglycan in gram-positive cells does not pose a significant barrier to the passage of low–molecular-weight compounds. Nutrients as well as many deleterious agents, such as antibiotics, dyes, and detergents, have direct access to the cytoplasmic membrane. Basic dyes or bile salts often are included in media designed for the detection of gram-negative enteric bacteria because these compounds selectively prevent growth of gram-positive bacteria. The porins in the outer membrane restrict the passage of these hydrophobic compounds and protect gram-negative bacteria against dyes, detergents, and many antibiotics. There are numerous examples of antibiotics (eg, erythromycin, novobiocin, and even some beta-lactams) that are effective against most gram-positive bacteria but are not active or at least not clinically effective against most gram-negative bacteria.

The presence of the outer membrane and the restricted passage of large or hydrophobic molecules is the basis for the inherent antibiotic resistance that is characteristic of many gram-negative bacteria. For example, the access of a nonpolar antibiotic such as penicillin G to its targets in the periplasmic space of *E coli* is sufficiently reduced by its restricted diffusion through the porin channels that this and related antibiotics are not clinically useful against the enteric bacteria, despite the fact that the isolated penicillin target enzymes are as sensitive to the drugs as are the corresponding enzymes from gram-positive bacteria. *Neisseria gonorrhoeae* is a gram-negative bacterium that is anomalously sensitive to these antibiotics and other agents, and its outer membrane exhibits high permeability properties, owing to its larger porin channels. *Pseudomonas aeruginosa* generally is resistant to many antibiotics because it lacks the usual high-permeability porins present in the enteric bacteria and has only an inefficient porin active at 1% of the rate of the usual porins. This bacterium takes up nutrients via a number of special porins, each active only for specific classes of compounds, allowing entry of only a limited number of compounds.

Many gram-positive bacteria are sensitive to lysozyme and other cell-wall lytic enzymes because their peptidoglycan is accessible from the medium. Most gram-negative bacteria are not affected by lysozyme unless their outer membrane barrier has been circumvented by exposure to metal ion chelators. On the other hand, specific antibody and complement does not kill gram-positive bacteria, because the attack complex of complement is formed on the exterior of the thick peptidoglycan layer, distant from the cytoplasmic membrane. For most gram-negative bacteria, the complement complex can assemble on the surface of the outer membrane and cause bacterial killing. A phenomenon called serum resistance is described later.

Many gram-positive bacteria secrete substantial numbers of proteins or enzymes that often behave as toxins; special wall-bound forms of the secreted protein are intermediates in the secretion process. In contrast, passage of proteins across the outer membrane requires special enzymatic machinery, and protein secretion is a less common feature, although certainly present, in gram-negative bacteria. Many proteins are located in the periplasmic space between the outer and cytoplasmic membranes, where they are involved in degradation of nutrients or their transport into the cell.

Serum Resistance

Serum resistance refers to the ability of bacteria to survive exposure to serum, specifically, their resistance to killing by the cytolytic C5b–9 terminal attack complex of complement (see Chap. 12). The importance of this trait can be seen from the observation that most isolates of *E coli* from blood are serum resistant, whereas isolates from stool or urine often are serum sensitive. There are numerous mechanisms for serum resistance in different organisms. A capsular protein of *Campylobacter fetus* blocks deposition of the C3 component of complement on the cell surface. In *N gonorrhoeae,* some factor prevents proper insertion of the attack complex into the outer membrane. Serum-resistant strains of *E coli, Salmonella typhimurium,* and *P aeruginosa* produce LPS with long, hydrophobic O-specific side chains. Perhaps the longer side chains cause the attack complex to be formed too far from the outer membrane surface to be lethal for that cell or where it is readily shed into the medium. LPS or capsules that contain sialic acid have a high affinity for serum protein H, which can bind to any complement C3 convertase and target its destruction by a serum protease.

External Structures

There are several types of external appendages and surface components that contribute to the virulence properties of bacteria in various ways, such as by increasing adherence to host cells or decreasing susceptibility to engulfment by phagocytic cells. Because these structures are exposed to the immune system of the animal host, they are under considerable selective pressure, and many of these structures are able to alter their immunologic character even during individual infectious episodes.

FLAGELLA

For most of the bacteria of medical interest, motility—or the ability to swim through liquid media—is conferred by a helical filament called a flagellum. Flagella can be found on both gram-positive and gram-negative bacilli. Most cocci are immotile, whereas about half of the bacilli and almost all of the spirilla possess flagella. Flagella are long, hollow, helical filaments, usually several times the length of the cell and with diameters of 10 to 20 nm, which is below the limit of resolution of the light microscope.

The number and location of flagella are distinctive for each genus. They may be distributed around the cell (peritrichous) or localized at one or both poles. Some examples are *Pseudomonas,* with a single polar flagellum, *Spirillum,* with tufts of flagella at both poles, *Escherichia,* with 6 to 10 flagella in peritrichous arrangement around the cell, and some *Proteus* strains, with over 100 peritrichous flagella (Fig. 17-11). In the spirochetes, the axial filament, around which the cell body twists, seems to be two polar tufts of flagella that do not extend into the medium but are trapped inside the periplasmic space.

Isolated flagella can be dissociated into a single polypeptide subunit (flagellin) by exposure to mildly acidic conditions (pH about 3). Neutralization of the solution

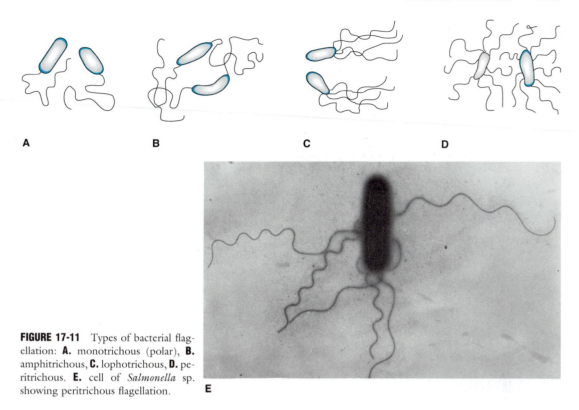

FIGURE 17-11 Types of bacterial flagellation: **A.** monotrichous (polar), **B.** amphitrichous, **C.** lophotrichous, **D.** peritrichous. **E.** cell of *Salmonella* sp. showing peritrichous flagellation.

results in the spontaneous reaggregation of flagellin subunits to form filaments with the characteristic diameter and helical periodicity of the original flagella.

In the immunologic classification of enteric bacteria, flagella are called H-antigens, from the German word *Hauch*, or breath. Cells treated with antiflagellar antibodies lose their ability to spread over the surface of a solid medium and form tight, compact colonies rather than the diffuse colony formed by motile cells, which appear like the haze seen when one breathes on a mirror.

The helical flagellar filaments are attached to the cell by means of a complex structure called the basal body (Fig. 17-12), which is embedded in the cytoplasmic membrane and has the appearance of a series of rods and rings. The resemblance to a turbine is more than structural: the basal body rotates within the cytoplasmic membrane, thereby causing the flagellar filament to rotate. Rotation is driven by the passage of protons from the exterior to the cytoplasm through the basal body; the entry of roughly 300 protons causes one complete rotation of the rotor. Thus, bacterial flagella cause cell movement by acting like a propeller, unlike the structurally more complex flagella of eucaryotic cells, which behave like an oar.

For cells with multiple flagella, some coordination must occur, because independent rotation of each filament could not result in any straight-line motion. When all flagella on a cell are rotating in the same relative direction, their helical filaments coalesce with one another to form a single, large, helical structure. Rotation of the individual flagella then results in the passage of a wave

down the length of the combined structure, and it is this wave that drives the cell in a straight line.

Chemotaxis

Bacterial motility is controlled by a process called *chemotaxis*, whereby cells tend to swim toward higher concentrations of certain nutrients (chemoattractants) or away from gradients of chemorepellents. This behavioral response and the direction of swimming is determined by the direction of flagellar rotation. Bacteria swim in a straight line when their flagella are rotating counterclockwise (viewed toward the cell) and tumble randomly when the flagella rotate in a clockwise direction. A bacterium normally swims for a short time (several seconds) in a straight line (counterclockwise rotation) followed by a period of tumbling (clockwise rotation), which is then followed by the cell swimming off in a new direction. The clockwise rotation causes the flagellar bundle to fly apart and reorient the cell into a new, random direction.

When a cell is moving up a gradient of a chemoattractant (or away from a repellent), tumbling occurs less frequently and straight-line motion predominates (ie, clockwise rotations are suppressed). Conversely, a cell that finds itself moving into a lowering concentration of attractant tumbles more frequently until it is headed in a more favorable direction. Bacteria sense and respond only to changes in chemical concentrations. If an attractant is present at a uniform concentration, bacteria swim as randomly as if the attractant were absent.

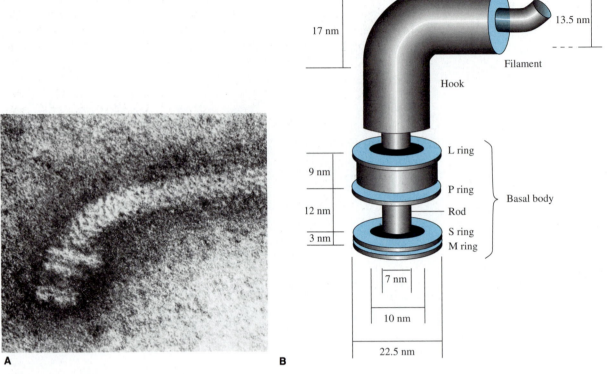

FIGURE 17-12 A. The electron micrograph and **B.** accompanying drawing illustrate the detailed structure of a flagellum and suggest how it is anchored to the bacterial cell. It is proposed that in *Escherichia coli*, the L and P rings are anchored to the outer membrane, and the S and M rings are anchored to the inner membrane. Gentler preparation procedures reveal addition protein components at the base of the basal body, which are involved in the control of the direction of flagellar rotation and the assembly of the flagellar filament. Flagella from *Bacillus subtilis*, which is gram-positive and has no outer membrane, lack the L and P rings.

The mechanism whereby bacteria sense and adapt to their environment is a fascinating example of sensory control, involving transmembrane signaling and protein methylation (Fig. 17-13). A major component in the process of chemotaxis is a family of transducer proteins that span the cytoplasmic membrane and have binding sites for specific chemoattractants and repellents on their exterior face. Binding of chemoeffectors transmits a signal to the cytoplasmic portion of the protein, and this change in protein conformation is the signal that provides the measure of the presence and concentration of specific chemoeffectors in the medium. This signal is transmitted to the flagellar basal body to control the frequency of switching of the direction of flagellar rotation. This information is transmitted through the cytoplasm rather than through a change in membrane potential. Several proteins (called CheA and CheY in *E coli*) are sequentially phosphorylated on a histidine and aspartate residue, respectively. The rate of autophosphorylation of CheA and correspondingly the degree of phosphorylation of CheY is reduced when the transducer proteins are in the activated conformation that results when an attractant is bound or when a repellent disappears. The phosphorylated form of CheY seems to foster clockwise rotation of the flagella, thus accounting for the decreased tumbling when attractants are added.

Chemotaxis senses a gradient of chemicals and, thus, must adapt to the presence of a constant concentration of any chemoeffector. The mechanism of adaptation involves the methylation of the transducer proteins. These proteins are termed methylated chemotaxis proteins (MCPs) because the extent of their methylation increases when attractants are present and decreases when they are removed. These MCPs are substrates for a methylation system that uses *S*-adenosyl-methionine as donor. The degree of methylation is determined by the conformation of the cytoplasmic domain of the protein, which is itself determined by the level of chemoeffector present at that time. Thus, the degree of methylation of the MCPs is a measure of the external concentration of specific chemoeffector specific for that protein at an earlier time. If the concentration has changed because the cell swam into a region of different concentration, then the conformation of the protein will be different from that which would be appropriate for its degree of methylation. The degree of methylation is continuously updated to reflect the concentration of chemoeffectors. In this way, the MCPs serve both as signal for the immediate presence of a specific

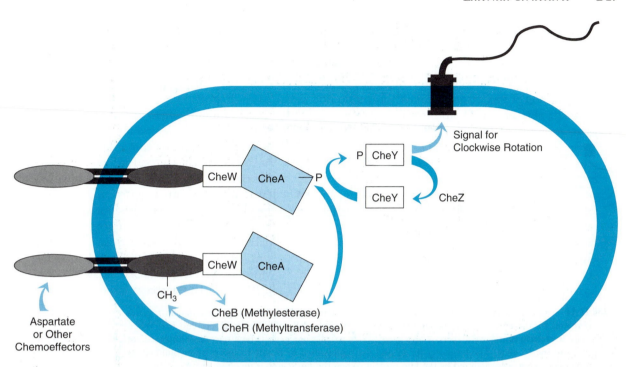

FIGURE 17-13   Signal transduction during bacterial chemotaxis. Chemoeffectors, such as the attractant aspartate, bind to a transmembrane transducer protein and thereby alter the conformation of a cytoplasmic domain of that protein. Somehow, this altered conformation results in decreased ability of the CheA protein to transfer a phosphate residue from itself to the CheY and CheB proteins. The phosphorylated form of CheY is necessary to trigger clockwise flagellar rotation, which leads to tumbling of the cell. The suppression of tumbling that results from attractant binding to its receptor is counteracted by the methylation of the receptor by CheR methyltransferase; methyl groups are removed, when the attractant concentration falls, by action of CheB methylesterase.

chemoeffector by affecting the CheA–CheY phosphorylation pathway and as the site for comparison, through the degree of methylation, with the concentration of the effector present earlier.

Phase Variation

Some bacteria are able to switch from the production of one antigenic type of flagella to another. This periodic alternation of a surface structure, called phase variation, was first observed in *Salmonella* (see Chap. 26) and helps the bacterium avoid elimination by the host's immune system. *Salmonella* strains can produce either of two antigenically distinct flagella, H1 and H2, and about 1 in 10^5 cells switch from production of H1 to H2, or the reverse (Fig. 17-14). This type of phase variation occurs through a reversible genetic change, in which a short stretch of DNA can invert itself. At one site on the bacterial chromosome are two adjacent genes encoding the H2 flagellin and a repressor that blocks expression of the gene for H1 flagellin. When these two genes are expressed, the cell produces only H2 flagellin. The promoter responsible for reading them is located nearby on a 914–base pair DNA segment that has the ability to invert itself by a site-specific recombination event. When this segment reorients at the low frequency characteristic of phase variation, neither the H2 nor the repressor of H1 gene is expressed, and the cell produces only H1 flagellin. Inversion of the promoter segment is reversible and occurs with roughly similar frequencies. Other examples of phase or antigenic variation are common, and some are described in Chapter 22.

FIMBRIAE (PILI)

Fimbriae are usually straight filaments, thinner and shorter than flagella, extending out from the surface of the cell (Fig. 17-15). The terms fimbriae and pili are used interchangeably, despite the proposal that the term pili be restricted to the filaments used to mediate bacterial cell contact during conjugation. They are present only on gram-negative cells and provide a means for adherence to other cells, either bacterial or animal. Fimbriae/pili are an example of a class of surface structures termed *adhesins* that allow attachment of a bacterial cell to other cells or surfaces. As clarified in the descriptions of pathogenic bacteria, fimbriae are extremely important for bacterial survival in an animal host. They originate in the cytoplasmic membrane and are composed of self-aggregating protein monomers (pilin).

labile) and the isoxazolyl penicillins (cloxacillin, oxacillin, and nafcillin), which are resistant to both penicillinases and acid. Other modifications can affect the antibacterial spectrum. Ampicillin and carbenicillin have charged side chains and are more hydrophilic than other penicillins and have increased activity against enteric bacteria and *Pseudomonas,* respectively. Changes in the side chain can also alter the protein-binding properties, which affects the lifetime of the antibiotic in serum, its ability to penetrate the blood–brain barrier, or the levels that are achieved in urine.

The penicillins have little toxicity for the host because they inhibit reactions unique to bacteria. The major side effect caused by the penicillins is the occurrence of allergic hypersensitivity. Although small molecules are normally nonimmunogenic, the antibacterial action of β-lactams involves their covalent attachment to target enzymes. When conjugated to its target proteins, the drug is a hapten to which an immune response can be generated.

Cephalosporins

Cephalosporin C, another β-lactam antibiotic structurally related to penicillin, was isolated in 1952 from the mold *Cephalosporium*. It was much more resistant to enzymatic inactivation, although it was also considerably less potent than penicillin. In 1961, a procedure was reported whereby the side groups of cephalosporin C could be removed chemically and, as with the semisynthetic penicillins, new groups could be added. This created a first generation of cephalosporins (cefazolin, cephalothin, and cephalexin) with increased potency and use against gram-

positive bacteria and some activity against gram-negative organisms. A second generation (cefamandole, cefuroxime, cefaclor, and the cephamycins, cefoxitin and cefotetan) lost some activity against gram-positive bacteria but had increased activity against many gram-negative bacteria. Figure 18-6 shows the structure of some of these semisynthetic cephalosporins.

In the late 1970s, a third generation of cephalosporins was developed by replacement of the sulfur atom in the cephalosporin nucleus with an atom of oxygen. These cephalosporins, termed *oxacephalosporins* or oxacephems, have a much broader specificity and higher potency than the previous types of cephalosporins, particularly for gram-negative organisms. Major third-generation cephalosporins in use include moxalactam, cefotaxime, ceftazidime, and ceftriaxone.

The basic mode of action of the cephalosporins is identical to that of penicillin in that they block peptidoglycan cross-linking and are bactericidal. They have a broad antimicrobial spectrum of activity and are destroyed by some β-lactamases but not others. Because of their structural similarities to penicillins, they engender an allergic reaction in 10% to 20% of individuals who are allergic to penicillin.

Other types of β-lactam antibiotics include the monobactam aztreonam, whose nucleus has only the single β-lactam ring and which exhibits good activity against many gram-negative bacteria. Thienamycins are carbapenem compounds different in structure from the penicillin and cephalosporins. Imipenem has broad activity against almost all medically important species.

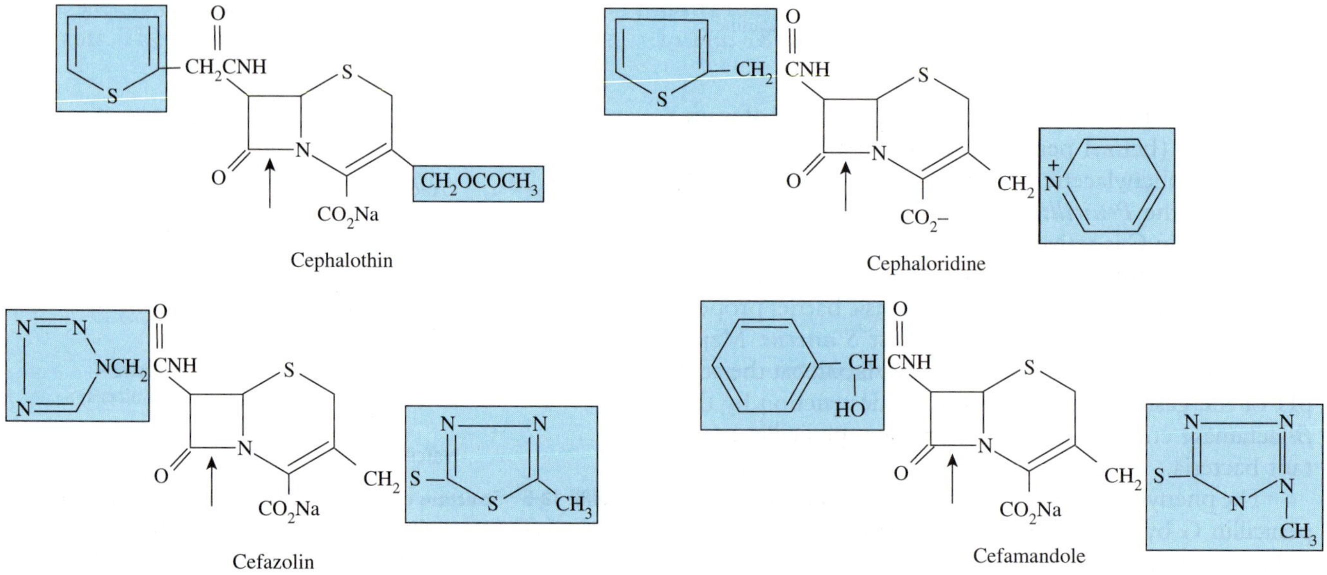

FIGURE 18-6 Structures of second-generation cephalosporins. The arrow points to β-lactam bond. The shaded areas represent chemical groups that were added to the cephalosporin nucleus. Some third-generation cephalosporins have substituted an oxygen atom for the sulfur atom.

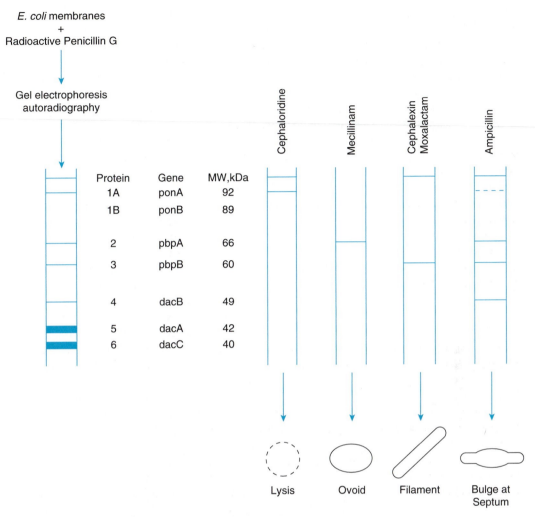

FIGURE 18-7   Properties of penicillin-binding proteins (PBPs). PBPs can be identified by incubating cell membranes with a radioactively labeled β-lactam antibiotic, such as penicillin G, to allow covalent reaction of the antibiotic with its target enzymes. Membrane proteins are separated by gel electrophoresis under protein denaturing conditions, and the radioactively labeled species are identified by autoradiography. At high β-lactam concentrations, seven major PBP species are seen in membranes of *Escherichia coli*, whereas at lower drug concentrations near their minimum inhibitory concentrations, different β-lactam antibiotics display preferential binding and reaction with only certain PBPs. Treatment of susceptible cells with these β-lactams have different outcomes, as revealed at the bottom of the figure. Thus, inhibition of PBP1AB leads to cell lysis, although inhibition of PBP2 leads to formation of ovoid cells, and inhibition of PBP3 leads to formation of long nonseptate filaments.

ACTION OF CELL-WALL INHIBITORS

Penicillin-Binding Proteins

Because β-lactam antibiotics can inhibit peptidoglycan synthesis in all eubacteria that have a cell wall, a specific target must exist for these antibiotics. The presence of a specific penicillin-binding protein (PBP) is detected by mixing cell membranes with a radioactively labeled β-lactam compound, followed by electrophoretic separation to identify the protein species to which the β-lactam is covalently bound. All bacteria possess several proteins that react covalently with penicillin but have different affinities and specificities for various β-lactams. Which of the multi-ple PBPs is the specific lethal target? The three to seven PBPs present in any species have different enzymatic activities and include glycosyltransferases, peptidyltransferases, transpeptidases, endopeptidases, and D-alanine carboxypeptidases.

In *Escherichia coli*, seven major PBPs occur whose functions have been identified by biochemical and genetic tests in which each individual PBP was inactivated by mutation or by treatment with a β-lactam having a high affinity for that PBP (Fig. 18-7). PBP5 and PBP6 are present in the greatest amounts. Their carboxypeptidase activity hydrolyzes the terminal D-alanine from the newly incorporated peptidoglycan pentapeptide, but neither enzyme is necessary for cell growth. PBP3 is involved in septum formation and the β-lactams (ampicillin, cephalexin, and furazlocillin), with the highest affinity for PBP3, cause formation of long filaments or bulged cells that lack a division septum. PBP2 seems to help determine cell shape because mutants lacking this activity or wild-type cells treated with mecillinam, a β-lactam specific for PBP2, form viable, ovoid-shaped cells. Treatment of *E coli* with a concentration of cephaloridine that will bind only to PBP1B results in cell lysis, indicating that this PBP is necessary for synthesis of an integral cell wall and is the lethal target for this antibiotic. PBP1A and PBP1B also are blocked by cefsulodin and are responsible for elongation or overall wall growth; these PBPs have both transpeptidase and transglycosylase activities. Thus, the various β-lactam antibiotics have the same mode of action by their covalent linkage to enzymes responsible for modifying the newly incorporated peptidoglycan subunits. β-Lactams can have different consequences for different bacteria because of their preference for different PBPs, which carry out different enzymatic reactions or act at different sites in the growing cell wall.

Mechanism of Penicillin Killing

Inhibitors of peptidoglycan synthesis normally are bactericidal for susceptible species, and many cause bacterial lysis when present at lethal concentrations (Fig. 18-8). Lysis results from the loss of the protective peptidoglycan layer and can be prevented by placing the cells in a medium of high osmolarity. Thus, treatment of sensitive cells with penicillin in a growth medium containing magnesium and an osmotic stabilizer (usually sucrose) results in the production of spherical, osmotically fragile forms called spheroplasts, if gram negative, and protoplasts, if gram positive.

Antibiotics that inhibit cell-wall synthesis are effective only on growing cells. If bacterial growth is prevented by starvation for a required nutrient or addition of a bacteriostatic antibiotic, cells are protected against killing by cell-wall synthesis inhibitors. An explanation for this effect is that during growth the incorporation of the peptidoglycan precursor molecules requires concomitant hydrolytic cleavage of the existing peptidoglycan to provide the sites for insertion of the precursors into the growing wall. If the action of the autolytic enzymes continues unabated when precursor synthesis is blocked or the cross-linking of incorporated precursors is inhibited, areas of weakened wall result, through which the cell bulges and ultimately bursts.

There are various conditions where β-lactam antibiotics block cell-wall synthesis and halt growth as effectively as under normal conditions, but do not cause lethality. Presumably the autolytic enzymes are less active, for

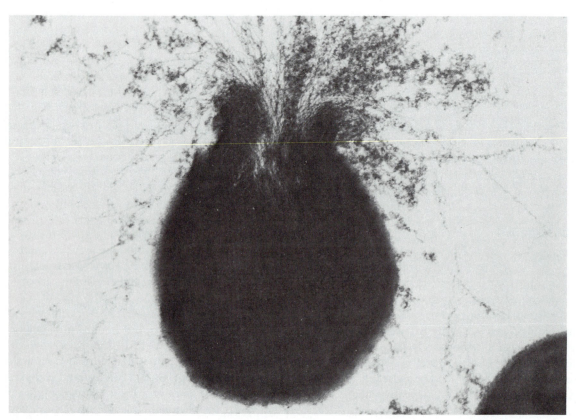

FIGURE 18-8   *Staphylococcus aureus* grown on medium containing fosfomycin. A similar lytic event occurs when cells are grown in the presence of any cell-wall inhibitor.

example, when *E coli* is at a lower pH (pH less than 6). Substitution of ethanolamine for the choline normally linked to lipoteichoic acid of *Streptococcus pneumoniae* also confers tolerance to the lytic effects of β-lactam antibiotics, although cell growth is inhibited by the drugs. This result suggests that teichoic acids may regulate the autolytic enzymes, and that inhibition of peptidoglycan synthesis is not lethal by itself. In addition, peptidoglycan isolated from cells starved for a required amino acid is resistant to the action of autolytic enzymes, suggesting that covalent modifications of the peptidoglycan might affect its ability to be acted on by the autolysins.

RESISTANCE TO β-LACTAM ANTIBIOTICS

The use and effectiveness of antimicrobial agents over the last 40 years has been continually complicated by the appearance and spread of bacterial variants resistant to individual or multiple antibiotics. In 1940, all isolates of *S aureus* were sensitive to benzyl penicillin, but by 1951 about 75% were resistant. Drug resistance is so widespread that antimicrobial susceptibility levels must be determined for almost all bacterial isolates before a definite choice of chemotherapeutic agent can be made.

Numerous mechanisms exist by which microorganisms become resistant to drugs, but these fall into two general categories: (1) modification of the target reaction so that it is no longer blocked by the antimicrobial agent, or (2) modifications that prevent access of the drug to its target reaction either by inactivating the drug or by decreasing its entry into the cell. These changes can result either from mutations in the bacterial chromosome or from acquisition of new genetic information, such as a plasmid.

Numerous mechanisms for resistance to β-lactam antibiotics are seen in different bacteria. In many cases, clinical resistance results from the production of β-lactamases, which are enzymes that catalyze the opening of the β-lactam ring and thereby prevent the antibiotic from being able to form a covalent bond with the target PBPs. Various types of β-lactamases exist with different relative activities against penicillins and cephalosporins. Although many β-lactamases are encoded by plasmids, some are encoded by chromosomal genes, and increased drug resistance can result from an increase in the copy number or rate of expression of that gene. Gram-positive bacteria usually produce penicillinase as an inducible enzyme that is secreted into the extracellular environment. Gram-negative β-lactamase producers usually synthesize the enzyme constitutively, but it remains localized in the periplasmic space adjacent to the target enzymes.

Many of the new classes of β-lactams have bulky side chains that decrease susceptibility to β-lactamases. Another solution to the clinical problems posed by this type of drug resistance makes use of certain β-lactams, such as clavulanic acid and sulbactam, which are them-

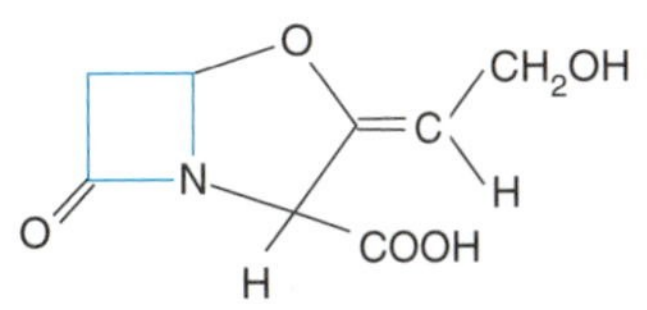

FIGURE 18-9 Structure of the β-lactamase inhibitor, clavulanic acid.

selves only weakly active as an antibiotic but are effective inhibitors of β-lactamases (Fig. 18-9). The combined administration of a β-lactamase–sensitive drug with such a β-lactamase inhibitor has proven to be effective, but forms of β-lactamase that are refractory to inhibition are emerging as a result of the extensive use of this drug therapy.

Several other mechanisms of resistance to β-lactams have appeared in bacterial types that have not acquired β-lactamase production. In gram-negative bacteria, the outer membrane poses an intrinsic barrier that nonspecifically retards antibiotic entry. Genetic changes in the properties of the porins in the outer membrane can have profound effects on drug susceptibility, especially in the case of large nonpolar molecules like the β-lactams. Another route of resistance is through mutations that affect the structure of a PBP to decrease its affinity for β-lactam antibiotics. These changes are rare in most clinical isolates but have been observed in *Neisseria gonorrhoeae* and *S pneumoniae*, and their origins are described in later chapters. The methicillin-resistant isolates of *S aureus* express a new PBP, called PBP2′, which carries out the functions of the three crucial PBPs of the bacterium and is resistant to inhibition.

In summary, the PBPs from most varieties of bacteria, including intrinsically resistant species like *P aeruginosa*, have similar affinities for β-lactams. The variations in susceptibilities of different organisms to β-lactams usually is not a consequence of the PBPs themselves, but of differences in the effective concentrations of the drugs at their site of action. Primary factors that determine the β-lactam level at the growing wall are the rate of diffusion of the drug through the cell envelope and the susceptibility of the drug to β-lactamases produced by the bacterium or its neighbors. The gram-positive wall poses little or no barrier, whereas the outer membrane represents a substantial intrinsic barrier.

Antibiotics That Affect Cell Membranes

The cytoplasmic membrane separates the cell from the exterior medium and is the site of essential functions, such as the regulation of the movement of metabolites into and out of the cell. Damage to this membrane has many detrimental effects, including the loss of metabolites and the disruption of essential biosynthetic functions. In contrast to other antibiotics, agents that affect bacterial cell membranes can be lethal even to nongrowing cells.

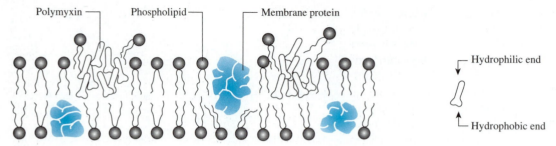

FIGURE 18-10   Schematic diagram illustrating how polymyxin distorts the cell membrane, destroying its effectiveness as a semipermeable barrier.

However, many of these agents also are injurious to mammalian cell membranes and, hence, have toxic side effects.

POLYMYXINS

Various polymyxins, designated A, B, C, D, and E, are produced by different strains of *B polymyxa,* but only polymyxins B and E (colistin) are used. Polymyxins are peptide derivatives in which one end of the molecule is a water-soluble and highly basic cyclic peptide with a high content of 2,4-diaminobutyric acid, whereas the other end is a hydrophobic fatty acid. The possession of both polar and nonpolar segments confers detergent activity, and polymyxins bind avidly to phospholipids and lipid A. Polymyxins interact specifically with the outer surface of membranes, with the water-soluble end remaining in the external medium and the hydrophobic tail embedded in the membrane. This detergent mode of action distorts the membrane bilayer (Fig. 18-10), allowing the passage of substances across the membrane in an unregulated manner.

Polymyxin is particularly effective against infections caused by members of the genus *Pseudomonas,* although it has also been used effectively against infections by *Brucella abortus, Klebsiella pneumoniae,* and *Bordetella pertussis.* Polymyxin usually is limited to topical use because of its toxic effects on the kidney and, to a lesser extent, on the central nervous system.

ANTIFUNGAL AGENTS

Fungal infections in humans range from localized cutaneous growth to invasive system spread, whose frequencies in immunosuppressed individuals represent a major cause of mortality. Few effective antifungal agents exist because of the difficulty of blocking a required step in the eucaryotic fungal cells without producing toxic effects on the host. The three major groups of antifungal agents in clinical use (polyene antibiotics, azole derivatives, and the allylamines-thiocarbamates) all act at or block the synthesis of ergosterol, the major sterol of fungal membranes.

Nystatin and Amphotericin B

Nystatin and amphotericin B are called polyene antibiotics because of their possession of large ring structures with a series of conjugated double bonds. They form a complex with sterols in the membranes of eucaryotic cells and the mycoplasmas, resulting in the disruption of the barrier properties of those membranes, probably because of the perturbation of the normal phase transition properties of the membrane lipids. These antibiotics have no effect on bacteria that lack sterols in their membranes. Their selective toxicity stems from their preferential binding to ergosterol of fungal cell membranes relative to the cholesterol derivatives in animal cell membranes. Amphotericin B is the primary antifungal agent used for treatment of systemic fungal infections; it does, however, produce a number of side effects, of which nephrotoxicity is the most serious. Nystatin is even more toxic than amphotericin B and is used only topically for infection with *Candida.*

Azoles and Allylamines

The synthetic azole derivatives (ketoconazole, fluconazole, and itraconazole) inhibit ergosterol biosynthesis at a cytochrome P450-dependent demethylation step to inhibit fungal growth. Their side reactions are primarily the result of their interference with the endocrine system in the cytochrome P450-dependent synthesis of steroid hormones. The allylamine (naftifine and binafine) and thiocarbamate (tolnaftate) antifungals inhibit squalene epoxidase, resulting in depletion of ergosterol. These compounds are less toxic than the azoles but are only useful against dermatophytes, mostly in topical application.

A Closer Look

Antibiotic Resistance: The Hidden Cost of Miracle Cures

Antibiotics are some of the wonder drugs of 20th century medicine, and they have played a remarkable and prominent role in the extension of the average human life expectancy and the improvement in the quality of life that has occurred since the 1940s. Antibiotics, together with some effective vaccines, have markedly reduced the impact of infectious diseases in developed nations. However, this considerable success has bred an unwarranted expectation in the public that bacterial infections are easily treatable and an equally unwarranted disregard by some clinicians in thinking that antibiotics can be indiscriminately and innocuously dispensed to fill the public's desires. It is crucial that medical students realize that antibiotics do have adverse effects, which can be either common but mild, or rare but severe. It is equally important to realize that the use of antibiotics carries a less-direct but more generally troubling consequence by affecting the distribution of antibiotic-resistant bacteria in the environment.

There are numerous reasons for the adverse side effects that can result from the use of an antibiotic by an individual patient. Effective antibiotics are those that inhibit some metabolic reaction or structure that exists in prokaryotic cells and not in eukaryotic cells. Some of the adverse side effects of antibiotics arise because antibiotics can inhibit a step of mitochondrial function that is related to the corresponding process in bacteria. Thus, some side effects result from interference with the function of host cells that are dividing frequently and are dependent on mitochondrial replication and protein synthesis. Chloramphenicol, for example, can cause a reversible but toxic depression of the hematopoietic system in the bone marrow, presumably through this mechanism.

Other adverse effects of antibiotic therapy arise because of interference with the normal bacterial flora, which provide considerable benefits to the human host. A major benefit of the normal flora is that it prevents other bacteria from colonizing or achieving significant numbers on any eposed body surface, by means of their competing for nutrients or producing metabolites or toxic proteins that restrict the growth of the pathogens. Hence, treatment of a patient with any antibiotic perturbs the normal bacterial flora with a concomitant reduction of its protective effect. If this perturbation is severe enough, superinfections with

organisms that are insensitive to the antibiotic can result. For example, treatment of chlamydial infections of the genitourinary tract with tetracycline sometimes results in overgrowth of a yeast, *Candida*, in the vagina.

Other adverse effects are idiosyncratic or only appear upon interaction with another pharmacological agent, and could not have been predicted. For example, sulfonamides can displace the heme-degradation product bilirubin from serum proteins. In neonates, this displaced bilirubin can pass into the central nervous system and cause kernicterus. Hence, sulfonamides should not be used in neonates or in pregnant women near term.

There is a less indirect but more generally worrisome adverse effect of antibiotic use, resulting from the role of antibiotics selected for the maintenance and spread of antibiotic resistance through the microbial populations. The indiscriminate use of antibiotics for treatment of mild and self-limiting diseases or as a prophylactic measure to reduce the threat of onset of a secondary bacterial infection in an individual suffering from a viral infection requires serious consideration and is not without major risk.

There seem to be cycles of microbial virulence, in the sense that the contact of an infectious agent with a human population does not have the same outcome as it had in the past, or may have in the future. The degree of illness suffered by the population is influenced by the virulence properties of the organism, which vary in poorly understood manners. The acquisition on mobile genetic elements of virulence determinants or mechanisms for evasion of the immune system can profoundly affect the degree of virulence of different isolates of bacteria that would appear identical by the usual criteria used for typing bacteria into genus and species. On the other hand, the immune status of the population, the degree of genetic diversity in the population, the state of nutrition and sanitation, the presence of other infectious agents in the environment, and many other subtle factors can affect the degree of virulence exhibited by a particular bacterial species. Recent examples of changing cycles of virulence are given by the reappearance of highly virulent and often rapidly fatal strains of group A streptococci, and the reemergence of the rheumatic fever, caused by the same species. On the other hand, influenza virus is now less virulent than the serotype that was active in the 1918 pandemic, and the virulence of *Yersinia pestis* appears reduced relative to the strains responsi-

A Closer Look *continued*

ble for the Black Plague that devastated Europe in the 1300s.

Given this cyclical nature of virulence patterns, it seems very short-sighted to dissipate the effectiveness of a useful antibiotic in treatment of mild, innocuous or self-limiting diseases in non-compromised individuals. This behavior runs the risk that that drug will not be available for use upon the emergence of some bacterium of increased virulence. Antibiotics do not affect only the bacterium causing the disease for which they were prescribed, but they provide selection for drug resistance in all of the bacteria carried by that patient. And it is clear that antibiotic resistance properties can be efficiently spread to other types of bacteria than the species in which the resistance first arose.

The appearance of antibiotic resistance in bacteria occurred from the beginning of the antibiotic era, in the 1940s. Even the discovery in 1974 of multiply antibiotic-resistant strains of *Shigella dysenteriae*, and the fact that all of these resistance traits were efficiently transmitted to other bacterial genera, was a cause for concern but did not affect the widespread use of antibiotics for human and agricultural animal consumption. During the 1990s, it has become glaringly apparent that the cost for this practice must now be paid and that the antibiotic era may be at an end. Antibiotic resistance is now very common in most human pathogens. The list of organisms that are still sensitive to the antibiotic that was the first choice for treatment 20 years ago is far shorter than the list of bacteria in which at least some isolates are insensitive to formerly effective antibiotics.

The basic mechanisms of antibiotic resistance have been described in this chapter and include mutational changes in the target enzyme that result in decreased binding of the antibiotic or acquisition of an alternative reaction that bypasses the antibiotic-sensitive step, usually by encoding a new enzyme with low affinity for the drug. A large number of resistance mechanisms involve production of enzymes that inactivate the antibiotic by covalent chemical modification, such as the opening of the β-lactam ring by β-lactamases, or acetylation of hydroxyl groups of chloramphenicol. Recently, the existence of multiple nonspecific efflux systems, which pump out foreign molecules of a general chemical type, have become apparent.

A few cases of generalized antibiotic resistance in gram-negative bacteria result from changes in the distribution of the outer membrane porins, with the production of a porin having a more restrictive channel than the normally expressed porin. A well-defined example of changes in porin function is seen in *E. coli*, which normally produces two general porins, called OmpF and OmpC. Several other porins with different substrate preferences are made under particular growth conditions, including the anion-preferring PhoE phosphoporin, made under conditions of phosphate limitation, the maltodextrin-preferring LamB maltoporin, made when grown with maltose, or the nucleoside-preferring Tsx porin. The general porins OmpF and OmpC have little substrate preference, but do favor polar neutral or cationic compounds. Their transmembrane channels are reported to have effective diameters of 1.2 and 1.1 nm, respectively, which allow the passage of molecules with a molecular weight around 600 (a trisaccharide or a tetrapeptide). Although the difference in effective diameter between the two porins is small, it is thought that production of OmpC with the smaller channel would be noticeably more restrictive to passage than with OmpF. Expression of the two porins is subject to strong and oppositely directed regulation such that OmpC synthesis is favored under conditions of high osmolarity and temperature, as would be encountered in the intestinal environment. OmpF synthesis is favored at low osmolarity and temperature, and the total amounts of OmpF + OmpC proteins made under any conditions are approximately constant. This differential expression of two porins may have developed to exclude the membrane-disruptive bile salts present in the intestine. However, expression of OmpC should also favor reduced uptake of antibiotics, especially larger ones whose size is near the exclusion limit of the OmpF porin. It is found that many conditions that result in genetic or transient physiological increases in antibiotic resistance display increased OmpC synthesis. These conditions include entry into stationary phase and mutations at the MAR (multiple antibiotic resistance) regulatory loci.

Continual selection for antibiotic-resistant bacteria is provided by the continual presence of antibiotics in the environment. This is particularly the case in the hospital setting, which brings together extensive usage of antibiotics with immunologically debilitated individuals. This strong selection pressure is resulting in a generation of new forms of antibiotic resistance, as well as the acquisition of novel and existing mechanisms of resistance by previously sensitive bacterial species. One example of new forms of resistance is the appearance of a β-lactam-resistant form of penicillin-binding protein-2 (PBP2), seen in *Neisseria gonorrhoeae* and *Streptococcus pneumoniae*. In both cases, it appears that this new enzyme arose as a result of homologous recombi-

A Closer Look *continued*

nation events that created a hybrid between the normal *pbp* gene native to that organism and the critical region from the homologous gene present in a naturally penicillin-resistant species of that bacterial genus present in the environment. It is likely that this genetic manipulation occurred as a result of genetic transformation, or the acquisition by the human parasites of the appropriate region of DNA from some natural source. Such a genetic experiment can occur naturally and the product is likely to be successfully retained only if they offer that cell a considerable growth advantage, as is the case in an antibiotic-laced environment. Another example of this genetic experiment has been shown to occur in the laboratory. Numerous strains of *Enterococcus* are resistant to the antibiotic, vancomycin, by their use of a peptidoglycan precursor and transpeptidase enzymes that are not affected by β-lactam antibiotics. Vancomycin is the only antibiotic that is clinically effective against some isolates of methicilin-resistant *Staphylococcus aureus*. It has been found in the laboratory that vancomycin resistance can be transferred from *Enterococcus* to *Staphylococcus*. If this transfer can occur in a laboratory, there is little reason to hope that it will not eventually occur in nature, resulting in the potential of a truly antibiotic-resistant and very serious pathogen.

Thus, there is no question that antibiotics have been miraculous tools that have greatly reduced the threat of disease and death from bacterial infections with relatively little risk to the patient. The hidden cost of the use of antibiotics is that the more a particular antibiotic is used, the more likely it is that resistance to that antibiotic will be established and proliferate throughout the microbial populations. Although there are many antibiotics available, many of them are minor modifications of a few basic types of antibiotic structures and mechanisms of action. Cross-resistance to all members of a type is usually the case. Finally, the accumulation of multiple antibiotic-resistance determinants on a single plasmid as a result of transposition or integron mobility means that selection for any one of those drug-resistances by use of that antibiotic is likely to maintain the presence of the entire plasmid and its multiple antibiotic resistances.

Bibliography

JOURNAL

Sanders CC. Chromosomal cephalosporinases responsible for multiple resistance to newer β-lactam antibiotics. Annu Rev Microbiol 1987;41:573.

BOOKS

Jackson GG, Thomas H, eds. The pathogenesis of bacterial infections: Bayer Symposium VIII. New York, Springer-Verlag, 1985.

Tipper DJ, ed. Antibiotic inhibitors of bacterial cell wall biosynthesis. Oxford, Pergamon Press, 1987.

Essentials of Medical Microbiology, Fifth Edition, edited by Wesley A. Volk, Bryan M. Gebhardt, Marie-Louise Hammarskjöld, and Robert J. Kadner. Lippincott-Raven Publishers, Philadelphia © 1996.

Chapter 19

Macromolecular Synthesis and Mechanisms of Antibiotic Action

The biosynthesis of bacterial macromolecules—including DNA, RNA, protein, and peptidoglycan—requires the action of enzymes that are different in structure from their counterparts in eucaryotic cells or involves the metabolism of biologically unique biosynthetic intermediates. These points of difference are the target sites at which antimicrobial agents can inhibit or kill procaryotic cells with little effect on eucaryotic cells. Selective toxicity is the prime requisite for any agent used in antimicrobial chemotherapy. This chapter describes the flow of genetic information in bacterial cells to define the site of action of the major classes of antibiotics. These topics are an extension of the material presented in Chapter 2, and the antimicrobial agents are listed according to their primary sites of action. A few clinically useful antimetabolites interfere with steps of intermediary metabolism. The action of agents that are useful for sterilization of surfaces or inanimate objects is briefly described. Finally, the mechanisms by which bacteria become resistant to antimicrobial agents are reviewed, along with information about the origin and development of antibiotic resistance.

Nucleic Acid Synthesis

As described in Chapter 2, the replication of DNA and its transcription into RNA require separation of the two strands of the DNA double helix. Several antibiotics block nucleic acid synthesis either by interfering with DNA strand separation or by inhibiting an enzyme necessary for replication or transcription.

STRUCTURE AND REPLICATION OF DNA

Agents that prevent strand separation are lethal for the cell because both replication and transcription of DNA will be blocked. As described later, *ultraviolet light* (lambda max = 260 nm) causes the formation of a bond between pyrimidines in the same DNA strand. The presence of pyrimidine dimers blocks the passage of both

DNA and RNA polymerases, and the cell dies unless the dimers are removed by excision repair or recombinational repair processes. *Mitomycin C* is lethal to most types of cells because it blocks DNA synthesis and causes extensive DNA breakdown. On entry into a cell, mitomycin is enzymatically converted into a reactive hydroquinone derivative that can form covalent cross-links between guanine residues on the same or opposite strands of DNA. The cross-links prevent separation of the strands, which blocks passage of polymerases and promotes the action of repair enzymes and endonucleolytic strand breakage. It is too toxic for clinical use.

METRONIDAZOLE. Metronidazole is an effective lethal agent for treatment of amoebic dysentery, trichomoniasis, and infections with anaerobic bacteria, but has little or no effect on aerobic organisms. Its key feature seems to be its nitro group, which is reduced under anaerobic conditions to produce reactive intermediates or radicals that cause DNA strand cleavage, primarily at thymine residues.

Supercoiling

A characteristic feature of procaryotic DNA is that it is negatively supercoiled (untwisted by three to nine turns per 1000 base pairs) by the action of *DNA gyrase*. This enzyme couples the hydrolysis of ATP to the unwinding of circular double-stranded DNA molecules, including the chromosome and any phages and plasmids in the bacterial cell. Negative supercoiling makes the DNA helix easier to unwind and is necessary for DNA replication, for many recombination processes, and for the transcription of some genes. DNA gyrase is an enzyme complex of two protein subunits, one possessing DNA strand nicking-closing activity similar to other topoisomerases and the other possessing ATPase activity. The nicking-closing activity by itself can allow the relaxation of negatively or positively twisted DNA topoisomers. In the presence of ATP, the enzyme complex introduces negative supercoils by unwinding the DNA two turns at a time. The two protein subunits responsible for the nicking-closing activity and the ATPase activity are encoded by the genes *gyrA* and *gyrB*. The DNA of eucaryotic cells is supercoiled by its wrapping around the histone cores.

QUINOLONES, NALIDIXIC ACID, AND NOVOBIOCIN. Several antibiotics inhibit the action of DNA gyrase and have multiple effects, the most prominent being the immediate cessation of bacterial DNA synthesis. Nalidixic acid and oxolinic acid, which share the 4-quinolone nucleus, bind to the GyrA subunit and inhibit its nicking-closing activity. These drugs are bactericidal to many gram-negative bacteria. Resistance to high levels of these drugs occurs by mutations in the *gyrA* gene to produce a subunit unable to bind them. Novobiocin and coumermycin bind to the GyrB subunit, and mutations in the *gyrB* gene confer

resistance to them. Inhibition of the ATPase activity catalyzed by this subunit results in cell killing.

Nalidixic acid has been used in the treatment of urinary tract infections caused by gram-negative enteric bacteria because it is excreted rapidly by the kidneys. Fluoroquinolones (norfloxacin, ciprofloxacin) are significantly more potent (100- to 1000-fold) than nalidixic acid. Advantages to the use of fluoroquinolones are that they are rapidly bactericidal and achieve inhibitory levels for treatment of infections in the respiratory tract, skin, bone, and gastrointestinal tract. They show minimal cross-resistance to other drugs, and their resistance results from chromosomal mutations rather than acquisition of plasmids. Although resistance can develop during therapy (as it has in *Staphylococcus aureus*), it is not rapidly transmitted to other bacteria or associated with multiple drug resistances.

Novobiocin does not enter most gram-negative bacteria efficiently because of its relatively large size and hydrophobic character. It is effective against gram-positive bacteria and has been used for treatment of infections caused by penicillin-resistant staphylococci, but its use is not indicated. The coumermycins are too toxic for clinical use.

TRANSCRIPTION OF DNA

No antibiotics act directly on the DNA replication enzymes, although antibiotics that bind to DNA inhibit its replication (but usually later than their inhibition of transcription). Antimetabolites that inhibit DNA replication include *N*-hydroxyurea, which blocks the formation of deoxyribonucleotides by the enzyme ribonucleotide reductase.

Actinomycin

Actinomycin D is the prototype of the actinomycins, comprised of a peptide linked to a planar chromogenic group. These antibiotics form complexes with guanine residues in helical DNA by intercalating their chromophore into the double helix or by binding along the helix in the minor groove. Actinomycin prevents RNA synthesis by blocking the passage of RNA polymerase on the DNA template. At higher concentrations, DNA replication also is inhibited. The actinomycins exhibit no selectivity and block both procaryotic and eucaryotic transcription. They are too toxic for clinical use but frequently are used as an experimental tool for the specific inhibition of DNA-directed RNA synthesis, as is the fungal toxin alpha-amanitin, an inhibitor of several eucaryotic RNA polymerases.

Rifamycins

The rifamycins compose a large family of antibiotics, of which the most widely used member is the semisynthetic derivative *rifampin*. It binds to the β subunit of bacterial RNA polymerase and inhibits an early step of transcription after synthesis of the first phosphodiester bond but before release of sigma factor. Rifampin seems to perturb the conformation of RNA polymerase so that the transition from initiation phase to elongation phase is blocked. There is little effect on chain elongation after the release of the sigma factor. Rifampin has a broad antibacterial spectrum and is especially active against gram-positive bacteria and mycobacteria. It is given orally for the treatment of tuberculosis, leprosy, and certain infections with *Staphylococcus*. The rifamycins have no effect on the RNA polymerases of eucaryotic nuclei, but do inhibit the replication of pox and adenoviruses, but not by inhibition of their RNA synthesis. Resistance to rifampin develops rapidly because of mutational alteration of a segment of the β subunit of RNA polymerase.

Among other antibiotics that affect transcription, streptovaricin seems to act identically to rifampin, whereas streptolydigin, which also binds to the β subunit of bacterial RNA polymerase, allows the initiation of transcription but blocks elongation of the RNA product.

Griseofulvin

Griseofulvin is used to treat superficial dermatophyte infections by fungi that destroy keratin structures in the host. It inhibits the growth of fungi possessing cell walls containing chitin and has no effect on fungi with cellulose cell walls, or on bacteria or yeasts. It seems to somehow inhibit the process of nuclear division.

Protein Synthesis

Although the basic steps of translation in procaryotic and eucaryotic cells are similar, they take place on ribosomes that are distinctly different in their size, protein content, and ability to bind and be inhibited by specific antibiotics. Antibiotics that inhibit translation in bacteria usually have no effect on the 80S ribosomes in the cytoplasm of eucaryotic cells, although many inhibit translation on the mitochondrial 70S ribosomes. Regarding ribosome structure, notice that the ribosomal RNA is not simply a scaffold for the attachment of the catalytically active proteins, but in addition is an active participant in some of the reactions of translation, particularly the step of peptide bond formation. Antibiotic action may thus be directed at a ribonucleoprotein complex, and resistance can occur through changes in either a specific ribosomal protein or at a specific site on the rRNA. Mutations affecting rRNA are not normally obtained among resistant mutants because most cells have several rRNA genes, each of which would have to be altered for cellular resistance. Resistance to some antibiotics is seen through production of enzymes that modify by methylation a single rRNA nucleotide. It

is thus difficult to identify unambiguously the target site on the ribosome for each antibiotic.

Sometimes mutations confer resistance to that agent because the antibiotic is no longer able to bind to a ribosomal protein. Binding of antibiotic to isolated proteins may not be a reliable indicator of the natural conformation of the protein in the assembled structure. Some antibiotics bind to several ribosomal proteins, although with different affinities. Antibiotic binding or mutational alteration affecting one protein can affect the function of adjacent proteins.

A useful approach to identifying the site of action of an antibiotic tests the drug sensitivity of hybrid ribosomes prepared by the reassembly of ribosomes from their isolated components. In this type of study, only one component (a ribosomal subunit, rRNA, or a ribosomal protein) is derived from a resistant mutant organism; the remainder are from the sensitive strain. In a simple example, reconstructed ribosomes, in which the 30S subunit is from a streptomycin-resistant bacterium, are resistant to streptomycin, regardless of the source of the 50S subunit. Reconstitution of the 30S subunit from the individual RNA and proteins obtained from sensitive or resistant strains reveals that the response to streptomycin is determined only by the origin of the 30S ribosomal subunit protein S12, showing that this protein is involved in the binding and response to this antibiotic. It is not always possible to define precisely the site and mode of action of many of the antibiotics that block protein synthesis.

Figure 19-1 is a schematic diagram showing the major steps of protein synthesis and the reactions that are blocked by representative antibiotics.

INHIBITORS OF THE 30S RIBOSOMAL SUBUNIT

The 30S subunit of the ribosome contains the sites for attachment of mRNA and for specific recognition of aminoacyl-tRNAs. Antibiotics acting on the 30S subunit interfere with protein synthesis by preventing attachment of the mRNA or tRNAs or by blocking the movement of the ribosome along the mRNA. Important antibiotics in this group include streptomycin and other aminoglycosides, and the tetracyclines.

Streptomycin

Streptomycin is an aminoglycoside, a family of antibiotic inhibitors of the 30S subunit that carry an amino-inositol group glycosidically linked to one or two more sugar-like moieties. In streptomycin, one of these moieties is streptidine, which is an inositol nucleus substituted with two guanidinium groups (Fig. 19-2). Aminoglycosides are bactericidal for gram-positive and gram-negative bacteria, including *Pseudomonas aeruginosa* and *Mycobacterium tuberculosis*. Their clinical use has decreased with the development of extended-spectrum β-lactams because of their renal toxicity and ototoxicity. They often are re-

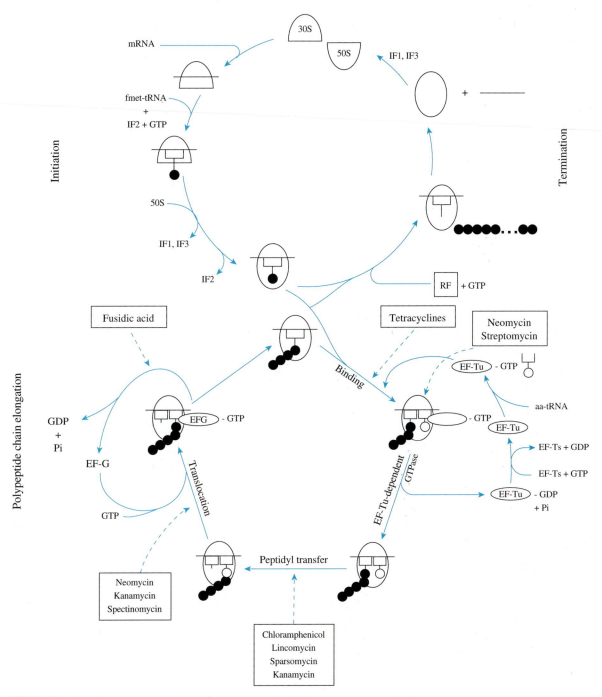

FIGURE 19-1 Protein synthesis in bacteria showing sites of inhibition by various antibiotics.

served for life-threatening diseases, but streptomycin remains the drug of choice for tularemia, plague, and brucellosis. Streptomycin is a basic molecule and has a variety of nonspecific effects, including the alteration of membrane permeability, with the loss of potassium and other small metabolites from the cell. Streptomycin binds irreversibly to a single protein (S12) in the 30S ribosomal subunit (binding is influenced by the presence of proteins S3, S5, S9, and S14) and this binding has two major effects on protein synthesis. The first effect is that initia-

tion complexes assemble on the ribosome-binding site of the mRNA, but streptomycin blocks further movement of the initiation complexes. As a result, only a single ribosome binds to the mRNA and remains stuck near the first codon. This explains why a cell containing both wild-type and streptomycin-resistant ribosomes is sensitive to streptomycin, because as soon as a wild-type ribosome binds to an mRNA molecule, it freezes in place, thereby preventing the subsequent translation of the mRNA by any resistant ribosomes.

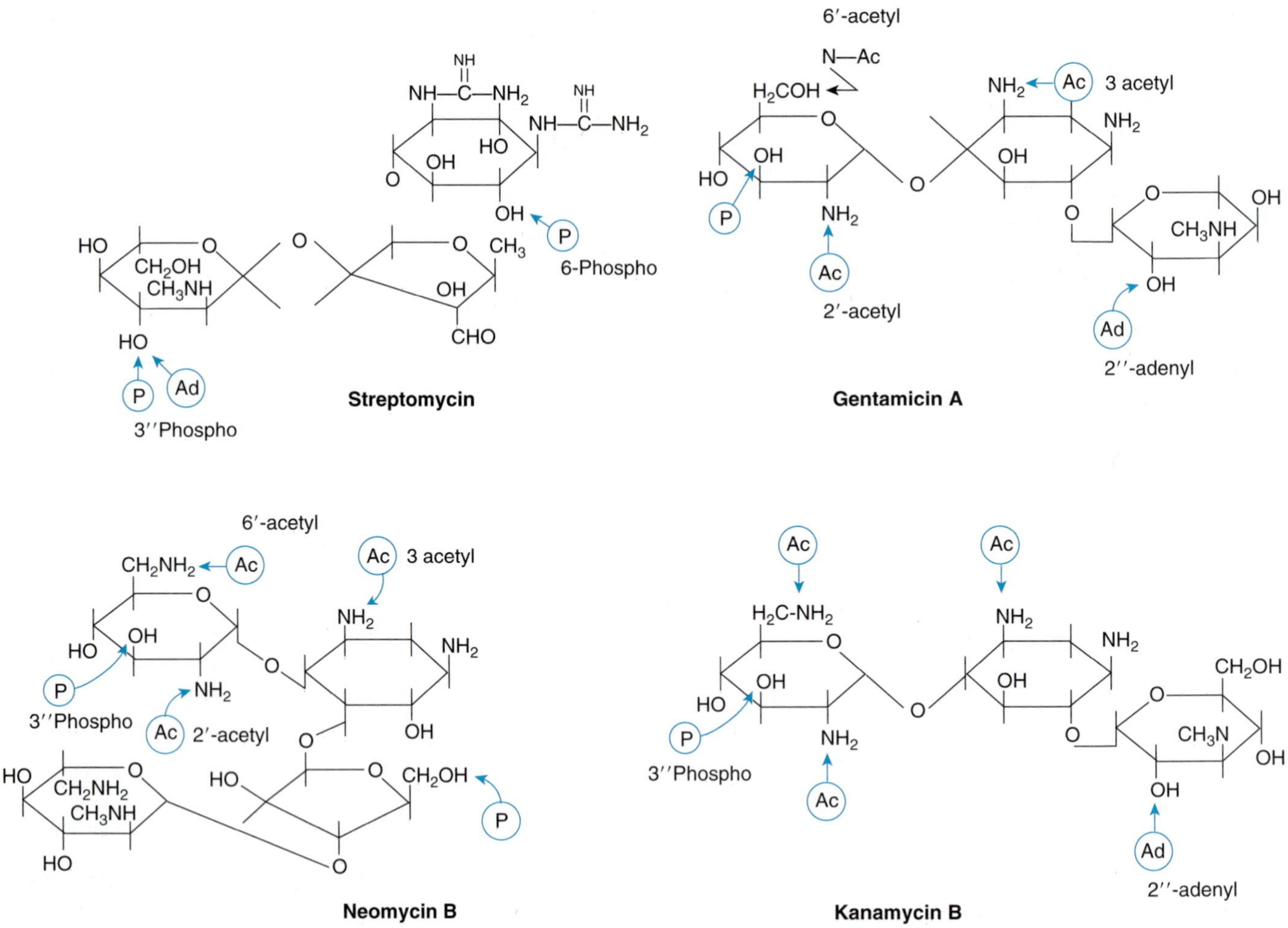

FIGURE 19-2 Structures of several aminoglycosides. The sites of modification by drug-resistance enzymes are indicated.

The second effect of streptomycin is that its binding to sensitive ribosomes that have already passed the initiation stage causes a moderate slowing of translation and a marked increase in misreading because of the binding of the wrong aminoacyl-tRNAs in response to a codon. Misreading is measured as the incorporation of inappropriate amino acids during the in vitro translation of artificial mRNAs that lack the proper initiation signals, such as the incorporation of isoleucine instead of phenylalanine specified by poly U as template. Misreading also is seen in vivo at sublethal concentrations of streptomycin and is apparent as streptomycin-induced suppression of missense or nonsense mutations. Misreading is not the cause of lethality, but it probably indicates that the binding of streptomycin distorts the ribosome in such a manner that the ribosomal functions that maintain the precise fidelity of translation are unable to operate.

Misreading seems to play an important role in the entry of streptomycin into the cell, a process which exhibits a paradoxical inducibility. Uptake of the drug begins at a low rate but then dramatically accelerates after an induction period, concomitant with loss of cellular metab-

olites. The apparent induction of high transport activity is blocked by other protein synthesis inhibitors and does not occur in streptomycin-resistant cells, but it can be engendered by any of the other aminoglycosides that cause misreading. Although it is possible that this process involves induction of a specific transport system for streptomycin, it is more likely that the misreading that occurs after initial entry of low levels of streptomycin leads to the synthesis of deranged membrane proteins whose insertion into the membrane disrupts its barrier properties. The leaky state of the membrane is responsible for both the loss of metabolites and the rapid access of external streptomycin to binding sites on the ribosomes.

Mutants resistant to streptomycin appear at low frequency as a result of chromosomal changes affecting the S12 protein. Some resistant mutants show no binding of the drug, but other mutants are actually dependent upon the presence of streptomycin for growth. The requirement for streptomycin can be satisfied by aminoglycosides that cause misreading; perhaps the mutation leading to streptomycin dependence has altered the ribosome in such a manner that it is too defective or too inexact at translation to allow the cell to survive unless the ribosome is distorted in a different manner by the presence of streptomycin. Mutations affecting other proteins in the 30S subunit can result in increased or decreased fidelity of translation.

Other Aminoglycoside Antibiotics

Other clinically important aminoglycosides include neomycin, kanamycin, gentamicin, tobramycin, amikacin, and netilmicin. All are bactericidal and all block initiation of translation irreversibly in a manner similar to that described for streptomycin, although they bind to different proteins in the 30S subunit. These antibiotics also induce misreading and can substitute for streptomycin in streptomycin-dependent mutants.

Spectinomycin also belongs to this group of antibiotics but differs by the absence of a glycosidic linkage and is more correctly called an aminocyclitol. Spectinomycin is only bacteriostatic and does not cause misreading, although it does inhibit protein synthesis by inhibiting the translocation step of the elongation process, as do many of the aminoglycosides. Resistance results from mutations affecting ribosomal protein S5. Spectinomycin is used to treat gonorrhea caused by penicillin-resistant gonococci.

All aminoglycosides have a relatively broad spectrum of activity but a narrow range of effectiveness before toxic levels are reached. The most serious adverse reactions are damage to the vestibular portion of the eighth cranial nerve, auditory toxicity, and renal damage. These antibiotics often are used in treating serious gram-negative infections (especially with the enterics and pseudomonads), and the appearance of resistant organisms is a problem. A functioning electron transport system seems to be necessary for the uptake of aminoglycosides, and they are essentially ineffective against anaerobic bacteria or even against sensitive bacteria cultured under anaerobic conditions.

AMINOGLYCOSIDE RESISTANCE. Chromosomal mutations to resistance to a specific aminoglycoside arise at low frequency (around 10^{-8}) and alter a specific ribosomal protein so that it no longer binds or is inhibited by its cognate aminoglycoside. Of greater impact are the considerable number of plasmid-coded enzymes, which modify certain aminoglycosides by acetylation of amino groups, phosphorylation of hydroxyl groups, or adenylation of hydroxyl groups. Different enzymes can carry out the same modification but at different sites, thereby rendering them specific for different aminoglycosides, which carry the susceptible group located at the appropriate position. The modified forms do not inhibit ribosome function and they may not enter the cell as effectively as the normal drug. Table 19-1 and Figure 19-2 provide summaries of the aminoglycoside-modifying enzymes.

Tetracyclines

The tetracyclines are a family of related antibiotics that differ in their side chains, as shown in Figure 19-3. All have a broad antibacterial spectrum and are bacteriostatic against all bacteria except the mycobacteria. The semisyn-

TABLE 19-1
Aminoglycoside-Modifying Enzymes

Enzyme	Bacterial Source	Modification
Kanamycin, amikacin, neomycin, tobramycin acetyltransferase AAC (6′)	R⁺ *Escherichia coli* *Pseudomonas aeruginosa*	6-Amino group of an amino hexose is acetylated
Gentamicin, tobramycin, kanamycin acetyltransferase AAC (3)	*Pseudomonas aeruginosa* *Klebsiella pneumoniae* *E coli*	3-Amino group of 2-deoxystreptamine is acetylated
Gentamicin, tobramycin acetyltransferase II AAC (2′)	*Providencia*	2-Amino group of an amino hexose is acetylated
Streptomycin-spectinomycin adenylyltransferase AAD (3″)	R⁺ *E coli*	Hydroxyl group of a D-*threo* methylamino alcohol moiety is adenylylated
Gentamicin, tobramycin, kanamycin adenylyltransferase AAD (2″)	R⁺ *E coli* R⁺ *K pneumoniae*	2-Hydroxyl group of an amino hexose is adenylylated
Streptomycin phosphotransferase (APH 3″)	R⁺ *E coli* *Staphylococcus aureus* *P aeruginosa*	3-Hydroxy group of *N*-methyl L-glucosamine is phosphorylated
Neomycin-kanamycin I phosphotransferase APH (3′)	R⁺ *E coli* *P aeruginosa* *S aureus*	3-Hydroxyl group of an amino hexose is phosphorylated
Lividomycin phosphotransferase APH (5″)	*P aeruginosa* R⁺ *E coli*	5-Hydroxyl group of D-ribose is phosphorylated

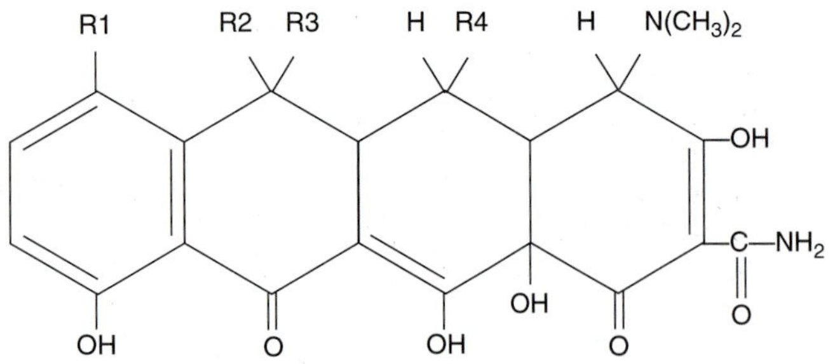

Antibiotic	R1	R2	R3	R4
Tetracycline	-H	-OH	-CH$_3$	-H
Oxytetracycline	-H	-OH	-CH$_3$	-OH
Chlortetracycline	-Cl	-OH	-CH$_3$	-H
Minocycline	-N(CH$_3$)$_2$	-H	-H	-H
Doxycycline	-H	-H	-CH$_3$	-OH

FIGURE 19-3 Structure of several tetracyclines.

thetic derivative doxycycline is used for treating infections with *Rickettsia* and *Chlamydia* and for treating early stages of Lyme disease. They inhibit protein synthesis on both bacterial and eucaryotic ribosomes, but bacterial growth is selectively prevented because bacteria actively accumulate these drugs by a transport process absent from eucaryotic cells. The tetracyclines bind to the ribosomal RNA and proteins S4 and S18 of the 30S subunit through magnesium salt bridges, and inhibit the binding of aminoacyl-tRNA to the acceptor site.

Undesirable side effects include inhibition of the intestinal flora and the outgrowth of drug-resistant organisms. This problem is reduced by use of the more hydrophobic tetracyclines, doxycycline and minocycline, which are almost completely absorbed from the intestinal tract. Some of the tetracyclines are deposited in bones and teeth and cause staining and possible structural impairment, thus precluding their use during pregnancy or childhood. They also tend to render their recipient sensitive to sunlight. As with other antibiotics, the appearance of resistant organisms is a serious problem. Nonetheless, the tetracyclines are an important collection of drugs for treating infections caused by penicillin-resistant bacteria and diseases caused by *Rickettsia* and *Chlamydia*.

There seems to be only a single mechanism by which *Escherichia coli* acquires resistance to tetracycline. Plasmids conferring resistance to this drug encode a new transport system that brings about the protonmotive force-dependent pumping of a tetracycline/divalent cation complex out of the cell, thereby reducing its effective concentration on the ribosomes. Tetracycline resistance can also result from changes in the ribosome or alteration of the drug.

Nitrofurans

Nitrofurantoin is used clinically to treat urinary tract infections. It and other nitrofurans, which are characterized by the presence of a 5-nitro-furan group, inhibit protein synthesis in vivo and in vitro at the stage of initiation of translation.

INHIBITORS OF THE 50S RIBOSOMAL SUBUNIT

Puromycin

Puromycin inhibits protein synthesis in all systems and is an important tool for study of translation and the site of action of other antibiotics. Puromycin is a structural analogue of the aminoacyl end of tRNA and is a substrate for the peptidyl transfer reaction catalyzed by the 50S subunit. When puromycin binds at a free A site on the ribosome, the nascent peptide chain is transferred from the tRNA in the P site onto the amino group of puromycin. After translocation of the ribosome to the next codon, the peptidyl–puromycin lacks the long tRNA chain that held the peptide stably on the ribosome and dissociates from the ribosome. As the concentration of puromycin is increased, translating ribosomes release increasingly shorter oligopeptides ending with a puromycin. The formation of peptidyl–puromycin oligopeptides provides an assay of peptidyl transfer activity and serves to indicate the presence of a free A site on the ribosome. If another antibiotic blocked the binding of aminoacyl-tRNA, resulting in a free A site, puromycin would be able to react with the peptide in the P site to a higher degree than if the first antibiotic were not present. Conversely, if the first antibiotic blocked the peptidyl transferase reaction

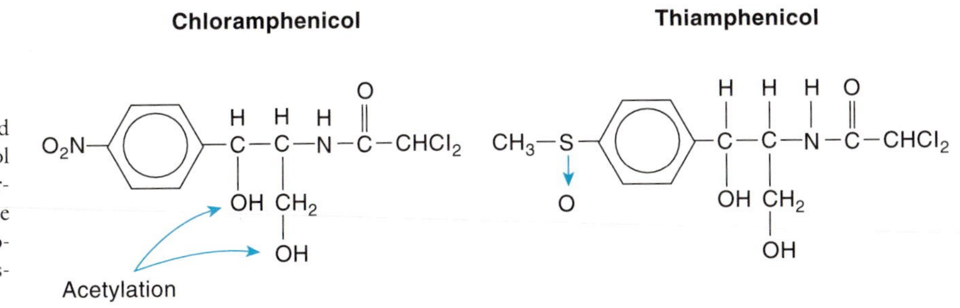

FIGURE 19-4 Structures of chloramphenicol and thiamphenicol. Inactivation of chloramphenicol occurs by the acetylation of the antibiotic. Chloramphenicol-3-acetate is formed first, and the 1,3-diacetate forms later. Neither the monoacetylated nor the diacetylated antibiotic possesses antibacterial activity.

In some cases, resistance results from ability of the organism to transport the cell, as in the cases of fosfomycin and D-c

In general, resistance to an antibiotic a mutational change occurs in nature duri of antibiotic therapy and not because the caused the disease was originally resistan alteration of a cellular reaction or enzyme in a less efficient enzyme and poorer growth If the selective pressure provided by the a moved, the mutant strains cannot grow a wild-type parents and will soon be lost fr lation.

TRANSPORT MECHANISMS AND DRUG RESISTANC

Transport activities are recognized as playin in determining the susceptibility or resistan to numerous antibiotics and to other toxi impact of the outer-membrane porin ch stricting access to large or nonpolar mole targets in gram-negative bacteria has be Some cases of low-level multiple drug resista bacteria, including *N gonorrhoeae*, are becau in porin channel size, which result from cl pattern of porin gene expression or of th residues that line the porin channel.

The expression of a transport system r the protonmotive force-dependent efflux c

or the translocation step to move the peptide from the A to the P site, reactivity with puromycin will be decreased.

Chloramphenicol

Chloramphenicol (Fig. 19-4) was first isolated from the actinomycete *Streptomyces venezuelae,* but it has since been prepared by chemical synthesis because of its relatively simple structure. It reversibly inhibits protein synthesis by binding to the 50S subunit and inhibiting the peptide transfer reaction carried out by the 23S rRNA. It competes with puromycin and the 3' end of aminoacyl-tRNA for binding to the A site. Chloramphenicol has a broad antimicrobial spectrum; it is effective against both gram-positive and gram-negative bacteria as well as mycoplasma, chlamydia, and rickettsia. It is bacteriostatic for most organisms, but has a lethal effect on *Haemophilus influenzae, Neisseria meningitidis,* and *Streptococcus pneumoniae*. It is rapidly absorbed and penetrates into all tissues.

There are serious side effects that demand caution in the clinical use of chloramphenicol. Its major toxicity on the hematopoietic system is through its inhibition of mitochondrial protein synthesis. Usually, the resultant bone marrow suppression is reversible, but, in rare cases (1 in 10,000 to 45,000), an irreversible (and usually fatal) aplastic anemia (loss of the stem cells that are precursors to red blood cells) occurs. Thiamphenicol, a structural analogue of chloramphenicol, seems not to give rise to this fatal complication. Chloramphenicol usually is reserved for meningitis caused by *H influenzae,* typhoid fever, rickettsial diseases, and serious infections by some anaerobic bacteria.

Resistance to chloramphenicol is mediated by a plasmid-coded enzyme, chloramphenicol acetyltransferase, that transfers acetyl groups from acetyl-CoA to either or both of the free hydroxyl groups on the drug. The acetylated species cannot bind to the ribosome or inhibit bacterial growth. Even though this drug is not extensively used clinically, chloramphenicol-resistant bacteria frequently are encountered because of the carriage of multiple drug resistance determinants on the same plasmid.

Erythromycin

Antibiotics of the macrolide family contain a large 12- to 22-carbon lactone ring bound to various sugars and includes erythromycin (the most effective), oleandomycin, carbomycin, and spiramycin (the least effective). Erythromycin binds to the L15 protein of the 50S subunit near the site at which chloramphenicol binds, but this drug does not inhibit the puromycin reaction. It is thought that macrolides interfere with the translocation step, possibly the release of the free tRNA from the P site. The effect of the drug is primarily bacteriostatic, and resistant organisms appear readily, often as a result of an alteration of the ribosomal protein L4 or L12. Organisms resistant to erythromycin as a result of mutational alteration of the ribosome are at a disadvantage when growing in competition with sensitive organisms in the absence of the drug because of their decreased rate of protein synthesis. Erythromycin is the drug of choice for pneumonia caused by *Legionella,* and an oral form is effective for pneumonia caused by *Mycoplasma, Chlamydia,* and *Streptococcus*; it is also useful for treatment of streptococcal and staphylococcal infections in patients who are allergic to penicillin. Clarithromycin extends the spectrum against other gram-positive bacteria. The large size of the macrolides reduces their rate of entry and their effectiveness against gram-negative bacteria.

Resistance to erythromycin can arise from mutations affecting ribosomal proteins L4 and L12. The mechanism of resistance associated with clinical isolates is plasmid mediated and is provided by an enzyme that methylates two sites on a A residue in the 23S rRNA. This modified ribosome also is resistant to lincomycin and other macrolides.

Lincomycin and Clindamycin

Lincomycin and the closely related derivative clindamycin have unusual structures, but their mode of action and antibacterial spectrum is similar to that of chloramphenicol and erythromycin. Lincomycin competes with chloramphenicol for binding to the 50S subunit and inhibits the peptidyl transfer reaction, probably by inhibiting binding of the incoming aminoacyl-tRNA. In contrast to

PABA permits the formation of fo
level of the inhibitor decreases. Th
sulfonamides is only bacteriostatic,
be continued for a sufficient period
host defenses to destroy the infecti

Resistance to sulfonamides occt
ularly in gram-negative organisms st
rhoeae, and *N meningitidis*. There at
for sulfonamide resistance. Plasmid
sults from production of a new ena
the inhibited reaction but that has z
for sulfonamides relative to PABA.
coded mechanisms of resistance inc
uptake, overproduction of PABA,
normal enzyme so that sulfonamide

TRIMETHOPRIM

Trimethoprim is an effective inhibit
drofolate reductase, an enzyme esse
The normal form of folic acid tha
units is the reduced tetrahydrofolat
synthetase makes thymine from ura
tetrahydrofolate serves as the donor
and is converted to dihydrofolate a
in any cell making DNA, dihydrofc
act continually to replenish the poo

Many dihydrofolate reductase
aminopterin, amethopterin, and met
enzymes from both bacterial and et
contrast, trimethoprim is a good inh
form of the enzyme but has 10^4 l
mammalian form. Subtle difference
the folate-binding sites of the two
enhance trimethoprim binding to the
not favoring its binding to the euc
19-6 summarizes the steps involved
tetrahydrofolic acid and shows the re
petitively inhibited by antimetabolit

Trimethoprim acts synergistica
amides because they inhibit sequent
metabolic pathway. The combinati
and sulfamethoxazole is useful in t
infections, salmonellosis, and chror
media, and pneumonia caused by *P*

Plasmid-coded trimethoprim re
the production of a new dihydrofola
low affinity for trimethoprim charac
malian form of the enzyme.

Other Analogues of Para-Aminobenzoic A

Dapsone (4,4'-diaminodiphenyl su
specificity against the genus *Mycoba*
primarily in treating leprosy.

Para-aminosalicylic acid is wea

duction, although conjugal plasmid transfer does occur in some streptococci and other strains.

Resistance involving plasmids can result either from a change in the target reaction or, more commonly, by altering the drug before it reaches its target. Prominent examples of drug inactivation include the numerous β-lactamases and the enzymes that acetylate chloramphenicol or that modify aminoglycoside antibiotics by phosphorylation, acetylation, or adenylation. When resistance occurs by these methods, the target reaction itself is still in place, and the price paid by the cell for resistance is fairly small. Thus, some drug-resistant organisms are at only a slight disadvantage in the absence of antibiotic selection compared with their drug-sensitive relatives. Chapter 22 describes some of the genetic mechanisms that lead to acquisition and dissemination of antibiotic resistance and other virulence determinants.

Measurement of Antibiotic Susceptibility

The widespread distribution of antibiotic resistance in bacteria has made it necessary to determine the drug-susceptibility patterns of almost every clinical isolate. The physician requires information on the concentration of the antibiotic needed for growth inhibition. The lowest level of a drug sufficient to prevent growth of a bacterial

isolate is termed the minimum inhibitory concentration (MIC). It is determined by inoculating, under controlled conditions, a defined number of bacterial cells into tubes containing specified growth medium with increasing concentrations of an antibiotic. The MIC is directly measured in the Kirby-Bauer tube dilution test by determining which is the lowest concentration of a drug that is sufficient to prevent growth in a defined time period; however, this assay requires considerable material and effort.

Routinely, drug susceptibility tests are performed by dropping paper disks impregnated with a particular concentration of antibiotic onto a bacterial lawn that was prepared by seeding the test organism onto the surface of a suitable agar medium. The larger the size of the zone of inhibition of bacterial growth, the more sensitive the organism is to the drug (ie, the lower its MIC). The size of the zone of inhibition is correlated to the MIC by calibrations in which a large number of isolates of a bacterial species are simultaneously examined by the tube dilution and the agar plate diffusion techniques (Fig. 19-7). The importance of the MIC value for a particular bacterial isolate lies in comparison to the antibiotic levels that can be attained in serum or tissues on administration of the drug. Even if an antibiotic can inhibit bacterial growth, it would not be clinically effective unless its levels at the site of infection exceed the MIC for a sufficient period of time.

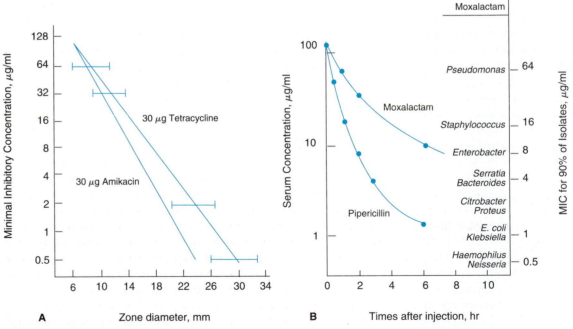

FIGURE 19-7   A. Comparison of antibiotic susceptibility of numerous bacterial isolates measured by tube-dilution method, in units of the minimum inhibitory concentration (MIC), versus the diameter of the zone of growth inhibition by the agar diffusion method. The thin line shows the correlation obtained with disks containing 30 μg of tetracycline, kanamycin, or cephalothin. The thick line was obtained with disks containing 30 μg of amikacin. The range of zone diameters seen with different isolates is indicated by the bars. **B.** Pharmacokinetics of two β-lactams, moxalactam and piperacillin, as a function of time after administration of 1 g of each antibiotic. Also shown are the levels of moxalactam needed to exceed the MIC of 90% of the isolates of the indicated genera.

Many antibiotics, including the inhibitors of cell-wall synthesis, can be bactericidal. The level of antibiotic effective for killing (at least a 100-fold decrease in viable cell numbers by 24 hours) is called the minimum bactericidal concentration (MBC). For effective bactericidal drugs, their MBC is near the MIC. Combinations of antibiotics frequently are administered, especially in seriously ill patients, before the invading pathogen has been identified. However, bacteriostatic drugs often are antagonistic to the bactericidal action of β-lactam and other antibiotics that can kill only growing cells. In contrast, combinations of bactericidal drugs, especially those with different targets, often are synergistic, giving a greater degree of killing than would either drug alone.

Physical and Chemical Methods for Sterilization

Bacteria and viruses are present on almost every exposed surface and must be eliminated from materials that will enter the human body or that have become contaminated by patients with contagious diseases. Their levels on other surfaces should be reduced by good housekeeping to reduce exposure to and transmission of infectious diseases. Sterilization is the general term for the absolute killing of all forms of life, whereas disinfection is a relative term referring to the inactivation or inhibition of growth of pathogenic microorganisms. The procedures to be employed depend on the nature of the object to be sterilized.

FACTORS AFFECTING KILLING OF MICROORGANISMS

The death of a microorganism is defined as the irreversible loss of its ability to reproduce and usually is determined by transferring the cells onto a rich agar medium and counting the number able to form colonies. Many lethal agents cause an exponential decrease in the number of survivors with time, such that a plot of the logarithm of the number of remaining viable cells versus time gives a straight line; in some cases, an initial lag occurs before onset of exponential killing. Exponential killing means that the probability of killing a given cell is constant and is independent of the number of other cells in the population that have already died. In other words, if half of the cells are killed by a certain dose of the lethal agent in a given time, then doubling the time of exposure will not kill all of the remaining cells, but only half of them. The death curve often deviates from this relationship as the number of survivors becomes small, perhaps because of the presence of a few variants having increased resistance to the lethal agent. This situation could be critical during the inactivation of a viral or bacterial culture for preparation of a vaccine, where complete sterilization is necessary, but prolonged use of the disinfectant impairs the immunogenicity of the vaccine.

The rate of killing by different agents can vary and some disinfectants show a linear relationship between concentration and killing, whereas other show more complex relationships, and a modest change in their concentration can have a dramatic effect on the rate of killing. The pH and temperature can have marked effects and it is not unusual for an increase of 10°C to double the rate of disinfection. Organisms more resistant to one lethal agent may not be more resistant to another one. The presence of organic material, such as serum, pus, or proteins, often protects bacteria against killing, perhaps because of the inactivation or dissipation of the disinfectant chemical by the extraneous proteins.

PHYSICAL AGENTS FOR STERILIZATION

Heat

Heat is the most frequently used method for killing microorganisms. It kills cells by damaging all macromolecular structures, particularly their nucleic acids and the cytoplasmic membrane. Moist heat is more rapid and effective at killing than dry heat. An autoclave provides a temperature of 121°C at 1.05 kg/cm^2 (15 lb/in^2) pressure. Such high temperatures are required to inactivate bacterial endospores, although temperatures of 80°C for 5 or 10 minutes are sufficient to kill essentially all vegetative cells. Moist heat is advantageous because the high heat conductivity of steam under pressure causes all parts of the sample to reach a lethal temperature rapidly. The autoclave should contain only pressurized steam, not air, and the steam should reach all parts of the object to be sterilized.

DRY HEAT. Dry heat kills cells by desiccation and by denaturation of their macromolecules. Dry heat is used to sterilize assembled objects whose interior parts could not be reached by steam, or powders or oily preparations that are either sensitive to water or are not permeable to steam. Sterilization with dry heat requires considerably higher temperatures than moist heat and usually is carried out at 160°C for 2 hours or more.

PASTEURIZATION. Because most vegetative cells are killed by lower temperatures than are required to kill spores, a variety of protocols collectively termed *pasteurization* are employed to rid heat-labile materials of certain undesired microorganisms. This approach was developed by Pasteur to prevent spoilage of beer and wine but is most commonly employed with milk. The milk is heated to 62.9°C for 30 minutes or to 71.6°C for 15 seconds, followed by rapid cooling. These treatments do not appreciably impair the taste of the product and do not sterilize the milk, but they do kill disease-producing bacteria commonly transmitted in milk, especially the agents of tuberculosis, brucellosis, and Q fever.

FREEZING. Although some bacteria are killed by cold, freezing is not a reliable method for sterilization. Repeated steps of freezing and thawing are more destructive than storage at freezing temperatures. Killing seems to be the result of the formation of icy crystals both inside and outside the cells. If ice formation is reduced by inclusion of glycerol or similar protectants, killing is greatly reduced, and freezing under these conditions provides a valuable method for the preservation of bacterial cultures.

Radiation

Several types of radiation can be used to kill microorganisms. Ionizing radiation includes x-rays (wavelengths from 0.1 to 40 nm) and gamma rays, which produce free radicals during the passage of high-energy photons through water. These free radicals form peroxides that act as powerful oxidizing agents. Other forms of damage are the denaturation of proteins and the breakage of DNA strands. Because of their great penetrating power, ionizing radiations are used for sterilization of a few pharmaceuticals and some plastic items. Food preservation has been attempted with ionizing rays, but changes in the quality of the food have prevented widespread acceptance.

ULTRAVIOLET LIGHT. Ultraviolet light refers to the wavelengths between x-rays and visible light, that is, from 40 to 390 nm. Maximal killing occurs at 260 nm, which is the wavelength for optimal absorption of light by nucleic acids (Fig. 19-8). Ultraviolet light causes the formation of cross-links that produce dimers between adjacent pyrimidine bases along a strand of the DNA. These dimers distort the structure of the DNA and interfere with the passage of the polymerases that catalyze its replication and transcription. All cells possess repair systems that eliminate the pyrimidine dimers, thereby promoting cell survival. The major limitation of ultraviolet light is its inability to penetrate glass, dirt, paper, pus, or more than a few layers of cells. Germicidal lamps (mercury vapor lamps) are used for control of airborne contamination in hospitals, food preparation establishments, and operating rooms.

Filtration

Solutions of heat-labile compounds that cannot be sterilized by heat or chemicals can be sterilized by filtration, which physically removes bacteria from the solution. Membrane filters are cellulose ester or polycarbonate membranes made with various pore sizes ranging from 8 to 0.025 μm. The filters can be sterilized by autoclaving. A pore size of 0.22 μm usually is effective in removing bacteria, but viruses and some mycoplasma can pass through this size pore.

Membrane filtration is used to quantitate the number of bacteria present in air or water samples. This is done by filtering a known quantity of the sample through the membrane and then placing the filter onto the surface of a nutrient agar medium (Fig. 19-9).

CHEMICAL AGENTS FOR STERILIZATION

Many chemicals have been used to kill or reduce the numbers of microorganisms. Vague terms such as antiseptic or disinfectant are applied to chemicals that are used topically or on inanimate objects, respectively, to destroy disease-producing microorganisms. The mechanisms by which the chemical agents affect microorganisms are diverse. Many of these agents have multiple modes of action, and the classifications given here are based on their major effect. The effectiveness of these agents is subject to many variables such as time of exposure, temperature, concentration, number and type of organisms present, and nature of the material being treated.

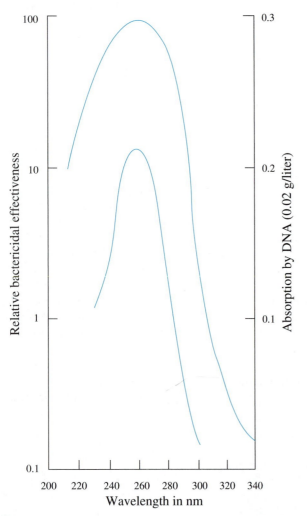

FIGURE 19-8 The top curve shows the bactericidal effectiveness of various wavelengths of ultraviolet light in killing bacteria. The bottom curve represents absorption by DNA. Notice that both curves peak at 260 nm, indicating that bacterial death caused by ultraviolet light is because of absorption by DNA.

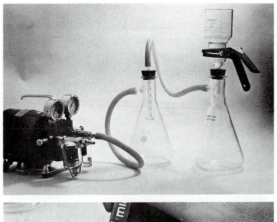

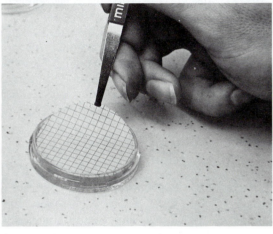

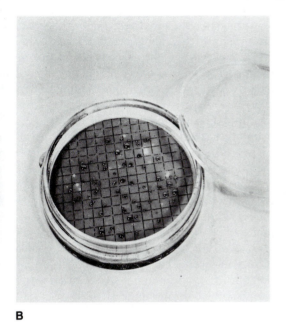

A   **B**

FIGURE 19-9 **A.** Membrane filter apparatus and membrane being laid on agar medium. **B.** Typical coliform colonies with metallic "sheen" on millipore filter.

Action on the Cytoplasmic Membrane

The cytoplasmic membrane provides for the retention of cellular constituents, and disinfectants that disrupt the arrangement of lipids and proteins in the membrane kill cells as a result of the release of metabolites and interference with active transport and energy metabolism. The most common agents for this task are soaps and detergents, which possess both polar hydrophilic and fat-soluble hydrophobic regions. The hydrophobic portions of the molecules are long-chain hydrocarbons, which insert into the nonpolar regions of the cell membranes. Detergents disrupt membranes by dissipating the forces that keep the nonpolar regions of the phospholipids out of the aqueous phase, thus allowing the membrane constituents to form into small vesicles rather than the large, organized structure. They have widespread use in the home and in industry as emulsifiers and wetting agents, and many have antimicrobial activity.

SURFACE-ACTIVE DISINFECTANTS. Many soaps and detergents are bactericidal, but their application in washing skin usually is too brief to allow appreciable killing of microorganisms on the skin surface, and their major effect is simply removal of bacteria along with dirt and oils. Much of the normal flora of the skin resides deep in the sweat glands and hair follicles. Fragile bacteria, such as gonococci, meningococci, and pneumococci, however, usually are killed by the action of even mild soaps or detergents.

Among the bactericidal surface-active agents, the quaternary ammonium detergents are the most effective. Their disruption of cell membranes is probably enhanced by the attraction between the positive charge on the detergent molecule and the negative charge on the cytoplasmic membrane; their effectiveness is greater at alkaline pH. Generally they are more effective against gram-positive bacteria, although at higher concentrations they also act against gram-negative organisms. Some anionic detergents (possessing a negative charge) display a rapid bactericidal activity, especially at acid pH, and are effective against most gram-negative organisms. Nonionic detergents are not useful, although some zwitterionic detergents having both positive and negative charges have been claimed to be as effective as, and less toxic than, the cationic detergents.

ALCOHOLS. Alcohols disrupt cellular membranes, the shorter chain homologues generally being the most effective. Ethanol is widely used at a concentration of 70%

and is lethal for all vegetative cells, provided a sufficient period of exposure is allowed. Alcohols are not useful, however, for inactivation of spores and should not be relied on for sterilization. Isopropyl and benzyl alcohols are more germicidal but have greater toxicity for humans than does ethanol.

PHENOLIC COMPOUNDS. Phenol and related compounds act primarily to cause membrane damage with loss of internal constituents, lysis, and death. Higher concentrations will inactivate proteins. Phenol (carbolic acid) was one of the first disinfectants to be used; it is effective in killing all vegetative cells but is less active against spores or nonenveloped viruses, and is toxic and highly caustic. Cresols, which are methyl substituted derivatives of phenol, are used in soap solutions as effective disinfectants for inanimate objects, although too irritating to be used on skin. They are sold as a 1% solution of cresol in soap under the trade name Lysol (L & F Products, Montvale, NJ).

Other substituted phenols are hexylresorcinol and the halogenated biphenyl hexachlorophene, which at one time was incorporated into many soaps and detergent preparations to increase their antimicrobial effectiveness. Hexachlorophene had been used for the daily bathing of infants and was effective in reducing colonization of the skin with *S aureus*. Studies showed that this compound was absorbed through the skin and caused significant neurotoxicity, and its use has since required a physician's prescription.

Agents That Act on Proteins

Many chemical agents act on enzymes or structural proteins. Acids, alkalis, phenols, and organic solvents denature proteins by disruption of their secondary and tertiary conformations. The widespread practice of using organic acids for preservation of food has been in long use and arose naturally through bacterial fermentation of plant sugars to the preservative lactic acid in such preparations as sauerkraut and pickles. Organic acids such as benzoic, acetic, citric, and propionic acids are added as food preservatives.

HALOGENS. Halogens, particularly iodine and chlorine, are widely used disinfectants. Both are bactericidal oxidizing agents that modify sulfhydryl, amino, indole, and phenolic groups. Chlorine and its derivative hypochlorites and chloramines react with water to form hypochlorous acid ($HClO$), which is a strong oxidizing agent. Hypochlorites are conveniently handled chemicals that dissociate to form hypochlorous acid:

$$Ca(OCl)_2 + 2\ H_2O \rightarrow Ca(OH)_2 + 2\ HOCl.$$

These chemicals are contained in household bleach products such as Clorox bleach (Clorox Co., Oakland, CA).

Iodine is widely used for disinfection of skin, especially in conjunction with alcohol swabbing. Iodine (I_2) is oxidized to form a reactive species that reacts with tyrosine and other residues on proteins. It can also form hypoiodous acid in a manner analogous to the reactions undergone by chlorine.

Iodine may be combined chemically with large carrier molecules, such as polyvinylpyrrolidone, to produce iodophors (*iodo*, iodine; *phor*, carrier). Iodophors are readily soluble in water and liberate free iodine slowly from the complex when dissolved. Commercially available iodophors, such as Betadine (Purdue Frederick Co., Norwalk, CT), Isodine, Ioprep, and Surgidine, are used as skin disinfectants, particularly for preparation for surgical procedures.

HYDROGEN PEROXIDE. Hydrogen peroxide is a weak, nontoxic antiseptic when used in 3% solutions. It is an oxidizing agent but has a short lifetime in tissues because of the presence of the enzyme catalase, which converts hydrogen peroxide to water and oxygen. The release of oxygen and free radicals may be part of the basis for its antibacterial action, especially in deep wounds where anaerobic bacteria are a problem.

SALTS OF HEAVY METALS. Salts of heavy metals, such as mercury, silver, arsenic, and others, can react with protein sulfhydryl groups. Various mercurials have been used for generations and include commercial preparations named Mercurochrome (Becton Dickinson & Company, Franklin Lakes, NJ). Phenylmercury salts also are fairly effective as disinfectants. The ability of mercurials to inhibit enzyme function is reversed by the presence of organic materials rich in sulfhydryl groups. Silver salts are widely used for the prophylactic treatment of newborn infants' eyes to prevent infection by gonococci. Other silver-containing preparations are employed in ophthalmic antiseptics and for topical application to burn patients. Arsenicals are widely used in wood preservation.

FORMALDEHYDE. Formaldehyde, glutaraldehyde, ethylene oxide, and β-propiolactone are alkylating agents that react irreversibly with sulfhydryl and amino groups on proteins:

$$R-SH + HCHO \rightarrow R-S-CH_2OH$$

$$R-NH_2 + HCHO \rightarrow R-NH-CH_2OH.$$

Formaldehyde is used in solutions for preservation of tissue samples and is effective against vegetative cells, fungi, viruses, and spores. It has been used in its gaseous phase for the decontamination of entire buildings. Glutaraldehyde is used increasingly as a sterilizing agent; it has an action similar to that of formaldehyde, but it is more effective.

ETHYLENE OXIDE. Ethylene oxide is an alkylating agent that is employed for sterilization. Given sufficient time to act, it is effective in killing vegetative cells spores and viruses.

Ethylene oxide   Beta-propiolactone

FIGURE 19-10 Chemical structures of gaseous disinfectants.

It is a gas above 10.8°C, and its vapors are able to penetrate even closed containers. It has proved useful for sterilizing heat-sensitive materials, including plastics and electronic and medical equipment. Some disadvantages include its potential toxicity and its high flammability unless diluted with an inert gas such as carbon dioxide.

The structures of ethylene oxide and the related β-propiolactone are shown in Figure 19-10. Their reactive oxide ring opens in the presence of a free amino, carboxyl, sulfhydryl, or hydroxyl group on a protein, resulting in the covalent attachment of a hydroxyethyl group to the protein. The chemical also reacts with nucleic acids and is mutagenic at sublethal doses. β-Propiolactone kills rapidly, and because it is quickly hydrolyzed to the volatile acrylic acid, it can be used to sterilize serum or bone grafts.

A Closer Look

Genetic Tricks for Immune Evasion: Changing Coats to Stick Around

It should be clear that pathogenic bacteria have evolved over many centuries to be effective parasites of their animal or human host. This successful parasitism must be accomplished in the face of the very powerful and multifaceted immune system of the host, whose nonspecific, humoral, and cell-mediated branches each bring highly efficient means for recognition and killing of invading organisms. Most encounters of a bacterium with a human result in the bacterium being rapidly eliminated, usually by the competition with the normal bacterial flora and by the action of the nonspecific defenses. Any successful parasite must be able to avoid or delay the immune elimination, both the nonspecific defenses and the very powerful specific immunity. Many mechanisms for evasion of the immune response are employed by different bacteria, and this section describes one of them.

Neisseria gonorrhoeae causes gonorrhea, a very common sexually transmitted disease responsible for at least 400,000 cases annually in the United States. The organism infects the cervix in women and the urethra in men and elicits a marked inflammatory response in most, but not all, of the colonized individuals. This inflammatory response results in a purulent (pus-filled) discharge, associated with pain during urination. The bacterium colonizes the columnar epithelial cells of the cervix and urethra, and can also colonize the mucosa of the throat and rectum. In women, the disease is usually limited to the cervix, and may be asymptomatic. Occasionally, the bacterial colonization can ascend into the uterus and fallopian tubes to cause salpingitis or pelvic inflammatory disease. This spread is quite serious, because the inflammatory response can result in scarring and irreversible blockage of the fallopian tubes. Consequences include infertility or ectopic pregnancy, which can be fatal. Further, in about 1% of colonized men or women, the bacteria can spread into the bloodstream, whence they commonly cause a crippling arthritis or, less commonly, endocarditis or meningitis. Thus, the bacterium must possess the ability to remain attached to the genitourinary tract or to release from them for passage through the epithelia to disseminate through the bloodstream. Several surface proteins are present on *N. gonorrhoeae* and undergo some very interesting alterations in their amount and their structure that appear to be related to these changes in bacterial location.

Adherence and invasion of epithelial cells is a feature of the disease. The bacteria attach to the cell surface by means of a filamentous pili, composed of a major protein subunit, encoded by the gene *pilE*. After the initial attachment via the pili, the bacteria adsorb tightly to the cell surface, forming an intimate association that can be followed by phagocytosis. The bacterial outer membrane protein called P.II or Opa is involved in this step. Variants of *N. gonorrhoeae* that have lost the ability to produce this protein arise upon growth in the laboratory and are detected owing to the change in opacity of their colonies. These variants are impaired in the ability to adhere to and invade epithelial cells. Another outer membrane protein, called P.I, serves as a general porin but also affects host cells that have phagocytosed the bacteria by blocking phago-lysosome fusion or attenuating the oxidative burst in neutrophils. Thus, there are at least three major surface proteins that contribute substantially to the process of bacterial infection. It would seem that antibody responses to these proteins would provide immunity against further infection, but such immunity does not occur.

All of these proteins exhibit phase variation, or the genetically reversible turning on and off of the genes for these proteins. Pili in particular also undergo a

A Closer Look *continued*

process called antigenic variation, in which pili of a different antigenic character are produced in random succession. A brief description of the mechanism of this antigenic variation of pilin structure follows. In most strains, there is a single gene that expresses the pilin protein subunit, and it is called *pilE*, indicating expression. Elsewhere on the chromosome are several clusters containing fragments of pilin genes having different sequences. These are not expressed and they are called the *pilS* loci, indicating silent genes. Occasionally, homologous recombination events bring about the transfer of the genetic information from one of the gene fragments in the silent loci to replace the sequences in the gene in the expressed gene, leading to a new DNA sequence at *pilE* and hence the production of a new pilin subunit with different antigenic character. The *pil* genes contain interspersed variable and constant regions, and any combination of the variable regions from any one of the silent genes can replace the corresponding portion at *pilE*, thereby greatly increasing the number of possible combinations of pilin sequences.

The homologous recombination can occur between the two distinct loci on the same chromosome. It is also proposed that recombination can occur following genetic transformation, or the uptake of free DNA from lysed cells or DNA that might be released as a normal process during bacterial growth. *N. gonorrhoeae* is continually competent to take up DNA that contains a specific recognition sequence. The frequency of antigenic variation is reduced but not eliminated by inclusion of DNase in the medium to degrade any transforming DNa, or in strains defective for transformation. The frequency of antigenic variation is fairly low, and one cell in 100 to 10,000 exhibit this variation. However, this frequency should be sufficient to allow the bacterial to continually evade the antibody response by allowing appearance of variants that do not bind the secretory antibody that will be generated to the dominant pilin and outer membrane protein epitopes that were expressed before the recombination event occurred.

Thus, the ability to vary the proteins on the bacterial surface by phase or antigenic variation provides a genetically efficient mechanism for continuous evasion of the humoral response. Other genes in other organisms are varied by different mechanisms. It is important to be aware of the existence of these processes of genetic variation, because their process has crucial consequences for the possibility of the development of effective vaccines.

Bibliography

JOURNALS

Davis BD. Mechanism of bactericidal action of aminoglycosides. Microbiol Rev 1987;51:341.

Matthews DA, Bolin JT, Burridge JM, Filman DJ, Volz KW, Kraut J. Dihydrofolate reductase: the stereochemistry of inhibitor selectivity. J Biol Chem 1985;260:392.

Shaw KJ, Rather PN, Hare RS, Miller GH. Molecular genetics of aminoglycoside resistance genes and familial relationships of the aminoglycoside-modifying enzymes. Microbiol Rev 1993;57:138.

Yunis AA. Chloramphenicol: relation of structure to activity and toxicity. Annu Rev Pharmacol Toxicol 1988;28:83.

BOOK

Bryan LE, ed. Antimicrobial drug resistance. Orlando, Academic Press, 1984.

Conte JE, Barriere SL. Manual of antibiotics and infectious diseases. ed 7. Malvern, PA, Lea and Febiger, 1992.

Franklin TJ, Snow GA, eds. Biochemistry of antimicrobial action. London, Chapman and Hall, 1989.

Moellering RC, ed. Frontiers in antimicrobial chemotherapy. Washington DC, American Society for Microbiology, 1993.

Essentials of Medical Microbiology, Fifth Edition, edited by Wesley A. Volk,
Bryan M. Gebhardt, Marie-Louise Hammarskjöld, and Robert J. Kadner.
Lippincott-Raven Publishers, Philadelphia © 1996.

Chapter 20

Bacteriophage

Viruses that infect bacteria are called *bacteriophages*, or simply phages. Any one phage can infect a limited number of bacterial species or types, but the vast number of different phages makes it likely that every type of bacterium is susceptible to some phage. Viruses are of interest because they provide easily studied systems of gene regulation and expression and the assembly of complex structures that can be models for cellular processes. They also play a role in the evolution of bacterial types and in the transmission of some virulence characters.

Chemical Composition and Structure

All phages consist of a nucleic acid enclosed by a protein coat, called a *capsid*. The structure of phages ranges from simple filaments and icosahedra, to complex forms, with tail structures that participate in phage attachment and nucleic acid injection into a host cell (Fig. 20-1).

The capsids of most phages exhibit icosahedral symmetry, which is the stable structure formed by 20 triangular sides; this is the pattern seen in geodesic domes and is described in more detail in Chapter 38. In some phages, the structure is elongated in one direction. Other phages have a filamentous or rod-shaped morphology, in which the monomeric units of a coat protein are wrapped around the nucleic acid in a helical fashion. There is considerable variability in the tail structures. Among the T phages that infect *Escherichia coli*, the tail of the T-even phages (T2, T4, T6) consists of a long hollow core surrounded by a contractile sheath that extends from an end plate to a collar immediately below the head. Attached to the base of the tail are six pins and six tail fibers that bind to specific receptor sites on the bacterial surface. In contrast, coliphages T1 and T5 do not possess a contractible sheath, and the tails of T3 and T7 are much shorter than those of the T-even phages.

The type of nucleic acid present in the phage particle varies, but no phage has more than one type. Although double-stranded DNA is the most common, single-stranded RNA or DNA is present in some phages; single-stranded phage DNA often is circular. The nucleic acids range in size from about 3000 bases, sufficient to encode

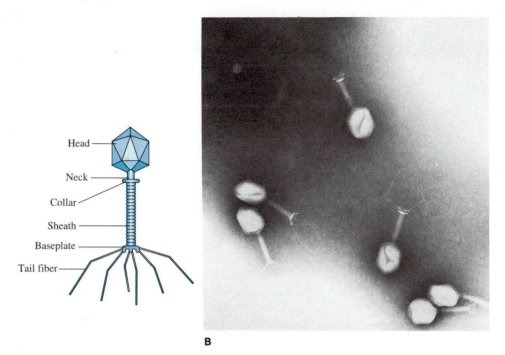

FIGURE 20-1   **A.** Anatomy of a T2 bacteriophage. **B.** Isolated, negatively stained T2 phages.

three or four proteins, up to 150,000 base pairs in the case of coliphage T4, which encodes more than 150 proteins.

Phage Multiplication

The basic sequence of events that occurs during viral replication is similar for most phages, although there is considerable variability with respect to the number of phage proteins made and the degree of takeover of host function. Much of the following description is applicable to any phage, but the specific details concern the life cycle of phage T4, one of the T-even phages and perhaps the most complex phage known and the one that exhibits the greatest degree of takeover of host function.

ADSORPTION

The ability of a particular phage to infect a cell is determined primarily by its ability to recognize and bind to specific receptor sites on the bacterial cell surface. Recognition occurs through structures present on the tip of the phage tail. Infection cannot occur in the absence of adsorption, and bacterial mutants unable to synthesize the specific phage receptor are resistant to infection by that type of phage. Any component on the bacterial surface can serve as receptor for some phage. Known receptors include specific sugars in the outer membrane lipopolysaccharide, capsules, pili, flagella, and specific proteins in the cell wall. Initial adsorption does not require the input of energy, although the subsequent steps of nucleic

acid entry usually are energy dependent, a system that is designed to reduce loss of phages by their adsorption to debris from dead cells.

PENETRATION

After adsorption, most phages inject their nucleic acid into the bacterial cytoplasm and leave their protein capsid outside. When the T-even phages adsorb to the receptor on a live bacterium, the sheath contracts, forcing the hollow interior tail tube through the bacterial cell wall. Because most other phages, including T1 and T5, do not possess a contractile sheath, the syringe-like mechanism of DNA injection is not a common feature. Many coliphages appear to inject their nucleic acid at adhesion sites where the inner and outer membranes are in contact, suggesting that these sites might allow the most efficient entry of the phage nucleic acid into the cytoplasm. Some idea of the magnitude of the injection task can be gained from the length of the T2 DNA molecule seen in Figure 20-2.

PHAGE DNA TRANSCRIPTION

The steps involved in the transcription of phage DNA vary considerably from one phage to another. Phage T4 transcription occurs in several distinct stages to form immediate-early, delayed-early, and late gene products. The total transcription and translation of T4 DNA produces almost 200 proteins, of which about a quarter are present

Some delayed-early genes code for enzymes that produce a new nucleotide base, 5-hydroxymethylcytosine (5-HMC), which substitutes for cytosine in the phage DNA. Another enzyme transfers a molecule of glucose to the hydroxyl group on the 5-HMC, and another enzyme is made that causes dephosphorylation of deoxycytidine triphosphate (dCTP) to deoxycytidine diphosphate (dCDP) and deoxycytidine monophosphate (dCMP) to ensure that no cytosine can be incorporated into the phage DNA. One reason these DNA modifications are important factors in the survival of the phage and in the takeover of the infected cell is because bacterial restriction enzymes cannot cleave phage DNA that contains glycosylated 5-HMC in place of cytosine. Moreover, phage-coded nucleases degrade any DNA that contains unsubstituted cytosine. Other delayed-early gene products include DNA polymerase and ligase to replicate the phage DNA and enzymes that modify the host RNA polymerase a second time to change its promoter specificity.

Late genes are expressed only after the phage DNA has replicated. Late gene products include the structural components for the new phage particles, including heads, tails, and fibers. Late products also include the phage lysozyme, which will degrade the bacterial cell wall to liberate the mature phage particles.

ASSEMBLY AND RELEASE

The phage structural proteins and nucleic acid are assembled in definite pathways to form the mature progeny phage particle, as outlined in Figure 20-3. Separate assem-

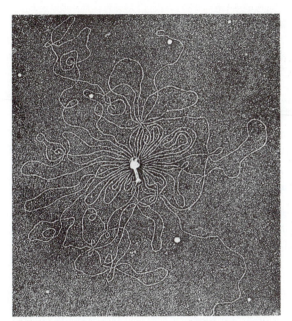

FIGURE 20-2 The DNA molecule of a T-even phage released from the head by osmotic shock. Note the empty phage capsid in the center of the electron micrograph and the two ends of the DNA molecule at the lower right and top center. (Approximate magnification ×60,000.)

in the completed phage particle. Immediate-early genes are transcribed using the existing host RNA polymerase; early genes encode nucleases that hydrolyze host cell DNA and enzymes that alter the bacterial RNA polymerase so that it preferentially transcribes the delayed-early group of phage genes.

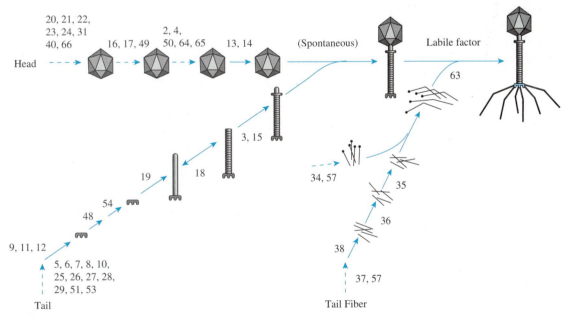

FIGURE 20-3 The morphogenetic pathway of phage T4 maturation has three principal branches leading independently to the formation of heads, tails, and tail fibers, which then combine to form complete phage particles. The numbers refer to the T-even phage genes whose products are involved at each step. The solid arrows indicate the steps that have been shown to occur in extracts.

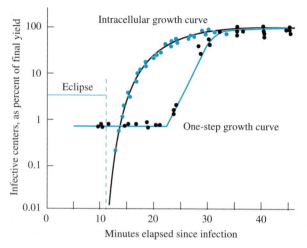

FIGURE 20-4 Intracellular growth kinetics of phage T4. Note that no intact phage exists during the eclipse, but intracellular phage particles can be detected by disruption of the bacterium after about 12 minutes (*open circles*). Without artificial disruption to release intracellular phages, the number of infective centers outside the cell follows the one-step growth curve, showing a sharp rise at the end of the burst time, when the bacterium is lysed and the phage liberated.

bly processes lead to the formation of subparticles such as the head, tail, and fibers. Mutational loss of any phage protein halts the synthesis of its subparticle, usually at the state where the missing protein should be added. Part of the assembly process is spontaneous and does not require the action of other enzymes, but some proteins are involved in assembly and are not present in the finished phage particle. These include a scaffolding protein that maintains the size and shape of the prehead before entry of the nucleic acid; this protein subsequently is degraded by a phage-coded protease. Note that the head does not assemble around the nucleic acid; rather, an empty head is produced first, and the nucleic acid is stuffed inside. Nucleic acid packaging remains an interesting topic, especially because the nucleic acid usually is packaged from a concatenate, that is, a long molecule containing multiple repeated lengths of viral chromosome.

Phage replication can be plotted as a one-step growth curve, as shown in Figure 20-4. During the first 10 minutes after phage DNA injection, no phage can be recovered, even after disrupting the infected cell. By the end of this eclipse period (the time between phage injection and the first appearance of completed phage inside the cell), mature phage particles accumulate inside the cell up to the time cell lysis occurs. The number of intracellular phages increases from about 12 minutes until 34 minutes after infection, but extracellular phages are not seen until lysis. The yield of phages per infected cell is called the *burst size* (100 to 300 phages), and the time from infection until lysis is called the *latent period* (20 to 40 minutes).

RNA PHAGES

Several RNA-containing phages adsorb to the F pilus of male bacteria (see Conjugation, Chap. 21). When the

phage RNA enters the cell, it is translated directly into proteins by the host ribosomes. One of the proteins thus formed is an RNA-dependent RNA polymerase that replicates the phage RNA by first forming a double-stranded RNA (replicative form) and then producing multiple progeny single strands of RNA using the replicative form as template. As the newly formed strands of RNA are released from the replicative intermediate, they assemble with the capsid proteins and are ready to be released.

ASSAY OF PHAGES

Phages usually are detected and counted by mixing a dilution of the phage sample with an excess of susceptible bacteria to ensure that only one phage infects any one cell. After adsorption has taken place, the mixture is plated on a solid growth medium to form a bacterial lawn. Each phage in the sample goes through many cycles of replication and causes lysis of the cells surrounding each originally infected cell. The result is a plaque, or clear area in the bacterial lawn, produced by each phage present in the original dilution (Fig. 20-5). The number of phages in the original sample can be calculated by multiplying the number of plaques by the dilution factor.

Phage Genetics

Genetic studies of viruses reveal the location of the genes for all phage-coded proteins, the effect of the loss of individual proteins on phage growth, and the regulation of each gene's expression. Some phage mutants can be identified on the basis of altered plaque size or shape, but most mutations prevent viral replication. Thus, to study

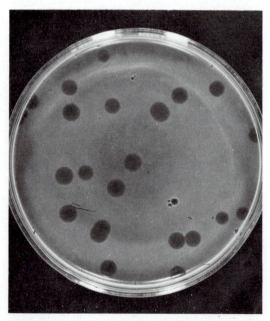

FIGURE 20-5 Plaques in a bacterial lawn are caused by lysis of the bacteria in the vicinity of a cell infected by a single bacteriophage.

phage genetics, conditional lethal mutants are used, which can complete a cycle of replication under some conditions but not under others. Temperature-sensitive mutants are unable to replicate at 42°C but can do so at 30°C. Other types of mutants are able to grow on one host bacterium but not on another strain, even though both strains support the growth of the wild-type phage. Phages carrying nonsense mutations can grow only in hosts carrying nonsense suppressor mutations.

Phage genetic crosses are carried out by simultaneously infecting a bacterium with two different phage mutants, neither of which can replicate in the host cell by itself. If the mutations in the two phages are located in different genes, each mutant phage provides the function the other phage lacks, resulting in the release of about normal numbers of phage particles from the infected cell. This procedure is called a *complementation test* and shows whether two mutations are in the same or different genes. In addition to the progeny phage of parental genotypes recovered from a cross, recombinant phage also is released, in which a homologous recombination event has occurred between the sites of the mutations in the two parental phages. Recombination results in the production of phage possessing a nondefective genome. The frequency of formation of recombinant molecules provides information about the distance between the two mutations and their order with respect to a third gene. The closer two mutations are to each other, the less likely it is that a recombination event will occur between them; thus, recombination frequency is related to physical distance between the two sites.

Temperate Phages and Lysogeny

The previous sections described virulent phages that invariably cause cell lysis. These phages form clear plaques, because every cell of the lawn in the vicinity of the original phage particle is likely to be lysed (with the exception of the rare bacterial mutants that are resistant to the phage because of their inability to produce the phage receptor). Many other phages produce turbid plaques, because not all the infected bacteria are killed. One example of this phenomenon includes the filamentous *E coli* phages fd and M13, whose genomes are circular single-stranded DNA molecules. These phages are not released from the cell by lysis but instead are continually extruded from the cell surface, although the infected bacterium remains viable but grows at a reduced rate. Thus, the plaques seen with these phages are not the result of cell lysis but of the slowed growth rate. This type of viral release also occurs with many animal viruses.

The most common group of phages that produce turbid plaques are called *temperate phages*. The infection of a cell by a temperate phage has two possible courses. In some infected cells (usually the majority), phage multiplication, assembly, and release occurs in a manner similar to that carried out by virulent phages. Alternatively, the lytic pathway can be turned off by the repression of most phage genes. The repressed phage genome remains within the cell as a *prophage*, replicating in synchrony with the bacterial chromosome, so that each progeny cell contains a prophage.

Bacteria that carry a prophage are termed *lysogens*, because the prophage retains the potential to lyse its host bacterium. Cultures of lysogenic bacteria contain free phage particles, as a result of the failure of repression in a few cells in the population (about one in 10^6), which return to the lytic process and release a normal burst of phage.

Lysogenic cells are immune to superinfection by the same phage, which explains their growth within the turbid plaque. Temperate phages commonly are found in clinical isolates of gram-positive and gram-negative bacteria and, in some cases, contribute to the pathogenicity of the organism.

MECHANISM OF LYSOGENY

The temperate phages possess a mechanism to repress their lytic functions. The choice of lysis or lysogeny is understood best for coliphage λ (Fig. 20-6). All temperate phages carry a gene encoding a repressor protein that blocks the expression of its replication and lytic functions. Genes that contribute to the control of the lysogenic state often are called *c* genes (*cI* in the case of λ), because a phage carrying a mutation affecting them can no longer repress its lytic expression and forms clear plaques. The repressor protein (also called *immunity repressor*) is specific for its own phage and will not prevent the multiplication of phages with different immunity specificity. The phage-coded repressor binds to specific operator sites on the phage genome. In coliphage λ, two promoter–operator sites, located on each side of the *cI* gene, are responsible for the transcription of the early phage genes and are necessary for the expression of all lytic functions. The λ *cI* repressor binds to specific sequences in these two operator regions and blocks the binding of RNA polymerase, thereby preventing transcription from those promoters. Repressor not only binds to the operator sites on the prophage that produced it, but also acts on any phage λ DNA that subsequently infects the cell. This is the basis for superinfection immunity.

Phage mutants that do not make a functional *cI* repressor form clear plaques on sensitive cells but do not form plaques on bacteria that are lysogenic for phage λ, because the mutant phage still has the operator sites and, therefore, is still repressed by the repressor present in the lysogenic cell. Phage mutants that can form plaques on lysogenic bacteria are called *virulent mutants*, and they are altered in both operator sites so that the repressor binds poorly.

The actual mechanism involved in the regulation of the choice of lysis or lysogeny in phage λ is much more

Transformation

Bacterial transformation is the genetic transfer process whereby cells take up free DNA from the medium. This system is of historical importance, because it provided the first demonstration that DNA is the genetic material of the cell. This story began with experiments carried out in 1928 by the English physician Frederick Griffith, who described the apparent transformation of one type of pneumococcus (*Streptococcus pneumoniae*) into another type of the same species. About 100 distinct types of pneumococci exist and are divided on the basis of the composition of their capsule (see Chaps. 17 and 23). Smooth, encapsulated pneumococci are extremely virulent for mice, whereas rough, nonencapsulated variants are avirulent. Griffith mixed live, nonencapsulated cells that originally had produced a capsule of one antigenic type with heat-killed, smooth cells of a different capsular type (Fig. 21-1). Neither preparation alone caused disease in mice, but injection of the mixture of the two preparations was lethal, and the blood of the mice infected with the mixture contained live pneumococci having a capsule of the same antigenic type as that of the heat-killed cells. Oswald Avery, Colin MacLeod, and Maclyn McCarty showed in 1942 that DNA was the transforming principle that was released from the heat-killed bacteria and was able to confer on a live recipient cell the ability to make a new type of capsule. The DNA that was taken up by the rough cells supplied the genetic information needed to make the missing enzyme needed for capsule synthesis.

Transformation, or the uptake of free DNA, occurs in numerous organisms other than *S pneumoniae*, including members of the genera *Bacillus, Haemophilus, Campylobacter, Neisseria,* and *Rhizobium.* There appear to be significant differences in the mechanism of transformation in the gram-positive and gram-negative bacteria.

NATURE OF THE DNA

The DNA released from a donor organism by cell lysis consists of fragmented double strands with molecular weights ranging from 300,000 to 10 million. Each fragment represents less than 1% of the donor genome. Several fragments can be taken up by any recipient cell, but the amount of genetic information acquired during transformation is small, even less than that obtained in transduction. The DNA must be double stranded to be taken into the recipient cell. In most bacterial cultures, not all cells in a population are able to assimilate DNA. Those that can are called *competent cells,* and the state of competence usually is exhibited only during a certain stage of the growth phase, often early stationary phase. The competent state is manifested by the presence of surface structures necessary for efficient binding and entry of DNA. Once inside the cell, the genetic information on the DNA fragment can be expressed. However, bacteria possess mechanisms that prevent the expression of heterologous DNA from organisms that are not closely related to the recipient species, thereby avoiding the inheritance of traits that might be incompatible with the recipient organism.

TRANSFORMATION IN GRAM-POSITIVE CELLS

In *Streptococcus* and *Bacillus,* double-stranded DNA binds to proteins on the surface of competent cells, and is taken into the cells by an energy-dependent process in which one of the DNA strands is broken down during uptake, leaving a molecule of single-stranded DNA inside the cell. The hydrolysis of one strand appears to be necessary for uptake of the other strand, and mutants lacking the surface-bound nucleases are deficient in DNA uptake. The genetic information carried on the single-stranded molecules cannot be expressed immediately. Instead, the trans-

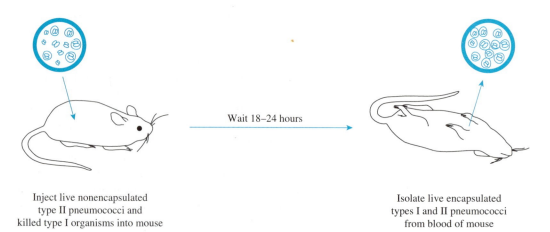

Inject live nonencapsulated type II pneumococci and killed type I organisms into mouse

Wait 18–24 hours

Isolate live encapsulated types I and II pneumococci from blood of mouse

FIGURE 21-1   Griffith's original transformation experiment. The isolation of living, encapsulated type I pneumococci from the mouse could occur only if some genetic substance from the killed type I organisms was able to enter the nonencapsulated type II cells. This genetic substance was subsequently shown to be DNA.

forming DNA molecule must integrate into the host-cell chromosome by homologous recombination to be converted to the double-stranded form and to be permanently integrated into the chromosome and genetic repository of the recipient cell. If the DNA taken up during transformation is not homologous with the recipient chromosome, the single-stranded piece will not be able to integrate or be expressed. Thus, the specificity for transformation is determined directly by the presence of homologous DNA sequences able to participate in genetic recombination.

TRANSFORMATION IN GRAM-NEGATIVE CELLS

In the gram-negative bacteria, *Haemophilus* (competent in stationary phase) and *Neisseria* (always competent), a different mechanism of DNA uptake occurs. Competent cells have special DNA-binding structures on the surface of the outer membrane. Both homologous and heterologous DNA can bind to this surface complex, but only DNA from closely related species is taken up efficiently, and the heterologous DNA is excluded. This specificity results from the fact that the uptake process recognizes a specific sequence of 10 to 14 base pairs, which is present about every 4000 base pairs in DNA of the same species, but is much less common in DNA from other organisms. The actual mechanism of DNA uptake from the membrane vesicles has not been fully elucidated.

SIGNIFICANCE OF TRANSFORMATION

It is difficult to judge whether transformation plays an important role in the transmission of traits involved in bacterial virulence. Free DNA is released from bacteria after their lysis, but it is susceptible to shearing forces and nuclease degradation. Moreover, only a small proportion of the cells in a population are competent, and the expression of transforming DNA requires that it come from a homologous organism, thereby reducing the spread of information among different organisms. In most cases, transforming DNA is released by lysis of the donor cell, meaning that transformation does not result in a net increase in the number of organisms having a particular genotype. Chapter 22 describes several genetic processes in which transformation has been suggested to be involved, namely, phase variation of the gonococcal pili and the development of chimeric penicillin-binding proteins that are resistant to β-lactam action.

Transformation has been useful for the genetic mapping of the bacterial chromosome, because the frequency of inheritance of two genetic characters is a measure of the distance between them on the chromosome. Transformation also is a critical tool for the introduction of recombinant DNA molecules into bacterial cells. This type of transformation was made possible by the finding that many bacterial species that do not naturally exhibit competence can become competent after treatment with solutions of $CaCl_2$ or other salts. These treatments appear to produce cracks in the surface membrane, providing a route for DNA entry. Another method for introduction of DNA into bacteria is called electroporation, in which cells are exposed in the presence of DNA to steep electrical gradients.

Restriction and Modification

Bacteria possess mechanisms to eliminate DNA that was taken up by genetic exchange with unrelated organisms. Some of the specificity comes from the nature of the homologous recombination pathways that integrate the newly acquired DNA into the recipient cell chromosome. In addition, almost all microorganisms produce *restriction endonucleases,* enzymes that cleave DNA at or near specific sequences. A cell's own DNA, and DNA from closely related species, is resistant to cleavage by the resident restriction endonucleases by virtue of specific modifications of the DNA, often methylation of a base within the recognition sequence. DNA that enters a cell by genetic transfer can be degraded, unless it is modified at the sites appropriate for the recipient cell, even though it is properly modified by the restriction—modification system of the donor cell.

Restriction does not present an absolute barrier, although it reduces the recovery of foreign DNA by a factor of 10^2 to 10^5. The restriction—modification system is effective against phage DNA, although some phages possess mechanisms to inactivate the restriction systems of recipient cells.

Conjugation

Conjugation is the transfer of DNA that occurs during contact between bacterial cells. This mechanism is much more efficient than transformation or transduction, and does not require the destruction of the donor cell. Transfer of DNA by conjugation is rare in gram-positive bacteria (and occurs by a fundamentally different mechanism) but common among gram-negative bacteria. It is the major mechanism for the transfer of drug resistance and can occur between unrelated genera. Conjugation is dependent on the presence in the donor cells of plasmids that code for DNA transfer functions. Plasmids are nonessential extrachromosomal genetic elements that provide additional useful genetic information. Not all plasmids confer the ability to serve as a donor in conjugation.

Conjugation was discovered in *Escherichia coli* by Joshua Lederberg and Edward Tatum in 1946, and most early work was concerned with the transfer of the bacterial

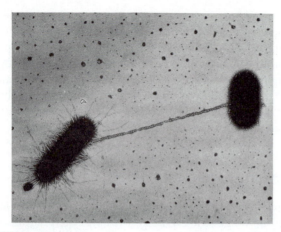

FIGURE 21-2 Initiation of conjugation in *Escherichia coli*. The male cell (with numerous short pili) is connected to the female bacterium by an F pilus, as described in the text. (Original magnification ×3000.)

chromosome from one cell to another. It is now clear that chromosome transfer is a relatively rare event mediated by only a few plasmids, whereas plasmid transfer occurs frequently.

PLASMID TRANSFER

DNA transfer during bacterial conjugation is a one-way process; there is no cell fusion and formation of diploid cells, as occurs in eucaryotes. Every donor cell contains a self-transmissible plasmid that bears the *tra* (for transfer) operon whose 20 to 25 genes encode the structures and enzymes necessary for conjugation. One essential structure on donor cells is the *traA*-encoded sex pilus, a long filament that is made up of a single polypeptide (called *pilin*) and protrudes from the cell surface. The sex pilus can be distinguished from the many other fimbriae a cell can possess because, in general, the sex pilus is longer, is present in few copies (3 to 10 per cell), and is the site of binding of male-specific phages that adsorb to the tip or sides of the pilus (Fig. 21-2). When a donor cell comes into contact with a recipient cell, plasmid transfer involves the following steps (Fig. 21-3):

1. The tip of the sex pilus has lectin activity, allowing it to bind to a polysaccharide on the surface of recipient cells. A donor cell has several sex pili and can interact simultaneously with several recipients, resulting in a mating aggregate.
2. Stimulated by the contact, the sex pilus appears to withdraw into the donor cell by dissolving its pilin subunits in the cytoplasmic membrane. Retraction of the pilus brings the recipient cell into intimate contact with the donor cell, leading to the formation of a conjugal bridge through which DNA, but few cellular proteins, can be transferred.

3. The *traYZ* gene-dependent endonuclease specifically cleaves one strand of the plasmid DNA at a site called the *origin of transfer*. The origin of transfer (*oriT*) is different from the origin (*oriV*) used during normal plasmid DNA replication.
4. The 5' end of the cleaved plasmid strand is covalently linked to *tra*-coded proteins and is threaded through the conjugation bridge into the recipient cell by the action of other *tra* gene-coded enzymes.
5. Although not essential for the DNA transfer process to occur, both the transferred strand and the strand remaining in the donor are copied by DNA polymerases, yielding double-stranded circular copies of the plasmid in both cells.
6. After DNA transfer, the conjugation bridge breaks down, and the two cells separate. The *tra* genes are expressed in the cell that acquired the plasmid, so that it too becomes a donor cell.

Unlike transformation and transduction, in which the transfer or expression of the donor DNA occurs only among closely related species, plasmid transfer by conjugation exhibits much less specificity. Some broad-host-range plasmids can transfer themselves into and out of many different species of gram-negative bacteria. The efficiency of plasmid transfer can be extremely high, approaching 100% of the donor cells. Because the recipient cell can express *tra* functions shortly after acquiring a self-transmissible plasmid, the number of cells that have inherited a plasmid during a period of mating can greatly exceed the original number of donor cells. In most cases, the expression of a plasmid's transfer functions is subject to regulation by a repressor, so that cells that have newly acquired a conjugal plasmid gradually reduce their transfer ability. A plasmid that has lost this autoregulation is the F plasmid.

CHROMOSOME TRANSFER

The best-studied self-transmissible plasmid or sex factor is called *F* (for fertility). The F plasmid is about 100 kilobases in size and its *tra* operon occupies about 33 kilobases. No other easily recognized traits are carried on this plasmid. Conjugation between an F+ donor cell carrying an F plasmid and a recipient (F−) cell results in the rapid and efficient transfer of the F plasmid to the recipient cell. F+ cells transfer the donor cell chromosome at a much lower frequency than plasmid transfer, and most chromosomal genes are transferred with the same low frequency. Rare variants, in which the F plasmid has integrated into the chromosome, can be isolated from a population of F+ cells. Such cells are able to transfer portions of the host chromosome at frequencies approaching that at which F+ cells transfer the F plasmid.

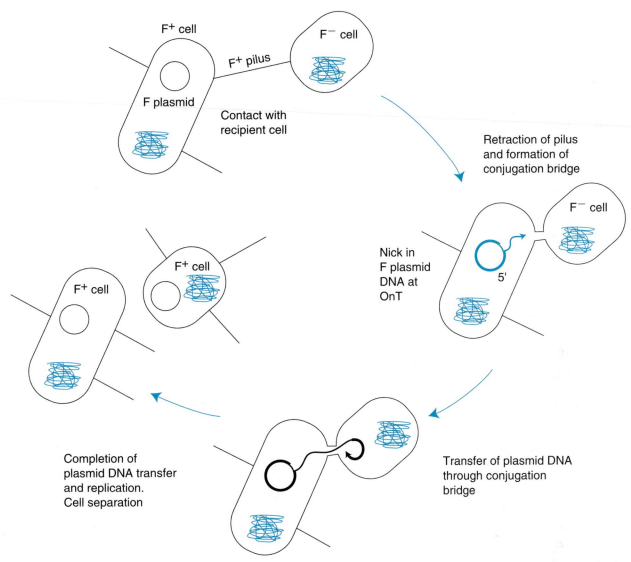

FIGURE 21-3 Simplified model of a sex pilus–dependent plasmid transfer. After the formation of a conjugation bridge, one strand of the plasmid DNA is nicked at a specific site (*oriT*) by a plasmid-encoded endonuclease. The 5′ end of the nicked DNA (possibly attached to a protein) then is transferred to the recipient. Both exposed single-stranded regions are replicated simultaneously (*dashed lines*) during the transfer process.

These cells are called *Hfr cells* to indicate that they give rise to a high frequency of chromosomal recombinants.

Transfer of the bacterial chromosome from an Hfr cell begins at the site of integration of the F factor (the origin of transfer) and proceeds around the chromosome in a fixed direction (Fig. 21-4). Chromosome transfer proceeds in exactly the same manner as F plasmid transfer, with nicking at *oriT* and 5′-to-3′ transfer of single-stranded DNA. Although the entire donor-cell chromosome can be transferred in about 120 minutes, this process is subject to spontaneous interruption, and the probability that a specific chromosomal gene will be transferred depends on the distance of that gene from the origin of

transfer. The constant rate of chromosome transfer allowed construction of the genetic map based on the time of mating required for the entry of the donor allele of a gene into the recipient cell; the mating process can be interrupted at defined intervals by vigorous agitation. The *E coli* chromosome map is divided into minutes, based on the rate of transfer of the genes. The map location of a gene also can be estimated from the frequency of inheritance of one gene relative to the frequency at which other known genes are acquired, because the likelihood of inheriting a donor-cell gene is an exponential function of the distance of that gene from the origin of transfer. The orientation of the integrated F factor is such that the

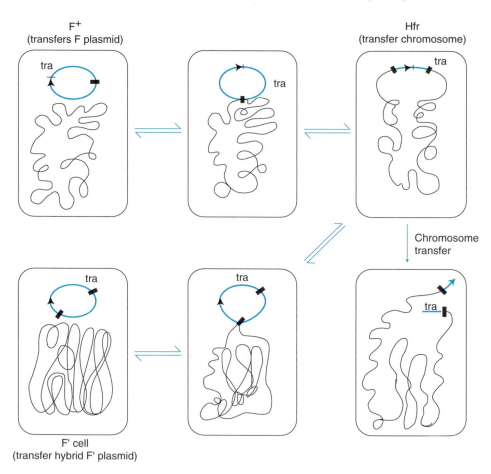

FIGURE 21-4   Transfer of the bacterial chromosome by Hfr cells containing an integrated F factor. DNA transfer to a recipient begins at *oriT* and proceeds to transfer the bacterial chromosome. The *tra* region of the F factor itself is transferred to the recipient only if the entire chromosome is transferred, a rare event. As described for phage λ, the integrated F plasmid can be excised from the chromosome in either a precise manner (reforming an F⁺ cell) or an imprecise manner, generating an F′ hybrid plasmid.

tra genes are the last to be transferred and, thus, few recipients of the transferred chromosome become donor cells.

F-PLASMID INTEGRATION

Integration of the F plasmid into the bacterial chromosome to form an Hfr strain does not occur at random locations. There appears to be a limited number of sites (less than 10) in any bacterial cell into which F can recombine and remain there in a stable state, and there are two mechanisms that determine the sites of integration. The first mechanism occurs by homologous recombination between short (800 to 1500 base pairs) sequences present on both the F plasmid and the chromosome. The regions of homology are called *insertion sequences,* and because they are capable of transposition (described later), they are found in various locations in the chromosomes of different isolates of the same bacterial species. The small size of the insertion sequences, relative to the entire plasmid, accounts for the low frequency at which the recombinational event occurs. The second mechanism for integration of F involves another region of the F plasmid called the *τδ transposon,* which mediates the integration of the F plasmid at random sites in the bacterial chromosome, as described in the section on transposons. Formation of a cointegrate that fuses the F plasmid and chromosome

also is a rare event, and the infrequent occurrence of both these mechanisms accounts for the rarity of F plasmid integration and the low degree of chromosome transfer in an F⁺ culture.

Excision of the F Plasmid

The circular F plasmid integrates into the bacterial chromosome by a single recombinational event similar to the integration of phage λ, and the reverse can occur to excise the F factor from the chromosome. Abnormal excision also can occur to create an F′ plasmid carrying bacterial genes from one or both sides of the site where the F factor had integrated, as shown in Figure 21-4. An F′ plasmid is capable of autonomous replication and conjugal transfer, thus providing another method by which chromosomal genes can be dispersed throughout a bacterial population. F′ plasmids have been useful in the formation of cells that are diploid for a portion of the chromosome.

CONJUGATION IN GRAM-POSITIVE BACTERIA

Cell-to-cell transfer of DNA occurs in some gram-positive bacteria by different mechanisms than in gram-negative organisms. One of these mechanisms that operates in *Enterococcus* (formerly *Streptococcus*) *faecalis* is associated with the presence of specific plasmids, but there is no indication of the existence of adhesive sex pili. Instead, donor cells produce an adhesive substance after they detect a pheromone produced by suitable recipient cells. The adhesive material causes the aggregation of donor and recipient cells, and DNA transfer occurs, but the mechanism for this is not clear.

Another transfer mechanism in gram-positive bacteria involves an unusual conjugative transposon, a genetic element that mediates its own transfer from cell to cell and its integration into random sites on the recipient cell's chromosome. This conjugative transposon can be transferred among a fairly wide range of bacterial genera.

Recombination

A chromosomal fragment that enters a recipient cell by any of the DNA transfer mechanisms cannot replicate or be inherited by progeny cells unless it integrates into the recipient-cell chromosome by homologous recombination (also called generalized, or *rec*-dependent, recombination). Recombination is an extremely important process and most recombination-deficient mutants grow poorly and have a multitude of defects. Homologous recombination is an essential step of meiosis in eucaryotic organisms and probably occurs by a similar mechanism as in bacteria.

HOMOLOGOUS RECOMBINATION

The homologous recombination system carries out crossover events between regions of DNA having similar or identical sequences. If the regions of homology are on the same DNA molecule, recombination results in either the deletion or the inversion of the region between the homologous regions, depending on the relative orientation of the recombining segments. Recombination between different DNA molecules requires one crossover event if the incoming fragment is circular, but two (or an even number) events for integration of a linear segment, so that the circular bacterial chromosome is not disrupted.

The reactions involved in the formation of a recombination joint are carried out by host enzymes encoded by the *rec* (for recombination) genes. The basic model for homologous recombination (Fig. 21-5), developed by Robin Holliday, begins with the synapsis or alignment of homologous DNA double helices. The longer the homologous regions, the higher the likelihood of recombination, and a minimum length of homology of about 50 base pairs is necessary for RecA-mediated recombination to occur. If a nick occurs on one duplex, the single-stranded end can invade the homologous region of the other duplex, displacing one of the double strands. Nicking and ligation of invading strands to resident strands results in a crossover junction structure, in which one strand of each duplex is linked to the corresponding strand of the other duplex. This crossover branch can move

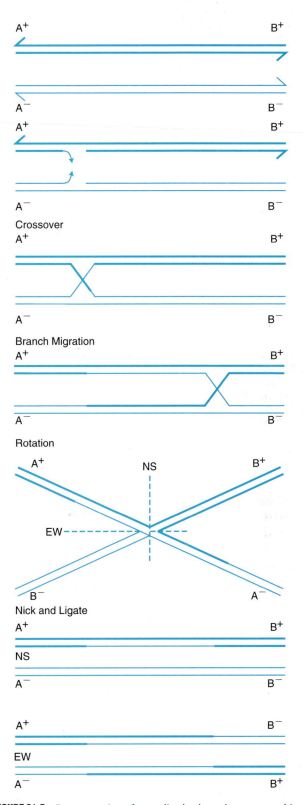

FIGURE 21-5 Representation of generalized or homologous recombination. The pairing of homologous chromosomes is followed by nicking and strand exchange to form the Holliday junction. Branch migration can occur readily to create regions of heteroduplex where two strands in a double helix came from different parents. Isomerization of the Holliday structure by rotation of the ends leaves the symmetric intermediate. The strands can be cleaved and ligated in either a north–south or an east–west direction to create products without or with crossover of the flanking markers, respectively.

rapidly along the helices by a spontaneous process called branch migration, which results in the formation of heteroduplex regions in which the two paired strands came originally from the two different parental DNA molecules. Action of an endonuclease and a DNA ligase can resolve the crossover structure to form duplex recombinant molecules.

The multifunctional RecA protein, encoded by the *E coli recA* gene, plays essential roles in homologous recombination, which is reduced by a factor at least 10^{-5} in the absence of the *recA* product. Single-stranded DNA binds to the RecA protein with high affinity and activates its coprotease function, which results in cleavage of the LexA repressor and induction of the expression of damage-inducible DNA repair and recombination proteins (the SOS response). In addition, the RecA protein carries out the first steps of the recombination process, namely, finding regions of double-stranded DNA that are homologous to the single-stranded DNA bound to the RecA protein and catalyzing the invasion of the homologous double helix by the single DNA strand from the homologous region of the other duplex. After this crossover structure is formed by the action of *recA* protein, it is resolved by the action of various nucleases, DNA polymerase, and DNA ligase. The levels of various exonucleases (exonucleases I, V, and VIII) influence the recovery of recombinant molecules by creating or destroying single-stranded DNA tails, which are necessary for recombination. In addition to *recA,* whose requirement is the hallmark of a homologous recombination process, there are at least eight other *rec* genes that are important in recombination with different types of substrates, such as circular plasmids or linear conjugally transferred DNA.

Carcinogen Testing

A practical application of the SOS response in bacteria was the development by Bruce Ames of a simple test for the carcinogenic potential of a chemical. One measures the effect of the presence of the chemical on the frequency of reversion of missense or frame-shift mutations in the *his* operon (for histidine biosynthesis) of *Salmonella typhimurium* to histidine independence (ie, ability to grow on a defined media that does not contain histidine). There is a correlation between the activity of most chemicals as mutagens in bacteria and their carcinogenic potential in rodents, although some chemicals violate this relationship. Most chemicals that are active as mutagens induce the bacterial SOS response and its error-prone repair systems, suggesting that many chemical carcinogens act by binding to DNA.

Transposable Elements

Early genetic studies of antibiotic resistance in bacteria revealed the puzzling finding that antibiotic resistance traits appeared to move from one plasmid to another, or to a phage, or to the bacterial chromosome. Around the same time, insertion sequences (IS elements) were identified as migratory genetic elements that caused mutations by inserting into any bacterial gene, or that provided the movable regions of homology for F plasmid integration. The general name *transposon* is used for such mobile genetic elements (coding for a wide range of characters, including drug resistance, toxins, or nothing) that can insert almost randomly into DNA by nonhomologous recombination. The term *transposition* does not indicate either that the transposon leaves its previous site to integrate into a new location or that it integrates into a new site while leaving a copy of itself at the previous location; both alternatives occur.

PROPERTIES OF TRANSPOSONS

Transposons are discrete, mobile genetic elements that possess the following common features:

1. Transposons are incapable of autonomous replication and must be integrated into a replication unit such as a phage, plasmid, or chromosome.
2. Transposons have special sequences at each end that are essential for their ability to integrate into another region of DNA. In most cases, these terminal sequences are inverted repeats of 8 to 40 base pairs in length, which means that the sequences at each end of the transposable element are identical. This means that along each DNA strand, the sequences at the end are inverted and complementary to each other. If DNA is melted to separate the strands, and if the inverted repeats are of sufficient length to form a stable duplex, the repeats along each single strand will reanneal to generate a stem-and-loop (lollipop) structure. Because the ends of the transposon remain intact during the movement of the element, they must be specifically recognized by the enzymes that carry out transposition.
3. A transposon can insert at many sites in the target DNA. Some transposons integrate completely at random; others prefer sites that have a sequence similar to that at the ends of the transposon. Integration of a transposon is accompanied by the duplication of 5, 9, or 11 base pairs of the target DNA on both sides of the newly inserted element. The length of the direct repeats is a characteristic feature of that transposon.
4. Transposon insertion is independent of *rec* function and requires at least one enzyme, called *transposase,* which is encoded by and is specific for each transposon. Transposase recognizes the ends of the transposon and catalyzes the ligation of the transposon into the target site after cutting the recipient DNA in a staggered manner.
5. Transposition can occur by two distinct pathways. One involves the formation of a cointegrate, in which the

DNA molecule carrying the transposon fuses with the target DNA molecule, with a copy of the transposon at each of the sites of fusion of the two pieces of DNA. This process requires duplication of the transposon. Such transposons encode a resolvase enzyme, which catalyzes a site-specific recombinational event between the two copies of the transposon in the cointegrate. The resolution process separates the cointegrate back into two replicons: the donor DNA molecule with the transposon in its original location and the target DNA with the transposon inserted at a new site. The second pathway is called *direct transposition,* in which the transposon integrates into the target DNA without

formation of a cointegrate. Direct transposition can occur without replication of the transposon, which is lost from its original site (Fig. 21-6).

6. Transposition usually occurs at a very low frequency (in the range of once per 10^6 cells). However, when a transposon enters a naive cell that did not carry that element, its transposition frequency is much higher and is reduced to the repressed level only after several cell doublings.

7. Transposable elements can be lost. Imprecise excision is fairly common, whereas precise removal of the element (measured by restoration of function of the gene disrupted by transposition insertion) is rare (usually

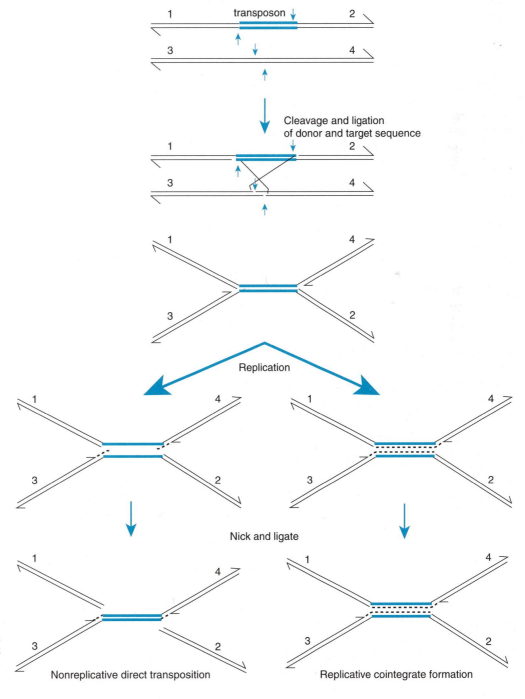

FIGURE 21-6 Transposition routes leading to replicon fusion (cointegrate formation) or to direct transposition.

less than 10^{-8} per division). The presence of a transposon often causes increased mutability of the surrounding chromosome and generates inversions, deletions, and other rearrangements.

8. Insertion of a transposon into a bacterial gene is likely to disrupt the function of that gene. Some transposons have a polar effect to block transcription from an upstream promoter of genes downstream from the site of insertion. Other transposons have a promoter that reads outward and, hence, can activate the transcription of adjacent bacterial genes.

TYPES OF TRANSPOSONS

There are three general types of transposons (Fig. 21-7). One type, called the Tn*3*-like transposons, is typified by transposon Tn*3*, an element of about 5 kilobases in length, which always moves as a discrete unit. It contains three genes: *tnpA*, which encodes the specific transposase; *tnpR*, which encodes the resolvase protein; and *bla*, which encodes a β-lactamase responsible for resistance to β-lactam antibiotics. Three sites are important for Tn*3* function. The two 37–base-pair inverted repeats at each end of Tn*3* are necessary for transposition, and the *res* site in

Tn3

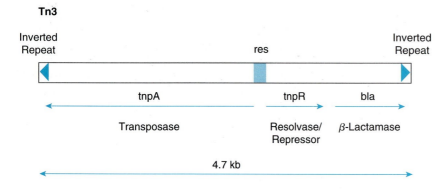

IS10

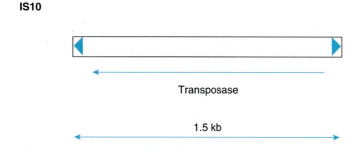

Tn10

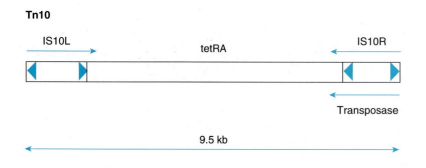

FIGURE 21-7 Genetic structure of two transposons. Transposon Tn*3* is about 5 kilobases (kb) in length and has 37 base pair inverted repeat sequences at its ends. It carries three genes: *tnpA*, transposase, which catalyzes the formation of cointegrates; *tnpR*, resolvase, which splits cointegrates into two separate replicons; and *bla*, β-lactamase, which confers resistance to β-lactam antibiotics. Transposon Tn*10* (9.5 kb) carries genes for tetracycline resistance flanked by two 1.5-kb insertion sequences (IS-10-L and IS-10-R), one of which encodes the transposase.

the middle of the element is the site of resolvase action and of repression of transposase synthesis. Transposition by Tn*3* is a replicative process that occurs by formation of a cointegrate catalyzed by TnpA transposase and host DNA replication enzymes. The cointegrate is resolved by a single site-specific recombination between the two *res* sites catalyzed by the TnpR protein to restore the two separate replicons, one with Tn*3* at its original site and one with Tn*3* at a new site.

The second type of transposon, called composite transposons, is characterized by the presence of *insertion sequences* flanking a central region of DNA. Insertion sequences are transposable elements that usually are 800 to 1500 base pairs in length, have short inverted repeat sequences at each end, encode only their own transposase, and generally are detected by their mutagenic effect on bacterial genes into which they insert. When two copies of an insertion sequence are inserted close to each other, they and the intervening DNA segment can transpose either as a unit or as individual insertion sequences. Many of the common transposons are of this type. Composite transposons such as Tn*5* and Tn*10* exhibit direct transposition, in which the element is excised from its original location and inserted without replication into the new site.

One implication of this behavior is that transposons can be readily created by transposition of insertion sequences to both sides of a chromosomal region to form a new transposon, which can transfer that chromosomal region to other sites on the chromosome or onto phages or plasmids. Another implication of the mobility of transposons is that the same toxin or drug-inactivating enzyme can be present in many different bacterial species or encoded on different plasmids or phages. For example, the same penicillin-inactivating enzyme is produced by resistant strains of *E coli, Neisseria gonorrhoeae,* and *Haemophilus influenzae,* although in each species the transposon resides on a different plasmid. Similarly, the *E coli* ST enterotoxin can be encoded on a plasmid or on a temperate phage.

A third type of transposon is typified by bacteriophage Mu, whose sole mode of replication is through transposition. The mechanism of transposition by phage Mu transposase begins with the attachment of the 3′ end of each strand of the transposon to the 5′ end of target DNA, in which a staggered cut was made by transposase. The resultant structure is acted on either by nuclease and ligase to give a direct transposition product without extensive replication, or by DNA polymerase and ligase to give a cointegrate with replication.

Transposable elements have been described in gram-positive and gram-negative bacteria, Archaebacteria, fungi, *Drosophila,* and plants. Many RNA tumor viruses (retroviruses) integrate into random sites in animal-cell chromosomes and, because their nucleic acid possesses terminal direct or inverted repeats, they also have the general properties of a transposon.

Plasmids

Plasmids are the vehicle for most of the nonessential functions a bacterial cell can acquire. They exist as covalently closed circular double-stranded DNA (Fig. 21-8). Plasmids can be classified by numerous properties, including their size, the number of copies present in the cell, the nature of the host enzymes required for their replication, their incompatibility with other plasmids, the functions they encode, and their ability to be transferred to other cells. We will consider each of these parameters, but note that there are numerous exceptions to the general picture drawn here; these examples refer primarily to plasmids in the enteric bacteria.

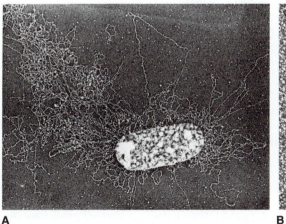
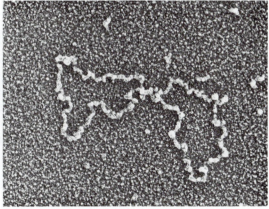

A   **B**

FIGURE 21-8   A. Disrupted cell of *Escherichia coli;* the DNA has spilled out, and a plasmid can be seen slightly to the left of the top center. **B.** Enlargement of a plasmid (about 1 μm from side to side). This plasmid provides the *E coli* cell bearing it with the ability to produce the bactericidal protein colicin E1 and with immunity from the action of this protein.

NONSELF-TRANSMISSIBLE PLASMIDS

Plasmids range in size from 2 million to greater than 200 million daltons, and in copy number from 1 to greater than 20 copies per cell. In general, nonself-transmissible plasmids tend to be relatively small (3 million to 20 million daltons) and to have high copy numbers. All plasmids must have a replicon function, namely an origin of replication and a mechanism to control the frequency of initiation of DNA replication. In many of the smaller plasmids, replication is dependent on DNA polymerase I and is not subject to the controls that regulate chromosome replication. Moreover, initiation of plasmid replication does not require a period of protein synthesis, and there is extensive multiplication of these plasmids after inhibition of protein synthesis by appropriate antibiotics. Despite the high frequency of their replication, these plasmids contain a special region of DNA that ensures their efficient partition into the progeny cells. They do not carry *tra* genes, but many can be transmitted by conjugation, if they are present in a cell that also contains a self-transmissible plasmid.

SELF-TRANSMISSIBLE PLASMIDS

Plasmids that are self-transmissible are relatively large (40 million to 100 million daltons), because they must carry almost 30 *tra* genes encoding the sex pili and DNA transfer enzymes. Most of these plasmids are replicated by the enzymes that control chromosomal replication and often are present in 1 to 3 copies per cell. Unlike many of the smaller plasmids mentioned earlier, these plasmids do not require DNA polymerase I activity for their maintenance.

Expression of the *tra* operon is regulated by a plasmid-coded repressor. A recipient cell that has just acquired a transmissible plasmid initially will be a good donor for that plasmid; after several doublings, however, such progeny cells express their transfer functions, including the sex pili, at a low level. This repression does not extend to other functions that might be carried on the plasmid, such as the drug resistance carried on many R (for resistance) plasmids. The F plasmid is unable to repress its own transfer functions and, therefore, is an effective sex factor.

Different plasmids can exist simultaneously in the same cell. Plasmids that cannot coexist are said to be in the same incompatibility group; they have closely related systems for the control of plasmid replication and interfere with one another's replication or partition.

PLASMID FUNCTIONS

Plasmids are widely distributed in nature, and most bacteria isolated from clinical materials possess between one and six different plasmids. They occur in both gram-positive and gram-negative bacteria and code for a wide range of different functions.

Antibiotic resistance frequently is carried on self-transmissible or nonself-transmissible plasmids. Self-transmissible plasmids that carry drug-resistance determinants are called R factors (Fig. 21-9). All have a *tra* operon similar to that of the F plasmid, although it usually encodes a different type of sex pilus. The remainder of the plasmid consists of various genes for antibiotic resistance and other functions, many of which are on transposable elements. Because many of the antibiotic resistance determinants are carried on transposons, it is easy to see how these determinants can move from one plasmid to

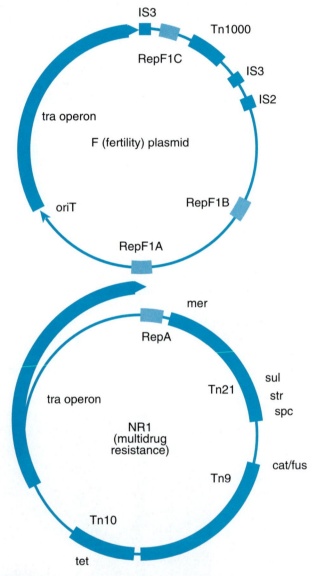

FIGURE 21-9 Diagrams of the self-transmissible plasmids F and NR1. The location of the closely related *tra* operons in the two plasmids is indicated, as are the *rep* regions that function for plasmid replication. The F plasmid has three independent *rep* systems. The R factor, NR1, confers resistance to numerous antibiotics. Note that these antibiotic-resistance genes are parts of transposons and are flanked by IS elements. In fact, one can deduce that there were three separate occurrences where one transposon inserted into another transposon resident on the plasmid.

another. Nonself-transmissible plasmids lack the *tra* operon, but many can be mobilized for efficient conjugal transfer when a self-transmissible plasmid resides in the same cell. Other medically important functions carried on plasmids include resistance to heavy metal salts (Ag, Hg), by encoding a metal reductase, and resistance to ultraviolet light, by encoding DNA repair enzymes. Some plasmids code for the production of fimbriae, which mediate adherence of bacteria to epithelial cells. *Salmonella* and *Shigella* species carry large plasmids that confer certain virulence traits. Production of hemolysin by *E coli*, enterotoxins responsible for gastroenteritis, and exotoxins such as those for botulism, tetanus, and scarlet fever are encoded by plasmids, as is the ability to metabolize new sugars and other carbon sources, capabilities that blur the biochemical distinctions between different species. Other plasmid-mediated properties include nitrogen fixation and root nodule formation in *Rhizobium*, the production of plant tumors by *Agrobacterium*, and the ability to metabolize petroleum hydrocarbons.

Another interesting group of plasmid-coded proteins are the bacteriocins, which are secreted proteins that are lethal for cells of the same or related species, but to which the producing strain is immune. Bacteriocins usually are named after the species producing them, such as colicins from *E coli*, megacins from *Bacillus megaterium*, and agrocins from *Agrobacterium*. There are several mechanisms whereby bacteriocins kill susceptible bacteria, such as their action as a nuclease (deoxyribonuclease or ribonuclease) or as an ionophore dissipating the membrane potential. A possible role for these proteins may be to maintain the normal flora of the host by killing incoming sensitive bacteria.

Site-Specific Recombination

Numerous nonhomologous recombinational events occur in bacteria, in which specific proteins carry out recombination between specific DNA sequences. The integration and excision of phage λ by the Int and Xis proteins, along with some host proteins, occurs by recombination between specific bases in the phage and bacterial *att* sites (see Chap. 20). The resolution of cointegrate structures formed during the transposition of Tn*3*-like transposons involves recombination between the directly repeated *res* sites of the two Tn*3* copies; this is catalyzed by the *tnpR* product.

Plasmids like F are present in a few copies per cell. If plasmid multimers were to form by homologous recombination, the copy number of discrete plasmids would decrease and the partitioning of the plasmid into progeny cells would be compromised. The plasmids and prophage P1 (see Chap. 20) carry out site-specific recombination to resolve such multimers.

The promoter region that controls expression of the flagellar genes in *S typhimurium*, a process subject to phase variation, undergoes a reversible inversion by site-specific recombination between two oppositely oriented short sequences (see Chap. 17). The enzyme responsible for this recombination (Hin, for H-inversion) is encoded within the invertible segment. Several site-specific recombination systems display rigid topologic constraints, in that the sequences to be recombined must be on the same piece of DNA in the proper orientation. This recognition is dependent on supercoiling to intertwine the sites appropriately.

Thus, bacteria present us with ever more fascinating examples of genetic rearrangements through recombination to increase their coding potential and allow them to respond to changing environments.

Bibliography

JOURNALS

Clewell DB, Gawron-Burke C. Conjugative transposons and the dissemination of antibiotic resistance in streptococci. Annu Rev Microbiol 1986;40:635.

Craig NL. The mechanism of conservative site-specific recombination. Annu Rev Genet 1988;22:77.

Foster PL. Adaptive mutation: the uses of diversity. Annu Rev Microbiol 1993;47:467.

Mazodier P, Davies J. Gene transfer between distantly related bacteria. Annu Rev Genet 1991;25:147.

Meyer TF, Gibbs CP, Haas R. Variation and control of protein expression in *Neisseria*. Annu Rev Microbiol 1990;44:451.

Mizuuchi K. In vitro transposition of bacteriophage Mu: a biochemical approach to a novel replication reaction. Cell 1983;35:785.

Novick RP. Plasmid incompatibility. Microbiol Rev 1987;51:381.

Reznikoff WS. The Tn5 transposon. Annu Rev Microbiol 1993;47:945.

Smith GR. Homologous recombination in procaryotes. Microbiol Rev 1988;52:1.

BOOKS

Clewell DB. Bacterial conjugation. New York, Plenum Press, 1993.

Helinski DR, Cohen SN, Clewell DB, Jackson DA, Hollaender, eds. Plasmids in bacteria. New York, Plenum Press, 1985.

Low KB, ed. The recombination of genetic material. San Diego, Academic Press, 1988.

Maloy SR, Cronan JE, Freifelder D. Microbial genetics, ed 2. Boston, Jones & Bartlett, 1994.

Smith-Keary PF. Molecular genetics of *Escherichia coli*. New York, Guilford Press, 1989.

Thomas CM, ed. Promiscuous plasmids of gram-negative bacteria. San Diego, Academic Press, 1989.

Essentials of Medical Microbiology, Fifth Edition, edited by Wesley A. Volk, Bryan M. Gebhardt, Marie-Louise Hammarskjöld, and Robert J. Kadner. Lippincott-Raven Publishers, Philadelphia © 1996.

Chapter 22

Molecular Genetic Aspects of Bacterial Virulence

Molecular genetic studies of pathogenic bacteria have revealed numerous important results and insights into the mechanisms by which bacteria respond to the actions of the host immune system, adapt to the presence of antibiotics, and cause many diseases. Understanding the virulence mechanisms of bacteria has become even more important with the widespread dissemination of antibiotic resistance among many bacterial types. This chapter presents several aspects of bacterial adaptation.

Antibiotic Resistance

Until this century, infectious diseases represented a major cause of death, from acute epidemics such as cholera, plague, and smallpox, to debilitating chronic diseases such as tuberculosis and malaria. The effects of these scourges were reduced by improvements in nutrition, sanitation, and vaccination. Development of vaccines and antibiotics starting in the 1940s further reduced the impact of bacterial infections, at least in the developed world. Interest in the development of new antibiotics and in bacterial pathogenesis waned with the assumption that pathogenic bacteria could be controlled easily with existing drugs. This sense of security was ill-founded and short-lived, and the development of antibiotic-resistant bacteria is proceeding at an alarming pace. Some fear the return of a preantibiotic era in which existing antibiotics will have little therapeutic value. Antibiotic resistance is rampant in clinical isolates of bacteria. The proportion of drug-resistant isolates has been increasing continually in most bacterial pathogens. How did antibiotic resistance develop, how did it spread, and what can be done about it?

It was unwise to presume that bacteria would not adapt to the presence of antimicrobial agents. It was generally recognized in laboratory experiments that bacteria could become resistant to most antibiotics through mutational processes. These were thought to be, and are, rare enough and debilitating enough to the bacterium that they are not major routes for development of the widespread drug resistance seen today. Other processes also are operative and are extremely important. The carriage of multiple drug resistance on plasmids has been recognized since 1956. Studies of bacterial strain collections from the preantibiotic era and analyses of populations that have never received medical care reveal the presence of antibiotic-resistant bacteria in the absence of any drug selection. The frequency of resistant organisms in these cases is low and multiple drug resistance is not seen, but the potential for an explosive increase in resistant organisms has always been present. Many antibiotics are natural products of soil organisms, and many bacteria have been exposed to these endogenous antibiotics during contact with soil samples. The widespread and almost indiscriminate use of antibiotics in medicine and animal husbandry has served to increase the number of resistant bacteria. The existence of multiply resistant bacteria or plasmids meant that selection with any single antibiotic to which the plasmid conferred resistance selected for retention of the resistance traits toward all other antibiotics.

ACQUISITION OF RESISTANCE TRAITS

What are the sources of antibiotic resistance? The bacteria that produce antibiotics possess mechanisms for self-protection against their own products, including transport systems to pump the antibiotic out of the cell and enzymes for covalent modification and inactivation of any antibiotic that remains inside. These inactivation enzymes are likely to have developed from enzymes used in normal metabolism by mutational alterations in the substrate-recognition sites of kinases, acetylases, and nucleotide-adding enzymes. There are some documented examples suggestive of gene transfer from antibiotic-producing bacteria to or from pathogenic bacteria. The type of tetracycline efflux system originally present in the drug-producing strain, *Streptomyces rimosus*, now is found in some mycobacteria. These and other results indicate that DNA-exchange processes occur in nature among distantly related bacteria and can account for the transmission of resistant determinants from antibiotic-producing organisms to pathogenic types.

Another route for the acquisition and transmission of resistance traits makes use of the ease with which novel transposable elements are constructed. The way in which the character of the composite transposons could lend itself to the formation of new, but stable, elements is described in Chapter 21. Whenever the same insertion sequence (IS element) inserts near another copy of itself, it can mediate the transposition or either or both IS elements, including the sequences between them. Integrons, other types of transposable elements that have been identified, acquire any random piece of DNA as a stable part of a new genetic element—but in a single step, without the need for two rare transposition events. These mechanisms would allow the movement of any region of DNA from one organism onto some mobile genetic element, such as a plasmid, and thence to another bacterial species.

Transfer of DNA from bacteria to yeast has been claimed and may be operative. Acquisition of genes from eucaryotic organisms could provide another mechanism of drug resistance. Some forms of resistance to sulfonamides and trimethoprim involve the synthesis of a replacement enzyme that is insensitive to that drug. It is possible that the trimethoprim-resistant form of dihydrofolate reductase might have a eucaryotic origin, although the source of the sulfonamide-insensitive dihydropteroate synthase is unknown.

CHANGE IN TRANSPORT ACTIVITY

Resistance also occurs to unnatural drugs, which are synthesized chemically and have novel structures without a source of inactivating enzyme. Resistance to these agents occurs not by drug inactivation, but by alteration of the target enzyme or by nonspecific means. One of the major nonspecific routes of resistance involves active transport systems that use metabolic energy to pump small molecules out of the cell. Many of these active efflux systems have been found in a wide range of bacteria, and they often have fairly broad substrate specificities. Transport systems used to pump toxic metals such as arsenite, cadmium, and calcium out of the cell may have been their progenitors. Another source of these efflux systems could be modification of the transporters that normally pump some normal cellular metabolite out of the cell; one promising candidate is a transporter for the release of iron-binding siderophores.

CHANGE OF TARGET

Antibiotic resistance also can arise from alterations of the target reaction itself. One interesting example comes from the study of beta-lactam–resistant forms of *Neisseria meningitidis*. The *Neisseria* possess three penicillin-binding proteins (PBPs), and both PBP1 and PBP2 are essential for growth. Although beta-lactamase production has occurred in *Neisseria gonorrhoeae*, it is not seen in *N meningitidis*. Forms of *Neisseria* that have penicillin-resistant forms of PBP2 produce a protein with a chimeric structure in which part of the usual penicillin-sensitive form of the enzyme has been replaced with sequences from other species, such as the commensal *Neisseria flavescens*, which has a lower inherent affinity for penicillin. It is suggested that the mosaic gene arose as the result of acquisition of the gene from the related species by transformation, followed by its replacement of the part of the normal gene by homologous recombination. A similar process of transformation and recombination is suggested for the appearance of mosaic PBP2B genes in penicillin-resistant *Streptococcus pneumoniae*.

Methicillin-resistant *Staphylococcus aureus* arose by a different process. These strains produce a new PBP2' protein with low affinity for all beta-lactams and can replace the function of all three of the essential PBPs in this species. It is not clear where this new PBP came from.

Adherence

In many situations, the virulence of a bacterium requires its ability to adhere to host cell surfaces to avoid being washed away by the flow of urine in the urinary tract or of food masses in the intestinal tract, or to enable the cell to recognize and invade a particular host tissue. The enterotoxigenic strains of *Escherichia coli* must express two functions to cause their characteristic diarrheal disease, often called travelers' diarrhea. These strains often produce two toxins, termed LT and ST, which induce substantial increases in cellular cyclic adenosine monophosphate and cyclic guanosine monophosphate, respectively, in the intestinal epithelial cells of the host and result in substantial loss of salts and water. Also necessary is a mechanism for adherence to the epithelial cells of the small intestine; this is generally called CFA, for colonization factor antigen. Without the adherence mechanism, toxin-producing strains do not cause significant disease, suggesting that the bacteria need to deliver the toxin at or near the susceptible cell surface for its action. For example, specific adherence is crucial in the attachment of *N gonorrhoeae* to urinary tract epithelial cells, of *Bordetella pertussis* to columnar cells of the respiratory tract, of *Streptococcus pyogenes* to various types of cells in the skin, and of certain *E coli* strains to urinary tract epithelial cells.

There are numerous types of adherence mechanisms, perhaps the most distinctive of which are the pili/fimbriae on many gram-negative bacteria. These are filamentous structures extending from the outer membrane into the medium. Their thickness, density, shape, and protein content are characteristic for each system. The properties and assembly of one of the best studied fimbrial systems, the pyelonephritis-associated pilus (Pap) structure, are described.

THE PYELONEPHRITIS-ASSOCIATED PILUS (PAP) STRUCTURE

Most community cases of urinary tract infection (70% to 80%) are caused by *E coli,* and at least 80% of the *E coli* isolates from these infections express on their surface the Pap, or P, pili. The P pilus mediates attachment to specific eucaryotic surface glycoproteins or glycolipids; its presence can be detected by the ability of the bacteria to promote hemagglutination of human erythrocytes that can be blocked by the addition of galactosyl-α(1-4)galactose. The P pilus is a long, straight filament, most of which is a hollow tube made up of thousands of copies of the PapA polypeptide (20 kilodaltons). High-resolution electron microscopic examination reveals that the tip of the P pilus is morphologically distinct, appearing as short, thin fibers that are made up of three polypeptides, PapE, PapF, and PapG. PapG is responsible for the lectin or carbohydrate-binding activity of the pilus. The presence of the lectin at the tip of the pilus is different from the situation in some other pili. For example, the common or type 1 pilus present in most *E coli* strains has a major pilin subunit forming the filament, with the lectin subunit interspersed, perhaps at random, along its length. In other pili, the major subunit is the lectin.

The eleven genes of the chromosomal *pap* operon are expressed as a unit in response to several environmental signals. Temperature is a particularly important signal in the expression of many bacterial virulence determinants because it clearly indicates to the bacterium whether it has found its way into a warm-blooded host or is out in the environment. Thus, the degree of Pap expression is much higher at or above 37°C than it is below 30°C. In addition, the *pap* operon is subject to phase variation, such that individual cells within a population can switch back and forth between Pap expression and nonexpression. The mechanism of phase variation is not presented here, but it involves reversible changes of the methylation of particular DNA sequences. Among the 11 products of the *pap* operon are two regulatory proteins, the major fimbrial subunit PapA, four minor pilin subunits whose incorporation starts or stops filament assembly, and the tip-associated lectin PapG. In addition, there are three proteins necessary for proper assembly of the structure. Two are periplasmic chaperones, especially PapD, which forms complexes with several of the subunits to maintain them in an assembly-competent state and to present them to the assembly site in the outer membrane. Proteins normally cannot pass across the gram-negative outer membrane without the assistance of specific export components. The outer membrane PapC protein carries out the assembly by picking from the pool of periplasmic complexes of the subunits and the PapD chaperone, the appropriate subunit to be added to the filament. PapC is known as the usher protein because of its responsibility for choosing the correct subunit at the proper point in the assembly process.

Phase and Antigenic Variation

Pathogenic bacteria are constantly exposed to attack by the immune system, which primarily recognizes surface structures (proteins or polysaccharides) and directs the synthesis of antibodies to coat those structures and result in either killing by complement or uptake by phagocytic cells. To avoid presenting such targets, bacteria have developed numerous mechanisms to turn off the synthesis of their surface structures (phase variation) or to continually alter their structure and change their antigenic profile (antigenic variation). These processes are of obvious importance for bacterial survival and for the development of effective vaccines. A few of these mechanisms are described briefly here.

FIMBRIAL PHASE VARIATION

The occurrence of phase variation of fimbriae is fairly common. Production of the type I fimbriae or common pili of *E coli* is turned on or off by a reversible switch involving inversion of a promoter-containing DNA segment, as described for the control of flagellar expression.

A more complex system operates in the case of *N gonorrhoeae*, in which many different antigenic types of the major adherence fimbriae, called the pili, are expressed in a reversible manner, or in which the synthesis of any pilus is turned on or off. These various changes occur by a process of intergenic recombination. On the chromosome, there is one complete pilin gene, with all the sequences necessary for expression, and numerous (12 to 16) nonexpressed partial pilin genes of different sequence. Recombination between these copies of pilin genes can change the sequence of the gene at the expression site by exchanging all or part of the sequence of one of the nonexpressed copies. By this means, only one pilin gene can be expressed at any time by a cell, but a wide variety of different pilin genes can be constructed in different cells of the population. In the pilus-negative variants, either the entire expression gene is lost (nonreverting) or the pilin gene that is present at the expression site encodes a truncated or unstable product. It is suggested that transfer of the DNA sequences from the silent loci into the expressed locus occurs after uptake of DNA fragments by transformation and a form of homologous recombinational event.

OTHER TYPES OF PHASE VARIATION

Similar recombinational switches are seen in phase variation of major surface proteins in other organisms. Trypanosomes routinely switch among numerous Variable Surface Glycoproteins by bringing different coding region cassettes to the single expression site through specialized recombinational events. Sequential expression of different genes for the Variable Major Protein of *Borrelia* is responsible for recurring episodes of relapsing fever. During afebrile periods, few spirochetes are present, and there is a high level of antibody against the previously expressed Variable Major Protein. In 1 in 10^3 to 10^4 cells, there is a recombinational event between this organism's unusual linear plasmids to exchange the genes for this surface protein at the single expression site. A bacterium with a new Variable Major Protein on its surface grows effectively in the bloodstream until the host mounts an immune response against this new organism. These are a few examples of how pathogenic bacteria use specialized recombinational events to vary the expression of a broad repertoire of surface coats or antigens and thereby evade the host's immune defenses.

Another example is provided by the gonococcal surface protein, originally called protein II, whose expression is associated with colony opacity, cell adherence, and serum resistance. There are multiple copies of the gene for this protein in the chromosome, but expression is not associated with major changes in the genome. Instead, the gene contains tandem repeats of the 5–base-pair sequence CTCTT in the region that encodes the signal sequence needed for export of the protein to the cell surface. The number of these 5–base-pair repeats can increase or decrease, probably by homologous recombination. When there are 9 copies of the repeat, they encode 15 amino acids, which are in frame with the rest of the protein and can serve as a signal sequence. However, if there are 7, 8, 10, or 11 repeats, the sequences are out of frame with the rest of the protein, and no protein can be produced. If there are 3 repeats, the protein would be made in frame, but the encoded 5 amino acids would be too short to serve as a functional signal sequence. This mechanism provides a clever way to turn on or off the expression of a surface protein without requiring specialized recombinational processes or other regulatory controls.

There are many more examples of clever ploys developed by bacteria to enable them to adapt rapidly to changes in the environment and to respond to the immune system and antibiotic pressure.

Bibliography

JOURNALS

Davies J. Inactivation of antibiotics and the dissemination of resistance genes. Science 1994;264:375.

Falkow S, Isberg R, Portnoy D. The interaction of bacteria with mammalian cells. Annu Rev Cell Biol 1992;8:333.

Hultgren SJ, Normark S, Abraham SN. Chaperone-assisted assembly and molecular architecture of adhesive pili. Annu Rev Microbiol 1991;45:383.

Macnab R. Genetics and biogenesis of bacterial flagella. Annu Rev Genet 1992;26:131.

Nikaido H. Prevention of drug access to bacterial targets: permeability barriers and active efflux. Science 1994;264:382.

Pugsley AP. The complete general secretory pathway in gram-negative bacteria. Microbiol Rev 1993;57:50.

Seifert HS, So M. Genetic mechanisms of bacterial antigenic variation. Microbiol Rev 1988;52:327.

Spratt BG. Resistance to antibiotics by target alterations. Science 1994;264:388.

BOOK

Salyers AA, Whitt DD. Bacterial pathogenesis: a molecular approach. Washington, DC, ASM Press, 1994.

Bacteria
and Fungi

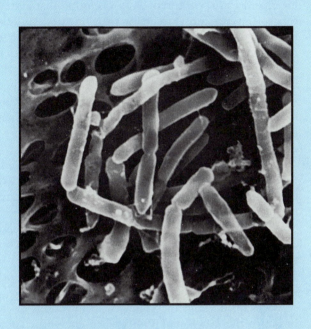

JUST a little more than a century ago, the germ theory of disease was finally accepted by scientists. Since then, the relationship between humans and pathogenic microorganisms has changed dramatically, mostly in our favor, but the conquest of one problem frequently results in the appearance of new challenges in the control of infectious organisms. Our hospitals are no longer the death traps of the 19th century, but new life-saving techniques have resulted in types of infections unheard of several decades ago.

During the past century, we learned that microorganisms cause diseases such as cholera, tuberculosis, typhoid fever, and anthrax. Moreover, it was found that a precise series of events must occur for such microorganisms to be transmitted from an infected person or animal to a noninfected host. This concept gave rise to the science of epidemiology, and the epidemiologist learned where to break the link in the chain of transmission. Thus, better sanitation of drinking water drastically curtailed typhoid fever and dysentery; control of mosquitoes eliminated urban yellow fever; and scrubbing and disinfectants reduced surgical infections.

During this century of rapidly developing knowledge, the science of immunology began with the discovery that individuals could be protected from many diseases caused by microorganisms by artificially inducing a specific immunity. By the middle of the 20th century, diseases such as smallpox, diphtheria, tetanus, and whooping cough could be prevented, and during the past quarter century, effective vaccines have become available for many other infectious diseases.

The third era in the conquest of infectious diseases began in the 1930s and 1940s when chemotherapeutic drugs and antibiotics appeared that seemed destined to eliminate bacterial infections. However, we soon learned that many microorganisms can mutate to antibiotic-resistant forms, so the microbiologist battles constantly to develop new antibiotics to replace those that are no longer effective.

So, where do we stand now? Many dreaded organisms have been curtailed to where they no longer cause important diseases, particularly in the Western world. However, recent medical knowledge and techniques have led indirectly to the occurrence of many previously rare or unknown infections caused either by organisms considered to be normal flora or by organisms previously thought of as nonpathogens. These infections result when host resistance is reduced to such a degree that normal flora or nonpathogens are able to grow and flourish in areas where they otherwise could not penetrate or, if they did invade, would be killed by our immune mechanisms. A few situations leading to this type of infection include (1) the use of immunosuppressants to prevent the rejection of organ transplants; (2) the use of kidney dialysis machines and heart pumps; (3) the frequent use of urethral catheters; (4) the use of antibiotics that destroy part of our normal flora; and, most important, (5) infection with the virus that causes acquired immunodeficiency syndrome. Any procedure that destroys the protection offered by an intact skin and mucosa, interferes with the immune system or cough reflexes, or changes the normal flora is conducive to serious infections by "harmless" organisms. Thus, to understand fully the numerous problems in the diagnosis and prevention of infections, it is vital that we know about those organisms that have a permanent home in some area of our body, that is, our normal flora.

Later in this unit, we shall learn that most major disease-producing microorganisms possess specific properties that enable them to cause disease, and that these properties can be categorized broadly as (1) the production of toxins or enzymes that destroy host cells or inhibit normal physiologic processes, and (2) the ability to inhibit the normal immune responses of the host. Most of the organisms constituting the normal flora of the body lack these properties and, under normal circumstances, are unable to produce disease. The past several decades, however, have seen a tremendous increase in the number of infections caused by organisms making up our normal flora, and, surprisingly, a large percentage of such infections are acquired during a hospital stay. Such hospital-acquired infections are known as *nosocomial infections*, and the microorganisms involved are called *opportunists*, because they normally produce infections only in the presence of one or more of the following conditions: (1) impaired immunity in the host; (2) burns, wounds, or surgeries that eliminate anatomic barriers; or (3) contaminated catheters, syringes, or respirators. It has been estimated by the Centers for Disease Control in Atlanta, Georgia, that about 2 million patients become infected each year during their hospital stays, and that such infections contribute to about 80,000 deaths annually in the United States.

The remainder of this unit is concerned with the organisms that cause human diseases and the properties they must possess to do so.

Essentials of Medical Microbiology, Fifth Edition, edited by Wesley A. Volk, Bryan M. Gebhardt, Marie-Louise Hammarskjöld, and Robert J. Kadner. Lippincott-Raven Publishers, Philadelphia © 1996.

Chapter 23

Normal Flora, Infections, and Bacterial Invasiveness

All of us are infected from our birth until our death. Our normal flora is actually an infection by microorganisms that have adapted to a specific habitat in our bodies where they can replicate without harming their hosts. However, should any one species of the microbes comprising our normal flora invade and grow in an area of our bodies where it is not adapted to a harmless coexistence with its host, it will cause *disease*. For instance, most urinary tract infections are caused by organisms that are normal flora of the intestinal tract. In addition, we frequently harbor organisms that, although they result in no disease to us, can provide a source of infection and disease to persons with whom we come in contact, particularly those who already are ill or debilitated, as in a hospital environment. For example, many of us peacefully coexist with staphylococci in our nose and throat, but if these staphylococci infect a burn or a wound, a severe disease can ensue.

This difference between infection and disease is important to the physician who must identify the causative agent of an infectious disease. To make this decision, the physician must know what organisms can be expected to occur in the various areas of the body. For example, it would not be unexpected to find *Escherichia coli* in a normal stool specimen, but if a large number of *E coli* were isolated from a catheterized urine specimen, it would unequivocally indicate a urinary tract infection and, hence, disease. Similarly, isolation of α-hemolytic streptococci from the throat would be a normal finding, whereas isolation of the same organisms from the blood could indicate serious disease.

In this chapter, we survey both the specific organisms that make up the normal flora of the various parts of our bodies and diverse kinds of infections. In addition, we discuss the general characteristics of organisms that permit them to cause disease and the ways in which they are transmitted to humans.

Relationships of Humans and Microbes

NORMAL FLORA

Before birth, the human body has no normal flora. During the birth process, the body comes in contact with microbes in the external environment. Later, with the initial feedings and exposure to an expanding environment, some microorganisms find their way to a permanent residence in many parts of the body.

Most organisms in the external environment apparently do not find the body to be a favorable habitat. Characteristic features of different body areas, such as temperature, oxygen availability, nutrient availability, natural inhibitors, and pH, influence the population that is able to survive and establish itself. Because these conditions vary from site to site in the body, different sites acquire considerably different organisms as their normal flora. Once the normal flora is established, it benefits the body by preventing the overgrowth of undesirable organisms. Destruction of the normal flora frequently disrupts the status quo, resulting in the growth of harmful organisms. This can be seen after the prolonged administration of broad-spectrum antibiotics. For example, if the normal flora of the intestinal tract and vagina are largely destroyed, the yeast *Candida albicans,* which is unaffected by these antibacterial antibiotics, can grow unchecked to become the major organism in these areas. It then can infect the mucous membranes and the skin, causing a severe inflammation. Another complication of antibiotic therapy is a severe gastroenteritis known as pseudomembranous colitis. This syndrome has been associated with several antimicrobial agents, but the antibiotics clindamycin and lincomycin have been incriminated most often. The mechanism of this diarrhea was elucidated when it was observed that the use of these antibiotics resulted in an overgrowth in the intestine of an organism identified as *Clostridium difficile.* This organism produces an enterotoxin that causes the gastroenteritis, but it can do so only when antibiotic therapy destroys much of the other normal intestinal flora, permitting it to grow unchecked.

Our normal flora can be categorized as helpful *(mutualistic symbionts),* harmless *(commensals),* or potentially harmful *(opportunists).* However, these groups are not mutually exclusive. Under certain circumstances, even a mutualist can cause harm and, thus, become a pathogen. Therefore, these categories are of value only in describing the usual role of the organism in relation to its host.

In a mutualistic relationship, the microbe and the host benefit one another. This type of relationship is common in the plant kingdom, and is essential in ruminants such as cattle, in which microbes are necessary for digestion of the cellulose in plant material. Few such relationships exist in humans, however. Probably the only good example of mutualism in humans is found in the normal flora of the large intestine, where enteric organisms synthesize vitamin K and the vitamins of the B complex, enabling them to be absorbed through the intestinal wall and contribute to human nutrition. However, considering that our normal flora provides us with protection by interfering with the growth of potentially harmful organisms, much of our normal flora could be considered mutualistic symbionts.

The microbe that lives on and benefits from its host without either benefiting or harming the host is called a commensal. Most of the organisms that make up the normal flora of a healthy individual could be categorized as commensals.

Opportunists (microbes that are potential pathogens) are of greatest interest to us. These organisms seem to lack the ability to invade and cause disease in healthy individuals, but may be able to colonize as pathogens in ill or injured persons. *Staphylococcus aureus* is a good example of an opportunist. Many people (about 25%) carry staphylococci in their nasopharynx without suffering any illness. However, if these people acquire respiratory tract infections such as measles or influenza, the staphylococci can invade the lung and cause severe pneumonia. Accidental contamination of the bladder with *E coli* or *Enterococcus faecalis* during a catheterization procedure also can lead to opportunistic infection. Both these organisms are part of the normal flora of the large intestine and usually do not produce urinary tract infections. However, if they gain access to the urethra or are transplanted mechanically to an environment in which they can grow, they can cause disease. The most startling examples of opportunistic infections are associated with the viral infection known as *acquired immunodeficiency syndrome* (AIDS). This syndrome is caused by a virus that destroys certain subsets of T cells, inhibiting the body's ability to mount an immune response. As a result, infection by the virus causing AIDS is characterized by severe and eventually fatal infections or malignancies that do not occur in individuals with functional immune systems.

Because much of our normal flora can cause disease under the proper conditions, these organisms could be considered opportunists. This is particularly true in elderly and debilitated individuals, and in patients receiving immunosuppressive drug therapy to prevent rejection of organ transplants. Opportunists are especially important as causes of nosocomial infections (ie, those acquired during hospitalization). Under appropriate circumstances, most of the organisms that constitute our normal flora can cause disease.

Another group of bacteria that is not really part of our normal flora consists of pathogenic organisms that can exist in a large percentage of the population without causing disease. This group includes such organisms as *Neisseria meningitidis* (also called the meningococcus), the causative agent of epidemic meningitis. Many individuals carry this organism in their respiratory tracts without ever having meningitis, yet they can spread the bacterium to nonimmune individuals and cause disease. *Streptococcus pneumoniae* (the pneumococcus), the major cause of lobar pneumonia, also is carried by 10% to 20% of normal, healthy individuals. Persons who harbor bacteria such as these without ever exhibiting overt symptoms of disease are referred to as *carriers.*

Thus, although our normal flora can be beneficial by preventing the growth of potential pathogens, it also can be a reservoir from which endemic and epidemic diseases are spread.

The Skin

The pH of the skin usually is about 5.6. This factor alone may be responsible for inhibiting the establishment of many bacterial species, although the skin (particularly on the hands) harbors a large population of transient organisms. Moist areas of the skin, such as the axilla, are populated far more densely than are relatively dry areas, such as the forearm. For example, it has been reported that under a moist dressing on the arm, the number of bacteria rises in 4 days from $1000/cm^2$ to almost 10 million/cm^2.

Although some organisms occur only superficially on the skin surface, much of the bacterial flora is located in the openings of the hair follicles. Consequently, to sterilize the skin effectively, an antiseptic must enter the openings of the hair follicles.

Even though the skin is exposed to the external environment, the number of genera routinely found are fewer than might be expected. *Propionibacterium acnes* constitutes part of the deep-seated skin flora, and the production of propionic acid by this organism appears to exert a bacteriostatic effect on many other organisms. Probably the greatest single population on the skin is *Staphylococcus epidermidis; S aureus* is present to a much lesser extent.

Other organisms commonly found on the skin include *Corynebacterium* sp, *Micrococcus* sp, *Peptostreptococcus* sp, and various *Neisseria* sp. Certain potentially pathogenic yeasts such as *C albicans, Pityrosporum ovale,* and *Pityrosporum orbiculare* also can be present. In addition, organisms from upper respiratory tract secretions can be deposited on the skin. The external ear, the axillae, and the genital region usually harbor nonpathogenic acid-fast mycobacteria.

The Eye

It is surprising that the eye is infected so seldom, because it seems to be particularly susceptible to disease. One explanation for this may lie in the fact that the secretions of the eye are rich in the enzyme lysozyme, which causes the lysis of many bacteria through its ability to cleave the bacterial cell-wall peptidoglycan (Fig. 23-1). This action, plus the washing action of tears, helps to eliminate many organisms from the eye.

However, several skin organisms are found in the normal conjunctiva. These include *S epidermidis, Haemophilus influenzae, Neisseria* sp, and *Corynebacterium xerosis.* Other organisms occasionally isolated from the healthy

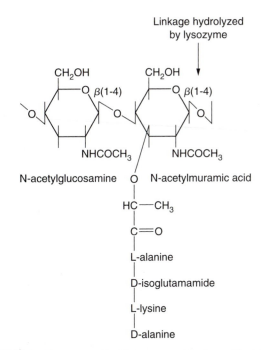

FIGURE 23-1 The action of lysozyme on peptidoglycan. Note that the bond cleaved is between *N*-acetylmuramic acid and *N*-acetylglucosamine, resulting in a breakdown of the peptidoglycan cell wall.

conjunctiva include *S pneumoniae,* enteric gram-negative rods, and the viridans streptococci.

The Respiratory Tract

In the course of normal breathing, many kinds of microbes are inhaled into the nose to reach the upper respiratory tract. Among these are normal soil inhabitants as well as pathogenic and potentially pathogenic bacteria. Some of these organisms are filtered out by the hairs in the nose, and some land on the moist surface of the nasal mucous membranes. Others migrate to the nasopharynx and take up residence there.

Bacteria routinely found in these areas include *Lactobacillus* sp, *Corynebacterium pseudodiphtheriticum,* and viridans streptococci. Obligate anaerobes include *Bacteroides* sp, *Fusobacterium* sp, *Bifidobacterium* sp, nonpathogenic *Treponema, Actinomyces israelii,* and *Veillonella* sp. Organisms that can cause disease but are carried asymptomatically by many persons include *S pneumoniae, Streptococcus pyogenes, S aureus, H influenzae,* and *N meningitidis.*

With the exception of an occasional organism that passes into the larynx, no normal inhabitants are found in the larynx, trachea, bronchi, or lungs. One reason for this is that organisms are filtered by the upper respiratory tract. Thus, when the upper respiratory tract is bypassed, as in a tracheostomy, a major defense against infection of the lower respiratory tract is no longer operating, and care must be exercised to prevent pathogenic or potentially pathogenic organisms from entering and contaminating the trachea.

The Digestive Tract

THE MOUTH AND OROPHARYNX. Microorganisms are taken into the mouth with food and drink, the hands, and various objects carrying dust and bacteria. Others are transmitted by chewed pencils or fingers.

Because of difficulties encountered in cultivation, some organisms present in the mouth probably have not been grown in the laboratory or even identified. However, microbes recognized as normal oral inhabitants include lactobacilli, streptococci, spirochetes, various cocci, spore-forming bacteria, coliforms, vibrios, and the fusiform bacilli. As this list indicates, the mouth has an extensive normal flora. Food left on and between the teeth causes a significant increase in the number of oral organisms. Moreover, both tooth decay and periodontal disease are a consequence of bacterial activity (see Chap. 37).

THE STOMACH. Although many microorganisms slip past the gastric barrier to become established in the intestinal tract, the healthy stomach has no natural flora. Its acid content is either inhibitory or destructive to swallowed organisms. Those that do pass into the intestinal tract probably have had only short contact with the gastric juice at a time when the acidity was temporarily lessened by food intake.

It has been established, however, that *Helicobacter pylori*, a curved, gram-negative bacterium, can colonize the mucus-secreting epithelial cells of the human stomach and cause peptic ulcers or chronic gastritis.

THE INTESTINES. Certain external factors, such as diet and antibiotic therapy, can influence the composition of the intestinal flora. With long-term antibiotic use, the normal flora can be so changed that organisms typically present in small numbers (ie, *Candida albicans, Clostridium difficile*) become the predominant microbes. However, in the absence of some unusual factor, the intestine has a fairly characteristic bacterial population.

THE SMALL INTESTINE. The stomach contents pass into the duodenum, which, like the stomach, has no natural flora. Organisms begin to appear in the jejunum and ileum, but large numbers of bacteria are not found until near the lower end of the ileum. The major bacteria present in this area are enterococci, staphylococci, lactobacilli, *Clostridium perfringens, Veillonella* sp, and, occasionally, *E coli*. Yeasts also can be present.

THE LARGE INTESTINE. The large intestine contains digested food and food wastes, providing excellent growth conditions for a diverse population of bacteria. As a result, this organ contains an incredible variety of microbes. The largest single group consists of obligately anaerobic gram-negative organisms. Of these, *Bacteroides* sp account for the majority, followed in frequency by *Fusobacterium* sp.

Many gram-positive anaerobes also are found, such as *Clostridium tetani, C perfringens, Clostridium sporogenes, Clostridium putrificum, C difficile, Clostridium histolyticum, Bifidobacterium* sp, and *Eubacterium* sp.

The lower intestinal tract also contains many facultative gram-negative organisms known as the *enteric bacteria*. They are much easier to grow than are the obligate anaerobes, but make up only about 5% of the intestinal flora. The most common of these are *E coli, Enterobacter aerogenes, Klebsiella pneumoniae*, and *Pseudomonas aeruginosa*. Also found are *E faecalis*, viridans streptococci, *Mycoplasma* sp, and lactobacilli. The major fungi present include *Candida, Geotrichum, Cryptococcus, Penicillium*, and *Aspergillus*. Some bacteria are found that are closely related to the pathogens, such as *Vibrio, Spirillum, Borrelia*, and *Treponema*.

The Genitourinary Tract

The urinary tract, except for the external urethra of the male, is normally sterile, although a few nonpathogenic cocci can be present in the female urethra.

Mycoplasma organisms have been isolated from the urethras of both men and women. Mycoplasmas are believed to account for many of the inflammatory infections of the urethra; they also are found in the urethras of a large percentage of healthy individuals. *Mycobacterium smegmatis*, an acid-fast rod, is present on the external genitalia in both sexes. This organism is morphologically similar to the tubercle bacillus, but can be differentiated easily on the basis of its rapid growth on laboratory media.

The female vaginal area has an acid pH between puberty and menopause, but the secretions are alkaline at other times. In an acid environment, lactobacilli predominate, but corynebacteria, yeasts, staphylococci, streptococci, and anaerobic cocci often are found in lesser numbers.

The Blood

As a rule, in the absence of disease, microorganisms are not found in blood or healthy tissue. Although bacteria can get into the blood through cuts or abrasions, dental manipulations, or even food in the intestine (situations sometimes referred to as transient bacteremias), they are quickly engulfed and destroyed by the white blood cells. There is always a risk, however, that a blood donor is unknowingly incubating some pathogen that could cause serious disease in a recipient. This is especially true of the virus that causes AIDS, but also applies to several other organisms.

Bacteremia refers to the presence of bacteria in the blood, and *septicemia* implies that the bacteria are multiplying in the bloodstream. *Viremia* has a similar meaning applied to viruses. The presence of microbes in the blood may be only transient, or the microbes may always be present during the acute stage of the disease.

Table 23-1 summarizes some of the common organisms that are part of the normal flora of the human body.

TABLE 23-1
Summary of Common Microbial Flora of the Human Body

Body Area	Microbial Flora	Body Area	Microbial Flora
SKIN		**GASTROINTESTINAL TRACT**	
General	*Acinetobacter* sp.	Stomach	No permanent normal flora
	Candida albicans and other yeasts	Intestines	
	Micrococcus sp.	Duodenum	Usually none
	Neisseria sp.	Jejunum and upper	Usually none or very few
	Peptostreptococcus sp.	ileum	*Achromobacter* sp.
	Propionibacterium acnes	Lower ileum and	*Bacteroides* sp.
		large intestine	*Bifidobacterium* sp.
External ear	*Corynebacterium* sp.		*Candida albicans* and other yeasts
	Mycobacterium sp.		*Clostridium* sp. including *C. tetani* and
	Staphylococcus aureus		*C. perfringens*
	Staphylococcus epidermidis		Enteric organisms included in the En-
			terobacteriaceae
Axilla and groin	*Corynebacterium* sp.		*Eubacterium* sp.
	Mycobacterium smegmatis		*Fusobacterium* sp.
	Staphylococcus epidermidis		*Lactobacillus* sp.
			Peptostreptococcus sp.
			Pseudomonas aeruginosa
EYE			*Staphylococcus aureus*
Conjunctiva	*Corynebacterium* sp.		Viridans streptococci
	Haemophilus influenzae		
	Neisseria sp.	**GENITOURINARY TRACT**	
	Staphylococcus epidermidis	Bladder	None
	Viridans streptococci	Urethra (anterior)	*Acinetobacter* sp.
			Candida albicans and other yeasts
RESPIRATORY			*Corynebacterium* sp.
Mouth and tonsils	*Actinomyces* sp.		Enteric organisms included in the En-
	Bacteroides sp.		terobacteriaceae
	Bifidobacterium sp.		*Mycobacterium* sp.
	Borrelia refringens		*Mycoplasma* sp.
	Candida albicans and other yeasts		*Neisseria* sp.
	Corynebacterium sp.		*Trichomonas vaginalis*
	Coliforms		
	Fusobacterium sp.	Vagina	*Candida albicans*
	Haemophilus sp.	Prior to puberty	*Corynebacterium* sp.
	Lactobacillus sp.	and after meno-	Enteric organisms included in the En-
	Micrococcus sp.	pause	terobacteriaceae
	Neisseria sp.		*Micrococcus* sp.
	Peptostreptococcus sp.		*Staphylococcus epidermidis*
	Staphylococcus aureus		Viridans streptococci
	Staphylococcus epidermidis		
	Streptococcus pneumoniae	Between puberty	*Acinetobacter* sp.
	Treponema denticum	and menopause	*Bifidobacterium* sp.
	Veillonella sp.		*Candida albicans* and other yeasts
	Viridans streptococci		*Clostridium* sp.
			Corynebacterium sp.
Nose and nasopharynx	*Corynebacterium* sp.		*Fusobacterium* sp.
	Haemophilus sp.		Group B streptococci
	Neisseria sp.		*Haemophilus vaginalis*
	Staphyloccus aureus		*Lactobacillus acidophilus* and other lac-
	Staphylococcus epidermidis		tobacilli
	Streptococcus pneumoniae		*Mycobacterium* sp.
			Mycoplasma sp.
			Peptostreptococcus sp.
Larynx, trachea, bron-	No permanent flora; transient flora de-		*Trichomonas vaginalis*
chi and lungs	stroyed		Viridans streptococci

Infections

TRANSMISSION

The division between bacteria that produce disease and those that do not is not a sharp demarcation. To cause a disease, an organism must be able (1) to get in or on the body, (2) to grow and avoid host immune reactions, (3) to cause damage, and (4) to spread to a new host. Some organisms routinely cause illness when they infect an individual, whereas others cause symptomatic infections in some persons but not in others. There are terms to describe such situations, but it is difficult to assign quantitative values to them. For example, *pathogenicity* is defined as the ability of a microorganism to cause disease, whereas *virulence* refers to the extent of pathogenicity. Thus, highly virulent organisms require fewer organisms to establish an infection and initiate disease. Therefore, some pathogenic organisms can be described as highly virulent, whereas others, which only occasionally cause disease, are referred to as weakly virulent.

Not all infectious diseases are spread from person to person. For example, in tetanus or gas gangrene, the infective agent is introduced through the skin and into the muscle after a wound such as a nail puncture or a gunshot. Other infectious diseases can be acquired from animals, either by direct contact (eg, handling infected meat) or by the ingestion of contaminated meat or milk products. On the other hand, many diseases are transmitted, either directly or indirectly, from one individual to another. Those diseases that are spread from an infected animal or person are called *communicable* or *contagious* diseases.

Infectious diseases also can be categorized on the basis of how often they occur. If a disease, such as the common cold, is constantly present within a stated geographic area, it is said to be *endemic*. An *epidemic* is present when the occurrence of a disease exceeds expected levels. It is difficult to assign numbers to an epidemic because we are concerned with disease occurrence over normal expectations. For example, four or five cases of yellow fever in a village in South America might not be considered an epidemic, whereas that many cases in a city in the United States clearly would be labeled as one. Diseases such as influenza and measles often spread as epidemics. When an epidemic of a disease becomes worldwide, it is considered to be *pandemic*. Pandemics of influenza have caused the deaths of millions of people. If a particular disease occurs only occasionally, it is said to be *sporadic*.

When a microorganism capable of producing disease gains entrance into a host, a period elapses before there is any manifestation of illness. This interval between infection and the appearance of the first symptoms is called the *incubation period*. It is constant and predictable for some diseases (eg, 11 days for measles) but variable for others (eg, 15 to 40 days for hepatitis A). The incubation period is followed by the period of *illness*, after which

occurs the period of *convalescence*. Even though no symptoms of disease are present during the periods of incubation and convalescence, the infectious disease organisms still can be spread to others. In some instances, individuals who have fully recovered from a disease harbor and spread the causative organisms for months or even years. Such individuals are called *carriers*. They apparently have acquired sufficient immunity to the disease-producing agent to prevent the occurrence of symptoms, but are unable to eliminate the agent from their bodies. The most common type of carriers are those who harbor disease-producing agents in their intestines, resulting in the spread of these organisms through contaminated food and water. Infectious agents typically spread by such carriers include those that cause typhoid fever, bacillary dysentery, amebic dysentery, bacterial diarrhea, and viral hepatitis. Other infectious agents linger in the macrophages of persons who, though not ill themselves, continue to carry the organisms in their bloodstream for months, years, or even a lifetime. This type of carrier is particularly dangerous if unwittingly used as a blood donor. Hepatitis B, hepatitis C, and AIDS are the most common examples of diseases transmitted through blood products and body secretions.

Infectious diseases also can be spread by individuals who have mild symptoms of an undiagnosed infection. One typical example is seen in the spread of tuberculosis. This disease usually begins with a mild but persistent cough, causing the organisms in the lungs to be expelled in an aerosol. By the time tuberculosis is diagnosed, the organisms may have been spread to many other people. Many infectious disease agents exist in reservoirs (eg, wild mammals, birds, or ticks) from which they are transmitted to humans. For instance, many rickettsial diseases exist in the wild animal population; the organisms that cause plague, tularemia, and brucellosis also exist primarily in both wild and domestic animals. Birds constitute the chief reservoir for several agents that cause viral encephalitis, and humans are the reservoir for many bacterial and viral diseases.

ACUTE AND CHRONIC INFECTIONS

Acute infections develop rapidly, usually cause fever, and generally are of short duration. Most hospitalized patients with infectious diseases are acutely ill. In contrast, chronic infections develop more slowly, with milder and longer-lasting symptoms. A chronic infection can become acute, and an acute infection can become chronic. Tuberculosis and leprosy are examples of infections that are frequently chronic, whereas scarlet fever and toxic shock syndrome generally are acute.

LOCAL AND SYSTEMIC INFECTIONS

A local infection is one in which the causative agent is limited to one site on the body, such as a boil (furuncle).

A systemic infection is one in which the infecting agent spreads throughout the body, as in Lyme disease or mumps. The clinical picture is never as simple as the examples given here, however, because a local infection can cause general symptoms similar to those resulting from a systemic infection. Local infections with general symptoms usually result from the elaboration of toxins by the microorganism. Such is the case with diphtheria, in which the organism remains localized in the throat and nasopharynx but produces a powerful toxin that is transported throughout the body. Tetanus and pertussis also are diseases of this type.

Occasionally, an infection occurring in one area of the body (particularly an abscess) acts as a nucleus for its spread to other areas. An example of this type of focal infection is a dental or tonsillar abscess that seeds organisms into the blood, resulting in endocarditis or widespread foci of infection. It frequently is necessary to find the area of focal infection and remove it surgically.

INAPPARENT INFECTIONS

It is difficult to differentiate between an inapparent infection and a mild, undiagnosed one. The term, *inapparent infection,* refers to an illness caused by a frank pathogenic organism in which the symptoms are either absent or so mild that they go undetected and undiagnosed. This category includes many human illnesses. Poliomyelitis and hepatitis A are excellent examples of diseases in which most cases go undiagnosed. We know this is true because many people who have no history of either infection have protective antibodies against both the viruses that cause these illnesses.

PROOF OF THE CAUSE OF A DISEASE

Isolation of a particular organism from an infected person does not prove it to be the causative agent of the disease. The organism may exist in or near a lesion merely as normal flora or a transient contaminant. Robert Koch faced this problem in the 1870s as he labored to establish the cause of anthrax. Consequently, Koch laid down a series of experimental steps that should be followed to establish unequivocally a causal relationship between an organism and a specific disease. These rules, known as *Koch's postulates,* can be summarized as follows:

1. The same organism must be found in all cases of a designated disease.
2. The organism must be isolated from the infected person and grown in pure culture.
3. The organisms from the pure culture must reproduce the disease when inoculated into a susceptible animal.
4. The organism then must be isolated again from the experimentally infected animal.

Although these postulates are effective in determin-

ing the causative agents of most diseases, there are a few exceptions. For example, neither *Mycobacterium leprae* nor *Treponema pallidum* has been grown in the laboratory, so they fit only the first postulate. Figure 23-2 provides an illustration of these postulates.

HOW PATHOGENS ENTER AND LEAVE THE BODY

Secretions and excretions from infected areas often contain the infective microbe. In some illnesses (eg, malaria), there is no obvious exit, because the organisms are present in the blood and require a vector (eg, a mosquito) for transmission. However, whether it is obvious or not, each organism capable of producing disease has its own portal or portals of entry as well as a means of escape (portal of exit) from the host. The infectious agent in discharges from infected areas must be destroyed to prevent transmission of the agent to a new host.

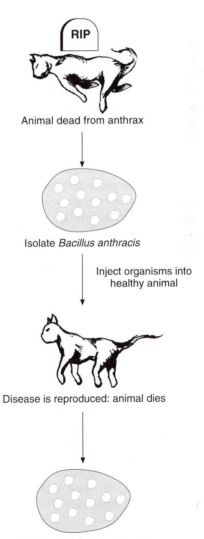

Animal dead from anthrax

Isolate *Bacillus anthracis*

Inject organisms into healthy animal

Disease is reproduced: animal dies

Reisolate *Bacillus anthracis*

FIGURE 23-2 The use of Koch's postulates to establish the causative agent of a specific infection, such as anthrax.

cus (the etiologic agent of epidemic meningitis), such capsules appear to be their most important virulence factor. Antibodies directed against the capsule induce a rapid phagocytosis and destruction of the invading organism by virtue of the fact that phagocytic cells possess Fc receptors on their surface. As a result, many vaccines are designed solely to stimulate the formation of specific anticapsular antibodies.

Group A streptococci have evolved a slightly different antiphagocytic capsule, which has been designated the *M protein*. This structure, made up entirely of protein, is an intimate part of the cell wall and prevents phagocytosis by blocking the alternate pathway of complement activation. Unlike the carbohydrate capsules, purified M protein displays considerable toxicity to polymorphonuclear leukocytes. As discussed in Chapter 24, group A streptococci possess a variety of virulence factors, but only antibodies to the M protein (which permits phagocytosis of the organism) are protective, providing another example in which an antiphagocytic structure is the major virulence factor for the invading microorganism.

Fimbriae

Fimbriae already have been categorized as virulence factors because of their role as colonization factors, but in many cases, they appear to serve also as antiphagocytic structures. Fimbriae impede phagocytosis through their ability to bind to a surface component of the phagocyte in such a manner that they prevent the bacterial cell from making the close contact necessary for phagocytosis to occur. In such cases, antibodies directed to the fimbriae neutralize the antiphagocytic effect, permitting engulfment of the organism. As discussed in Chapter 25, *Neisseria gonorrhoeae* possesses multiple genes encoding fimbriae structures and, through a process of genetic recombination, is continually changing the antigenic composition of its fimbriae. (Historically, these structures on *Neisseria* have been referred to as *pili*, but they are morphologically similar to fimbriae on other gram-negative bacteria and should be referred to as fimbriae.) Thus, by the time an individual mounts an immune response to one set of fimbriae, a population possessing antigenically different fimbriae already is present, allowing the organisms to continue growing. An analogous system occurs with other surface structures. For example, members of the genus *Borrelia* possess multiple genes for a cell-surface protein, which results in the appearance of new antigenic types, thwarting the opsonic effect of a humoral immune response. Similarly, the parasitic trypanosomes have been shown to possess thousands of different genes encoding surface glycoproteins, resulting in frequent surface changes and preventing any effective antibody-dependent phagocytosis.

SIDEROPHORES

Vertebrates have evolved some ingenious ways of retaining iron in a soluble state so that this highly insoluble metal is available for the synthesis of new cell components. This is accomplished by binding iron to high-affinity glycoproteins, which not only keep it soluble, but serve to transport it throughout the body. One of these, termed *lactoferrin*, is found primarily in secretions such as milk, tears, saliva, mucus, and intestinal fluid. The other major iron transporter is called *transferrin* and is found most commonly in plasma. Microorganisms also require iron for growth, and unless they are able to "steal" the bound iron from transferrin or lactoferrin, they cannot reproduce within the body. This is exactly what many pathogenic microorganisms are able to do through the production of siderophores and membrane receptors for the siderophore–iron complex.

Siderophores are low-molecular-weight compounds with a high affinity for iron. Many have higher affinities than transferrin and, thus, are able to capture iron, permitting growth within the host. After accepting a molecule of iron, the siderophore can bind to specific membrane receptors on the bacterium, releasing the iron for microbial growth. There are many different siderophores, but they all fall into one of two types: (1) catechols, or (2) hydroxymates. In both types, the ferric ion is chelated between two hydroxyl groups or, sometimes, between a hydroxyl group and an amino group (Fig. 23-5).

Thus, the ability to produce a siderophore that can compete successfully for host iron is an important virulence factor. Many organisms synthesize more than one siderophore, and many others are able to bind siderophores that they are unable to synthesize. Their importance has been demonstrated in experiments with animals

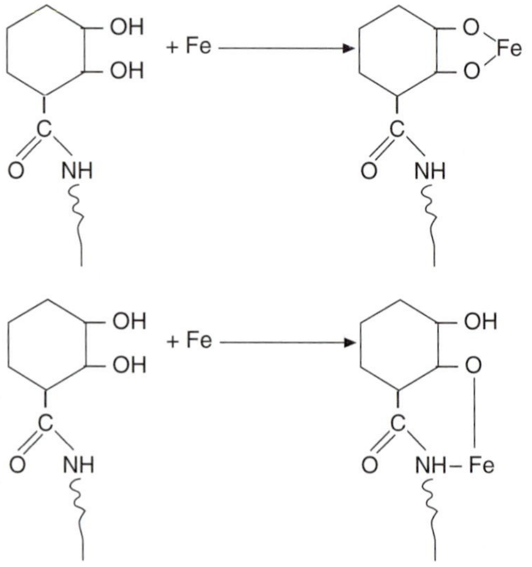

FIGURE 23-5 Iron is chelated either between two hydroxyl groups or between a hydroxyl group and an amino group. This illustration shows only the part of the siderophore molecule that chelates the iron.

and various microorganisms, which showed that a genetic loss in the ability to synthesize a siderophore is correlated with a reduction in virulence, and vice versa.

EXOTOXINS

Toxic substances that are excreted from the bacterial cell or released after lysis of the bacterium are called *exotoxins.* Some organisms, such as the streptococci and the staphylococci, form many of these toxins, whereas others, such as the etiologic agents of tetanus, diphtheria, and cholera, appear to synthesize a single exotoxin that is responsible for the symptoms of the disease. In addition, the food poisoning caused by *Clostridium botulinum, S aureus,* and *Bacillus cereus* results from the liberation of an exotoxin into the food. Because the ability to produce an exotoxin can be the only property that allows some organisms to cause disease, loss of this ability results in a complete loss of pathogenicity. Exotoxins can be thought of as toxins that act outside the host cell, at the host cell surface, or inside the host cell.

TOXINS THAT ACT OUTSIDE THE CELL

Hyaluronidase

Various pathogenic bacteria excrete an enzyme capable of breaking down hyaluronic acid, the intracellular material of connective tissue. The hydrolysis of this material would seem to help in the spread of the organisms; based on this belief, hyaluronidase sometimes has been referred to as *spreading factor.* Experimentally, it is difficult to measure the value of hyaluronidase in microbial invasiveness, but it probably aids in penetration and in the spread of certain organisms in host tissues.

Streptokinase

By activating a proteolytic enzyme called plasmin, which is normally present in the host's plasma, streptokinase causes the dissolution of blood clots and, thus, allows the spread of streptococci. An essentially identical substance produced by the staphylococci is refferred to as *staphylokinase.*

Coagulase

The principal organism producing coagulase is the familiar staphylococcus. The result of the action of coagulase is the coagulation of plasma, which produces a fibrin clot. It is postulated that this ability allows the organisms to lay down a thin fibrin layer around each individual cell, thus preventing or inhibiting phagocytosis by the host's leukocytes. Furthermore, it is thought by many investigators that coagulase is responsible for the fibrin barrier, typical of an abscess, that walls off the local infection from the host's defense mechanisms. In any case, it is certainly true that of all the properties associated with the virulence of staphylococci, the production of coagulase is the most constant.

Collagenase

Collagenase is formed by some of the clostridia that cause gas gangrene. Collagenase causes the breakdown of collagen, which is the ground substance of bone, skin, and cartilage. Thus, collagenase helps in the spread of organisms from the initial site of infection.

TOXINS THAT ACT AT THE CELL SURFACE

Many different *hemolysins* are produced by bacteria that induce the lysis of the host's red blood cells. However, hemolytic anemia is not a normal result of infection, even by organisms that produce large amounts of hemolysin, and it is likely that the real purpose of hemolysin is to kill leukocytes. Such hemolysis does, however, provide iron essential for growth from liberated hemoglobin and, as a result, contributes to the virulence of the hemolysin-producing organisms.

Many hemolysins also are capable of causing membrane damage to many kinds of eucaryotic cells. Damage to phagocytic cells may enhance the survival of the invading organism.

Leukocidins

Leukocidins, little-studied, nondescript substances, kill the host's leukocytes. It is easy to evaluate their role in the invasiveness of the organism because leukocytes are so important in the defense mechanisms of the body that any substance that is toxic to them gives an advantage to the invading organism.

TOXINS THAT ACT WITHIN THE CELL

The symptoms of many diseases are directly attributable to one or more specific exotoxins produced by the infecting organisms. The mechanism of action of such exotoxins is described in chapters dealing with the organism, and only the major types associated with human disease are categorized here.

Enterotoxins

Enterotoxins are exotoxins that interact with the gastrointestinal system to cause diarrhea or dysentery (bloody diarrhea). Although there are several different enterotoxins, they generally can be grouped into two types: (1)

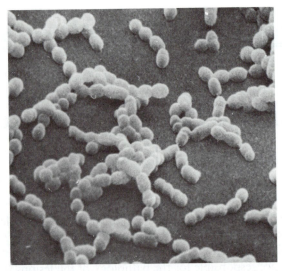

FIGURE 24-1 Chains of *Streptococcus mutans.* As discussed later in the chapter, this streptococcus uses sucrose to produce an acid capable of eroding tooth enamel. (Original magnification ×5000.)

Obviously, such a complex synthetic medium would be used only in a research laboratory. For routine culturing of streptococci, a complex, undefined medium containing peptones, meat infusion, salts, glucose, and agar for solidification is used. To this is added 5% sterile defibrinated blood before the medium is poured into Petri dishes. The resulting plates usually are referred to as blood-agar plates, valuable both for growing and for identifying the streptococci.

Most streptococci are aerotolerant anaerobes, although there are obligately anaerobic streptococci that are normal inhabitants of the female genital tract. The term *aerotolerant aerobe* is used, because the streptococci obtain all their energy requirements from the fermentation of sugars to lactic acid, whether they are growing aerobically or anaerobically. They have no aerobic metabolism because they are unable to synthesize heme, a necessary prosthetic group of the cytochromes. Thus, they have no mechanism for an aerobic metabolism requiring the transport of electrons through a cytochrome system to molecular oxygen. Their growth in the presence of air also is limited because of the spontaneous aerobic oxidation of reduced pyridine nucleotides (NADH or NADPH). In the absence of cytochromes, this results in a two-electron transfer to oxygen to form H_2O_2. Aerobic bacteria can protect themselves from the killing effect of H_2O_2 because they synthesize the enzyme catalase, which quickly converts H_2O_2 to H_2O and O_2. However, the streptococci are unable to synthesize the heme prosthetic group for this enzyme and, as a result, can form lethal amounts of H_2O_2 during aerobic growth. In laboratory practice, the streptococci are grown on blood-agar plates, and red blood cells provide a good source of catalase for the destruction of any H_2O_2 formed during aerobic metabolism.

HEMOLYSINS

As streptococci grow, they secrete a large number of toxins and enzymes. The exact role of some of these products in the development of disease is unknown, but several are used for the identification of the streptococci and, occasionally, for the diagnosis of a possible recent streptococcal infection. Among these secreted products can be one or more hemolysins that cause the lysis of red blood cells in the medium. Although there is no evidence that the lysis of red blood cells plays any part in the disease syndrome, it is well established that these hemolysins are important in the infection through their ability to destroy other types of cells. Moreover, they are used to divide the streptococci into three groups based on the presence or absence of hemolysis and on the type of red blood cell destruction that occurs during growth on a blood-agar plate.

When grown on a blood-agar plate, the *α-hemolytic* streptococci produce an incomplete hemolysis of the red blood cells, resulting in a greenish brown discoloration surrounding the colony. The partially opaque area contains unlysed red blood cells and a green, unidentified, reduced product of hemoglobin. (Both viridans streptococci and *S pneumoniae* are α-hemolytic.)

The *β-hemolytic* streptococci cause a hemolysis of red blood cells surrounding the colony, resulting in a completely clear zone in which no color remains. This β-hemolysis results from the secretion by the streptococci of one or both of two different hemolysins, designated *streptolysin S* and *streptolysin O.* Streptolysin S was so named because early work with this hemolysin showed that it could be extracted from the streptococci with serum. However, because it is stable in the presence of atmospheric oxygen (streptolysin O is not), the S could represent "stable" as well as "serum-extractable." Streptolysin O is reversibly inactivated in the presence of oxygen, and the β-hemolysis seen on the surface of a blood-agar plate is primarily the result of streptolysin S rather than streptolysin O. If the streptococci are grown anaerobically, however, both hemolysins produce β-hemolysis.

The third major group of streptococci produces no hemolysins and, hence, has no effect on blood cells in an agar medium. Members of this group of streptococci are sometimes called the *γ-hemolytic streptococci,* although the term is really a misnomer because they are not at all hemolytic.

CLASSIFICATION

Until the 1930s, the classification of the streptococci was confusing. Many streptococci were considered specific for the disease entity from which they were isolated and were given names based on that type of infection. Examples of such names include *Streptococcus erysipelatis* for an organism isolated from the skin infection erysipelas and

TABLE 24-1
Major Criteria Used in Sherman's Biochemical Classification of the Streptococci

Group	Characteristics
Pyogenic (all Lancefield groups except D and N)	Mostly β-hemolytic; will not grow at 45°C or in the presence of 6.5% NaCl
Viridans (not classifiable in Lancefield's classification)	α-Hemolytic; will grow at 45°C but not in the presence of 6.5% NaCl
Lactic (Lancefield's group N)	Nonhemolytic; will not grow at 45°C or in the presence of 6.5% NaCl; will grow at 10°C in the presence of 0.1% methylene blue in milk
Enterococcus (Lancefield's group D)	Usually not hemolytic; will grow at 45°C in the presence of 6.5% NaCl; will grow at pH 9.6

Streptococcus scarlatinae for one isolated from scarlet fever. A biochemical classification system, proposed by J.M. Sherman in 1937 (Table 24-1), proved valuable in the overall classification of this genus. However, because essentially all acute infections were caused by organisms in Sherman's pyogenic group, this classification was of little value to the medical epidemiologist. The present classification of the streptococci still uses the criteria proposed by Sherman but, in addition, uses antigenic properties to subdivide most of the streptococci into groups and types. This latter classification system originally was proposed by Rebecca Lancefield in 1933, and it made it clear that a single streptococcal species could be responsible for a variety of disease entities.

Lancefield found that if streptococci are placed in dilute acid (pH 2) and heated at 100°C for 10 minutes, a soluble carbohydrate antigen is extracted from their cell walls. This carbohydrate, which she called *C carbohydrate,* also can be extracted with formamide by heating the cells at 150°C for 15 minutes.

All streptococci except the viridans group and *S pneumoniae* (see Table 24-1) are classified on the basis of their C carbohydrate. When the C carbohydrate from many different streptococcal isolates was categorized using antibodies obtained by immunizing rabbits with the streptococci, it was found that there were 13 different antigenic C carbohydrates. Based on these antigenic differences, Lancefield divided the streptococci into groups designated by letters. Table 24-2 lists some of the properties of those serogroups associated with human illnesses. Thus, the organisms in group A all possess the same antigenic C carbohydrate, and the organisms in group B all possess another C carbohydrate. The C carbohydrate from group A has been shown to consist of a long polymer of rhamnose, to which are attached residues of *N*-acetyl-glucosamine (Fig. 24-2). Furthermore, it soon became apparent that each group had a more or less specific habitat, that is, group A were primarily human pathogens, group B were primarily cattle and human pathogens, and so on (Table 24-3). Although common, these habitats are not rigid.

In addition to the carbohydrate used to classify the streptococci into groups, other antigens are present in each group. Some of these antigens are not involved in the virulence of the streptococci, nor are they of value in a specific classification; thus, they are not discussed here.

TABLE 24-2
Lancefield's Serogroups Associated With Human Illnesses

Group	Species Name	Type of Hemolysis	Major Types of Infections
A	*Streptococcus pyogenes*	β	Pharyngitis, scarlet fever, impetigo, toxic shock-like syndrome
B	*Streptococcus agalactiae*	β	Neonatal pneumonia, sepsis, meningitis
D	*Enterococcus faecalis, Streptococcus bovis*	Variable	Urinary tract infection, endocarditis

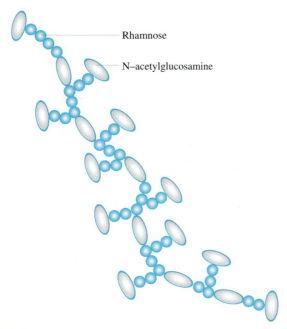

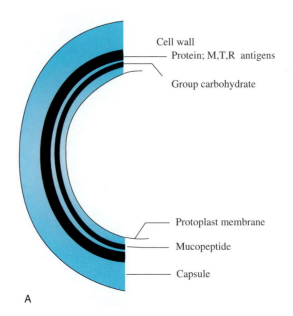

FIGURE 24-2 Diagrammatic representation of the streptococcal group A carbohydrate.

However, each Lancefield group does contain a type-specific substance that allows a further subdivision of each group into specific types. The type-specific antigen in some groups is a second carbohydrate (different from the C carbohydrate), whereas in group A, which contains the major human pathogens, it is a cell-wall protein called the *M protein*. Figure 24-3*A* shows a schematic representation of a typical group A streptococcus cell; Figure 24-3*B* shows a section through a cell possessing M protein; and Figure 24-3*C* is without the M protein.

TABLE 24-3
Lancefield's Group Classification and Normal Habitat of Streptococci

Group	Normal Habitat
A	Humans
B	Cattle and humans
C	Wide variety of animals and humans
D	Intestinal tract of humans and animals (enterococci)
E	Swine
F	Humans
G	Humans and dogs
H	Humans
K	Humans
L	Dogs
M	Dogs
N	Dairy products (never hemolytic on blood agar)
O	Humans

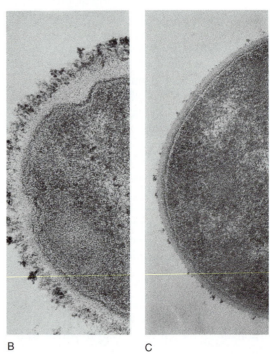

FIGURE 24-3 A. Layers of the cell wall and capsule of a group A streptococcus. **B.** Section through a streptococcal cell showing fimbriae of M protein. (Original magnification ×100,000.) **C.** Section through a type of streptococcal cell without M protein; compare with **B.** (Original magnification ×80,000.)

GROUP A β-HEMOLYTIC STREPTOCOCCI

Cellular Components

Although human infections can be caused by organisms from several Lancefield groups, group A contains most of the streptococci known to produce acute disease; members of group A (*Streptococcus pyogenes*) also can lead to late nonsuppurative (non–pus-forming) complications such as rheumatic fever, acute glomerulonephritis, and erythema nodosum. All these organisms are β-hemolytic. On the basis of antigenic differences in the M protein, the group is subdivided into more than 60 types designated by numbers. The M protein also is important in the virulence of group A streptococci, for several reasons. First, it is antiphagocytic by virtue of its ability to block the alternate pathway of complement activation; as a result, organisms possessing M protein are able to resist phagocytosis and maintain an infection in the absence of specific antibodies. Second, many of the M proteins act as superantigens. Third, the M protein is the antigen that induces type-specific immunity. Thus, even though antibodies are formed against many streptococcal antigens, including the C carbohydrate, only the type-specific anti-M protein antibodies provide immunity, because these antibodies act as opsonins to allow the virulent organisms to be phagocytosed.

Many group A streptococci also possess a capsule of *hyaluronic acid,* but anticapsular antibodies are not formed because hyaluronic acid is a normal component of connective tissue. The capsule could provide additional antiphagocytic protection; however, because the M protein actually extends through the capsule as fine fimbriae, the presence of the capsule does not protect the cell from the opsonic effect of anti-M protein antibodies. An additional type-specific protein called the *T antigen* is found in many group A organisms. Unlike the M protein, the T antigens are not involved in the virulence of the organisms, nor are they related to type-specific immunity. It is not customary, therefore, to determine the T-antigenic specificity of a streptococcus except in the event that the isolate is one of those rare group A streptococci that does not possess an M protein.

Like many pathogenic organisms, the group A streptococci must be able to adhere to eucaryotic cells to produce an infection. They do this through the mediation of several different *adhesins,* which are cellular constituents that bind to specific eucaryotic glycoproteins. *Lipoteichoic acid* is a streptococcal product that will bind to fibronectin, forming a weak hydrophobic link to human epithelial cells. It has been proposed that once this interaction has occurred, M protein binds to an epithelial receptor, resulting in a firm attachment of the bacterium to the pharyngeal cells. A second cell-wall protein, termed *streptococcal F protein,* has been reported to bind to fibronectin even more strongly than lipoteichoic acid.

Extracellular Products

The group A streptococci excrete numerous enzymes and toxins, most of which appear to have some role in the production of disease. The enzyme *streptokinase* promotes the lysis of fibrin blood clots and is thought by some to be at least partially responsible for the rapid spread of streptococcal infections by preventing the formation of a fibrin barrier around the infected site. However, antibodies to streptokinase do not seem to influence the infection, and the role of streptokinase is vague. Streptokinase acts by catalyzing the conversion of an inactive plasma component, *plasminogen,* into the active proteolytic enzyme, *plasmin.* It is interesting to note that group A streptococci will bind specifically to the activated plasmin, and that this cell-bound plasmin retains its proteolytic activity. Moreover, such bound plasmin is no longer regulated by its specific inhibitor; as a result, it has been postulated that plasmin-bound streptococci have a greater potential for tissue invasion by virtue of their ability to hydrolyze connective tissue and basement membranes. Streptokinase also has been given to patients immediately after a myocardial infarction to prevent the formation of blood clots. However, this has been superseded in part by the use of a cloned human tissue plasminogen activator.

Hyaluronidase depolymerizes hyaluronic acid. It is believed to play a role in the spread of streptococci through tissues by hydrolyzing the host's hyaluronic acid and, therefore, has been called *spreading factor.*

Streptodornase is a general name given to the four streptococcal enzymes that degrade DNA, the deoxyribonucleases. They are capable of degrading the viscous DNA resulting from the disintegration of the host's leukocytes and may contribute to the more rapid spread of the infection.

Streptolysin O is an oxygen-labile hemolysin that binds to cholesterol in the cell membrane and causes the lysis of erythrocytes. However, because anemia is not a usual result of streptococcal infections, it is not this function that contributes to the virulence of the organisms, but rather the ability of streptolysin O to react with sterols in the host's leukocyte membranes, where it forms toxin oligomers, resulting in large transmembrane pores. This causes the release of the enzymes in the cell's lysosomes, resulting in degranulation and death of the leukocyte (see Chap. 4). The release of these hydrolytic enzymes also can destroy adjacent tissue and contribute further to the streptococcal infection. In addition, streptolysin O binds naturally occurring IgGs to form immune complexes with potent complement-activating capacity, perpetuating local tissue damage. Furthermore, streptolysin O is capable of suppressing chemotaxis and leukocyte mobility. The fact that streptolysin O is antigenic and that antistreptolysin O will prevent the hemolysis of erythrocytes provides an important tool for detecting a recent group A streptococcal infection. Such information is a valuable aid in the diagnosis of the late complications of streptococcal infections, which usually occur after the organisms have been eliminated from the host.

Streptolysin S is a small polypeptide of about 28 amino acid residues that is active only when bound to a nonspecific carrier such as RNA or streptococcal cell wall. In addition to causing β-hemolysis, it is able to inhibit chemotaxis and phagocytosis as well as exert a cytotoxic effect on various types of eucaryotic cells. It is believed to act by binding to phospholipid in the target-cell membrane, and it has been shown that mere external contact of group A streptococci with leukocytes is sufficient to kill the phagocytic cells. It seems clear, therefore, that this hemolysin is an important virulence factor of group A streptococcal infections. Unlike its O counterpart, streptolysin S is not antigenic—probably because of its small size.

Most group A streptococci also produce a surface-bound *C5a peptidase* that specifically cleaves six amino acids from the carboxy terminus of the C5a component of complement. This results in a drastic inhibition in its ability to bind to polymorphonuclear leukocyte (PMN) receptors, thus destroying much of the effectiveness of complement components to act as chemoattractants.

Essentially all group A streptococci produce one or more of the three serotypes of *pyrogenic toxins* (A, B, and C). These toxins are part of a large family of toxins that have been classified as superantigens because they bind to the major histocompatibility complex of antigen-presenting cells, stimulating certain subsets of T cells to divide. They also induce the macrophage to synthesize and secrete tumor necrosis factor-α (TNF-α) and interleukin-1 (IL-1; see Chap. 23 for a review of superantigens).

Interestingly, serotypes A and C are carried by a temperate phage and serotype B is chromosomally encoded. As a result, one survey of a large number of group A strains showed that the A and C serotypes were produced by 15% and 50%, respectively, whereas the B serotype was produced by 100%. However, when all strains were compared with those isolated from patients with scarlet fever or rheumatic fever, the A serotype was found in 53% and 51%, respectively. No such enrichment of serotypes B and C were noted, leading to the conclusion that only serotype A production has a significant correlation with disease.

Pathogenicity

STREPTOCOCCAL PHARYNGITIS. Streptococcal pharyngitis is the most frequent manifestation of group A infections. This condition can be acute, in which case the mucous membranes of the tonsils and pharynx are red and edematous (filled with fluid) with a purulent exudate; the cervical lymph nodes can be enlarged, and the temperature usually is high. The infection typically is self-limiting, with symptoms lasting less than 5 days. Complications include spread of the organisms to the middle ear or, rarely, to the meninges. Pneumonia is not usual but might occur in conjunction with a viral respiratory tract infection such as influenza or measles. Epidemics of streptococcal pharyngitis usually are the result of personal contact with either infected persons or healthy carriers. Epidemiologic studies have shown that, commonly, school-age children

bring the infections home and spread them within the family.

SCARLET FEVER. Scarlet fever can be caused by any type of group A streptococcus that produces a *pyrogenic toxin* (also called an *erythrogenic toxin*). It appears to be associated most frequently with organisms that produce pyrogenic toxin A. Therefore, scarlet fever generally is the result of a streptococcal sore throat caused by a pyrogenic toxin-producing organism. Although the bacteria can remain localized in the throat, the dissemination of the toxin causes the appearance of a diffuse rash.

The severity of scarlet fever appears to have waxed and waned over the centuries. During the mid-19th century, pandemics of scarlet fever occurring in Europe and the United States were the most common infectious childhood disease, causing a case fatality rate of over 30%. In Kunming, China, 50,000 of a total population of 200,000 persons died of scarlet fever between 1921 and 1923. Many died within 24 hours after manifesting the initial symptoms of the disease. From 1890 to 1987, however, strains of streptococci causing such severe disease seemed to have disappeared from the Western world and case fatality rates remained less than 3%. Recently, however, group A streptococci have been isolated more and more frequently from serious and fatal infections involving pneumonia and bloodstream invasion. Such infections are really a manifestation of scarlet fever, but they usually are referred to as *streptococcal toxic shock-like syndrome*. It is noteworthy that the sudden death of "muppeteer" Jim Hensen in 1990 resulted from a pneumonia caused by a pyrogenic toxin-producing group A streptococcus, and that it occurred less than 24 hours after the initial appearance of symptoms. Interestingly, rare cases of toxic shock-like syndrome have been reported to occur after infections by groups B, C, F, and G streptococci.

The streptococcal pyrogenic toxins are part of a large family of toxins that includes staphylococcal pyrogenic toxins A and B, staphylococcal enterotoxins A through E, staphylococcal exfoliatin, staphylococcal toxic shock syndrome (TSS) toxin, and certain M proteins. All the toxins in this group share numerous biologic properties, such as pyrogenicity (induction of fever), immunosuppression, mitogenicity for lymphocytes, and the ability to greatly enhance the lethality of endotoxic shock.

The streptococcal pyrogenic toxins are low-molecular-weight proteins possessing two functional parts: (1) a heat-labile domain that carries the immunologic determinants used to differentiate the three serotypes, A, B, and C; and (2) a heat-stable domain that is common to all three serotypes. The heat-labile portion of the molecule induces fever and suppresses the immune system, whereas the heat-stable part of the molecule enhances the pyrogenicity and lethality of the toxin. Moreover, the rash that is characteristic of scarlet fever is the result of a hypersensitivity reaction to this part of the molecule. Thus, a person could be infected with a group A, scarlet fever–producing streptococcus and not have the characteristic rash, if that person possessed neutralizing antibodies to the heat-labile part of the toxin or lacked a hypersensitivity to the heat-stable portion of the molecule.

Even more interesting is the ability of these pyrogenic toxins to increase the sensitivity of the host to other products, such as streptolysin O and endotoxin (see staphylococcal toxic shock syndrome toxin). Rabbits have been shown to be as much as 100,000 to 1 million times more sensitive to endotoxin after they have been injected with streptococcal pyrogenic toxin. In addition, low levels of endotoxin have been shown to be fatal to monkeys who previously received sublethal amounts of pyrogenic toxin. It seems probable that a mixed infection with group A streptococci and a gram-negative organism could explain the severity of symptoms associated with scarlet fever, and it is not surprising that several cases of typical TSS (see Staphylococcal Infections) have been ascribed to infections caused by group A streptococci. In one study of severe group A streptococcal infections associated with a toxic shock-like syndrome (mortality rate 30%), cultures from affected patients predominantly produced pyrogenic toxin A, and most were associated with a soft tissue infection. Therefore, it seems that strains producing toxin A largely disappeared during much of the 20th century but now are coming back. This is exemplified by the observation that 8% of all invasive streptococcal infections between 1988 and 1989 in Pima County, Arizona caused a toxic shock-like syndrome. No toxic shock-like illness had occurred there during the preceding 3 years.

NECROTIZING FASCIITIS. This is a rapidly spreading infection that occurs in planes of tissue under the skin, particularly in the fascia. Nerve cells and blood vessels are destroyed and, as a result, skin is deprived of blood and dies. The organisms causing this syndrome appear to be a newly evolved strain of group A streptococci and have been dubbed by some scientists as the "flesh eating bacteria". Treatment requires the removal of all tissue down to the muscle layer and frequently involves amputation of an infected limb. The infection spreads extremely rapidly and has a mortality rate of 50% to 80%.

STREPTOCOCCAL IMPETIGO. Impetigo is a skin infection that occurs most often in young children, particularly those living in crowded, low-socioeconomic conditions. Streptococcal impetigo is characterized by the occurrence on the skin of small vesicles that eventually form a thin, amber crust. The group A streptococci that cause impetigo frequently are nephritogenic, that is, they lead to acute glomerulonephritis.

OTHER GROUP A STREPTOCOCCAL INFECTIONS. Puerperal sepsis is a postpartum infection of the uterus that has claimed the lives of many women. Modern aseptic techniques and

A Closer Look

At long last, some data are surfacing to explain why superantigens and endotoxins cause a lowering of blood pressure, resulting in irreversible shock and death.

The sequence of events begins when a superantigen binds to a macrophage, inducing it to synthesize TNF-α and IL-1. As described in Chapter 23, many biologic effects are initiated by TNF-α, one of the most interesting of which is its ability to increase the transcription of various genes. Of these, an inducible form of NOS may be the crucial enzyme involved in TSS or septic shock.

NOS removes and oxidizes an amino group from L-arginine, producing NO, and it is this NO molecule that has been shown to be critical in blood pressure regulation. NO accomplishes this by relaxing blood vessel smooth muscle cells, leading to the dilation of the vessel and a lowering of blood pressure. When too much NO is released because of a bacterial infection, the blood pressure becomes too low and the patient dies of septic shock or TSS.

It also has been amply demonstrated that this same molecule functions as a neurotransmitter in sexual excitement. A message from the brain induces the synthesis of NO, which then acts to dilate blood vessels within the penis, allowing blood to flow in to produce an erection.

It seems fairly obvious, therefore, that when we learn how to control either the synthesis of NO or the activity of NOS, we can develop procedures for reducing the mortality of septic shock or, perhaps, even discover a treatment for some cases of impotence. And this is exactly what is being done. Initial trials using analogues of L-arginine or NO inhibitors are encouraging, and researchers are racing to develop chemicals that can control the synthesis or activity of NO.

antibiotics have eliminated much of this type of infection from developed countries.

Wound infections, as well as postpartum infections, can be caused by the obligately anaerobic streptococci that are part of the normal flora of the intestinal tract and the female genital tract. Such infections usually occur in conjunction with some of the other obligately anaerobic organisms from those areas (ie, *Bacteroides*).

Pathogenesis of Group A Streptococcal Infections

Because pharyngitis is the most common manifestation of a group A streptococcal infection, it can be concluded logically that streptococci usually are spread through the respiratory tract secretions of an infected individual. Before the pasteurization of milk and the availability of adequate refrigeration, food-borne streptococcal outbreaks were common. Such outbreaks still occur, as exemplified in 1992 when 71 persons acquired a group A pharyngitis that eventually was traced to a macaroni and cheese dish prepared by a food handler whose hand had a skin lesion infected by a group A streptococcus. Thus, food contaminated by an infected person should be considered by an investigator faced with the clustering of a large number of cases of acute streptococcal sore throat.

Streptococcal impetigo appears to be transmitted mechanically from an infected person to another individual.

Late Nonsuppurative Complications of Group A Streptococcal Infections

Complications of group A streptococcal infections are rheumatic fever involving the heart and joints, acute glomerulonephritis involving the kidney, and, perhaps, erythema nodosum involving the skin.

RHEUMATIC FEVER. Rheumatic fever occurs in a small percentage of patients 2 to 3 weeks after the onset of an untreated pharyngeal infection caused by a β-hemolytic group A streptococcus. During World War II, about 1 million streptococcal infections occurred among sailors in the United States Navy, and more than 21,000 of these infections resulted in acute rheumatic fever. Most cases occurred in training camps, and in 1944, acute rheumatic fever ranked second only to fractures as a cause of time lost due to sickness or noncombat duty. In the Western world, however, the incidence of rheumatic fever declined dramatically during the 1950s and 1960s, possibly because of the frequent use of penicillin. Now, however, for unknown reasons, all major hospitals are seeing a substantial increase in the number of patients admitted with acute rheumatic fever. Some believe that this might be due to a resurgence of rheumatogenic strains of group A streptococci. The disease remains a major problem in developing countries, where it still accounts for 25% to 40% of all cardiovascular disease. Early studies suggested that rheumatic fever could be a sequelae to infection with any type of group A streptococcus, but the evaluation of more recent epidemics of rheumatic fever indicates that it may be linked to only a few group A serotypes that have unknown rheumatogenic properties. Recovery from rheumatic fever occurs without residual injury to the joints, but the involvement of the heart is important, because permanent damage can occur there. The mechanism by which streptococci produce rheumatic fever is still obscure, but much circumstantial evidence indicates that it is the result of an immunologic reaction. Various theories have been postulated that streptococcal antigens, such as the M protein, might be deposited in the joints and heart. In addition, there have been many reports that

a common cross-reacting antigen exists in some group A streptococci and in the heart. In this case, antibodies synthesized in response to the streptococcal infection could react with antigens in the heart, causing cellular destruction and permanent damage. This concept is supported by the observation that even sera from patients with uncomplicated streptococcal infections can contain antibodies that bind to heart tissue, although at lower levels than those seen in patients with rheumatic fever. The theory that rheumatic fever is the result of an immunologic reaction also is supported by postmortem studies showing large deposits of immunoglobulins and the C3 component of complement within the heart. More recent data have implicated superantigen (M-protein) expansion of T cells as a factor in rheumatic fever. This is supported by the observation that M proteins from high rheumatic fever–producing strains (3, 5, 6, 14, 18, 19, 24, and 27) all stimulate T-cell division.

GLOMERULONEPHRITIS. Acute glomerulonephritis, an inflammation of the glomeruli in the kidney, is less frequently a consequence of streptococcal infection than is rheumatic fever. Most cases of glomerulonephritis occur about 1 week after group A, type 12 pharyngeal infections or skin infections by nephritogenic types such as 2, 6, 49, 55, 57, and 60. In this condition, bloody urine (hematuria) is the predominant symptom, often accompanied by hypertension.

Glomerulonephritis also is believed to be an immunologic disease, in which the streptococci possess or synthesize an antigen that cross-reacts with glomerular basement membranes of the kidney, or they deposit streptococcal antigen–antibody complexes on the basement membranes. Interestingly, monoclonal antibodies to human renal glomeruli will cross-react with streptococcal M protein types 6 and 12 (nephritogenic strains), but not with M protein types 1, 3, 5, 19, or 23 (nonnephritogenic strains). In either case, the activation of the C3 and C5 components of complement would lead to tissue destruction.

ERYTHEMA NODOSUM. Erythema nodosum is a type of skin lesion that can occur after diseases such as tuberculosis or coccidioidomycosis (a fungal infection discussed in Chap. 35), as well as occasional group A streptococcal infections. The explanation for this syndrome is even more vague than that for the other poststreptococcal complications, but it has been proposed that the streptococcal cell wall might be the toxic agent.

Laboratory Diagnosis of Group A Streptococcal Infections

To prevent rheumatic fever, it is essential that β-hemolytic streptococcal infections be diagnosed promptly and treated adequately. The best way to make a diagnosis is to isolate and serologically identify the causative organism. To accomplish this, material from the patient (usually a throat swab) is streaked on a blood-agar plate. After about 24 hours' incubation at 37°C, the plate is examined for the presence of β-hemolytic streptococci, indicated by tiny, compact, dull colonies surrounded by areas of clear hemolysis. If a Gram stain of such a colony reveals gram-positive cocci occurring in chains, a tentative diagnosis is made. A specific identification can be accomplished in about 30 minutes using commercially available latex beads that have been coated with antibodies that are specific for the group A carbohydrate. The C substance is extracted from a loopful of the isolated culture (using a commercially available extraction solution) and, on a slide, one drop of the extracted material is mixed with a drop of latex beads that have been coated with antibodies to group A carbohydrate. Agglutination of the beads within 1 minute provides confirmatory evidence that the unknown organism is a group A streptococcus.

Commercial kits also are available, which permit an identification of group A streptococci directly from a pharyngeal swab of the inflamed area. The overall procedure is as described earlier, except that the group A carbohydrate is extracted directly from the throat swab into about 150 μL of extraction solution. Depending on the intensity of the infection, this provides sufficient group carbohydrate to cause agglutination of the coated latex beads. Serologic identification of the M protein is not routinely done.

Because group A streptococci are more sensitive to the antibiotic bacitracin, presumptive evidence that a β-hemolytic streptococcus belongs to group A also can be obtained by using commercially available disks containing a calibrated amount of bacitracin, which will inhibit the growth of group A streptococci but not other groups of streptococci (Fig. 24-4). Fluorescence labeled antibody

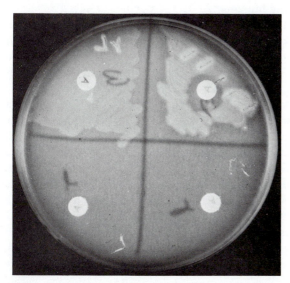

FIGURE 24-4 Streptococcal growth in the presence of disks containing bacitracin. (*Upper left*) Growth right up to the edge of the disk indicates resistance and, thus, a streptococcus not of group A. (*Upper right*) A zone of inhibition around the disk indicates sensitivity to bacitracin by a group A streptococcus.

against the C substance of group A also can be used for definitive identification of these organisms.

Immunologic procedures are useful in the diagnosis of the late, nonsuppurative complications that generally occur when it is no longer possible to isolate the infecting streptococcus. In these cases, the amount of antibody present against streptolysin O can be determined. A high antistreptolysin O titer indicates a recent infection by β-hemolytic streptococci.

Treatment of Group A Streptococcal Infections

Fortunately, all group A streptococci are sensitive to a wide variety of therapeutic drugs. The sulfonamides suppress their growth, but do not prevent the occurrence of the late, nonsuppurative complications. Penicillin, which is bactericidal, is the antibiotic of choice, and most experts agree that therapeutic levels of penicillin should be maintained for at least 8 to 10 days to ensure complete eradication of the organisms. It is extremely important to remember that adequate treatment during the acute infection will prevent the complications of rheumatic fever. Penicillin therapy for 10 days also is effective in eradicating streptococci from skin infections, but is not always capable of preventing the subsequent occurrence of acute glomerulonephritis.

Persons who have recovered from rheumatic fever are particularly vulnerable to a recurrence if they again become infected with a group A streptococcus. These individuals usually continue to take low doses of oral penicillin for many years to prevent such an infection. Persons who have recovered from glomerulonephritis usually are not given prophylactic penicillin, because the chances of reinfection with a nephritogenic strain (capable of inducing kidney inflammation) are low.

It is almost impossible to control the spread of streptococci, because there are so many asymptomatic carriers of β-hemolytic strains. Depending on the season, 5% to 30% of apparently healthy persons may carry these potentially pathogenic organisms.

GROUP B STREPTOCOCCI

Group B streptococci (*Streptococcus agalactiae*) are the etiologic agents of bovine mastitis; until a decade or two ago, they were not believed to cause serious human disease. However, it has been established that group B streptococci are present in the vaginal flora of about 25% of all women and, although it is uncommon for these organisms to cause overt disease in healthy adults, cases of bacteremia (bacteria in the blood) and meningitis (infection of the membranes surrounding the brain and spinal cord) have occurred in patients with diabetes and cancer, and in individuals taking immunosuppressive drugs. In the United States, these organisms also are responsible for about 45,000 cases per year of postpartum endometritis (infection of the endometrium). Group B streptococci also have been isolated frequently from rectal swabs and less frequently from the throat and male urethra.

Surprisingly, a group B streptococcus was isolated in 1993 from the vagina of a 27-year-old woman who had a typical toxic shock-like syndrome. A previously undescribed toxin was purified from the isolate and was shown to possess all the attributes of the pyrogenic group A superantigens. Subsequent work has identified additional group B strains that produce a pyrogenic toxin, and it must be concluded that either a new strain of group B streptococcus capable of producing a toxic shock-like syndrome has evolved or these cases are relatively rare and have been overlooked in the past.

It is in the newborn that serious group B streptococcal infections most commonly occur. Bacteremia and pneumonia develop within the first 5 days of life in about 1% of children born to mothers infected with group B streptococci (about 9600 neonates per year in the United States). In spite of intensive antibiotic therapy, such infections carry a mortality rate of 30% to 50%. Meningitis also occurs, with about a 15% mortality rate, but this complication usually is seen between the 10th and 60th days of life. Group B streptococci are divided into seven types based on antigenic differences in their carbohydrate capsule. All seven serotypes (Ia, Ib, II, III, IV, V, and VI) are involved in the early infections. However, type III is associated more frequently with the late meningeal infections of neonates. These infants come from mothers without type III antibody, suggesting that the mother is not the source of the infection. It has been proposed that many cases of group B meningitis could be prevented by immunizing expectant mothers to the type III polysaccharide, thus providing their newborns with protective maternal antibodies. To test this theory, a group of pregnant volunteers was vaccinated with 50 μg of purified type III capsular polysaccharide. The results were not spectacular, but 80% of the infants born to these mothers still had protective antibodies to type III group B streptococci at 1 month of age. A newer experimental vaccine consisting of a conjugate of type III carbohydrate to tetanus toxoid appears to be effective in animals. Such a conjugate also converts the carbohydrate vaccine from a T-independent to a T-dependent antigen. Interestingly, type III capsules consist of a linear backbone with short side chains ending with residues of sialic acid. Such side chains block the activation of the alternate pathway of complement, and mutants unable to synthesize sialic acid are avirulent.

Group B streptococci are exceedingly difficult to eradicate from a colonized woman, perhaps because the real reservoir is the lower gastrointestinal tract. However, several attempts have been made to control the incidence of neonatal disease. In one study involving 22,738 infants, penicillin was given to half the newborns within 60 minutes of birth. Of those receiving penicillin, one infant had an early-onset group B infection, compared with 12 such infections in the control group. In another study,

ampicillin was administered during labor to mothers known to be colonized with group B streptococci. Of those infants born to ampicillin-treated mothers, 8 of 85 (9%) were colonized with group B streptococci, as compared with a control group of colonized mothers not receiving ampicillin, in which 40 of 75 (53%) of the infants became colonized with group B streptococci.

Specific identification of group B streptococci is accomplished most easily using latex beads that have been coated with antibodies to group B carbohydrate in a procedure analogous to that described for identification of the group A streptococci.

OTHER STREPTOCOCCI

Group G Streptococci

Group G streptococci are commonly found in humans on the skin, in the female genital tract, and in the respiratory tract. Group G streptococci do not routinely cause acute infections but are isolated occasionally in cases of bacteremia and endocarditis, particularly in long-term drug abusers. Elderly patients, especially those with malignancies, also are highly prone to group G streptococcal infections.

Viridans and Group D Streptococci

The viridans streptococci are α-hemolytic organisms that are normal flora in the throat and nasopharynx of humans. They are a heterogeneous group that cannot be classified using Lancefield group-specific carbohydrates. Some, such as *Streptococcus parasanguis* and *Streptococcus mutans*, are involved in dental caries and periodontal disease, but none appear to produce acute infections in normal healthy humans.

Group D streptococci usually are α-hemolytic and, unlike other Lancefield groups, they can be divided into two distinct subsections, namely the enterococci and the nonenterococci. Enterococci are normal flora in the human intestine and are characterized by their ability to grow in the presence of 6.5% NaCl at 45°C. These organisms were classified with the streptococci for many years, but now have been placed in the genus *Enterococcus*. The three species within this newly established genus are *Enterococcus faecalis*, *Enterococcus faecium*, and *Enterococcus durans*. The enterococci, especially *E faecalis*, are found as secondary invaders in urinary tract or wound infections, but rarely are involved in acute infections such as described for groups A and B streptococci. Most urinary tract infections occur in hospitalized patients, particularly those who have undergone urinary tract catheterization.

Nonenterococci, notably *Streptococcus bovis* and *Streptococcus equinus*, also routinely are found as normal intestinal flora and, like the enterococci, can be involved in genitourinary tract infections.

The one infection in which all these streptococci unquestionably are involved is *subacute bacterial endocarditis*. This infection can be caused by many different bacteria, but the viridans streptococci and the group D organisms are the most common etiologic agents. The infection occurs most often in individuals who already have an injured heart valve, although about 40% of enterococcal 5 BE occurs in patients with no underlying heart abnormalities. On reaching the valve, the organisms multiply frequently releasing a shower of emboli (foreign particulate matter) from the valve. The characteristic findings in such infections are fever, heart murmurs, enlarged spleen, and anemia. Once the disease is suspected, the diagnosis is made by obtaining blood cultures from which the bacteria are isolated. Left untreated, this condition is almost invariably fatal.

Subacute bacterial endocarditis can be difficult to treat, because the bacteria are enmeshed in a vegetative growth on the heart valve. In addition, some strains of viridans streptococci produce a glycocalyx of a mostly glucose polymer, which appears to impede entry of the antibiotic into the bacterium. In experimental endocarditis in rabbits caused by such organisms, treatment with penicillin plus dextranase was far more effective than treatment with penicillin alone. However, most viridans streptococci and nonenterococci are sensitive to penicillin, and an intensive course of penicillin therapy for 2 weeks usually is effective. When an enterococcus (which is identified by its ability to grow at 45°C in a medium containing 6.5% NaCl) is the infecting organism, a combination of vancomycin and gentamicin typically is used.

Streptococcus anginosus (Streptococcus milleri)

The taxonomic designation of *Streptococcus anginosus* (older designation, *Streptococcus milleri*) reflects a serologically heterogeneous group of streptococci that share several physiologic characteristics. Most are nonhemolytic, forming small colonies on blood agar. A few, however, are β-hemolytic, and many of these are typeable in Lancefield groups A, C, F, or G.

Most of these streptococci are found as normal commensals of the oral cavity, throat, intestinal tract, and vagina. They have been implicated as etiologic agents of brain and liver abscesses, as well as infections of the mouth and teeth. Their vague taxonomic status makes it difficult to decide whether to assign to this species a status of commensal, opportunist, or pathogen.

Streptococcus pneumoniae

S pneumoniae, commonly called the *pneumococcus*, was isolated in 1881 by Pasteur and later was shown to be the major cause of lobar pneumonia in humans (infecting one or more lobes of the lung). Perhaps no other bacterium was as important to the early development of immunology and molecular genetics. Studies of pneumococcal pneumonia initiated specific serum therapy, which was the primary therapy for a variety of infectious diseases until the discovery of antibiotics. Research work with pneumococcal transformation provided the initial proof that DNA alone was the carrier of genetic information.

MORPHOLOGY AND METABOLISM. Pneumococci are lancet-shaped organisms usually arranged in pairs, although short chains also can be seen (Fig. 24-5). They are gram-positive, nonmotile, and non–spore-forming, but virulent organisms are encapsulated. They are particularly sensitive to lysis by an autolytic enzyme that cleaves the bond, linking the L-alanine peptide to the muramic acid of the peptidoglycan wall. This enzyme, L-alanine-muramyl amidase, routinely becomes activated after the culture enters the stationary phase of growth, and eventually causes lysis of the entire culture. The enzyme also can be activated by numerous surface-active agents (including detergents), but because bile salts (such as sodium taurocholate) were used originally, the pneumococci are spoken of as *bile soluble,* a term that is a misnomer.

Pneumococci require choline for growth, and the choline becomes a constituent of teichoic acid in the cell wall. If ethanolamine is substituted for choline, the pneumococci will grow, but they are no longer sensitive to lysis and cannot be genetically transformed. Apparently, the incorporation of ethanolamine in place of choline causes steric differences that result in major changes in cell properties.

Nutritionally, the pneumococci need an enriched medium for growth and, like other streptococci, they lack both cytochromes and catalase. All pneumococci produce α-hemolysis when growing on a blood-agar medium and, therefore, closely resemble the viridans streptococci in colonial appearance and morphology.

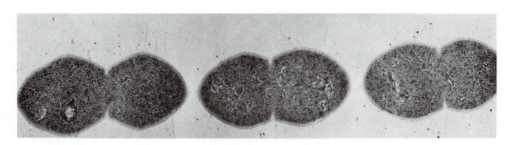

FIGURE 24-5 *Streptococcus pneumoniae.* Note the diploid arrangement of cells and the lancet shape of individual cells. Capsules are not visible in this electron micrograph. (Original magnification about ×46,000.)

ANTIGENIC STRUCTURE. The pneumococci can be subdivided into more than 80 serologic types on the basis of antigenic differences in their polysaccharide capsule. (The ability to transform one type of *S pneumoniae* to a new type using purified DNA is discussed in Chap. 22.) They also contain a C carbohydrate analogous to that used by Lancefield to group the streptococci, as well as a type-specific M protein. Unlike the group A streptococci, however, pneumococcal M protein is not antiphagocytic, nor are antibodies to the M protein protective.

PNEUMOCOCCAL INFECTIONS. The pneumococci are α-hemolytic and excrete a sulfhydryl-activated cytolytic toxin called *pneumolysin* that binds to cholesterol in host-cell membranes. The role of pneumolysin in the pathogenesis of pneumococcal infections is obscure, but preliminary reports indicate that it may function by inhibiting the antimicrobial properties of neutrophils and the opsonic activity of serum. It also has been reported to be a cytotoxin for pulmonary endothelial cells, and it may be an important factor in the pathogenesis of alveolar hemorrhages in pneumococcal infections. It appears, however, that the pneumococcus can survive and produce disease in the host primarily because of its capsule. Once a strain loses its capsule, it can be readily phagocytosed and destroyed. Thus, immunity is the result of humoral antibody directed against the capsule and, therefore, is type specific.

Interestingly, *S pneumoniae* is carried as part of the normal flora of the respiratory tract in many healthy individuals. It is not clear why carriers do not have pneumonia, but it appears that the normal lung is resistant to infection and that pneumococcal pneumonia occurs most frequently in conjunction with viral infections of the upper respiratory tract. The disease also occurs in persons whose respiratory tract drainage is impaired, such as bedridden patients, heavy smokers, and individuals who have inhaled toxic irritants.

PNEUMOCOCCAL PNEUMONIA. The estimated incidence of pneumococcal pneumonia varies considerably according to an individual's age, conditions of crowding, and occupation. In the United States, the incidence is thought to be 300,000 to 400,000 cases per year, with an overall mortality of 15,000 to 60,000. Military personnel living in a closed group have an incidence 10 to 20 times higher per 1000 population; the rate of pneumococcal pneumonia in African gold miners is about 100-fold greater than that of the general population.

The disease is characterized by an acute lung inflammation that tends to be lobar in adults (ie, involving the tissues in one or more lobes of the lungs) but frequently causes a more restricted bronchopneumonia in children or the elderly. It usually is sudden in onset and is characterized by chills, fever, and pleural pain (in the area surrounding the lung). The alveoli fill with exudate and, in about 25% of cases, bacteremia is found early in the course of the disease.

Pneumococci also can invade other tissues, particularly the sinuses, the middle ear, and the meninges. It is noteworthy that 5% to 10% of upper respiratory tract infections in early childhood are complicated by acute sinusitis. *S pneumoniae* is responsible for about 30% to 40% of cases of sinusitis caused by bacteria. Other possible secondary complications include septicemia; endocarditis (inflammation of the heart and valves); pericarditis (inflammation of the pericardium, the membrane surrounding the heart); and empyema (an infection of the pleural cavity).

Recovery is characteristically abrupt and coincides with the appearance of circulating anticapsular antibodies.

MENINGITIS. The pneumococcus is the second most common cause of bacterial meningitis in adults. Meningitis can arise as a complication of pneumonia or sinusitis, in which the bacteria reach the meninges through the bloodstream, or it can result from a skull fracture or other injury, permitting organisms from the nasopharynx to enter the meninges.

OTITIS MEDIA. At least 75% of all children have middle ear infections by the age of 6 years, and the pneumococcus is the etiologic agent for about half these cases; such infections are rare in adults. Children experiencing an initial middle ear infection during the first year of life are likely to have recurrent otitis media during early childhood, resulting in reduced hearing acuity. Surprisingly, not all pneumococcal types cause this infection; only types 6, 14, 19, and 24 can be isolated from more than half the cases of pneumococcal otitis media.

LABORATORY DIAGNOSIS. Direct smears of sputum can be stained and observed for gram-positive encapsulated pneumococci. In addition, a quellung test can be performed either directly on sputum samples or on the cultured organisms. This test is based on the fact that if encapsulated bacteria are mixed with type-specific antibodies, the capsule swells to a size considerably larger than normal (see Chap. 4, Fig. 4-1). The capsular swelling is diagnostic; before the advent of penicillin therapy, it was always necessary to determine which pneumococcal type was causing the infection to ascertain which antiserum should be administered. In current practice, the quellung test rarely is used for specific typing, but the use of an omni-antiserum, which contains antibodies against all types, is helpful in providing a definite identification of pneumococci in the sputum.

Because a bile solubility test requires prior growth of the organisms, this technique has been supplanted by a much simpler method in which commercially available optochin disks (impregnated with ethylhydrocupreine hydrochloride) are laid down on the surface of an agar plate that has been inoculated with the unknown organism. The pneumococci are exceedingly sensitive to this compound and will fail to grow in the proximity of the disk.

The α-hemolytic viridans streptococci are insensitive to optochin and will grow adjacent to the implanted disk.

In addition, sputum or spinal fluid can be injected through the peritoneum into a white mouse; because mice are sensitive to most types of pneumococci (as contrasted with other streptococci), the injection of only a few organisms will result in the death of the mouse—usually within 1 to 2 days. The organisms then can readily be seen and cultured from blood drawn from the mouse's heart.

In cases of suspected pneumococcal meningitis, essentially the same diagnostic procedures are followed, except that a spinal tap is performed and the spinal fluid (rather than the sputum) is observed. In addition, it is routine to withdraw and culture blood from a patient suspected of having either pneumonia or meningitis to provide another means of isolating the organism for a definite diagnosis.

TREATMENT OF PNEUMOCOCCAL INFECTIONS. The most effective treatment of all pneumococcal infections is the administration of penicillin G. For individuals sensitive to penicillin, cephalothin or erythromycin can be used for pneumonia, but pneumococcal meningitis should be treated with chloramphenicol.

Multiple antibiotic-resistant pneumococci first were reported in 1977 when *S pneumoniae* type 57 was isolated from patients in South Africa. This strain was resistant to penicillin, tetracycline, chloramphenicol, erythromycin, and clindamycin, but was sensitive to vancomycin. In another instance, a penicillin-resistant pneumococcus, type 14, was recovered from the blood of a 5-year-old child in Minneapolis, Minnesota. This child had received oral penicillin and ampicillin daily since 16 months of age. Unfortunately, antibiotic-resistant pneumococci are being seen more and more commonly.

PREVENTION OF PNEUMOCOCCAL INFECTIONS. Despite intensive antibiotic therapy, the case fatality rate for pneumococcal pneumonia averages between 5% and 10%, and for individuals older than 70 years of age, it approaches 60%. For this reason, considerable effort has been expended over the past 50 years to develop an effective vaccine. The desirability of a vaccine that protects against the more than 80 types of pneumococci was somewhat lessened by the observation that 23 pneumococcal types are responsible for over 90% of the infections. A vaccine is now available that contains 50 μg each of purified capsular polysaccharides from the most prevalent 23 types, that is, types 1 through 5, 8, 9, 12, 14, 17, 19, 20, 22, 23, 26, 34, 43, 51, 54, 56, 57, 68, and 70.

The administration of this vaccine is reported to give between 75% and 95% protection in normal adults, although infants and young children do not respond as well. Data from the Centers for Disease Control (CDC) suggest that the vaccine is effective and should be used for persons older than 10 years of age who are at high risk of death from infection with the pneumococcus. This group includes individuals with sickle cell anemia and other splenic malfunctions. In addition, the vaccine is recommended for all persons with chronic underlying diseases such as congestive heart failure, alcoholism with cirrhosis, and diabetes mellitus, and for elderly persons in closed populations such as nursing homes and long-term care facilities. Persons older than 60 years of age also should be vaccinated, because mortality rates for pneumococcal infections rise dramatically beginning at that age.

Staphylococci

Members of the genus *Staphylococcus* are hearty organisms that cause a myriad of infections ranging from localized furuncles (boils) and carbuncles (deeper and larger than boils, discharging pus from multiple points) to food poisoning, pneumonia, meningitis, and disseminated infections involving any organ of the body. Controlling these organisms is particularly difficult, because virulent strains are carried asymptomatically in the nasopharynx of 10% to 50% of normal adults.

MORPHOLOGY AND METABOLISM

Members of the genus *Staphylococcus* are spherical cells, about 1 μm in diameter. In stained smears, they appear singly, occasionally in pairs, and most frequently as irregular, grape-like clusters (Fig. 24-6*A*). They are gram-positive, nonmotile, non–spore-forming, facultative anaerobes. Their appearance on a gram-stained smear usually is sufficient to distinguish them from the streptococci, because the latter are much more prone to form chains of cells (see Figs. 24-1 and 24-6 for comparison). If doubt exists, these two genera can be separated easily on the basis of the enzyme catalase. Catalase will break down hydrogen peroxide to form water and oxygen, and, if a loopful of staphylococci is mixed on a slide with a drop of 3% hydrogen peroxide, bubbles of oxygen will be visible to the naked eye. Because streptococci do not form catalase, they do not cause bubbles. In addition, staphylococcal colonies are considerably larger than those formed by the streptococci.

Staphylococci are facultative anaerobes and ferment a wide variety of sugars to form acid but no gas. This property permits their differentiation from the large number of avirulent but morphologically similar members of the genus *Micrococcus*. All micrococci are obligate aerobes and, although they oxidize many sugars, they do not produce acid.

Staphylococci grow well on most meat-infusion laboratory media, with or without added sugar; however, synthetic media capable of supporting their growth must contain at least 14 amino acids and 2 B vitamins, thiamine and nicotinic acid.

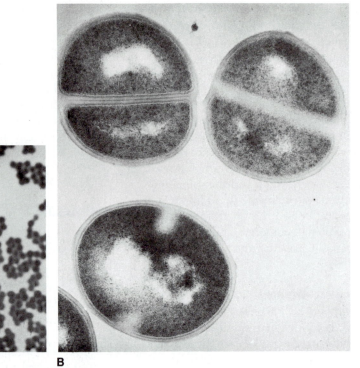

A   **B**

FIGURE 24-6 A. Clusters of gram-stained *Staphylococcus aureus*. (Original magnification about ×4500.)
B. Electron micrograph of cells of *S aureus*. (Original magnification ×49,000.)

CLASSIFICATION

Under the present classification, there are three species of staphylococci associated with humans: *Staphylococcus aureus, Staphylococcus epidermidis,* and *Staphylococcus saprophyticus.* Of these, *S aureus* represents the major pathogen, although the other two species also can cause human infections.

Staphylococcus aureus

S aureus can be differentiated from other staphylococcal species by the fact that it normally produces a light golden pigment and possesses a species-specific antigenic determinant called *polysaccharide A*. Polysaccharide A is a component of the cell wall consisting of a ribitol-type teichoic acid that is esterified with *N*-acetylglucosamine. However, it is the ability of *S aureus* to ferment mannitol and produce coagulase (an enzyme inducing the clotting of plasma) that is used to delineate this species.

About 90% of *S aureus* strains produce a cell-wall protein, called *protein A,* that has the unusual property of binding to the Fc region of normal IgG. Protein A possesses four Fc-binding sites on each molecule, and it has been suggested that this property imparts antiphagocytic activity by competing with leukocytes for the Fc portion of specific opsonins. Protein A can be covalently linked to an insoluble matrix, and this commercial preparation has proven to be a valuable tool for the specific absorption of antibodies from a mixture of other proteins.

Further division of *S aureus* uses *phage typing* to assign an unknown strain to one of four phage groups. In practice, a small drop of each phage group is placed into a plate previously seeded with the unknown strain of *S aureus*. After overnight incubation, clear plaques of lysis allow the unknown strain to be ranked in one of the phage groups shown in Table 24-4. Additional breakdown can be accomplished through the use of individual phages within the assigned group.

The serologic typing of *S aureus* into subtypes is difficult, and ordinarily only large diagnostic centers such as the CDC are set up for this procedure.

EXTRACELLULAR TOXINS AND ENZYMES. The ability of *S aureus* strains to produce disease depends on their resistance to phagocytosis and their production of extracellular toxins

TABLE 24-4
Lytic Phage Groups of *Staphylococcus Aureus*

Group	Phage Numbers
I	29, 52, 52A, 79, 80
II	3A, 3C, 55, 71
III	6, 42E, 47, 53, 54, 75, 77, 83a, 84, 85
IV	42D
Not grouped	81, 187

TABLE 24-5
Classification of Hemolysins by Type of Erythrocyte Lysed

Type of Hemolysin	Red Blood Cell Lysed	Usual Source
alpha	Calf, rabbit, sheep	Human
beta	Human, ox, sheep (effective only as hot–cold lysis, i.e., 37°C for 1–2 hr followed by overnight in refrigerator)	Animal
gamma	Guinea pig, horse, human, ox, rabbit, rat, sheep	Human
delta	Guinea pig, horse, human, rabbit, rat, sheep	Human

and enzymes. The role of some of the following products is obvious, whereas others do not appear to be involved in the production of disease.

COAGULASE. *Coagulase* is an extracellular enzyme that activates a coagulase-reacting factor normally present in plasma (possibly prothrombin), causing the plasma to clot by the conversion of fibrinogen to fibrin. All coagulase-producing staphylococci are, by definition, *S aureus;* as a result, coagulase production is considered the best laboratory evidence for the potential pathogenicity of a staphylococcus. Seven antigenically different extracellular coagulases have been identified from various staphylococci, but the pathogenic role suggested for the enzyme is obscure. It is thought that the coating of the organisms with fibrin may inhibit their phagocytosis, and also that the fibrinopeptides released may cause increased capillary permeability and smooth muscle contraction.

Coagulase can be readily detected by mixing 0.5 mL of broth culture or a loopful of organisms with 0.5 mL of citrated rabbit plasma. In the presence of coagulase, a clot will develop, usually in 3 to 4 hours.

Although the presence of coagulase provides good evidence for the potential pathogenicity of a staphylococcal isolate, its absence does not indicate a lack of pathogenicity, because coagulase-negative strains are known to cause infections.

In addition to extracellular coagulase, *S aureus* also possesses a bound coagulase that causes the organisms to clump when mixed with plasma. This *clumping factor* can convert fibrinogen directly to fibrin and does not require the presence of coagulase-reacting factor for activity.

STAPHYLOCOCCAL HEMOLYSINS. Because of their varied effect on many types of cells, the staphylococcal hemolysins are referred to more frequently as toxins. There are four such toxins, designated α, β, γ, and δ. These can be differentiated from each other by antigenic distinctions and, as shown in Table 24-5, by the type of erythrocytes that they preferentially will lyse.

α *Toxin (α hemolysin)* has been studied extensively and shown to be toxic to numerous cell types. This toxin

is known to damage smooth muscle as well as to kill skin cells (dermonecrotic), and it is lethal when injected into mice or rabbits. In addition, α toxin is toxic for human macrophages and platelets, and it causes degranulation of PMNs through disruption of their lysosomes. Its reaction with erythrocytes results in a prelytic release of K^+, followed by complete lysis of the cell.

The ability of α toxin to destroy eucaryotic cells appears to result from the formation of 2- to 3-mm ring-shaped hexamers in the membranes of susceptible cells. In the presence of Ca^{2+}, sublytic amounts of α toxin will induce PMNs to generate and release leukotriene B4. It has been suggested that the release of leukotriene B4 may be widespread in staphylococcal disease, augmenting PMN adhesion to epithelial cells as well as being chemotactic for PMNs.

β *Toxin (β hemolysin)* has been referred to as a hot–cold hemolysin, because its lysis of erythrocytes requires an initial incubation at 37°C followed by an incubation at refrigerator temperature. The toxin is an enzyme that reacts with sphingomyelin to split off phosphorylcholine, and the subsequent chilling of the cells leads to their disruption. Those cells rich in sphingomyelin are most susceptible to β toxin.

Little is known about the mechanism of action of γ *toxin (γ hemolysin)*. It will readily lyse several animal erythrocytes, including human erythrocytes, and its activity is inhibited by the presence of phospholipids. It might be deduced, therefore, that membrane phospholipids are the targets for γ toxin.

δ *Toxin (δ hemolysin)* damages many types of cells, including erythrocytes, PMNs, macrophages, lymphocytes, and platelets. Damage appears to result from the reaction of its hydrophobic amino acids with the phospholipids in the cell membrane.

LEUKOCIDIN. *Leukocidin* activity, which is separable from the hemolysins, can be demonstrated in many pathogenic staphylococci. The toxin is made up of two separable components that act synergistically to damage PMNs and macrophages. The mechanism by which leukocidin exerts its effect is complex and unclear. It has been proposed

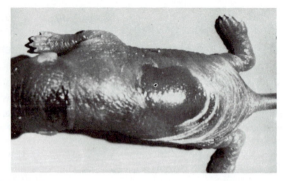

FIGURE 24-7 Neonatal mouse injected 24 hours earlier with 1×10^9 staphylococci from phage group II. The staphylococci were obtained from a patient with scalded skin syndrome.

that leukocidin stimulates a membrane acylphosphatase, which carries out a dephosphorylation of membrane triphosphoinositide, resulting in membrane damage and inactivation of the leukocyte. Leukocidin also causes a degranulation of PMNs similar to that described for streptolysin O.

EXFOLIATIN. *Exfoliatin* is an exotoxin, encoded in a plasmid, that causes an acute exfoliative dermatitis called *staphylococcal scalded skin syndrome*. Staphylococci from phage group II are involved more frequently than are other phage groups, and the syndrome can be caused by either or both of two serotypes of exfoliatin. It is characterized by a wrinkling and peeling of the epidermis, resulting in considerable fluid loss from the denuded skin (Fig. 24-7). Because the epidermal sloughing is caused by a diffusible exotoxin, the infecting staphylococci may or may not be present at the dermal site. This disease is seen most commonly in newborn infants, but it has occurred in adults receiving immunosuppressive therapy. In fact, the rarity of this syndrome is surprising; about 5% of randomly isolated strains of *S aureus* are reported to produce exfoliatin.

STAPHYLOCOCCAL ENTEROTOXINS. *Enterotoxins*, which are exotoxins, cause food poisoning (intoxication) that is characterized by severe diarrhea and vomiting. Enterotoxins are excreted by about one third of all clinical isolates of staphylococci. Five antigenically distinct enterotoxins, designated A, B, C, D, and E, have been described, which in some cases are encoded in a lysogenic phage. Enterotoxin C has been subdivided further into enterotoxins C1, C2, and C3 on the basis of minor serologic differences. The usual incubation period ranges from 2 to 6 hours after the ingestion of food in which the staphylococci have grown and produced enterotoxin. The duration of the acute symptoms usually is less than 24 hours, but an individual may feel debilitated for several days. The illness rarely is fatal, but patients may be hospitalized for the infusion of intravenous fluids to replace the fluids lost through diarrhea and vomiting.

One important property of staphylococcal enterotoxins is their heat stability. Once formed, enterotoxins might not be destroyed even if the food harboring them is heated sufficiently to kill all viable staphylococci. This undoubtedly accounts for the increase in cases of staphylococcal food poisoning observed around Thanksgiving and Christmas due to the ingestion of contaminated turkey and turkey dressing.

The diarrhea caused by these organisms is related to their ability to enhance fluid secretion in the small intestine, but the molecular basis of this effect is unknown. It is known, however, that staphylococcal enterotoxins can bind to class II major histocompatibility complex molecules on antigen-presenting cells, causing the expansion of certain sets of T cells.

It also has been known for more than 25 years that staphylococcal enterotoxins greatly augment the sensitivity of animals to irreversible shock and death by endotoxins. This is supported by current molecular data, which has established that the staphylococcal enterotoxins are part of a large family of toxins that act as superantigens.

PYROGENIC TOXINS. Coagulase-positive staphylococci produce one or more antigenically distinct *pyrogenic toxins*. These toxins are biologically analogous to the pyrogenic toxins produced by the group A streptococci and, as such, they act as superantigens. Thus, they are pyrogenic, they enhance susceptibility to endotoxic shock, they stimulate the expansion of certain T-cell clones, and they can cause a scarlet fever–type erythematous rash.

OTHER STAPHYLOCOCCAL PRODUCTS. Staphylococci also can excrete enzymes such as *penicillinase* (which destroys penicillin), *hyaluronidase* (spreading factor), *lipases*, and a *staphylokinase* (which causes the lysis of fibrin clots in a manner analogous to that of streptokinase). In addition, an extracellular staphylococcal product designated *staphylococcal decomplementation antigen* has been described that causes the rapid consumption of early-reacting complement components up to and including C5 in human serum. This factor appears to suppress the normal opsonizing role of host complement by inducing its destruction. All these products may play a role in the pathogenesis of staphylococcal infections.

PATHOGENESIS OF STAPHYLOCOCCAL INFECTIONS. *S aureus* is found in the nasopharynx of 20% to 40% of adults at any given time, and this carrier rate can increase to 50% to 70% in a hospital setting. Such carriers provide the reservoir for the spread of staphylococcal infections, most frequently through the hands. In spite of the fact that most persons either carry or are exposed frequently to coagulase-positive staphylococci, overt disease (with the exception of staphylococcal food poisoning) in a healthy individual is not a frequent event. Persons most susceptible to serious staphylococcal infections include those whose ability to phagocytose and destroy the staphylococci is not completely developed or is significantly inhibited. Such persons can include newborns, surgical or burn patients, individuals receiving immunosuppressive drugs, and persons with immunodeficiency diseases such as chronic granulomatous disease (see Chap. 4). Patients with lower respiratory tract viral infections (eg, influenza), measles, and diabetes also are more susceptible to staphylococcal infections.

SKIN INFECTIONS. Infection of a hair follicle by staphylococci resulting in a localized superficial *abscess* or boil is undoubtedly the most frequent manifestation of staphylococcal disease. These lesions usually heal spontaneously but, particularly if irritated, can spread to the subcutaneous layers of the skin to produce a furuncle. Such lesions can continue to spread to include multiple contiguous lesions, which then are referred to as *carbuncles*. The lesions are painful and can require surgical draining for healing to take place.

S aureus also is a major cause of *impetigo,* either alone or in conjunction with group A streptococci. Such infections are seen most frequently in school children, often beginning around the nose and spreading over the face.

TOXIC SHOCK SYNDROME. A seemingly new syndrome, *TSS,* was first described in 1978, with almost all reported cases (96%) occurring in women aged 12 to 52 years, during their menstrual periods. Initial epidemiologic and microbiologic studies revealed that the disease usually resulted from a vaginal colonization with *S aureus* associated with the use of tampons during the menstrual period. Moreover, these initial data suggested that one particular brand of tampon was the most likely to contribute to the occurrence of TSS, forcing that manufacturer to withdraw those tampons from the market. What do we know today about the symptoms, cause, and epidemiology of this disease?

TSS is characterized by an abrupt onset, with symptoms of fever, erythematous rash, desquamation (particularly of the palms and soles), and hypotension, often leading to irreversible shock; diarrhea and vomiting also are common. The mortality rate appears to be between 5% and 12% of confirmed cases.

The etiologic agent of TSS is known to be strains of *S aureus* that secrete a specific exotoxin that is responsible for the symptoms of the disease. Such a toxin has been isolated and characterized independently by Merlin Bergdoll and his associates at the University of Wisconsin and by Patrick Schlievert and his associates at the University of Minnesota. It generally is accepted that *toxic shock syndrome toxin-1 (TSST-1)* enhances the susceptibility to

endotoxin by many thousand-fold, which explains in part the hypotension and fatal shock associated with this disease. TSST-1 is similar to the streptococcal pyrogenic toxins, suggesting that TSS actually may be a staphylococcal scarlet fever. TSST-1 appears to be produced by all vaginal strains causing TSS, but many nonvaginal cases of TSS have yielded strains of staphylococci that produce enterotoxin B and, to a lesser extent, enterotoxins A and C.

Some insight into the mechanism of action of TSST-1 was gained when it was found that TSST-1 binds to class II major histocompatibility complex antigens on monocytes; in the presence of certain subsets of T cells, this results in the formation of both IL-1 and TNF-α. Like the pyrogenic toxins, TSST-1 and endotoxin are synergistic in their ability to induce the synthesis of TNF-α and IL-1. These two observations explain how TSST-1 causes the fever and irreversible shock seen in TSS. Moreover, it has been reported that TNF-α induces the transcription of the gene encoding nitric oxide synthetase (NOS), and the resulting nitric oxide (NO) contributes to the hypotension seen in this disease.

The ubiquity of TSST-1–producing strains of staphylococci was illustrated in a report in which 24 strains of *S aureus* were isolated from 44 asymptomatic men. Of these, 9 produced TSST-1 and, surprisingly, all persons still carried the same strain 3 months later.

Thus, it seems clear that the symptoms of TSS are initiated by colonization with a strain of *S aureus* capable of producing TSST-1 or one or more enterotoxins, and the primary question remaining unanswered is: Who is most likely to develop TSS?

The answer is still incomplete, but a retrospective review of medical records indicates that between 15% and 35% of all cases of TSS occur in men and nonmenstruating women. These nonmenstrual cases occur after cutaneous and subcutaneous infections, childbirth or abortion, and surgical procedures (particularly nasal surgery and the subsequent use of nasal tampons for packing), and there are many instances in which the site of *S aureus* colonization is unknown. Surprisingly, a major cause of TSS in children is staphylococcal infection of a chickenpox lesion. In some cases, this has caused disseminated intravascular coagulation that resulted in limb loss. Nonmenstrual TSS is most often due to the secretion of enterotoxin rather than TSST-1.

One of the curious aspects of this disease is the relatively recent occurrence of large numbers of tampon-associated cases, in spite of the fact that tampons have been in use for more than 40 years. One possible explanation came from the work of Edward Kass and his associates at Harvard University. They reported that low concentrations of Mg^{2+} stimulated the synthesis of TSST-1. Furthermore, they provided data demonstrating that fibers within the newer, superabsorbent tampons bound Mg^{2+}

from vaginal fluids, thereby stimulating TSST-1 production. On the other hand, Patrick Schlievert from the University of Minnesota has presented data indicating that staphylococci require O_2 to produce TSST-1, and he has proposed that the larger tampons provided the O_2 necessary for the production of the toxin. It is probable, however, that the sequence of events leading to this syndrome begins with contamination of the tampon with the fingers.

Women can almost eliminate their risk of TSS by not using tampons at all, or they can reduce their risk by not using tampons continuously during the menstrual period.

The recurrence of TSS appears to be restricted to menstrually associated disease. This can run as high as 65% in untreated cases, but is reduced substantially after antibiotic treatment or the noncontinuous use of tampons during the menstrual period.

PNEUMONIA. Staphylococcal pneumonia is rarely a primary event in an otherwise healthy individual. Infection with influenza virus, however, predisposes to a serious, and frequently fatal, pulmonary infection by staphylococci. Persons with cystic fibrosis also are particularly susceptible to staphylococcal pneumonia. Many believe that the millions of deaths resulting from periodic epidemics of influenza (a viral disease) may be due to a subsequent bacterial pneumonia caused by a TSS-producing staphylococcus.

OSTEOMYELITIS. *S aureus* exceeds all other microorganisms as an etiologic agent of human osteomyelitis (an infection of the bones). It occurs most frequently in boys younger than 12 years of age and, if untreated, can have a mortality rate of 25%. The source of such infections may be adjacent tissue infections, or it may be spread through the bloodstream to the traumatized bone.

WOUND INFECTIONS. Staphylococcal wound infections are less common now than they were in the preantibiotic era, but they are still the single most common hospital-acquired surgical or wound infection. Such infections most often appear to arise from endogenous strains carried by the patient, but they also can be transmitted by medical personnel or by contaminated bedding or equipment.

ENTERITIS. Staphylococcal enteritis is a severe infection of the small or large intestine, which can occur after gastrointestinal surgery or intensive antibiotic therapy, which destroys much of the normal intestinal flora. The necrotic lesions in the intestinal wall are believed to result from the secretion of enterotoxin by the invading staphylococcus.

Other manifestations of *S aureus* infections include acute bacterial endocarditis and meningitis.

LABORATORY DIAGNOSIS OF STAPHYLOCOCCAL INFECTIONS. Because staphylococci are found so frequently on the skin and in the nasopharynx, diagnosis can be complicated by the fact that it may not always be clear whether one is dealing with the true etiologic agent of the disease or with a contaminating parasitic staphylococcus. Exudates or blood specimens should be streaked on blood-agar plates and, after growth, observed for pigment production and hemolysis. Isolated cultures also must be assayed for the production of coagulase, because it is this property that is correlated most consistently with pathogenicity. Commercially available kits also are widely used for the rapid identification of *S aureus*. Such kits use latex beads, which are coated with both fibrinogen and IgG. About 97% of human isolates of *S aureus* possess protein A on their surface, which will bind to IgG. Therefore, if a culture of *S aureus* is emulsified on a card with a drop of such coated latex beads, visible agglutination will occur within 20 seconds. It should be noted, however, that false-positive and false-negative reactions do occur in such tests.

Animal inoculation usually is not of value, but the subcutaneous or intraperitoneal injection of an exfoliatin-producing staphylococcus into a newborn mouse will result in a diffuse sloughing of the epidermis.

TREATMENT AND CONTROL OF STAPHYLOCOCCAL INFECTIONS. *S aureus* appears to be consistently adaptable in becoming resistant to drug therapy; as a result, many antibiotics soon become ineffective for the treatment of staphylococcal infections. Many strains of staphylococci-producing penicillinase can be treated successfully with the penicillinase-resistant semisynthetic penicillin, methicillin (see Chap. 19), but strains resistant to this antibiotic are being encountered more often. Vancomycin has proven to be effective for many methicillin-resistant strains. However, any isolated staphylococcus must be assayed for antibiotic sensitivity as soon as possible, even though therapy usually should commence before such results are available. Once therapy has begun, it should be intensive to kill all organisms before mutation to a slightly higher level of drug resistance can occur.

Control is directed primarily at those individuals who are most susceptible to staphylococcal infections. Thus, the newborn nurseries of hospitals and surgical operation rooms are particularly dangerous areas where rigid aseptic procedures must be followed. In the event of a hospital outbreak, the etiologic staphylococcus should be phage-typed and all attending personnel should be cultured to locate the possible source of the organism.

Coagulase-Negative Staphylococci

Although *Bergey's Manual* lists 18 different species of coagulase-negative staphylococci, *S epidermidis* is by far the most important human opportunist.

S epidermidis is widely distributed on human skin and is found universally within human nares. It can be differentiated from *S aureus* by its white colonies, a glycerol-type teichoic acid, and the absence of coagulase. It also lacks α toxin and protein A, and is unable to ferment mannitol.

S epidermidis causes primarily nosocomial infections and, because of its wide distribution, it frequently is difficult to ascertain whether it is the true infectious agent or merely a skin contaminant. *S epidermidis* is among the most prevalent causes of sepsis in neonatal nurseries. This is a fairly recent phenomenon, probably due to new invasive procedures for maintaining and monitoring infants, and to prolonged stays in the neonatal intensive care unit. It is the organism most often isolated from indwelling foreign devices such as prosthetic joints, prosthetic heart valves, peritoneal dialysis catheters, intravascular catheters, and cerebrospinal fluid shunts. The property that these opportunistic organisms share is their ability to produce a polysaccharide capsule that adheres to a variety of prosthetic materials.

Treatment of infections caused by coagulase-negative staphylococci frequently necessitates removal of the infected foreign body. Antibiotic treatment requires susceptibility testing, because *S epidermidis* strains often are resistant to multiple antibiotics. Such treatments frequently are lengthy, especially for those strains that possess resistance to methicillin, and can entail the use of vancomycin plus rifampin and gentamicin for 2 weeks, followed by vancomycin and rifampin for an additional 4 weeks.

Staphylococcus saprophyticus

It is unclear whether *S saprophyticus* represents a new species or is merely a variant of *S epidermidis*. *S saprophyticus* is characterized as being coagulase-negative, deoxyribonuclease-negative, unable to ferment glucose, and resistant to novobiocin.

S saprophyticus causes 7% to 20% of all bacteriologically confirmed cases of urinary tract infection in women, particularly those aged 16 to 30 years. It seldom is observed in men. In one study, it was reported to be present in the urine of 42.3% of all women aged 16 to 25 years who had bacteriuria (bacteria in the urine).

The source of these infections is obscure because this organism is isolated only rarely from the urine, rectum, or skin of uninfected individuals. However, because of the frequency of urinary tract infections, it is possible that many women carry this organism in their genitourinary tract. This concept is supported by the fact that bacteriuria with *S saprophyticus* has been shown to occur after sexual intercourse. It also can be isolated from the skin of a variety of animals, and from lesions on the hands of persons handling animals.

S saprophyticus is routinely resistant to novobiocin, but usually is sensitive to a wide variety of antibiotics, such as penicillin, ampicillin, methicillin, and erythromycin.

Bibliography

JOURNALS

Bisno AL. Group A streptococcal infections and acute rheumatic fever. N Engl J Med 1991;325:783.

Culotta E, Koshland DE Jr. NO news is good news. Science 1992;258:1862.

Demers B, et al. Severe invasive group A streptococcal infections in Ontario, Canada: 1987-1991. Clin Infect Dis 1993;16:792.

Fischetti VA. Streptococcal M protein: molecular design and biological behavior. Clin Microbiol Rev 1989;2:285.

Kloos WE, Bannerman TL. Update on clinical significance of coagulase-negative staphylococci. Clin Microbiol Rev 1994;7:117.

Moellering RC Jr. Emergence of enterococcus as a significant pathogen. Clin Infect Dis 1992;14:1173.

van der Poll T, et al. Release of soluble receptors for tumor necrosis factor in clinical sepsis and experimental endotoxemia. J Infect Dis 1993;168:955.

Essentials of Medical Microbiology, Fifth Edition, edited by Wesley A. Volk,
Bryan M. Gebhardt, Marie-Louise Hammarskjöld, and Robert J. Kadner.
Lippincott-Raven Publishers, Philadelphia © 1996.

Chapter 25

Neisseriaceae

The gram-negative pyogenic cocci (Neisseriaceae), like their gram-positive counterparts, are able to cause disease because of their ability to resist phagocytosis. However, unlike many of the gram-positive pyogenic cocci, none of the Neisseriaceae appear to produce extracellular products that could aid in disease production.

Two species of gram-negative cocci cause serious disease in humans: (1) *Neisseria meningitidis,* the etiologic agent of epidemic meningitis; and (2) *Neisseria gonorrhoeae,* the cause of the sexually transmitted disease, gonorrhea. Members of other genera of this family that either are normal flora or occasionally cause disease in humans are found among *Acinetobacter* and *Moraxella.*

Morphology and Nutrition of the *Neisseria*

Bacteria in the genus *Neisseria* are nonmotile, gram-negative diplococci whose stained cells appear characteristically kidney-shaped with their concave sides adjacent to each other. As a result, the pairs of stained diplococci sometimes look like small doughnuts (Fig. 25-1).

The nonpathogenic *Neisseria* (part of the normal flora of the nasopharynx) are slightly larger and considerably easier to grow than the pathogenic species; they are able to multiply at 22°C on ordinary laboratory media such as nutrient broth, whereas the pathogens grow poorly below 37°C and not at all at 22°C. Furthermore, the pathogens are extremely sensitive to fatty acids and trace metals present in peptones and agar. This inhibitory effect can be eliminated by the addition of serum or blood to the growth medium. Moreover, if the blood is heated to 80°C for 10 minutes, it is even more effective. This procedure turns the agar medium a dark brown, and the resulting medium is commonly called *chocolate agar.* The pathogens also require a higher concentration of CO_2 for optimal growth than is present in the atmosphere. It is customary, therefore, to culture newly isolated pathogenic *Neisseria* either in a special incubator containing excess CO_2 or in a jar in which a candle has been lit before

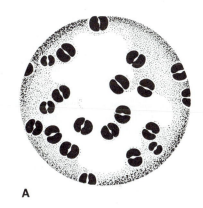

A

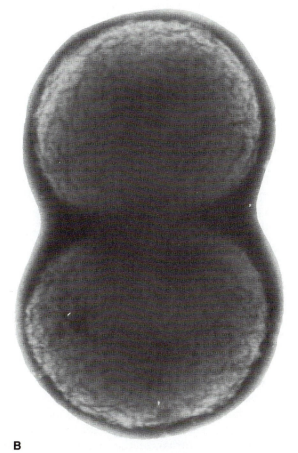

B

FIGURE 25-1 A. Drawing of doughnut-shaped diplococci of *Neisseria gonorrhoeae* as they sometimes appear under the microscope. **B.** Electron micrograph of a negatively stained pair of *N gonorrhoeae* cells. (Original magnification ×49,140.)

it is closed. The candle uses about half the oxygen and releases CO_2, resulting in a final concentration of about 10% CO_2.

The pathogenic *Neisseria* are fragile organisms and will readily undergo autolysis unless their autolytic enzymes are destroyed by heating at 65°C for 30 minutes or by the addition of formalin. These techniques are used to preserve cell suspensions for serologic tests.

Another unusual property of the pathogenic *Neisseria* is their ability to secrete a protease whose only known

substrate is human immunoglobulin of the IgA1 subclass. This protease has no effect on the IgA2 subclass of antibodies. Its role in the pathogenesis of infection is unknown, but the observation that all strains of *N meningitidis* and *N gonorrhoeae* secrete this protease suggests that it may be of value to the invading organism.

All *Neisseria,* including the nonpathogens, are *oxidase positive,* that is, they are able to oxidize dimethylparaphenylene and tetramethylparaphenylene diamine. This property can be used to distinguish colonies of *Neisseria* from colonies of other bacteria growing on the same plate. The oxidase test can be carried out by spraying either dimethylparaphenylene or tetramethylparaphenylene diamine onto the colonies and observing color changes. Colonies that are oxidase positive turn pink, then dark red, and finally black (Fig. 25-2); oxidase-negative colonies are unchanged. The reagent eventually kills the cells, but if the colony is restreaked on fresh media before it turns dark, it can be grown again. A piece of filter paper can be wetted with the reagent, and part of a suspected bacterial colony can be smeared on the wet filter paper. A positive reaction is indicated by the development of a dark purple color within 10 to 15 seconds. It should be noted that although the oxidase test is an aid in the isolation and identification of *Neisseria,* any organism that possesses cytochrome oxidase in its respiratory chain will be oxidase positive.

NEISSERIA MENINGITIDIS

N meningitidis, commonly called the *meningococcus,* was first described in 1887 as occurring in the spinal fluid of

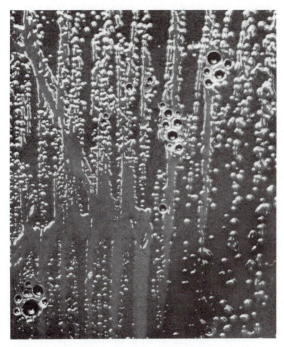

FIGURE 25-2 Black colonies of *Neisseria meningitidis* on chocolate agar indicate a positive oxidase test result.

TABLE 25-1
Chemical Composition of Meningococcal Capsular Polysaccharides

Serogroup	Chemical Composition
A	N-acetyl O-acetyl mannosamine phosphate
B	2-8-α-N-acetylneuraminic acid
C*	2-9-α-N-acetylneuraminic acid
X	2-acetamido-2 deoxy-D-glucose 4-phosphate
Y	D-glucose and N-acetylneuraminic acid 1:1
W135	D-galactose and N-acetylneuraminic acid 1:1
L	N-acetylglucosamine-phosphate

* In some variants of group C, the neuraminic acid is partially O-acetylated.

patients with meningitis. Subsequently, it has been shown to be the etiologic agent for epidemic meningitis in humans and also to cause a fulminating, frequently fatal septicemia resulting in lesions, primarily of the skin, bones, and adrenal glands.

Antigenic Classification

Meningococci can be classified into numerous groups based on common antigens. Current serogroups are designated A, B, C, D, X, Y, Z, 29E, and W135. Rare isolates also have been reported, which are placed in serogroups H, I, K, and L. It is groups A, B, and C, however, that are the causes of epidemics of meningitis.

The group-specific antigen for the meningococci is a polysaccharide capsule that surrounds the organisms. The capsular polysaccharides occurring on most of these serogroups have been purified, and their chemical composition is listed in Table 25-1.

Each group of meningococci can be subdivided further into distinct serotypes based on the antigenicity of their major outer membrane proteins. Frasch and his colleagues have assigned the outer membrane proteins of the meningococci to one of five classes according to the

TABLE 25-2
Outer Membrane Proteins of *Neisseria meningitidis* Used for Serotyping

Class of Protein	Major Properties
1	Trypsin sensitive; not found in all strains; quantitatively variable
2	Trypsin resistant; functions as a porin; quantitatively predominant
3	Similar to class 2 proteins but mutually exclusive
4	Trypsin resistant; found in all strains
5	Highly variable in expression and size; single strain can express more than one class 5 protein

various properties listed in Table 25-2. Classes 2 and 3 (also called PorB) make up the major outer membrane proteins, but both are never found in the same strain of meningococcus. Because of their stability within a strain, these classes are used to establish subtypes of meningococci. Class 5 proteins are analogous to the PII proteins found in the outer membrane of *N gonorrhoeae* in that they may not be expressed at all, or several different ones may be expressed simultaneously.

Epidemiology and Pathogenesis of Meningococcal Infections

The meningococcus is a strict parasite of humans and can be cultured routinely from the nasopharynx of asymptomatic carriers. In periods between epidemics, civilian carrier rates range from 2% to 8%, depending on the season, whereas in a closed society such as a military camp, the average carrier rate has been reported to exceed 40%, with more than 90% of the personnel becoming carriers at some time during 10 weeks of observation.

Therefore, it is obvious that the organism is spread from person to person through the respiratory route, and that, even in a situation in which most individuals are carrying the virulent organisms in their nasopharynx, few ordinarily get sick. However, if we follow the fate of the infecting organism, meningococcal infections can be categorized into three stages.

1. First in occurrence is the nasopharyngeal infection, which usually is asymptomatic but might result in a minor inflammation. This state can last for days to months and induces the formation of protective antibodies within a week, even though the infection remains asymptomatic.

2. In a small percentage of cases, the meningococci enter the bloodstream from the posterior nasopharynx, probably through the cervical lymph nodes. This stage, called *meningococcemia,* can be explosive, resulting in death within 6 to 8 hours, or it can begin more gradually with fever, malaise, and a petechial rash (minute, rounded skin hemorrhages), the lesions of which contain the cocci. The organisms also can cause lesions in the joints and lungs and, rarely, can cause massive hemorrhages in the adrenals (Waterhouse-Friderichsen syndrome).

   The hemorrhagic lesions occurring in both the skin and the internal organs, particularly the adrenals, are believed to result from the release of endotoxin. Electron micrographs show that the meningococcus possesses pili, which allows intimate contact with host cells, and that the organisms appear to release blebs of endotoxin (Fig. 25-3).

   Because patients with meningococcemia can develop severe shock within a few hours even if intensive treatment is initiated immediately, one hospital in the Netherlands has begun treating all patients who have meningococcal disease and hypotension with plasma-

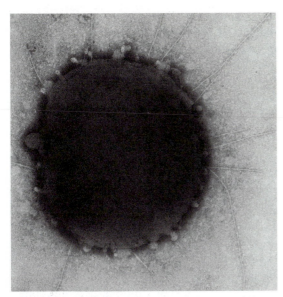

FIGURE 25-3 A negatively stained cell of *Neisseria meningitidis* group B, showing pili and surface blebs of cell-wall lipopolysaccharide, or endotoxin. (Original magnification ×39,000.)

A Closer Look

Bacterial meningitis is an important cause of permanent neurologic disability. Some concept of the magnitude of such sequelae can be appreciated by reports that 20% to 30% of patients recovering from bacterial meningitis have permanent developmental handicaps. Of these disorders, hearing loss seems to be the most frequent deficit, followed by epilepsy, mental retardation, partial paralysis, and blindness. The mechanism behind this damage is unclear, but evidence points to the release of large amounts of cytokines, particularly TFN-α, as a prime mediator of neurologic disorders. For example, a large study carried out at Northwestern University Medical School revealed that an initial cerebrospinal fluid concentration of TNF-α greater than 1000 pg/mL was associated with a high level of seizure activity. Moreover, the occurrence of TNF-α in the bloodstream of patients with meningococcal meningitis had a strong association with mortality; patients with a serum TNF-α concentration greater than 140 pg/mL invariably died.

It also is interesting that the concentration of platelet activating factor (PAF) in the cerebrospinal fluid is significantly higher in children with bacterial meningitis. This is not surprising, because both TNF-α and IL-1 are potent inducers of PAF, and it is noteworthy, because PAF recruits white blood cells to the site of inflammation, providing an additional source for the release of inflammatory cytokines.

pheresis or whole-blood exchange. This treatment can be repeated every 12 hours, and the results obtained in 25 patients show mortality rates of 60% for control subjects and 20% for treated patients.

Meningococcemia also can result in a condition known as *disseminated intravascular coagulation*. In such situations, blood clots can block circulation to the extremities, necessitating amputation. The initiation of disseminated intravascular coagulation is not a specific property of the meningococcus, but can occur anytime the body is subjected to large amounts of endotoxin, causing the synthesis of tumor necrosis factor-α (TNF-α) and the activation of clotting factor XII.

3. In the third stage of meningococcal infection, the organisms can cross the blood–brain barrier and infect the meninges, causing the major symptoms of severe headache, stiff neck, and vomiting accompanied by delirium and confusion. Interestingly, levels of intrathecal TNF-α, (but not interleukin-1 [IL-1]), correlate with the degree of blood–brain barrier disruption and disease severity, suggesting that TNF-α is related to blood–brain damage in bacterial meningitis. It also is possible that the presence of such cytokines accounts for the fact that about one third of newborns and children recovering from bacterial meningitis have neurologic sequelae.

Therefore, the major virulence factors of the meningococcus are its ability to resist phagocytosis due to its polysaccharide capsule, and its release of prodigious amounts of endotoxin.

Surprisingly, meningococci also are isolated occasionally from areas of the body usually considered to be the domain of gonococci. Such infections as acute urethritis (inflammation of the urethra), epididymitis (inflamma-

tion of the epididymis), vulvovaginitis (inflammation of the vulva and vagina), or cervicitis (inflammation of the cervix of the uterus) would be labeled as gonococcal infections in the absence of a complete laboratory identification of the etiologic agent.

Laboratory Diagnosis of Meningococcal Infections

Spinal fluid, blood, and nasopharyngeal tissue, as well as smears and cultures from skin lesions, can be sources of meningococci. Nasopharyngeal tissue is obtained most effectively using a cotton swab on a bent wire, so that the posterior nasopharynx can be reached without contamination by the normal flora of the mouth.

Frequently, the gram-negative diplococci can be directly observed in, or adhering to, white blood cells sedimented from freshly obtained spinal fluid.

Final identification requires both sugar fermentations (Table 25-3) and serologic tests using group-specific antisera for the agglutination of the unknown isolate. Kits are

TABLE 25-3
Growth Characteristics and Sugar Fermentations by *Neisseria* and Morphologically Similar Human Parasites

Organism	Growth in the Absence of Blood	Glucose	Maltose	Sucrose	Lactose	Fructose
Neisseria meningitidis	−	+	+	−	−	−
Neisseria gonorrhoeae	−	+	−	−	−	−
Neisseria flavescens	+	−	−	−	−	−
Neisseria sicca	+	+	+	+	−	+
Branhamella catarrhalis	+	−	−	−	−	−

available that provide microcupules (containing glucose, maltose, lactose, sucrose, DNA, and penicillin). Each of these cupules can be rehydrated with a heavy suspension of the isolated bacterial culture suspended in physiologic saline. The fermentation results can be read after 2 hours of incubation at 37°C. Counterimmunoelectrophoresis also has been used successfully to detect the presence of meningococcal antigens in spinal fluid. In addition, either a quellung reaction or latex particles to which a group-specific polysaccharide has been adsorbed can be used in an agglutination procedure to detect antibody to the group polysaccharides.

Tissue from throat swabs usually is streaked on blood agar or chocolate agar, but the selective Thayer-Martin medium frequently is used because it contains polymyxin, vancomycin, and nystatin. These inhibit the growth of many bacteria and yeast contaminants, while allowing the growth of the pathogenic *Neisseria*.

Treatment and Prevention of Meningococcal Infections

Until the early 1960s, the sulfonamides were the main drugs used to treat infections caused by *N meningitidis,* because they readily penetrated the blood–brain barrier. However, the incidence of organisms resistant to sulfonamides has increased to the point where these agents are rarely used for meningococcal infections today. Fortunately, penicillin is effective, and it is the current drug of choice. Erythromycin and chloramphenicol also are effective and can be used in individuals who are hypersensitive to penicillin.

Prevention of meningococcal infections has been approached in two different ways: (1) by the elimination of carriers, and (2) by the use of vaccines.

During World War II, entire military camps of thousands of men were given sulfonamides as an effective method of eliminating meningococci from carriers and stopping epidemics. Now that many strains are sulfonamide-resistant, this treatment probably would be of little value. The close personal contacts of a patient should be treated with 600 mg of rifampin every 12 hours for 2 days. Occasional rifampin-resistant mutants are being found, however, and it may be necessary to use other antibiotics.

A quadrivalent vaccine, consisting of purified capsular polysaccharides, is commercially available for groups A, C, Y, and W135. In 1974, a group A and C vaccine was used to stop a major epidemic in São Paulo, Brazil, where more than 20,000 cases and 3000 deaths caused by both group A and group C meningococci occurred. The efficacy of these vaccines also has been shown in American and Finnish military recruits. After immunization with group A polysaccharide, most children by the age of 3 months can form some bactericidal antibodies, but their response is markedly weaker than that of young adults. The ability to form antibodies to groups C, Y, and W135 polysaccharide is even more age restricted, because children younger than 2 years of age respond poorly or not at all.

Purified group B polysaccharide is not immunogenic in humans, and there is no commercial vaccine for group B meningococci. Experimental vaccines in which the group B polysaccharide is noncovalently complexed with outer membrane proteins induce only the short-lived IgM antibodies to the polysaccharide. Other experimental vaccines have conjugated the oligosaccharides (obtained by the mild acid hydrolysis of the cell-wall lipopolysaccharides) to tetanus toxoid. Such vaccines do induce the formation of bactericidal antibodies, but such antibodies are, for the most part, type specific and not group specific.

In 1991, more than 90,000 Norwegian adolescents were immunized with an outer membrane vesicle vaccine prepared from a serogroup B strain of *N meningitidis.* Follow-up studies showed that the vaccine induced IgG antibodies to the 5C protein that were bactericidal to strains expressing large amounts of 5C protein. However, because many strains express little or no 5C protein, the search for an effective vaccine for group B meningococci continues.

NEISSERIA GONORRHOEAE

During the past decade, gonorrhea has grown to epidemic proportions that are second only to the sexually transmitted chlamydial infections. About 1 million cases are reported annually in this country, and this undoubtedly

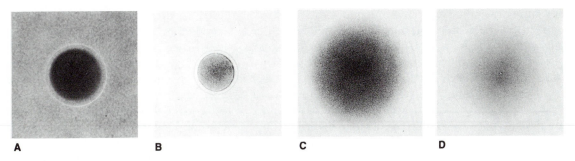

FIGURE 25-4 Colony type of *Neisseria gonorrhoeae*. **A.** Type 1 (T1). **B.** Type 2 (T2). **C.** Type 3 (T3). **D.** Type 4 (T4). (Original magnification about ×180.)

represents only a portion of the total number of cases that actually occur.

Antigenic Classification

N gonorrhoeae, routinely called the *gonococcus,* appears to consist of an antigenically heterogeneous group of organisms, and no successful immunologic classification is available. However, serotypes have been proposed based on different electrophoretic mobilities of the major outer membrane proteins. The organisms also are divided into four types based on their colonial appearance (Fig. 25-4), but these morphologic variations are a result of mutations occurring within a single strain. Thus, types 1 and 2 are pathogenic for humans, but, after growing on laboratory media overnight, at least half of any culture will show the colonial morphology of type 3 or 4, and,

after more prolonged cultivation, all organisms will appear as the avirulent types 3 and 4.

PILI. On a microscopic level, the most obvious difference between the various colonial types is that the virulent types 1 and 2 possess pili (Fig. 25-5*A*), whereas the avirulent types 3 and 4 do not (see Fig. 25-5*B*). Because it is well established that pili are involved in the attachment of microorganisms to cells, it appears probable that the gonococcus requires close attachment to produce disease. Furthermore, the pili are antiphagocytic, perhaps in part because the organisms are attached so intimately to host cells. Removal of pili from virulent cells by treatment with trypsin results in their phagocytosis and destruction.

Because pili not only mediate the attachment of the gonococci to epithelial cells, but also are instrumental in

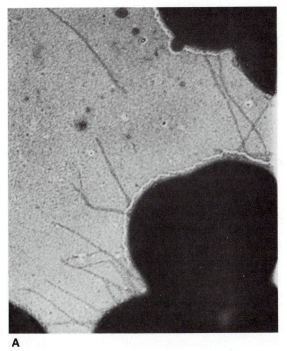
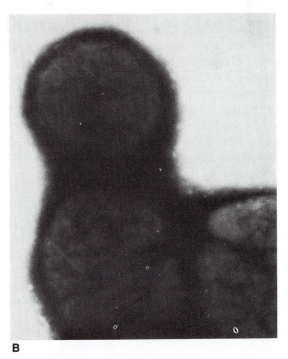

FIGURE 25-5 Negatively stained cells of *Neisseria gonorrhoeae*. **A.** Cells from a T1 colony showing numerous pili. **B.** Cells from a T4 colony lacking pili. (Original magnification about ×34,000.)

preventing their phagocytosis, it might be postulated that purified pili could serve as an effective vaccine for the prevention of gonorrhea. Unfortunately (for humans), pili isolated from different strains of gonococci display a wide variation in their amino acid composition and, as a result, extensive antigenic heterogeneity. Moreover, it has been shown conclusively that even a single strain of the gonococcus possesses multiple genes for pilus production, resulting in many antigenic types within a given clone. These genes, as characterized by Per Hagblom and co-workers, consist of one or two expression loci, designated *pil*E1 and *pil*E2. Both genes carry intact pilin-coding sequences and their own promoters. As a result of single or multiple recombinational events between repeated sequences that exist within these loci, deletions occurring in either of these genes convert the organism from a p⁺ to a p⁻ cell, even though the other pilin expression gene remains unchanged.

In addition to the pilin expression genes, the chromosome of the gonococcus also contains six or seven silent sequences (*pil*S loci), which lack their own promoters and, hence, are not expressed. These silent loci, however, contain multiple sequences, which correspond to the variable part of pilin, and it appears that the antigenic diversity of the pilus is due to recombinational events between the two expression genes, *pil*E1 and *pil*E2, and between the expression genes and the silent loci. Thus, the gonococcus not only changes from p⁺ to p⁻, but also switches from p⁻ back to a different p⁺. That such events happen in nature was clearly demonstrated by an analysis of pilin genes obtained from isolates whose origin could be traced to a single source during an epidemic of gonorrhea. Nucleotide sequence determination of a series of genes located within one *pil*S locus has provided some insight into how gene conversion of the expression *pil*E genes occurs. It appears that the semivariable and highly variable domains are interspersed with short, highly conserved regions that flank areas of variable sequence information. Such areas, termed *minicassettes,* are duplicated and readily exchanged among both silent and expressed pilus genes by virtue of the homology of the conserved regions surrounding them.

OUTER MEMBRANE PROTEINS. The three major outer membrane proteins of the gonococci have been named proteins I, II, and III. (It has been suggested that these designations be changed to Por, Opa, and Rmp, respectively.) Protein I is the predominant species in the outer membrane and, although antigenically constant within a given strain, varies considerably among the diverse strains of gonococci. It appears to act as a porin and serves as a basis for serotyping the gonococci.

Based on tryptic and chymotryptic peptide maps and on differences in susceptibility to protease cleavage when present in intact gonococci, two different groups of protein I molecules, designated PIA and PIB, have been described. Serotypes 1 through 3 are associated with PIA,

and serotypes 4 through 9 are found in PIB. Strains possessing PIA are resistant to killing by normal human serum and, hence, are the strains involved in disseminated infections. Because of the limited number of serotypes, protein I is being investigated for use as a vaccine to prevent gonorrhea. Protein II consists of a large, related family of proteins that appears to be associated with the adherence of the gonococci to various types of host cells. Protein II also has been termed the *opacity protein,* because its presence is correlated with a dark, opaque colony; most light, translucent colonies of gonococci lack protein II.

Because antibodies induced by protein II act as opsonins, it would appear that this protein might serve as an effective vaccine. Unfortunately, the gonococcus has evolved mechanisms to circumvent this possibility. Thus, a strain of gonococci can produce 1 or 2 types of protein II simultaneously; it can cease to produce protein II or, as described for gonococcal pili, can switch to form an antigenically different protein II. As many as six antigenically distinct types of protein II have been found within a single strain of gonococci. It has been estimated that about 1 cell in each 1000 generations will switch to make a different protein II.

The mechanism whereby the gonococcus controls the expression or antigenic variation of protein II is an ingenious example of evolution. Sequence analysis of several variant opacity genes revealed that each of these genes possessed a highly repetitive sequence made up of identical pentameric pyrimidine units (CTCTT) within the 5′-terminal section of the open reading frame. The number of repeating units varied from 7 to 28, and it appeared that many protein II genes were constitutively transcribed, even though some were not translated into protein. Anne Stern and her colleagues showed that the actual expression of a protein II is controlled at the translation level through the loss or gain of one or two CTCTT sequences, causing the mRNA to become out of frame and, hence, not translatable. For example, the loss or gain of three repeating sequences (15 nucleotides) did not affect the reading frame, permitting translation of the mRNA, but it is easy to see that the loss or gain of one or two repeating pyrimidine sequences will throw the mRNA out of frame, resulting in the loss of protein II. However, a loss or gain that returns the mRNA to the proper frame will result in the expression of the protein II gene. Preliminary data suggest that the class 5 proteins in the meningococcus are under a similar type of control mechanism. It is apparent that the pathogenic *Neisseria* have evolved some complex genetic mechanisms to ensure their survival.

Protein III appears to be identical in all gonococci, and it has not been associated with any specific virulence factor.

A more recently described surface antigen, termed H.8, is, like protein I, homologous within a given strain. Because this antigen is a lipoprotein, a newer nomenclature refers to it as Lip. This antigen is found on all strains of *N gonorrhoeae* and *N meningitidis* and, because mono-clonal antibodies to H.8 are bactericidal, it is being ac-tively investigated for use as a potential vaccine.

Virulence Factors

Pili are an essential virulence factor because in their ab-sence, the organisms are rapidly phagocytosed and de-stroyed. *Protein II* also is involved in the adherence of the gonococci to various types of host cells. However, because neither pili nor protein II are cytotoxic, there must be other factors taking part in the disease process.

Gonococci release fragments of peptidoglycan that are cytotoxic for ciliated epithelial cells. These fragments are termed *tracheal cytotoxin* and are responsible for the fallopian tube damage and resulting sterility associated with gonorrhea. Tracheal cytotoxin appears to stimulate ciliated epithelial cells to make IL-1. This is supported by the observation that adding IL-1 to hamster tracheal organ cultures produces the same effect as adding tracheal cytotoxin to the cultures. An identical cytotoxin is re-leased by the organism that causes whooping cough (*Bor-detella pertussis*) and, in this case, it appears to be responsi-ble for the destruction of the ciliated respiratory cells.

All gonococci also produce an *IgA protease* that spe-cifically inactivates the IgA1 subclass of antibodies.

Epidemiology and Pathogenesis of Gonorrhea

Gonorrhea is a sexually transmitted disease that, with few exceptions, is acquired through sexual contact with an infected individual. The organisms penetrate the mucous membranes of the genital tract, causing a localized infec-tion initially. In men, the infection can be asymptomatic, but it usually causes an acute urethritis, resulting in a purulent discharge and painful urination. The gonococci also can infect the prostate gland and epididymis. In women, the infection is much more likely to be asymp-tomatic or accompanied by a minor discharge that may go unnoticed. However, the organisms can infect the urethra, vagina, cervix, and fallopian tubes, causing a *pel-vic inflammatory disease (PID)* resulting in sterility. Dis-seminated gonococcal infection also occurs in 1% to 3% of cases, leading to lesions in the skin, heart, eye, menin-ges, or joints, and resulting in gonococcal arthritis.

Until recently, it was unclear why some individuals succumbed to the disseminated disease. It now appears likely that the strains of gonococci that are capable of hematogenous spread are resistant to killing in the ab-sence of specific antibodies, whereas those organisms that cause local infections are more readily eliminated in the presence of normal human serum. An explanation for these differences is based on the following observations:

Normal human serum contains bactericidal antibodies that bind to gonococci, initiating the complement cascade.

Serum-resistant gonococci, but not serum-sensitive strains, also bind blocking antibodies present in normal human serum.

The bound blocking antibodies appear to inhibit the binding of the bactericidal antibodies or to prevent the complement attack complex from correctly in-serting into the bacterial cell wall.

It is possible that there is more than one surface structure capable of binding such blocking antibodies. In one case, however, transfection of a gene obtained from a serum-resistant strain conferred resistance on a serum-sensitive strain. Phenotypically, this resistance was seen as a new 29-kilodalton surface protein capable of binding blocking antibodies.

Ophthalmia neonatorum is a gonococcal infection of the eye acquired by a newborn during passage through the birth canal of an infected mother. Such infections often result in blindness but have been largely eliminated in the developed world by the legal requirement that silver nitrate, which is bactericidal for these organisms, be dropped into a baby's eyes at birth. Tetracycline and erythromycin also are used and appear to be at least as effective as $AgNO_3$. Unfortunately, eye prophylaxis is not widely used in some developing countries because of the mild chemical conjunctivitis induced by the silver nitrate. This is particularly disquieting, because in many such areas, 9% to 10% of women in labor have gonorrhea, resulting in considerable visual loss or blindness in their newborns.

Laboratory Diagnosis of Gonorrhea

In the purulent stage, particularly in infected men, a stain of the urethral exudate will show numerous leukocytes associated with or containing intracellular gram-negative diplococci, but a positive laboratory diagnosis of gonor-rhea requires that the organism be grown and identified as an oxidase-positive, gram-negative diplococcus that ferments glucose but fails to ferment maltose or sucrose.

Chronic gonorrhea, particularly in women, can be difficult to diagnose by smear, because there is little or no discharge and few organisms. Fluorescence labeled antibody can be used to identify organisms in smears, but gonococci often cannot be observed or isolated from such cases. Significant effort is being directed toward the dis-covery of serologic techniques that will demonstrate the presence of specific antibodies in infected persons. Com-plement fixation has not been successful. However, in some cases, the use of an indirect immunofluorescence test, in which the patient's serum is reacted with known type 1 gonococci, followed by fluorescence labeled rabbit antihuman γ-globulin, appears to be of value for sero-logic diagnosis.

A new DNA probe is commercially available and, according to Y.A. Jean Louis of the University of Wash-ington, it is 100% specific and 99% sensitive for *N gonor-rhoeae*.

Bibliography

JOURNALS

Durand ML, et al. Acute bacterial meningitis in adults: a review of 493 episodes. N Engl J Med 1993;328:21.

Gray LD, Fedorko DP. Laboratory diagnosis of bacterial meningitis. Clin Microbiol Rev 1992;5:130.

Quagliarello VJ, Scheld WM. New perspectives on bacterial meningitis. Clin Infect Dis 1993;17:603.

Tunkel AR, Scheld WM. Pathogenesis and pathophysiology of bacterial meningitis. Clin Microbiol Rev 1993;6:118.

Wetzler LM, et al. Gonococcal porin vaccine evaluation: comparison of por proteosomes, liposomes, and blebs isolated from *rmp* deletion mutants. J Infect Dis 1992;166:551.

Essentials of Medical Microbiology, Fifth Edition, edited by Wesley A. Volk,
Bryan M. Gebhardt, Marie-Louise Hammarskjöld, and Robert J. Kadner.
Lippincott-Raven Publishers, Philadelphia © 1996.

Chapter 26

Enterics and Related Gram-Negative Organisms

The organisms forming the enormous heterogeneous group of gram-negative bacteria that are either part of the normal flora of the intestine or may cause systemic infections, urinary tract infections, or gastrointestinal diseases are called collectively the *enterics*. In this designation are included the facultatively anaerobic bacteria in the families Enterobacteriaceae and Vibrionaceae, the obligately aerobic Pseudomonadaceae, and the obligately anaerobic gram-negative organisms in the family Bacteroidaceae.

ENTEROBACTERIACEAE

Some members of the Enterobacteriaceae are always considered to be pathogens, whereas others are routinely found as part of the normal flora of the intestinal tract or as saprophytes living on decaying matter. However, most seem to have the potential to produce disease under

TABLE 26-1
Classification of the Enterobacteriaceae

Ewing and Martin		Bergey's Manual
Tribe	Genera	Genera
Eschericheae	Escherichia	Escherichia
	Shigella	Shigella
Edwardsielleae	Edwardsiella	Edwardsiella
Salmonelleae	Salmonella	Salmonella
	Arizona	Citrobacter
	Citrobacter	Klebsiella
Klebsielleae	Klebsiella	Enterobacter
	Enterobacter	Hafnia
	Serratia	Serratia
Proteeae	Proteus	Proteus
		Providencia
		Morganella
	Providencia	Yersinia
Erwineae	Erwinia	Erwinia
	Pectobacterium	

appropriate conditions and must be considered opportunists.

The Enterobacteriaceae contain gram-negative rods which, if motile, are peritrichously flagellated. Because members of this family are morphologically and metabolically similar, much effort has been expended to develop techniques for their rapid identification. In general, biochemical properties are used to define a genus, and further subdivision frequently is based on sugar fermentation and antigenic differences. Yet, many paradoxes exist; for example, more than 2200 species of *Salmonella* have been named, whereas the equally complex species *Escherichia coli* is divided into more than 1000 serotypes. Over the years, many taxonomists with different ideas have been involved in the classification of these bacteria, and disagreement still exists concerning family and generic names. Table 26-1 gives an outline of the taxonomic scheme proposed by Ewing and Martin for the Enterobacteriaceae, compared with that proposed in *Bergey's Manual of Systematic Bacteriology*. As shown, *Bergey's* has eliminated all tribes in the taxonomic division of this large family. Both schemes are used in various diagnostic laboratories, but this chapter adheres more closely to the Bergey classification.

Biochemical Properties Used for Classification

Early taxonomic schemes relied heavily on the organism's ability to ferment lactose, and numerous differential and selective media have been devised to allow one to recognize a lactose-fermenting colony on a solid medium. The effectiveness of such differential media is based on the fact

that organisms fermenting the lactose form acid, whereas nonlactose fermenters use the peptones present and do not form acids in these media. The incorporation of an acid–base indicator into the agar medium thus causes a color change around a lactose-fermenting colony (Fig. 26-1). This has been a valuable technique for selecting the major nonlactose-fermenting pathogens that cause salmonellosis or shigellosis; under special conditions, however, many lactose fermenters also cause a variety of infectious diseases.

Furthermore, many enterics ferment lactose only slowly, requiring several days before sufficient acid is formed to change the indicator. They all synthesize beta-galactosidase, (the enzyme that splits lactose into glucose and galactose) but lack the specific permease necessary for the transport of lactose into the cell. One can easily determine whether an organism is a slow lactose or nonlactose fermenter by mixing a loopful of bacteria with ortho-nitrophenol-beta-galactoside (ONPG) dissolved in a detergent. The linkage of the galactose in ONPG is the same as its linkage in lactose; inasmuch as the ONPG can enter the cell in the absence of a permease, an organism possessing beta-galactosidase will hydrolyze ONPG to yield galactose and the bright yellow compound, ortho-nitrophenol. Thus, only the absence of a specific lactose permease differentiates the slow lactose fermenters from the normal lactose fermenters.

In addition, a number of selective media have been devised that contain bile salts, dyes such as brilliant green and methylene blue, and chemicals such as selenite and bismuth. The incorporation of such compounds into the growth of medium has allowed for the selective growth of the enterics while inhibiting the growth of gram-positive organisms.

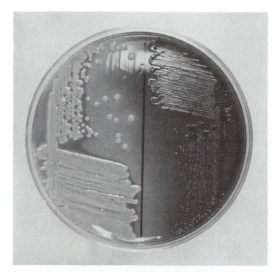

FIGURE 26-1   Lactose-positive (*left*) and lactose-negative (*right*) enteric organisms grown on Hektoen enteric agar plates. Lactose-positive colonies are larger and become salmon to orange in color, whereas lactose-negative colonies remain colorless on the green agar medium.

Some other biochemical properties used to classify members of the Enterobacteriaceae include the ability to form H_2S; decarboxylate the amino acids lysine, ornithine, or phenylalanine; hydrolyze urea into CO_2 and NH_3; form indole from tryptophan; grow with citrate as a sole source of carbon; liquefy gelatin; and ferment a large variety of sugars.

LABORATORY IDENTIFICATION OF THE ENTERICS

The complete identification of one of the enterics requires the use of dozens of different types of media. The modern clinical laboratory, which may have many isolates at one time, has devised a number of ingenious procedures to accomplish an identification in the shortest possible time. One procedure uses a plastic strip with about two dozen microwells containing different kinds of dehydrated media. A single isolated colony is suspended in 5 mL of saline, and this is used both to rehydrate and to inoculate the microwells. After 18 to 24 hours, positive reactions are read and an identification is made by referring to a standard chart.

An automated system also is available that uses a plastic card containing 30 microwells of various kinds of dehydrated media. The wells are simultaneously rehydrated and inoculated with a suspension of the unknown organism. The card then is placed in a special incubator where, after about 8 hours, it is automatically read and results are transmitted from the reader–incubator to a programmed computer, which prints the identification of the unknown organism.

Serologic Properties Used for Classification

No other group of organisms has been so extensively classified on the basis of cell-surface antigens as the Enterobacteriaceae. These antigens can be divided into three types, designated O, K, and H antigens.

O ANTIGENS

As described in Chapter 16, all gram-negative bacteria possess a lipopolysaccharide (LPS) as a component of their outer membrane. This toxic LPS (also called endotoxin) is composed of three regions: *lipid A*, *core*, and a repeating sequence of carbohydrates called the *O antigen* (Fig. 26-2). Based on different sugars, alpha- or beta-glycosidic linkages, and the presence or absence of substituted acetyl groups, *Escherichia coli* can be shown to possess at least 173 different O antigens, and 64 have been described in the genus *Salmonella*.

Sometimes, after continuous laboratory growth, strains will, through mutation, lose the ability to synthesize or attach this oligosaccharide O antigen to the core region of the LPS. This loss results in a change from a smooth colony to a rough colony type, and it is referred to as an S to R transformation. Interestingly, the R mutants have lost the ability to produce disease.

K ANTIGENS

K antigens exist as capsule or envelope polysaccharides and cover the O antigens when present, inhibiting agglu-

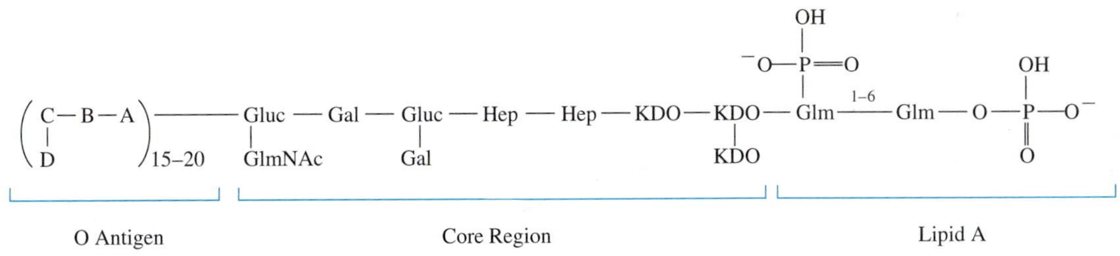

Glm — Glucosamine
KDO — Ketodeoxyoctonic acid
Hep — Heptose
Gluc — Glucose
Gal — Galactose
GlmNAc — *N*-acetyl glucosamine
A,B,C,D — Monosaccharides such as mannose, galactose, rhamnose, fucose, glucose, abequose, and colitose. These sugars exist in a repeating sequence of 15 to 20 units of 3 or 4 sugars.

FIGURE 26-2 Schematic structure of one unit of *Salmonella* cell-wall lipopolysaccharide (endotoxin). The structure of the cell-wall lipopolysaccharide may vary slightly from one genus of gram-negative organisms to another but, as far as is known, all contain three general regions, as shown here. Although not shown, all free hydroxyl groups of the glucosamines in lipid A are esterified with fatty acids. The serologic differences between different strains within a genus lie in the kinds of sugars and their linkages that exist in the O-antigen region.

tination by specific O antiserum. Most K antigens can be removed by boiling the organisms in water.

H ANTIGENS

Only organisms that are motile possess H antigens because these determinants are in the proteins that make up the flagella. However, to complicate matters, members of the genus *Salmonella* alternate back and forth to form different H antigens. The more specific antigens are called phase 1 antigens and are designated by lower-case letters (a, b, c, and so on), whereas the less-specific phase 2 H antigens are given numbers. The mechanism of this phase variation reveals an interesting way in which a cell can regulate the expression of its genes. In short, *Salmonella* possesses two genes: H1 encoding for phase 1 flagellar antigens, and H2 encoding for phase 2 flagellar antigens. The transcription of H2 results in the coordinate expression of gene *rhl*, which codes for a repressor that prevents the expression of H1. About every 10^3 to 10^5 generations, a 900–base-pair region, containing the promoter for the H2 gene, undergoes a site-specific inversion, stopping the transcription of both H2 and *rhl*. In the absence of the *rhl* gene product, the H1 gene is then transcribed until the 900–base-pair region in the H2 promoter is again inverted, resulting in the expression of H2 and *rhl*.

After obtaining the serologic data, an antigenic formula can be written, such as *E coli* 0111 : K58 : H6, meaning this *E coli* possesses O antigen 111, K antigen 58, and H antigen 6. The formula *Salmonella togo* 4,12 : l,w : 1,6 indicates this serotype of *Salmonella* possesses O antigens 4 and 12, phase 1 H antigens l and w, and phase 2 H antigens 1 and 6.

Coliforms

The meaning of the term coliform is arbitrary, but it usually refers to members of the Enterobacteriaceae that are normal inhabitants of the intestinal tract. With certain exceptions, these do not cause gastrointestinal-type diseases and, using this definition, the coliforms can be separated into two major groups: (1) *Escherichia*, and (2) *Klebsiella, Enterobacter, Serratia,* and *Hafnia*.

ESCHERICHIA COLI

Escherichia coli is an obligate intestinal parasite that cannot live free in nature, and its presence in water supplies is, therefore, evidence of recent fecal contamination.

Presumptive Test for *Escherichia coli*

To determine the presence of *E coli* in water, test tubes of nutrient broth containing lactose are inoculated with measured quantities of water samples. These tubes also

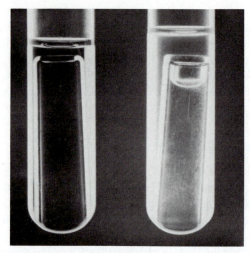

FIGURE 26-3 Fermentation tubes with inverted vials and acid indicator to test for *Escherichia coli*. Notice the light color (actually yellow) in the right-hand tube, because of the presence of acid, and the bubble in the vial, because of the evolution of gas.

contain an inverted vial to trap gas produced and an acid–base indicator to show acid production (Fig. 26-3). Because *E coli* ferments lactose, the presence of acid and gas in the inoculated tubes after 24 hours of incubation is presumptive evidence for its presence. If the lactose is not fermented, it is concluded that *E coli* is not present and that the water is free from recent fecal contamination. The fermentation of lactose may, however, result from nonenteric organisms and, for a positive conclusion of fecal contamination, it is necessary to show that the lactose-fermenting organisms are of fecal origin.

Confirmed Test

Because fecally derived *E coli* can grow at 44.5°C and nonfecal coliforms cannot, differential agar media (containing lactose as a carbon source) can be streaked with known amounts of water and incubated at both 37°C and 44.5°C. A comparison of the number of lactose-fermenting colonies growing at 37°C and 44.5°C will provide information concerning the origin of the coliforms. More precise results, however, can be obtained by carrying out the following test: eosin methylene blue agar is streaked from the positive lactose broth fermentation grown at 37°C. *E coli* grows as a characteristic small, flat colony that has a definite metallic green sheen.

Completed Test

Colonies from the confirmed test that show a metallic green sheen are reinoculated into lactose broth and, if acid and gas are produced, the organism is identified as *E coli*.

Membrane filters also can be used to detect the presence of bacteria in water. The membrane of cellulose acetate permits water to pass easily, but it traps bacteria on its surface. Coliform counts can be made by filtering a known volume of water through the membrane followed by incubation of the membrane in a special differential medium. Colonies growing on the surface of the membrane can be counted and observed for the characteristic appearance of *E coli* on the differential medium.

Pathogenicity of *Escherichia coli*

Although *E coli* is part of the normal flora of the intestinal tract, it is also the most common gram-negative pathogen responsible for nosocomially acquired septic shock, meningitis in neonates, cystitis and pyelonephritis in women, and for several distinct forms of diarrheal disease and dysentery affecting populations throughout the world. Strains of *E coli* capable of causing such diseases possess one or more virulence factors that are not found in *E coli* strains comprising the normal flora. Such virulence factors can be characterized as follows: the capacity to adhere to specific mammalian cells; the ability to invade and grow intracellularly in intestinal epithelial cells; the secretion of one or more enterotoxins that cause fluid loss, resulting in diarrhea; the formation of a cytotoxin that blocks protein synthesis, causing a hemorrhagic colitis; and the possession of an antiphagocytic capsule that is responsible, at least in part, for the bacteremia and meningitis caused by *E coli*. In addition, the ability to obtain iron from transferrin or lactoferrin by the synthesis of iron-binding siderophores markedly enhances the virulence of such strains through their ability to grow in host tissues. No one strain of *E coli* possesses all of these properties but, as is discussed later, all pathogenic strains must have one or more virulence factors to produce disease.

Diarrheal Diseases

It is estimated that during the American Revolutionary War there were more deaths from diarrhea than from English bullets, and during the American War between the states, over 25% of all deaths were because of diarrhea and dysentery. Diarrhea kills more people worldwide than AIDS and cancer, with about five million diarrheal deaths occurring annually primarily because of dehydration. Most of these occur in neonates and young children, and a large number are caused by pathogenic *E coli*. The disease in adults, known by many names such as traveler's diarrhea or Montezuma's revenge, may vary from a mild disease with several days of loose stools to a severe and fatal cholera-like disease. Such life-threatening *E coli* infections occur throughout the world but are most common in developing nations.

The virulence factors responsible for diarrheal disease are frequently encoded in plasmids, which may be spread from one strain to another either through transduction or by recombination. As a result, various combinations

of virulence factors have occurred, which has been used to place the diarrhea-producing strains of *E coli* into various groups based on the mechanism of disease production.

Enterotoxigenic *Escherichia coli*

Enterotoxin-producing *E coli*, called enterotoxigenic *E coli* (ETEC), produce one or both of two different toxins: a heat-labile toxin called LT and a heat-stable toxin called ST. The genetic ability to produce both LT and ST is controlled by DNA residing in transmissible plasmids called *ent* plasmids. Both genes have been cloned, and the ST gene has been shown to possess the characteristics of a transposon (see Chap. 21).

HEAT-LABILE TOXIN. The heat-labile toxin LT, which is destroyed by heating at 65°C for 30 minutes, has been extensively purified, and its mode of action is identical to that described for cholera toxin (CT). LT has a molecular weight of about 86,000 daltons and is composed of two subunits, A and B. Subunit A consists of one molecule of A_1 (24,000 daltons) and one molecule of A_2 (5000 daltons) linked by a disulfide bridge. Each A unit is joined noncovalently to five B subunits.

Like CT, LT causes diarrhea by stimulating the activity of a membrane-bound adenylate cyclase. This results in the conversion of ATP to cyclic AMP (cAMP) as shown below:

$$ATP \rightarrow cAMP + PPi$$

Minute amounts of cAMP induce the active secretion of Cl^- and inhibit the absorption of NaCl, creating an electrolyte imbalance across the intestinal mucosa, resulting in the loss of copious quantities of fluid and electrolytes from the intestine.

The mechanism by which LT stimulates the activity of the adenylate cyclase is as follows: (1) The B subunit of the toxin binds to a specific cell receptor, GM_1 ganglioside (see Fig. 26-7); (2) the A_1 subunit is released from the toxin and enters the cell; and (3) the A_1 subunit cleaves nicotinamide-adenine dinucleotide (NAD) into nicotinamide and ADP-ribose and, together with a cellular ADP-ribosylating factor, transfers the ADP-ribose to a GTP-binding protein. The ADP-ribosylation of the GTP-binding protein inhibits a GTPase activity of the binding protein, leading to increased stability of the catalytic complex responsible for adenylate cyclase activity. This results in an amplified activity of the cyclase and a corresponding increase in the amount of cAMP produced.

Two antigenically distinct heat-labile toxins are produced by various strains of *E coli*. LT-I is structurally and antigenically related to CT to an extent that anti-CT will neutralize LT-I. LT-II has, on rare occasions, been isolated from the feces of humans with diarrhea, but it is most frequently isolated from feces of water buffalos and cows. LT-II is biologically similar to LT-I, but it is not neutralized by either anti–LT-I or anti-CT.

LT will bind to many types of mammalian cells, and its ability to stimulate adenylate cyclase can be assayed in cell cultures (see Fig. 26-8).

A report has also shown that CT stimulated an increase in prostaglandin E (PGE), and that PGE1 and PGE2 caused a marked fluid accumulation in the ligated lumen of rabbit intestinal segments. The mechanism whereby CT induces PGE release is unknown.

HEAT-STABLE TOXIN. The heat-stable toxin STa consists of a family of small, heterogeneous polypeptides of 1500 to 2000 daltons that are not destroyed by heating at 100°C for 30 minutes. STa has no effect on the concentration of cAMP, but it does cause a marked increase in the cellular levels of cyclic GMP (cGMP). cGMP causes an inhibition of the cotransport of NaCl across the intestinal wall, suggesting that the action of STa may be primarily antiabsorptive compared with that of LT, which is both antiabsorptive and secretory.

STa stimulates guanylate cyclase only in intestinal cells, indicating that such cells possess a unique receptor for STa. The cell receptor for STa is known to be either tightly coupled to, or a part of, a particulate form of guanylate cyclase located in the brush border membranes of intestinal mucosal cells. Also, intimately associated with this complex is a cGMP–dependent protein kinase that phosphorylates a 25,000-dalton protein in the brush border. It has been proposed that this phosphorylated protein might be the actual mediator for the toxin-induced ion transport alterations that lead to fluid loss. The usual assay for STa is to inject the toxin intragastrically into a 1- to 4-day-old suckling mouse and measure intestinal fluid accumulation (as a ratio of intestinal/remaining body weight) after 4 hours. STa may also be assayed directly by measuring its effect on the increase in guanylate cyclase in homogenized intestinal epithelial cells.

A second heat-stable toxin that is produced by some strains of *E coli* has been termed STb. This toxin is inactive in suckling mice but will produce diarrhea in weaned piglets. STb producers have not been isolated from humans. It does not seem to increase the level of adenylate or guanylate cyclase in intestinal mucosal cells, but may stimulate the synthesis of prostaglandin E2. The end result is to enhance net bicarbonate ion secretion.

COLONIZATION FACTORS. Animals also are subject to infections by their own strains of ETEC, and such infections in newborn animals may result in death from the loss of fluids and electrolytes. Extensive studies of strains infecting newborn calves and piglets (as well as humans) have revealed that, in addition to producing an enterotoxin, such strains possess one of several fimbriate surface structures that specifically adhere to the epithelial cells lining the small intestine. These antigens (K-88 for swine

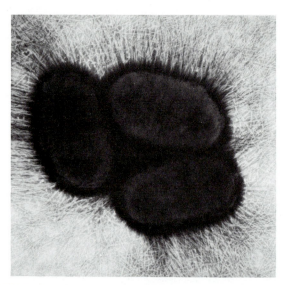

FIGURE 26-4 Cells of enterotoxigenic *Escherichia coli* isolated from a patient with diarrhea and bearing a large number of pilus-like structures, or fimbriae. (Original magnification ×8000.)

strains, and K-99 for cattle) usually are fimbriate structures that cause the toxin-producing organisms to adhere to and colonize the small intestine. The need for this colonizing ability is supported by the fact that antibodies directed against the colonizing fimbriae are protective.

Analogous human ETEC strains also possess fimbriate structures that have been designated as colonization factors (CFA) (Fig. 26-4). At least five such serologically different factors, CFA/I, CFA/II, CFA/III, E8775, and CFA/V, have been described. Interestingly, these colonization factors also are plasmid mediated, and single plasmids have been described that carry genes for both CFA/I and STa.

Interestingly, during the Gulf War in 1990, there were about 100 cases of diarrhea per week per 1000 personnel. Of these, 55% resulted from ETEC.

Enterohemorrhagic *Escherichia coli*

The enterohemorrhagic *E coli* (EHEC) were first described in 1982 when they were shown to be the etiologic agent of hemorrhagic colitis, a disease characterized by severe abdominal cramps and a copious, bloody diarrhea. These organisms are also known to cause a condition termed hemolytic-uremic syndrome (HUS), which is manifested by a hemolytic anemia, thrombocytopenia (decrease in the number of blood platelets), and acute renal failure. HUS occurs most frequently in children.

Although most initially recognized EHEC belong to serotype O157:H7, other EHEC serotypes such as 026, 0111, 0128, and 0143 have been recognized. These organisms are not invasive, but they do possess a 60-megadalton plasmid that encodes for a fimbrial antigen that adheres to intestinal epithelium. In addition, the EHEC are lysogenic for one or more bacteriophages that encode for the production of one or both of two antigenically distinct toxins. These toxins are biologically identical and antigenically similar to the toxins formed by *Shigella dysenteriae* (Shiga's bacillus), and are designated as Shiga-like toxin I (SLT-I) and Shiga-like toxin II (SLT-II). Because the Shiga-like toxins initially were characterized by their ability to kill Vero cells, a cell line developed from African green monkey kidney cells, they also are called Verotoxin I and Verotoxin II.

SLT-I consists of an A subunit and five B subunits. The sequence of the B subunit from *S dysenteriae* type 1 is identical to that of the B subunit of SLT-I. The B subunit binds specifically to a glycolipid in microvillus membranes, and the released A subunit stops protein synthesis by inactivating the 60S ribosomal subunit. This inactivation results from the *N*-glycosidase activity of the toxin, which cleaves off an adenine molecule (A-4324) from the 28S ribosomal RNA, causing a structural modification of the 60S subunit, resulting in a reduced affinity for EF-1 and, thus, an inhibition of aminoacyl-tRNA binding. The consequence of toxin action is a cessation of protein synthesis, the sloughing off of dead cells, and a bloody diarrhea. Notice that SLT-1 carries out the same reaction as the plant toxins ricin and abrin.

SLT-II is biologically similar to SLT-I, but because only a 50% to 60% homology exists between the two toxins, it is not surprising that they are antigenically distinct. Interestingly, both STL-I and STL-II can be transferred to nontoxin-producing strains of *E coli* by transduction.

Outbreaks of hemorrhagic colitis have been traced to contaminated food as well as to person-to-person transmission in nursing homes and day-care centers. Contaminated, undercooked hamburger meat seems to be the most frequently implicated source of food-borne illnesses followed by contaminated milk and water, indicating that cattle are a common reservoir for EHEC. Of note is that *E coli* O157:H7 has been shown to survive up to 9 months at −20°C in ground beef.

Thus, the EHEC are able to cause hemorrhagic colitis as a result of their ability to adhere to the intestinal mucosa, and they presumably destroy the intestinal epithelial lining through their secretion of Shiga-like toxins. The mechanism whereby the EHEC cause HUS is unclear but seems to follow bloodstream carriage of SLT-II to the kidney. Experimental results have shown that human renal endothelial cells contain high levels of receptor for SLT-2. Moreover, in the presence of interleukin (IL)-1β, the amount of receptor increases, enhancing the internalization of the toxin and the death of the cell.

The highlighted section, "A Closer Look," describes several epidemics of hemorrhagic colitis that have occurred in the United States and techniques that are used for the identification of this serotype.

Enteroinvasive *Escherichia coli*

The disease produced by the enteroinvasive *E coli* (EIEC) is indistinguishable from the dysentery produced by members of the genus *Shigella*, although the shigellae seem to be more virulent because considerably fewer shigellae are required than EIEC to cause diarrhea. The key virulence factor required by the EIEC is the ability to invade the epithelial cells.

EIEC INVASION. The specific property that provides these organisms with their invasive potential is far from understood. It is known, however, that this ability is encoded in a plasmid and that the loss of the plasmid results in a loss of invasive ability and a loss of virulence. Moreover, the shigellae seem to possess the same plasmid, because Western blots show that shigellae and EIEC plasmids express polypeptides that are similar in molecular weight and antigenicity.

EIEC TOXINS. Although the primary virulence factor of EIEC strains is the ability to invade intestinal epithelial cells, they also synthesize varying amounts of SLT-I and SLT-II. Based on the severity of the disease, however, it could assumed that the amount of toxin produced is considerably less than that formed by the highly virulent shigellae or the EHEC. Other enterotoxic products produced by the EIEC are under study.

EIEC can be distinguished from other *E coli* by their ability to cause an inflammatory conjunctivitis in guinea pigs, an assay termed a Sereny test. A DNA probe that hybridizes with colony blots of EIEC and all species of *Shigella* also has been used to identify organisms producing Shiga-like toxins.

Enteropathogenic *Escherichia coli*

The enteropathogenic *E coli* (EPEC) are diffusely adherent organisms that are particularly important in infant diarrhea occurring in developing countries, where they may cause a mortality rate as high as a 50%. They comprise a mixture of organisms that seem to produce diarrhea by a two-step process. The classic EPEC exist among a dozen or so different serotypes, all of which are characterized by the possession of a 55- to 65-megadalton plasmid that encodes for an adhesin termed EPEC adherence factor (EAF). EAF causes a localized adherence of the bacteria to enterocytes of the small bowel, resulting in distinct microcolonies. This is followed by the formation of unique pedestal-like structures bearing the adherent bacteria. These structures have been termed attaching and effacing lesions. The ability to form the effacing lesion resides in an attaching and effacing gene (*eae*). The lesions are characterized by a loss of microvilli and a rearrangement of the cytoskeleton, with a proliferation of filamentous actin beneath areas of bacterial attachment.

A Closer Look

In January 1993, the Childrens Hospital in Seattle notified the Washington State Health Department of an outbreak of hemorrhagic colitis. This epidemic eventually involved over 500 persons living in the Pacific Northwest, of whom 125 were hospitalized, 41 developed acute renal failure, and 4 died. The cause of this outbreak was quickly linked to *Escherichia coli* O157:H7, an enterohemorrhagic strain of *E coli* that was acquired by eating undercooked hamburgers obtained from a fast food chain.

Symptoms of hemorrhagic colitis are characterized by diarrhea that is frequently bloody and a kidney involvement, which is termed hemolytic uremic syndrome (HUS). HUS occurs in 3% to 7% of these infections, particularly in children younger than 5 years of age. In about 90% of cases, HUS results in renal failure that often requires dialysis; approximately 10% will require a kidney transplant, and 3% to 5% will die.

Such infections were initially described in 1982 when epidemics of *E coli* O157:H7 occurred in Oregon and Michigan. These also were attributed to the ingestion of undercooked hamburger from fast food restaurants. Another outbreak, occurring in a nursing home during 1984, resulted in 34 cases; 14 patients were hospitalized and 4 died. This also was traced to undercooked hamburger, as have a number of similar outbreaks that have been reported throughout the last decade.

Not all such epidemics, however, are traced to undercooked beef. One major outbreak involving 243 cases—32 patients were hospitalized and 4 died—was traced to a municipal water supply whose distribution system had become contaminated with sewage. Others are thought to result from person-to-person spread because, after recovery, one becomes an asymptomatic carrier for 3 weeks to 2 months.

The primary reservoir of *E coli* O157:H7 is the intestinal tract of animals, particularly cattle, where it may exist completely asymptomatically. Thus, it is not surprising that outbreaks of this infection have been traced to unpasteurized milk and undercooked beef that had been contaminated in the slaughter house. If such contaminated beef is cooked in a single piece (steaks or roasts), it probably can be safely eaten rare because contamination by *E coli* is limited to the surface of the meat. After grinding to make hamburger, however, any contaminating organisms are spread throughout the meat, and cooking to 68°C (155°F) is the only safe procedure to avoid ingesting viable organisms.

There is considerable pressure for meat inspectors to sample all beef at the slaughter houses to detect contamination with *E coli* O157:H7. This is accomplished by growing a sample on sorbitol-MacConkey agar plates. Because *E coli* O157:H7 usually does not ferment sorbitol, colonies not producing acid can be selected for a serologic determination of O or H antigens. A single nonsorbitol-fermenting colony can be mixed with commercially available latex beads to which anti-O157 antibodies have been absorbed. There is also a polymerase chain reaction (PCR) available to test for the genes encoding Shiga-like toxins I and II.

All in all, it seems to require an incredible amount of work to ensure that rare hamburger is safe to eat. An alternative might be to subject all beef to sufficient γ-irradiation to eliminate all contaminating organisms.

Thus, the ability of the EPEC to cause diarrhea involves two distinct genes, EAF and *eae*. The end result is an elevated intracellular Ca^{2+} level in the intestinal epithelial cells and the initiation of signal transduction, leading to protein tyrosine phosphorylation of at least two eucaryotic proteins.

EPEC strains routinely have been considered noninvasive, but data have indicated that such strains can invade epithelial cells in culture. However, EPEC strains do not typically cause a bloody diarrhea, and the significance of cell invasion during infection remains uncertain.

Other Diarrhea-Producing *Escherichia coli*

All possible combinations, deletions, or additions of the various virulence factors responsible for intestinal fluid loss result in diarrhea-producing strains that do not fit the categories already described. Such has been found to be the case.

The most recent of these has been termed the enteroaggregative *E coli*. These strains seem to cause diarrhea through their ability to adhere to the intestinal mucosa and possibly by yet a new type of enterotoxin. It seems possible that the acquisition of other virulence factors may result in the discovery of additional pathogenic strains of *E coli*.

E coli Urinary Tract Infections

Escherichia coli is the most common cause of urinary tract infections of the bladder (cystitis) and, less frequently, of the kidney (pyelonephritis). In either case, infections usually are of an ascending type (enter the bladder from the urethra and enter the kidneys from the bladder). Many infections occur in young female patients, in persons with urinary tract obstructions, and in persons requiring urinary catheters, and they occur frequently in otherwise healthy women. Interestingly, good data support the postulation that certain serotypes of *E coli* are more likely to cause pyelonephritis than others. Thus, the ability to produce P-fimbriae (so called because of their ability to bind to P blood group antigen) has been correlated with the ability to produce urinary tract infections, seemingly by mediating the adherence of the organisms to human uroepithelial cells. Of note is that the rate of nosocomial urinary tract infection per person-day was significantly greater in patients with diarrhea, particularly in those with an indwelling urinary catheter.

In addition to fimbrial adhesins, a series of afimbrial adhesins has been reported. Their role in disease is not yet firmly established, but it has been demonstrated that at least one afimbrial adhesins mediated specific binding to uroepithelial cells.

Recurrent urinary tract infections in premenopausal, sexually active women frequently can be prevented by the postcoital administration of a single tablet of an antibacterial agent such as trimethoprim-sulfamethoxazole, cinoxacin, or cephalexin.

E coli Systemic Infections

About 300,000 patients in United States hospitals develop gram-negative bacteremia annually, and about 100,000 of these persons die of septic shock. As might be guessed, *E coli* is the most common organism involved in such infections. The ultimate cause of death in these cases is an endotoxin-induced synthesis and release of tumor necrosis factor-α and IL-1, resulting in irreversible shock (see Endotoxins, Chap. 16).

The newborn is particularly susceptible to meningitis, especially during the first month of life. A survey of 132 cases of neonatal meningitis occurring in the Netherlands reported that 47% resulted from *E coli* and 24% from group B streptococci. Notice that almost 90% of all cases of *E coli* meningitis are caused by the K1 strain, which possesses a capsule identical to that occurring on group B meningococci.

Table 26-2 summarizes the virulence factors associated with pathogenic *E coli*.

KLEBSIELLA PNEUMONIAE

Klebsiella pneumoniae can be isolated from the respiratory or intestinal tracts of about 5% of healthy individuals. The organism is nonmotile and can be subdivided into at least 77 types based on the antigenic difference in its capsule. *K pneumoniae* (types 1 and 2) may cause a severe and destructive bacterial pneumonia, but klebsiellae, in gen-

TABLE 26-2
Escherichia coli **Virulence Factors**

Diarrhea-producing E coli	
Enterotoxigenic *E coli*	Heat-labile toxin (LT)
	Heat-stable toxin (ST)
	Colonization factors (fimbriae)
Enterohemorrhagic *E coli*	Shiga-like toxin (SLT-I)
	Shiga-like toxin II (SLT-II)
	Colonization factors (fimbriae)
Enteroinvasive *E coli*	Shiga-like toxin I (SLT-I)
	Shiga-like toxin II (SLT-II)
	Ability to invade epithelial cells
Enteropathogenic *E coli*	Adhesin factor for epithelial cells
Urinary trace infections	P-fimbriae
Meningitis	K-1 capsule

eral, more frequently are involved in hospital-acquired urinary tract infections, burn wound infections, or as secondary invaders in other respiratory infections. In fact, the *Klebsiella* organism is the most frequently encountered gram-negative pathogen causing nosocomial infections of the lower respiratory tract and is second only to *E coli* as a cause of primary bacteremia by gram-negative organisms. Immunization of human volunteers with purified capsular material seems to provide protection, but because this protection is serotype specific, its use may be of minimal value unless it can be established that only a few of the 77 serotypes are involved in nosocomial bacterial infections. It is also not surprising that there have been some reports linking this genus to epidemics of diarrhea, because some strains of *Klebsiella* seem to have acquired the plasmids from *E coli* that code for the heat-labile or heat-stable enterotoxins. Another important virulence factor of *K pneumoniae* is the production of aerobactin, a siderophore that can obtain iron from transferrin.

ENTEROBACTER

The bacteria in the genus *Enterobacter* can be differentiated from those in *Klebsiella* by the fact that they are motile. They occur as normal flora of the intestinal tract but also are found on plant material as free-living organisms. *Enterobacter* is rarely a primary pathogen except in hospital-acquired urinary tract infections.

SERRATIA

The genus *Serratia* was, in the past, considered to be totally innocuous, and because many strains synthesize a bright red pigment, the organisms were used to demonstrate bacteremia after dental extraction or the spread of organisms through a room by shaking hands. However,

Serratia organisms are known to cause serious hospital-acquired infections, particularly in the newborn, the debilitated, or the patient receiving immunosuppressive drugs, and these organisms must be considered as opportunistic pathogens.

HAFNIA

Some taxonomists believe that all organisms in the *Hafnia* genus should be included as a species of *Enterobacter,* particularly because the distribution and disease potential of their 197 serotypes are essentially identical to those of *Enterobacter.*

EDWARDSIELLA AND CITROBACTER

Edwardsiella is a newly established genus of motile, H_2S-producing, nonlactose-fermenting enterics. They are occasionally isolated from the stools of humans with diarrhea, but they are also found in healthy humans. Metabolically, they are similar to *Salmonella.*

Citrobacter is a genus of the Enterobacteriaceae that contains citrate-using bacteria; they may be either slow or fast lactose fermenters. They seem to be antigenically similar to the *Salmonella* but usually are involved as opportunistic pathogens in compromised hosts. A survey of *Citrobacter* infections at a large veterans hospital showed that these organisms could be isolated from urinary tract infections, superficial wound infections, osteomyelitis, and cases of gastroenteritis. Heat-stable toxin, heat-labile toxin, and SLT-II have been reported to occur in strains of *C freundii* isolated from cases of diarrheal disease, but none of them seem to be widespread in this genus. Also, a number of cases of neonatal meningitis has been ascribed to species of *Citrobacter.* In most cases, however, isolates were obtained from elderly and debilitated patients who had acquired them during their hospital stays.

PROTEUS, PROVIDENCIA, AND MORGANELLA

The *Proteus, Providenica,* and *Morganella* genera consist of motile, nonlactose fermenters that possess the ability to deaminate phenylalanine to phenylpyruvic acid.

Proteus is distinguished from *Providencia* by its capacity to hydrolyze urea to CO_2 and NH_3. Also, because the previous species *Proteus morganii* had a G + C ratio that was considerably higher than that of the other members of the genus *Proteus,* it has been placed in a new genus named *Morganella.* As can be seen, the taxonomy of this group still is in a fluid state.

In general, bacteria in these genera are noted for their rapid motility, which may result in their "swarming" over an agar plate rather than forming distinct colonies. Some strains of *Proteus,* designated OXK, OX2, and OX19, have antigens in common with some of the pathogenic

rickettsia; therefore, the presence of antibodies to these strains of *Proteus* is used as a diagnostic aid for the diseases caused by certain rickettsia (see Chap. 34).

Proteus is found in feces, sewage, and soil. Its species elicit a number of opportunistic infections and probably rank close to *E coli* as a cause of urinary tract infections. *Proteus mirabilis* is the most frequent agent of *Proteus* bacteremia, perhaps because it produces an adhesin that binds to uroepithelial cells. *Providencia* and *Morganella* most often are found to be the cause of nosocomial urinary tract infections, but they also cause sepsis, pneumonia, and wound infections.

TREATMENT AND CONTROL OF THE NORMAL FLORA ENTERICS

Because of the many recombinations and transductions that occur among the members of the Enterobacteriaceae, susceptibility to any specific antibiotic will vary from strain to strain. In general, ampicillin has been effective for the treatment of many of the infections mentioned above. However, kanamycin, gentamicin, chloramphenicol, cephalothin, polymyxin, and streptomycin also are used in situations in which the organisms are resistant to ampicillin.

Because many of these organisms found as "normal flora" are opportunists, control measures are directed more toward the prevention of nosocomial infections in the individual who is most susceptible to infection.

The brief descriptions of these enterics indicate that all can initiate disease under certain circumstances and that these circumstances occur most frequently in hospitalized patients whose specific and nonspecific immune systems are no longer fully functional. Most persons will probably go through a large portion (if not all) of their lives without experiencing an infection caused by these organisms. The following two genera of the Enterobacteriaceae, *Salmonella* and *Shigella,* cannot, however, be considered normal flora at any time.

SHIGELLA

Members of the genus *Shigella* are pathogens that cause a serious disease known as bacillary dysentery. The genus is divided into four species, and, as shown in Table 26-3, each species may be additionally divided into serotypes. Because all *Shigella* are nonmotile, H antigens are not involved in their serologic classification. *Shigella sonnei* is a slow lactose fermenter, but no other species of *Shigella* can ferment lactose. *Shigella* organisms are unable to form H_2S.

Shigellae are serologically related to *E coli,* probably because of the intergeneric conjugation resulting in considerable genetic mixing. Both carry out a mixed-acid fermentation of glucose, but the *Shigella* do not metabolize the formic acid produced and, hence, do not form gas.

TABLE 26-3
Classification of *Shigella*

Species	No. of Serotypes
Shigella dysenteriae	10
Shigella flexneri	8
Shigella boydii	15
Shigella sonnei	1

Epidemiology and Pathogenesis of Shigellosis

Humans seem to be the only natural hosts for the shigellae, becoming infected after the ingestion of contaminated food or water. Unlike *Salmonella*, the shigellae remain localized in the intestinal epithelial cells, and the debilitating effects of shigellosis are mostly attributed to the loss of fluids, electrolytes, and nutrients and to the ulceration that occurs in the colon wall.

It has been known for many years that *Shigella dysenteriae* type 1 secreted one or more exotoxins (called Shiga toxins), which would cause death when injected into experimental animals and fluid accumulation when placed in ligated segments of rabbit ileum. These toxins are essentially identical to the Shiga-like toxins produced by the EIEC and the EHEC. Thus, Shiga toxin consists of one A subunit and five B subunits and seems to kill an intestinal epithelial cell by inactivating the 60S ribosomal subunit, halting all protein synthesis. Moreover, although all virulent species of *Shigella* produce Shiga toxins, there seems to be a wide variation in the amount of toxin formed.

The mechanism whereby Shiga toxin causes fluid secretion is thought to occur by blocking fluid absorption in the intestine. In this model, Shiga toxin kills absorptive epithelial cells, and the diarrhea results from an inhibition of absorption rather than from active secretion.

Of note is that, like the EHEC, *Shigella* species can cause HUS. Moreover, Shiga-like toxins have been detected in certain strains of *Vibrio cholerae* and *Vibrio parahaemolyticus* that were associated with HUS, indicating an important role of Shiga toxin in this malady. There has also been a report indicating that tumor necrosis factor-α acts synergistically with Shiga toxin to induce HUS.

To cause intestinal disease, shigellae must invade the epithelial cells lining of the intestine. After escaping from the phagocytic vacuole, they multiply within the epithelial cells in a manner similar to that described for EIEC strains. Thus, *Shigella* virulence requires that the organisms invade epithelial cells, multiply intracellularly, and spread from cell to cell by way of finger-like projections to expand the focus of infection, leading to ulceration and destruction of the epithelial layer of the colon. Interestingly, for *Shigella* to be fully invasive, both plasmid and chromo-

somally encoded products seem to be required. The invasion plasmid is identical for the *Shigella* and the EIEC and contains at least four genes, *IpaA*, *IpaB*, *IpaC*, and *IpaD* that encode for a series of proteins termed invasion-plasmid antigens, which are involved in the virulence of these organisms. Interestingly, *IpaB* acts both as an invasin that triggers phagocytosis of the bacterium and as a cytolysin that allows escape from the phagocytic vacuole. The elaboration of toxic products causes a severe local inflammatory response involving both polymorphonuclear leukocytes and macrophages, resulting in a bloody, mucopurulent diarrhea.

During 1990, over 27,000 cases of shigellosis were reported to the Centers for Disease Control (CDC) and, of these, the most prevalent species in the United States was *S sonnei*. The disease produced by this species is transmitted by a fecal–oral route, and most of patients are preschool-age children, particularly those in day-care centers.

Laboratory Diagnosis of Shigellosis

Isolation and identification of the etiologic agent are necessary for a definitive diagnosis of shigellosis. The organisms are not particularly hearty, and best results are obtained when a direct swab of the ulcerative lesions is streaked out on selective media, such as MacConkey or eosin methylene blue plates.

Shigellae and EIEC also have been detected using a polymerase chain reaction to amplify genes on the invasion plasmid. Using the polymerase chain reaction (PCR), shigellae sequences were detected in some cases after treatment with ciprofloxacin when it was no longer possible to isolate viable organisms.

Treatment and Control of Shigellosis

Intravenous replacement of fluids and electrolytes plus antibiotic therapy are used for severe cases of shigellosis. Ampicillin frequently is not effective, and alternative therapies include sulfamethoxazole/trimethoprim and, with increasing sulfamethoxazole/trimethoprim resistance, the quinolone antibiotics such as nalidixic acid and ciprofloxacin. In the Far East, India, and Brazil where shigellosis is more common than in the United States, multiple antibiotic resistance because of the acquisition of plasmids has become common (see Chap. 20). Shigellosis also is common in Latin America.

Efforts to control the disease usually are directed toward sanitary measures designed to prevent the spread of organisms. This is particularly difficult in view of the fact that many persons remain asymptomatic carriers after recovery from an overt infection. Such individuals provide a major reservoir for the spread of the shigellae.

The injection of killed vaccines is worthless, because humoral IgG does not seem to be involved in immunity to the localized intestinal infection. Live vaccines that cannot grow in the absence of streptomycin (ie, streptomycin-dependent vaccines) have been developed and used in clinical trials, but success has been equivocal. It seems that the organisms must invade and colonize the intestine to induce a local immunity. An engineered vaccine designed to induce this type of immunity used an avirulent *E coli* K12 into which was transferred a 140-megadalton plasmid obtained from a virulent strain of *Shigella flexneri*. The transfected plasmid endowed the *E coli* K12 strain with the ability to invade intestinal epithelial cells, and its use as an oral vaccine in monkeys conferred significant protection against oral challenge with virulent *S flexneri*. Acquired immunity seems to result from both a cell-mediated immune response and an IgA antibody production.

Interestingly, human milk contains a globotriaosylceramide that binds to Shiga and Shiga-like toxins. This suggests that human milk could contribute to a protective effect by preventing these toxins from binding to their intestinal target receptors.

SALMONELLA

The term *salmonellosis* may be used to describe any infection caused by members of the genus *Salmonella*. This is an extremely large group of gram-negative rods that can be distinguished from the normal flora of the intestine using biochemical and antigenic criteria.

The Kauffman-White scheme is a complex antigen classification system, in which each *Salmonella* is assigned to a group based on the O antigens present in its cell-wall LPS. Thus, each organism possessing O antigen 2 is placed into group A, all those possessing O antigen 4 are in group B, and so on; groups are lettered A to Z, and then the remaining groups are numbered. Table 26-4 lists a few examples of some of the more frequent human pathogens, showing their group placement and O-antigen designation. As can be seen from this table, the group designation is based on the presence of one dominant antigen, even though other O antigens are present in the organism. Also, notice the subgroups that depend on the overall complement of O antigens possessed by a species.

The salmonellae in any one group can be further divided into serotypes on the basis of the H antigens that occur in both phase 1 and phase 2. Also, some salmonellae form a polysaccharide antigen on the outer surface of the cell that covers up the O-antigen layer of the organism. Because this antigen has been found most frequently in isolated virulent organisms, it is called the Vi antigen, indicating virulence. Because the Vi antigen surrounds the O antigen, organisms possessing a Vi antigen will not

TABLE 26-4
Kauffman-White Classification of Selected *Salmonellae*

Species or Serotype	O Antigens*	H Antigens Phase 1	Phase 2
Group A			
S paratyphi	1, **2**, 12	a	—
Group B			
S schottmuelleri	1, **4**, 12	b	1, 2
Group C₁			
S choleraesuis	**6**, 7	c	1, 5
S montevideo	**6**, 7	g, m, s	—
Group C₂			
S manhattan	**6**, 8	d	1, 5
Group D₁			
S typhi	**9**, 12, (Vi)	d	—
S panama	1, **9**, 12	l, v	1, 5
Group D₂			
S strasbourg	**9**, 46	d	1, 7
Group E₁			
S anatum	**3**, 10	e, h	1, 6
Group E₂			
S new-brunswick	**3**, 15	l, v	1, 7
Group E₃			
S minneapolis	**3**, 15, 34	e. h	1, 6
Group H			
S florida	1, 6, **14**, 15	d	1, 7

* O antigen in bold type is common to all members of the group.

agglutinate in specific O antiserum unless the Vi antigen is first destroyed by placing the bacteria in a boiling water bath.

Salmonellae do not ferment lactose, but most form H_2S and gases from carbohydrates and will decarboxylate lysine. *Salmonella typhi,* the cause of typhoid fever, is an exception in that it produces little H_2S or gas from carbohydrate fermentation. *Salmonella arizonae,* which consists of more than 300 serotypes, is a second exception in that these organisms are slow lactose fermenters. Many taxonomists prefer to place this group of organisms into a separate genus called *Arizona.*

Originally, the salmonellae were given species' names that were descriptive of the disease they caused, the animal they customarily infected, or in honor of the individual who originally isolated a particular species. Later, as more antigenic types were described, a system of nomenclature was used that named each new antigenic type according to the geographic area where it was isolated. So, there are names such as *S typhi, Salmonella choleraesuis, Salmonella minneapolis,* and *S arizonae.* Clinical practice, however, tends to use only three species of *Salmonella:* (1) *S typhi,* (2) *S choleraesuis* and (3) *Salmonella enteritidis.* More than 1700 additional antigenic types are listed as serotypes of *S enteritidis,* such as *S enteritidis* serotype alabama or *S enteritidis* serotype miami.

The most recent taxonomic scheme for the *Salmonella* genus divides these organisms into five subgroups based on DNA hybridization studies. However, because the CDC, as well as essentially all clinical laboratories, use the older designations, that terminology is used in this text.

Epidemiology and Pathogenesis of Salmonellosis

The primary reservoir for the salmonellae is the intestinal tracts of many animals, including birds, farm animals, and reptiles. Humans become infected through the ingestion of contaminated water or food. Water, of course, becomes polluted by the introduction of feces from any animal excreting salmonellae. Infection by food usually results either from the ingestion of contaminated meat or by way of the hands, which act as intermediates in the transfer of salmonellae from an infected source. Thus, the handling of an infected—although apparently healthy—dog or cat can result in contamination with salmonellae. Another major source of *Salmonella* infections has been pet turtles. In the early 1970s, almost 300,000 cases of turtle-associated salmonellosis were estimated to occur annually in the United States and, as a result, it is illegal to import turtles or turtle eggs or even to ship domestic turtles with shells less than 4 inches in diameter across state lines.

In the United States, poultry and eggs increasingly comprise the most common source of salmonellae for humans. This occurs because a large percentage of chickens routinely are infected with salmonellae. Thus, humans

can acquire these organisms through direct contact with uncooked chicken or by the ingestion of undercooked chicken. And, because the organisms may occur both on the outer shell and in the yolk and egg white, consuming anything containing raw eggs (caesar salad, hollandaise sauce, mayonnaise, homemade ice cream) could result in a *Salmonella* infection. The CDC even cautions against eating eggs sunny-side up and recommends that eggs be boiled for 6 to 7 minutes before being served.

On an industrial scale, slaughterhouse workers are faced with salmonellosis as an occupational hazard, primarily from poultry and pigs. Because humans can become asymptomatic carriers of *Salmonella,* infected food handlers also are responsible for the spread of these organisms.

Virulence Factors of *Salmonella* Organisms

It is surprising that virulence factors for organisms that have caused so much disease still are largely unknown. However, the ability to invade and grow inside of nonphagocytic cells undoubtedly comprises the major virulence determinant of the *Salmonella* because this intracellular location provides a compartment where they can replicate and avoid host defenses. The mechanism whereby these bacteria accomplish this invasion is complex and only beginning to unfold.

Using various mutants of *Salmonella typhimurium,* John Pace and colleagues at the State University of New York determined that invasion of a host cell occurs in two separable steps: (1) adhesion to the host cell, and (2) invasion of the host cell. Furthermore, they found that invasion required that the organisms activate a growth factor receptor on the host cell known as epidermal growth factor receptor (EGFR). Mutants that could adhere, but not invade, were unable to activate EGFR. However, if EGF was added to the host cell–bacterium mixture, the EGFR was activated and the noninvasive mutant was internalized.

When EGFR is activated, a signal transduction process occurs, which results in at least two major events: (1) a rapid rise in the internal Ca^{2+} level occurs, and (2) enzymes are activated that lead to the synthesis of leukotriene D_4 (LTD_4). It is unclear how these events trigger the entry of *Salmonella* into the cell, but it is known that the Ca^{2+} level increase is essential because the addition of Ca^{2+} chelators blocked entry of the bacterium into the cell. It is also known that the addition of LTD_4 to cultured cells causes an increase in intracellular Ca^{2+} levels, permitting the internalization of an invasion-deficient mutant.

One can postulate, therefore, that the mediation of Ca^{2+} influx by LTD_4 results in the opening of a Ca^{2+} channel, which, in turn, causes a reorganization of the host cell cytoskeleton, permitting entry of the bacterium.

It is also of note that the inflammatory diarrhea produced by the *Salmonella* may result from its ability to induce leukotriene synthesis because leukotrienes are well-known mediators of inflammation.

It is also known that a number of *Salmonella* serotypes carry plasmids that greatly increase virulence in experimentally infected mice. Although many of these plasmids are distinct, all have a highly conserved 8-kb region that has been named the *spv* regulon. Interestingly, *spv* genes are not expressed during logarithmic growth in vitro but seem to enhance the growth of salmonellae within host cells. In experimentally infected mice, the expression of *spv* by intracellular salmonellae in vivo has been postulated to lead to an increased rate of bacterial growth, resulting in early bacteremia and death before the infected mice can develop immunity.

The general types of infections that may be caused by the salmonellae usually are grouped into three categories: enterocolitis, enteric fevers, and septicemia.

Enterocolitis (Gastroenteritis)

Salmonella enterocolitis is one of the most frequent cause of food-borne outbreaks of gastroenteritis in the United States. It may be caused by any one of the hundreds of serotypes of *Salmonella,* and it is characterized by the fact that organisms do not cause an appreciable bacteremia. The hallmark of all *Salmonella* infections lies in the ability of the *Salmonella* to invade the intestinal epithelial cells, which are normally nonphagocytic. Those species involved in gastroenteritis may reach the bloodstream early in the disease but are rapidly taken up and killed by phagocytic cells. In general, bacteremia occurs only in persons having an impaired phagocyte system, AIDS, or chronic granulomatous disease. In the average case, symptoms of diarrhea may occur 10 to 28 hours after ingesting contaminated food, and the headache, abdominal pain, nausea, vomiting, and diarrhea may continue for 2 to 7 days.

A search for salmonella toxins has not been as conclusive as one might wish, but there are multiple reports that many *Salmonella* species secrete a cholera-like enterotoxin that induces increased levels of cAMP, and that some strains produce a heat-stable enterotoxin. In addition, a cytotoxin that inhibits protein synthesis in intestinal epithelial cells has been described. This toxin, characterized by its ability to kill Vero cells, is immunologically distinct from both Shiga toxin and the Shiga-like toxins produced by strains of *E coli* and *Shigella*. The observation that those species of *Salmonella* causing the more severe enteric symptoms and inflammatory diarrhea also produce the highest levels of cytotoxin suggests that this toxin may be of paramount importance in the pathologic manifestations of gastrointestinal salmonellosis. Neither the molecular structure, its specific mechanisms of blocking protein synthesis and causing cell death, nor the number of such *Salmonella* cytotoxins is known.

Most cases of *Salmonella* enterocolitis formerly had not been treated with antibiotics because such treatment did not seem to shorten the duration of the infection. There have been reports, however, that the fluoroquinolones do decrease the period of illness but, interestingly, they do not eradicate the organisms from the intestinal tract.

Enteric Fevers

There are about 400 to 500 cases of typhoid fever each year in the United States (as contrasted to about 500,000 cases of typhoid fever reported in the United States in 1909). This disease, caused by *S typhi,* is the classic enteric fever. After an incubation period of 1 to 3 weeks after ingestion of the organisms, inflammation occurs in the small intestine followed by invasion of the regional lymph nodes. From the lymphatic system, the organisms enter the blood and infect various organs and tissues, including the liver, kidneys, spleen, bone marrow, gall bladder, and sometimes the heart. Reinvasion of the Peyer's patches in the intestinal mucosa may cause a severe inflammation characterized by bleeding. Enlargement of the spleen is characteristic, and multiplication of the organisms in the skin may result in the presence of rose spots, particularly on the abdomen. Symptoms also may include headache, loss of appetite, abdominal pain, weakness, stupor, and a continued fever. *S typhi* possesses the unusual ability to grow intracellularly in monocytes by virtue of the fact that it is able to prevent the phagosome–lysosome fusion. While the phagocyte fills with organisms, it lyses, releasing the *Salmonella* to be taken up again by the macrophages.

Other species of *Salmonella* also cause enteric fevers, but usually these *paratyphoid* fevers are milder than those caused by *S typhi.*

LABORATORY DIAGNOSIS OF TYPHOID FEVER. The organisms can be isolated from the blood during the first 2 weeks of the illness and from the urine, usually between the first and fourth week. Stool specimens may remain positive for indefinite periods of time. Preincubation in selenite or tetrathionate broth is occasionally used to enrich the growth of the *Salmonella* over the coliforms before streaking the organisms on various selective and differential media.

A DNA probe is available that recognizes the DNA coding for the production of Vi capsular antigen. This probe, which is said to be highly specific and sensitive, makes possible a rapid identification of *S typhi* from isolated colonies.

In addition, a retrospective diagnosis can be made by demonstrating a rise in agglutinating antibodies to *S typhi*. To be valid, this test (known as the Widal test) must show at least a fourfold increase in titer between the acute and the convalescent phase serum. Negative results on the Widal test are not, however, conclusive because, in untreated cases, only about 50% of patients recovering from typhoid fever showed a fourfold increase in agglutinating antibodies.

TREATMENT AND CONTROL OF TYPHOID FEVER. Chloramphenicol is the major antibiotic effective against *S typhi*. It causes a reduction in the febrile period but, because many organisms grow intracellularly in monocytes, the administration of chloramphenicol must be continued for at least 2 weeks to avoid recurrent febrile attacks. However, aplastic anemia (inability to make red blood cells because of a defect in the stem cells) can result from the use of this antibiotic, and many physicians are reluctant to prescribe it unless it is absolutely necessary. Ampicillin or trimethoprim-sulfamethoxazole also may be effective, but results may not be as dramatic as those seen with chloramphenicol. In addition, the new 4-fluoroquinolones and third-generation cephalosporins seem to be effective and are used for strains that have become increasingly resistant to ampicillin, chloramphenicol, and trimethoprim-sulfamethoxazole.

Because humans are the only reservoir of *S typhi*, proper sewage disposal and the periodic examination of food handlers to ascertain that they are not carriers remain the best methods of control of typhoid fever. Between 1% and 5% of persons recovering from typhoid fever become asymptomatic carriers. The most famous carrier was a Swiss immigrant to the United States in 1868 who took the name of Mary Mallon. This woman, who later became known as Typhoid Mary, served as a cook and domestic primarily in the New York area. It is estimated that either directly or indirectly, she was responsible for dozens of cases of typhoid fever. In 1989, there was an outbreak in New York that involved about 70 cases of typhoid fever. This outbreak occurred in persons having breakfast in a local hotel and was traced to orange juice that presumably was contaminated by an asymptomatic food handler. The number of typhoid carriers is thought to be about 2000 in the United States, but in Latin America or South America, carriers may comprise 1% to 10% of the population, depending on the area. High doses of ampicillin or amoxicillin, as well as sulfamethoxazole/trimethoprim with or without rifampin, have been used to treat carriers, but such treatments have been successful in curing only slightly more than half of the typhoid carriers. Ciprofloxacin or norfloxacin have been used with much greater success.

Active immunization against *S typhi* has been carried out for years, using a killed vaccine containing *S typhi* and two additional paratyphoid organisms; but, the procedure is only moderately effective, and it is not used routinely in the United States. However, because immunity to typhoid fever seems to be primarily cell mediated, a living vaccine would be expected to be more effective than killed vaccines. To this end, a living, avirulent, galactose epimerase–negative, Vi antigen–negative mutant of *S typhi* (strain Ty 21a) has been approved for use in the United States by the Food and Drug Administration. This vaccine, given orally on 3 successive days, confers approximately 95% protection against typhoid fever. Another experimental vaccine that has proved to be effective in animal studies consists of a galactose epimerase–negative *S typhi* containing a recombinant plasmid that encodes only the B subunit of LT. When given orally to animals, a good antibody response to both *S typhi* and the B subunit of LT was obtained. In still another vaccine trial in Nepal, a single immunization with 25 μg of purified Vi antigen was reported to give a 75% protection against typhoid fever.

Salmonella Septicemia

Septicemia caused by *Salmonella* is a fulminating blood infection that does not involve the gastrointestinal tract. Most cases are caused by *S choleraesuis* and are characterized by suppurative lesions throughout the body. Pneumonia, osteomyelitis, or meningitis may result from such an infection. *Salmonella* osteomyelitis is especially prevalent in persons who have sickle cell anemia, and focal infections, particularly on vascular prosthesis, also are common.

VIBRIONACEAE

Vibrio cholerae

Vibrio cholerae is a small, curved (comma-shaped) gram-negative organism possessing a single polar flagellum (Fig. 26-5). The organisms have many similarities to the members of the Enterobacteriaceae but can be readily differentiated by their positive oxidase reaction and their ability to grow at a pH between 9 and 9.5.

A number of serologic types of *V cholerae* have been reported, based on differences in their O antigens. Those causing the classic epidemic cholera traditionally have belonged in the 01 serogroup, and it has been generally believed that only the 01 serogroup was associated with cholera outbreaks. In 1993, however, a newly identified strain of *V cholera*, designated as serogroup 0139, was shown to cause a major epidemic of cholera in India

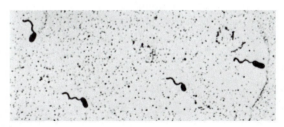

FIGURE 26-5 *Vibrio cholerae*, Leifson flagellar stain. (Original magnification ×1000.)

involving thousands of cases and hundreds of cholera-related deaths; other serologically distinct vibrios frequently have been referred to as non-01 *V cholerae*, but it may be necessary to call them non-01, non-0139 strains. In addition, some 01 strains produce a soluble hemolysin, and they have been designated as the El Tor biotype of *V cholerae*. Within these two biotypes, three serotypes have been given specific names: Inaba, Ogawa, and Hikojima. Other vibrios, however, that are either serologically unrelated or share partial antigenicity with the above strains also may cause serious diarrheal disease.

EPIDEMIOLOGY AND PATHOGENESIS OF CHOLERA

Cholera is undoubtedly the most dramatic of the waterborne diseases. As far as is known, cholera was confined to India for the almost 2000 years between its first description by Hindu physicians in 400 B.C. and its spread to Arabia, Persia, Turkey, and Southern Russia in the early 1800s. There were six major pandemics of cholera during the 1800s covering the entire world, killing millions wherever it struck. During one such outbreak in London during 1849, the famous physician, John Snow, traced the spread of the disease to a Broad Street pump from which area residents obtained their water. The spread of cholera in this area was stopped when Snow recommended that the handle of the pump be removed. This is particularly remarkable when one remembers that the germ-theory of disease had not yet been formulated.

Cholera is spread as a fecal–oral disease, and people acquire the infection by the ingestion of fecally contaminated water and food. The organisms do not spread beyond the gastrointestinal tract, where they multiply to high concentrations in the small and large intestines. Unlike the shigellas, they do not penetrate the epithelial layer but remain adhered to the intestinal mucosa (Fig. 26-6).

The major symptom of cholera is a severe diarrhea in which a patient may lose as much as 10 to 20 L or more of liquid per day. The feces contain mucus, epithelial cells, and large numbers of vibrios and have been referred to as *rice-water stools*. Death, which may occur in as many as 60% of untreated patients, results from severe dehydration and loss of electrolytes.

V cholerae produces diarrhea as a result of the secretion of an enterotoxin, choleratoxin, which acts identically to *E coli* LT to stimulate the activity of the enzyme adenyl cyclase. This, in turn, converts ATP to cAMP, which stimulates the secretion of Cl^- and inhibits the absorption of NaCl. The copious fluid that is lost also contains large amounts of bicarbonate and K^+. Thus, the patient has both a severe fluid loss and an electrolyte imbalance.

The enterotoxin has been shown to bind specifically to a membrane ganglioside designated GM_1 (Fig. 26-7). Interestingly, *V cholerae* produces a neuraminidase that is unable to remove the *N*-acetylneuraminic acid from GM_1, but it is able to convert other gangliosides to GM_1, thus synthesizing even more receptor sites to which its enterotoxin can bind. Like the LT of *E coli*, choleragen is composed of five B subunits that react with the cell receptor, an A_1-active subunit that enters the cell and, together with a cellular ADP-ribosylating factor, carries out the ADP-ribosylation of the GTP-binding protein, and a small A_2 subunit that seems to link the A_1 subunit to the B subunit. Interestingly, unlike LT, the DNA encoding choleragen is not plasmid mediated but is on the chromosome of *V cholerae*.

CT (as well as the LT produced by *E coli*) can be quantitated by a number of in vivo, cell culture, or immunologic assay units. In one method, a segment of rabbit small intestine is tied to form a loop. Enterotoxin is serially diluted, and an aliquot of each dilution is injected into a loop. The highest dilution that stimulates fluid accumula-

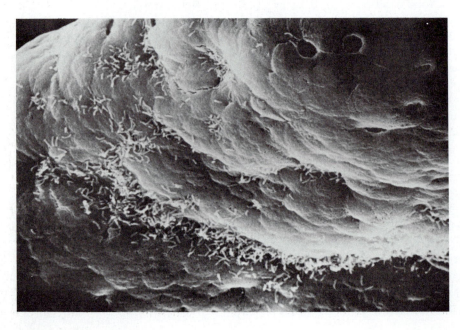

FIGURE 26-6 Numerous cells of *Vibrio cholerae* attached to rabbit intestinal villus. (Original magnification ×1400.)

$$\left(\text{Cer} \longrightarrow 1 \text{ gluc } 4 \xrightarrow{\ \beta\ } \underset{\underset{\underset{2 \text{ NANA}}{\uparrow \alpha}}{3}}{1 \text{ gal } 4} \xrightarrow{\ \beta\ } 1 \text{ gal NAc } 3 \xrightarrow{\ \beta\ } 1 \text{ gal} \right)$$

FIGURE 26-7 Repeating sequence of the ganglioside GM$_1$. Although other gangliosides also bind cholera toxin in varying amounts, GM$_1$ is at least 35-fold more efficient than the next best. Cer, ceramide; gluc, glucose; gal, galactose; NANA, *N*-acetylneuraminic acid; galNAc, *N*-acetylgalactosamine.

tion in the loop is recorded as the titer of the enterotoxin. A second method takes advantage of the fact that cAMP causes a morphologic response in cultured Chinese hamster ovary cells, and that enterotoxin will induce such cells to produce cAMP. Figure 26-8 illustrates the changes induced by a toxigenic strain of *E coli*. To quantitate enterotoxin using this assay, a standard curve is established (with purified enterotoxin) that can be used subsequently to assay an unknown enterotoxin from *E coli* or *V cholerae* (Fig. 26-9).

As is true with essentially all diarrhea-producing bacteria, *V cholerae* must specifically colonize the intestinal epithelial cells to produce disease. In this case, however, the pili binding the bacteria to the host cells seem to be under the same regulator as choleragen production and, as a result, are termed toxin-coregulated pili. Mutants unable to bind to intestinal cells are avirulent in spite of their ability to produce choleragen. Moreover, antibody directed to toxin-coregulated pili are protective.

Remember that non-01 and non-0139 strains of *V cholerae* also cause a wide spectrum of infections, ranging from mild diarrhea to one indistinguishable from classic cholera. Some of these serotypes are known to produce a choleratoxin that is identical to that of the classic biotypes,

whereas others produce a heat-stable enterotoxin analogous to the ST of *E coli*.

LABORATORY DIAGNOSIS OF CHOLERA

The organisms can be viewed directly in the stools, particularly with a dark-field microscope. Additionally, because *V cholerae* is able to grow at a higher *p*H than other enterics, selective media at alkaline *p*H values are used. Fluorescently labeled antiserum can be used to confirm the identification of the observed organisms.

TREATMENT AND CONTROL OF CHOLERA

The mortality rate of cholera can be reduced to less than 1% by the adequate replacement of fluids and electrolytes. The observation that the inclusion of glucose in the salt solution allows oral replacement of electrolytes has made treatment of this disease (particularly in rural areas) much more effective. In fact, the use of any metabolizable carbohydrate together with NaCl seems to be effective for electrolyte replacement. Thus, a well-cooked and salted rice soup is recommended for diarrheal patients who are unable to obtain a glucose–salt solution plus fruit juices for the replacement of K$^+$. The efficacy of the oral replacement therapy can be seen by comparing the mortality of an epidemic before and after such therapy was used. A 1947 epidemic in Egypt involved about 33,000 cases and caused 20,000 deaths. An epidemic in South America beginning in 1991 had over 391,000 cases by the end of the year but less than 4000 deaths. Antibiotics, particularly tetracycline, reduce the number of intestinal vibrios and should be used along with fluid replacement.

Control of cholera requires proper sewage disposal and adequate water sanitation as well as the detection and

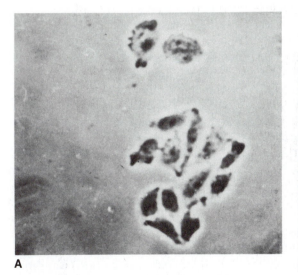
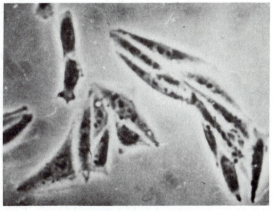

A   **B**

FIGURE 26-8 Giemsa stain of Chinese hamster ovary cells 24 hours after exposure to the culture filtrate of **A** nontoxigenic control *Escherichia coli* and **B** of the enterotoxigenic *E coli* strain 334. (Original magnification ×500.)

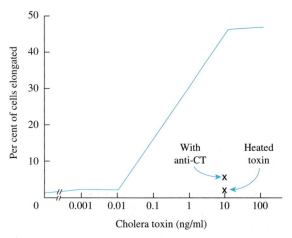

FIGURE 26-9 A standard curve to equate *Escherichia coli* enterotoxin with purified cholera toxin. The percentage of Chinese hamster ovary cells that have elongated after growing 24 hours in the presence of cholera toxin in 1% fetal calf serum is plotted against the concentration of cholera toxin present in the culture. As shown, heated toxin or toxin preincubated with antitoxin (anti-CT) have no effect on the morphologic features of the cells.

treatment of carriers. The disease is rare in the developed world, but occasional cases are acquired in the Texas–Louisiana coastal area from eating raw or undercooked shellfish or crabs. Cholera is still endemic, however, in parts of Asia and India.

Immunization with heat-killed cholera organisms seems to give some protection, and recovery from the disease imparts immunity of an unknown degree or duration. Killed whole cells of *V cholerae* given orally along with purified B subunits of the toxin induced immunity in about 85% of persons who received it. Another experimental engineered oral vaccine consists of a live attenuated *V cholerae* El Tor Ogawa strain. This mutant no longer expresses the A subunit of the toxin but does produce B subunits. It seemed to provide good immunity in volunteers but it has not been used in large-scale field trials.

A experimental vaccine that induces toxin-neutralizing antibodies in mice uses an ingenious technique in which a 45–base-pair oligonucleotide encoding an epitope of the B subunit of CT is inserted into the flagellin gene of an avirulent *Salmonella*. This 15–amino acid insert was expressed at the flagellar surface without abolishing flagellar function. The concept of placing an immunogen in a prominently displayed position on the bacterial surface could be used as a cholera vaccine as well as for inserting a number of other epitopes from both bacteria and viruses.

Remember, however, that none of these vaccines offer any protection against the newly described 0139 strain of *V cholera*, and it is necessary to develop new vaccines for these organisms.

Vibrio parahaemolyticus

Vibrio parahaemolyticus is a marine bacterium that requires a high NaCl concentration for growth. It has attained major importance as the etiologic agent of food poisoning after the ingestion of uncooked or partially cooked seafood, particularly shellfish.

The organisms are normal flora of coastal and estuary waters throughout most of the world and have caused a multitude of cases of acute enteritis in the United States. In countries such as Japan where seafood constitute a high percentage of the normal diet, *V parahaemolyticus* is estimated to be the etiologic agent of about half of all cases of bacterial food poisoning. The best means of prevention is to eat only seafood that is well cooked.

The nature of the *V parahaemolyticus* virulence factors is unknown, but almost all strains isolated from cases of gastroenteritis produce a heat-stable hemolysin that produces β-hemolysis on a special blood agar medium called Wagatsuma agar. This hemolysin has been designated thermostable direct hemolysin, or Kanagawa hemolysin, and strains producing it are designated Kanagawa positive.

In addition to food poisoning and gastroenteritis, *V parahaemolyticus* may cause a bacteremia after the ingestion of contaminated food or may infect soft tissue after handling of contaminated seafood.

Other Pathogenic Vibrios

Vibrio vulnificus is a halophilic organism that characteristically produces an overwhelming primary sepsis without an obvious source of infection, or an infection of a preexisting wound followed by a secondary sepsis. The primary sepsis seems to follow the ingestion of undercooked or raw seafood, particularly raw oysters. The number of *V vulnificus* infections totals fewer than 100 per year in the United States, but the mortality rate is 45% to 60%, particularly in individuals with liver disease, or those with diabetes, kidney disease and other ailments affecting the immune system. As a result, the CDC have strongly recommended: "Don't eat raw oysters if you suffer from any kind of liver disease." Secondary sepsis may also occur after the exposure of wounds to salt water or infected shellfish.

Vibrio fluvialis is another halophile that has been isolated from the diarrheal stools of many patients in Bangladesh. It has also been found in coastal waters and shellfish on the east and west coasts of the United States. This organism has been reported to produce both enterotoxin-like substances and an extracellular cytotoxin that kills tissue cells.

Vibrio mimicus, an organism similar to certain non-01 *V cholerae* strains, also produces a cholera-like disease, and reports indicate that it produces an enterotoxin that is indistinguishable from choleragen.

Campylobacter

Members of the genus *Campylobacter* are gram-negative, curved, spiral rods possessing a single polar flagellum. Four acknowledged species of *Campylobacter* exist, and several additional species have been termed Campylobacter-like organisms. All seem to be inhabitants of the gastrointestinal tract of wild and domestic animals, including household pets. Transmission to humans occurs by a fecal–oral route, originating from farm animals, birds, cats, dogs, and particularly processed poultry. Fifty percent to 70% of all human infections result from handling or consuming improperly prepared chicken. Because the organisms often are found in unpasteurized milk, many epidemics of campylobacteriosis have been spread via milk. Some epidemics have occurred in school children who were given unpasteurized milk during field trips to dairies. The Food and Drug Administration has, therefore, specifically recommended that children not be permitted to sample raw milk during such visits.

Campylobacter jejuni ranks along with rotaviruses and ETEC as the major cause of diarrheal disease in the world, particularly in developing countries. Clinical isolates of this organism have been shown to produce a heat-labile enterotoxin that raises intracellular levels of cAMP. Furthermore, the activity of this enterotoxin is partially neutralized by antiserum against *E coli* LT and CT, demonstrating that *Campylobacter* enterotoxin belongs to this same group of adenylate cyclase-activating toxins. The production of this cholera-like toxin does not, however, explain the mechanism by which *C jejuni* causes an inflammatory dysentery or bloody diarrhea. Analysis of strains producing such infections have revealed the presence of an additional cytotoxin that is biologically distinct from Shiga-like and *Clostridium difficile* toxins. The role of this toxin as a cause of inflammatory colitis, however, remains unknown. As is true for most intestinal pathogens, *C jejuni* has been shown to possess an adhesin for intestinal mucosa.

A number of reports have also indicated a close association between certain serotypes of *C jejuni* and Guillain-Barré syndrome, but the nature of this relationship is completely unknown. In one study of 46 patients with Guillain-Barré syndrome, *C jejuni* was isolated from 30% of patients compared with 1% of controls. Of these, 83% were serotype 19 and 17% were serotype 2.

Campylobacter fetus also causes human diarrheal disease, but this species is more likely to progress to a systemic infection resulting in vascular necrosis.

The incubation period for the diarrheal disease usually is 2 to 4 days. The organisms can be grown readily on an enriched medium under microaerophilic conditions (6% O_2 and 10% CO_2). Gentamicin, erythromycin, and a number of other antibiotics may be used successfully for the treatment of *Campylobacter* infections.

Helicobacter

A new species of gram-negative curved rods, named *Helicobacter pylori*, was first described in 1983. This organism was found growing in gastric epithelium, and it is accepted by most investigators that *H pylori* is the primary etiologic agent of chronic gastritis and duodenal ulcers in humans. Symptoms of chronic gastritis include abdominal pain, burping, gastric distention, and halitosis. The disease can be reproduced in gnotobiotic piglets and in human volunteers after the ingestion of *H pylori*. The observation that their eradication by antibacterial treatment results in normalization of the gastric histology and prevents the recurrence of peptic ulcers strongly supports the role of a this agent in chronic gastritis and peptic ulcer disease. Notice that *Helicobacter mustelae* can be routinely isolated from both normal and inflamed gastric mucosa of ferrets, and *H felis* routinely colonizes the gastric mucosa of cats.

Surprisingly, *H pylori* infection is widespread, particularly in developing countries where it occurs at a younger age than in developed countries. For example, the prevalence of *H pylori* infection in Guangdong Province in China was 52.4%, and it has been suggested that early acquisition and, hence, long-term infection may be an important factor predisposing to gastric cancer.

Adhesins, proteases, and cytotoxins all have been reported as virulence factors for *H pylori*. One adhesin that has definitely been characterized is the blood group antigen, Lewis[b], (Le[b]) which, if present, is found on the surface of gastric epithelial cells in the stomach. Gastric tissue lacking Le[b] antigen or antibodies to the Le[b] antigen inhibited bacterial binding. Thus, because Le[b] is part of the antigen that determines blood group A, individuals with blood group O run a greater risk for developing gastric ulcers. A second adhesin reported to occur on the surface of *H pylori* binds specifically to the monosaccharide sialic acid, also found on glycoproteins on the surface of gastric epithelial cells.

The production of a cytotoxin that induces vacuolation of eucaryotic cells has been reported to occur in about 50% of all isolates. Interestingly, one small study suggested that infection with toxin-producing strains was associated with increased antral inflammation.

All wild-type strains of *H pylori* do produce the enzyme urease, and a number of reports have indicated that urease may protect the organisms from the acidic environment of the stomach by the release of ammonia from urea. Urease may also function as a cytotoxin, destroying gastric cells that are susceptible to its activity.

Notice that over-the-counter medications containing bismuth salts have been used for years to treat gastritis (Pepto-Bismol, Procter & Gamble Pharm., Norwich, NY) and the fact that *H pylori* is sensitive to bismuth may explain its efficacy for the relief of gastric symptoms.

Plesiomonas shigelloides

Plesiomonas shigelloides has been implicated as a cause of diarrhea in the United States as well as in tropical and subtropical countries. The mechanism by which this organism causes diarrhea is unknown, but a report indicated that sterile filtrates of growth medium obtained from 24 different strains of *P shigelloides* induced the synthesis of cAMP in Chinese hamster ovary cells. Moreover, this effect was eliminated by either heating the filtrates or by preincubation of them with cholera antitoxin, suggesting that the diarrhea produced by *P shigelloides* results from the formation of a cholera-like toxin.

These organisms have been isolated from surface waters, the intestines of fresh water fish, pet shop aquariums, and many animals, particularly dogs and cats. It is more common in tropical and subtropical areas, and isolations from Europe and the United States have been rare and usually associated with foreign travel or consumption of raw oysters.

Aeromonas

Aeromonas species are gram-negative, facultatively anaerobic bacteria that are found in soil, fresh and brackish water, and as pathogens of fish, amphibians, and mammals; symptoms range from diarrhea in piglets to fatal septicemia in fish and dogs and abortion in cattle. Human infections are most commonly seen as a gastroenteritis but *Aeromonas* organisms have also been recovered from wounds and soft tissue abscesses that have been contaminated with soil or aquatic environments.

In 1988, California became the first state to make infections by *Aeromonas* a reportable condition and during that year 280 infections were reported, of which 81% were gastroenteritis and 9% were wound infections. Others were isolated from blood, bile, sputum, and urine, occurring mostly in persons with chronic underlying diseases.

Virulence factors that have been reported for *Aeromonas* include cholera-like and heat stable enterotoxins and at least two hemolysins, one or both of which may be cytotoxic or enterotoxic. *Aeromonas hydrophila* and *Aeromonas sobria* probably are the only clinically important species.

PSEUDOMOMADACEAE

Most members of *Pseudomonas,* a vast genus of obligately aerobic gram-negative rods of the Pseudomomadaceae family, are free-living organisms; others are plant pathogens, and only a few species are associated with human diseases. Before the 1940s, *Pseudomonas* infections were rare, but these organisms have become among the more common opportunists that infect debilitated, burned, or immunosuppressed individuals.

Human diseases have been caused by *Pseudomonas cepacia, Pseudomonas multivorans, Pseudomonas fluorescens, Pseudomonas putida, Pseudomonas pseudomallei, Pseudomonas stutzeri,* and *Pseudomonas maltophilia,* but by far the most common human pathogen is *Pseudomonas aeruginosa.*

Pseudomonas aeruginosa

Pseudomonas aeruginosa is found in the stools of 5% of healthy individuals, but this figure may approach 50% among hospital patients. The organism usually produces two water-soluble pigments: a bluish pigment named pyocyanin; and a greenish, fluorescent pigment called fluorescein. Both pigments are lethal for many other bacteria, but there is no evidence that either plays a major role in human infections.

TOXINS AND ENZYMES PRODUCED BY *PSEUDOMONAS AERUGINOSA*

Pseudomonas aeruginosa produces several exotoxins, a cytotoxin, a phospholipase-C, and several proteases. Of these, the product that has been most extensively studied is exotoxin A. The potency of this toxin can be attested to by the fact that it has an LD_{50} (lethal dose for 50% of the population) of less than 1 μg for the mouse and, on a weight basis, shows a similar LD_{50} for monkeys, dogs, and cats. It has been shown to inhibit protein synthesis, as illustrated in Table 26-5. Notice that protein synthesis is markedly inhibited as the time the cells are in contact with the toxin increases. Exotoxin A is also lethal for various cell cultures, as shown in Table 26-6, because of inhibition of protein synthesis. Surprisingly, the mechanism of action of exotoxin A is identical to that of diphtheria toxin (see Chap. 30), in which the toxin acts enzymatically to cleave the nicotinamide moiety from NAD, and then to catalyze the transfer of the resulting ADP-ribose to form a covalent bond with elongation factor 2. Because elongation factor 2 is required for the ribosome to move to the next codon, its inactivation freezes the ribosome, and protein synthesis stops.

Although exotoxin A from *P aeruginosa* is reported to act by the same intracellular mechanism as diphtheria toxin, the two toxins are not identical. Antisera to either

TABLE 26-5
Protein Synthesis in the Liver of Normal and Toxin-Treated Mice

Injection	Time After Injection (h)	Amino Acid Incorporation*	Percent Toxin-Treated Saline-Treated
Saline	1–3†	2765 ± 252	
Toxin		1822 ± 304	66.0
Saline	2–4	2933 ± 444	
Toxin		1418 ± 508	48.3
Saline	16–18	2989 ± 354	
Toxin		564 ± 41	18.8

* Mean counts per min per mg of protein ± the standard deviation.
† First no. indicates the time of amino acid injection posttoxin; second no. indicates the end of pulse.

toxin will neutralize the homologous product, but, as shown in Table 26-7, no cross-reaction occurs between exotoxin A and diphtheria toxin, nor is there any evidence that the production of exotoxin A occurs as a result of lysogenic conversion, as occurs in diphtheria. Another major difference is that exotoxin A affects primarily cells in the liver whereas diphtheria toxin affects the heart, indicating that the molecular receptors for the two toxins are different.

Exotoxin A also has been reported to function as a superantigen in that it will bind to MHC class II molecules and, after processing by an accessory cell protease, will bind to V_β thymoctes, inducing their proliferation.

Exoenzyme S is another ADP-ribosylating enzyme that contributes to the pathogenicity of *P aeruginosa*. Mutants unable to produce exoenzyme S are unable to cause a disseminated infection, whereas exoenzyme S–producing strains readily spread via the bloodstream to infect other tissues. Exoenzyme S exerts its activity by the hydrolysis of NAD and the subsequent ADP-ribosylation of a number of GTP binding proteins, particularly one termed p21[ras]. It is not known why this specifically enhances a disseminated infection. Exoenzyme S also acts as an adhesin to bind the bacteria to the host cells.

Phospholipase C also contributes to the pathogenicity of the organisms. This enzyme causes a marked inflammation, apparently by stimulating host cells to metabolize arachidonic acid to form leukotrienes, a known inflammatory substance.

P aeruginosa also elaborates two proteases that may be involved in disease production. One, an elastase, digests elastin, a component of arterial walls. Elastase also inactivates some of the components of complement. In addition, elastase cleaves transferrin, enhancing iron removal from this protein by the *P aeruginosa* siderophore pyoverdin. The other is a collagenase that hydrolyzes collagen. Both proteases could aid in the spread of the organisms within the body. Some strains of *P aeruginosa* secrete an exopolysaccharide that is antiphagocytic and also acts as an adhesion. Such strains are frequent causes of pneumonia in persons with cystic fibrosis.

P AERUGINOSA INFECTIONS

In spite of its lack of invasiveness, *P aeruginosa* does cause infections and severe disease under the following circumstances:

TABLE 26-6
Effect of *Pseudomonas aeruginosa* Toxin on Various Mammalian Cell Cultures

Cell Line	Percent of ^{14}C Amino Acid Uptake After 5-h Exposure	Percent Viable Cells After 24-h Exposure
L cells	20	0–10
Vero	25	0–10
PSY-15	60	40–60
HeLa	72	20–30
KB	85	Not done

TABLE 26-7
Effect of Specific Antiserum on the NAD Trnasferase Activity of Fragment A of Diphtheria Toxin and *Pseudomonas aeruginosa* Exotoxin

Preincubation Serum	*Acid-Insoluble Radioactivity (CPM)*		
	H_2O	*0.02 µg of Fragment A*	*0.02 µg of Exotoxin A*
H_2O	164	1328	1651
Normal rabbit serum		1556	1080
Rabbit anti-fragment-A serum		284	1545
Normal horse serum, 1:10		1684	1309
Pony anti-exotoxin A serum, 1:10		1544	168

It can cause infections when it is mechanically placed into the urinary tract during catheterization or into the meninges during a lumbar puncture, trauma, or a neurosurgical procedure.

It is able to infect respiratory ventilators and deliver large numbers of organisms directly into the lungs of an already debilitated person.

It has been responsible for a number of cases of whirlpool-associated dermatitis.

It may cause a fatal sepsis in persons with leukemia or persons who are receiving immunosuppressive drugs, or it may cause a septic arthritis or endocarditis in heroin addicts.

Because of its resistance to many antibiotics, it can cause severe infections in persons receiving antibiotic therapy for burns, wounds, cystic fibrosis, and so forth.

In addition, *P aeruginosa* will colonize the respiratory tract of over 70% of individuals with cystic fibrosis and, as such, is responsible for over 90% of deaths from this disease. Table 26-8 provides data for the incidence of *P aeruginosa* infections in a large number of hospitalized individuals. As can be seen, burn patients are the most susceptible, in that about 25% of them become infected.

Therapy for *P aeruginosa* infections uses tobramycin, carbenicillin, gentamicin, and ticarcillin. In addition, the quinolones, such as ciprofloxacin, seem to have good antipseudomonal activity. However, because of the frequency with which these organisms become resistant to antibiotics, new antimicrobials will, undoubtedly, soon become the therapy of choice. Also notice that antibodies directed against exotoxin A seem to provide considerable protection. To this end a number of experimental vaccines have been constructed, the most interesting of which was prepared by deletion of a residue in the active site of the toxin. This recombinant toxin has lost all of its ADP-ribosyltransferase activity, but its use as a vaccine provides significant protection to mice that have been challenged with authentic exotoxin A.

Pseudomonas cepacia

During the last decade, clinicians have seen an increasing number of infections with *P cepacia*. These infections are seen most frequently in burn patients and in individuals with cystic fibrosis or who are debilitated or immunosuppressed. This organism is particularly troublesome because it is resistant to many of the antibiotics used to treat other gram-negative infections but may be susceptible to sulfa-trimethoprim.

TABLE 26-8
Risk of Infection From *Pseudomonas aeruginosa* in 90,000 Patients Under Surveillance in Community Hospitals

Hospital Service or Area	Site of Infection	Patients at Risk per 1000
Burn unit	Burn	246
Burn unit	Urinary tract	16
Burn unit	Surgical wound	11
Urology	Urinary tract	6
Burn unit	Lower respiratory tract	5
General surgery	Surgical wound	4
Medicine	Urinary tract	4
General surgery	Urinary tract	4
General surgery	Lower respiratory tract	3
Gynecology	Urinary tract	2

OBLIGATELY ANAEROBIC ENTERICS

It may seem paradoxical that most of organisms composing the normal flora in humans are so obligately anaerobic that short periods of exposure to air may result in their death. It may seem that the coliforms make up the majority of normal intestinal flora but, in truth, they are outnumbered more than 100 to 1 by the obligately anaerobic gram-negative rods in the family Bacteroidaceae. Two genera of this family, *Bacteroides* and *Fusobacterium,* also are found to a lesser extent in the mouth, in the vagina, and on the external genitalia.

Bacteroides

Bacteroides fragilis is the major human pathogen of the genus *Bacteroides,* producing abscesses in a variety of organs. It is one of the rare gram-negative organisms whose cell wall seemingly lacks the biologic activities associated with endotoxin. Yet it does possess a capsule that seems to be a major virulence factor, because only encapsulated organisms are capable of producing abscesses.

Bacteroides melaninogenicus is found as part of the normal flora of the oropharynx, vagina, external genitalia, and large intestine. It also produces a capsule, but it is serologically distinct from that of *B fragilis.* Its name is derived from the fact that it produces a brownish black pigment when grown 5 to 7 days on a blood-agar plate.

HUMAN INFECTIONS

The major lesion produced by members of the genus *Bacteroides* is the abscess and, although these organisms can be considered as opportunists with little invasive ability, they can be extremely virulent, causing widespread tissue destruction. In most lesions, they exist as mixed flora, usually along with facultative organisms.

Intraabdominal abscesses follow contamination of the peritoneal cavity by fecal contents, resulting either from trauma or surgical procedures. *B fragilis* is the leading pathogen, being found in at least two thirds of such infections. Pelvic abscesses are also frequently caused by *B fragilis.* Such infections may follow trauma during delivery, induced abortion, malignancy, or the use of intrauterine contraceptive devices.

B fragilis is also known to produce an enterotoxin; enterotoxigenic strains have been isolated from about 15% of individuals with diarrhea. However, because such strains could also be isolated from 7% of matched controls without diarrhea, it is difficult to assign *B fragilis* a major role as a diarrhea-producing organism.

B melaninogenicus is found in pulmonary abscesses, where it apparently arrives as a result of the aspiration of mouth flora. *B melaninogenicus,* along with spirochetes and other anaerobes, is also a serious etiologic agent of periodontal disease. Such infections, together with intraabdominal abscesses, provide a source for *Bacteroides* bacteremia, resulting in the spread of the organisms throughout the body and a mortality rate of about 32%. *B fragilis* is the most frequent *Bacteroides* species isolated from such blood cultures. Brain abscesses may result from bacteremia or from the contiguous spread from a middle ear or sinus infection. Other major infections in which members of the genus *Bacteroides* are involved include liver abscesses, endocarditis, and urinary tract infections.

Fusobacterium

A number of species of *Fusobacterium* are found as normal flora of the mouth, large intestine, and female genital tract. They are characteristically obligately anaerobic gram-negative organisms that appear as long, slender rods with tapered ends.

The fusobacteria are principal causes of sinus infections, otitis media, and dental infections. They are also involved in brain abscesses and are a major anaerobic organism involved in lung infections. *Fusobacterium necrophorum,* the most common pathogen of this genus, frequently is associated with *Bacteroides* species in liver abscesses, intraabdominal abscesses, and peritonitis.

Anaerobic Gram-Positive Cocci

Anaerobic gram-positive cocci comprise a large part of the normal flora of the mouth, large intestine, and female genital tract. *Peptostreptococcus* grows as chains of cocci, whereas *Peptococcus* is seen as irregular clumps resembling the staphylococci.

Both organisms frequently are found along with other obligate anaerobes in wound infections, particularly those associated with abdominal surgery. They are also seen in liver abscesses, brain abscesses, lung infections, and female pelvic tract infections, particularly after a septic abortion.

LABORATORY ISOLATION OF THE OBLIGATE ANAEROBES

All of these organisms must be grown anaerobically in one of several ways. A simple anaerobic Gas Pak jar will suffice for many anaerobes. Such jars contain a package that, after the addition of water, will remove oxygen. More sophisticated techniques involve the use of prereduced anaerobically sterilized media. Notice that many of the obligately anaerobic bacteria are exquisitely sensitive to the presence of oxygen, and such organisms must be transported from the patient to the laboratory under anaerobic conditions and processed as soon as possible after collection. Others, such as *B fragilis,* are tolerant of the presence of oxygen and can survive for some time if kept moist.

Most of the anaerobes can be identified by determining the kinds of fatty acids produced during the fermentation of carbohydrates. To accomplish this, a small amount of culture fluid is esterified to form the methyl esters of the fatty acids, and the methyl esters are then injected into a gas chromatograph. In this manner, separation and identification of the fatty acids can be accomplished in 30 to 60 minutes.

TREATMENT OF INFECTIONS CAUSED BY OBLIGATE ANAEROBES

Treatment of obligate anaerobe infections almost always requires surgical drainage in conjunction with antibiotic therapy. Most anaerobes are susceptible to erythromycin, clindamycin, lincomycin, and chloramphenicol. Penicillin also may be effective, but many strains of *Bacteroides*, particularly *B fragilis*, elaborate a β-lactamase that destroys the penicillin.

Bibliography

JOURNALS

Bone RC. Gram-negative sepsis: a delemma of modern medicine. Clin Microbiol Rev 1993;6:57.

Donnenberg MS, Kaper JB. Enteropathogenic *E. coli*. Infect Immun 1992;60:3953.

Finegold SM, Goldstein EJC, eds. Proceedings of the First North American Congress on Anaerobic Bacteria and Anaerobic Infections. Clin Infect Dis 1993: 16(Suppl 4).

Goldberg MB, Sansonetti PJ. Minireview. *Shigella* subversion of the cellular cytoskeleton: a strategy for epithelial colonization. Infect Immun 1993;61:4941.

Hale TL. Genetic basis of virulence in *Shigella* species. Microbiol Rev 1991;55:206.

Lee A, Fox J, Hazell S. Minireview. Pathogenicity of *Helicobacter pylori*: a perspective. Infect Immun 1993;61:1601.

Johnson JR. Virulence factors in *Escherichia coli* urinary tract infection. Clinical Microbiol Rev 1991;4:80.

Martin MA, Silverman HJ. Review article. Gram-negative sepsis and the adult respiratory syndrome. Clin Infect Dis 1992;14:1213.

Parrillo JE. Pathogenetic mechanisms of septic shock. N Engl J Med 1993;328:1471.

Spangler BD. Structure and function of cholera toxin and the related *Escherichia coli* heat-labile enterotoxin. Microbiol Rev 1992;56:622.

Essentials of Medical Microbiology, Fifth Edition, edited by Wesley A. Volk,
Bryan M. Gebhardt, Marie-Louise Hammarskjöld, and Robert J. Kadner.
Lippincott-Raven Publishers, Philadelphia © 1996.

Chapter 27

Brucella, Yersinia, Francisella, and Pasteurella

All of the organisms discussed in this chapter are animal pathogens with which humans become infected through contact with an infected animal or animal product or from the bite of an infected insect or arthropod vector. Thus, with the possible exception of epidemics of human plague by *Yersinia pestis,* these bacteria reach the end of the line when they infect humans, because transmission between humans is unusual.

BRUCELLA

At one time, there were a number of synonyms for infections with *Brucella,* including Malta fever, Mediterranean fever, Gibraltar fever, Cyprus fever, and undulant fever, but all infections by species of *Brucella* usually are referred to as brucellosis.

The causative agent of brucellosis was first characterized during the late 1800s on the island of Malta, a British base where troops from England were acclimated en route to India. At the time that Dr. David Bruce arrived from Scotland to take care of the troops, about 1000 cases of Malta fever (military and civilian) occurred each year, resulting in 75 to 80 deaths. In 1887, Bruce isolated the etiologic agent from the spleens from four cases of fatal disease and fulfilled Koch's postulates by transmitting the disease to monkeys.

Shortly afterward, a young Maltese physician named Zammit showed that many of the more than 20,000 goats on Malta were excreting the disease organisms in their milk, so exclusion of goats' milk and cheeses essentially eliminated the disease from the military base. This organism from goats has been named *Brucella melitensis.*

Meanwhile, a Danish veterinarian named Bang isolated a related organism that caused abortions in infected cows and was excreted in the cows' milk. This organism has been given the name *Brucella abortus.* Still later, a third organism was isolated that normally infects swine, and this species has been designated *Brucella suis.*

Three additional species of *Brucella* have been isolated: *Brucella canis* from dogs, *Brucella ovis* from sheep, and *Brucella neotomae* from the wood rat.

In the United States, usually fewer than 200 cases occur per year, but the World Health Organization reports that worldwide there are about 500,000 cases of brucellosis annually, most of which are caused by *B melitensis*.

Classification and Antigenic Structure

All *Brucella* are gram-negative aerobic organisms and can be differentiated on the basis of metabolic and antigenic properties, as shown in Table 27-1. The three major species can be subdivided into varying numbers of biotypes, based primarily on their production of H_2S, their ability to grow in a medium containing the dyes basic fuchsin or thionin, and their agglutination by monospecific antiserum.

The three major species of *Brucella* contain two antigens (designated A and M) as surface determinants, but the relative proportion of each antigen varies considerably from one species or biotype to another. Thus, monospecific A and M antiserum can be prepared by adsorbing out cross-reacting antibodies (Fig. 27-1), and differences in the agglutination reactions among the various brucellae can be shown (see Table 27-1).

Epidemiology and Pathogenesis of *Brucella* Infections

The portal of entry for most human infections with *Brucella* is the skin or conjunctiva, after direct contact with infected animals or aborted fetuses. Some persons contract the disease by the ingestion of contaminated dairy products, but since the organisms are sensitive to the acidity of the stomach, infection probably occurs by way of the mucous membranes of the throat.

TABLE 27-1
Differential Characters of the Species and Biotypes of the Genus *Brucella*

BIOTYPE	CO_2 Required	H_2S Produced	Basic Fuchsin b.	Thionin a	Thionin b	Monospecific Sera A	Monospecific Sera M	Antirough Serum	Lysis by Phage Tb, RTD	L-Alanine	L-Asparagine	L-Glutamic acid	L-Arabinos	D-Galactose	D-Ribose	D-Glucose	L-Erythritol	D-Xylose	L-Arginine[+]	L-Lysine
B melitensis																				
1	–	–	+	–	+	–	+	–	–	+	+	+	–	–	–	+	+	–	–	–
2	–	–	+	–	+	+	–	–	–	+	+	+	–	–	–	+	+	–	–	–
3	–	–	+	–	+	+	+	–	–	+	+	+	–	–	–	+	+	–	–	–
B abortus																				
1	d‡	+	+	–	–	+	–	–	+	+	+	+	+	+	+	+	+	–	–	–
2	d	+	–	–	–	+	–	–	+	+	+	+	+	+	+	+	+	–	–	–
3	d	+	+	+	+	+	–	–	+	+	+	+	+	+	+	+	+	–	–	–
4	d	+	+	–	–	–	+	–	+	+	+	+	+	+	+	+	+	–	–	–
5	–	–	+	–	+	–	+	–	+	+	+	+	+	+	+	+	+	–	–	–
6	–	–	+	–	+	+	–	–	+	+	+	+	+	+	+	+	+	–	–	–
7	–	d	+	–	+	+	+	–	+	+	+	+	+	+	+	+	+	–	–	–
8	+	–	+	–	+	–	+	–	+	+	+	+	+	+	+	+	+	–	–	–
9	–	+	+	–	+	–	+	–	+	+	+	+	+	+	+	+	+	–	–	–
B suis																				
1	–	+	–	+	+	+	–	–	–	–	–	+	+	+	+	+	+	+	+	+
2	–	–	–	+	+	+	–	–	–	–	+	+	+	–	+	+	+	+	+	–
3	–	–	+	+	+	+	–	–	–	–	+	+	–	–	+	+	+	+	+	+
4	–	–	+	+	+	+	+	–	–	–	+	+	–	+	+	+	+	+	+	+
B neotomae	–	+	–	–	+	+	–	–	–	–	+	+	+	+	d	+	+	+	–	–
B ovis	+	–	+	+	+	–	–	+	–	+	+	+	–	–	–	–	–	–	–	–
B canis	–	–	+	+	+	–	–	+	–	–	–	–	–	–	–	+	+	d	+	+

RTD, routine test dilution.

* Certified dyes (National Aniline Division, Allied Chemical and Dye Co., New York) at concentrations a = 1:25,000; b = 1:50,000.

+ Same reactions with DL-citrulline and DL-omithine.

‡ 11%–89% strains positive.

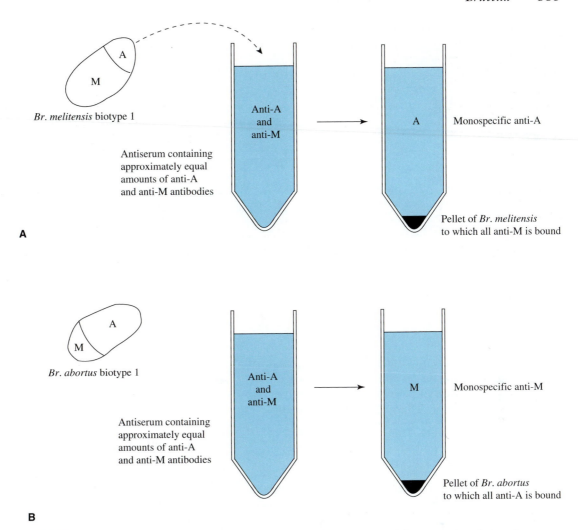

FIGURE 27-1 Preparation of *Brucella* monospecific antiserum. Antiserum containing approximately equal amounts of anti-A and anti-M antibodies is used with *Brucella* organisms that possess considerably more of one antigen than the other. The addition of limiting amounts of organisms to the antiserum results in the complete reaction of the antibody directed to the major antigen and leaves the antibody to the minor antigen unreacted in the serum. **A.** The organism thus contains far more M than A antigen and will, as a result, react with more anti-M antibodies, leaving pure anti-A antiserum; **B.** The opposite situation results in pure anti-M antiserum.

Primary invasion spreads by way of the lymphatics, with localization in the regional lymph nodes. The organisms undergo phagocytosis by macrophages but are able to survive and multiply within this protected environment (Fig. 27-2).

Bloodstream invasion follows and the brucellae eventually become localized in the mononuclear phagocytic system where their intracellular existence provides protection from both antibodies and antibiotics. The brucellae are able to survive in this intracellular environment because they inhibit the myelo-peroxidase-H_2O_2-halide antibacterial system by blocking degranulation. They accomplish this by releasing 5′-guanosine monophosphate and adenine, both of which prevent degranulation. After activation of the monocytes, however, the immune monocytes are able to kill the ingested bacteria. In some mammals (but not humans), the organisms may infect the mammary glands and be shed in the milk. The brucellae also infect the placenta in cows, sheep, pigs, or goats (but again, not humans) and cause abortions. Animals that are susceptible to this type of abortion contain large amounts of the four-carbon sugar alcohol erythritol in their placentas, and erythritol markedly stimulates the growth of brucellae.

In humans, the incubation period may vary from 1 to 6 weeks, followed by malaise, weakness, and an undulating diurnal fever (undulant fever). Other symptoms include backache, headache, and loss of appetite. Relapses during a 2- to 4-month convalescence are frequent and, in rare cases, the disease is thought to become chronic, extending over periods of many years, resulting in variable symptoms of weakness and malaise, and characterized by emotional disturbances.

Brucellosis is endemic in Saudi Arabia where it is

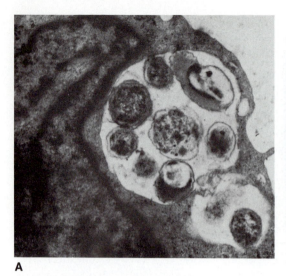 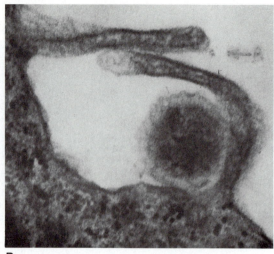

A   B

FIGURE 27-2   A. Phagocyte infected with *Brucella abortus* for 48 hours. The brucellae are in a large vacuole. (Original magnification ×21,170.) **B.** Phagocytosis of *B abortus* by a phagocyte in a 48-hour infection mix. Pseudopodia engulf the brucella. (Original magnification ×75,300.)

contracted by drinking raw milk from goats, sheep, or camels. Neurobrucellosis in which involvement of the central nervous system or peripheral nervous system has been reported occurs in 2% to 5% of these patients.

Laboratory Diagnosis of Brucellosis

A definitive diagnosis of brucellosis requires the isolation and identification of the etiologic agent. Most human cases are caused by *B abortus, B melitensis,* and *B suis,* although human infections with *B canis* have been reported.

Blood or biopsy material from bone marrow, liver, or lymph nodes should be inoculated into trypticase soy broth and incubated at 37°C in a candle jar or a CO_2 incubator with an aerobic atmosphere containing 10% CO_2. An evaluation of diagnostic methods used on 50 patients who were eventually shown to have brucellosis indicated that brucellae could be grown from bone marrow aspirates considerably more often than from blood. In either case, the initial isolates may grow slowly, and it may require as long as 6 weeks before organisms can be subcultured on solid media.

The presence of agglutinating antibodies may aid the diagnosis of brucellosis but, because other organisms contain antigens that induce cross-reacting antibodies, one should obtain an agglutinating titer of at least 1:160 or, ideally, see at least a fourfold increase in the agglutination titer arising during the convalescent phase of the disease.

A few patients will form high levels of nonagglutinating serum IgA, which inhibits the agglutination of the test suspension. The interference of these blocking antibodies may be eliminated by diluting the patient's serum with saline or albumin to the point where the blocking antibodies are ineffective and the IgG antibodies will agglutinate the organisms.

Because the brucellae induce a cellular-type immunity, a protein extract of the organisms, called brucellergin, will give a delayed-type skin reaction in persons who are hypersensitive to the antigens of the brucellae. However, a positive reaction does not mean active disease but only a past history of exposure to brucellosis. Based on antibody studies, many abattoir workers and veterinarians apparently have had asymptomatic or undiagnosed brucellosis. Furthermore, because brucellergin is itself antigenic, repeated skin tests may induce a positive skin reaction.

Treatment and Prevention of Brucellosis

Acquired immunity to brucellosis appears to involve humoral antibodies as well as CD4 and CD8 T cells. Moreover, cytokines are probably also involved because the addition of interferon-γ or interleukin-2 results in a large decrease in cultured, viable intracellular bacteria.

The incidence of brucellosis in the United States has decreased during the last several decades from a common infection to about 200 reported cases annually. This drop has been primarily because of an extensive program of testing and immunization of cattle by the U.S. Department of Agriculture. It is required that all cattle be immunized with a living, attenuated strain of *B abortus* (strain 19), and brucellergin-positive animals that have not been immunized are destroyed. Pasteurization of milk also is designed to kill brucellae, and this procedure alone has undoubtedly prevented many human infections.

Researchers at Texas A & M University received approval in 1989 from the Agricultural Biotechnology Research Advisory Committee to field test a newly bioengineered vaccine. Their organism is the result of a transposon mutagenesis that inactivated normal outer membrane lipopolysaccharide synthesis in *B abortus*. Initial studies indicate it does not cause disease in mice or goats, and it is being evaluated in cattle to compare its efficacy with the vaccine.

Most human cases in the United States occur in workers (such as slaughterhouse employees, veterinarians, and farmers) who have direct contact with infected animals, or result from eating unpasteurized dairy products or imported cheeses (Table 27-2). Active immunization of humans has not been done in the United States, although some eastern European countries have used attenuated avirulent strains to immunize high-risk groups of individuals.

Treatment of brucellosis is difficult, probably because the organisms exist intracellularly in the monocytes (see Fig. 27-2) and are protected from the effect of antibiotics. However, use of a combination of doxycycline and rifampin is the treatment of choice. Interestingly, the use of multilamellar vesicles containing entrapped aminoglycosides proved effective for the treatment of *Brucella*-infected mice and guinea pigs. The superiority of these liposome-entrapped antibiotics over free antibiotics is, in all likelihood, because of the ability of a liposome to fuse with the cell membrane, depositing its antibiotic into the cytoplasm of the infected cell.

YERSINIA

In 1970, the genus *Yersinia* was created in commemoration of Yersin, the discoverer of the plague bacillus. It had been shown that yersiniae could conjugate with *Escherichia coli* and accept various plasmids such as resistance transfer factors. In addition, *Yersinia* organisms have several antigens in common with some of the enterics and thus appear to be better positioned taxonomically as a members of the Enterobacteriaceae.

The genus *Yersinia* contains three species that are pathogenic for humans: *Yersinia pestis*, the etiologic agent of bubonic plague, and *Yersinia enterocolitica* and *Yersinia pseudotuberculosis*, which are primarily responsible for a mild-to-severe gastroenteritis. All are pathogens that humans acquire directly or indirectly from infected animals, and all share a number of virulence factors.

Yersinia pestis

Bubonic plague, caused by *Y pestis,* is an ancient disease that has killed millions of people over the centuries. For example, it is believed to have killed more than 100 million persons in an epidemic in the sixth century. Another epidemic in the 14th century killed one fourth of the European population, and the London plague in 1665 killed more than 70,000 persons. In 1893, an epidemic began in Hong Kong and spread to India where more than 10 million individuals died over a 20-year period. This epidemic eventually reached San Francisco in about 1900, and the disease is firmly established in the southwestern United States (eg, in prairie dogs, ground squirrels, wood rats, chipmunks, and mice; Fig. 27-3), as well as in many other areas of the world.

MORPHOLOGY AND VIRULENCE FACTORS

Yersinia pestis is a small, gram-negative, nonmotile coccobacillus that becomes pleomorphic if grown under suboptimal conditions, such as a high salt concentration. The organisms have a tendency for bipolar staining (in which the ends of the bacilli stain darker than the central part; Fig. 27-4) but are not particularly fastidious; they can easily be grown in a routine peptone medium.

The important virulence factors of *Y pestis* seem to be directed toward two goals for the organisms: (1) invasion and proliferation within host cells, and (2) resistance to killing by the host. The incredibly high fatality rate of bubonic plague is probably primarily because of septic shock resulting from the bacteremia occurring in the disease.

Y pestis produces a variety of different virulence factors, but only a few have been characterized sufficiently well to postulate their role in production of disease: (1) a capsular antigen, designated Fraction 1 (F1), is antiphagocytic, and antibodies to F1 seem to be protective; (2) V/W antigens, consisting of a protein (V) and a lipoprotein (W), are produced together, but their role as virulence factors is unclear, although there are data that V-antigen suppresses the production of interferon-γ and tumor necrosis factor-α, thus suppressing granuloma formation with the resulting delayed-type hypersensitivity to the organisms; and (3) an intracellular murine toxin that is lethal for the mouse ($LD_{50} < 1$ μg) and rat but is essentially inert in other hosts. Also described has been a bacteriocin, Pesticin I, that has a lethal effect on *Y pseudotuberculosis* and some *E coli* strains through an *N*-acetylglucosaminidase–mediated hydrolysis of peptidoglycan. It is always produced coincidentally with coagulase and fibrinolysin. Mutants unable to synthesize fibrinolysin have a million-fold higher LD_{50} than wild-type strains if the mutant is injected subcutaneously, but not if the organisms are injected into deeper tissues. It is postulated that the ability of fibrinolysin to convert plasminogen to plasmin is essential for the invasion of deeper tissues after the superficial inoculation of the host by an infected flea bite. Interestingly, these factors are encoded on a small plasmid not found in the other pathogenic yersiniae. Other determinants that are associated with virulence include the ability to synthesize purines

TABLE 27-2
309 Cases of Brucellosis by Occupation and Most Probable Source of Infection, United States 1975

Classification	Occupation	Domestic Animals				Wild Animals			Unpasteurized Dairy Products		Accidents		Unknown	Total	% of Total
		Swine	Cattle	Swine or Cattle	Unspecified Farm Animals	Deer	Caribou	Feral Swine	Domestic	Foreign	Strain 19 Vaccine	Laboratory			
Meat processing industry	Packing house employee	77	47	44	2	—	—	—	—	—	—	—	—	170	55.2
	Government inspector	2	6	4	1	—	—	—	—	—	—	—	—	13	4.2
	Rendering plant employee	—	—	1	1	—	—	—	—	—	—	—	—	2	0.6
Livestock industry	Livestock market employee	—	1	—	—	—	—	—	—	—	—	—	—	1	0.3
	Livestock producer	11	39	1	—	—	—	—	2	—	1	—	—	54	17.5
	Veterinarian	—	2	1	—	—	—	—	—	—	1	—	—	4	4
Other categories	Laboratory worker	—	—	—	—	—	—	—	—	—	—	1	—	1	0.3
	Homemaker	—	1	—	—	—	—	—	2	1	—	—	1	5	1.6
	Student or child	—	2	2	—	—	—	—	2	5	—	—	3	14	4.5
	Other	3	6	—	2	1	—	4	2	9	—	—	9	36	11.6
	Unknown	1	—	—	—	—	1	—	—	1	—	—	6	9	2.9
Total		94	104	53	6	1	1	4	8	16	2	1	19	309	100.0
% of Total		30.5	33.7	17.2	1.9	0.3	0.3	1.3	2.6	5.2	0.6	0.3	6.1	100.0	

Most Probable Source of Infection

and the property to absorb and store hemin and certain basic aromatic dyes to form colored colonies. It is not possible to associate these characteristics with any specific virulence determinant, but mutants unable to synthesize purines or store iron to form colored colonies display a decreased virulence for experimental animals.

Probably the most confusing virulence factors are encoded on a plasmid termed the low calcium response (Lcr) plasmid. This plasmid is expressed only at 37°C (not at 26°C) and in the presence of low Ca^{2+} levels as would be present in mammalian intracellular fluid. Expression of the plasmid results in (1) a reduced adenylate charge; (2) shutoff of stable RNA synthesis; (3) synthesis of V and W antigens; and (4) synthesis of a number of

new outer membrane proteins, which have been termed YOPs. The importance of the Lcr plasmid in the pathogenesis of infection with *Y pestis* is apparent in that Lcr-negative mutants are avirulent.

Some of the YOPs have been shown to be virulence factors. YOP E disrupts actin filaments and may be involved in the internalization of the bacteria into epithelial cells. YOP H is a protein tyrosine phosphatase, and it has been proposed that this protein may be secreted into the cytoplasm of the infected cell where it could cause dephosphorylation of protein tyrosines that are important in signal transduction pathways. YOP H also has been shown to inhibit phagocytosis. Mutants lacking YOPs K and L were rapidly cleared from organs, and it is assumed

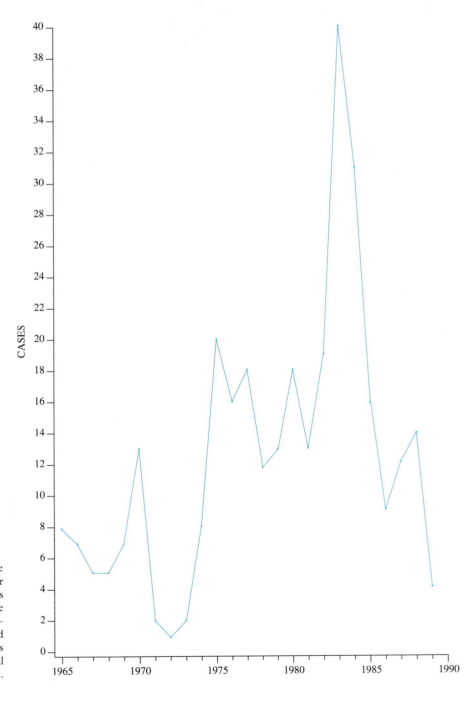

FIGURE 27-3 Thirty-nine cases of plague were reported in 1983, the largest number in a single year in over a half century. Cases occurred in the southwestern part of the United States, predominantly in New Mexico. These figures represent the scope and intensity of rodent plague. The drop in cases during 1989 hopefully reflects educational efforts about the transmission of this disease.

epidemic of 28 cases of tularemia in North Dakota, it was shown that ticks collected from 8 of 46 dogs were infected with *F tularensis*. Domestic cats that have eaten infected animals have provided a source of human infection.

In general, three major manifestations of tularemia exist, depending, in part, on the route of entry of the organisms: ulceroglandular, pneumonic, and typhoidal.

Ulceroglandular tularemia, which follows direct contact with infected animals or the bite of an infected arthropod, is the most common type of this disease. It is characterized by the appearance of a primary lesion at the point of entry, which may become an open ulcer after 7 or 8 days. The primary lesion in tick-borne cases usually is on the lower extremities or, less commonly, on the trunk. In cases in which the eye has been the portal of entry, a severe conjunctival ulcer may develop, and the disease may be referred to as *oculoglandular tularemia*. The organisms reach the regional lymph nodes, which become swollen and tender and may on occasion break open and drain. They can then spread by way of the bloodstream to cause lesions in other organs, particularly the liver and spleen, and, occasionally, the lungs.

When the organisms reach the lungs, whether by hematogenous spread or by the respiratory route, the infection is called *pneumonic tularemia*. About 10% to 15% of ulceroglandular infections become pneumonic, but it is not unusual for an individual to acquire primary pneumonic tularemia by skinning an infected rabbit. This manifestation of tularemia can result in the direct spread from person to person and is associated with a high mortality rate.

Tularemia also can be acquired by ingesting contaminated food or by drinking water contaminated by animals that have died from tularemia. In these instances, no primary lesion occurs, and the disease, known as *typhoidal tularemia*, has many of the gastrointestinal and high-fever symptoms associated with typhoid fever.

There are two biologic varieties of *F tularensis*. Biovar *tularensis* causes about 80% of human cases in North America and is distinguished from biovar *palaearctica* by its ability to ferment glycerol and by the possession of the enzyme, citrulline ureidase. Biovar *tularensis* is found only in North America where it is usually associated with ticks and rabbits. Biovar *palaeartica*, which is found worldwide, causes a much milder disease than biovar *tularensis*. Although also found in ticks, biovar *palaeartica* is more frequently associated with aquatic animals and contaminated water.

F tularensis is considered to be among the most virulent organisms that infect humans, but other than an antiphagocytic capsule, it is not possible to pinpoint the factors that contribute to this virulence. Certainly, its ability to grow and survive in monocytes and polymorphonuclear neutrophils protects the organisms from destruction and from lysis by humoral antibody and comple-

ment. However, no toxic factors have been described that can explain the extreme virulence of these organisms.

Laboratory Diagnosis of Tularemia

Smears from skin lesions can be stained with fluorescently labeled specific antibody to provide a diagnosis, or one can determine the agglutination titer of the patient's serum to the specific organisms for a retrospective diagnosis. An enzyme-linked immunosorbent assay also has been described that uses a sonicate of tularemia vaccine as an antigen.

Ideally, the causative organisms should be grown and identified using fluorescent antibody or agglutination with specific antiserum but, to do so, a special cystine–glucose blood medium is required. In actual practice, many diagnostic laboratories are reluctant to grow this organism because of the danger to laboratory personnel. As a consequence, most diagnoses of tularemia are based on the history, the clinical picture, and either examining the exudate with labeled antibody or noticing the appearance of agglutinins 8 to 10 days after the initial symptoms.

Treatment and Control of Tularemia

Treatment with any antibiotic is difficult, probably because of the intracellular existence of the organisms. However, streptomycin seems to be the antibiotic of choice, although the tetracyclines, gentamicin, or chloramphenicol also are efficacious. Relapses are common, and prolonged treatment may be necessary.

Both phenol-killed and -attenuated vaccines have been used, but, because immunity is primarily cell mediated, the inactivated vaccine seems to be of little value. An attenuated vaccine is available from the Centers for Disease Control and should be given to persons whose risk of exposure is high.

Control is virtually impossible in the wild animal population but, because many human cases result from direct contact with infected rabbits, one should either use plastic gloves when cleaning wild rabbits or, for absolute protection, follow the advice given in Leviticus XI, verses 6 to 8, which, in part, states, ". . . and of the hare . . . of their flesh shall ye not eat, and their carcass shall ye not touch; they are unclean to you."

PASTEURELLA MULTOCIDA

Pasteurella multocida exists as part of the normal flora of the respiratory tract of many animals and birds. Members of this species are small, gram-negative coccobacilli that seem to cause disease in animals, primarily when the animals are under stress, such as while being shipped to market. The manifestations of disease usually are pneumonia or hemorrhagic septicemia, and this is referred to as *shipping fever* or *fowl cholera*.

Humans can become infected, particularly after the bite by an animal such as a dog or cat, resulting in localized tissue infection or systemic septicemia or meningitis. Also, chronic respiratory infections occur in humans with pre-existing pulmonary disease.

Interestingly, *P multocida* colonizes the nasopharynx of the cat in a manner analogous to that of *Streptococci viridans* in humans, which undoubtedly accounts for the fact that about 65% of human infections result from cat bites.

Killed vaccines have been used for animal protection, and most strains are sensitive to penicillin and tetracycline.

Bibliography

JOURNALS

Brubaker RR. Factors promoting acute and chronic diseases caused by yersiniae. Clin Microbiol Rev 1991;4:309.

Fortier AH, et al. Activation of macrophages for destruction of *Francisella tularensis*: identification of cytokines, effector cells, and effector molecules. Infect Immun 1992;60:817.

Goldstein EJC. Bite wounds and infection. Clin Infect Dis 1992;14:633.

Jiang S, Baldwin CL. Effects of cytokines on intracellular growth of *Brucella abortus*. Infect Immun 1993;61:124.

Miller VL. *Yersinia* invasion genes and their products. ASM News 1992;58:26.

Nakajima R, Brubaker RR. Association between virulence of *Yersinia pestis* and suppression of gamma interferon and tumor necrosis factor alpha. Infect Immun 1993;61:23.

Rankin S, Isberg RR, Leong JM. The integrin-binding domain of invasin is sufficient to allow bacterial entry into mammalian cells. Infect Immun 1992;60:3909.

Straley SC, et al. Minireview: YOPs of *Yersinia* spp. pathogenic for humans. Infect Immun 1993;61:3105.

Essentials of Medical Microbiology, Fifth Edition, edited by Wesley A. Volk,
Bryan M. Gebhardt, Marie-Louise Hammarskjöld, and Robert J. Kadner.
Lippincott-Raven Publishers, Philadelphia © 1996.

Chapter 28

Haemophilus, Bordetella, and Legionella

Organisms included in the genera *Haemophilus* and *Bordetella* frequently are referred to as the hemophilic bacteria, because they either require fresh blood or are stimulated if blood is added to their growth medium. The major pathogen in each genus is characterized by its ability to cause respiratory or meningeal infections, primarily in young children. *Haemophilus influenzae* is the principal etiologic agent of meningitis in children younger than 3 years of age, and *Bordetella pertussis* is the cause of whooping cough.

Legionella pneumophila is unrelated to either *Haemophilus* or *Bordetella* but is included in this chapter because its portal of entry is also the respiratory tract, causing systemic involvement and respiratory illness.

HAEMOPHILUS

The generic name *Haemophilus* evolved from the fact that, for growth, these organisms have an absolute requirement for blood-containing medium. This need for red blood cells is based on two essential substances: (1) a heat-stable material originally designated as X factor, and (2) a heat-labile component that was given the name V factor. Subsequent research has shown that X factor is hematin, which is required for the synthesis of *Haemophilus'* heme-containing cytochrome system and the enzyme catalase. The V factor can be replaced by either nicotinamide-adenine dinucleotide (NAD) or nicotinamide-adenine dinucleotide phosphate (NADP), although if nicotinamide riboside is supplied, the organisms can synthesize their own NAD and NADP. Not all species of *Haemophilus* need both factors, but (as suggested by Table 28-1) all species require the addition of at least one of these components for growth. Notice that although red blood cells contain the required X and V factors, only *Haemophilus hemolyticus,* a nonpathogen of the respiratory tract, is beta hemolytic and able to lyse the erythrocytes. The other *Haemophilus* species do not grow well on blood-agar media unless the medium has been heated

TABLE 28-1
Growth Characteristics of Some Species of *Haemophilus* and *Bordetella*

Organism	Requires X (Hematin)	Requires V (NAD)	Beta-Hemolytic
Haemophilus influenzae	+	+	−
Haemophilus parainfluenzae	−	+	−
Haemophilus hemolyticus	+	+	+
Haemophilus suis	+	+	−
Bordetella pertussis	−	−	+

NAD, nicotinamide-adenine dinucleotide.

to 80°C for 15 minutes to lyse the red blood cells and inactivate enzymes that may destroy V factor. As noted elsewhere in this text, the resulting brown-agar medium is commonly called chocolate agar.

Haemophilus influenzae

Haemophilus influenzae is a small, gram-negative, pleomorphic coccobacillus (Fig. 28-1) and a facultative anaerobe that prefers aerobic conditions. These organisms use carbohydrates poorly, and differential sugar fermentation reactions are of no value for their identification.

ANTIGENIC STRUCTURE

The organisms in *H influenzae* are divided into six types, designated a, b, c, d, e, and f on the basis of antigenic differences in their capsular material. Antibodies to the capsules are protective; they enhance phagocytosis as well

as stimulate a complement-requiring bactericidal effect. Type b (frequently designated *Hib*), the type associated with almost all serious disease in children, possesses a capsule that is a polymer of ribose and ribitol phosphate (commonly called PRP). Nonencapsulated strains of *H influenzae* (also termed nontypeable *H influenzae*) are antigenically heterogeneous and can be separated into a number of biovars based on various biochemical properties. Like the pneumococcus, transformation of capsular types, as well as transfer of streptomycin resistance, has been accomplished with free DNA.

EPIDEMIOLOGY AND PATHOGENICITY OF *H INFLUENZAE* INFECTIONS

Encapsulated Type B Strains

The somewhat misleading name *H influenzae* stems from uncertainty about the role of this organism as the etiologic agent of the influenza pandemics of 1890 and 1918. It

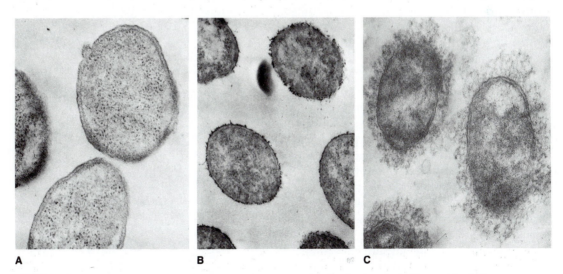

A   **B**   **C**

FIGURE 28-1 Electron micrographs of thin sections of nonencapsulated and encapsulated *Haemophilus influenzae* type b. **A.** Nonencapsulated cells. (Original magnification ×38,000.) **B.** Encapsulated cells with dense matted capsular antigen visible on their surfaces. (Original magnification ×27,000.) **C.** Encapsulated cells exposed to type b specific antiserum before fixation. Notice the complete enveloping of the cells and the fibrillar nature of the antigen–antibody complex, which seems to emanate from discrete points in the cell wall. (Original magnification ×30,000.)

is recognized that influenza is a viral disease (see Chap. 48), but the fact that this organism is a common secondary invader of viral influenza victims led to the erroneous conclusion that *H influenzae* was the etiologic agent. There is a possibility that this organism can act synergistically with the human influenza virus, but this hypothesis is supported primarily by the observation that a combination of *Haemophilus suis* and swine influenza virus produce a swine disease more severe than that which either agent could cause alone.

H influenzae is an obligate human parasite that is passed from person to person by way of the respiratory route. Thirty percent to 50% of all children carry nontypeable *H influenzae* asymptomatically in the nasopharynx, whereas only 2% to 3% carry encapsulated type b organisms. Asymptomatic carriage of encapsulated *H influenzae* induces a protective immunity.

Meningitis is the most severe type of infection caused by *H influenzae,* and most of such infections occur in children between the ages of 6 months and 3 years. In fact, *H influenzae* is the chief cause of meningitis in the young, and until the vaccine was introduced, it had an annual attack rate of about 1 in 2000 in children between the ages of 3 months and 6 years, resulting in 8000 to 11,000 cases annually in the United States, with a mortality rate of 3% to 7%. With the advent of an effective vaccine, however, the incidence of invasive infections with *H influenzae* has decreased considerably: 1113 cases reported in the United States in 1994.

The pathogenesis of the disease is like that of meningococcal meningitis, in which the organisms travel from the nasopharynx to infect the regional lymph nodes, enter the bloodstream, and invade the meninges. Neurologic sequelae occur in many children who recover from *H influenzae* meningitis. For example, approximately 10% experience hearing loss and a much larger percentage seem to be mentally retarded. The brain damage is believed to result from the combined deleterious effects of the microorganisms and of the host's inflammatory response, particularly the increased concentration of tumor necrosis factor-α and interleukin-1 (IL-1) in the spinal fluid. One study using rabbits as experimental animals demonstrated significantly lower levels of tumor necrosis factor-α in spinal fluid when dexamethasone was administered simultaneously with the antibiotic, ceftriaxone. Other studies using dexamethasone therapy in 260 infants with bacterial meningitis demonstrated that the steroid-treated patients had a statistically significant reduction in meningeal inflammation and in the incidence of moderate-to-profound hearing impairment compared with those given a placebo. The precipitating event that determines whether an individual will be an asymptomatic carrier or succumb to an overt infection is not understood, but this may be initiated by other respiratory infections. As shall be seen, the severity of the infection is inversely

A Closer Look

Although many viruses and bacteria are capable of invading the central nervous system (CNS), it is not always clear just how these agents cross the blood–brain barrier. Some may spread contiguously from an adjacent site of infection, whereas others may move along peripheral nerves (Herpes simplex, rabies, *Listeria monocytogenes*). Still others may cause damage to the blood–brain barrier, permitting ready access to the CNS. For many others, however, such damage is absent early in the course of the disease and one must postulate yet another mechanism for entry into the CNS. One proposal, dubbed the "Trojan horse mechanism," suggests that some organisms are carried into the CNS while growing intracellularly in monocytes. What data is available to support this theory?

The CSF compartment possesses a population of resident macrophages that are similar to macrophages in other organs. The monocytic origin of such macrophages has been difficult to prove, but monocytes labeled with colloidal carbon or fluorescent latex particles have been shown to enter the CSF compartment. There have also been at least two separate reports that monocytes could carry bacteria-sized particles into the CNS or the CSF, or both. So, it seems fairly well established that monocytes possess the potential of transporting biologic material into the CNS/CSF and, in a couple of cases this has been reported to occur. The first case was *Streptococcus suis* type 2, the most common cause of generalized meningitis in pigs and also a cause of meningitis in humans. The Trojan horse concept has also been proposed for the Lentiviruses, which include Visna virus (causing a chronic progressive encephalitis in sheep) and human immunodeficiency virus.

How about *Haemophilus influenzae* type b (Hib)? It has been established that although encapsulated Hib are resistant to antibody-independent, complement-mediated lysis, they can undergo phagocytosis by macrophage populations of the liver and spleen. Moreover, they can survive and replicate within these macrophages. Such observations have led to the proposal that these sequestered bacteria are able to enter the CNS while in their intracellular environment. Thus, it appears that the Trojan horse mechanism of entry may account for the entry of a number of different pathogens into the CNS.

proportional to the presence of circulating antibodies to the specific capsular carbohydrate.

Interestingly, encapsulated *H influenzae* organisms are able to survive and replicate within macrophages, and it is thought by some investigators that they may enter the cerebrospinal fluid while inside a macrophage.

Acute epiglottitis is another serious disorder produced by type b *H influenzae*. In this case, an apparently healthy child suddenly has acute respiratory distress and may need immediate hospitalization for relief from the obstruction of the air passages. Usually, the epiglottis is markedly swollen, red, and edematous (filled with fluid). If acute epiglottitis is not treated promptly, commonly by tracheotomy, the child may suffocate. Acute epiglottitis also occurs in adults, and of 56 cases reported in Rhode Island over an 8-year period, 4 died from acute airway constriction.

H influenzae also is the most common cause of septic arthritis in children younger than 2 years of age and of cellulitis, which occurs in children younger than 2 years of age but rarely in adults.

Nonencapsulated Strains of *Haemophilus influenzae*

The nontypeable strains of *H influenzae* are well established as an important pathogen in adults and children. Such strains rarely cause systemic disease, but mucous membrane infections are common, including sinusitis, bronchitis, alveolitis, bronchiolitis, conjunctivitis, and otitis media. Infection of the female genital tract with nontypeable strains is common, and *H influenzae* neonatal sepsis with about a 50% mortality rate is being seen more often in neonates born to infected mothers. Pneumonia also occurs, particularly in the elderly and in adults with chronic bronchitis.

VIRULENCE FACTORS OF *HAEMOPHILUS INFLUENZAE*

The ability to resist phagocytosis seems to be the most obvious characteristic that differentiates virulent from avirulent strains of *H influenzae* and, like many other pathogenic bacteria, this property is manifested in a capsule. However, there must be additional factors intrinsic within the type b capsule inasmuch as essentially all systemic disease occurring in otherwise healthy persons is because of *H influenzae* type b. Some clinical isolates of *H influenzae* possess fimbriae that extend out beyond the capsule. These fimbriae promote bacterial adherence to oropharyngeal epithelial cells, and antibodies to the homologous fimbriae prevent adherence. Multiple serotypes are known to occur, and a monovalent fimbriae vaccine confers protection against only the homologous strain. The role of fimbriae as a virulence factor in establishing meningitis is unclear because most of the isolates from nasopharynges of children with invasive disease are non-

fimbriated. Moreover, all strains isolated from blood and cerebrospinal fluid lack detectable fimbriae.

There are also several outer membrane proteins that may serve some function in adhesion or in invasion of host tissues because, in some cases, antibodies directed against these proteins may be protective. Moreover, nonencapsulated strains are able to cause a chronic bronchitis in adults and otitis media in children. Such strains have been reported to possess fimbriae that adhere to nasopharyngeal epithelial cells, and in experimental animals, it has been shown that a fimbriae vaccine confers protection against otitis media when animals are challenged with a strain carrying homologous fimbriae.

H influenzae also produces a protease that specifically cleaves the heavy chain of IgA1. It is not known just how this contributes to its virulence, but it is curious that *Neisseria meningitidis* and *Neisseria gonorrhoeae* are also able to carry out this hydrolysis.

LABORATORY DIAGNOSIS OF *H INFLUENZAE* INFECTIONS

Suspected cases of *H influenzae* meningitis must have immediate treatment because untreated cases have a high mortality rate. Survivors have a high incidence of neurologic disorders, including mental retardation, blindness, hydrocephalus, and convulsions. Gram stains of sedimented spinal fluid specimens that show pleomorphic gram-negative rods are assumed to be *H influenzae*, but they should be mixed with specific type b antiserum and observed for a positive quellung reaction. Fluorescently labeled antibodies also are of value for identifying *H influenzae* in sedimented spinal fluid specimens.

The spinal fluid specimens may also be subjected to countercurrent electrophoresis against specific antiserum to the polysaccharide capsule. The formation of a line of precipitate provides evidence for the presence of *H influenzae* capsular material. Enzyme-linked immunosorbent assay (ELISA), as well as latex particle agglutination using beads that have been coated with antibodies to the type b capsule, also provide a mechanism for the rapid identification of soluble capsular material in spinal fluid.

Both blood and spinal fluid should be cultured on chocolate agar and incubated at 37°C in a candle jar or in a CO_2 incubator. Isolated organisms can be assayed for X and V factor requirements: a trypticase-soy-agar plate is streaked; and sterile disks containing X factor, V factor, and a combination of X and V factors (available commercially) are placed onto the surface of the agar. Growth limited to the vicinity of the paper disks will make obvious any X or V factor requirement (Fig. 28-2). A satellite phenomenon also can be demonstrated if a blood-agar plate is streaked with the unknown organisms, and a small loopful of *Staphylococcus aureus* is pinpointed on the plate. The hemolytic staphylococci will release both X and V factors from the red blood cells, and satellite

TABLE 28-2
Characteristics of *H influenzae* Type b Conjugate Vaccines

Vaccine (Producer)	Protein Carrier
HbOC, HibTITER (Lederle-Praxis Biologicals)	CRM$_{197}$ mutant *Corynebacterium diphtheriae* protein
PRP-OMP, PedvaxHIB (Merck Sharpe & Dohme)	*Neisseria meningitidis* outer membrane protein complex
PRP-T, ActHIB Pasteur Merieus Serum et Vaccins	Tetanus toxoid conjugate

growth of the *Haemophilus,* occurring only in the vicinity of the *Staphylococcus* colony, will be seen.

TREATMENT AND CONTROL OF *H INFLUENZAE* INFECTIONS

Because of the ubiquity of *H influenzae*, most persons acquire protective antibodies between the ages of 3 and 8 years. The newborn is usually protected for 3 to 6 months by passively acquired maternal antibody, and the danger period begins at about 6 months and lasts until the acquisition of bactericidal antibody. Most individuals acquire such antibody either by becoming asymptomatic carriers or from an undiagnosed respiratory disease.

Vaccines consisting of the purified type b capsule material have been shown to be nontoxic and to stimulate the formation of protective antibodies in children older than 18 months of age. Because such vaccines are poor immunogens in children younger than 18 months of age, considerable effort has been expended to produce a vaccine that will induce the formation of antibodies to type b polysaccharide in children aged 2 to 18 months. This has been accomplished by conjugating the capsular polysaccharides capsular material to large protein molecules. Three such vaccines are licensed for use in the United States to be given at 2 months of age. In controlled trials, these vaccines provided protection to 93% to 100% of the recipients. Table 28-2 shows the composition of the conjugate vaccines and Table 28-3 lists the recommended vaccination schedule.

Another report also demonstrated that women who were immunized with *H influenzae* type b polysaccharide capsule during their eighth month of pregnancy secreted

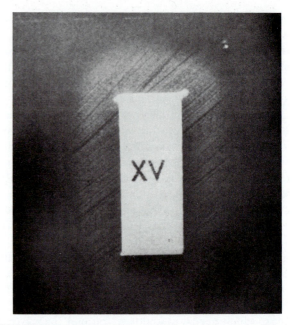

FIGURE 28-2 In this preparation, colonies of *Haemophilus influenzae* on tryptic soy agar grow only around a paper strip impregnated with X and V factors.

in their breast milk more than 20 times as much antibodies to *H influenzae* as did nonimmunized women. Moreover, the level of antibody in breast milk remained high during the 6-month study, indicating that this procedure could also be an important control of neonatal *H influenzae* infections.

Passive immunization using hyperimmune human serum also has proved effective in infants as young as 2 months of age. Such treatment, however, should probably be reserved for high-risk children or immunodeficient infants.

Rifampin has been used successfully as a prophylaxis for children who are exposed at home or in day-care centers, and it is recommended for *H influenzae* contacts of all ages who develop symptoms of invasive disease, such as fever or headache, in a household with another child younger than 4 years of age.

Formerly, ampicillin was the therapy of choice for infections with *H influenzae*; with the increase in reported ampicillin-resistant organisms, however, ampicillin sensitivity is no longer reliable. Chloramphenicol also is usually

TABLE 28-3
Recommended *H influenzae* Vacinnation Schedule

Vaccine	2 mo	4 mo	6 mo	12 mo	15 mo
HbOC	Dose 1	Dose 2	Dose 3		Booster
PRP-OMP	Dose 1	Dose 2		Booster	
PRP-T	Dose 1	Dose 2	Dose 3		

effective and is used when ampicillin resistance is suspected. Chloramphenicol-resistant strains have, however, been reported. Moxalactam also may be effective.

Haemophilus aegyptius

Haemophilus aegyptius is the etiologic agent of a common conjunctivitis informally referred to as *pink-eye*. Because of its similarity to *H influenzae*, this organism is also called *Haemophilus influenzae* biotype *aegyptius*. The illness may be mild or severe, varying from vascular infection of the conjunctiva with a slight discharge to severe irritation with lacrimation, swelling of the lids, photophobia, and a mucopurulent discharge.

The infection can be diagnosed by microscopic examination of smears and growth of the organism on chocolate agar. Topical application of tetracycline ointment usually provides effective treatment.

A series of severe and frequently fatal infections from *H influenzae* biotype *aegyptius* was described in Brazil. Termed Brazilian purpuric fever, this invasive disease characteristically begins with a purulent conjunctivitis, which in a small percentage of patients progresses to an overwhelming endotoxemia resulting in irreversible shock. The clinical presentation is similar to that of meningococcemia.

Haemophilus ducreyi

Haemophilus ducreyi is the cause of the sexually transmitted disease chancroid (soft chancre), which is characterized by an ulcer on the genitals, with marked swelling and pain. Regional lymph nodes swell and may become suppurative. Autoinoculation may occur, resulting in multiple lesions.

The diagnosis is confirmed by smears and cultures. Both sulfamethoxazole/trimethoprim and oral erythromycin have been used to treat infections.

Gardnerella (Haemophilus) vaginalis

Gardnerella vaginalis frequently is found in the vaginal discharge of women whose diagnosis is nonspecific vaginitis. The disease is characterized by a foul-smelling discharge that does not result from other known causes of vaginitis such as *Trichomonas* or *Candida*. This organism also is isolated from the normal female genitourinary tract, and it has been suggested that the vaginitis may result from a mixed infection with *G vaginalis* and vaginal anaerobes. An initial diagnosis can be postulated by a microscopic examination of the vaginal discharge and noticing the presence of "clue" cells, which are vaginal epithelial cells studded with tiny coccobacilli. *G vaginalis* does not

require either the X or V factor, prompting its recent exclusion from the genus *Haemophilus*.

BORDETELLA

Bordetella pertussis

Bordetella pertussis, the causative agent of whooping cough, was isolated and described in 1906 by bacteriologists Jules Bordet and Octave Gengou. It is a fragile, gram-negative coccobacillus that is nonmotile but may be encapsulated.

B pertussis does not require either the X or V factors to grow, but it does need an enriched medium to which have been added such substances as blood or starch. The organisms are most commonly grown on a potato blood glycerol agar called Bordet-Gengou medium.

EPIDEMIOLOGY AND PATHOGENESIS OF WHOOPING COUGH

Whooping cough is an acute infection of the respiratory tract involving primarily the ciliated epithelial cells of the bronchi and trachea. After an incubation period, the disease begins with a catarrhal stage characterized by sneezing and a mild, but irritating, cough. After 1 to 2 weeks, it enters the paroxysmal stage, in which the cough may become violent. These episodes of violent coughing are often followed by a "whoop" on inspiration, and it is this characteristic whoop that gives the disease its name. The paroxysms of coughing may be so severe that cyanosis, vomiting, and convulsions follow, completely exhausting the patient. The paroxysmal state may be prolonged (8 to 10 weeks) and is followed by a convalescent state that lasts an additional 2 to 4 weeks.

The incubation period usually is 7 to 10 days after contact with the respiratory discharges of an infected individual. The organisms may be transmitted either by direct contact, by droplets, or from freshly contaminated articles. Major spread probably occurs in the catarrhal stage before the disease is diagnosed. In this stage, the organisms are present in the nasopharynx, and, when the individual coughs (even though the cough is not severe), the organisms are expelled and sprayed through the air. Unfortunately, a person is isolated only after whooping begins, past the stage at which an individual is an important source of spread of the disease. Healthy carriers have not been recognized, but it is generally believed that adults who have lost much of their immunity become infected and are the primary source of infection for children. This was substantiated when 34 of 130 university students with a persistent cough of at least 6 days were shown to have evidence of *B pertussis* infection. In another outbreak in a nursing home, 38 of 105 elderly people with persistent coughs became seropositive for *B pertussis*.

VIRULENCE DETERMINANTS

Few organisms have been studied as intensely as *B pertussis* to understand virulence at a molecular level. The results have been the isolation and characterization of a host of protein fractions that have been given names such as histamine-sensitizing factor, lymphocytosis-promoting factor, mouse protective factor, and islet-activating factor. These organisms also possess a gram-negative endotoxin that may be involved in the symptomatology of the infection.

Although gaps still exist in the knowledge of the pathogenesis of *B pertussis*, it is possible to categorize the primary virulence factors as (1) pertussis toxin, (2) extracytoplasmic adenylate cyclase, (3) filamentous hemagglutinin (FHA), (4) pertactin, and (5) tracheal cytotoxin. Other factors that may be associated with virulence but have not been well characterized include a pertussis heat-labile toxin (PEHLT) and a hemolysin.

Pertussis Toxin

As is described for many other bacterial toxins, pertussis toxin (PT) can be dissociated into A and B subunits. The A subunit, designated S-1, contains the enzymatic activity; four nonidentical subunits, termed S-2, S-3, S-4, and S-5, are combined to form the B oligomer, which functions to bind the toxin to specific cell receptors. After binding to the cell, the A subunit (S-1) crosses the cell membrane, hydrolyzes NAD to nicotinamide and ADP-ribose, and then transfers the ADP-ribose to the α subunit of several G regulatory proteins involved in the control of adenylate cyclase, phospholipase-C, and ion channels.

These membrane-bound G proteins act as regulatory elements to carry a message from a hormone-receptor complex to the enzyme, adenylate cyclase. There seems to be a number of such G proteins, but this chapter focuses on only those two that have been directly implicated in adenylate cyclase activity and that are modified by bacterial toxins, namely, G_s and G_i. In the basal state, both G_s and G_i have the nucleotide GDP tightly bound to their subunits. After binding to the appropriate agonist or inhibitory agent, GDP is released, and GTP is bound to the α subunit. It is at this point that the action of the stimulatory G_s and the G_i differ.

$G_{s\alpha} \cdot$ GTP appears to react directly with the catalytic unit of the adenylate cyclase, stimulating its activity to form more cAMP. This will continue until a GTPase hydrolyzes the GTP to GDP, leaving the $G_{s\alpha}$ in an inactive state. As described for choleragen and *Escherichia coli* labile toxin (LT), ADP-ribosylation of $G_{s\alpha}$ stabilizes the $G_\alpha \cdot$ GTP, resulting in a continual stimulation of adenylate cyclase.

G_i, the inhibitory component of adenylate cyclase stimulation, seems to function through G_s. Thus, when confronted with an inhibitory stimulus such as α_2-adrenergic or muscarinic agonists, G_i dissociates into $G_{i\alpha}$ and $G_{i\beta\gamma}$ subunits, increasing the available pool of $\beta\gamma$ subunits. These interact with free $G_{s\alpha} \cdot$ GTP reconstituting the complete, but inactive, G_s complex. Then, when G_s again becomes stimulated through its stimulatory agonists, the $\beta\gamma$ subunits are again released and bind to $G_{i\alpha} \cdot$ GTP to form the inactive G_i.

So, where does PT fit into this complex scheme? PT can ADP-ribosylate the α subunit of several G proteins. However, because little is known about G_o and because G_t is confined to retinal rods, this discussion is limited to the effect of PT on G_i.

The ADP-ribosylation of G_i results in a stabilization of the G_i complex, even in the presence of inhibitory agonists. There are, therefore, insufficient free $\beta\gamma$ subunits to bind to the activated $G_{s\alpha} \cdot$ GTP, leaving them in a continual stimulated state. Thus, even though PT ADP-ribosylates G_i, it is the activated G_s that continues to stimulate adenylate cyclase, leading to a sustained elevation of cAMP. This increased level of cAMP results in the activation of protein kinases, which in turn phosphorylate a number of cellular proteins that are involved in the regulation of cell growth. Other major effects of PT include a histamine-sensitizing effect, resulting in a high susceptibility to anaphylaxis; an islet-activating effect observed by insulin synthesis, resulting in hypoglycemia; and a lymphocytosis-promoting effect. These effects may, in part, be a result of the increased levels of cAMP, but it is possible that some may be because of a polyclonal activation of T cells induced by PT.

Extracytoplasmic Adenylate Cyclase

The procaryotic adenylate cyclase that is produced by virulent *B pertussis* possesses the novel property that it can be activated as much as 1000-fold by the eucaryotic calcium-dependent regulatory protein calmodulin. When taken into eucaryotic cells, this enzyme synthesizes cAMP from cellular ATP. Interestingly, the *B pertussis* adenylate cyclase seems to function independently of normal cellular regulatory mechanisms.

Many types of cells are affected by the bacterial adenylate cyclase and in each instance the biologic response is correlated with the elevated cAMP levels. Insofar as *B pertussis* virulence is concerned, it is the cAMP-induced inhibition of phagocytic cell response that may be most important. This is manifested in polymorphonuclear neutrophils by blocking chemotaxis and by preventing the myeloperoxidase-dependent production of H_2O_2, as well as by inhibiting the generation of superoxide. It has been shown that *B pertussis* is able to enter into macrophages and epithelial cells, and it seems possible that the extracytoplasmic adenylate cyclase is delivered directly into the cytoplasm of the infected cell.

Filamentous Hemagglutinin

Whooping cough is the result of a noninvasive infection in which the bordetellae display a marked trophism for respiratory cilia. It follows, therefore, that the ability to produce the disease is absolutely dependent on adhesins that will bind the organisms to the cilia. Two such adhesins are involved, and it seems that both are necessary for efficient binding of the organisms to the cilia. One adhesin, FHA, exists as filamentous rods extending from the cell surface of the bacterium. FHA is a protein that acquired its name through its ability to agglutinate erythrocytes, but its role as a virulence factor is to bind the bordetellae to the respiratory cilia. Antibodies directed against FHA are protective.

The second adhesin required for bacterial binding to respiratory cilia is the PT described in the previous section. The exact mechanism whereby PT acts as an adhesin is not fully understood, but mutants lacking PT are unable to bind to cilia even though FHA is present. Surprisingly, mutants lacking FHA are also unable to adhere, even if they are PT-positive organisms. Thus, it seems that these two adhesins must act in concert to form a bivalent bridge between the bacterium and the carbohydrate receptors on the cilia. Interestingly, organisms lacking either FHA or PT could be reconstituted to adherence by incubating them in the presence of the exogenous surface component they were missing, demonstrating that either FHA or PT could bind to the bordetellae and restore their ability to adhere to respiratory cilia.

Virulent *B pertussis* organisms also possess fimbriae which are distinct from FHA. These fimbrial components are agglutinogens that may contribute to adherence in addition to serving as serotyping antigens.

Pertactin

Pertactin is a 69-kd surface protein that promotes the attachment of the bacterium to mammalian cells; mutants unable to make pertactin adhere 30% to 40% less efficiently to such cells. Cell invasion occurs when pertactin recognizes and binds to a class of integrins on macrophages and epithelial cells. This is similar to that described for cell invasion by members of the genus *Yersinia*. Its importance in the virulence of the organism is suggested by the observation that antibodies to pertactin are protective in animal studies.

Tracheal Cytotoxin

One of the characteristic symptoms of an infection by *B pertussis* is the severe cough, from which the respiratory illness gets its name. The severity of the cough is probably correlated with the destruction of the ciliated respiratory epithelial cells, resulting in an accumulation in the lungs of mucus, bacteria, and inflammatory debris. The nature of this cell destruction came to light only within the last decade, and the activity that causes the specific killing of ciliated respiratory epithelial cells has been termed tracheal cytotoxin (TCT).

Although *B pertussis* produces a variety of toxins, TCT is the only one able to reproduce the respiratory epithelial cytopathology that is characteristic of pertussis. The nature of TCT has been shown by William Goldman at Washington University (St. Louis) to be a building block or breakdown product of gram-negative cell-wall peptidoglycan (Fig. 28-3). The observation that this toxin accumulates in culture supernatants of *B pertussis* during logarithmic growth suggests that it may originate from peptidoglycan precursors that were not incorporated into preexisting peptidoglycan chains. The mechanism whereby TCT accomplishes cell destruction seems to result from its ability to induce the intracellular production of IL-1 in the ciliated epithelial cells. This is supported by the observation that exogenously added IL-1 could reproduce the pathology of TCT in hamster tracheal organ cultures. Moreover, the addition of TCT to respiratory epithelial cells stimulated the production of intracellular IL-1. A similar toxin also has been shown to be produced by the gonococcus and, in cases of pelvic inflammatory disease, it is probably involved in damage to the ciliated cells of the fallopian tubes.

Also, notice that TCT is structurally identical to the human slow-wave sleep-promoting factor, FS_u, and it has been postulated that muramyl peptides of bacterial origin may play a role in the normal regulation of mammalian sleep. Interestingly, the time courses of sleep effects stimulated by recombinant IL-1 or TCT in rabbits are consistent with the hypothesis that muramyl peptides modulate sleep by triggering the production of IL-1. The presence of TCT in whole cell pertussis vaccines might also explain

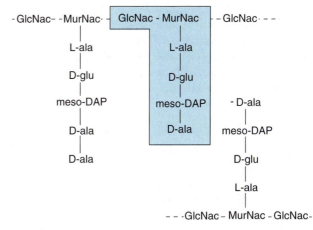

FIGURE 28-3 Tracheal cytotoxin shown within box. Notice its relationship to that of peptidoglycan from gram-negative cells. GlcNac, *N*-acetylglucosamine; MurNac, *N*-acetylmuramic acid; L-ala, L-alanine; D-Glu, D-glutamic acid; meso-DAP, mesodiaminopimelic acid.

the drowsiness that characteristically follows pertussis immunization.

Heat-Labile or Dermonecrotic Toxin

All species of *Bordetella* produce a toxin, the PEHLT or dermonecrotic toxin, which produce a necrotic lesion when injected intradermally into an experimental animal such as the guinea pig. The role of this toxin in human disease is unknown, but it is postulated to cause a severe inflammation in swine that have *Bordetella bronchiseptica* colonized on their nasal mucosa. Purified PELHT displays a 50% lethal dose for mice of about 0.3 μg, and the minimal cytotoxic dose for embryonic bovine lung cells is about 2 ng/mL. PELHT is a poor antigen that does not stimulate the production of antibodies in humans.

PHASE CHANGES IN *BORDETELLA PERTUSSIS*

It has been known for many years that freshly isolated, virulent organisms undergo a series of changes when cultivated in the laboratory. These modifications were manifested by changes in colonial morphologic features and a loss of virulence and were designated as phases 1, 2, 3, and 4, with phase 1 being highly virulent and phase 4 avirulent. Because phase 4 organisms had lost the ability to produce most of the virulence factors, it was assumed that this change resulted from a series of mutations and, as a result, was irreversible.

This assumption has been shown by Alison Weiss and Stanley Falkow to be incorrect. Their data, obtained by transposon mutagenesis, support the conclusion that a single gene, termed *vir,* produces a product that acts as a positive inducer for the virulence-associated genes. Thus, single mutations could eliminate any one of the virulence determinants, or a single mutation in the inducer gene could prevent the synthesis of all virulence determinants. The observation that organisms in phase 4 could revert to phase 1, as well as the fact that the insertion or loss of a single transposon could turn "off" or "on" these virulence factors, supports their conclusion. The ability to effect such phase changes might serve as a defense mechanism to escape immune detection.

LABORATORY DIAGNOSIS OF WHOOPING COUGH

Cultures for pertussis are collected by using a swab of calcium alginate (cotton is inhibitory for growth of the organisms) on a fine, flexible wire. The swab is inserted into one nostril and gently pushed in until it reaches the posterior nares, where it is left while the patient coughs. The swab is then plated on Bordet-Gengou medium and incubated for several days. The organisms die off rapidly, and best results are obtained if the plate is inoculated immediately after the nasal swab. Because *B pertussis* is

resistant to penicillin, the swab may be dampened with a drop of penicillin to limit the growth of throat contaminants.

Organisms growing on the culture plates may be identified by using specific antiserum for an agglutination test or by staining with fluorescently labeled specific antibody. This latter staining technique can also be used to stain smears taken from the nasopharynx.

TREATMENT AND CONTROL OF WHOOPING COUGH

Several antibiotics are used in the treatment of whooping cough, although results are not entirely satisfactory. Erythromycin is the antibiotic of choice, and its use eliminates the organisms from the nasopharynx in 3 to 4 days. Reversion to a positive culture occurs occasionally, possibly because of the intracellular location of some organisms. Tetracycline and chloramphenicol also can be used. Antibiotic therapy also lessens the number of secondary infections, such as bronchitis or pneumonia, and decreases the severity of the disease.

The introduction of an effective vaccine has markedly reduced the incidence of whooping cough. Formerly, almost every child had this disease during the early years of life, whereas in 1994, only 3590 cases of pertussis were reported in the United States. The vaccine used in the United States consists of heat-killed or thimerosal-treated phase-1 *B pertussis* organisms that are usually incorporated with diphtheria and tetanus toxoids (commonly called DPT). This vaccine contains PT, adenylate cyclase, and FHA, as well as structural components of the cell such as pertactin, endotoxin, and outer membrane agglutinogens. Unfortunately, it may cause a local reaction in many infants and, on rare occasions, can cause serious systemic toxic reactions, including brain damage and death. For example, a government report indicates that over the last 10 years, 5 to 20 children died annually after DPT immunization, and about 50 had permanent brain damage each year. These figures are statistically small compared with the many thousands of infant deaths that occurred before the advent of pertussis immunization, but they have been the cause of considerable concern for parents, vaccine producers, and legislatures.

In 1984, two of the three vaccine manufacturers in the United States announced that because of legal liabilities, they were ceasing to produce the pertussis vaccine. This prompted Congress in 1986 to pass a no-fault vaccine injury compensation bill that awards monetary damages from a trust fund formed from excise taxes on vaccines. As a result, the price of a dose of pertussis vaccine went from 11 cents in 1982 to $11.40 in 1986, of which $8.00 per dose was added to the insurance reserve.

On the other side of the argument, however, are the epidemics of pertussis that have ensued in Japan and England when they stopped using DPT because of fears of severe reactions. England experienced outbreaks of pertussis between 1977 and 1979 that resulted in thousands of cases and 36 deaths, effecting a mortality rate significantly higher than when the vaccine was in use.

The best solution, of course, is to produce a less toxic vaccine that would be used by everyone. One possible example of this is a component vaccine consisting of formalin-treated purified PT and FHA, which has been used in Japan since 1981. This vaccine seems to be effective and less toxic than the killed vaccine. However, in a prospective study of a pertussis outbreak in Japan involving 19 children younger than 2 years of age, they concluded that there was no difference in infection between unimmunized and immunized individuals, but a significant difference existed in the symptoms shown by these two groups. They reported that 8 of 9 immunized children acquired the infection, but only 1 developed typical symptoms, compared with 6 of 10 unimmunized children who developed typical symptoms of whooping cough.

At least six companies are producing an acellular pertussis vaccine. Most of these vaccines contain formalin-treated PT and FHA, although one tried in Sweden contained only detoxified PT. Such vaccines were only 54% to 69% effective, but they did prevent severe disease. In addition, experimental results have demonstrated that the purified B oligomer of PT induces antibodies in the mouse that seem to be protective. Moreover, the gene coding for the five subunits of PT have been cloned in *E coli*, and it seems probable that some day a vaccine will be developed using components arising from cloned sequences from *B pertussis*.

In 1991, the FDA licensed one acellular vaccine for use in the United States, but has recommended that it be used only in the fourth and fifth doses of the DPT series of immunizations. This vaccine is a four-component vaccine containing pertussis toxoid, FHA, pertactin, and type 2 fimbriae. The FDA recommends that DPT vaccine containing whole-cell pertussis vaccine be given at 2, 4, and 6 months of age, and a DPT vaccine containing the acellular pertussis vaccine be given at 15 months and 4 to 6 years of age.

Other *Bordetella* Species

Bordetella parapertussis is a human pathogen that causes a whooping cough syndrome that is milder than that normally seen with *B pertussis*. *Bordetella bronchiseptica* is primarily an animal parasite, and its association with human respiratory disease is unclear. It has, however, been isolated from a nonrespiratory infection in an immunocompromised host. Interestingly, neither of these two species produce PT (even though they contain a nonfunctional gene for PT), but both excrete an extracytoplasmic adenylate cyclase and the PEHLT.

LEGIONELLA

In 1976, a number of fatal cases of pneumonia occurred in individuals attending an American Legion convention in Philadelphia. This disease, subsequently named legionnaires' disease, brought panic to that city and resulted in the closing of one of the city's largest hotels (where the convention was held). The frightening aspect of this sudden epidemic was that it could not be attributed to any known agent.

Legionella pneumophila

Legionella pneumophila eventually was cultured and shown to be the etiologic agent of legionnaires' disease (legionellosis). It is a gram-negative, pleomorphic rod (Fig. 28-4) that does not stain easily with routine stains, explaining the fact that it was first visualized using a silver impregnation technique.

L pneumophila can be grown in guinea pigs, chick embryos, cell cultures, and on Mueller-Hinton medium containing 1% hemoglobin and 1% Isovitalex (a vitamin and amino-acid supplement prepared by BBL Microbiology Systems, Cockeysville, MD) in an atmosphere containing 5% CO_2. The organism has an absolute requirement for cysteine (supplied by the Isovitalex) and for iron (supplied by the hemoglobin).

Legionella organisms contain considerably more branched-chain fatty acids and phosphocholine than other gram-negative bacteria. Using DNA hybridization techniques (see Chap. 2), it has not been possible to identify any other species of bacteria to which it is related, and it can truly be considered a new organism that had never been described before the 1976 epidemic in Philadelphia.

It is known that *L pneumophila* is a facultative intracellular parasite that replicates within alveolar macrophages. The detailed mechanism whereby it prevents a phagolysosomal fusion in infected macrophages is unknown, but it does appear probable that a cellular-type immunity is necessary for recovery.

Fourteen distinct serogroups of *L pneumophila* have been isolated. Antiserum to the serogroup antigen seems to be protective, and each serogroup shows little cross-reactivity with any of the other serogroups. The serogroup-specific antigen is a positively charged polysaccharide (designated the F1 fraction), and it seems to exist as a capsule.

VIRULENCE DETERMINANTS

Legionella pneumophila possesses an endotoxin and produces a hemolysin and a cytotoxin that is lethal for Chinese hamster ovary cells. However, the role of these products in the development of disease is unknown.

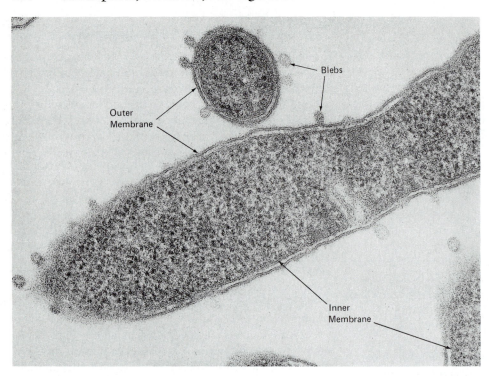

FIGURE 28-4 Electron micrograph of the bacterium causing legionnaires' disease (*Legionnella pneumophila*) prefixed with 1.25% glutaraldehyde, 0.75% formalin, and 0.002% creosol. Both inner (cytoplasmic) and outer membranes can be seen along with several evaginations (blebs) at the outer membrane. (Original magnification ×105,000.)

A series of reports have implicated several proteases secreted by *L pneumophila* as important virulence determinants. These investigators demonstrated that the pathologic changes of legionnaires' disease pneumonia could be reproduced experimentally in guinea pigs by instillation of one of the proteases into their lungs, suggesting that this protease may play an important role in in vivo infections by *L pneumophila*. This organism also secretes a zinc metalloprotease that is both hemolytic and cytotoxic. Moreover, this protease has been cloned in *E coli* and shown to degrade interleukin-2 and to cleave CD4 from human T cells, suggesting that it may contribute to the pathogenesis of *L pneumophila* by impeding T-cell activation and immune function.

It is fairly well-established that infection and pulmonary disease require the intracellular multiplication of the legionellae in alveolar macrophages. Genetic studies have demonstrated a *mip* gene (for macrophage infectivity potentiator), which encodes a 24-kd surface protein that enhances the abilities of *L pneumophila* to parasitize human macrophages and causes pneumonia in experimental animals. In addition, it has been demonstrated that specific antibodies to the *mip* gene product combined with complement promoted the phagocytosis of *L pneumophila*. Many of the legionellae also are taken up by neutrophils, but the role of such organisms in the production of disease is less well understood.

A number of other factors have been described, but none has been sufficiently characterized to pinpoint its role in the production of disease. A summary of such factors include: (1) two peptides which are cytotoxic and lethal for animals and which appear to inhibit phagocytic activation; (2) a phosphatase which blocks superoxide anion (O_2^-) production by stimulated neutrophils; and (3) a hemolysin which has been termed legolysin.

PATHOGENESIS OF LEGIONELLOSIS

After the organism was isolated, it was possible to check for antibodies to *L pneumophila* among survivors of several previous outbreaks for which a cause had never been determined, and it was soon found that this organism causes infections on a worldwide basis. A description of two such epidemics demonstrates the spectrum of illness caused by *L pneumophila*.

Pontiac Fever

In 1968, 144 people, representing 95% of the people working in the county health department in Pontiac, Michigan, developed fever, headache, diarrhea, vomiting, muscle aches, and chest pain. All recovered within 3 or 4 days. Investigation by the Centers for Disease Control demonstrated that guinea pigs exposed to the air in the building contracted pneumonia, but none became ill when the air conditioner was turned off. It was concluded that a defect in the air conditioner, which permitted mist from the cooling condenser to circulate, carried the causative organisms throughout the building. Serum specimens subsequently collected from the exposed guinea pigs were all shown to contain antibodies to *L pneumophila*.

St. Elizabeth's Hospital Epidemic

In 1965, 81 patients at St. Elizabeth's Hospital in Washington, D.C. developed a severe pneumonia, and 14 died. In 1977, a serologic check among the survivors revealed that most possessed antibodies to *L pneumophila,* and it was concluded that the 1965 epidemic was caused by the same organism that caused Pontiac fever and legionnaires' disease.

EPIDEMIOLOGY OF LEGIONELLOSIS

It seems that serologically related strains of *L pneumophila* can cause a spectrum of illnesses ranging from legionnaires' disease, with a 20% mortality rate from pneumonia and shock, to Pontiac fever, in which all infected persons recovered in 2 to 5 days. It has been proposed that Pontiac fever is produced by *Legionella* strains that are unable to invade human cells. Extrapulmonary infections that involve *L pneumophila* include cutaneous abscesses, perirectal abscesses, postoperative wound infections, hepatic abscesses, pericarditis, myocarditis, and bacteremia.

Organisms have been isolated from a number of air-conditioning cooling towers, and such contaminated water is believed to be a source of infection for those inhaling mist from these towers. Mist machines designed to keep produce fresh in supermarkets have also been responsible for a number of cases of legionellosis, some of which were fatal. Strains have also been isolated from creek water in the areas where epidemics have occurred. Outbreaks also have occurred in areas where excavation has taken place, and it is thought that the organisms may reside in the soil, being transmitted to humans on contaminated dust. Most surprising was the report that *Legionella* had been isolated from a large number of hot water systems in hospitals, apartment houses, and homes. A survey of 95 apartments and homes in the Chicago area revealed that 32% of the hot water systems were contaminated with *L pneumophila*. Another survey found *L pneumophila* in 9 of 16 shower heads examined in a Chicago hospital where three persons had contracted legionellosis while they were patients there. This has been an extremely serious problem in hospitals, where reports have indicated that *Legionella* can be responsible for as much as 10% of nosocomial infections in some areas. Nosocomial legionellosis has also been traced to the use of medication nebulizers that had been rinsed with tap water. Eradication of these organisms from hot water systems has required periodic superheating (80°C) followed by flushing and intermittent or continuous hyperchlorination.

In the environment, it seems that the legionellae frequently exist, growing intracellularly in free-living amoebae of the genera *Acanthamoeba* and *Naegleria*; it may well be that such contaminated water supplies are the primary source of community-acquired infections. These organisms seem to be both widespread and hardy in our environment, and it seems that undiagnosed or asymptomatic infections are common. Individuals who are at especially high risk of acquiring overt legionellosis include those who are receiving immunosuppressive drugs and patients who are undergoing surgical procedures requiring general anesthesia.

Paradoxically, even though legionellosis is a respiratory disease and the lung is the only organ consistently involved in fatal infections, person-to-person spread has not been demonstrated. Risk factors that seem to increase the likelihood of infection include immunosuppression, cigarette smoking, chronic pulmonary disease, alcohol consumption, and endotracheal intubation.

Immunity is primarily cell-mediated and activation of the infected macrophage is probably an essential host response to legionellosis. The major macrophage activating factor seems to be IFN-γ, which is released by stimulated lymphocytes.

LABORATORY DIAGNOSIS AND TREATMENT OF LEGIONELLOSIS

A definitive diagnosis of legionellosis requires the isolation and identification of the organism. However, the organism is difficult to isolate, and the diagnosis frequently is based on serologic evidence. Such tests have included both a direct immunofluorescent assay to detect organisms in tissue and an indirect immunofluorescent assay for determining antibody titers to *L pneumophila*. Furthermore, a microagglutination test and a micro-ELISA test have been developed for the detection of antibodies to *L pneumophila*. Detection of *L pneumophila* antigens in the urine is also a convenient and sensitive method of diagnosing the infection. This is performed with a commercial radioimmunoassay kit. Its major disadvantage is that it will detect only disease caused by *L pneumophila* serogroup 1, but because this serogroup causes 70% to 90% of all cases of legionnaires' disease, it would detect the great majority of infections.

Erythromycin is the drug of choice, but isolates are also sensitive to rifampin, and a combination of these two drugs is recommended for severe disease. In addition, a fluoroquinolone antimicrobial a good alternative to a combination of erythromycin and rifampin. Cephalosporin and penicillin are not effective, because the organisms produce a β-lactamase that inactivates them.

Other *Legionella* Species

The isolation of *L pneumophila* in 1976 spurred investigators to look for similar etiologic agents of pneumonia. Thirty-two such species have been isolated and placed in the family Legionellaceae. All are aerobic, flagellated bacilli that are weakly gram-negative, and all can be grown in embryonated eggs or on special media containing cysteine and iron. Sixteen of these species have been implicated in human infections. Of human infections, approximately

85% of cases of legionellosis are due to *L pneumophila* with about 70% of all disease resulting from serogroup 1 and about 10% resulting from serogroup 6.

One organism, originally termed the *Pittsburgh pneumonia agent*, has been given the name *Legionella micdadei*. *L micdadei* is weakly acid-fast and does not share any antigenic determinants with *L pneumophila*. This organism has been isolated from moist environments, such as respiratory therapy equipment and cooling towers, and the fact that most adults possess some antibody to this agent suggests that it is ubiquitous in nature and that inapparent or undiagnosed infections are common. Serious and frequently fatal pneumonia has occurred only in individuals who are immunocompromised because of renal transplants, leukemia, or some infection for which corticosteroids were given. *L micdadei* is sensitive to both erythromycin and rifampin, and those individuals in whom an early diagnosis was made responded to treatment with erythromycin.

Little is known concerning the other species of Legionella. First termed the Wiga agent,* *L bozemanii* originally was isolated from the lung of a patient with fatal pneumonia by inoculation of the lung tissue into a guinea pig. It has been isolated from another fatal case of pneumonia, grown on artificial media, and shown to be morphologically and metabolically related to the members of Legionellaceae.

Legionella dumoffii was first grown from organisms found in air-conditioning cooling towers, and it has since been isolated from a patient with fatal pneumonia.

Thus, is seems that there is a large family of these organisms widespread in nature. Their ubiquity is attested to by reports that about half of the air samples (containing airborne water droplets) near the erupting Mount Saint Helens showed abundant levels of various *Legionella* bacteria. *L pneumophila* obviously can cause disease in normal healthy adults, whereas the other species of *Legionella* appear to be only weakly virulent, causing overt disease only in immunocompromised individuals or in persons who may be subjected to an overwhelming initial contact with the organisms.

Bibliography

JOURNALS

Aoyama T, et al. Efficacy of acellular pertussis vaccine in young infants. J Infect Dis 1993;167:483.

Bart KJ. National vaccine program and national vaccine injury compensation program. ASM News 1991;57:125.

Catlin W. *Gardnerella vaginalis*: characteristics, clinical considerations, and controversies. Clin Microbiol Rev 1992;5:213.

Dowling JN, Saha AK, Glew RH. Virulence factors of the family Legionellaceae. Microbiol Rev 1992;56:32.

Edelstein PH. Legionnaires' disease. Clin Infect Dis 1993;16:741.

Heiss LN, et al. Interleukin-1 linked to the respiratory epithelial cytopathology of pertussis. Infect Immun 1993;61:3123.

Morse SA. Chancroid and *Haemophilus ducreyi*. Clin Microbiol Rev 1989;2:137.

Odio CM, et al. The beneficial effects of early dexamethasone administration in infants and children with bacterial meningitis. N Engl J Med 1991;324:1525.

---

* *L bozemanii* was isolated in 1959 from a patient named Wiga, who died 2 days later from bronchopneumonia.

Essentials of Medical Microbiology, Fifth Edition, edited by Wesley A. Volk,
Bryan M. Gebhardt, Marie-Louise Hammarskjöld, and Robert J. Kadner.
Lippincott-Raven Publishers, Philadelphia © 1996.

Chapter 29

Gram-Positive Spore-Forming Bacilli

Five different genera of bacteria produce endospores (see Chap. 16), but only two are of medical importance: *Bacillus* and *Clostridium.*

Bacillus

The genus *Bacillus* contains a heterogeneous group of organisms that are gram-positive, endospore-forming rods whose metabolism is either aerobic or facultatively anaerobic. Metabolically, some species carry out a homolactic fermentation, some a butanediol fermentation, and others a modified mixed-acid fermentation. In all likelihood, future taxonomists will subdivide this genus into several genera, but because *Bacillus anthracis* and *Bacillus cereus* are the only species that are pathogenic for humans, additional subdivisions should not provide undue hardship for the medical microbiologist.

BACILLUS ANTHRACIS

Bacillus anthracis, the causative agent of anthrax, is a large, facultatively anaerobic rod (Fig. 29-1). Its isolation by German bacteriologist Robert Koch in 1877 marked the beginning of modern medical microbiology, because it was, in part, Koch's work with this organism that was responsible for the development of the well-known Koch's postulates.

Antigenic Classification

There is only one antigenic type of *B anthracis,* and it contains three major types of cell antigens: (1) a cell-wall polysaccharide made up of equimolar amounts of *N*-acetylglucosamine and D-galactose, (2) a capsular polypeptide that is a polymer of γ-D-glutamic acid, and (3) a complex of protein toxins. The capsule is unusual in that it contains only the D (or unnatural) isomer of the amino acid; furthermore, the virulence of the organism depends, in part, on the antiphagocytic activity of this capsular material.

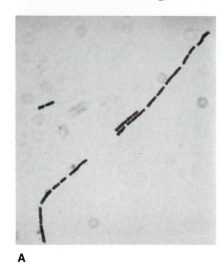

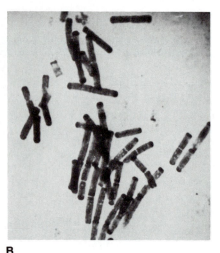

A   B

FIGURE 29-1 Giemsa-stained cells of *Bacillus anthracis*. (Original magnification about ×2000.) **A.** Chains of cells after 18 hours in nutrient broth. **B.** *B anthracis* as it appears when growing in animals (media was supplied with all constituents necessary for antigen production). Notice the broader cells, square corners, and irregularly stained cytoplasm.

Epidemiology of Anthrax

Anthrax is primarily a disease of sheep, goats, cattle, and, to a lesser extent, other herbivorous animals. Although in the United States it is found only in a few areas (Louisiana, Texas, California, Nebraska, and South Dakota), it is a worldwide problem, especially in parts of Europe, Asia, and Africa. Once the disease is established in an area, bacterial endospores from infected or dead animals are able to contaminate the soil and, because of the resistant endospores, the pasture areas remain infectious for other animals for many years. In most animal infections, the spores enter the body by way of abrasions in the oral or intestinal mucosa, and after entering the bloodstream, they germinate and multiply to tremendous numbers, causing death in 2 to 3 days.

Humans become infected through the skin by contact with hides of infected animals or by inhaling the spores from infected hides. Because the pulmonary form of the disease occurs frequently in those persons engaged in sorting sheeps' wool or goats' hair, it has been referred to as *woolsorter's disease*. The lesion from a skin inoculation (cutaneous infection route) is sometimes called a malignant pustule.

Cutaneous infection is an occupational hazard for persons who handle livestock or work with items derived from contaminated wool or hides. An initial lesion occurring at the site of entry soon develops into a black necrotic area (Fig. 29-2). If the lesion is not treated, the organisms may invade the regional lymph nodes and bloodstream, causing death. The pulmonary form of the disease occurs less frequently than the cutaneous form but is more serious and carries a higher mortality rate.

A seemingly rare source of anthrax infection came to the fore in 1979 when an epidemic of anthrax occurred in Sverdlovsk in the Soviet Union. This epidemic, which is believed to have killed almost 100 people, supposedly originated as gastric anthrax caused by eating anthrax-infected meat. In such cases, it is assumed that the organisms enter the bloodstream from the intestine. Although gastric anthrax is rare in the western world, Soviet textbooks have described previous epidemics of gastric anthrax that resulted in 100% mortality.

Pathogenesis of Anthrax

Until 1955, it was believed that anthrax caused death by its ability to resist phagocytosis, allowing it to grow to tremendous numbers of bacilli that clogged capillaries. This explanation had been termed the "log jam" theory. It is known that this concept is incorrect and that *B anthracis* secretes a highly toxic exotoxin.

The toxin consists of a complex of proteins that has been isolated as three components named edema factor (EF), lethal factor (LF), and protective antigen (PA). None of these factors has any biologic activity by itself. An insight into the mechanism of action of this toxin complex was provided by Stephen Leppla when he discovered that EF is an inactive form of adenylate cyclase, which is activated by eucaryotic calmodulin, and that PA is required to facilitate the entry of EF into cells. Thus, it is similar to other A–B toxins in that PA is analogous

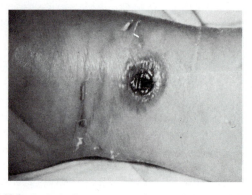

FIGURE 29-2 Lesion of cutaneous anthrax (eighth day of illness) on the arm of a woman who had been a carder in a wool factory.

TABLE 29-1
Components of Anthrax Toxin

Component	Function
EF	Inactive adenylate cyclase activated by calmodulin
LF	Causes pulmonary edema and death in rats; cytolytic for macrophages
PA	Required for the binding of both EF and LF to host cell

EF, edema factor; LF, lethal factor; PA, protective antigen.

to what is termed the B subunit, with EF acting as the A subunit of this toxin. It differs in that unlike the A–B toxins already discussed, PA and EF are secreted as separate components. The end result is an increase in cAMP in polymorphonuclear neutrophils, inhibiting their ability to carry out normal phagocytosis. Thus, as described for *Bordetella pertussis*, the phagocyte impotence seen in anthrax infections results from the secretion of an extracellular adenylate cyclase and its effect on host leukocytes. Table 29-1 summarizes the effects of these components.

Interestingly, PA also is required to show a biologic effect of LF, indicating that PA acts as a common binding subunit for both EF and LF. No enzymatic activity is known for LF, but when injected together with PA, LF causes severe pulmonary edema and death in Fisher 344 rats. PA and LF together are also rapidly cytolytic for macrophages.

When PA binds to a specific receptor on a host cell, a cell-surface protease cleaves off a peptide of about 20 kd to generate a cell-bound 63-kd PA, which possesses a new binding site to which LF and EF bind with high affinity. The resulting complexes of PA_{63}–LF and PA_{63}–EF are then internalized by receptor-mediated endocytosis. Mutants lacking LF produced edema when injected subcutaneously but were not lethal. Mutants missing EF but still producing LF were lethal when injected into susceptible animals.

Notice that the virulence of *B anthracis* is dependent on two separate plasmids, one of which codes for the D-glutamic acid capsule, and the other for the three separate genes of the secreted toxin.

Laboratory Diagnosis of Anthrax

Direct smears and cultures from cutaneous lesions may aid in making a diagnosis; sputum is not usually a good source of organisms. Blood should be cultured from a patient with a suspected case of either cutaneous or pulmonary anthrax. Blood can be injected into a guinea pig or a mouse, and the chains of gram-positive rods can be isolated from the animal's blood in 24 to 36 hours.

Prevention and Control of Anthrax

Ever since Pasteur's celebrated field trial, in which animals were successfully immunized with a living attenuated suspension of *B anthracis*, efforts have been directed toward the production of effective vaccines that possess little or no toxicity. Because killed vaccines are of little value, two different approaches for the stimulation of artificial immunity have been undertaken: (1) the isolation and use of the protective antigenic component of the anthrax toxin, and (2) the use of attenuated living bacteria to induce antitoxic immunity.

Recovery from anthrax provides an animal with a good immunity against subsequent infections; therefore, the use of attenuated vaccines stimulates a more effective and longer-lasting immunity than does the use of toxin preparations. However, all effective living vaccines possess some toxicity, and they have not been used in the United States for humans. The vaccine licensed in the United States for use in humans is an aluminum hydroxide-adsorbed supernatant material from fermentor cultures of a toxigenic, but nonencapsulated strain of *B anthracis*. Unfortunately, it induces a short-lived immunity and requires annual boosters.

PA seems to be the only effective component of the vaccine because neither EF nor LF induced protection. It has been cloned in *Bacillus subtilis*, and guinea pigs immunized by the intramuscular injection of the *B subtilis* cell suspension were protected against challenge by *B anthracis*. PA also has been cloned in vaccinia virus, where it induced at least partial immunity to challenge in guinea pigs and mice. It is, therefore, possible that a cloned source of PA will be used in future anthrax vaccines for humans. The vaccine used in domestic animals consists of a living spore culture, which is designated the Sterne strain. It still carries the plasmid encoding for PA, EF, and LF, but its avirulence is attributed to the loss of the plasmid encoding the antiphagocytic capsule.

Control of anthrax in humans is, therefore, not a

TABLE 29-2
Bacillus anthracis Culture Results for Haitian Goatskin Products imported Into the United States, 1974

Item	No. Cultured	No. Positive	% Positive
Drums	219	22	10
Rugs	58	45	78
Mosaic pictures	55	20	36
Voodoo dolls	13	3	23
Goatskins	10	4	40
Purses	10	1	10
Stool	1	1	100
Hat	1	0	0
Bottle holder	1	0	0
Total	368	96	26

simple matter, particularly for those who are occupationally exposed, but sterilization of wool, hair, and other animal materials capable of transmitting the disease does prevent the spread of the bacilli to persons not normally exposed to infected hides. However, not all such products are sterilized, as exemplified by the person who contracted anthrax from contaminated goat hair fringe on a souvenir drum purchased in Haiti. Other Haitian products using goat hair have been found contaminated with anthrax spores (Table 29-2), and the Centers for Disease Control in Atlanta has recommended that all such items be considered potentially contaminated and that they be given to local health authorities for disposal.

BACILLUS CEREUS

Bacillus cereus is an aerobic, spore-forming, gram-positive rod that is the etiologic agent of a food-borne intoxication.

Pathogenesis of *B cereus* Intoxication

Bacillus cereus produces two distinct clinical forms of food poisoning: (1) an illness with an incubation period of 10 to 12 hours, which is characterized by abdominal pain, profuse diarrhea, and nausea, lasting 12 to 24 hours; and (2) an illness with an incubation period of 1 to 6 hours characterized by vomiting, with or without a mild diarrhea.

These two clinical entities result from the production of two different enterotoxins by *B cereus*. The first, like cholera enterotoxin and LT from *Escherichia coli*, stimulates the adenylate cyclase–cyclic AMP system in intestinal epithelial cells. When fed to rhesus monkeys, this heat-labile toxin causes only diarrhea. The second enterotoxin does not stimulate the synthesis of cAMP, and this heat-stable toxin causes only vomiting when fed to rhesus monkeys.

Epidemiology and Control of *B cereus* Intoxication

Bacillus cereus is readily found in soil and on raw and dried foods, including uncooked rice, a major source of *B cereus* food poisonings. The spores may not be killed during cooking, and will germinate when the boiled rice is left unrefrigerated (to avoid clumping of grains). Brief warming or flash frying does not always destroy the elaborated enterotoxins, particularly the heat-stable toxin. Meat or meat products, as well as cream or pudding preparations, also have been sources of *B cereus* food poisoning. A diagnosis usually is based on finding 10^5 organisms per gram of the incriminated food.

Prevention is best accomplished by the prompt refrigeration of boiled rice and other dried foods that have been cooked. Because the symptoms are mediated by preformed enterotoxins, antibiotic therapy is of no value.

Clostridium

The clostridia are large, gram-positive, endospore-forming rods that are unable to use molecular oxygen as a final electron acceptor. They are also unable to synthesize the prosthetic heme component necessary for a cytochrome system and the enzyme catalase, or superoxide dismutase and must, therefore, be grown under anaerobic conditions. A number of techniques have been devised to grow anaerobic bacteria. One common method adds a reducing agent, such as sodium thioglycolate or dithiothreotol, that will react with the free oxygen in the medium. In other cases, special cultural equipment is employed to remove the oxygen mechanically and to replace the atmosphere with nitrogen, hydrogen, and carbon dioxide. This may be done in a small anaerobic jar or, for laboratories involved in a large amount of anaerobic bacteriology, a large glove box may be used, in which the atmosphere is maintained free of oxygen (Fig. 29-3).

The natural habitats of the clostridia are soil and the intestinal tracts of humans and animals. Some are saccharolytic and will ferment carbohydrates to form products such as butyric acid, butanol, isopropanol, and acetone, whereas others are proteolytic and will metabolize proteins, often yielding foul-smelling amines as end products.

In general, the clostridia are not invasive organisms, and those that produce disease do so as a result of the formation and liberation of destructive enzymes and exotoxins.

CLOSTRIDIUM TETANI

Clostridium tetani, the causative agent of tetanus, is widely distributed in the soil and feces of many animals,

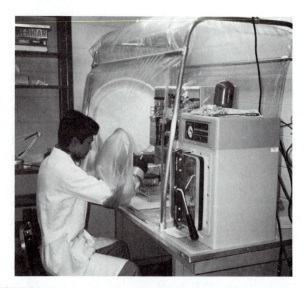

FIGURE 29-3 Anaerobic glove box containing an atmosphere of 85% N_2, 5% CO_2, and 10% H_2. The enclosed gases are constantly circulated through a screen of palladium-coated pellets, which catalyzes a reaction between the H_2 in the atmosphere and any O_2 within the glove box.

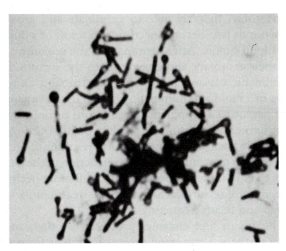

FIGURE 29-4 Cells of *Clostridium tetani* after 24 hours on a cooked-meat glucose medium. Notice spherical terminal endospores. (Original magnification ×4500.)

including humans. The organisms are morphologically characterized by swollen, terminally located endospores that give the spore-forming organism a drumstick appearance (Fig. 29-4).

Antigenic Classification

Clostridium tetani can be divided into a number of serologic types, but the exotoxin released by all of them is serologically identical. Because immunity is directed only against the exotoxin, the antigenic characterization of the species is of little value.

Epidemiology and Pathogenesis of Tetanus

Although widely distributed in soil, *C tetani* essentially has no invasive abilities. To produce tetanus, the spores must be introduced into the body by way of a wound such as a puncture, gunshot, burn, or even an animal bite.

Once inside the body, the presence of necrotic cells (cells no longer receiving oxygenated blood) provides a sufficiently anaerobic environment to allow the germination of the tetanus spores and the subsequent formation of the toxin. The incubation period may vary considerably, and it is possible for the endospores to remain dormant for long periods of time before germinating and producing toxin.

Tetanus toxin (also termed tetanospasmin) is synthesized in the bacterium as a single polypeptide chain, but after its release by lysis of the organism, a bacterial protease cleaves one peptide bond to yield two chains that remain linked together through a disulfide bond. The larger chain (H chain) has a molecular weight of 100,000 daltons, and it possesses the specific receptors that bind the toxin to the neuronal gangliosides. The smaller peptide (L chain) has a molecular weight of 50,000 daltons and is thought to exert the biologic effect of the toxin.

The mechanism of action of the toxin is not fully understood, but it is known that the toxin is first bound to neuronal cells at the neuromuscular junction. The complete toxin then crosses the nerve cell membrane and is transported retrogradely to the inhibitory interneurons. There, by an as yet unknown mechanism, the toxin enters the interneurons and blocks the exocytosis of inhibitory transmitters, namely, glycine and γ-aminobutyric acid. In an analogous situation, tetanus toxin has been reported to inhibit the secretion of lysosomal contents from stimulated human macrophages. The final effect is a spastic paralysis characterized by the convulsive contractions of voluntary muscles. Because the spasms frequently involve the neck and jaws, the disease had been referred to as *lockjaw*. Death ordinarily results from muscular spasms affecting the mechanics of respiration.

Interestingly, all toxin-producing strains of *C tetani* possess a large plasmid, which encodes for the synthesis of the toxin. Loss of the plasmid converts the cell to an avirulent, non–toxin-producing organism.

A second toxin produced by *C tetani* is called tetanolysin. This toxin is related functionally and serologically to streptolysin O and belongs to a large group of oxygen-sensitive hemolysins from a variety of bacteria. In addition to erythrocytes, tetanolysin lyses a variety of cells such as polymorphonuclear neutrophils, macrophages, fibroblasts, ascites tumor cells, and platelets. It is unknown, however, whether it plays any significant role in infections by *C tetani*.

Laboratory Diagnosis of Tetanus

A clinical picture of tetanus with a history of injury usually is sufficient to provide a working diagnosis. A more specific diagnosis requires the isolation and identification of the organisms, as well as the demonstration of tetanus toxin production by the bacterium. However, because the clinical picture is usually conclusive, a complete laboratory diagnosis is not routinely done.

Prevention and Control of Tetanus

Characteristically, tetanus can occur after wounds that are so minor they are soon forgotten. Untreated tetanus may have a fatality rate as high as 60%, and even with therapy, the mortality may be 20% to 30%.

Prevention relies almost entirely on the presence of antibodies that can neutralize the toxin before it enters the interneurons. Good, active immunity can be acquired by the injection of a formalin-inactivated toxin (tetanus toxoid) that may or may not be precipitated with alum. The initial immunization requires three injections (usually begun at about 3 months of age along with diphtheria toxoid and pertussis vaccine). Booster doses are not necessary for 5 to 10 years. Rarely, some persons do form an IgE response, and excessively frequent boosters are, therefore, not recommended.

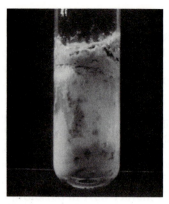

FIGURE 29-6   Stormy fermentation in coagulated milk caused by *Clostridium perfringens.*

lecithin in an egg yolk medium, breaking down the lipid emulsion and, in turn, causing an opaque area to appear around the colony. Individual clostridial species are identified by a series of biochemical tests.

Prevention and Control of Gas Gangrene

Surgical cleansing of wounds to eliminate extraneous material or necrotic tissue is, undoubtedly, the most important control mechanism for gas gangrene. Additionally, antitoxin against the bacterial filtrates can be used when complete surgical debridement is not possible. Antibiotics, such as penicillin or the tetracyclines, are effective in tissues still receiving a blood supply but are of little value in necrotic areas. Hyperbaric oxygen chambers, in which an infected area is placed in a chamber containing pure oxygen under pressure, have been used with some success to stop the growth of these obligate anaerobes.

CLOSTRIDIUM PERFRINGENS AND FOOD POISONING

In addition to being the major etiologic agent in wound infections, *C perfringens* also is an important cause of food poisoning. Most outbreaks follow the ingestion of meat or gravy dishes that are heavily contaminated with vegetative cells of *C perfringens*. Interestingly, *C perfringens* type A strains produce a heat-labile enterotoxin only when the vegetative cells form spores in the small intestine, releasing the newly synthesized enterotoxin. Symptoms of acute abdominal pain and diarrhea begin 8 to 24 hours after ingestion of the contaminated food and usually subside within 24 hours. The toxin appears to bind to specific receptors on the surface of intestinal epithelial cells in the ileum and jejunum. The entire molecule then is inserted into the cell membrane, but does not enter the cell. This induces a change in ion fluxes, affecting cellular metabolism and macromolecular synthesis. As the intracellular Ca^{2+} levels increase, cellular damage and altered membrane permeability occurs, resulting in the loss of cellular fluid and ions.

Rare, but severe, cases of food poisoning, characterized by hemorrhagic enteritis and a high mortality rate, usually are caused by *C perfringens* type C. Such cases have been reported primarily from Germany and New Guinea. Those in New Guinea (known as pig-bel) have been associated with the eating of pork or other high-protein foods. Type C organisms produce a sporulation enterotoxin indistinguishable from that produced by *C perfringens* type A, but they also produce large amounts of α toxin and the lethal necrotizing β toxin. It seems that the severe hemorrhagic enteritis is primarily a result of the action of the β toxin.

C perfringens type C has been reported to occur in the feces of over 70% of the villagers in Papua, New Guinea. Because of a diet low in protein, the organisms in the gut do not ordinarily grow and produce sufficient toxin to cause any pathologic manifestations. Meat and other high-protein foods (which are seldom eaten), however, stimulate growth and toxin production by the clostridia. The disease occurs primarily in young children because of their poor immunity to β toxin. Also, because of a diet low in proteins, such children have an abnormally low level of intestinal proteases that could destroy the toxin before intestinal damage occurs. Furthermore, even this low level of protease activity is inhibited by protease inhibitors present in sweet potatoes that are consumed in large quantities at New Guinea feasts.

Because of the severity and high incidence of this disease, a program of active immunization with *C perfringens* β toxoid was initiated in 1980. Data indicate that the use of this vaccine has resulted in a dramatic decrease in the incidence of pig-bel in the New Guinea highlands.

C perfringens also has been reported to cause an infectious diarrhea, in which the organisms seem to be spread from person to person. Such infections are characterized by large numbers of *C perfringens* and high titers of enterotoxin in stool specimens, as well as a considerably longer duration of illness.

CLOSTRIDIUM DIFFICILE

Pseudomembranous colitis, a severe, necrotizing process that may occur in the large intestine after antibiotic therapy and produces severe diarrhea, has been associated with a number of antimicrobial agents, but the antibiotics clindamycin, ampicillin, amoxicillin, and the cephalosporins have been incriminated most often. One mechanism of this diarrhea was elucidated in 1978, when it was observed that the use of these antibiotics resulted in an overgrowth of an organism in the intestine identified as *Clostridium difficile*. *C difficile* can cause a spectrum of symptoms, ranging from asymptomatic carriage, mild to severe cholera-like diarrhea with 20 or more watery stools per day, and, in its most serious form, pseudomembranous colitis. Evidence indicates that *C difficile* is responsible for virtually all cases of pseudomembranous colitis and for up to 20% of cases of antibiotic-associated diarrhea without colitis. *C difficile* seems to be part of the normal intestinal flora of about 7% to 10% of adults; but only when antibiotic-sensitive organisms are eliminated from the intestine is it able to grow to sufficient numbers to produce disease. Interestingly, as many as 50% to 75% of neonates may become colonized with *C difficile* acquired as a nosocomial infection. Fortunately, most infants remain asymptomatic, but they do serve as a reservoir for the spread of toxigenic *C difficile* to others both in the hospital and at home.

To demonstrate the nosocomial acquisition of this organism in adult patients, the University of Washington (Seattle) carried out a study in which 428 consecutive patients were cultured for *C difficile* over an 11-month period. They reported that 7% had positive results on admission, but of the patients with negative culture results, 21% acquired the organism during their hospital stay. Of these, 37% had diarrhea. Moreover, of the hospital personnel carrying for the patients, 59% were positive for *C difficile*.

C difficile produces disease by the elaboration of two distinct exotoxins, which have been designated as A and B. Toxin A is an enterotoxin that is primarily responsible for the diarrhea associated with this disease. Its mechanism of action seems to result from tissue damage after an inflammatory process induced by the toxin. Toxin A acts as a strong chemoattractant for neutrophils, and it is thought that the release of inflammatory cytokines from these cells results in altered membrane permeability, fluid secretion, and hemorrhagic necrosis. Toxin B is a cytotoxin that demonstrates a lethal effect on cultured tissue cells. Its cytotoxic action is thought to involve depolymerization of filamentous actin, resulting in a change in the cell cytoskeleton and a rounding of the cell.

In addition, an enzyme with ADP-ribosylating activity has been described in one strain of *C difficile*. This toxin has been shown to modify cell actin in a manner similar to that of *Clostridium botulinum* C_2 and *C perfringens* ι toxin.

The diagnosis of *C difficile* diarrhea usually is based on the demonstration of the presence of toxin A, toxin B, or both. Toxin B can be detected by its effect on cell cultures, but this requires 18 to 24 hours. Latex beads coated with antibody to toxin A also are commercially available, as is an enzyme-linked immunosorbent assay kit, for detecting both toxins A and B.

The primary treatment is to discontinue the implicated antibiotic. Most patients then recover spontaneously. An agent can be substituted that is unlikely to cause an antibiotic-associated diarrhea such as a quinoline, sulfonamide, parenteral aminoglycoside, metronidazole, or trimethoprim-sulfomethoxazole.

Clostridium sordellii occasionally is one of the etiologic agents of clostridial myonecrosis. It is mentioned here because pathogenic strains of *C sordellii* produce two toxins that share biologic and immunologic properties with toxins A and B of *C difficile*, and it may be responsible for some cases of antibiotic-associated diarrhea.

CLOSTRIDIUM BOTULINUM

Clostridium botulinum is the causative agent of a highly fatal food poisoning that usually follows the ingestion of a preformed toxin produced by the organisms growing in the food. A total of 80 cases of botulism occurred in the United States in 1993. This included 21 cases of infant botulism, 54 cases of food-borne botulism, and 5 cases designated as *classification undetermined*.

Antigenic Classification

Seven immunologically distinct toxins are produced by different types of *C botulinum* and are indicated by capital letters. Types A, B, E, and, to a lesser extent, F, are responsible for most cases of human botulism, whereas type C is found most often in ducks and fowl, and type D is found in cattle, horses, and sheep. Type G has been isolated from soil and, although it does produce toxin, it has only rarely been reported to cause human botulism.

Curiously, the toxins seem to be secreted as progenitor toxins which, even though some have been crystallized, are composed of two polypeptide subunits linked by disulfide bonds. Also, the toxicity of those toxins that have been extensively studied can be increased from fourfold to 250-fold by treatment with trypsin. This phenomenon is not understood at the molecular level.

Additionally, it has been shown that the toxins produced by types C, D, and E are a result of a lysogenic conversion. Moreover, type C organisms can be cured by heating their spores at 70°C for 15 minutes, after which they are no longer toxin producers. Reinfection of these cured bacteria with phage 3C restores type C toxigenicity, but reinfection with phage 1D converts the cured type C organism into a toxigenic *C botulinum* of type D. Moreover, reinfection of the cured type C organisms with phage NA1 (isolated from *C novyi*) converts the *C botulinum* into a toxigenic *C novyi* type A, which then produces the lethal α toxin characteristic of the gas gangrene group. Reports of botulism caused by *Clostridium butyricum* and *Clostridium barati* indicate that the genes encoding botulism toxin are transferable to other closely related species of *Clostridium*.

Epidemiology and Pathogenesis of Botulism

Clostridium botulinum is distributed in soil, lake bottoms, and decaying vegetation; thus, many foods, both vegetables and meats, become contaminated with these organisms. Numerous animals die each year after ingestion of fermenting grains. This is especially true of ducks (the disease is called *limber neck*) and cattle (particularly in South Africa).

The endospores of *C botulinum* are resistant to heat and may withstand boiling-water temperatures for several hours. Thus, botulism in humans usually occurs in food that has been inadequately sterilized and placed in an anaerobic environment where the surviving spores can germinate and produce toxin.

Most cases of food-borne botulism in Europe have resulted from eating smoked, salted, or spiced meats and fish; botulism in the United States frequently follows the ingestion of home-canned vegetables. Botulism in commercially prepared foods is rare, and when it occurs it is a result of human error. During the last several decades, botulism has occurred in commercial cheese, tuna fish, vichyssoise, mushrooms, smoked white fish, and commercially canned cherry peppers.

The toxins produced by *C botulinum* are among the most toxic compounds known. It is estimated that 1 mL of culture fluid is sufficient to kill 2 million mice, and that the lethal dose for humans may be in the range of 1 μg of toxin.

Human symptoms usually begin after an incubation period of 18 to 36 hours and may include nausea and vomiting in addition to double vision, difficulty in swallowing, and some muscle paralysis. This may be followed by muscle weakness, blurred vision, and death as a result of respiratory failure.

The toxin acts primarily as a neurotoxin, inducing paralysis in three basic steps: (1) binding of the toxin to a receptor on the nerve synapse, (2) entrance of the toxin (or possibly one polypeptide subunit) into the nerve cell, and (3) blocking of the release of acetylcholine from the cell, resulting in a flaccid muscle paralysis.

C botulinum type C produces two distinct toxins that have been designated C1 and C2. The C1 toxin functions like other botulism toxins to block the release of acetylcholine at the myoneural junction. C2 toxin, however, is a binary complex consisting of two unlinked components designated as I and II. Component II recognizes the cell receptor and thus facilitates the entrance of component I into the cytoplasm. The C2 toxin causes a necrotic enteritis, which seems to result in an increase in vascular leakage of the intestinal mucosa. Its mechanism of action is unclear, but it has been shown to ADP-ribosylate G-actin as well as the synthetic substrate, homo-poly L-arginine.

C botulinum organisms, types C and D, also produce an additional toxin which has been termed exoenzyme C3. The DNA encoding C3 is located on both phage C and phage D, the phages that also encode for botulism toxins C and D, respectively. Its function is to ADP-ribosylates Rho protein, a eucaryotic member of the *ras* superfamily of proteins. Because the *ras* superfamily of proteins are GTP-binding proteins involved in enzyme regulation, this exoenzyme could function as a virulence

A Closer Look

With the knowledge that botulism toxin is probably the most toxic substance on earth, it is a little difficult to imagine anything good about such a substance. However, as stated over 100 years ago by physiologist Claude Bernard, "Poisons can be employed as a means for the destruction of life or as agents for the treatment of the sick." His predictions have become a reality for the use of botulism toxin in controlling involuntary muscle contractions.

Many individuals experience dystonia, which is defined as "involuntary sustained muscle contraction that results in twisting, repetitive, and sometimes painful movements or abnormal postures." Such disorders had been considered psychological in origin, and little was accomplished in their treatment. However, as recently as 1981, Alan B. Scott, an ophthalmologist, reasoned that the muscle paralysis caused by botulism toxin could be taken advantage of in treating certain forms of dystonia. His initial use was to use the toxin to treat strabismus (crossed-eyes), a condition in which the muscles controlling eye movement of one eye are hyperactive. Success in treating this disorder led the U.S. Food and Drug Administration in 1989 to license the use of botulism toxin type A for the treatment of a number of human muscle disorders.

In addition to strabismus, botulism toxin is being used to treat blepharospasm (uncontrolled blinking), hemifacial spasms (facial twitching and spasms), and eyelid disorders. In general, toxin injection relieves the muscle contractions for several months, but then the undesired movement returns and repeated injections are required. However, in some cases, patients have received repeated injections for over 7 years without experiencing any long-term adverse effects. Because of the infinitely small doses of toxin used, it seems unlikely that immunity to treatment would become a major problem.

Tetanus toxin also is being investigated for use in clinical medicine. This toxin (unlike botulism toxin) possesses the ability to enter the central nervous system by retrograde intraaxonal transport through motor nerves. Much research is directed toward the isolation of nontoxic fragments of the toxin that possess this property. Such fragments could be chemically linked to drugs that could then transport them to the central nervous system.

Other toxins also are being investigated for use in treating a variety of neurologic disorders, and it seems likely that the next few decades will see important breakthroughs in this field.

factor, but the exact consequence of the C3 ADP-ribosylation is unknown.

Laboratory Diagnosis of Botulism

Even after a person develops symptoms of botulism, free toxin may exist in the bloodstream. Mice are incredibly sensitive to the toxin, and the intraperitoneal injections of a patient's serum may result in death of the mouse. Usually, the implicated food is no longer available, but if it is, extracts should also be injected into mice and aliquots cultured anaerobically to grow the organisms.

Prevention and Control of Botulism

Anyone suspected of having botulism should be given antitoxin to types A, B, and E. The antiserum cannot neutralize any fixed toxin but can react with free residual toxin. All others who possibly could have eaten the same food also should be administered antitoxin.

In contrast to the endospores of the organism, botulism toxin is heat labile; thus, home-canned vegetables (particularly nonacid ones such as corn, peas, and beans) should be boiled for about 10 minutes before eating. Such treatment would inactivate toxin that might be present. Home-canned foods that are prepared in a pressure cooker, where temperatures of 120°C are reached, should be completely sterile; however, to be effective, the cooking temperature must be maintained for sufficient time to bring all of the food to that temperature for at least 15 minutes.

Whereas home-canned vegetables are a major source of botulism in the United States, other less noted foods also have been implicated. For example, over a 40-year period, 59 outbreaks involving 156 cases of botulism occurred in Alaska from eating seafood that had been fermented, dried, and frozen. Other outbreaks have resulted from the ingestion of stews, turkey loaf, or commercial meat pies that had been cooked and then allowed to remain at ambient temperature for 1 to 2 days before eating. It is obvious that customary cooking does not necessarily kill spores of *C botulinum* and that under appropriate conditions, such spores can germinate, grow, and produce toxin.

Toxoids stimulate solid immunity but, because of the rarity of the disease in humans, their use would be unwarranted. Toxoids have, however, been used successfully for the prevention of botulism in cattle, particularly in South Africa.

Although *C botulinum* is described as an organism with essentially no invasive abilities, several cases of wound botulism are reported in the United States each year. Usually, the wounds themselves were not serious, but wound botulism should be suspected in any persons with even minor wounds who present the typical symptoms of botulism: blurred vision, weakness, and difficulty in swallowing.

Infant Botulism

A new variety of botulism was recognized during 1976 with the report of five cases of infant botulism. These cases occurred in babies as young as 5 weeks, some of whom were breast fed, although all had had some exposure to other foods. Since then, hundreds of additional cases of infant botulism have been diagnosed, and it has become a significant pediatric clinical entity.

EPIDEMIOLOGY AND PATHOGENESIS OF INFANT BOTULISM. Infant botulism has been diagnosed in infants ranging from 3 to 35 weeks of age. It is well-established that the disease is acquired by the ingestion of *C botulinum* spores that subsequently germinate in the intestine and produce botulism toxin. Such spores are ubiquitous and, in fact, soil and dust samples from many homes have been shown to contain such spores. Thus, even breast-fed infants are susceptible through contaminated dust. Honey also has been shown to contain spores of *C botulinum*, and a number of cases of infant botulism have followed the ingestion of honey.

The major initial symptom of infant botulism is 2 to 3 days of constipation followed by flaccid paralysis, resulting in difficulty in nursing and a generalized weakness that has been described as "overtly floppy."

The mortality rate of infants admitted to the hospital has been about 3%, and some patients have required mechanical respirators because of respiratory distress. Death, however, may occur more frequently in undiagnosed cases, and considerable data link infant botulism to at least some cases of the sudden infant death syndrome.

Because, by definition, infant botulism is the result of toxin production by organisms that have colonized the gut, it is not surprising that there have been a few cases of adult–infant botulism that occurred after antibiotic therapy or gastric surgery. Even in cases of food-borne botulism, it is usual for the gut to be colonized with *C botulinum*, providing a continuing source of toxin.

DIAGNOSIS AND TREATMENT OF INFANT BOTULISM. A tentative clinical diagnosis of botulism can be made for an infant with several days of constipation, an unexplained weakness, difficulty in swallowing, or respiratory distress. A laboratory diagnosis, however, requires the demonstration of botulism toxin in the feces, which is determined by the injection of fecal extracts intraperitoneally into a mouse. Death of the mouse within 96 hours (which did not occur in controls in which the fecal extracts were first neutralized with botulism antitoxin) is taken as positive evidence for the presence of the toxin.

Infants are not usually treated with antitoxin, primarily because it is a horse product and may induce lifelong hypersensitivity. Attempts to eradicate the bacteria are not recommended because of the fear that the organisms might lyse in the intestine, releasing large amounts of toxin. Treatment thus far has been mostly symptomatic, requiring an average of 1 month of hospitalization.

Bibliography

JOURNALS

Drobniewski FA. *Bacillus cereus* and related species. Clin Microbiol Rev 1993;6:324.

Hatheway CL. Toxigenic clostridia. Clin Microbiol Rev 1990;3:66.

Iacono-Connors LC, et al. Expression of the *Bacillus anthracis* protective antigen gene by baculovirus and vaccinia virus recombinants. Infect Immun 1990;58:366.

Jankovic J, Brin MF. Review article. Therapeutic uses of botulinum toxin. N Engl J Med 1991;324:1186.

Kelly CP, et al. Review article. *Clostridium difficile* colitis. N Engl J Med 1994;330:257.

Knoop FC, et al. *Clostridium difficile*: clinical disease and diagnosis. Clin Microbiol Rev 1993;6:251.

Masure HR, et al. Mechanisms of bacterial pathogenicity that involve production of calmodulin-sensitive adenylate cyclases. Microbiol Rev 1987;51:60.

Rood JI, Cole ST. Molecular genetics and pathogenesis of *Clostridium perfringens*. Microbiol Rev 1991;55:621.

Schantz EJ, Johnson EA. Properties and use of botulinum toxin and other microbial neurotoxins in medicine. Microbiol Rev 1992;56:80.

Titball RW. Bacterial phospholipases C. Microbiol Rev 1993;57:347.

Essentials of Medical Microbiology, Fifth Edition, edited by Wesley A. Volk,
Bryan M. Gebhardt, Marie-Louise Hammarskjöld, and Robert J. Kadner.
Lippincott-Raven Publishers, Philadelphia © 1996.

Chapter 30

Corynebacterium and Listeria

CORYNEBACTERIUM

Although diphtheria no longer is common in the United States, it still occurs as sporadic individual cases or small outbreaks (one reported case in 1988 and two in 1989). Table 30-1 provides the annual case rate for the period 1980 to 1989. Although the morbidity rate is small, few areas of the country are completely free of the disease.

Corynebacterium diphtheriae

Corynebacterium diphtheriae was isolated in 1883 by T.A.E. Klebs, and in 1884 it was shown to be the etiologic agent of diphtheria by his colleague, A.J. Loeffler. The generic name *Corynebacterium* is derived from the Greek stem *kory*, meaning "club shaped." Diphtheria bacilli are gram-positive, non–spore-forming, nonmotile rods that can be described as pleomorphic. Some may be straight, whereas others are curved or club-shaped. When they have divided by binary fission, the newly formed bacteria have a tendency to snap apart. Stained smears show many cells forming sharp angles with each other (Fig. 30-1).

Another outstanding characteristic of the diphtheria bacillus is its granular and uneven staining. When stained with methylene blue or toluidine blue, the granules in the cell take on a reddish appearance. These refractive granules have a variety of names, such as Babès-Ernst bodies, metachromatic granules, and volutin; they are composed of a polymer of inorganic polyphosphate. The granules are not seen during active growth, but start to appear toward the end of the logarithmic growth period. It seems that they represent storage depots for materials needed to form high-energy phosphate bonds; the bacteria possess enzymes which phosphorylate glucose to form glucose-6-phosphate and phosphorylate ADP to form ATP, using the phosphate and energy present in the storage granules.

C diphtheriae grows well on blood-agar medium. However, because most other bacteria in the throat also

TABLE 30-1
Diphtheria in the United States, 1980–1989

Year	No. of Cases
1980	5
1981	4
1982	3
1983	5
1984	1
1985	2
1986	0
1987	3
1988	1
1989	2

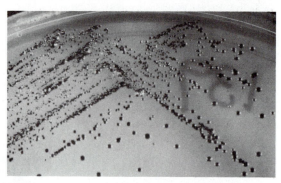

FIGURE 30-2   Gray–black colonies of *Corynebacterium diphtheriae* from a throat swab streaked on cystine tellurite medium.

grow under these conditions, media have been devised that favor the growth of the diphtheria bacillus and restrict the growth of some of the normal flora of the throat. Two media are useful for this purpose: (1) Loeffler's coagulated blood serum, and (2) blood agar or chocolate agar, to which potassium tellurite (K_2TeO_3) has been added. On the latter medium, colonies of *C diphtheriae* become dark gray to black (Fig. 30-2). This staining occurs because the tellurite or tellurous ions are able to diffuse through the cell wall and membrane and are reduced to tellurium metal, which is precipitated inside the cell.

The organisms in this species have been divided into three biotypes, based primarily on the appearance of their colonies on tellurite media. Originally, it was thought that there was a correlation between the severity of the disease and the colony type. This is known to be untrue, but the names *gravis, intermedius,* and *mitis* are still used to refer to the three types of *C diphtheriae.*

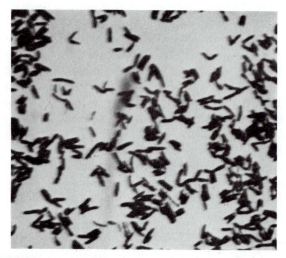

FIGURE 30-1   Gram-stained culture smear of *Corynebacterium diphtheriae.* (Original magnification ×4200.)

EPIDEMIOLOGY AND PATHOGENESIS OF DIPHTHERIA

Basic comprehension of diphtheria came in 1888 when bacteriologists Pierre Roux and Alexandre Yersin discovered that diphtheria culture filtrates (free from diphtheria bacilli) are lethal for animals. Furthermore, the symptoms and the pathogenic changes that result from the injection of the toxic filtrates are the same as those from the disease itself. Notice that the report of Roux and Yersin comprised the first description of a bacterial toxin. In brief, then, diphtheria is an acute infection in which the causative organisms remain in the respiratory tract, even though on some occasions (especially in the tropics) the organisms produce wound infections. The site of infection, usually the throat, becomes inflamed as the bacteria grow and excrete a powerful exotoxin. Dead tissue cells, along with the host's leukocytes, red blood cells, and the bacteria, form a dull gray exudate called a diphtheritic pseudomembrane. If this pseudomembrane extends into the trachea, the air passages may become blocked; in such cases, a tracheotomy may be necessary to prevent suffocation.

Although there is no doubt as to the role of the toxin in the production of diphtheria, there are unknown virulence factors that also contribute to the ability of the diphtheria bacillus to cause infections. One such substance, known as cord factor, is a toxic glycolipid consisting of two molecules of mycolic acid esterified to trehalose. The fact that an analogous cord factor is closely associated with the virulence of *Mycobacterium tuberculosis* supports its role as a virulence factor for *C diphtheriae.* Thus, it is possible for non–toxin-producing strains of *C diphtheriae* to be involved in a local infection with pseudomembrane formation, but these cases are mild. The severe symptoms and frequent death from diphtheria are the result of the action of the diphtheria toxin, which is transported by way of the bloodstream to all parts of the body. Lesions may occur in the kidney, heart, and nerves, resulting in acute nephritis and serious cardiac weakness. The incubation period is 2 to 5 days.

TOXIGENICITY OF *CORYNEBACTERIUM DIPHTHERIAE*

The ability to produce toxin is the major difference between avirulent and virulent diphtheria organisms. In 1951, Freeman discovered that this ability to synthesize toxin was possessed only by organisms that are lysogenic for phage β or a closely related bacteriophage. Thus, all strains of diphtheria organisms that produce toxin are lysogenic, and avirulent strains of diphtheria bacilli can be made into virulent, toxin-producing strains by infecting them with the temperate bacteriophage. As seen in previous instances, this change in the properties of a bacterial cell as a result of becoming lysogenic is called lysogenic conversion (see Chap. 21).

In the commercial production of diphtheria toxin for vaccine, the amount of iron present in the growth medium is critical. Good toxin production is obtained only at low concentrations of iron (2 μmol/L). At concentrations as low as 10 μmol/L, toxin production becomes negligible. Evidence suggests that, normally, the bacterium forms a repressor which prevents the expression of the phage *tox*⁺ gene, and that this repressor is an iron-containing protein. Thus, when the concentration of iron is abnormally low, the complete repressor is not formed, and the *tox*⁺ gene is transcribed, ultimately yielding toxin.

Mode of Action of Diphtheria Toxin

Because diphtheria toxin is effective against many cells, the use of tissue cultures provides a model for studying its mode of action. Early studies reported that, although toxin had no effect on the respiration of HeLa cells (human cervical carcinoma tissue culture cells), all protein synthesis stopped about 1 to 1.5 hours after the addition of the toxin. Surprisingly, dialyzed, cell-free, protein-synthesizing systems were entirely insensitive to the action of the toxin, unless oxidized nicotinamide-adenine dinucleotide (NAD) was added to the reaction.

Subsequent research has shown that the toxin possesses enzymatic activity that cleaves nicotinamide from NAD and then catalyzes the ADP-ribosylation of elongation factor 2 (EF-2; Fig. 30-3). EF-2 is required for the translocase reaction of polypeptide synthesis, in which the ribosome is moved to the next codon on the mRNA after the peptide bond is formed to the most recent amino acid to be added to the chain. When EF-2 is inactivated by the addition of ADP-ribose, the ribosome is frozen, and protein synthesis stops. Insofar as is known, EF-2 from all eucaryotic cells (those studied include vertebrate, invertebrate, wheat, and yeast) is inactivated in the presence of diphtheria toxin and NAD, whereas the corresponding factor, EF-G (which occurs in bacteria), or the analogous factor from mitochondria, is not affected. The ADP-ribose is transferred to a histidine-modified residue on the EF-2 molecule. This modified amino acid (com-

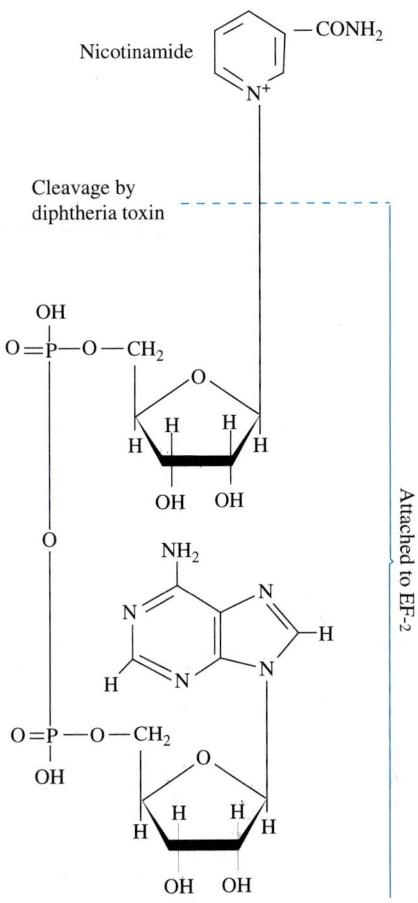

FIGURE 30-3 Structure of NAD showing bond cleaved by diphtheria toxin.

monly called diphtheramide) does not exist in bacterial or mitochondrial elongation factors.

Structure of Diphtheria Toxin

Diphtheria toxin is excreted from the bacterium as a single polypeptide chain of about 61,000 daltons with two disulfide bridges. Although highly toxic for cells or animals, the pure, intact toxin is inert in cell-free protein systems, even when NAD is present. Thus, the secreted toxin is actually a *proenzyme* which, in cell-free systems, must be activated before it can function as an enzyme. This activation, as shown in Figure 30-4, is accomplished in two steps: (1) treatment with trypsin hydrolyzes a peptide bond between the disulfide-linked amino acids; and (2) reduction of the disulfides to sulfhydryl groups using a reducing agent such as mercaptoethanol yields two smaller peptides, which have been designated fragment A (21,150 daltons) and fragment B (40,000 daltons).

Fragment A is active in cleaving the nicotinamide moiety from NAD and in catalyzing the transfer of ADP-ribose from NAD to EF-2 when added to cell-free, protein-synthesizing systems, but it has no effect when given

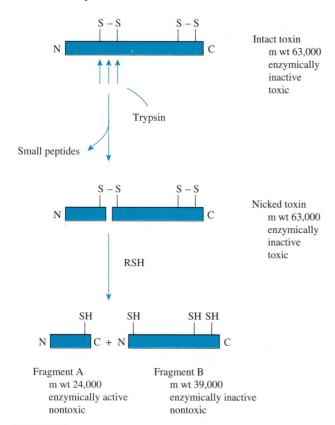

FIGURE 30-4 Sequence of events in the expression of enzymatic activity (ADP ribosylation of EF-2) in diphtheria toxin. Fragment A is nontoxic because it cannot cross the cell membrane, except when it is linked to the fragment B portion of the molecule.

to animals or to intact HeLa cells. Thus, although fragment A is the activated enzyme (and hence contains all the toxic properties), it cannot get into intact cells.

Fragment B, on the other hand, has no enzymatic activity, but it is needed for attachment of the toxin to specific receptor sites on cells. Cells possess specific glycoprotein receptor sites for the diphtheria toxin, as suggested by the following observation: Rats and mice are over 1000 times more resistant to the intact toxin than are other susceptible animals, but their cell-free protein-synthesizing system is equally sensitive to the enzymatic action of fragment A. Moreover, toxin that is defective in its A fragment (and is, therefore, nontoxic) but retains a normal B fragment, will competitively inhibit the action of normal toxin on HeLa cells.

The question of whether the phage genome itself codes for the toxin or merely derepresses a bacterial gene, which could then synthesize the toxin, originally was solved using a series of mutant phages that induced the synthesis of mutant toxins. Moreover, the *tox* gene has been completely sequenced and unequivocally shown to exist in the phage genome.

Also, different toxigenic strains of *C diphtheriae* vary considerably in the amount of toxin produced under identical conditions. This is, in part, because of subtle differences in the regulation of the *tox* gene expression, but a more obvious explanation for this observation was shown by Rino Rappuoli and his colleagues. Using specific DNA probes, they conclusively demonstrated that high–toxin-producing strains had two or even three *tox* genes inserted into their genome. Thus, the quantity of toxin produced was correlated to the amount of *tox* DNA within the toxin-producing strain of *C diphtheriae*.

In summary, the usual series of events leading to toxin action is as follows: (1) the toxin binds to specific receptor sites on susceptible cells; (2) the toxin enters the cell (perhaps through a phagocytic vesicle that can then fuse with a lysosome), and lysosomal proteases hydrolyze the toxin into fragments A and B; and (3) reduction of the disulfide bridges (perhaps by glutathione) releases fragment A from fragment B; and (4) fragment A can then enzymatically inactivate EF-2.

LABORATORY DIAGNOSIS OF DIPHTHERIA

Diagnosis of diphtheria is based on isolating *C diphtheriae* from the infected area and demonstrating its toxin-producing ability. Specimens are inoculated on Loeffler's coagulated serum slants, tellurite plates, and blood-agar plates. Direct smears are stained with methylene blue and observed for volutin granules.

A definitive laboratory diagnosis requires the differentiation between the avirulent, non–toxin-producing strains and the virulent toxin-producing organisms. This can be done by the intracutaneous injection of a suspension of organisms into a guinea pig. After 5 hours, diphtheria antitoxin is injected intraperitoneally, followed 30 minutes later by a second intracutaneous injection of the suspension of organisms. A toxigenic strain will cause an area of necrosis at the site of the first injection and only a small nodule at the control site. There is also an in vitro virulence assay (termed an Elek test), in which the unknown organism is compared with a known toxin-producing diphtheria bacillus. In this case, antiserum absorbed to strips of filter paper is placed vertically across the streaks of the organisms on a Petri dish. If toxin is produced by the unknown organisms, a line of precipitate will occur at the optimal concentration of the toxin and antitoxin, forming a line of identity with the adjacent, known toxin-producing organisms (Fig. 30-5).

TREATMENT AND CONTROL OF DIPHTHERIA

In treating diphtheria, antitoxin must be administered promptly to neutralize the toxin being produced. This is because antitoxin is ineffective if given after the toxin is bound to cell receptor sites. Thus, the initial diagnosis must be made from the clinical picture, because it would be unsafe to wait for a bacteriologic confirmation before starting treatment. Most physicians agree that it is safer to err by occasionally administering antitoxin to someone

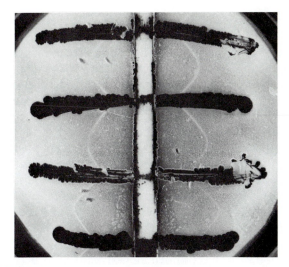

FIGURE 30-5. Curved lines of identity (precipitate) are visible between the dark streaks of organisms that cross a paper strip saturated with antitoxin. In this case, then, all four streaks are *Corynebacterium diphtheriae.*

who was clinically misdiagnosed than to wait for a more positive confirmation.

Most diphtheria organisms are sensitive to penicillin and other antibiotics, but the antibiotics do not neutralize circulating toxin and, therefore, are of value only when used concurrently with antitoxin.

The fact that there were over 200,000 cases and about 10,000 deaths annually from diphtheria in the United States during the early 1920s, and only 1 reported case in 1994, attests to the fact that mass immunization provides an effective control for this disease. Children are injected with a nontoxic toxoid prepared by treating the diphtheria toxin with formalin. This is usually administered along with tetanus toxoid and pertussis vaccine (DPT) at 2, 4, 6, and 18 months of age, with the final DPT injection being given at 4 to 6 years of age. Thereafter, it is recommended that a person be given a booster of tetanus and diphtheria toxoid (Td) every 10 years, particularly if the person travels overseas to Asia, Africa, or Central and South America where the incidence of diphtheria is higher than that seen in the United States.

Reports show that only antibodies to the fragment B portion of the toxin molecule are capable of neutralizing the toxin, supposedly by preventing the attachment of toxin to the specific receptor sites on the cell surface. Treatment of the toxin with formalin, however, both detoxifies the toxin and protects fragment B from the action of proteolytic enzymes, resulting in better protective antibody production than that obtained by using untreated fragment B or defective toxins possessing a normal fragment B.

A Schick test may be used to determine whether an individual is susceptible to diphtheria. This test is carried out by the intradermal injection of a small amount of diphtheria toxin. A person without antibodies to the toxin (and, hence, susceptibility to diphtheria) will develop an inflamed area at the site of injection that will reach a maximum level in about 48 hours. In contrast, persons who have antibodies will neutralize the toxin and will not develop an inflammation at the site of the toxin injection. In actual practice, a control substance—in which the toxin has been inactivated by heating—is injected intradermally into the other arm to make certain that any inflammatory response is because of the toxin and is not a result of a hypersensitivity reaction to some extraneous component in the toxin preparation.

Other Corynebacteria

Many species of *Corynebacterium* exist in the soil; a few cause animal diseases, and a large number are plant pathogens. Such species, however, are only rare causes of human diseases. Interestingly, both *Corynebacterium ulcerans* and *Corynebacterium pseudotuberculosis* are known to cause occasional diphtheria-like illnesses. Moreover, selected isolates of these species have been shown to produce a toxin that is indistinguishable from that of *C diphtheriae.* The fact that human disease by these species is both rare and mild suggests that even though toxigenic, they may lack some virulence factor possessed by *C diphtheriae.*

LISTERIA

A decade or two ago, listeriosis was considered a rare disease in humans, but reports indicate an increasing frequency of human infections. This may be because past diagnoses were missed, but it is more likely because years ago individuals most susceptible may not have survived their primary illness long enough to become infected with *Listeria.* For example, data show that about 70% of human listeriosis occurs in individuals who have an underlying immunosuppressive illness, a primary hematologic cancer, or are receiving immunosuppressive drugs, usually corticosteroids. Because many cancer patients fall into one of the above categories, it is not surprising that *Listeria* is the leading cause of meningitis in persons with cancer. However, neonates and pregnant women also are particularly susceptible to infections by *Listeria* and, if the organisms are ingested in heavily contaminated foods, essentially anyone may become infected.

Listeria monocytogenes

Listeria monocytogenes is a small, gram-positive, motile diphtheroid. The organisms are facultatively aerobic and produce a narrow band of beta hemolysis when growing on blood-agar plates. Colonies growing on a clear tryp- tose agar appear blue green when viewed with an oblique light held at an angle of about 45 degrees.

After it is isolated, *L monocytogenes* is easily subcul- tured, but initial isolation may be difficult. One unusual enrichment technique is to store specimens at 4°C for extended periods of time. This may be done by inoculat- ing blood or spinal fluid into a tenfold excess of blood- culture medium. This is then stored at 4°C and subcul- tured at weekly intervals for 3 to 6 months by streaking onto a blood-agar plate. Tissue or fecal suspensions may also be stored in screw-cap tubes at 4°C and subcultured at weekly intervals. The organisms demonstrate a tumbling type of motility if grown at 18° to 20°C.

At least 13 serotypes have been described, but 90% of clinical listeriosis infections are caused by types 1a, 1b, and 4b.

EPIDEMIOLOGY OF LISTERIOSIS

Listeria monocytogenes causes about 1700 cases of menin- gitis and sepsis in the United States each year, with a case-fatality rate of 25%. It appears that it is primarily an animal pathogen, and it is likely that most infections of adults are food borne. *L monocytogenes* can be isolated from stool specimens of 5% to 10% of normal asympto- matic adults, and it has also been isolated from soil, water, and sewage, and from the feces of a number of rodents, swine, and poultry. In fact, one can cultivate *L monocyto- genes* from about 80% of raw poultry, accounting for the fact that undercooked chicken provides a major reservoir of infection for humans. Large numbers of *L monocyto- genes* also have been found in raw milk obtained from infected cows, and, when they are present in such high numbers, normal pasteurization procedures will not al- ways eliminate all of these organisms. This became appar- ent in 1985, after an epidemic in which 49 patients seemed to have contracted listeriosis after the ingestion of pasteurized milk, resulting in a 29% fatality rate. It is probable that the intracellular existence of these orga- nisms in leukocytes present in the milk contributes to their higher heat resistance, permitting some to escape the normal pasteurization process.

Another epidemic in 1985, which caused about 90 deaths, resulted from eating a Mexican-style cheese that was contaminated with *L monocytogenes*. In this instance it is not known whether the milk used to make the cheeses (queso fresco and cotija) was properly pasteurized, but both of these epidemics clearly illustrate that *L monocyto- genes* can be spread by contaminated milk.

Foods from store delicatessens also have been in- volved and have included a wide variety of prepared meat products. A survey during the summer of 1993 found that about 20% of all hot dogs tested were contaminated with *L monocytogenes*, and people were advised to be sure that all hot dogs were well cooked before being eaten. In another epidemic involving over 40 persons, coleslaw was identified as the vehicle of transmission, and investiga- tors concluded that listeriosis could be spread readily by vegetables that are consumed uncooked, particularly if raw manure had been used to fertilize the fields.

VIRULENCE FACTORS OF LISTERIOSIS

Listeria monocytogenes is an intracellular bacterium capa- ble of growing and surviving inside of mononuclear phagocytes as well as epithelial cells. The primary viru- lence factor permitting this type of growth is a hemolytic cytolysin termed listeriolysin O (LLO). This hemolysin is produced by all pathogenic *Listeria*, and its function

TABLE 30-2
Age and Sex Distribution for Human Listeriosis in the United States, 1968–1969

Age Group	Male	Female	Total	Percentage of Total	Fatalities	Group Fatality Rate
0–4 wk	11	21	32	27.3	5*	15.2
4 wk–9 y	3	4	7	6.0	1	3.0
10–19 y	1	4	2	1.7	1	3.0
20–29 y	2	5	7	6.0	0	0
30–39 y	2	2	4	3.4	0	0
40–49 y	8	7	15	12.8	5	15.2
50–59 y	12	11	23	19.7	8	24.2
60–69 y	9	5	14	12.0	6	18.2
70+ y	12	1	13	11.1	7	21.2
Total	60	57	117	100.0	33*	28.2
Percentage of total	51.3	48.7	100.0	—	28.2	—

* Does not include one aborted 5-mo fetus or one death in which age and sex were unknown.

is to enable the phagocytized organisms to escape from the phagosome and grow in the cytoplasm of the invaded cell. Mutants lacking LLO are unable to escape the phagosome. It is sulfhydryl activated and shows considerable homology to streptolysin O. Transposon insertion into the gene encoding LLO causes the organisms to become nonhemolytic and avirulent for mice; loss of the transposon restores both hemolysis and virulence. Moreover, when the LLO gene was transfected into *Bacillus subtilis*, these organisms acquired the ability to grow in the cytoplasm of a macrophage-like cell line.

Another important virulence determinant resides in the ability of the intracellular organisms to spread directly from cell to cell, a process which shields them from coming into contact with humoral antibodies or complement. As the organisms divide in the cytoplasm of the host cell, they acquire a tail made up of actin filaments. It seems that these actin filaments direct the movement of the bacterium to the surface where it can leave the host cell and penetrate neighboring cells.

Surprisingly, *L monocytogenes* has been reported to possess a lipopolysaccharide-like component in its cell wall that experimentally produces many of the symptoms associated with gram-negative endotoxins. The occurrence of such a complex in a gram-positive organism is highly unusual but, if it is able to induce the synthesis and release of tumor necrosis factor-α and interleukin-1, it would explain many of the symptoms associated with listeriosis.

Other virulence factors that are not well characterized include the following: (1) the ability to induce their own phagocytosis; (2) the ability to mobilize iron from transferrin; (3) the ability to overcome the nonspecific immune responses mediated by activated phagocytes; and (4) a Zn-dependent phospholipase C whose loss results in impaired virulence. Interestingly, *L monocytogenes* binds C1q and this mediates enhanced uptake by C1q-binding receptors on macrophages.

PATHOGENICITY OF LISTERIOSIS

L monocytogenes has a propensity to infect pregnant women, as well as the immunosuppressed, perhaps because pregnancy causes a depression of cell-mediated immunity.

Listeriosis can mimic a number of infectious diseases, but meningitis is the most common manifestation, occurring in more than 75% of infections. In fact, *L monocytogenes* is the most common cause of bacterial meningitis occurring in renal transplant recipients, undoubtedly associated with the immunosuppression of such patients. *Listeria* also may cause endocarditis, urethritis, conjunctivitis, and abortions, but the majority of infections occur in the newborn. All age groups are susceptible to infection, but, as shown in Table 30-2, the fatality rate is much

A Closer Look

It has long been a puzzle as to why some organisms induce a humoral-type immunity, whereas others call forth a cell-mediated immune response. The answers to this conundrum are beginning to unfold as a result of studies on how organisms such as *Listeria monocytogenes* induce a specific subset of CD4$^+$ T cells.

It has been amply demonstrated that two distinct subsets of T helper cells are involved in our immune responses. T helper 1 (T$_H$1) cells produce interleukin (IL)-2 and interferon-γ and are responsible for cell-mediated immune responses (delayed-type hypersensitivity and macrophage activation). T helper 2 (T$_H$2) secrete IL-4, IL-5, and IL-10 and are necessary for a T-dependent humoral antibody response. The question, then, is, "What specifically causes a naive T cell to differentiate into a T$_H$1 cell rather than a T$_H$2 cell during an infection?"

Using *Listeria*-infected macrophages, Chyi-Song Hsieh and his colleagues at Washington University School of Medicine linked the capacity of *Listeria* to induce a cell-mediated immune response with the organism's ability to induce the infected macrophage to secrete IL-12. IL-12, in turn, drives the differentiation of T cells toward T$_H$1 development and the resulting cell-mediated immunity. If IL-12 was depleted by adding antiserum to IL-12, T$_H$1 differentiation did not occur.

Thus, certain pathogens seem to preferentially induce a cell-mediated immunity as a result of their ability to stimulate IL-12 production. This opens up a whole field for managing the type and intensity of the immune response, and it seems possible that by using IL-12, one could steer the body toward a cell-mediated response to almost any antigen.

There are a number of situations where this might be a great advantage to the individual. For example, *Leishmania major* infections in different mouse strains induces either a T$_H$1 or a T$_H$2 cell response. If a T$_H$1 response occurs, it is protective and the mouse recovers. If, however, a T$_H$2 response occurs, the mouse dies. IL-12 also could be of value in the treatment of certain allergies resulting from a T$_H$2 response. It could also be of value in treating AIDS patients who experience a loss in T$_H$1 cells.

So, another example is seen of how the unfolding of the molecular biology of the immune system opens the way for greater manipulation of the system to the benefit of all humankind.

higher for the newborn younger than 4 weeks of age and for persons older than 50 of age.

Neonatal listeriosis occurs in two forms: early onset and late onset. In the early onset disease, the infant is critically ill at birth or becomes so during the first day or two of life. The most common manifestation is pneumonia and sepsis, and it seems that the infection is acquired either in utero or from the vagina at the time of delivery.

Late onset listeriosis occurs between 1 and 4 weeks after birth and is seen as a meningitis. In such cases, it is probable that the infection was acquired after birth.

The parallel between neonatal listeriosis and neonatal group B streptococcal infections is interesting. Either organism may cause early or late onset infections. An early onset infection is acquired from the mother in utero or during birth, whereas the late form of both diseases is probably acquired through person-to-person contact. Both infections also have a serotype specificity in that most early onset listeriosis is caused by serotype 1a or 1b, whereas the late onset form most often results from serotype 4b.

Immunity to infection by *L monocytogenes* is primarily a cell-mediated event in which the eradication of the organisms is the result of immune T cells that enhance the bactericidal function of effector macrophages. The observation that *Listeria*-infected mice displayed an en-hanced ability to synthesize interferon-γ suggests the possibility that interferon-γ secreted by immune T cells may activate the listericidal mechanism of the macrophage.

TREATMENT AND CONTROL OF LISTERIOSIS

L monocytogenes is sensitive to penicillin, ampicillin, and the tetracyclines, and many investigators report that the tetracyclines are the drugs of choice.

Because of the ubiquity of the organisms, prevention of infections is difficult. Control seems limited to the early recognition and treatment of listeriosis.

Bibliography

JOURNALS

Broome CV. Listeriosis: Can we prevent it? ASM News 1993;59:444.

Farber JM, Peterkin PI. *Listeria monocytogenes*: a common food-borne pathogen. Microbiol Rev 1991;55:476.

Kleinman LC. To end an epidemic: lessons for the history of diphtheria. N Engl J Med 1992;326:773.

Portnoy DA, et al. Minireview: molecular determinants of *Listeria monocytogenes* pathogenesis. Infect Immun 1992;60:1263.

Schuchat A, Swaminathan G, Broome CV. Epidemiology of human listeriosis. Clin Microbiol Rev 1991;4:169.

Essentials of Medical Microbiology, Fifth Edition, edited by Wesley A. Volk,
Bryan M. Gebhardt, Marie-Louise Hammarskjöld, and Robert J. Kadner.
Lippincott-Raven Publishers, Philadelphia © 1996.

Chapter 31

Mycobacterium

The most obvious characteristic of the mycobacteria is the large amount of lipid present in their cell walls—approximately 40% of the total cell dry weight—causing them to grow as extremely rough, hydrophobic colonies. Mycobacteria also are difficult to stain, but, once stained, they resist discoloration, even when washed with 95% ethanol containing 3% hydrochloric acid. Organisms with the ability to retain a stain in spite of washing with acid alcohol are referred to as *acid fast*. Only the members of the genus *Mycobacterium* and a few species of *Nocardia* possess this property, and this characteristic helps in detecting mycobacteria in body fluids such as sputum or gastric washings.

There are many nonpathogenic mycobacteria, as well as many pathogens whose range of host animals is narrowly restricted. The major human mycobacterial infections have been grouped primarily into two basic types: (1) tuberculosis, usually a respiratory infection but occasionally acquired by ingestion of the organisms; and (2) leprosy, primarily a disease of the skin. Both of these diseases are chronic infections that may last for many years, causing destructive lesions as a result of a cellular immune response to the organisms and their products. The advent of AIDS and the use of immunosuppressive drugs have brought to the forefront a third critical type of human mycobacterial disease, namely, a systemic nontuberculous disease caused by organisms grouped into the *Mycobacterium avium* complex. There also are other mycobacterial infections involving the lungs, lymph nodes, and skin.

Mycobacterium tuberculosis

In 1882, *Mycobacterium tuberculosis* (commonly called the tubercle bacillus) was shown by bacteriologist Robert Koch to be the causative agent of tuberculosis. This human disease may occur as a brief, completely asymptomatic incident in the life of one person, whereas in another it may produce a chronic, progressive pulmonary disease that results in the loss of almost all functional lung tissue.

induces neither fever nor a regional lymphadenopathy. Moreover, unlike other mycobacterial infections, *M ulcerans* is only rarely found inside macrophages. An explanation for these observations became available when it was shown that culture filtrates of *M ulcerans* suppressed T-cell proliferation and phagocytosis by murine macrophages. The mechanism of tissue destruction is unknown, but unlike other mycobacterial infections, it is not because of the host's immune response.

Treatment frequently requires surgical intervention and skin grafting.

Atypical Mycobacteria

During the last several decades, it has become obvious that there is an extremely large group of mycobacteria that are apparently normal inhabitants of soil and water. In the United States, such organisms are found predominantly in the South, where, as judged by specific tuberculin reactions (using tuberculin prepared from these organisms), between one third and one half of the population has been infected with them. The pulmonary disease in diagnosed cases usually is milder than that caused by *M tuberculosis* and, strangely, does not seem to be communicable from person to person.

This overall group of organisms has had several names, such as the *anonymous mycobacteria* (because no one knew enough about them to name them) or the *atypical mycobacteria* (because, unlike *M tuberculosis* or *M bovis,* they are completely avirulent for guinea pigs). The popular classification divides them into the following three groups: (1) photochromogens, which produce a yellow pigment only if grown in the light; (2) scotochromogens, which produce an orange pigment whether grown in the light or dark; and (3) nonchromogens, which do not produce pigment under any circumstances. All are acid-fast bacilli, but infection does not usually induce a strong skin reaction to the usual tuberculin prepared from *M tuberculosis*. However, tuberculin prepared from the atypical mycobacteria reacts intensely when injected into persons with the homologous infection. Such purified tuberculin is available and is designated as shown in Table 31-1. Infections caused by most of the atypical mycobacteria respond to treatment with rifampin in combination with streptomycin or cycloserine, although some skin infections may require years of therapy.

PHOTOCHROMOGENS

Mycobacterium kansasii is the most prevalent human pathogen in the photochromogen group. Antigenically, it is similar to *M tuberculosis,* and PPD prepared from either organism shows considerable cross-reaction.

In the United States, infections by *M kansasii* occur most frequently in Texas and, to a lesser extent, in Chi-

TABLE 31-1
Tuberculins Prepared From Various Species of Mycobacteria

Mycobacterium Species	*Tuberculin Designation*
M avium	PPD-A
M intracellularis	PPD-B
M fortuitum	PPD-F
M scrofulaceum	PPD-G
M kansasii	PPD-Y
M tuberculosis	PPD-S
M marinum	PPD-platy
M phlei	PPD-ph
M smegmatis	PPD-sm

cago, California, Oklahoma, and North Carolina. The human disease is like that described for the tubercle bacillus and may occur as both pulmonary and extrapulmonary infections.

Mycobacterium marinum, another photochromogen, has been isolated from swimming pools and lakes. Infections occur at traumatized areas in the skin and are manifested by draining ulcers.

SCOTOCHROMOGENS

Mycobacterium scrofulaceum seems to be the most prevalent human pathogen of the scotochromogen group. The organism has been found worldwide, probably existing primarily as a soil saprophyte. Its most common clinical manifestation is a cervical adenitis. The fact that many such infections are asymptomatic or undiagnosed is confirmed by the observation that several large surveys show that about 50% of those tested gave a positive skin reaction to specific PPD prepared from *M scrofulaceum* (ie, PPD-G).

NONPHOTOCHROMOGENS–MAC COMPLEX

The organisms in the nonphotochrome group are heterogeneous, and their classification is still in a state of flux. The two major pathogens, *M avium* and *Mycobacterium intracellularis,* are so closely related that many refer to them as the *M avium–M intracellularis* complex (MAC).

The organisms are found worldwide and infect a variety of birds and animals. Both cause a pulmonary infection in humans similar to that caused by the tubercle bacillus, but such infections are seen most often in elderly persons with preexisting pulmonary disease.

The MAC has acquired a new significance in those individuals with AIDS in whom it is found to be the most common cause of a systemic bacterial infection. It usually is seen as a late opportunistic infection occurring after one or more episodes of *Pneumocystis carinii* infections. Such individuals often also experience an intestinal infection with these organisms.

Members of the MAC can be isolated from sputum, blood, and aspirates of bone marrow. Acid-fast stains of stools also may be valuable in making a diagnosis. Treatment is difficult because the MACs generally are resistant to the usual antituberculosis drugs. However, many physicians use a four- to six-drug regimen that includes INH, rifampin, ethambutol, and streptomycin. Experimentally, it has been reported that streptomycin that was encapsulated in liposomes was 50 to 100 times more effective in treating MAC infections in mice than was free streptomycin.

RAPIDLY GROWING MYCOBACTERIA

This group of mycobacteria has a generation time of less than 1 hour, and colonies become visible after 2 to 3 days of growth. The group includes nonpathogens such as *Mycobacterium phlei* and *Mycobacterium smegmatis,* as well as several species that do cause human infections. Pathogens include *Mycobacterium fortuitum, Mycobacterium chelonei,* and *Mycobacterium abscessus,* but, because of uncertainty about their classification, these three organisms are frequently grouped in an *M fortuitum* complex.

Members of the *M fortuitum* complex are most frequently involved in wound infections, which may occur as skin abscesses or as deeper infections after surgery. One surprising postoperative wound infection caused by this group occurred when 24 patients became infected after open heart surgery. Cultures of equipment used in the operating room all gave negative results, and the source of these organisms remains unknown.

Mycobacterium leprae

Leprosy has been one of the most feared chronic infectious disease known. About 13 million persons are infected worldwide, and over 100 new cases are diagnosed each year in the United States. Even though it is an ancient disease of humans, the etiologic agent has never been grown in an artificial medium. Moreover, the epidemiology of the disease is still unclear, and only during the last few years has there been a good comprehension of the events involved in the pathogenesis of leprosy.

The etiologic agent of leprosy is morphologically similar to *M tuberculosis.* The organisms appear in lesions as acid-fast rods 3 to 5 μm long and 0.2 to 0.4 μm in diameter.

Scores of attempts to infect human volunteers with *Mycobacterium leprae* have been unsuccessful. It does, however, grow in the foot pad of the mouse, and it has been shown to produce a generalized, progressive, systemic infection in the armadillo.

EPIDEMIOLOGY AND PATHOGENESIS OF LEPROSY

Little is known about the epidemiology of leprosy, but it is a disease in which infection may depend largely on the susceptibility of certain persons. Children seem to be more susceptible than adults and, on a worldwide basis, leprosy is twice as common in male as in female persons. In general, it seems that infection requires only relatively brief contact for "susceptible" persons, but most persons probably cannot be infected by any means.

It has been generally believed that humans constitute the only source of *M leprae* and that it may be acquired by a susceptible person by way of skin-to-skin contact. In cases of lepromatous leprosy, however, the nasal discharge may contain over 10^8 organisms per milliliter, and it appears that such discharges provide the major means of spread for this disease. Evidence suggests that exposure to wild, infected armadillos also may be a source of infection for some Mexican patients.

Clinically, the disease may occur in either of two major forms: lepromatous leprosy or tuberculoid leprosy. Considerable information has been reported that suggest that HLA genes determine the type of leprosy that develops by controlling leprosy-specific immune responses. There is, however, a continuum of responses between these two manifestations of leprosy, and a five-group system of classification is used that includes tuberculoid (TT), borderline tuberculoid (BT), borderline (BB), borderline lepromatous (BL), and lepromatous (LL).

Tuberculoid Leprosy

Tuberculoid leprosy is frequently a self-limiting disease that may even regress spontaneously. Skin lesions occur, and nerve involvement producing areas of anesthesia is the most conspicuous feature of this form of leprosy. Unlike the lepromatous form of leprosy, organisms are extremely rare and may not be seen in skin scrapings or biopsy specimens. The major characteristic accounting for this form of the disease is a vigorous cellular immune response mounted against the leprosy bacillus, which is associated with severe, local peripheral nerve destruction. Thus, nerve damage (which occurs much more rapidly than in the lepromatous form) actually results from inflammation that occurs during a cellular immune response to the bacilli in the nerves. Table 31-2 summarizes the characteristics of both forms of leprosy.

Lepromatous Leprosy

This form is progressive and malignant, which, if untreated, routinely ends in death. The organisms are found in essentially every organ of the body, although the major pathologic changes occur in the skin, nerves, and testes. Skin lesions may be hypopigmented or nodular, and lesions of mucous membranes may involve the nose, causing severe nasal deformities because of the destruction of of the cardiolipin. Another widely used nonspecific test is the rapid plasma reagin (RPR) card test. The RPR is performed by adsorbing the cardiolipin on carbon particles and mixing this modified antigen with the patient's serum on a card. In a positive test result, the flocculation of the carbon particles is visible to the naked eye. None of the tests employing cardiolipin as an antigen is completely specific, and about 1% of normal adults will give rise to antibodies resulting in false-positive reactions. A more specific test to evaluate positive results is essential.

SPECIFIC TESTS. A number of specific tests are available for the definite diagnosis of syphilis. All require either live *T pallidum,* grown in the testes of a rabbit and, in some cases, the Reiter strain of *Treponema,* which is thought to be an avirulent form of *T pallidum* and can be grown on artificial media. The *Treponema pallidum* immobilization test uses live, testes-grown treponemes. If suspended anaerobically in the presence of specific antibody and complement, the organisms will lose their motility. The test is positive for any of the treponemal diseases (including yaws and pinta), but it requires specialized equipment and 18 hours to complete. By far the most widely used serologic test for specific treponemal antibodies is an indirect fluorescent antibody test, the *fluorescent treponemal antibody-absorption test.* The absorption step in this test is necessary to eliminate nonspecific reactions that occur as a result of antibodies to common antigens shared by both pathogenic and saprophytic treponemes. The absorption is accomplished by mixing the patient's serum with a standardized extract from nonpathogenic Reiter treponemes. (This sorbant can be purchased commercially.) The absorbed serum is then used to cover a smear of pathogenic, testes-grown treponemes (Nichols strain, which can be purchased commercially as lyophilized organisms). After 30 minutes at 37°C, the slide is thoroughly rinsed to remove unreacted serum proteins, and the slide is then covered with a fluorescently labeled antihuman gamma globulin. This again is allowed to react for 30 minutes before rinsing, and the slide is examined microscopically (with an ultraviolet light source) for the presence of fluorescently stained treponemes. Because the fluorescently labeled antihuman gamma globulin could bind to the treponemes only if the organisms were coated with human antibody, the presence of fluorescently labeled treponemes signifies the presence of specific antibodies to *T pallidum.* On occasions when lesions are present, expressed material can be stained directly with specific antibodies to *T pallidum* that have been conjugated to a fluorescent dye (direct fluorescent antibody test for *T pallidum*).

The microhemagglutination test for *T pallidum* also assays for specific treponemal antibodies. This method employs specially treated sheep's erythrocytes that have been coated with antigen from *T pallidum.* The test has been automated and adapted to a microvolume proce-dure. A positive result is signified by the agglutination of the red cells.

There are a number of other procedures for determining specific treponemal antibodies, such as the *T pallidum* agglutination, *T pallidum* immune adherence, and whole-body *T pallidum* complement fixation tests. None of these, however, is used in diagnostic laboratories; they serve primarily as research tools.

The choice of which test to use may, in part, be dictated by personal preference. The Veneral Disease Research Laboratory or RPR test is less expensive than procedures for determining specific antibodies and is, therefore, used in screening low-risk populations such as persons having premarital serologic testing. Positive results can be confirmed with one of the specific tests. When it becomes possible to grow the pathogenic treponemes in an artificial medium, the availability of an inexpensive antigen will undoubtedly influence the choice of tests used to diagnose syphilis serologically.

Treatment and Control of Syphilis

Before the turn of the century, the only treatment for syphilis was mercury, which was usually applied in an ointment to the lesions occurring during secondary syphilis. In 1909, Paul Ehrlich was carrying out his systematic search for a "magic bullet" that would selectively attack microorganisms without undue toxicity to the host. Although Ehrlich never found his universal weapon, he did develop an arsenical compound, arsphenamine, that, together with bismuth, was relatively effective in treating syphilis. Such treatment was painful and long (at least 1 year) and has not been used since the advent of penicillin.

Syphilis could, theoretically, be eradicated because the organisms are sensitive to low levels of penicillin. Even the tertiary stage may be arrested with adequate penicillin therapy, but, in these cases, therapy must be prolonged for several weeks, probably because the organisms are growing so slowly. Erythromycin and tetracycline are also effective antibiotics, but they do not cross the placenta in sufficient concentrations to cure congenital syphilis. However, in spite of the ease with which the disease may be cured, public health authorities have reported a rising incidence since 1960.

An interesting phenomenon called the Jarisch-Herxheimer reaction occasionally occurs 1 to 2 hours after treatment with penicillin. This systemic reaction results from the release of endotoxin after lysis of the spirochetes. It is self-limiting and persists for only 12 to 24 hours.

T pallidum is exceptionally adept at evading host immune killing mechanisms, perhaps because its outer membrane contains so little protein (ie, about 100-fold less than *Escherichia coli*). However, in spite of its nearly naked lipid bilayer membrane, humoral antibodies to syphilis do appear several weeks after the occurrence of the primary lesion. However, a cellular immune response is believed to cause the eventual regression of the lesions of secondary syphilis. This conclusion is based on the observation that animals that were given immune syphilitic serum were protected from a subsequent infection, but animals that were first infected could not be cured with humoral antibodies. Persons with a latent infection cannot be reinfected, and, even if treated, persons with long-standing infections seem to retain their immunity. Therefore, it seems theoretically possible to produce an effective vaccine, and considerable effort is being expended toward this objective. Toward this end, the gene for a 47-kd surface protein of *T pallidum* has been cloned in *E coli*. This protein is present also as a surface protein of *T pallidum* subsp *endemicum* and *T pallidum* subsp *pertenue,* but it is absent in nonpathogenic treponemes. Moreover, it is highly immunogenic in humans. Antibodies to this pathogen-specific treponemal protein exert a complement-dependent treponemicidal activity. It is thus a prime candidate both for a vaccine and for use in an enzyme-linked immunosorbent assay for the diagnosis of syphilis.

Bejel (Endemic Syphilis)

A nonvenereal disease known as bejel occurs in Africa and the Middle East. The etiologic agent is similar to that causing syphilis and is called *Treponema pallidum* subsp *endemicum.*

The disease occurs primarily in rural children living under poor standards of personal hygiene and is spread from person to person, usually through the use of common drinking and eating utensils.

Initial lesions are most common in the oral mucosa, followed by additional, secondary lesions on the oral mucosa and at the corners of the mouth. Tertiary lesions are more widespread and consist of syphilitic gummata on the skin, bone, and nasopharynx.

The infection can be eliminated by a single injection of long-acting penicillin, and it seems probable that this disease may be eradicated.

TREPONEMA PALLIDUM SUBSPECIES *PERTENUE*

Treponema pallidum subsp *pertenue*, the etiologic agent of yaws, is morphologically indistinguishable from the causative agent of syphilis. DNA hybridization studies show complete homology, indicating that they are closely related organisms.

Epidemiology and Pathogenesis of Yaws

Yaws is restricted to the tropics, where it seems to be spread from person to person either by direct contact with open ulcers or by vectors such as flies. An initial lesion occurs 3 to 4 weeks after exposure, and, after ulcerating, spontaneously heals. Several months later, secondary lesions appear, which ulcerate, heal, and reappear in crops over a period of several years. The disease may become quiescent, only to reappear as tertiary lesions of the skin and bones, frequently resulting in considerable disfigurement of the face.

Laboratory Diagnosis, Treatment, and Control of Yaws

In all likelihood, the average diagnosis is based on the clinical picture occurring in an area where yaws is endemic. However, all of the serologic tests for syphilis described earlier will yield positive results. *T pallidum* subsp *pertenue* is sensitive to penicillin, and, like syphilis, this severely disfiguring disease could be easily controlled if it were possible to give adequate penicillin therapy to infected persons. Such eradication programs have been under way in the Western Hemisphere since 1950. At that time, Haiti was estimated to have 1 million cases of yaws. After a house-to-house survey and treatment of infected persons, the disease has been essentially eliminated from that country. A similar program was undertaken in Brazil and in the Lesser Antilles, leaving few infected areas in the Americas.

TREPONEMA CARATEUM

Pinta is a disease that occurs mainly in Central and South America. *Treponema carateum*, the etiologic agent, also is indistinguishable from *T pallidum*, but the skin lesions produced are flat red or blue areas that do not ulcerate and ultimately become depigmented. Lesions are usually confined to the skin.

Transmission seems to require direct person-to-person contact, and, like the other species of *Treponema, T carateum* is sensitive to penicillin. Eradication programs in Mexico and Colombia, similar to those for yaws, have considerably reduced the incidence of pinta in these areas.

TREPONEMA VINCENTII

Treponema vincentii (the older name was *Borrelia vincentii*) and *Bacteroides melaninogenicus* have been thought to be involved in a fusospirochetal (caused by both fusiform bacteria and spirochetes) disease. It is commonly referred to as Vincent's angina, or acute necrotizing ulcerative gingivitis, as well as "trench mouth," because it was prevalent among the infantry during World War I. *T vincentii* is an active, motile spirochete, and *B melaninogenicus* is a nonmotile, gram-negative, straight or slightly curved rod that frequently occurs in pairs, with the outer ends pointed and the blunt ends together. Both organisms are obligate anaerobes.

Vincent's angina is characterized by ulcerative lesions of the mouth or tonsilar area. There is a possibility that the real etiologic agent is a herpes virus and, for reasons not understood, the two bacteria, which are normal flora of the mouth, multiply during the active disease.

TABLE 33-1
Partial List of Mycoplasms That Infect Animals

Organism	Host	Disease
M bovigenitalism	Cattle	Mastitis and vulvovaginitis
M bovirhinis	Cattle	Respiratory disease (?)
M mycoides	Cattle	Pleuropneumonia
M ovipneumoniae	Lambs	Pneumonia
M conjunctivae	Goats and sheep	Conjunctivitis
M gallisepticum	Poultry	Respiratory disease and encephalitis
M pulmonis	Mice and rats	Respiratory disease
M arthritidis	Rats	Polyarthritis
M hyorhinis	Swine	Arthritis
M hyosynoviae	Swine	Arthritis and synovitis
M orale	Humans	Parasite of oropharynx
M pneumoniae	Humans	Primary atypical pneumonia
M salivarium	Humans	Parasite of oropharynx
M hominus	Humans	Pelvic inflammatory disease
Ureaplasma	Humans and other animals	Urethritis

terol for growth. The exact function of the cholesterol is not known, but it is adsorbed to a preformed constituent in the cell membrane and is thought to be necessary for the pliability and tensile strength of the cell membrane. Members of the genus *Acholeplasma* (in the family Acholeplasmataceae) do not require added sterols for growth but, instead, synthesize carotenoids, which they deposit in their cell membrane. There have been reports that *Mycoplasma* can be grown in a medium employing carotenoids as substitutes for cholesterol.

Growth of *Mycoplasma* on a solid medium routinely results in the formation of colonies so small that they cannot normally be seen with the naked eye. When cul-

tures are viewed under the low power (10×) of the light microscope, diphasic colonies with a "fried-egg" look frequently appear. Such colonies are formed when cells in the center of the colony grow down into the medium (Fig. 33-2).

A number of strains of *Mycoplasma* will also grow in the amniotic sac or yolk of chick embryos, or as contaminants of cell cultures, causing various cytopathic effects.

CLASSIFICATION

Immunologic techniques provide the primary basis for the classification of mycoplasmas, and growth inhibition

TABLE 33-2
Generic Classification of Mollicutes

Families and Genera	Major Characteristics
MYCOPLASMATACEAE	All require cholesterol
Genus 1 *Mycoplasma*	Pathogenic for animals and humans; colonies may be 600 μm diameter
Genus 2 *Ureaplasma*	Proposed name for urea-using T strains; pathogens or parasites; tiny colonies 10–30 μm diameter
ACHOLEPLASMATACEAE	None require cholesterol
Genus 1 *Acholeplasma*	Saprophyte or parasite for mammals and birds
Genus 2 *Thermoplasma*	Saprophyte having an optimum growth temperature of 59°C at pH 1 to 3
Genus 3 *Anaeroplasma*	Saprophyte obligately anaerobic isolated from rumen of cattle and sheep
SPIROPLASMATACEAE	
Genus 1 *Spiroplasma*	Plant/animal pathogen possessing helical and branched filaments

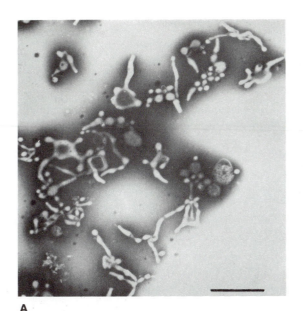
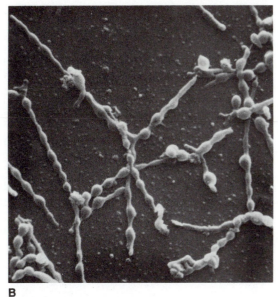

A **B**

FIGURE 33-1   **A.** Electron micrograph of a negatively stained preparation of *Mycoplasma pneumoniae*. The variable morphologic features, ranging from rings with lobes to beaded filaments, is evident. (Scale = 1 μm). **B.** Scanning electron micrograph of *M pneumoniae*; notice the coccoid structures within the filaments. (Original magnification ×10,000.)

by specific antisera seems to be the easiest and most specific method for their identification. The test can be carried out using one of a variety of techniques, such as (1) incorporating dilutions of antiserum directly into the agar medium, placing a filter-paper disc that has been soaked in antiserum onto an inoculated area of a culture plate, and subsequently observing for inhibition of mycoplasma growth around the disc; or (2) adding dilutions of antiserum to plastic cylinders embedded in the agar of the culture plate.

Complement fixation or agglutination tests also can be conducted, but studies have shown that growth-inhibition tests provide better correlations with accepted mycoplasma species.

MYCOPLASMA PNEUMONIAE

During the 1940s, clinical and laboratory observations provided a description of a type of pneumonia distinct from typical bacterial pneumonia. Using human volunteers, it was shown that this type of pneumonia was caused by an infectious agent and, because no bacterium could be isolated, it was assumed to be caused by a virus. The organism was named Eaton's agent for the scientist who first reported that the disease was caused by a filterable agent that could be grown in chick embryos. Not until 20 years later was Eaton's agent found to be a mycoplasma, subsequently named *Mycoplasma pneumoniae*.

M pneumoniae will adsorb to a number of different kinds of erythrocytes and mammalian cells, especially tracheal epithelial cells. The cell receptor is a glycoprotein that contains terminal neuraminic acid residues that are α 2–3 linked. *M pneumoniae* will also bind to glycophorin from red blood cells. Treatment of cells with neuraminidase removes the neuraminic acid, destroying the receptor, rendering the cells incapable of adsorption. (Influenza virus, which also causes a respiratory infection, adsorbs to a similar type of cell receptor.) One obvious virulence determinant of *M pneumoniae* is a specific receptor protein, which is located in a knobbed tip of the cell.

FIGURE 33-2   Colonies of *Mycoplasma fermentans* show "fried egg" appearance; growth was on agar for 14 days. (Original magnification ×185.)

Removal of this protein with trypsin or treatment with monoclonal antibodies specific for this tip protein completely prevents attachment of the mycoplasma to host cells, indicating it is a critical virulence determinant. The structural gene for this cytadhesin, termed *P1*, has been cloned and shown to encode for a 170-kd protein.

M pneumoniae causes beta hemolysis on a number of different types of erythrocytes, and the factor responsible for the hemolysis has been shown to be hydrogen peroxide–produced by the metabolism of *Mycoplasma*. Because erythrocytes possess an active catalase, their lysis by H_2O_2 is unusual, and it has been suggested that it occurs because of the close association of *Mycoplasma* when it is bound to a specific receptor site on the red blood cell. It also has been postulated that tracheal epithelial cell destruction may occur by the same mechanism.

Epidemiology and Pathogenesis of Primary Atypical Pneumonia

Primary atypical pneumonia (PAP) occurs most frequently in school children and in people who live in close confines, as in military camps. Mycoplasmas are found in the respiratory tracts of infected persons, and the disease spreads by the respiratory route. The incubation period is 2 to 3 weeks; symptoms vary from an inapparent or mild disease to a severe pneumonia characterized by headache, chills, fever, and general malaise. Chest x-rays usually show a patchy pneumonitis that frequently appears worse than anticipated from the physical examination. Major symptoms disappear between the 3rd and 10th days of illness, but chest infiltration and coughing may continue for 1 to 2 months. The disease rarely is fatal.

Interestingly, serologic surveys indicate that infections with *M pneumoniae* are common in persons 5 to 20 years of age, but only a small percentage of these individuals have had a diagnosed lower respiratory infection. Thus, it seems that many infections must be mild or inapparent. Surprisingly, the more severe disease seems to occur in persons older than 20 years of age. Because recovery does not result in solid immunity to reinfection, it has been proposed that the more severe manifestations of this disease are the result of an autoimmune reaction occurring during a second infection with *M pneumoniae*. This model suggests that after attachment of the mycoplasma to a host cell, their membranes fuse, and the mycoplasma membrane proteins are integrated into the host-cell membrane. A subsequent infection induces a humoral as well as a cell-mediated response directed against these foreign antigens. This concept is supported by two lines of evidence: (1) repeated infections in animals produce an accelerated and exaggerated pulmonary histopathologic result; and (2) immunosuppressed animals and patients with immune deficiencies may be infected without the occurrence of pulmonary disease.

Laboratory Diagnosis of Primary Atypical Pneumonia

Before the discovery that PAP was caused by a mycoplasma, diagnosis was based on the clinical picture, chest x-rays, and two laboratory findings: (1) the development of cold hemagglutinins (antibodies that will agglutinate human type-O erythrocytes when incubated at 0° to 4°C, but not at 37°C); and (2) the presence of antibodies to a bacterium named *Streptococcus mg,* apparently resulting from cross-reactions with glucosyl glycerides.

M pneumoniae from sputum can be grown in a medium containing serum, with penicillin added to inhibit the growth of contaminants. Conclusive identification is obtained by staining the organisms with a specific fluorescently labeled antibody or by growth inhibition in the presence of specific antibody.

Treatment and Control of Primary Atypical Pneumonia

Erythromycin and the tetracyclines are effective for the treatment of PAP. Many physicians prefer to use erythromycin, because it is also effective for the treatment of legionellosis. Experimental formalin-inactivated vaccines have been shown to give about 50% protection against pneumonia, and such vaccines may be of value in military camps. Live, attenuated vaccines have been tried experimentally in humans and animals, but many persons experienced some illness from the vaccine. Temperature-sensitive vaccines that are able to grow only in the upper respiratory tract also have been used with moderate success.

MYCOPLASMA HOMINIS AND MYCOPLASMA GENITALIUM

Mycoplasma hominis can be isolated from the genital tracts of 30% to 50% of asymptomatic humans, and the species also has been isolated from a variety of pelvic abscesses. As a result, a great deal of controversy exists over the potential of this organism to cause pelvic inflammatory disease. Opinions can be summarized as follows: (1) *M hominis* probably does cause occasional pelvic abscess but, in all likelihood, is rarely involved in lower genital-tract infections such as cervicitis, vaginitis, or urethritis; and (2) in most instances, *M hominis* exists in the genital tract as a nonpathogenic parasite.

Mycoplasma genitalium also has been isolated from a number of cases of nongonococcal urethritis, but its role as an etiologic agent of disease still is equivocal. Notice, however, that *M genitalium* possesses a 140-kd cytadhesin, which is morphologically similar to the knobbed receptor described for *M pneumoniae*, suggesting that *M genitalium* may possess a virulence factor analogous to that described for *M pneumoniae*.

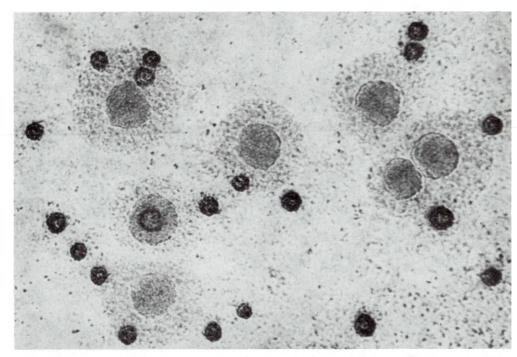

FIGURE 33-3 This micrograph demonstrates the size difference between colonies of the T-strain mycoplasma *Ureaplasma urealyticum* (small, dark colonies) and the "fried egg" colonies of the classic large-colony *Mycoplasma hominis*. This is a standard agar culture on which the direct spot test for urease was applied: the dark urease-positive T-strain colonies show the specific development of manganese reaction product, which positively identifies them as members of the genus *Ureaplasma*. The larger, lighter, urease-negative *M hominis* colonies have been counterstained with a blue dye. (Original magnification ×195.)

UREAPLASMA (T-STRAIN MYCOPLASMAS)

T strains of mycoplasma are so named because they grow as exceptionally tiny colonies, usually 10 to 20 μm in diameter. Such colonies cannot be seen with the naked eye; they are much smaller than normal mycoplasma colonies and barely visible with the light microscope using 10× magnification (Fig. 33-3).

T strains require both cholesterol and urea for growth, and the incorporation of 10% horse serum into a medium will supply both requirements. The organisms contain a urease that hydrolyzes urea to ammonia and carbon dioxide. Because of this absolute requirement for urea, the generic name *Ureaplasma* is used for these organisms.

There is only one species of *Ureaplasma*, *Ureaplasma urealyticum*; its role as a pathogen has been debated for two decades. As mentioned earlier, these organisms can be isolated from the genital tract of up to 50% of asymptomatic persons, and they can also be found in 50% to 80% of persons with nongonococcal urethritis. There have also been a number of claims that mycoplasmas can be isolated from the joints of patients with arthritis, but other researchers have been unsuccessful in attempts to repeat such isolations. There seems little doubt, however, that

Ureaplasma is transmitted by sexual contact, because it has been shown that after puberty, colonization results primarily from sexual contact.

An investigation into the role of the mycoplasmas on perinatal morbidity and mortality reported that *U urealyticum, M hominis,* or both were isolated from 21% of the placentas of premature and full-term infants who died in the perinatal period, 25% of those admitted to intensive care, and only 11% of controls. Gestational age and low birth weight also were related to the isolation of *Ureaplasma*.

The role of *U urealyticum* as an etiologic agent of nongonococcal urethritis also seems well established, but the paradox of many asymptomatic genital carriers of *Ureaplasma* is difficult to explain. It has been suggested that disease may occur only on initial exposure, and that subsequent immune reactions permit colonization but prevent overt disease.

The role of T strains with respect to human arthritis is less clear. Some mycoplasmas are known to cause arthritis in other animals, and reports that they have been occasionally isolated from human joint fluid and synovial tissue provide circumstantial evidence for their involvement in this human disorder. However, the failure of qualified investigators to routinely isolate mycoplasmas

A Closer Look

The observation that 40% to 80% of sexually experienced, asymptomatic women carry *Ureaplasma urealyticum* in their vagina and cervix has made it exceedingly difficult to correlate the presence of these organisms with disease. However, it is well established that in at least some individuals *U urealyticum* is associated with spontaneous abortion, chorioamnionitis, and premature birth. Moreover, it appears that *U urealyticum* is responsible for a significant number of cases of mortality, particularly in premature infants of low birth rate. The question one would like to answer is which of the large percentage of colonized women are likely to experience difficulties during pregnancy?

First, numerous studies have shown that infection by *U urealyticum* of the upper genital tract (chorioamnionitis), but not the lower genital tract (vagina and cervix), is associated with premature birth and perinatal morbidity and mortality. Such data have also documented that infection of the amniotic fluid can result in an in utero fetal infection.

One would like to ask what series of events must happen for an upper genital infection to occur, and why does it occur only in a small percentage of pregnant women who are colonized with *U urealyticum*? Unfortunately, there is no unequivocal answer to this question. It is known that the endometrium can become infected in nonpregnant females and, if infected, could result in an infection of the amniotic sac after conception. It is also known that bacterial vaginitis occurs in 15% to 20% of pregnant women, and such persons have an increased prevalence of *Gardnerella vaginalis*, certain anaerobic bacteria, *Mycoplasma hominis*, and about a 100-fold intravaginal increase in *U urealyticum*. Circumstantial evidence suggests that the

bacterial vaginitis and the increased *U urealyticum* may produce an additive effect, leading to uterine contraction and premature birth.

So, what can happen to the premature infant born to a mother with an upper genital infection with *U urealyticum*? The most common effect is either a congenital pneumonia or a pneumonia acquired during birth. Such infections carry a high mortality rate in low birth weight neonates. Survivors of the acute pneumonia may then die from a bronchopulmonary dysplasia termed *chronic lung disease*, which has a 15% to 38% mortality rate in those with birth weights less than 1500 g. Several studies have shown a significant association of *U urealyticum* pneumonia before presenting with chronic lung disease.

Do men become infected with *Ureaplasma* and, if so, what are the results? The answer is yes and, although the infection may be asymptomatic, it does have consequences. Electron micrographs from infected men showed sperm coated with *Ureaplasma* that imparted a rough texture and seemed to slow the motility of the sperm. In a second study, 161 men who were infected with *Ureaplasma* were treated along with their wives with doxycycline for 4 weeks. At the end of this period, 129 men had negative semen culture results for *Ureaplasma*. The rate of successful pregnancies after therapy was 60% for those in which *Ureaplasma* had been eradicated and 5% for the group still infected with *Ureaplasma*.

So, it seems obvious that this supposedly innocuous bacterium may be an important sexually transmitted disease, and the physician should be aware of its potential for harm.

from arthritic patients casts doubt on their role in this disease.

L-Forms of Bacteria (Cell-Wall–Defective Organisms)

L-forms are bacterial variant growth forms that no longer produce rigid peptidoglycan cell walls. Thus, they are in many ways analogous to mycoplasmas (Fig. 33-4).

The first isolation of a naturally occurring L-form took place at the Lister Institute (hence, the "L"), and it was characterized by Louis Dienes in 1939. He found that the L-forms (which produced tiny colonies on solid media) arose spontaneously from the bacterium *Strepto-*

bacillus moniliformis, and that after prolonged incubation in broth, some of the L-forms would revert to the parent bacterium. Subsequently, L-forms were isolated from various sources by studying freshly isolated cultures of bacteria from pathologic specimens. Still later, it was discovered that growth in the presence of penicillin could be used to select or induce the appearance of L-forms and, that under appropriate conditions, some strains in almost all studied species of bacteria can develop into L-forms. The terms *protoplast, spheroplast,* and *L-form* might be confusing, but one can define an L-form as any bacterium that has lost its ability to synthesize a peptidoglycan cell wall but that can still multiply.

The similarities between L-forms and mycoplasmas have prompted speculation as to whether mycoplasmas

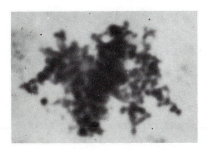

FIGURE 33-4 L1 phase variant of *Streptobacillus moniliformis*; notice the pleomorphism and the rounded appearance of individual cells, which lack peptidoglycan cell walls. (Original magnification ×2250.)

might represent stable L-forms of bacteria, because they form structurally similar colonies and seem to reproduce in a similar manner. However, after much immunologic research and studies of nucleic acid homology, the general consensus is that mycoplasmas are not related to L-forms. If mycoplasmas arose originally from bacteria, their genesis must have occurred long ago on the evolutionary scale.

No actual situation is known in which an L-form, by itself, can produce disease. *Streptobacillus moniliformis,* an organism that spontaneously forms L-forms, is the etiologic agent of rat-bite fever, but there is no evidence that the L-form is involved in the disease process.

There is, perhaps, a much more important potential role for L-forms: they might function as antibiotic-resistant cells during treatment of a disease with antibiotics that inhibit cell-wall synthesis. Because L-forms do not possess a peptidoglycan cell wall, they are not sensitive to cell-wall–inhibiting antibiotics such as penicillin, and it has been proposed that the formation of L-forms during antibiotic therapy could explain relapses after treatment. The isolation of L-forms after the termination of penicillin treatment supports this proposal, and, theoretically, such L-forms could revert to their original bacterial forms after cessation of therapy, resulting in a relapse of disease.

Bibliography

JOURNALS

Cassell GH, Waites KB, Watson HL, Crouse DT, Harasawa R. *Ureaplasma urealyticum* intrauterine infection: role in prematurity and disease in newborns. Clin Microbiol Rev 1993;6:69.

Henrich B, et al. Cytoadhesins of *Mycoplasma hominis.* Infect Immun 1993;61:2945.

Thirkill CE, Tyler NK, Roth AM. Circulating and localized immune complexes in experimental *Mycoplasma*-induced arthritis-associated ocular inflammation. Infect Immun 1992;60:401.

Essentials of Medical Microbiology, Fifth Edition, edited by Wesley A. Volk, Bryan M. Gebhardt, Marie-Louise Hammarskjöld, and Robert J. Kadner. Lippincott-Raven Publishers, Philadelphia © 1996.

Chapter 34

Rickettsiae and Chlamydiae

RICKETTSIAE

The rickettsiae are smaller than most other bacteria, but stained smears can be readily seen using an ordinary light microscope. It is not size, however, that sets them apart from other bacteria, but rather the fact that (with exception of species in the genus *Rochalimaea*), they grow only inside animal cells; in other words, they are obligate intracellular parasites. Thus, rickettsiae cannot be grown in the laboratory on artificial media as can most bacteria, but require living cells for growth. Moreover, with the one exception of Q fever, all rickettsial diseases are transmitted from animal to animal (humans included) by the bite of an infected arthropod vector.

Rickettsiae seem to be closely related to the gram-negative bacteria. Typically, they are coccoid to rod-shaped, with average dimensions of 0.3 to 0.7 μm by 1.5 to 2.0 μm (Fig. 34-1). Electron microscopic study reveals a cell wall consisting of an inner membrane and an outer membrane, a structure characteristic of gram-negative cells. Furthermore, when stained with Gram's stain, they appear as gram-negative bacteria. Rickettsiae also have been shown to contain muramic acid (a substance existing only in procaryotic cells) and diaminopimelic acid and 2-keto-3-deoxyoctulosonic acid (KDO) (compounds found only in the cell walls of gram-negative bacteria). Thus, it seems that rickettsiae are really a unique type of gram-negative bacteria.

Why, then, are rickettsiae obligate intracellular parasites? If they originally descended from gram-negative bacteria, what have they lost that would allow them to grow extracellularly? Not all of the answers to these questions are known, and various theories propose to explain this restricted growth. Rickettsiae seem able to synthesize their own proteins, nucleic acids, and any other macromolecules necessary for their structural components. Moreover, they are able to oxidize glutamic acid, as well as a number of intermediates of the citric acid cycle, and they are able to trap the energy released by these oxidations as ATP. However, rickettsiae are not able to metabolize glucose as a substrate.

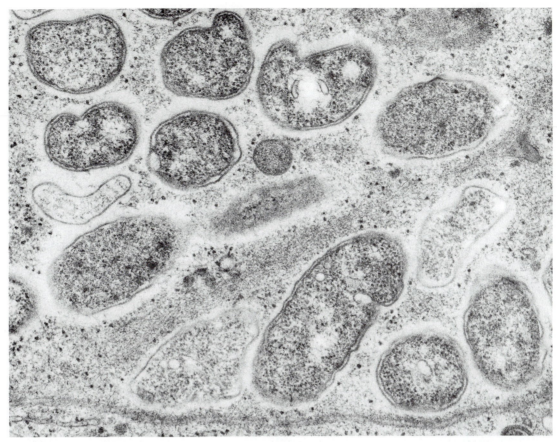

FIGURE 34-1 *Rickettsia prowazekii* in experimentally infected tick tissue. Notice the double-layered cell wall similar to that of gram-negative bacteria. (Original magnification ×45,000.)

Scientific information makes it possible to speculate about the parasitic, intracellular life-style of rickettsiae: if the rickettsiae are removed from their intracellular environment and placed in a balanced salt solution, they rapidly lose viability and infectivity. This seems to be correlated with the loss of intracellular metabolites, because they can be restored to infectivity by the addition of compounds such as nicotinamide-adenine dinucleotide, coenzyme A, ATP, and inorganic ions such as K^+ and Mg^{++}. Because most organisms are unable to take up such large molecules, this observation led to a "leaky membrane" explanation for the obligate intracellular requirement of the rickettsiae. This postulation, however, seems to be incomplete, based on the work of Herbert Winkler and associates at the University of South Alabama College of Medicine (Mobile, AL). They have shown that rickettsiae possess an unusual transport system that exchanges ADP for ATP across their cell membranes. These investigators have cloned this gene for the ADP/ATP translocator into *Escherichia coli,* and, based on their data, they suggest that the leaky membrane and the obligate intracellular parasitism of the rickettsia is because of their unusual transport systems. Interestingly, the rickettsial ADP/ATP translocator is functionally identical to the one present in mitochondria and in the chlamydiae, even though they do not share sequence homology. Uridine 5′-diphosphoglucose has been shown to be also transported across the rickettsial cell membrane.

Techniques for the Culture of Rickettsiae

In view of these characteristics, how can rickettsiae be propagated in the laboratory? One way is to infect susceptible animals such as guinea pigs; rickettsiae also can be grown in cultures of living animal cells. The method most commonly used during the last several decades involves the inoculation of rickettsiae into the yolk sac of a chick embryo. For this purpose, fertile hen eggs are incubated for 6 days, until the chick embryo is well advanced in its development. The rickettsiae are then injected into the yolk sac, where they grow in the cells of the membrane surrounding the yolk. After an additional 8 days of incubation, the egg is opened, and the yolk sac membrane is removed. The rickettsiae can then be partially purified by several techniques that usually involve disruption of the yolk sac cells followed by differential centrifugation.

Disease	OX-19	OX-2	OX-K
Epidemic typhus	++++	+	0
Endemic typhus	++++	+	0
Brill-Zinsser disease	Variable, often negative		0
Scrub typhus	0	0	+++
Spotted fever group	{ ++++ +	{ + +++	{ 0 0
Q fever	0	0	0
Rickettsialpox	0	0	0

Antigenic Characteristics of the Rickettsiae

All rickettsiae produce soluble group antigens that are released into the surrounding environment. These antigens are characteristic for each group of rickettsial infections: those from the typhus group can be differentiated from the group antigens produced by the spotted fever group or the scrub typhus group, and so forth. In addition, each strain of *Rickettsia* produces a type-specific antigen that is attached to the cell wall and can be used to distinguish both species and strains within a species. Both the group-specific and type-specific antigens give rise to antibodies that can be measured using an enzyme-linked immunoassay.

A more general serologic test for certain rickettsial diseases is called the **Weil-Felix test.** In this classic test, the patient's antibodies are measured (preferably during acute illness and again after convalescence) for the ability to agglutinate certain strains of a gram-negative rod in the genus *Proteus*. *Proteus* organisms have nothing whatsoever to do with causing rickettsial diseases, but certain strains of these bacteria have an antigen on their cells that is also present in the rickettsiae. Three different strains of *Proteus,* designated *Proteus* OX-2, *Proteus* OX-19, and *Proteus* OX-K, have been used in this test. As seen in Table 34-1, not all rickettsial diseases induce a positive Weil-Felix test result, and the test is not specific for infections that do cause a positive reaction. Moreover, the test is unreliable and is no longer used in many clinical laboratories. However, a positive result, when interpreted in conjunction with the clinical illness and history, can be a valuable aid in diagnosis.

Spotted Fever Group

Diseases of the spotted fever group have received common names from the areas of the world where they are found. A few examples of rickettsial diseases in the spotted fever group are Rocky Mountain spotted fever (RMSF), Queensland tick spotted fever, Boutonneuse spotted fever, and rickettsialpox. Organisms in the spotted fever group grow in both the nucleus and the cytoplasm of infected cells. When growing in the cytoplasm, these rickettsiae induce the polymerization of F-actin to form long polar tails. By analogy with the spread of *Shigella flexneri* and *Listeria monocytogenes,* it has been proposed that these actin filaments play a role in a direct cell-to-cell transmission of these organisms, permitting an evasion of host immune responses. The spotted fever rickettsiae share a common group antigen, but they also induce the formation of type-specific antibodies.

ROCKY MOUNTAIN SPOTTED FEVER

Rocky Mountain spotted fever was first recognized in the Bitterroot Valley in Montana, but the disease has been reported in almost every one of the United States. The causative organism, *Rickettsia rickettsii,* is named for Howard Taylor Ricketts, an early pioneer in the study of rickettsial diseases, who died as a result of his investigations of typhus.

EPIDEMIOLOGY AND PATHOGENESIS. Humans invariably contract RMSF from the bite of an infected tick. In the western United States, the wood tick, *Dermacentor andersoni,* carries the disease, whereas the dog tick, *Dermacentor variabilis,* serves as the vector in the eastern United States (Fig. 34-2). Notice that these hard-shelled, slow-feeding ticks are distinct from the soft-shelled, fast-feeding ticks that are vectors for relapsing fever. About 500 cases are reported in the United States each year, with most occurring in children living in the "tick belt" of Maryland, Virginia, North Carolina, South Carolina, Oklahoma, and Georgia.

Reports have shown that dogs are readily infected and that rickettsiae can be isolated from their blood for at least 2 weeks after infection. Thus, even though infected dogs do not seem to be ill, they may serve as an important reservoir for these organisms.

RMSF is characterized by fever, severe headache, and usually a maculopapular rash (discolored spots—some may be elevated above the skin and others not) that usually appears first on the palms and soles. The incubation period is variable but averages about 1 week. The organisms proliferate in the endothelial cells that line small blood vessels and capillaries, causing small hemorrhages and, occasionally, areas of necrosis. If untreated, the patient may die (usually during the second week of illness), or recovery will occur after an illness of about 3 weeks' duration. Surprisingly, a serologic survey of 368 sixth-grade students in Texas showed that between 9% and 21% had prior exposure to *R rickettsii,* suggesting that a large percentage of persons may experience RMSF as an inapparent or undiagnosed infection.

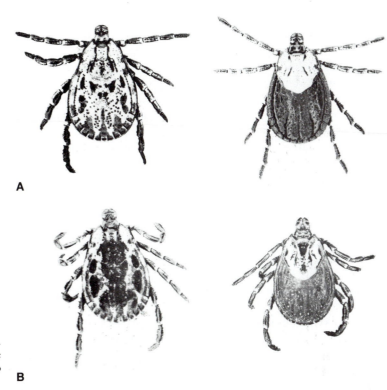

FIGURE 34-2 Tick vectors of Rocky Mountain spotted fever. **A.** *Dermacentor andersoni;* on the left is the male and on the right is the female. **B.** *Dermacentor variabilis;* the male is to the left, the female to the right.

The organisms are widespread in the wild mammalian and bird population as well as in the ticks themselves. A tick may become infected either as a result of a blood meal from an infected animal or by the transovarial passage of rickettsiae from mother to offspring. The disease does not harm ticks, and it has been estimated that about 3% of ticks are infected (although this figure varies greatly from one geographic area to another). Interestingly, the average mortality from untreated cases of RMSF varies from 90% in areas of Montana to as low as 5% in eastern parts of the United States. This variation in severity is likely the result of different strains of the etiologic agent in separate geographic areas.

LABORATORY DIAGNOSIS. The diagnosis of RMSF usually is made on the basis of the clinical picture and a history of a tick bite. Notice, however, that in the absence of a rash and history of a tick bite, an early diagnosis can be difficult to make. The Weil-Felix test, demonstrating a rise in titer to *Proteus* OX-19 organisms, can be used during convalescence to aid in making a retrospective diagnosis. The rickettsiae also can be grown in the yolk sac of embryonated hen eggs, and specific serologic tests can be done using the washed rickettsial organisms. Such a procedure, however, would be restricted to specialized laboratories. Staining of skin biopsy material with fluorescently labeled antibody can provide an early diagnosis, but this procedure also requires considerable talent and is not routinely done in most hospitals. RMSF can also be identified using a polymerase chain reaction, but it is available in only a few specialized rickettsial laboratories.

TREATMENT AND CONTROL. Control of RMSF is possible, in part, by frequent examination of one's body for the presence of ticks when in areas where ticks are likely to be found. Fortunately, a tick is unable to infect a person until about 4 hours after it has attached itself for a blood meal; this period is sometimes referred to as the rejuvenation period. Thus, a periodic removal of ticks, even though they may be infected with rickettsiae, is effective in preventing the disease.

Formalin-inactivated *R rickettsii* have been used in the past as a vaccine for individuals who are likely to be exposed to tick bites in endemic areas. Such vaccines, however, failed to provide significant protection, and they have been withdrawn from the commercial market. However, Gregory McDonald and associates have succeeded in cloning a gene from *R rickettsii* into *E coli* that encodes for a 155-kd surface protein. Immunization of experimental animals with this recombinant protein seems to be protective, indicating that a purified version of this vaccine may be used in humans.

Specific treatment with chloramphenicol or tetracyclines is effective against RMSF, particularly if started early in the illness, and immunity after recovery seems to be permanent.

RICKETTSIALPOX

Rickettsialpox was first described in 1946 after an epidemic in apartment houses in New York City. Subsequently, the causative organism, *Rickettsia akari,* has been found to have a worldwide distribution.

EPIDEMIOLOGY AND PATHOGENESIS. The reservoir of *R akari* is the common house mouse, and humans become infected from the bite of infected mites from mice. The infection varies considerably in severity from one person to another, but usually it is a mild disease. A primary lesion (termed an eschar), similar to that seen in scrub typhus, develops at the location of the bite of the mite. After an incubation period of 10 to 24 days, fever and chills occur, and about 3 or 4 days later a rash, like the rash in chickenpox, appears. The illness lasts 10 to 14 days, after which recovery is routine.

LABORATORY DIAGNOSIS, TREATMENT, AND CONTROL. The diagnosis of rickettsialpox may be based primarily on the clinical symptoms and history; however, the organisms can be readily isolated by inoculation of acute-phase blood into mice, guinea pigs, or the yolk sac of a chick embryo. Organisms can be identified by serologic tests using known serum.

Tetracycline and chloramphenicol are used for specific treatment; efforts to control the disease are directed toward elimination of rodents from areas proximal to humans.

Typhus Group

There are two major diseases in the typhus group: epidemic typhus and endemic typhus. The etiologic agents for both infections share a common group antigen, but they can be differentiated on the basis of specific complement-fixing antigen and on the basis of the epidemiology of the respective diseases.

EPIDEMIC TYPHUS

Rickettsia prowazekii is the causative agent of epidemic louse-borne typhus fever. Epidemic typhus has probably been more important than any other disease in shaping world history. The disease is associated with filth, and no major war has escaped its ravages. Supposedly, Napoleon's retreat from Russia was started by a louse, and his was not the first army to suffer such an ignominious defeat. Moreover, it has been estimated that there were over 30 million cases of epidemic typhus in Russia after World War I, resulting in more than 3 million deaths.

Epidemic typhus still is with us as evidenced by over 20,000 cases reported worldwide during the 1980s, a number that probably represents a small percentage of actual cases. Of these, 69% occurred in Ethiopia and 23% in Nigeria.

EPIDEMIOLOGY AND PATHOGENESIS. Epidemic typhus is usually a disease of substandard living conditions and poor sanitation. It was believed for many years that humans were the sole reservoir for this organism and that the human

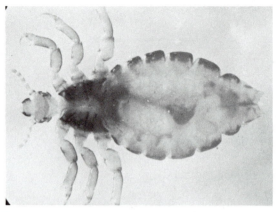

FIGURE 34-3   Micrograph of *Pediculus humanus,* the human louse that is the vector for epidemic typhus.

body louse served as the only arthropod vector (Fig. 34-3). Although this is true during large epidemics, it is known that flying squirrels in the southern part of the United States also serve as a reservoir for *R prowazekii.* Sporadic cases tend to occur during the winter months when flying squirrels nest in accessible attics. Fleas from the infected squirrel occasionally feed on humans, causing sporadic cases of this disease.

In the case of the louse-borne disease, the rickettsiae are present in the alimentary canal of the infected louse and may be introduced when an infected louse bites a human. The organisms are usually introduced by feces, vomitus, or a crushed louse that is scratched into the skin.

The incubation period usually is about 12 days, but it varies from 6 to 15 days. Interestingly, the rickettsiae are not passed transovarially in the louse as they are in the tick, and a louse dies several weeks after becoming infected.

The manifestations of epidemic typhus are the result of an overwhelming bacteremia, with growth of the rickettsiae in the endothelial cells of the blood vessels. The patient's temperature rises to about 40°C (104°F), and, after the fifth or sixth day of illness, a macular rash erupts on the trunk of the body and spreads to the extremities. Neurologic changes characterized by delirium and stupor also may occur. In cold weather, gangrene of feet and fingers may be seen. Other symptoms include headache, chills, fever, malaise, and general aches and pains. Recovery or death occurs within 2 to 3 weeks after the initial symptoms.

LABORATORY DIAGNOSIS. Diagnosis of epidemic typhus usually is not difficult when the disease occurs in epidemics. However, the sporadic cases originating from infected flying squirrels requires that the physician consider epidemic typhus in situations where the patient could have come into contact with an infected vector. Complement-fixing antibodies to both group and specific antigens show a positive reaction about 1 week after initial symptoms, as does the Weil-Felix test (as measured by agglutinins to *Proteus* OX-19).

TREATMENT AND CONTROL. Efforts to control epidemic typhus are directed toward sanitation and the eradication of human lice. Impressive results were obtained during World War II when epidemics were controlled immediately by spraying a susceptible population with DDT to kill human lice. Vaccines originally were prepared using rickettsiae obtained by washing out the intestines of infected lice, but they are now prepared from organisms grown in the yolk sac of chick embryos. The Cox vaccine, containing formalin-inactivated *R prowazekii,* was effectively used during World War II; however, a newer, living attenuated vaccine grown in yolk sacs seems to provide a longer, more solid immunity.

Both the tetracyclines and chloramphenicol are effective for the treatment of epidemic typhus.

BRILL-ZINSSER DISEASE

Brill-Zinsser disease (Brill's disease) occurs rarely, but it demonstrates an important property of the rickettsiae that cause epidemic typhus. It was first observed in the United States in 1898 in immigrants from eastern Europe. The disease was moderately mild, and, because these people were not infested with lice, it was originally thought to be endemic (flea-borne) typhus. However, subsequent work by American physician Nathan E. Brill established that the infections were identical to the louse-borne epidemic typhus. Bacteriologist Hans Zinsser correctly postulated that these illnesses occurred in persons who had recovered from epidemic typhus many years before their current disease, but who had carried the virulent rickettsiae in their bodies in a latent state. Under conditions that are not understood, the organisms may break latency, multiply, and produce overt disease. However, as might be expected, cases of Brill's disease usually are mild, because the afflicted person already possesses a partial immunity and responds with an anamnestic immunologic response. The most important aspect of Brill's disease is that these persons provide a reservoir for epidemic typhus during interepidemic periods.

ENDEMIC TYPHUS

Rickettsia typhi is the etiologic agent of endemic flea-borne typhus. This disease, also called murine typhus, occurs sporadically, not in epidemics like the louse-borne type.

EPIDEMIOLOGY AND PATHOGENESIS. *R typhi* is closely related to the etiologic agent of epidemic typhus, and either disease confers immunity to both. The infection is considerably less severe than the epidemic form, but in other details it is clinically indistinguishable from epidemic typhus. The rat serves as the primary reservoir for *R typhi,* although

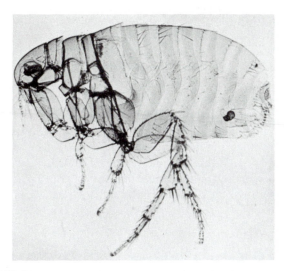

FIGURE 34-4 Micrograph of *Xenopsylla cheopis* (female), the rat flea that acts as the arthropod vector for endemic typhus.

in the southwestern United States, other wild rodents, such as ground squirrels, also may carry the disease. In the normal sequence of events, the disease is transmitted from rat to rat by the rat flea, *Xenopsylla cheopis* (Fig. 34-4). Only when a person accidentally interrupts this cycle by being bitten by the infected rat flea is this disease acquired. Because neither the rat nor the rat flea becomes ill as a result of the infection (in contrast to the death of the louse in epidemic typhus caused by *R prowazekii*), they constitute the reservoir and vector, respectively, for endemic typhus. Moreover, it has been demonstrated that *R typhi* is passed transovarially in the rat flea, thus making the flea a reservoir as well as a vector.

The disease begins after an incubation period of 1 to 2 weeks and is characterized by fever, headache, and generally a macular or maculopapular rash, appearing the third to fifth day of the illness.

LABORATORY DIAGNOSIS. The diagnosis of endemic typhus makes use of the Weil-Felix test, as measured by an increase in agglutinins to *Proteus* OX-19. In addition, the more specific complement-fixation test can be used to distinguish between these organisms and the etiologic agent of epidemic typhus. Intraperitoneal inoculation of male guinea pigs with *R typhi* causes severe scrotal swelling and testicular lesions, whereas *R prowazekii* causes only a mild disease with no testicular involvement.

Although it is not usually necessary, epidemic and endemic typhus can be differentiated by use of an indirect immunofluorescent test using the patient's serum after it has been absorbed with shared antigens of *R prowazekii* and *R typhi.*

TREATMENT AND CONTROL. Broad-spectrum antibiotics, particularly the tetracyclines and chloramphenicol, are effective for the treatment of endemic typhus.

Control measures are directed against both the rodent and the flea populations in an endemic area. DDT has been effective in reducing the flea population in rat-infested areas, and even though the use of DDT is markedly curtailed by law, it would probably be used after a cluster of sporadic cases of endemic typhus. However, as is true in plague-infected rats, DDT should be used before exterminating the rat population to preclude the infected fleas from leaving dead rats to bite people.

Because of the sporadic nature of endemic typhus, vaccines are used only for those persons who run a particularly high risk of becoming infected (such as laboratory workers).

Other Rickettsial Diseases

TSUTSUGAMUSHI FEVER (SCRUB TYPHUS)

Rickettsia tsutsugamushi is the causative agent of scrub typhus, a disease found in Asia and the Southwest Pacific. It achieved particular importance for the United States during World War II and in Vietnam, when large numbers of U.S. troops were infected with these organisms. The death rate varied according to the prevalent strain of the organism, ranging from 0.6% to 35%.

EPIDEMIOLOGY AND PATHOGENESIS. Scrub typhus normally occurs in rodents and is transmitted from rodent to rodent by a mite. Mites lay their eggs in the soil, and the larvae (chiggers) hatch later and feed on animals, including humans. After feeding, the larvae drop off and eventually develop into adult mites. Infected mites transmit the rickettsiae to their eggs, resulting in infected larvae. Thus, the mite can act both as a vector and as a reservoir for scrub typhus.

Humans acquire the disease from the bite of an infected chigger. Initial symptoms, which occur 7 to 14 days after the person has been bitten, include severe headache, chills, and fever; the disease is characterized by a primary lesion, called an eschar, which occurs at the location of the bite of the mite. Within a few days, a dull maculopapular rash appears; this may be accompanied by stupor and prostration. Recovery begins about 3 weeks after the initial symptoms, but convalescence may last for several months.

LABORATORY DIAGNOSIS. Agglutinins to *Proteus* OX-K, but not to OX-19 or OX-2, can be measured during the second week of illness. However, not all strains of *R tsutsugamushi* induce antibodies to the OX-K strain of *Proteus*. Immunofluorescent antibodies and complement fixation are available for some strains. Isolation of the rickettsiae by inoculation of infected blood into white mice will result in death of the mice within 2 weeks, at which time the rickettsiae can be observed as intracytoplasmic organisms in the mouse spleen cells.

TREATMENT AND CONTROL. Both tetracyclines and chloramphenicol are highly effective in the treatment of scrub typhus. However, because rickettsiae in general seem to cause latent infections (as in Brill's disease), relapses are common unless treatment is prolonged.

Control is directed against the mite. During World War II, a mitocide was used effectively both as a repellent on clothing and to kill mites within a given geographic area.

Vaccines have not been successful because of the large number of immunologically different strains of *R tsutsugamushi*.

TRENCH FEVER

Trench fever was first described in men engaged in trench warfare in Europe during World War I. The disease is spread from human to human by the body louse, and the etiologic agent, *Rochalimaea quintana*, can be grown on artificial media in the absence of living host cells.

The disease is associated with filth and poor sanitation, and seems to occur only during periods of war. Prominent symptoms are fever, headache, exhaustion, and a roseolar rash. Recovery is frequently followed by relapses occurring at 5-day intervals (hence, the species name, *quintana*). Fatalities are rare, but recovery is slow.

Broad-spectrum antibiotics, particularly chloramphenicol, are effective in eliminating the symptoms of the disease, but prolonged therapy is required to eliminate the carrier state in humans.

Efforts to control trench fever are obviously directed at the louse, and because the disease seems to reappear only in unsanitary situations prevalent in warfare, the most effective—but probably excessively idealistic—method of control would be to eliminate wars.

CAT SCRATCH DISEASE

Not until 1950 was cat scratch disease (CSD) firmly established as a clinical entity. It is estimated that about 24,000 cases (mostly children) occur annually in the United States and that about 2000 of them require hospitalization. Surprisingly, during the 40 years after its establishment, no etiologic agent was isolated, and the diagnosis remained clinical based on (1) a history of animal contact (usually cats, but dogs may also be involved); (2) characteristic histopathologic characteristic of the draining lymph nodes: (3) negative results of laboratory studies for other causes of lymphadenopathy; and (4) a positive skin test after the injection of an antigen obtained from lesions of an individual with CSD.

In 1988 a gram-negative, motile, oxidase-positive organism (subsequently named *Afipia felis*) was isolated from the tissues of a patient with CSD and was assigned as the putative etiologic agent of CSD.

In 1992, however, a second agent was isolated from

the lesions of CSD and shown to be a rickettsia belonging to the genus *Rochalimaea*. This organism has been named *Rochalimaea henselae* and, like other members of this genus, it can be grown on artificial media.

To summarize a long and confusing story, it seems that at least 90% of the cases of CSD are caused by *R henselae*. The evidence that *A felis* is involved is less solid, but it is thought that it may account for some or all of the cases of CSD when serologic measurements for *R henselae* give negative results.

Notice that this newly described species, *R henselae*, also has been isolated from several types of infections in immunocompromised AIDS patients. One of these, termed bacillary angiomatosis, is characterized by multiple subcutaneous nodules, and the other, bacillary peliosis hepatis, involves the liver of HIV-infected individuals.

Q FEVER

Coxiella burnetii is the etiologic agent of Q fever. Like other rickettsiae, *Coxiella* organisms require living cells for growth, but unlike other rickettsiae, an arthropod vector is not essential for transmission of the disease to humans. Furthermore, *Coxiella* organisms are exceptionally stable outside of host cells and can maintain their viability in dried excretions for extended periods of time.

In addition, *Coxiella* is heat resistant, being able to survive a temperature of 60°C for 1 hour; and, because the organisms may occur in cow's milk, pasteurization temperatures have been routinely raised to 62.9°C to inactivate this organism.

All of this began to make sense when Thomas McCaul and Jim Williams, from the Rocky Mountain Laboratories in Hamilton, Montana, discovered that suspensions of *C burnetii* contain two morphologic variants, which they termed large cell variant and small cell variant. Electron micrographs of these organisms strongly suggest that the small cell variant is a type of endospore that is formed at the polar end of the large cell variant, much as described for the members of the family Bacillaceae. Thin sections of *C burnetii* are shown in Figure 34-5, demonstrating endospore formation in these organisms. McCaul and Williams also have evidence suggesting that, after entry into a cell, the acid pH of the phagolysosome activates the general metabolism of the endospore, permitting it either to undergo binary fission or to differentiate into the vegetative cell variant. These observations have solved the mystery of the unusual stability and heat resistance of *C burnetii*, thus clarifying the uncharacteristic epidemiology of this disease. Notice that, unlike the other rickettsiae, *C burnetii* is acidophilic and, as such, remains and multiplies within the phagolysosome of the infected host

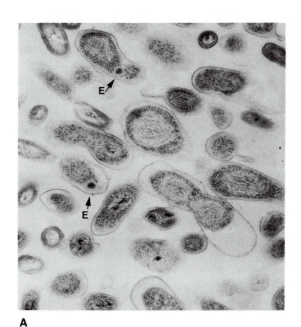

A

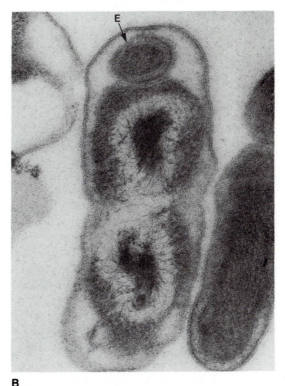

B

FIGURE 34-5 **A.** An electron micrograph of thin sections of *Coxiella burnetii* shows two large cell variants with endospores (E). **B.** Complete formation of the endospore (E) in large cell variant of *C burnetii* undergoing unequal cell division. Notice the nuclear regions of the dividing cell and the separation of the spore from the cytoplasmic contents by the membranes of the endospore.

cell. The organisms have little metabolic activity at neutral pH.

If one grows freshly isolated strains of *C burnetii* in the yolk sac of embryonated eggs, the organisms undergo a phase shift that is analogous of a S → R transformation of gram-negative enterics. The virulent phase I strains seem to lose a large part of their cell-wall lipopolysaccharide when they shift to the avirulent phase II status.

EPIDEMIOLOGY AND PATHOGENESIS. Although ticks serve as both vector and reservoir, they are not usually the direct source of human Q fever infections. Many human infections originate from cattle carcasses, and it is thought that the inhalation of dried tick feces from cattle hides is one mechanism of infection for slaughterhouse workers. Moreover, infected cattle and sheep do not appear ill, but shed large numbers of infectious organisms, particularly in their placental products. Thus, when infected cattle and sheep give birth, aerosols containing billions of organisms contaminate the surrounding area, where they remain viable in dust and hides for extended periods of time. That this is true for other infected animals is illustrated by the fact that all 15 people sleeping in a house in New England became infected when their cat gave birth to kittens during the night. In addition, many dairy herds are infected with *C burnetii,* and it is estimated, for example, that 10% of such herds in the Los Angeles area shed these organisms in their milk. However, even though the organism seems to be highly virulent when inhaled, the ingestion of contaminated milk does not often cause disease.

Among the acute symptoms of Q fever in humans are chills, headache, malaise, weakness, and severe sweats. Pneumonia, with a mild cough, occurs in most cases, and the condition is, in many ways, clinically similar to primary atypical pneumonia. The incubation period usually is 2 to 3 weeks, and the usual untreated infection resolves in 10 to 14 days.

C burnetii also can exist asymptomatically for periods of months or years, and these latent infections may become activated naturally or by the use of x-ray treatment or multiple cortisone injections. Such chronic infections also have been demonstrated by the isolation of *C burnetii* from the placentas of women who had recovered from Q fever more than 3 years previously. In some such cases, the organism has been reported to cause abortion and stillbirth. Valvular heart disease is the most common late manifestation of Q fever, although hepatitis is a frequent finding. Heart involvement usually follows a previously damaged heart valve and, if untreated, has a high mortality rate. In addition, osteomyelitis, bone marrow necrosis, and a variety of neurologic syndromes may be associated with chronic Q fever.

It seems that the chronic infections are caused by specific strains of *C burnetii.* Of the six strains that can be differentiated by genomic restriction fragment length polymorphisms, only organisms from the biotzere strain and the corazon strain have been isolated from chronic cases of Q fever. Moreover, a plasmid-encoded surface protein has been found in chronic-disease isolates of *C burnetii,* making it possible to predict which cases will self-resolve and which may result in a chronic infection.

LABORATORY DIAGNOSIS. Because the clinical symptoms are similar to those of many other infectious diseases, an unequivocal diagnosis requires the isolation and identification of the causative agent or a demonstration of a rise in specific complement-fixing antibodies during the patient's convalescence. The organisms can be grown in the yolk sacs of embryonated eggs or in tissue cultures of mouse fibroblasts, and can be identified by direct immunofluorescent antibody staining. Inoculation of blood or sputum into hamsters also is an effective method for isolation of the organisms.

TREATMENT AND CONTROL. Broad-spectrum antibiotics such as the tetracyclines are effective in treating Q fever, and relapses after adequate therapy are rare. In view of the seriousness of the myocardial and hepatic involvement, it has been suggested that patients with Q fever be treated with a combination of lincomycin and tetracycline for at least 12 months, with continued careful monitoring after withdrawal of antibiotics. It seems possible, however, to identify those strains that will completely resolve and those that may cause a chronic infection, making it unnecessary to treat all cases of Q fever for such extended periods.

Control of the disease is exceedingly difficult for individuals whose occupations result in frequent exposure to infected animals. A killed rickettsial vaccine can be administered to persons such as laboratory personnel and stockyard employees, whose occupations bring them into contact with the agent, but many such vaccines induce granulomas or sterile abscesses in recipients, and there has been considerable effort to prepare less toxic fractionated vaccines. One vaccine tried consisted of a single injection of 30 µg of highly purified inactivated phase I organisms. There were no cases of Q fever among the 3000 vaccinated workers at a South Australian abattoir compared with over 90 cases among the unvaccinated controls.

EHRLICHIOSIS

Rickettsiae that characteristically grow intracellularly in leukocytes are placed in the genus *Ehrlichia* and, until recently, it was believed that each species was host specific. Thus, *Ehrlichia risticii* is the etiologic agent of equine ehrlichial colitis or, as it is sometimes called, Potomac horse fever, a disease with a mortality rate for horses of about 30%. Similarly, *Ehrlichia canis,* the cause of canine ehrlichiosis, has been responsible for a high mortality in dogs. In this case, the organisms are spread from dog to dog by the brown dog tick, *Rhipicephalus sanguineus.* The only human agent was *Ehrlichia sennetsu,* the cause of a human mononucleosis-like syndrome that occurs only in Japan and Malaysia.

Strong evidence, however, suggests that *E canis* may be spread via tick bites to humans, mimicking RMSF. Major symptoms include headache, anorexia, leukopenia, and a rash in about 20% of infected patients. Essentially all cases have been diagnosed by demonstrating a rise in antibodies specific for *E canis,* and it is suggested that ehrlichiosis be considered for any febrile illness after a history of a tick bite and displaying negative serologic findings for RMSF, Lyme disease, or tularemia. A retrospective study in Oklahoma showed that 11% of 144 patients who had been suspected of having RMSF actually demonstrated at least a fourfold rise in antibodies to *E canis* in paired serum samples. Treatment with tetracycline has been shown to reduce the severity of the illness in both humans and dogs.

Chlamydiae

The chlamydiae, like the rickettsiae, comprise a group of obligately intracellular procaryotic parasites, which, before 1952, were referred to as large viruses or as the psittacosis–lymphogranuloma venereum–trachoma group of agents. It is known, however, that the chlamydiae are not viruses but likely are distantly related to the gram-negative bacteria. There are only three species, but they are responsible for a variety of diseases (Table 34-2).

Multiplication of Chlamydial Agents

The characteristic that best delineates the chlamydiae as a distinct group of organisms is their complex method of reproduction. The developmental cycle occurs as follows:

1. A small, dense cell about 0.3 μm in diameter, called an elementary body (Fig. 34-6), is taken into a host cell by phagocytosis.
2. During the next 8 hours, the elementary body undergoes a reorganization into a large, less-dense cell called an initial or reticulate body.
3. The initial body, about 1 μm in diameter, grows in size and divides by binary fission.
4. After 24 to 48 hours, the initial bodies (which, by themselves, are noninfectious) reorganize into small, dense elementary bodies, and the developmental cycle is completed when the host cell liberates the small, dense, infectious cells.

It is not known what triggers the reorganization of the large cells back into small cells, but it is known that this reduction in size is accompanied by the loss of a great deal of RNA from the large cell (the RNA-to-DNA ratio in the small elementary body is about 1:1, whereas that of the large, initial body is about 4:1). The high content of RNA in the dividing large cells is undoubtedly responsible for the high rate of reproduction of the initial bodies—and, hence, protein synthesis—taking place in the large cells. Because the small cells do not divide, a high concentration of RNA is not necessary for their maintenance. Interestingly, multiplication takes place within the host-cell phagosome, and the chlamydiae are able in some way to prevent fusion of the phagosome with lysosomes until late in the developmental cycle.

In spite of their complex method of reproduction, the chlamydiae are probably distant descendants of the gram-negative bacteria. Their cell walls do not, however, seem to contain muramic acid, and peptidoglycan cannot be detected, although the cell walls do possess an inner and outer membrane.

The extracellular survival of the elementary bodies may be possible as a result of the rigidity and strength provided by the high degree of disulfide bond linkage among the major outer membrane proteins. They reproduce by binary fission, they contain both RNA and DNA, and their DNA is not surrounded by a nuclear envelope. The question remains, however, as to why these organisms can grow only inside host cells. They are able to metabolize a few intermediates of the tricarboxylic acid cycle and can metabolize glucose through a portion of the pentose cycle to pyruvic acid. The presence of cytochromes and flavoproteins has not been demonstrated, and so it seems that the chlamydiae grow as anaerobic organisms.

TABLE 34-2
Classification of *Chlamydia* Organisms

	Major Disease	*Natural Host*	*No. of Serovars*
C trachomatis	Trachoma, inclusion conjunctivitis, infantile pneumonia, STD, LGV	Humans	18
C psittaci	Pneumonia	Birds	Unknown
C pneumoniae	Pneumonia, bronchitis	Humans	1

LGV, lymphogranuloma venereum; STD, sexually transmitted disease.

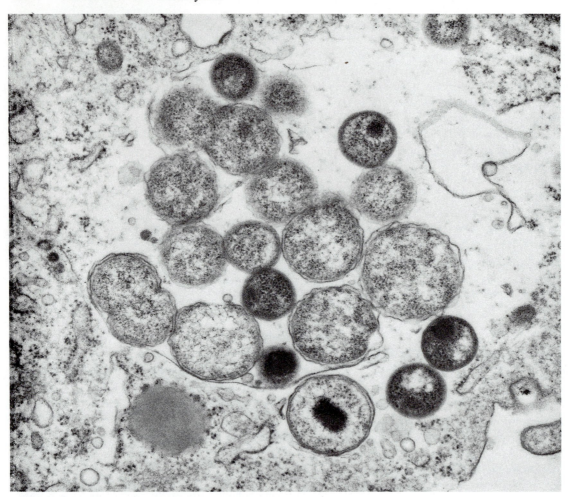

FIGURE 34-6 Microcolony of *Chlamydia psittaci* in a McCoy cell. In this electron micrograph, both small, dense, infectious elementary bodies (two at *lower right*) and larger, thin-walled, noninfectious initial bodies are shown. The initial body on the left is dividing. (Original magnification ×34,000.)

Chlamydiae also are able to arrest the host-cell cycle in the G-1 phase of division, inhibiting host-cell synthesis of macromolecules. They can synthesize their own proteins, lipids, and macromolecules, but these syntheses require energy, and the chlamydiae seem to be metabolically defective in that they have no mechanism for the production or trapping of energy. Thus, they are energy parasites, unable to synthesize their own ATP.

It is known that, like the rickettsiae, these organisms possess an ADP/ATP translocator, which is mandatory for their existence, because it provides their only source of ATP by transporting ATP from the host eucaryotic cell into the chlamydiae.

Classification and Antigenic Structure of the Chlamydiae

During the last several decades, there have been numerous attempts to classify this complex group of organisms. Early schemes assumed the chlamydiae were large viruses, and classification was, for the most part, restricted to a clinical description of the disease syndrome. Later, taxonomists tended to group the chlamydiae with the rickettsiae, because both groups are made up of procaryotic organisms that are obligately intracellular parasites. However, it is apparent that the complex developmental cycle and metabolic pathways of the chlamydiae clearly separates this group of organisms from other procaryotic cells.

MORPHOLOGIC AND CHEMICAL DIFFERENTIATION

The chlamydiae are divided into three species based on the morphologic appearance of their intracellular inclusion bodies, the presence or absence of glycogen in the inclusion, their sensitivity to sulfonamides, and the extent of DNA homology between related organisms. *Chlamydia trachomatis* contains the etiologic agents of trachoma, inclusion conjunctivitis, infantile pneumonia, nongonococcal urethritis (NGU) and cervicitis, and lymphogranuloma venereum. These organisms form compact inclusion bodies containing glycogen (Fig. 34-7) and are inhibited by sodium sulfadiazine. *Chlamydia psittaci* produces a

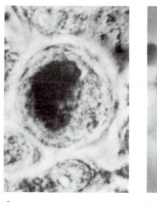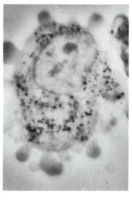

A   **B**

FIGURE 34-7 **A.** Compact inclusion body of *Chlamydia trachomatis* in a McCoy cell. The glycogen-containing inclusion appears dark after staining with 5% iodine-potassium iodide (I-KI). **B.** Diffuse inclusion of *Chlamydia psittaci* in a mononuclear mouse cell. The chlamydiae are the small, dark bodies distributed about the cytoplasm in this phase-contrast micrograph of a fresh wet mount.

diffuse inclusion body that does not contain glycogen and, because it requires preformed folic acid, is resistant to the presence of sulfonamides. Moreover, there is considerable DNA homology within each species, but little interspecies homology.

These two species also seem to differ in the manner in which they exit the host cell. *C psittaci* and the lymphogranuloma venereum strain of *C trachomatis* induce lysis of the host cell, whereas the other strains of *C trachomatis* seem to multiply and exit without killing the host cell. In such cases, it is suggested that the membrane surrounding the inclusion body fuses with the cytoplasmic membrane of the host cell, resulting in an extrusion of the inclusion body contents into the extracellular environment.

Chlamydia pneumoniae strain TWAR is a species that causes an acute respiratory disease in humans. This species seems to be genetically homogeneous and differs from both *C psittaci* and *C trachomatis*.

ANTIGENIC CHARACTERISTICS

All chlamydiae possess heat-stable, group-specific antigens that can be detected by complement fixation, agglutination, hemagglutination inhibition, and intradermal tests. These group-specific antigens apparently contain carbohydrate, inasmuch as they are readily destroyed by periodate oxidation. Most group-specific antigens are assumed to be associated with the cell-wall structure.

Species-specific antigens stimulate the formation of infectivity-neutralizing antibodies. These antigens are resistant to periodate oxidation and are, for the most part, heat labile. Antibodies directed against species-specific antigens react only with the homologous or closely related strains of chlamydiae, and, on the basis of species-specific

antigens, the chlamydiae have been subdivided into a series of subgroups. Curiously, antibodies to these cell-wall, type-specific antigens seem to prevent infection of host cells but have little effect on chlamydiae that have already established an intracellular existence. In fact, many of the chlamydial diseases can remain chronic for long periods of time, and the existence of a detectable immune response may not always be effective in eliminating the chlamydiae from the host.

A hemagglutinin has been found associated with many chlamydial strains. It is soluble and can readily be disassociated from the elementary bodies during centrifugation. Based on antigenic specificity, the hemagglutinin seems to be related to the group-specific antigens.

Chlamydia trachomatis

Chlamydia trachomatis is the specific name for the etiologic agents of trachoma, inclusion conjunctivitis, infantile pneumonia, NGU and cervicitis, and lymphogranuloma venereum. With the exception of an aberrant strain causing pneumonitis in mice, all of the chlamydiae classified as *C trachomatis* are solely human pathogens. However, this name does not imply a single entity, because various diseases may be caused by different strains of *C trachomatis*. For example, there are eight serotypes involved in the inclusion conjunctivitis syndrome (normally sexually transmitted in the adult), and they are responsible for a number of different clinical manifestations in both infants and adults.

TRACHOMA

Trachoma has been known for over 3000 years, and it was at one time listed as one of the three most important diseases of humans. The World Health Organization estimates that about 400 million persons are infected with trachoma, and 6 million to 10 million of these are totally blind as a result of this disease.

EPIDEMIOLOGY AND PATHOGENESIS. Trachoma occurs only in humans, where it grows exclusively in the conjunctival cells. It is transmitted by direct contact with fingers or contaminated towels and clothing, and in many areas of the world (eg, Egypt and the Middle East), it is so prevalent that children routinely become infected during early childhood. There are four immunologic variants of trachoma, designated A, B, Ba, and C, and all four serotypes may be endemic within a given geographic area. The infections occur primarily in geographic areas where poverty is common, and in the United States, the American Indians have probably been the most frequent victims.

The overt disease usually is seen as a chronic inflammation of the conjunctiva. Leukocytes enter the area and form follicles under the conjunctiva. Healing of initial lesions frequently occurs, but repeated reinfections result in vascularization and infiltration of the cornea, eventually causing scarring of the conjunctiva. It seems probable that the chronic inflammation may, at least in part, be because of a delayed-type hypersensitivity reaction.

Over a period of years, the scars contract, causing the upper eyelid to turn inward. Damage to the cornea results from a mechanical abrasion from the turned-in eyelashes, which, together with secondary bacterial infections, induces the lesions leading to blindness. Secondary infections are rare in the United States, and blindness from trachoma is not a major problem.

LABORATORY DIAGNOSIS. Trachoma usually is diagnosed on the basis of the pathologic findings associated with the disease. However, the agent may be grown by the inoculation of conjunctival scrapings into cell cultures or the yolk sacs of chick embryos, or it may be identified by staining the characteristic inclusion bodies with fluorescein-labeled antibody.

TREATMENT AND CONTROL. Treatment of trachoma with both systemic and topical sulfonamides and tetracycline usually is effective in alleviating the overt signs of the disease. However, advanced or chronic infections may be difficult to cure, and relapses are common. Relapses may result in part from the fact that the *C trachomatis* also causes a systemic infection, and topical treatment of the eye may fail because of a reinfection from other body sites.

In endemic regions, most infected persons recover spontaneously, probably as a result of IgA antibody and a cellular immune response. Immunity does not seem to be long-lasting, because reinfection or relapses may occur; however, chlamydiae characteristically produce latent infections, and so it also seems possible that relapses may result from a reactivation of the latent state.

INCLUSION CONJUNCTIVITIS

The etiologic agent of inclusion conjunctivitis is so similar to that of trachoma that the two organisms are frequently called the trachoma-inclusion conjunctivitis agents. However, the pathogenesis and the pathologic course of the conjunctivitis are considerably different from those of trachoma. The prevalence of such infections is manifested by the fact that 5% to 12% of all pregnant women have a chlamydial infection of the cervix, and 50% of infants born to such mothers will develop conjunctivitis. Moreover, it is estimated that there are 3 million to 10 million new cases of genital chlamydial infections each year in the United States and that 10% of all college students will become infected during their college careers.

EPIDEMIOLOGY AND PATHOGENESIS. The agent of inclusion conjunctivitis is most commonly found in the human genitourinary tract, from which it is passed from human to human by sexual contact. As a sexually transmitted disease (STD), the organisms grow in the epithelial cells of the female cervix or in the lining of the urethra of both sexes. Genital symptoms may be mild or absent, and many cases may be undiagnosed.

However, as the name of the agent implies, infections of the conjunctiva are not so benign. They are seen most frequently in the newborn about 5 to 12 days after birth. In such cases, the infection is acquired from the mother as the infant moves through the birth canal. The symptoms usually begin with an acute purulent conjunctivitis, which starts to subside after several weeks and spontaneously disappears in a few months. Inclusion conjunctivitis does not result in blindness.

Adult infections of the conjunctiva also may occur, and before the use of chlorine in swimming pools, such infections were often called *swimming pool conjunctivitis*. Most conjunctival infections of adults, however, occur through contamination by fingers or towels.

LABORATORY DIAGNOSIS, TREATMENT, AND CONTROL. Diagnosis of inclusion conjunctivitis may rely heavily on the history and clinical findings. However, laboratory confirmation requires the isolation of the agent or the demonstration of cellular inclusions that will stain with fluorescently labeled specific antibody.

Both the conjunctivitis and the genital infection respond to treatment with tetracycline and the sulfonamides. Nevertheless, reinfections can occur, and it is not clear whether specific immunity is ineffective or subsequent infections are caused by a different one of the eight specific serotypes of inclusion conjunctivitis (serotypes D through K).

A number of studies concluded that the instillation of a 1% tetracycline ointment or a 0.5% erythromycin ointment into the conjunctiva of the newborn was effective for the prophylaxis of both gonococcal ophthalmia and chlamydial inclusion conjunctivitis. These conclusions have, however, been challenged and one could probably conclude that such prophylaxis is beneficial, but does not offer absolute protection.

INFANT PNEUMONITIS

It is estimated that the same serotypes of *C trachomatis* responsible for inclusion conjunctivitis cause 30% to 40% of all pneumonias in hospitalized infants younger than 6 months of age. The newborn acquires the organism from an infected mother during birth, although its lower respiratory infection may have originated from a conjunctival infection. This is particularly disquieting, because the usual ocular prophylaxis with silver nitrate does not appear to kill *C trachomatis*.

To prevent chlamydial pneumonitis in the newborn, 152 women who were positive for cervical *C trachomatis* were given 400 mg/day of erythromycin for 7 days during the 36th week of gestation. Only 7% of the infants born to erythromycin-treated mothers acquired a chlamydial infection compared with 50% of the untreated controls.

Chlamydial infant pneumonia usually is not a severe disease, but it may last several weeks and lead to long-term respiratory complications. Infants with this disease also may have chlamydial infections of the middle ear (*C trachomatis* has been isolated from infants with otitis media).

Erythromycin or the sulfonamides are the drugs of choice, because tetracyclines are contraindicated for this pediatric group.

GENITAL-TRACT INFECTIONS

As is obvious from the preceding sections, *C trachomatis* (serotypes D through K) is spread among adults primarily as a STD. Chlamydiae have been isolated from almost one third of all women attending venereal disease clinics and from two thirds of those with gonorrhea; in men, about 20% of those with gonorrhea also have a chlamydial infection.

URETHRITIS AND CERVICITIS. *C trachomatis* seems to cause the most common STD occurring in the United States. Some 3 million to 10 million new cases are estimated to occur each year, and the rapid spread of this infection is probably partly because of the minimal nature or absence of symptoms, particularly in women. The disease is especially prevalent among sexually active adolescent girls (10% to 20%) and pregnant women. In spite of the paucity of symptoms, the Centers for Disease Control have estimated that over 100,000 American women may be rendered infertile each year from this infection, primarily from a scarring of the fallopian tubes. Fallopian tube scarring by *C trachomatis* also is a major cause of ectopic pregnancies. This organism is also the most common cause of NGU in men, and because many such men are dually infected with *Neisseria gonorrhoeae,* it also is responsible for most postgonococcal urethritis infections. Both infections are usually recognized by the failure of penicillin therapy to relieve the symptoms of urethritis. Although NGU usually is less severe than gonococcal urethritis, NGU cannot be differentiated on a clinical basis. Adequate treatment with tetracycline is effective for both *C trachomatis* and for *Ureaplasma urealyticum.* In addition, doxycycline given for 1 week is effective for the eradication of *C trachomatis* from the cervix, urethra, or rectum. It has also been reported that a single dose of azithromycin was equally effective.

CHLAMYDIAL EPIDIDYMITIS. Acute infections of the epididymis have long been known to be caused by the gonococcus, coliforms, and pseudomonads. However, for at least one half of all cases of acute epididymitis, no etiologic agent had been isolated, and such infections were termed *idiopathic epididymitis.*

Data have convincingly established that *C trachomatis* is the major cause of such idiopathic epididymitis.

Such infections seem to be transmitted sexually, because they occur primarily in sexually active men younger than 35 years of age. Epididymitis in older men usually is the result of a coliform infection.

FEMALE GENITAL-TRACT INFECTIONS. It seems that chlamydial infections are more prevalent in women than in men, possibly because many such infections are asymptomatic. The cervix seems to be the most common site of infection, but *C trachomatis* may also cause an acute infection of the fallopian tubes (salpingitis) and, as such, is thought to be a major etiologic agent in female pelvic inflammatory disease. Many such infections result in infertility in spite of the fact that the pelvic inflammatory disease was entirely asymptomatic. In addition, these organisms have been isolated from the rectum, from infections of Bartholin's gland, and from female urethritis.

LABORATORY DIAGNOSIS. Growth of the organisms on cell cultures is the most definitive means for the diagnosis of chlamydial infections. Procedures that enhance growth include centrifugation of clinical specimens directly onto the cell culture or pretreatment of the cell culture with a polycation such as DEAE dextran. Many laboratories, however, are not set up for growing chlamydiae and, as a result, serologic techniques are more often employed for the identification of these organisms. There are commercially available kits that contain fluorescently labeled polyclonal antibodies that will bind to elementary bodies. These antibodies can be used to stain smears taken from potentially infected persons and, if results are positive, will show the greenish fluorescently labeled elementary bodies against a reddish background of counterstained cells. There is also available an enzyme-linked immunoassay for detecting chlamydial antigens in scrapings or swab specimens of infected sites. This procedure uses known anti-chlamydia antibodies that have been linked to horseradish peroxidase. Sensitivities of greater than 90% have been claimed for both of these procedures.

In situ DNA hybridization of cervical scrapings may also be used. This procedure uses radioactively labeled probes, which will hybridize with a cryptic plasmid that has been shown to be present in all 15 serovars of *C trachomatis.* Sensitivities of over 90% have been reported for this technique.

The presence of humoral antibodies to *C trachomatis* cannot differentiate between past and present infection. Thus, in one study of 491 college women, 37% were seropositive, whereas only 7.9% were culture positive.

LYMPHOGRANULOMA VENEREUM

The etiologic agent of lymphogranuloma venereum is closely related to the trachoma-inclusion conjunctivitis agents (serotypes L-1, L-2, and L-3), but this disease is thought to be spread only through sexual contact. It is

A Closer Look

At least one million women in the United States experience an episode of symptomatic pelvic inflammatory disease (PID) each year. Such infections greatly increase the likelihood of a subsequent ectopic pregnancy. This is substantiated by a survey showing that after a single episode of PID, a woman's risk of ectopic pregnancy increases sevenfold compared with women who have no history of PID. In addition, approximately 12% of such women are rendered infertile after this single episode of PID. Moreover, the risk of infertility increases with subsequent occurrences of PID, being 25% after two episodes and 50% after three episodes.

Also notice that many women with a tubal infertility have experienced no symptoms characteristic of PID. Such women, however, frequently have serologic evidence of a previous sexually transmitted infection, indicating that "silent PID" may also lead to infertility.

Multiple organisms have been implicated as etiologic agents of PID, and most cases of PID are associated with more than one organism. *Chlamydia trachomatis* and *Neisseria gonorrhoeae* are the two most common causes of PID, but anaerobic bacteria in the genera *Bacteroides*, *Peptococcus*, and *Peptostreptococcus* also are frequently involved in PID. Facultative bacteria associated with PID include *Gardnerella vaginalis*, *Streptococcus* species, *Escherichia coli*, and *Haemophilus influenzae*.

The clinical diagnosis of PID is difficult because of the variation in signs and symptoms among infected women. As a result, many episodes of PID are unrecognized until after extensive scarring of the fallopian tubes has occurred. The Centers for Disease Control have, therefore, recommended that treatment for PID should be instituted on the basis of minimum clinical criteria for PID. Such criteria would included lower abdominal tenderness, bilateral adnexal tenderness, and cervical motion tenderness.

Prevention of PID involves avoiding acquisition of a sexually transmitted disease.

most prevalent in the tropics, but is seen also in the United States, particularly in the South.

Laboratory acquired infections, in which an aerosol of the lymphogranuloma venereum serotypes was inhaled, have resulted in severe pneumonia.

EPIDEMIOLOGY AND DIAGNOSIS. About 7 to 12 days after sexual contact, the infection becomes manifest by the appearance of a small erosion or painless papule in the genital area. The organisms migrate to the regional lymph nodes, and most symptoms result from this lymph node involvement. The original papule soon heals, but after 1 to 2 months, the regional lymph nodes become enlarged and tender and may break open and drain. These enlarged lymph nodes are called buboes, and as they enlarge, the draining lymph channel may be completely obstructed. Such restriction can cause a tremendous enlargement (elephantiasis) of the genitalia, and rectal strictures may occur as an effect of perirectal scarring.

LABORATORY DIAGNOSIS. The diagnosis of lymphogranuloma venereum is made from the clinical picture, history, complement-fixation test for antibodies, biopsy of infected nodes for isolation of the organisms, and Frei skin test. The Frei test is conducted by injecting the killed organisms into the skin and observing for a delayed-type skin reaction. The Frei test, however, is not specific and will give positive results in persons with psittacosis.

TREATMENT AND CONTROL. Control measures are, in general, the same as for other STDs. It is not known whether infection induces a lasting immunity but, like syphilis, there seems to be an infection immunity that will prevent lymph node involvement from a second contact in an already infected person. Moreover, the frequency of relapses and the usual life-long delayed-type hypersensitivity to the organism has led to the postulation that in many persons a spontaneous "cure" may represent only a latent state of the infection.

Both tetracycline and sulfonamides are effective for the treatment of lymphogranuloma venereum.

Chlamydia psittaci

In the early 1900s, reports described a disease acquired from contact with parrots and other psittacine birds. This infection, called psittacosis, has since been found to exist in at least 130 species of birds, and there is a trend toward changing the name to ornithosis. Another proposal, which has not yet gained wide acceptance, is to call the disease chlamydiosis.

ORNITHOSIS (PSITTACOSIS)

One of the characteristics of the avian form of ornithosis is its propensity to exist as an asymptomatic, latent infection that can become overt after stresses such as crowding, unsanitary conditions, and bacterial infections—all of which are likely to occur during shipment of birds. Once activated, the chlamydiae cause a generalized infection in which the organisms can be found in essentially every organ of the bird. Fecal excretions contain many organisms and provide the major source of infection for humans and other birds.

EPIDEMIOLOGY AND PATHOGENESIS. Humans usually acquire ornithosis by the inhalation of dried, infected feces, and, as in birds, the disease in humans may be asymptomatic or mild. However, in many cases, a severe and frequently fatal pneumonia develops after an incubation period of 1 to 3 weeks. In severe cases, organs other than the lungs may be involved, occasionally resulting in jaundice and acute thyroiditis. Meningitis accompanied by delirium may occur, and in the terminal stages, death may result from pulmonary insufficiency and a generalized toxemia.

LABORATORY DIAGNOSIS. Diagnosis of ornithosis requires the isolation of the etiologic agent. Injection of acute-stage blood or sputum into cell cultures or embryonated eggs is followed by identification with fluorescently labeled specific antibody, complement-fixation tests, or neutralization of infectivity by the use of specific antibody.

TREATMENT AND CONTROL. Tetracycline is the drug of choice for the treatment of ornithosis, and adequate therapy with this antibiotic seems to produce a rapid and permanent cure.

Control is difficult, because the disease prevails so widely as a latent infection of birds. Infection is an occupational hazard for workers in poultry slaughterhouses, particularly turkey abattoirs, although ducks and pigeons also provide a reservoir for ornithosis. Obviously, exclusion of parakeets as pets would also reduce sources of infection.

Chlamydia pneumoniae

Before 1986, it was assumed that essentially all chlamydial pneumonias occurring in adults were caused by *C psittaci* and resulted from exposure to infected birds. However, J. Thomas Grayston and associates at the University of Washington (Seattle) have reported the isolation of a new species, which has been designated *C pneumoniae* strain TWAR (first isolated in Taiwan, causing an acute respiratory disease) and which seems to be spread from person to person without the intervention of an avian host. This organism causes an acute lower respiratory infection similar to that of the avian strains, and it seems to be an important etiologic agent of pneumonia and bronchitis in adolescents and adults. Pharyngitis and sinusitis often are present also with the pneumonia and bronchitis. Most cases are relatively mild and rarely require hospitalization, but recovery is slow and a cough and malaise may continue for weeks or months after recovery from the acute symptoms. Some data also indicate that *C pneumoniae* may be responsible for coronary artery disease and endocardi-

tis, but data indicate that this is a rare manifestation of this infection.

Using specific serologic tests for antibodies, it has been shown that almost one half of the adults from five different parts of the world had been infected at one time or another with *C pneumoniae* strain TWAR, making it the most prevalent chlamydial infection occurring in humans. It seems probable that the reason this pathogen had not been previously recognized was because of the difficulty in cultivating the organism.

Potential Chlamydial Infections of Humans

Chlamydial infections of animals are widespread. For example, *C psittaci* causes pneumonitis and conjunctivitis in cats, dogs, goats, calves, lambs, horses, rabbits, and swine; fatal enteritis in cattle and wild hares; polyarthritis in calves, lambs, and piglets; and placentitis leading to abortion in cattle and sheep. Much of the premise that chlamydiae can produce any of these symptoms in humans is either preliminary or circumstantial. However, chlamydial agents have been isolated from the conceptuses of women in California and France, and the isolation of chlamydiae from the joints of patients with Reiter's syndrome (which is characterized by polyarthritis, conjunctivitis, and urethritis) has been reported. However, even though such isolations undoubtedly occurred, any causal relationship is purely circumstantial. Nevertheless, the similarity of human and animal symptoms makes it tempting to incriminate chlamydiae in these human disorders.

Bibliography

JOURNALS

Anderson B, et al. Detection of *Rochalimaea henselae* in cat-scratch disease skin test antigens. J Infect Dis 1993;168:1034.

Raoult D, Stein A. Q Fever during pregnancy: a risk for women, fetuses, and obstetricians. N Engl J Med 1994;330:371.

Reimer LG. Q Fever. Clin Microbiol Rev 1993;6:193.

Rikihisa Y. The tribe Ehrlichieae and ehrlichial diseases. Clin Microbiol Rev 1991;4:286.

Rynkiewicz DL, Liu LX. Human ehrlichiosis in New England. N Engl J Med 1994;330:292.

Sexton DJ, Corey GR. Rocky mountain "spotless" and "almost spotless" fever: a wolf in sheep's clothing. Clin Infect Dis 1992;15:439.

Spach DH, et al. Review article: tick-borne diseases in the United States. N Engl J Med 1993;329:936.

Walker DH. Rocky mountain spotted fever: a disease in need of microbiological concern. Clin Microbiol Rev 1989;2:227.

Essentials of Medical Microbiology, Fifth Edition, edited by Wesley A. Volk, Bryan M. Gebhardt, Marie-Louise Hammarskjöld, and Robert J. Kadner. Lippincott-Raven Publishers, Philadelphia © 1996.

Chapter 35

Medical Mycology

Mycology is defined as the study of fungi (commonly called yeasts and molds), and medical mycology is the study of fungi that cause disease in humans and other animals. The fungi discussed later in this chapter are eucaryotic organisms unrelated to bacteria; however, a large group of procaryotic organisms that are smaller than, but morphologically similar to, fungi is first discussed. These organisms are termed the *actinomycetes*.

Actinomycetes

Actinomycetes is the collective name for eight different families of bacteria that grow as frequently branched, long or short filaments of cells (hyphae: unbranched; mycelia: branched). They divide by binary fission and may or may not produce external spores. By far, most of these organisms are soil and water saprophytes (organisms living on decaying organic matter), and they are exceedingly important for their roles in the cycles of nature, such as the decomposition of organic material and the fixation of nitrogen.

Although sometimes mold-like in outward appearance, actinomycetes truly are bacteria, as judged by all the criteria for a procaryotic cell (Fig. 35-1). They contain muramic acid in their cell walls, they lack mitochondria, they contain 70S ribosomes, they lack a nuclear envelope, the diameter of their cells ranges from 0.5 to 2 μm, and they are killed or inhibited by many antibacterial antibiotics. Because of these characteristics, it is difficult to imagine a direct phylogenetic link between the procaryotic actinomycetes and the eucaryotic fungi.

Of the many different genera classified in the order Actinomycetales, only a few produce disease in humans, and this discussion is confined to the medically important actinomycetes.

ACTINOMYCES

The genus *Actinomyces* contains obligately anaerobic or microaerophilic, gram-positive organisms that grow in the form of a vegetative mycelium, which readily breaks up into bacillary and coccoid forms. They do not form

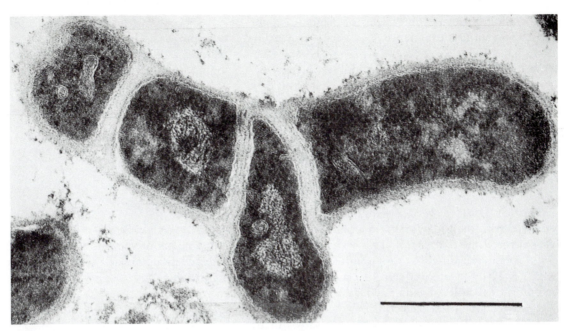

FIGURE 35-1 Electron micrograph of cells of *Actinomyces odontolyticus* showing basic procaryotic features; the downward-pointing cell is budding. (Scale = 0.5 μm.)

spores, and several species are of major medical importance. Both *Actinomyces bovis,* the causative agent of lumpy jaw in cattle, and *Actinomyces israelii,* the etiologic agent of actinomycosis in humans, cause similar types of infections. *Actinomyces viscosus, Actinomyces naeslundii, Bifidobacterium eriksonii,* and a closely related organism named *Arachnia propionica,* also may be involved in cases of human actinomycosis. All are part of the normal human oral or gastrointestinal flora. In addition, several gram-negative organisms such as *Eikenella corrodens, Bacteroides* species, and *Fusobacterium* also are frequently found in the actinomycotic lesions, and it has been proposed that actinomycosis may result from a synergistic reaction between these organisms and the *Actinomyces* species. Data from studies of actinomycosis in experimental animal models support this postulation.

In addition, several species of *Actinomyces* (primarily *A viscosus*) have been isolated frequently from dental plaques and are believed to cause dental caries and periodontal disease.

Epidemiology and Pathogenesis of Human Actinomycosis

Actinomyces israelii, as well as several other species of *Actinomyces,* occur as part of the normal flora in the oral cavity and the alimentary tract. Thus, infections caused by these organisms are thought to originate from an endogenous source, and the initial lesions usually occur after the organisms gain entry by means of trauma. Cervicofacial and abdominal lesions may arise by direct inoculation, but thoracic infections result from an extension from a cervicofacial or abdominal lesion, or from the aspiration of the organism from the oral cavity.

CERVICOFACIAL ACTINOMYCOSIS. Cervicofacial actinomycotic infection may occur as a result of trauma to the mucous membranes of the mouth or tonsils, or it may begin as a dental abscess caused by poor oral hygiene. Initial symptoms include minor pain, together with a hard nodular or lumpy swelling of the jaw. Later, the swelling softens, and the organisms spread and eventually extend through the skin, forming multiple draining abscesses. Advanced cases show considerable bone destruction, and, in rare instances, the organisms may penetrate the cranium, causing fatal brain lesions.

The skin abscesses discharge a purulent material containing firm microcolonies of *Actinomyces israelii, A viscosus,* or *Arachnia propionica* and cellular debris with associated microorganisms. Because of the yellow color of these granules, they are usually referred to as sulfur granules, and their appearance in a draining abscess provides good presumptive evidence for a diagnosis of actinomycosis.

ABDOMINAL ACTINOMYCOSIS. The primary source of abdominal actinomycosis is a diseased appendix, but infection also may follow penetrating abdominal wounds, perforated intestinal ulcers, or even blunt trauma without apparent perforation. The lesions may also extend to infect various internal organs, such as the viscera, the liver, and the urinary system; involvement of the spinal column can cause destructive bone lesions. Penetration of the abdominal wall, yielding draining abscesses containing so-called sulfur granules, provides the means of diagnosis in the absence of a surgical exploration.

THORACIC ACTINOMYCOSIS. Thoracic actinomycosis may occur as a primary lesion in the lung after aspiration, or it may result from an extension of the disease from either a cervicofacial or an abdominal infection. The initial symptoms resemble a mild pneumonia with fever and cough and a purulent sputum. The lesions eventually spread through the thoracic wall, causing external draining abscesses. Rib destruction may occur in advanced cases.

PELVIC ACTINOMYCOSIS. Pelvic actinomycosis is almost always associated with the use of an intrauterine device (IUD). Actinomycetes are normal flora of the vagina and therefore, it is not surprising that they eventually colonize up to 25% of IUDs. Moreover, approximately 2% to 4% of such individuals will subsequently have a serious actinomycotic infection. These data point out the problems that must be faced when a Papanicolaou smear shows that a patient with an IUD has an asymptomatic actinomycotic infection. Some physicians would replace the IUD immediately; others would simply remove it; and still others would remove the IUD and follow this with antibiotic treatment. Interestingly, few patients with a proven actinomycotic infection have had an IUD in place for less than 3 years.

Diagnosis, Treatment, and Control of Actinomycoses

The presence of sulfur granules in a draining abscess provides reasonable evidence for the diagnosis of actinomycosis. Crushing and staining a granule on a microscope slide shows gram-positive filaments, as well as bacillary and coccoid forms of the organism (Fig. 35-2). The isolation and identification of the organisms provide an absolute diagnosis, but because of the associated microorganisms, it is difficult to obtain pure cultures. However, *A israelii* can be grown anaerobically on a brain–heart infusion blood agar plate.

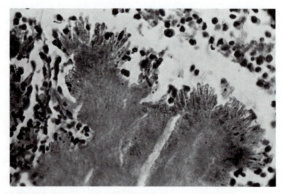

FIGURE 35-2 Hematoxylin and eosin stain of an *Actinomyces israelii* sulfur granule; notice the peripheral "clubs." (Original magnification × 1900.)

Penicillin is the drug of choice for the treatment of actinomycoses, but therapy must be continued for periods as long as 12 to 18 months, and surgical excision may be necessary in cases of advanced disease. Tetracycline and erythromycin also may be used to treat actinomycosis.

Control is especially difficult because the etiologic agent is part of the normal human flora. Good oral hygiene seems to lessen the possibility of actinomycosis, although many cases occur in apparently healthy young adults.

Periodontal Disease

Both *A viscosus* and *A naeslundii* have been shown to produce periodontal bone disease when inoculated into experimental animals. This is discussed in greater detail in Chapter 37.

NOCARDIA

Members of the genus *Nocardia* are distributed worldwide in the soil. However, only three species, *Nocardia asteroides, Nocardia brasiliensis,* and *Nocardia caviae,* are considered valid pathogens of humans.

The organisms grow aerobically on simple media, forming long filaments that easily fragment into rather pleomorphic bacillary and coccoid-shaped cells. The pathogenic species are gram positive and partially acid fast; as a result, the fragmented hyphae can be mistaken for tubercle bacilli.

Epidemiology and Pathogenesis of Human Nocardioses

Although species of *Nocardia* occasionally may be found in healthy persons, they are not considered normal flora. Nocardiosis occurs most frequently as a pulmonary disease in immunosuppressed or debilitated persons after the inhalation of the fragmented mycelium. In the usual course of events, one or more lung abscesses may develop and enlarge to form cavities similar to those seen in chronic tuberculosis. By far, most cases of pulmonary nocardiosis are caused by *N asteroides*. From the lung, the organisms may spread by way of the bloodstream; they have the potential to establish lesions in any area of the body, particularly the brain and kidneys. Unlike actinomycosis, bone destruction is rare; however, both *N asteroides* and *N brasiliensis* (and to a lesser extent *N caviae*) may form mycetomas (chronic subcutaneous infections identified with fungi), in which the abscesses extend by the destruction of soft tissue and bone to eventually erupt through the skin.

Diagnosis, Treatment, and Control of Nocardioses

Pulmonary nocardiosis can mimic many other infections, such as tuberculosis, carcinoma, actinomycosis, or fungal

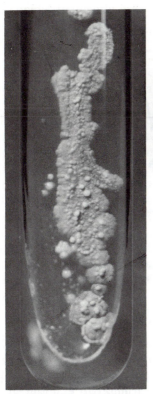

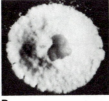

FIGURE 35-3 **A.** Colonies of *Nocardia asteroides* grown on Sabouraud's dextrose agar. **B.** Single colony of *N asteroides* grown on an inorganic salts–yeast, extract-glycerol agar medium in a humid atmosphere at 37°C.

infections of the lung. Thus, a definitive diagnosis requires the visualization of long, branching, gram-positive filaments and fragmented bacillary bodies that are partially acid fast. The organisms are easily grown, and the classic wrinkled, frequently pigmented colonies of *Nocardia* are easily recognized (Fig. 35-3).

The drug of choice for treating nocardiosis is sulfadiazine, but the prognosis is poor, particularly if the organisms have metastasized to other organs of the body.

Because of the widespread occurrence of species of *Nocardia,* control is impossible. However, humans undoubtedly possess considerable resistance to infection by these forms, because most cases occur in debilitated or immunosuppressed patients. Notice, however, that *N brasiliensis* possesses considerably higher virulence and may cause primary pulmonary infections in otherwise healthy individuals, as well as infections of the skin and soft tissue, acquired by means of cutaneous inoculation.

ACTINOMYCOTIC MYCETOMA (ACTINOMYCETOMA)

Actinomycetoma is a relatively painless, locally invasive, indolent, deforming infection characterized by swollen lesions with numerous draining sinus tracts. Lesions most commonly involve the feet, back, and head. Granules,

analogous to sulfur granules, may be expressed from sinus tracts or observed on the cut surface of tissue obtained for biopsy; the color of the granule can be correlated with the causative agent. Regional differences have been noticed for the actinomycetes most often isolated from infections. In equatorial Africa, the most common agents are *Actinomadura pelletieri* and *Streptomyces somaliensis,* but in Mexico, most infections are caused by *N brasiliensis.* This infection most commonly occurs in developing countries and rarely is seen in the United States and Europe. In developed countries, eumycotic mycetoma, an infection similar in appearance but caused by several genera of true fungi, is more common. It is important to differentiate between the actinomycotic and eucaryotic forms, because the latter require complete excision (amputation) to effect cure, but the former may respond to aggressive medical treatment and conservative surgical excision.

STREPTOMYCES

The genus *Streptomyces* includes an extremely large group of organisms distributed worldwide. Like other organisms in the Actinomycetales, they grow in long, branched filaments, but unlike members of the genera *Actinomyces* and *Nocardia,* they form long chains of aerial spores called conidia. Members of the genus *Streptomyces* are only rarely pathogenic, but occasional cases of actinomycetoma have been attributed to these organisms.

Members of the genus *Streptomyces* have achieved prominence as a result of their ability to produce antibiotics. Streptomycin and actinomycin were the first to be isolated and characterized, but since 1940, over 500 different antibacterial compounds, including many of the antibiotics in use today, have been isolated and characterized from organisms classified as *Streptomyces.*

Medically Important Fungi

The fungi, being eucaryotic organisms, differ from the actinomycetes in their cell-wall composition, nuclear structure, ribosome structure, and size. Included among the fungi are such macroscopic organisms as mushrooms, toadstools, and puffballs, as well as the microscopic organisms known as molds and yeasts.

It is estimated that over 100,000 different species of fungi participate in the cycles of nature, but, fortunately, only a few of these cause disease in humans.

CHARACTERISTICS

Fungi lack chlorophyll, are nonmotile (with the exception of certain spore forms), and may grow as single cells (yeasts) or as long, branched, filamentous structures (mycelia; Fig. 35-4). Fungi are classified by the type and method of sexual reproduction. Fungi not known to re-

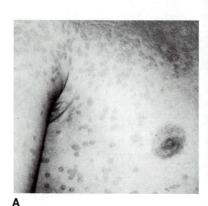

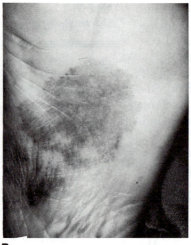

A   **B**

FIGURE 35-5   A. Hyperpigmented lesions of tinea versicolor on shoulder and chest. **B.** Tinea nigra on the side of a patient's foot.

sunlight) and on the appearance of the scaly lesions (Fig. 35-5*A*). A more definitive diagnosis can be obtained by observing a KOH preparation of skin scrapings for the characteristic yeast cells or by examining the affected area under an ultraviolet light (Wood's lamp) for a yellow fluorescence.

Infections caused by these organisms are treated with one of several topical agents such as salicylic acid, mild fungicides, 2% sulfur in an ointment base, or 1% selenium sulfide in a water-miscible ointment or as a shampoo. Oral ketoconazole or topical miconazole have also been used successfully to treat this infection. Unfortunately, recurrences are common.

Tinea Nigra

Tinea nigra, caused by *Exophiala werneckii* (a new designation of *Phaeoannellomyces werneckii* has been proposed), results in dark brown to black, painless, mottled areas on the skin, usually on the palms of the hands or soles of the feet (see Fig. 35-5*B*). The disease occurs primarily in the tropics, but it is being seen with greater frequency in the United States.

Skin scrapings dispersed in 10% KOH reveal septate hyphal filaments, and these can be grown on Sabouraud's glucose agar. The organism is slow to grow and may require as long as 3 weeks' incubation on a suitable medium before visible growth appears. The growth is at first yeast-like, but later develops into a mycelium.

Treatment as described for *M furfur* is effective in eliminating the infection.

Black Piedra and White Piedra

The agents responsible for black piedra and white piedra infections are unrelated and are grouped together here only because they are restricted to growth on the hair shaft.

Black piedra is characterized by hard, black nodules, which usually occur on the scalp hair and are composed of a hyphal mass cemented together by a capsule. The etiologic agent, *Piedraia hortae,* infects humans and other primates in the tropical areas of Asia, Africa, and South America.

White piedra, caused by *Trichosporon beigelii,* is seen less frequently than black piedra, but it occurs in both temperate and tropical areas of the world. This fungus may infect hairs on the face and the genital areas in addition to hairs on the scalp.

Both infections weaken the hair shaft, causing the hair to be easily broken. Diagnosis is based on the microscopic examination of infected hairs in a 10% KOH solution. Shaving the head or cutting off the infected hair usually provides an effective cure, but daily shampooing with an antifungal agent also is recommended.

DERMATOPHYTOSES

The etiologic agents of the dermatophytoses are closely related organisms that use keratin for growth. These organisms share antigenic and physiologic properties, and, for the most part, cause similar types of infections, even though the same species of dermatophyte may cause different symptoms in varying anatomic sites. Thus, the major differentiation between the three genera of dermatophytes (*Trichophyton, Microsporum,* and *Epidermophyton*) is based on the kinds and the appearance of conidia and hyphae (Fig. 35-6). In spite of the fact that the dermatophytes usually are considered members of the Deuteromycetes, sexual spores characteristic of Ascomycetes have been observed in about half of the known species of *Trichophyton* and *Microsporum*. As a result, sexual species of *Trichophyton* also are classified in the genus *Arthroderma,* and species of *Microsporum* known to produce sexual spores are additionally placed in the genus *Nannizzia.*

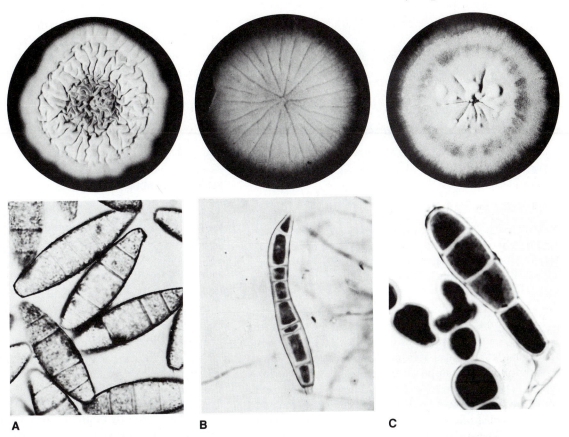

FIGURE 35-6 **A.** Colony and macroconidia of *Trichophyton gallinae*. **B.** Colony and macroconidium of *Microsporum audouinii*. **C.** Colony and macroconidium of *Epidermophyton floccosum*.

Dermatophytes invade only keratinized tissues, such as hair, nails, and the stratum corneum of the skin, causing an infection that does not extend into the subcutaneous areas of the body. In general, dermatophyte infections begin in the horny layer of the skin and spread in a centrifugal pattern showing a "ringworm" appearance.

The major clinical infections are termed (1) tinea pedis (ringworm of the feet), (2) tinea corporis (ringworm of the smooth skin), (3) tinea capitis (ringworm of the scalp), and (4) tinea unguium (ringworm of the nails). In addition, a further breakdown can be used, which includes (1) tinea cruris (ringworm of the groin), (2) tinea barbae (ringworm of the beard), and (3) tinea manuum (ringworm of the hand). All genera of dermatophytes may cause any of these clinical entities. However, species of *Microsporum* usually invade the hair and skin but not the nails; *Epidermophyton floccosum* invades the skin and nails but not the hair; and species of *Trichophyton* infect the hair, skin, and nails.

Tinea Pedis

Tinea pedis, also known as athlete's foot, is a common fungal disease of humans. Most cases are caused by *Trichophyton rubrum, Trichophyton mentogrophytes,* and *E floccosum*; because the infection seems to require warmth

and moisture to progress, the disease usually is found primarily in persons who wear shoes.

It is estimated that 30% to 70% of the population of the Western World is infected; however, most cases exist subclinically. The infection usually begins between the toes, and symptoms may vary from a chronic disease with peeling and cracking of the skin to an acute ulcerative form of the infection. It is thought that initial contact with the organisms probably occurs in places such as common shower stalls and bathing facilities, and that genetic factors may provide predisposing conditions for overt infections.

Chronically infected persons frequently develop a hypersensitivity to the fungus, which may cause an allergic response. This is called a *dermatophytid* (usually abbreviated *id*) *reaction,* and is manifested by the appearance of vesicles, usually on the hands. Such persons will also strongly react to an extract of the fungus (called trichophytin) to give a delayed-type skin reaction.

Tinea Corporis

Tinea corporis, or ringworm of the body, may be produced by any of the species of dermatophytes, although *T rubrum* and *T mentagrophytes* are the most common etiologic agents. Invasion of the horny layer of the skin

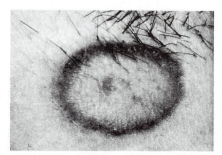

FIGURE 35-7 Tinea corporis (ringworm of the body) showing characteristic ring of inflammation.

is followed by the centrifugal spread of the organism, causing characteristic rings of inflammation (Fig. 35-7). Healing begins in the center of the ring. In the usual course of events, such infections will spontaneously clear within a few months.

Tinea Capitis

Tinea capitis can appear as noninflamed scaly red lesions or with loss of hair (alopecia) on the scalp, eyebrows, and eyelids. The most common etiologic agents in the United States are *Trichophyton tonsurans, Microsporum canis,* and *Microsporum audouinii.* Other geographic areas of the world may have different organisms as the prevalent cause of tinea capitis. Infections appear as expanding rings on the scalp with organisms growing in and on the hair. Inflammatory reactions may cause deep ulcers, which heal with scarring and permanent loss of hair.

Tinea capitis appears almost exclusively in children; it was formerly believed that healing occurred only at puberty, but it is apparent that spontaneous healing can occur after less than 1 year and well before the age of puberty. Obviously, some mechanism other than pubescent change is operative.

Tinea Unguium

Tinea unguium, an infection of the nails, is commonly associated with dermatophyte infections of other areas of

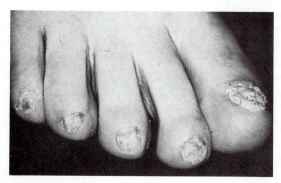

FIGURE 35-8 Tinea unguium (ringworm of the nails, or onychomycosis) in the toenails of a 61-year-old man.

the body. Almost all species of dermatophytes have been involved as etiologic agents, but *T rubrum* is found most commonly. The disease is characterized by thickened, discolored, brittle nails and may continue for years as a chronic infection (Fig. 35-8). An infection that is similar in appearance but caused by fungi other than dermatophytes is called *onychomycosis.* Common environmental saprophytic fungi, including *Scopulariopsis, Fusarium,* and *Aspergillus,* cause this infection.

Epidemiology of Dermatophytoses

The course of infection for the dermatophytes may be human to human (anthropophilic), animal to human (zoophilic), or soil to human (geophilic). Tinea pedis and tinea capitis are believed to spread from human to human indirectly through contaminated floors, towels, combs, theater seats, bed linens, and similar objects coming into contact with areas of the body. Other types of dermatophytoses seem to arise most frequently from human contact, but animal sources may be involved. Soil abounds with keratinophilic fungi with the potential to infect humans, but infections of geophilic origin are infrequent. When geophilic dermatophytes cause infections in humans, they are usually mild or chronic in contrast to infections caused by zoophilic and anthropophilic fungi, which are frequently highly inflammatory.

Treatment of Dermatophytoses

Topical applications of long-chain fatty acids, salicylic acid, selenium sulfide, sulfur in ointment, and many other compounds have for years been used to treat the dermatophytic fungal infections. However, the treatment of choice is a topical preparation containing one of the newer imidazole drugs. Griseofulvin often is used in conjunction with a topical agent for the treatment of tinea capitis, or it may be used alone for severe nail infections or extensive skin lesions. Given orally, it becomes incorporated into newly synthesized keratin layers, rendering them resistant to fungal infection, but has little effect on keratin structures that are already infected. Thus, depending on the site of the body involved and the causal organism, therapy can consist of daily treatment for several weeks with griseofulvin or topical agents (for tinea capitis caused by *M audouinii*) to use for many months (for nail infections caused by *T rubrum*).

In 1992, there was a report of a series of patients with either tinea corporis or tinea pedis that were treated once each week with 150 mg of fluconazole for up to 4 weeks. They reported a long-time cure of 95% for tinea corporis and 70% for tinea pedis.

PATHOGENIC YEASTS

It is, perhaps, a misnomer to set aside a section entitled "Pathogenic Yeasts," because the separation of yeasts from the filamentous fungi frequently is based on conditions of growth. Many pathogenic fungi grow as single-celled yeasts under one circumstance and as long, filamentous hyphae when growth conditions are changed. (This ability to grow as two distinct forms—either as yeast cells or as filamentous fungi—is an example of the phenomenon known as dimorphism.) This section is concerned with pathogenic fungi that appear only as yeasts or that only rarely form a true mycelium.

Candidiasis

Although the genus *Candida* contains a number of species, *Candida albicans* is by far the species most frequently encountered in candidiasis. Other important members of this genus are *Candida tropicalis, Candida parapsilosis,* and *Candida krusei.* Under normal conditions, members of *Candida* occur in small numbers in the alimentary tract, mouth, and vaginal area, and disease results only when a major change in other normal flora or a disturbance of the normal immune response occurs. Under such conditions, *Candida* is capable of invading every tissue and cavity of the body. These include infections of the oral cavity, vagina, intestinal tract, skin, and, less frequently, systemic infections of the kidney, eye, liver, biliary tract, and brain. All of these occur primarily in individuals who have physiologic defects, such as endocrine disorders, or in persons with an altered normal flora or suppressed immune defense. Patients with AIDS are highly susceptible to infection with *Candida.*

Newer therapeutic measures likely are responsible for the increase in *Candida* infections seen over the last two decades. The use of antibiotics, which suppress the normal flora, undoubtedly is, in part, responsible for the increased number of infections, particularly gastrointestinal candidiasis. The use of polyethylene catheters and implanted prosthetic devices also is associated with increased *Candida* infections.

C albicans usually appears as oval, yeast-like cells that reproduce by budding (Fig. 35-9); however, in infected areas, filamentous hyphae plus pseudohyphae (which consist of elongated yeast cells that remain attached to each other) also may be seen. The yeast is easily grown at 25° to 37°C on Sabouraud's glucose agar, and, if grown on cornmeal agar at 25°C, the *C albicans* can produce many characteristic thick-walled chlamydoconidia.

ORAL CANDIDIASIS. Oral candidiasis (also called thrush) occurs most frequently in the newborn and probably is acquired during passage through an infected or colonized vagina. The yeast appears as a creamy, gray membrane covering the tongue and seems able to produce disease only because of the absence of other resident flora. If thrush has not occurred by the third day of life, it is unlikely that it will appear, but if it should occur, it is treated with oral nystatin.

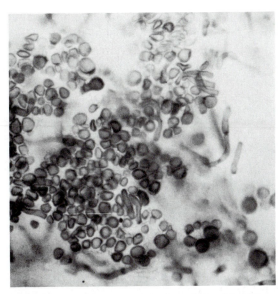

FIGURE 35-9 Yeast cells and pseudohyphae of *Candida albicans* on a skin scale. (Original magnification ×675.)

Oral thrush in older children or adults may occur as a result of endocrine disturbances or avitaminosis (particularly a deficiency of riboflavin), as a complication of diabetes, as a result of poor oral hygiene, or after the administration of corticosteroids or antibiotics. It is also reported to occur as an early manifestation of AIDS.

VAGINITIS. Of the 20 million cases of vaginal candidiasis occurring annually, most are seen in women with diabetes mellitus, during pregnancy, after antibiotic therapy, or with the use of oral contraceptives. The prominent symptom is a yellow, milky vaginal discharge. Yeast cells and pseudomycelium can be found on the mucous membranes, and such infections may result in an intense inflammation of the entire inguinal area.

Vaginal candidiasis can be difficult to eradicate, and many women experience recurrent infections. In one study, only a 50% cure rate was observed in women with recurrent vulvovaginal candidiasis who had been given low doses of oral ketoconazole daily for 6 months. Because the organism survives laundering in detergent at the usual washing temperatures, it has been suggested that some recurrent infections might result from a reinfection from contaminated underwear. This can be prevented, according to Professor Byron J. Masterson of the University of Florida (Gainesville, FL), by "zapping" freshly laundered, but still damp, underwear in the microwave for 5 minutes on high. This procedure will kill the organisms, but he cautions that only cotton undergarments should be so treated.

ALIMENTARY CANDIDIASIS. Alimentary candidiasis may follow essentially any of the predisposing conditions listed for adult oral thrush; however, most cases occur as a result of prolonged, broad-spectrum antibiotic therapy, which destroys a large part of the normal flora of the intestine. The organisms also may cause intense inflammation of the perianal region (the region around the anus) and may spread to the buttocks and thighs.

CUTANEOUS AND SYSTEMIC CANDIDIASIS. Infection of the skin by *Candida* usually occurs in those with metabolic disorders, in those whose obesity results in continuously moist folds of skin, or in persons in whom parts of the body are kept moist under surgical dressings. *Candida* also may cause diaper rash.

Systemic candidiasis seems to be increasing in incidence, and in debilitated persons or those receiving immunosuppressive drugs, *C albicans* can cause urinary tract infections, endocarditis, and meningitis. Chronic mucocutaneous candidiasis is a rare syndrome in which the skin, mucous membranes, hair, and nails become infected. Such infections seem to occur in persons with T-cell defects manifested by their inability to respond to *Candida* antigens.

TREATMENT OF *CANDIDA* INFECTIONS. A variety of agents are available for treating the different types of *Candida* infections. Systemic or internal organ involvement can be treated successfully with amphotericin B, flucytosine or fluconazole. Unfortunately, patients with immune deficiencies routinely become reinfected. Nystatin usually is effective for the treatment of mucocutaneous candidiasis, such as thrush or vaginitis. Other antibiotics used for the treatment of mucocutaneous candidiasis include miconazole, ketoconazole and clotrimazole. Interestingly, treatment of immunosuppressed patients with fluconazole has resulted in an increase of infections caused by resistant strains of *C krusei*.

Cryptococcosis

Cryptococcosis is caused by *Cryptococcus neoformans*. This yeast is distributed worldwide in soils, but most human infections are thought to be acquired by the inhalation of the fungus in dried pigeon feces. Curiously, pigeons are not infected, but the organisms grow well in bird droppings and, hence, are frequently found in high concentrations in such enriched areas.

C neoformans characteristically produces a large polysaccharide capsule, and, based on antigenic differences in the capsule, the species is divided into four serotypes: A, B, C, and D. Mating experiments have been used to divided these serotypes into two different varieties (ie, *C neoformans* var *neoformans* for serotypes A and D, and *C neoformans* var *gatti* for serotypes B and C). Serotype A is found most commonly in the eastern and central sections of the United States, whereas serotypes B and C cause most human infections in southern California. In-

terestingly, serotypes B and C have not been found in pigeon feces but have been isolated from soil in Australia.

CLINICAL CRYPTOCOCCOSIS. Because cryptococci are acquired by inhalation, primary infection occurs in the lungs. Based on skin tests using a cryptococcal antigen called cryptococcin, it seems that most infections are either asymptomatic or undiagnosed, and the resolution of the primary lesions usually occurs spontaneously. Fulminating (intense or sudden) pneumonia may result in spread of the organisms by way of the bloodstream, causing infections in various areas of the body, but the most frequent complication is involvement of the brain and meninges.

Cutaneous and mucocutaneous cryptococcosis is seen in about 10% of cases, curiously, more frequently in Europe than in the United States. Some investigators believe that the cutaneous lesions usually result from the mechanical seeding of injured sites in the skin. Primary cutaneous cryptococcosis is, however, seen more commonly in immunosuppressed individuals.

Immunity is cell mediated and probably is expressed through activation of macrophages. As might be expected, AIDS victims are highly susceptible, and cryptococci can be readily isolated from the spinal fluid of 10% to 15% of such individuals.

DIAGNOSIS AND TREATMENT OF *CRYPTOCOCCUS* INFECTIONS. *Cryptococcus neoformans* grows primarily as a yeast that produces a large capsule, but several strains now known can form a mycelium. An India-ink wet mount provides an easy method to visualize this encapsulated yeast (Fig. 35-10), and the presence of characteristic organisms in a sediment of cerebrospinal fluid provides a tentative diagnosis. The organisms can be readily grown but are sensitive to cycloheximide, which is frequently incorporated into some fungal media. Specific identification of *C neoformans* requires physiologic tests.

Commercial kits are available for the detection of capsular material in spinal fluid or blood. Such kits contain latex beads that have been coated with rabbit antibodies to the capsules. Agglutination of the beads after mixing

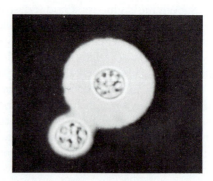

FIGURE 35-10   India-ink wet mount of *Cryptococcus neoformans* demonstrating the capsule around a yeast cell.

with dilutions of spinal fluid or blood are indicative of a cryptococcal infection.

Untreated meningitis resulting from *C neoformans* is invariably fatal; however, combined administration of amphotericin B and 5-fluorocytosine usually is effective and is the therapy of choice.

Miscellaneous Yeast Infections

Torulopsis glabrata, a member of the human normal flora, only rarely causes torulopsis, an infection occurring in persons receiving long-term antibiotics, cortisone, or immunosuppressive drugs. The most common site of infection is the genitourinary tract, although infections of the mouth, lungs, and kidneys have been reported.

Rhodotorula rubra also has occasionally been isolated from the lungs, kidney, and central nervous system of a debilitated patient. The yeast is a common contaminant of skin and feces, and has been isolated from soil and a number of food sources. Infections are usually attributed to contaminated catheters, heart–lung machines, and other invasive medical devices, and usually spontaneously resolve when the source of infection is removed.

Treatment with amphotericin B is effective for infections caused by both *T glabrata* and *R rubra.*

SUBCUTANEOUS MYCOSES

Subcutaneous mycoses are mycotic infections that gain entrance to the body as a result of trauma to the skin. Once established, these mycoses usually remain localized in the traumatized area, but may extend by way of draining lymph channels to regional lymph nodes. Fungi involved in subcutaneous types of mycoses are normal soil inhabitants whose localized infection and slow progression cause them to be considered organisms of low virulence.

Sporotrichosis

Sporothrix schenckii, the etiologic agent of sporotrichosis, is found in soil and plants in a worldwide but sporadic distribution. It also occurs in wood and moss, and infections frequently result from inoculation by splinters, thorn pricks, sphagnum moss, grasses, or garden soil. Thus, infection is an occupational hazard for gardeners and greenhouse workers. This is illustrated by the large outbreak of 84 cases of cutaneous sporotrichosis that occurred during the spring of 1988. All infected persons had handled seedlings that had been packed in sphagnum moss that had been harvested in Wisconsin and shipped to nurseries in more that 15 states. It is also frequently seen in South America in persons gathering grass or cultivating house plants. Curiously, endemic areas have shifted over the years, and it has been proposed that nutritional

deficiencies might explain the high incidence of sporotrichosis in areas of rural South America.

EPIDEMIOLOGY AND PATHOGENESIS. Sporotrichosis usually is a localized infection of the skin, subcutaneous tissues, and regional lymphatics that gains entrance to the body after trauma or through open wounds. After an incubation period varying from 1 week to 6 months, a subcutaneous nodule appears and develops into a necrotic ulcer. The initial lesions heal as new ulcers appear in adjacent areas. Lymphatics in the area develop nodules and ulcers along the lymph channels, and these may persist for months or years.

In highly endemic areas, many persons develop a cellular immunity to the organism; this can be demonstrated as a delayed-type skin reaction to sporotrichin. Such persons seem able to localize the initial infection to the original site of invasion. Rarely, *S schenckii* may invade the blood and spread to various organs of the body; occasionally, the fungi may enter the host by way of the respiratory tract, resulting in a primary pulmonary sporotrichosis.

Because of the widespread occurrence of *S schenckii,* protective clothing, especially gloves, should be worn when handling potentially infectious material.

DIAGNOSIS AND TREATMENT. *Sporothrix schenckii* is a dimorphic fungus that grows in culture, soil, or plant material as septate, branching hyphae with both rosettes and single, tear-shaped conidia formed laterally or at the ends of the branches. In contrast, the organisms appear in infected tissues as cigar-shaped yeast cells that reproduce by budding (Fig. 35-11).

A definitive diagnosis requires the growth and identification of the infecting organism, even though lymphocutaneous sporotrichosis with lymph channel ulceration can be diagnosed clinically with reasonable confidence. Few organisms are present in the lesions, and so a histologic examination frequently may be negative. The mycelial form from a Sabouraud's glucose agar medium grown

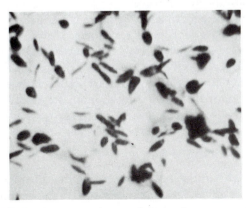

FIGURE 35-11 Gram stain of yeast cells in pus from a mouse infected with *Sporothrix schenckii.*

at 25°C can be transformed to the yeast phase by growth in moist blood-agar tubes at 37°C.

Oral potassium iodide administered over a period of weeks is the most common treatment for localized sporotrichosis; however, amphotericin B is used for relapsing cases, as well as for pulmonary and disseminated sporotrichosis.

Chromoblastomycosis

Chromoblastomycosis (also known as chromomycosis and verrucous dermatitis) is a term applied to a clinical infection that may be caused by any one of several different dermatiaceous (pigmented) fungi. The taxonomy of this group of agents is far from firm, but the principal genera involved in chromomycosis are *Phialophora* and *Cladosporium*.

EPIDEMIOLOGY AND PATHOGENESIS. The causative agents of chromoblastomycosis are soil saprophytes found in decaying vegetative matter and rotting wood. Most infections seem to originate from puncture wounds, and most of these occur in the tropics, particularly in Mexico and South America.

Most infections occur on the feet and legs in rural areas where shoes are rarely worn. The original lesion appears as a small, raised, violet papule, and, over a period of months to years, additional lesions appear in adjacent areas. The lesions are hard, dry, and usually raised 1 to 3 mm above the skin surface; clusters of such growths resemble florets of cauliflower.

The infection generally remains localized without involving bone or muscle or even causing particular discomfort to the patient. Lesions may become secondarily infected with bacteria, resulting in a purulent exudate. Rarely, a spreading may occur by way of the bloodstream to involve other areas of the body, including various organs such as lungs and brain; occasional blockage of lymph channels may result in elephantiasis. Skin scrapings mounted in KOH or biopsy tissue can reveal copper-colored sclerotic bodies that are pathognomonic for chromoblastomycosis. However, the specific identification of the etiologic agent usually requires culture and the use of botanical keys of fungal taxonomy.

Choices for therapy are limited, with no drug giving satisfactory results. 5-Flucytosine and excision are favored when lesions are not too extensive. Surgical excision of the lesion, particularly during the early stages of the disease, has also proved effective.

THE SYSTEMIC MYCOSES

The fungi causing systemic diseases (also called the deep mycoses) are all dimorphic: they exist as filamentous organisms in nature and as yeast cells or spherules with endospores in infected tissue. Moreover, in most cases, their distribution is extremely limited, occurring mostly within limited geographic areas. The diseases begin as lower respiratory infections resulting from the inhalation of fungal conidia. It seems that most cases are asymptomatic or undiagnosed, and only a small percentage progress to serious systemic manifestations.

Blastomycosis

Blastomycosis (formerly called North American blastomycosis or Gilchrist's disease) is caused by a single organism, *Blastomyces dermatitidis*. The disease seems to be endemic in the Southeastern part of the United States, extending north into Minnesota, Wisconsin, Michigan, and western New York; cases have been reported in Mexico and Africa. A sexual stage for the organism, described in 1967, allows the fungus to be technically classified in Ascomycetes as *Ajellomyces dermatitidis*.

EPIDEMIOLOGY AND PATHOGENESIS. Although all evidence indicates that the human disease is initiated by inhalation of the fungal conidia, attempts to isolate the etiologic agent from its natural habitat usually have failed. Rare successful isolations from soil have been followed by failure when subsequent samples are cultured from the same sites, and this has led to the postulate that the organism may be dormant except under specific environmental conditions. Some insight was gained, however, after an epidemic of 48 cases of blastomycosis in Wisconsin during June 1984. All of the infected individuals were attending a camp and had walked on an abandoned beaver lodge. Cultures from the lodge and decomposed wood near the beaver dam grew *B dermatitidis*. Notice that the isolations were made from moist soil with a high organic content, and which had been exposed to animal excreta. *B dermatitidis* also has been isolated from five sites near Augusta, Georgia, all of which were associated with animal excreta.

Blastomycosis has been divided into pulmonary, cutaneous, and systemic conditions, but generally it is believed that all three types originate in the lung from a primary pulmonary blastomycosis. The pulmonary lesions are like those of tuberculosis, carcinoma, or histoplasmosis, and misdiagnoses based on x-ray findings are typical. Unresolved pulmonary infections progress to acute lobar pneumonia accompanied by spread of the organisms by way of the bloodstream to other internal organs, bone, and skin.

Skin lesions, which eventually evolve into ulcerated granulomas, are the most common symptom of the disease. Such lesions may progress over a period of years, eventually involving large areas of the body. Bone invasion, causing arthritis and bone destruction, occurs in 25% to 50% of reported cases. Multiple internal organs may become infected, the most common of which is the genitourinary system and the rarest of which is the central nervous system.

Interestingly, it seems that most infections by *B der-*

matitidis are asymptomatic because a number of studies have shown that many individuals with immune markers of infection have experienced no signs or symptoms characteristic of blastomycosis. It thus seems that blastomycosis has patterns of subclinical infections comparable with that known to occur in histoplasmosis and coccidioidomycosis.

DIAGNOSIS AND TREATMENT. There is no specific serologic skin test for blastomycosis. Blastomycin, a filtrate extracted from *B dermatitidis* grown on a liquid medium, cross-reacts so strongly with histoplasmin and coccidioidin that skin tests are of little value. A specific, fluorescently labeled antibody has been prepared that will react with the yeast cells in histologic tissue sections. After the epidemic of blastomycosis in Wisconsin, three different serologic tests were evaluated in 47 patients for their ability to detect antibodies to the A antigen of *B dermatitidis,* namely, enzyme immunoassay, immunodiffusion, and complement fixation. Of these, the enzyme immunoassay was the most sensitive, detecting antibody in 77% of the patients compared with 28% and 9% for the immunodiffusion and complement fixation, respectively. Definitive laboratory diagnosis, however, is best accomplished by the growth and identification of the etiologic agent.

When cultured on Sabouraud's glucose agar at 25°C, the organism grows as a white fungus that darkens with age and bears spherical conidia from the sides of the hyphae. The conida are the infectious elements of this organism. Specific identification requires either growth at 37°C with conversion of the hyphal form to the yeast phase or an immunoidentification of the mold using water-soluble antigens in an immunodiffusion test (exoantigen test). The yeast cells are large, thick-walled, spherical cells, which can be readily identified by the single buds that arise from the parent cell on a broad base (Fig. 35-12).

Intravenous amphotericin B has been the treatment of choice for all forms of blastomycosis, and relapses occur only after inadequate therapy. It remains, therefore, the treatment of choice for seriously ill patients. However,

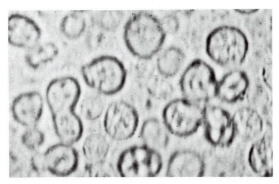

FIGURE 35-12 Yeast cells, many with buds, of *Blastomyces dermatitidis* in a culture of sputum.

the doses of amphotericin B used are usually toxic, and additional drugs to control nausea, pain, and headache may be required. Ketoconazole also has been used successfully in treating blastomycosis. This drug can be taken orally and may be useful for patients with less severe infections. Itraconazole, a drug with a low rate of toxic effects, has also proven to be effective for the treatment of blastomycosis and it may supplant ketoconazole for nonlife-threatening infections.

Notice, however, that only 9 of 44 patients who were infected during the epidemic in Wisconsin received antifungal therapy. Moreover, none of the remaining 35 untreated patients experienced relapses or had progressive infections.

Histoplasmosis

Histoplasma capsulatum, the etiologic agent of histoplasmosis, is distributed worldwide, although certain areas such as the central and mideastern United States seem to be the most heavily contaminated with this fungus. It is certainly one of the more common mycoses in humans; it has been estimated that 40 million persons in the United States have been infected and that 200,000 new cases occur annually. In 1972, this dimorphic organism was shown to have a sexual stage and, as a result, it is also classified with the Ascomycetes and placed in the genus *Ajellomyces*; its sexual state is properly referred to as *Ajellomyces capsulatus*. It seems likely, however, that medical mycologists will continue to use its imperfect name of *Histoplasma capsulatum*.

EPIDEMIOLOGY AND PATHOGENESIS. *Histoplasma capsulatum* is widely distributed in soil and preferentially grows in association with bird and bat feces. Thus, highly infectious areas may be found in chicken coops, bat caves, bird roosts, or any environment extensively inhabited by birds. It has even been proposed that there may be a correlation between the highly endemic places of the United States and the enormous numbers of starlings that inhabit these areas. When growing in soil, *H capsulatum* is found only as branched hyphal filaments that form small, single conidia and larger, spiny macroconidia referred to as tuberculated macroconidia (Fig. 35-13*A*). Infection follows inhalation of the small microconidia into the lung, where they germinate and are transformed into budding yeast cells.

The yeast cells are distributed from the lungs throughout the internal organs by way of the bloodstream, and, in most cases, the organisms are destroyed or sequestered by the host's immune responses. The lung lesions heal, followed by a fibrosis and calcification similar to healed calcified tuberculous lesions. For individuals possessing a normal immune response, the symptoms can be correlated with the extent of exposure. About 95% of infected persons give no history of infection, indicating the disease had been unapparent or mild. There have,

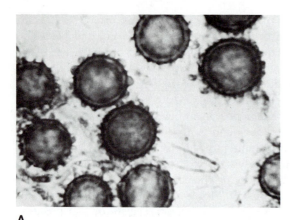

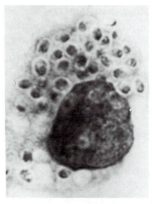

FIGURE 35-13   A. Tuberculated macroconidia of *Histoplasma capsulatum*. **B.** Yeast cells of *H capsulatum* in a macrophage are shown in this example from a Giemsa-stained tissue smear (human case).

however, been serious epidemics of histoplasmosis in individuals who were exposed to large quantities of conidia acquired while cleaning chicken coops or entering bat-infected caves. In such persons, the symptoms may be acute, with high fever and severe pneumonia. However, even in severe epidemics of histoplasmosis, the mortality rate is only about 1%, and most of the remaining cases are resolved.

A small percentage of infected persons develop a disseminated form of histoplasmosis that is usually seen in individuals with immune deficiencies or who are taking immunosuppressive drugs. This may occur as a fulminating disease, which is rapidly fatal if untreated, or as a chronic disease, which is frequently characterized by mucosal ulcers. The mild form of chronic disseminated histoplasmosis may involve only a single organ, whereas the more serious disease encompasses widespread infection.

Chronic pulmonary histoplasmosis may be pathologically similar to the cavitation of chronic tuberculosis. These patients frequently have emphysema or other underlying lung disease. The disease is most often seen in adult men and may be characterized by recurrent episodes of a productive cough accompanied by fever and weakness, or it may resolve spontaneously in a few weeks. When the disease develops some years after the primary infection, it is generally believed that the organisms came from the reactivation of a latent lesion, as was described for the recrudescence of tuberculosis. This is particularly true for AIDS patients.

DIAGNOSIS AND TREATMENT. Histoplasmosis is an intracellular disease in which the yeast cells generally exist and grow within the reticuloendothelial system and macrophages. Histologic examination of the buffy coat (containing the white blood cells) of centrifuged blood samples, or biopsy material from lesions, particularly during the acute disease, may reveal many yeast cells within the macrophages (see Fig. 35-13*B*). Such material, as well as sputum, can be readily cultured on Sabouraud's agar and on blood agar. Colonies of *H capsulatum* showing hyphal growth at 25°C produce characteristic tuberculated macroconidia that should appear within 4 to 6 weeks. Growth of these

organisms on blood agar at 37°C will produce ovoid, budding yeast cells. Identification can be accomplished by the morphologic conversion of the typical mold phase to a yeast or by an exoantigen test.

Concentration of the filtrates of broth cultures of *H capsulatum* yields a material called histoplasmin, analogous to tuberculin. Injection of dilutions of histoplasmin (usually 1:100 or 1:1000) intradermally will cause a delayed-type skin reaction in persons who have developed a cellular-type immunity to the organisms. However, a positive skin test result may not be of actual diagnostic value, because it may represent only a past contact with the organism. Skin testing with histoplasmin also may interfere with the complement-fixation tests for histoplasmosis and coccidioidomycosis. Histoplasmin should not, therefore, be used for general screening.

Other serologic tests used for the diagnosis of histoplasmosis include complement fixation and double immunodiffusion using histoplasmin as the antigen; the latter is preferred. Specific fluorescently labeled antibody also has been used as a diagnostic aid in the absence of cultures.

Most cases of histoplasmosis are undiagnosed, and recovery is spontaneous. Even moderately severe cases of primary histoplasmosis can be adequately treated with bed rest. However, disseminated or systemic disease requires antimicrobial therapy. Amphotericin B, ketoconazole, and itraconazole often are effective, and recovery is rapid, but relapses have occurred with each drug.

A separate form of this disease, known as *African histoplasmosis*, occurs in equatorial Africa. This infection is more commonly manifested by cutaneous lesions, and the yeast cells are somewhat larger than those seen in North America. These differences have resulted in the designation of the causative agent as *H capsulatum* var *duboisii*.

Coccidioidomycosis

Coccidioides immitis, the etiologic agent of coccidioidomycosis, is found in soil only in arid regions, and one of the most highly endemic areas includes the southwestern United States and northern Mexico. Endemic areas exist also in Central and South America.

EPIDEMIOLOGY AND PATHOGENESIS. *Coccidioides immitis* grows in soil as a septate, filamentous fungus that characteristically produces thick-walled arthrospores in alternating cells of a hyphal filament. The mature hyphae easily fragment, and the liberated arthrospores are readily carried on surrounding dust particles. It is estimated that as many as 100,000 individuals are infected in the United States each year.

Human infection follows inhalation of the arthrospores, and, like histoplasmosis, it may result in an asymptomatic or mild to severe respiratory infection. Infection also may produce either a chronic progressive disease or an acute disseminated infection. Epidemiologic studies have led to the conclusion that about 60% of all primary infections are asymptomatic, about 40% produce a mild to severe pulmonary disease, and 0.2% to 0.5% result in chronic or acute disseminated infections. Interestingly, the down-regulation of cell-mediated immunity that occurs during the latter stages of pregnancy leaves such women particularly susceptible to the disseminated forms of the disease.

After inhalation, the arthrospore differentiates into a large, round, thick-walled structure, 30 to 60 μm in diameter, which becomes multinucleate and, eventually, forms several hundred uninucleated endospores that are 2 to 5 μm in diameter (Fig. 35-14). This rounded structure, called a *spherule*, breaks open when mature, liberating the enclosed endospores. The morphologic events of spherule and endospore formation are recognized to be analogous to sporangium and sporangiospore production as found in the Zygomycotina, but no sexual stage has been observed. On the other hand, the saprophytic form of *Coccidioides* possesses septate hyphae and produces arthroconidia, thus closely resembling several members of the Ascomycotina. In most infections, the liberated spores undergo phagocytosis and are killed, and, in the absence of a positive coccidioidin skin test (analogous to histoplasmin), there would be no evidence that an infection had occurred.

Symptomatic pulmonary infections are characterized by fever, chest pain, a mild cough, headache, and loss of appetite. X-rays show small nodules in the lung like those seen in primary tuberculosis. Such lesions may form cavities, which usually become fibrotic and later calcify. Curiously, in about 5% to 10% of such cases, allergic reactions (as manifested by sterile, erythematous lesions and nodules) may appear, usually on the legs, within a few days after the beginning of the initial symptoms. These lesions ordinarily disappear in about 1 week, but in endemic areas of coccidioidomycosis, their occurrence is strongly suggestive of this disease.

Coccidioidomycosis may also take the form of a benign, chronic disease in which the organisms remain localized in the lung, causing enlarged cavities that are usually filled with spherules of *C immitis*. Such cavities may fibrose (grow white fibrous connective tissue) and calcify, or may require surgical removal. This condition may remain chronic for years.

The disseminated form of the disease occurs in about 1% of individuals infected with *C immitis*. It may be manifested soon after the primary infection, particularly in dark-skinned persons, or it may occur after years of chronic pulmonary disease. Disseminated coccidioidomycosis may produce an acute or chronic meningitis, or a generalized disease characterized by lesions in many internal organs. Cutaneous lesions appear as granulomas that may eventually heal or that, in advanced disease, may form draining ulcers.

AIDS patients living in endemic areas are particularly susceptible to symptomatic coccidioidomycosis, and the total number of coccidioidal infections occurring in HIV-infected persons has risen dramatically.

DIAGNOSIS AND TREATMENT. Direct examination of sputum, pus, or gastric washings frequently reveals the presence of mature spherules of *C immitis*. Culture of the organisms is dangerous and should be done only by experienced personnel using special precautions, because the arthroconidia produced are extremely infectious. The organism is, however, readily grown on Sabouraud's medium, and the presence of typical arthroconidia (in a formalized preparation) is indicative of *C immitis*. Spherule formation has been accomplished in vitro by growing the organisms at 40°C in an atmosphere of 20% CO_2, and it is easily demonstrated by injection of the organisms into mice.

Coccidioidin is the most useful of the skin-test materials. It can be used as a diagnostic aid and as a screening test. An immunodiffusion test using the patient's serum and extracts of the mycelium has proved both easy to use and moderately sensitive. Latex particle agglutination is also used as a rapid assay for the presence of IgM antibodies to *C immitis*. It is fairly sensitive but produces a num-

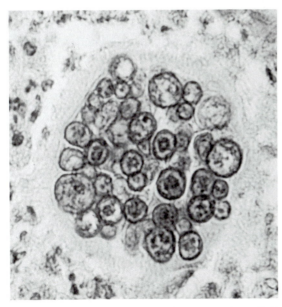

FIGURE 35-14 Endospore-filled spherule from a case of coccidioidomycosis.

ber of false-positive results. Other serologic tests include a tube precipitin test, in which dilutions of the patient's serum are mixed with coccidioidin and observed for precipitation. This test is both sensitive and reasonably specific for IgM. A complement-fixation test for IgG antibodies also is a reasonably sensitive test for the diagnosis of coccidioidomycosis.

A primary infection, even though asymptomatic, induces a solid immunity to reinfection. As in other mycotic infections, amphotericin B has been the therapy of choice for chronic pulmonary or disseminated disease; however, itraconazole, ketoconazole, and fluconazole also have been shown to be effective. Surgical removal of lung cavities may be required in cases of advanced pulmonary disease.

Paracoccidioidomycosis

Paracoccidioidomycosis (formerly South American blastomycosis) is caused by *Paracoccidioides brasiliensis*. The disease is found only in Central and South America, where 80% of reported cases occur in Brazil.

EPIDEMIOLOGY AND PATHOGENESIS. Despite the restricted geographic location of paracoccidioidomycosis, the natural habitat of the etiologic agent is not evident, although it has, on rare occasions, been isolated from soil samples in endemic areas.

P brasiliensis is a dimorphic organism that seems to exist in soil as a filamentous fungus, producing a variety of conidia types: single microconidia, chlamydoconidia, and arthroconidia. Primary infection was long believed to result from the direct implantation of the organisms into the oral mucosa, but it is apparent that, like the other systemic mycoses, paracoccidioidomycosis originates as a pulmonary infection.

Initial infection probably results from the inhalation of conidia of *P brasiliensis* that subsequently differentiate into the yeast form of the organism. Skin testing in endemic areas of the disease indicates that most infections occur as asymptomatic or undiagnosed cases, and that progressive pulmonary disease and secondary lesions from disseminated infections are rare. Primary infections usually resolve spontaneously and may result in the occurrence of calcified pulmonary lesions. When chronic progressive pulmonary disease does occur, considerable areas of the lung may become fibrosed.

More commonly, the pulmonary involvement is subclinical, and the invading yeast cells are disseminated (possibly by macrophages) to the oropharyngeal mucosa. The characteristic ulcerative lesions occurring in the mouth and nose frequently are the first symptom, and so it is understandable that the initial pulmonary aspect of this infection was not appreciated initially. Lymph nodes may become infected, ulcerate, and drain.

Disseminated organisms also may infect other organs such as the spleen, liver, and adrenals, resulting in a spread of the lesions and a corresponding involvement of the regional lymph nodes.

One of the real curiosities concerning this disease has been the high ratio of male to female patients who become infected (ratios in some areas are as high as 150:1). Interestingly, paracoccidioidin skin tests in healthy individuals from the same areas do not reveal sex differences, indicating that both sexes acquire subclinical infections but overt disease occurs more frequently in male patients. This mystery seems to have been solved by Angela Restrepo and colleagues, who showed that the presence of the female hormone, 17-estradiol, and to a lessor extent, diethylstilbestrol, inhibited the mycelium-to-yeast transformation of *P brasiliensis*. This transition was not affected by male hormones such as testosterone.

DIAGNOSIS AND TREATMENT. Direct examination of sputum, draining lymph nodes, or biopsy material reveals large, round yeast cells that may possess from one to two buds surrounding the parent yeast (Fig. 35-15). These cells can be readily differentiated from *B dermatitidis*, which forms a single bud on a broad base.

Culture at 25°C yields the mycelial form, which is difficult to identify; however, incubation at 37°C on blood agar promotes the conversion of the organism to the yeast with typical morphologic features.

A skin-testing antigen, termed *paracoccidioidin*, can be used to evaluate total infections in an endemic area, but a positive skin reaction does not necessarily indicate active disease. Complement fixation, immunodiffusion, and fluorescently labeled antibody have all been used with varying success.

Sulfonamide therapy results in remission of symptoms, but treatment must be continued on a daily basis for 3 to 5 years. Amphotericin B also is an effective chemotherapeutic agent for paracoccidioidomycosis, although more recent data suggest that the imidazoles, itraconazole, or ketoconazole may be the treatment of choice.

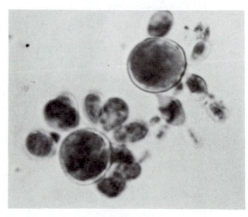

FIGURE 35-15   Yeast cells of *Paracoccidioides brasiliensis* with multiple buds.

Geotrichosis

Geotrichum candidum, the etiologic agent of geotrichosis, seems to be one of the more ubiquitous of the fungi that occasionally infect humans. It has been isolated from the stools, urine, and vaginal secretions of about one third of all persons checked, having caused no apparent disease. It has also been found in decaying plant material, in dairy products, and on normal skin.

EPIDEMIOLOGY AND PATHOGENESIS. Because of the widespread occurrence of *G candidum,* human contact with this fungus must occur frequently. The fact that it only rarely causes disease indicates that it possesses little virulence for animals or humans. Diagnosed infections most frequently are pulmonary and may be secondary to tuberculosis. Oral infections, clinically identical to thrush caused by *C albicans,* also may occur.

DIAGNOSIS AND TREATMENT. The diagnosis of *G candidum* as the etiologic agent of disease is difficult because of its ubiquity. One should find the organism frequently and in large numbers in sputum or in oral lesions to support the diagnosis. Growth and the demonstration of characteristic rectangular arthrospores (Fig. 35-16) are required for a culture confirmation of geotrichosis. Treatment may include iodides, aerosol nystatin, or amphotericin B.

OPPORTUNISTIC FUNGI

Many of the mycotic agents discussed in this chapter could be considered as opportunistic fungi, because they may commonly occur in endemic areas and yet rarely produce progressive disease. However, the fungi considered briefly here are of worldwide distribution and, under normal circumstances, do not usually cause even asymptomatic infections in humans. However, they may cause serious disease in debilitated persons, in diabetics, in patients with leukemia or lymphoma, in immunosuppressed persons, and in persons who are heavily exposed to large numbers of spores.

Aspergillosis

Persons who are heavily exposed to conidia from the genus *Aspergillus* may develop IgE and IgG antibodies, as well as a delayed-type hypersensitivity, and much of the resulting pulmonary disease may produce an asthmatic allergy to the fungus. In progressive disease, the growth of the hyphae may seriously interfere with normal gas exchange.

By far, most *Aspergillus* infections occur in debilitated and immunocompromised persons, particularly among those whose primary disease is leukemia or lymphoma. *Aspergillus fumigatus* and *Aspergillus flavus* are the major species involved, and infections usually are acquired by inhalation of *Aspergillus* conidia. In some cases, *Aspergillus* "balls" may develop in tuberculous cavities and par-

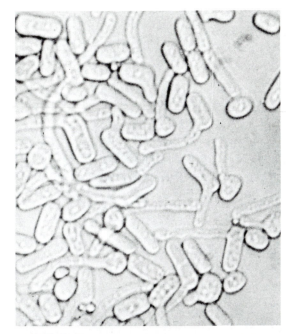

FIGURE 35-16 Arthrospores of *Geotrichum candidum.*

tially fill them with tangled masses of mycelium. Also, hyphae may invade adjacent blood vessels, causing the production of bloody sputum. Species of *Aspergillus,* especially *A flavus,* also may infect the nasal sinuses or may become widely disseminated, particularly after corticosteroid therapy or treatment with immunosuppressive drugs.

The diagnosis of aspergillosis is difficult because of the universality of species of *Aspergillus.* Direct examination of sputum should show branching hyphal filaments in a characteristic Y shape, and fungal balls may show the conidia still attached to the conidiophore (Fig. 35-17). *A fumigatus,* the most common pathogen, is somewhat thermophilic and will grow readily at 45°C.

Certain types of infections caused by members of the genus *Aspergillus* may remain chronic for years, but invasive aspergillosis normally is fatal if untreated. Prednisone has proved of value for the treatment of allergic bronchopulmonary aspergillosis, but pulmonary cavities filled with mycelia frequently must be removed surgically. Amphotericin B seems to be the most effective chemotherapeutic agent for disseminated infections.

Zygomycosis

Zygomycosis (formerly called phycomycosis or mucormycosis) is caused by members of the class Zygomycetes and occurs in diseased and debilitated patients. Human disease is most frequently caused by species of *Rhizopus,* but the genera *Mucor, Absidia,* and others are also involved.

As a result of the usually poor physical condition of the patient, infection with these agents frequently is a fulminating and fatal disease. The form that the disease takes depends on the condition of the patient, but infec-

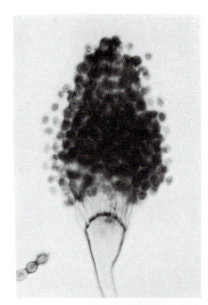

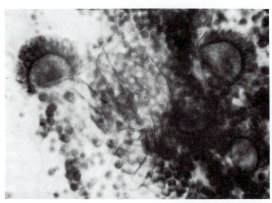

FIGURE 35-17   Conidiophores of *Aspergillus fumigatus.*

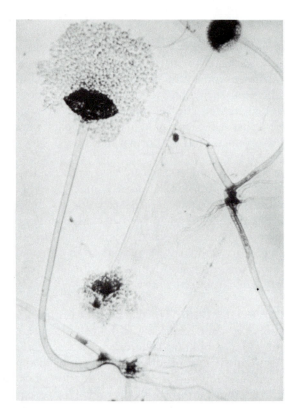

FIGURE 35-18   Two ruptured and one intact sporangia and nonseptate hyphae are shown in this micrograph of *Rhizopus arrhizus.*

tion frequently involves the rhinocerebral area, lungs, central nervous system, and viscera. Infections are associated particularly with diabetes when a ketoacidotic episode has recently occurred.

The organism is easily visualized in infected tissues, because it extends through contiguous cells and blood vessels. Identification of the fungi can be done by staining with hematoxylin-eosin and observing the large, nonseptate hyphae (Fig. 35-18).

Mortality is usually high, because the infection spreads rapidly, the diagnosis can be difficult to make, and there may be poor drug penetration to areas of necrosis. However, amphotericin B, often in conjunction with radical surgical excision, has been used to treat the disease with some success.

Mycotoxicosis

Mycotoxicosis is any disease that is induced by the consumption of food that has been made toxic by fungal toxins. These toxins, called *mycotoxins*, are found in a wide variety of foodstuffs consumed by humans and animals, and in all likelihood the diseases resulting from the ingestion of mycotoxin-contaminated food are sometimes more serious than are the fungal infections discussed earlier in this chapter. Table 35-3 shows a partial list of known mycotoxins; any detailed discussion of the chemical structure and the biologic action of mycotoxins is beyond the scope of this text. Nevertheless, a few highlights deserve mention.

AFLATOXIN

The discovery of aflatoxin in 1961 occurred as a result of a fatal disease in turkeys, which was tentatively named *turkey X* disease. Autopsies of afflicted turkeys revealed severe liver necrosis resembling alkaloid poisoning. Examination of turkey feed failed to show alkaloids but did show the toxic material in a Brazilian groundnut meal in the feed. Subsequent studies reported that ingestion of the meal for a few days caused liver necrosis in ducklings and liver cancer in rats and trout. In 1961, it was found that the toxic material in the groundnut meal was produced by the saprophytic mold *A flavus,* and for that reason, the toxin was named aflatoxin. Research in the following decade led to the isolation and chemical characterization of a family of 16 different aflatoxins.

Biologic Effects of Aflatoxins

The ability of aflatoxins to cause liver damage has been demonstrated in many mammals, fish, and birds, and

TABLE 35-3
Partial List of Mycotoxins and Mycotoxin-Producing Fungi

Mycotoxin	Mycotoxin-Producing Fungi
Aflatoxin	*A flavus, A parsiticus,* etc
Ascladiol	*A clavatus*
Butenolide	*F tricinctum, F nivale, F equiseti*
Citreoviridin	*P citreoviride, P ochrosalmoneum*
Citrinin	*P citrinum, P implicatum, P citreoviride, A terreus,* etc
Cyclopiazonic acid	*P cyclopium*
Ergot alkaloid	*Claviceps* sp
Fumigatin	*A fumigatus*
Chlorine-containing peptide	*P islandicum*
Luteoskyrin	*P islandicum, Mycelia sterilia*
Maltoryzine	*A oryzae* var *microsporus*
Muscarine, etc.	*Amanita muscaria,* etc
Ochratoxin A	*A ochraceus*
Patulin	*P urticae, A clavatus, P claviforme, P expansum, A giganteus,* etc
Penicillic acid	*P puberulum, P cyclopium, P thomii,* etc
Phalloidine	*Amanita phalloides*
Psilocybine	*Psilocybe* sp
Psoralens	*Sclerotinia sclerotiorum*
Rubratoxin B	*P rubrum, P purpurogenum*
Regulosin	*P rugulosum, P brunneum, P tardum, P variabile,* etc
Scirpenols (nivalenol, fusarenon)	*F nivale, F tricinctum*
Sporidesmolides	*Pithomyces chartarum*
Sterigmatocystin	*A versicolor, A flavus* (O-methyl-)
Xanthocillin X	*A chevalieri*

A, Aspergillis; F, Fusarium; P, Penicillium.

initiation of liver carcinoma by aflatoxin is known to occur in ducklings, trout, rats, and ferrets. Evidence of the role of aflatoxins in human disease is mostly circumstantial, but the fact that many foods consumed by humans are contaminated with *A flavus* is cause for grave concern. Peanuts and peanut butter are one of the main sources of aflatoxins for humans, but these toxins also have been found in rice, cereal grains, beans, dried sweet potatoes, African beers, and cow's milk. The fact that half of all cancers occurring in Africa south of the Sahara are liver tumors may be correlated with a report that 40% of the foods screened in Uganda contained measurable quantities of aflatoxin. The considerably higher incidence of childhood liver cirrhosis in tropical countries (where the warm, moist climate provides ideal conditions for the growth of *A flavus*) also can be correlated with the presence of aflatoxins in foods such as breast milk. Moreover, of 50 urine samples taken from children with liver cirrhosis, 18 were shown by thin-layer chromatography to contain aflatoxins.

The data linking aflatoxins with human liver disease are still circumstantial, but the fact that these toxins produce liver damage in essentially all experimental animals certainly makes them highly suspect. A report has shown that 50% of hepatocellular carcinomas from southern Africa had a specific mutation in an anti-oncogene designated p53. Almost all of these were G-to-T substitutions, suggesting exposure to a specific carcinogen. The primary suspect in these cases is *aflatoxin B$_1$*, a common food contaminant in Africa that is both a mutagen that induces G to T substitutions and a liver-specific carcinogen.

OCHRATOXINS

Two mycotoxins, ochratoxin A and B, are produced by *Aspergillus ochraceus*. These toxins occur in corn, grains, peanuts, Brazil nuts, fermented fish, and cottonseed meal, as well as in many other human and animal foods.

In ducklings, the LD$_{50}$ (the amount that comprises a lethal dose for 50% of the test animals) for ochratoxin A is 25 μg, whereas that for ochratoxin B is about 150 μg. Both mycotoxins produce liver necrosis, but neither seems to be carcinogenic. There is no proven evidence that the ochratoxins contribute to human disease, but their hepatotoxic (toxic to the liver) properties in other animals and their widespread occurrence in moldy food products make it likely that they are involved in human disease.

MISCELLANEOUS MYCOTOXINS

A number of mycotoxin-producing species of *Penicillium* are often are found on moldy rice. Two mycotoxins, luteoskyrin and cyclochlorotine, have been isolated as metabolites of *Penicillium islandicum*. In experimental animals, both toxins produce severe liver damage, varying from cirrhosis to liver carcinoma.

Some mycotoxins produce effects other than liver damage. The injection of crude extracts from moldy rice on which *Penicillium toxicarum* is growing causes paralysis, blindness, and death in experimental animals. Animals fed corn infected with *Penicillium rubrum* showed intense inflammation of the stomach, the large and small intestines, and the liver. Another mycotoxin (produced by the mold *Fusarium graminearum*) is an estrogen. Female animals ingesting food contaminated with this mold experience a severe inflammation of the vulva and vagina, an increase in size of the uterus, and growth and lactation of the mammary glands. The effect in young male animals is a feminizing one, with atrophy of the testes and an enlargement of the mammary glands.

There are many other mycotoxins, but the last one discussed here causes a disease known as alimentary toxic aleukia (ATA). This disease has occurred in the Soviet Union, including Siberia, in endemic forms. The symptoms of ATA include fever, bleeding from the nose, throat, and gums, a hemorrhage rash, and a marked reduction in the number of circulating leukocytes. The mortality rate may be as high as 60%, and frequently whole

A Closer Look

During the last decade, considerable data have accumulated showing that cancer cells have mutations in genes that regulate cell growth. Such mutations can be categorized into two distinct types: (1) those which result in an alteration or increased synthesis of an oncogene product, and (2) those having mutations in tumor-suppressor genes. In the former case, one has gained a function that signals the cell to divide, and in the latter case, one has lost a function that controls cell growth.

A number of tumor-suppressor genes have been described, and a mutation in a gene known as p53 is the single most common gene change seen in human cancer. This change has been documented in 70% of colon cancers, 30% to 50% of breast cancers, 50% of lung cancers, and 100% of small cell lung cancers.

The general mechanisms whereby a tumor-suppressor gene functions to prevent uncontrolled growth are obscure, but information concerning the p53 gene product has provided some interesting possibilities. These data suggest that the p53 gene product functions only in response to DNA damage in a normal cell. In such cases, the p53 protein binds to specific DNA sequences, blocking the progression of the cell through the cell cycle late in the G_1 phase of replication. This provides time to repair the DNA or to allow the cell to die by apoptosis.

Various point mutations in p53 result in a gene product that is unable to bind to the specific DNA sequences. In such cases, the damaged cell may die, or it may accumulate mutations and chromosomal rearrangements at an increased rate, leading to the selection of a malignant clone. This is precisely what is being seen in cases of human hepatocellular carcinoma (HCC), and good circumstantial data implicate an aflatoxin as the inducer of these p53 mutations.

As described in the section on mycotoxins, HCC is a prevalent cancer in sub-Saharan Africa, and it has been shown that these HCC cells have a high frequency of p53 mutations. Moreover, almost all cases of African HCC are characterized by a G-to-T substitution at codon 249 of the p53 gene, whereas non-African carcinomas showed a range of p53 mutations that were scattered between codons 132 and 309. This suggests a single cause for the genesis of African HCC.

Aflatoxins are known to induce HCC in animals and, because of their prevalence in sub-Saharan Africa, they have been suspect in such human malignancies. It has been shown that aflatoxin B_1 will bind to G + C–rich regions of DNA, inducing almost exclusively a G-to-T substitution. Sequence data of the p53 gene show that codon 249 lies in such a G + C–rich region. This certainly supports the proposal that an aflatoxin B_1-induced mutation at codon 249 of the p53 gene is responsible for the induction of HCC. Experiments with susceptible animals should provide data that will support this hypothesis.

---

families and villages have been affected. The etiology of ATA is that of a mycotoxicosis caused by eating grains that have overwintered under snow. The disease was particularly severe during the 1940s when famine forced many persons to collect and eat such overwintered grain. There are several genera of fungi implicated in the production of this particular mycotoxin, of which *Fusarium* and *Cladosporium* are observed most frequently. Like all other mycotoxicoses, prevention is accomplished only through education.

Bibliography

JOURNALS

Brummer E, Castaneda E, Restrepo A. Paracoccidioidomycosis: an update. Clin Microbiol Rev 1993;6:89.

Como JA, Dismukes WE. Oral azole drugs as systemic antifungal therapy. N Engl J Med 1994;330:263.

Einstein HE, Johnson RH. State-of-the art clinical article. Coccidioidomycosis: new aspects of epidemiology and therapy. Clin Infect Dis 1993;16:349.

Hsu IC, et al. Mutational hotspot in the p53 gene in human hepatocellular carcinomas. Nature 1991;350:427.

Jones JM. Laboratory diagnosis of invasive candidiasis. Clin Microbiol Rev 1990;3:32.

Meyer KC, et al. Overwhelming pulmonary blastomycosis associated with the adult respiratory distress syndrome. N Engl J Med 1993;329:1231.

BOOKS

Rippon JW. Medical mycology: the pathogenic fungi and the pathogenic actinomycetes, ed 3. Philadelphia, WB Saunders, 1988.

Webster J. Introduction to the fungi, ed 2. Cambridge, Cambridge University Press, 1980.

Essentials of Medical Microbiology, Fifth Edition, edited by Wesley A. Volk, Bryan M. Gebhardt, Marie-Louise Hammarskjöld, and Robert J. Kadner. Lippincott-Raven Publishers, Philadelphia © 1996.

Chapter 36

Diagnostic Bacteriology

The most important aspects of diagnostic bacteriology are (1) the collection of an adequate amount of the correct specimen, and (2) communication between the physician and the microbiologist, outlining the clinical diagnosis and suggesting any unusual organisms that could be the causative agent of the disease in question. Provided with a specimen and the clinical evaluation of the disease, it is the job of the microbiologist to isolate the etiologic agent of the disease, supply a profile of antibiotic susceptibilities to the physician, and identify the organism as quickly as possible. However, even after the isolation and identification of organisms present in a laboratory specimen, it is not always possible to determine whether such organisms are the etiologic agents of the disease in question or merely contaminants from the normal flora. As shown in Table 36-1, many organisms that can be present without causing disease or symptoms of any kind also can produce serious infections under special conditions.

It is not always clear why an organism sometimes causes disease and sometimes does not. It is known that organisms of the genera *Fusobacterium* and *Bacteroides* rarely cause disease when confined to their normal habitat in the large intestine, but cause severe abscesses when introduced into wounds. In this chapter, little is said in regard to this question beyond acknowledging its existence. Rather, this section is designed to furnish a brief outline of the steps involved in the isolation and identification of the organisms causing bacterial infections.

Collection and Culturing of Specimens

The collection of an adequate specimen is useless if the time between collection and culturing allows the disease-producing organism to die or to be overgrown by normal flora that may contaminate or normally be present in the specimen. It is of utmost importance that specimens be transported quickly to the diagnostic laboratory, where they can be processed promptly to ensure the best possible chance of growth, isolation, and identification of the dis-

TABLE 36-1
Bacteria Frequently Present as Normal Flora, Occasionally Causing Overt Disease

Organisms	Usual Locale	Infectious Disease Process
Staphylococcus aureus	Nose, skin	In all areas of the body; nosocomial diseases, food poisoning
Staphylococcus epidermidis	Skin, nose, vagina	Endocarditis, nosocomial phlebitis, acne
Enterococci	Feces	Blood, wounds, urinary tract; endocarditis
Viridans streptococci	Saliva	Endocarditis
Peptostreptococcus sp	Mouth, feces, vagina	Abscess formation, gangrene
Neisseria sp	Throat, mouth, nose	Meningitis
Veillonella sp	Mouth, vagina	Bacterial endocarditis, abscesses
Lactobacillus sp	Mouth, feces, vagina	Bacterial endocarditis (rare), lung abscess (1 report)
Corynebacterium sp	Nasopharynx, skin, vagina	Bacterial endocarditis
Mycobacterium (not *Mycobacterium tuberculosis*)	Prepuce, clitoris, lung, feces, tonsils, food, skin	Suspected in some infectious disease processes
Clostridium sp	Feces, skin, environment, including food, vagina	Clostridial myositis, cellulitis, food poisoning
Enterobacteriaceae	Feces, vagina, mouth, urethra	Urinary tract, wounds, pneumonia, nosocomial enteritis, abscesses, meningitis, blood, peritonitis, abscesses, etc.
Moraxella sp	Nose, genitourinary tract	Conjunctivitis, etc.
Achromobacter sp	Nose, genitourinary tract, skin	Meningitis, blood, urethritis, burns
Pseudomonas sp	Feces, skin	Blood, burns, wounds, urinary tract, respiratory tract, meningitis
Alcaligenes faecalis	Feces	Blood, urinary tract, conjunctiva, respiratory tract, meningitis
Haemophilus sp	Nasopharynx, conjunctiva, vagina	Laryngotracheobronchitis, meningitis, pyarthrosis, conjunctivitis, genitourinary tract
Fusobacterium sp	Mouth, saliva, feces	Infected human bites, gangrene
Bacteroides sp	Feces, mouth, throat	Bacterial endocarditis, abscesses, mixed infections

ease-producing organism. In some situations, it is recommended that the growth medium be inoculated immediately after obtaining the specimen from the patient, and that the inoculated medium then be taken to the laboratory to be incubated and the bacteria identified. In other cases, material can be protected in a buffered transport medium and then transported to the laboratory to be grown. In all cases, quick processing of specimens aids in providing the fastest and most reliable identification of the disease-producing organism.

BLOOD

Bacteremia—bacteria in the blood—frequently is accompanied by the onset of chills and fever, an increase in pulse rate, and a drop in blood pressure. Even in infections in which bacteremia is a major aspect of the disease, the organisms in the bloodstream are not always constantly present in sufficient numbers to be grown from a single blood specimen. Patients with such infections may have to provide several blood specimens before the causative agent can be isolated. When an intermittent bacteremia is suspected, it is routine to obtain three 10- to 20-mL blood samples over a 24-hour period to maximize chances for isolation of the organism.

Collection of a Blood Specimen

In taking a blood specimen for culture, one should be aware that although blood is normally sterile, the skin that must be penetrated is not sterile. Routinely, the skin should be cleansed first with 70% to 95% alcohol to remove dirt, lipids, and fatty acids. The site then should be scrubbed with a circular, concentric motion (working out from the starting point) using a sterile gauze pad soaked in an iodophor. The iodine should be allowed to remain on the skin for at least 1 minute before it is removed by wiping with a sterile gauze pad soaked with 70% to 95% alcohol. It must be emphasized, however, that all this will be useless if the person drawing the blood palpates the vein after the cleaning process, thereby contaminating the very site that had been cleaned.

After cleansing the penetration site, the blood can be withdrawn using either a sterile needle and syringe or a commercially available, evacuated blood-collection tube.

Media Inoculated With Blood Specimens

Blood always should be inoculated into the appropriate medium at the bedside. Partially evacuated, commercially available, blood-culture bottles, which contain 30 to 100 mL of a rich, liquid medium such as brain–heart infusion or trypticase soy broth, are routinely used.

If possible, 10 to 20 mL of blood should be taken from the patient and inoculated into an approximately 10-fold excess of the blood-culture medium. When possible, two such bottles should be inoculated. One is vented to permit the growth of aerobic bacteria (by inserting a sterile, cotton-plugged needle through the rubber stopper until the bottle has filled with air), and the other is not vented to allow the growth of anaerobic organisms. Special media for aerobic and anaerobic culture are available. Some commercially available bottles are provided with a venipuncture set, which allows the blood to be injected into the medium.

Identification of Blood Isolates

Blood cultures are incubated at 36°C and observed daily for at least 1 week for evidence of turbidity or hemolysis. Gram's stains, streak plates, and antibiotic susceptibility tests should be carried out as quickly as possible after the observation of visible growth in the original broth culture. In the absence of obvious growth in 1 or 2 days, blind subcultures on chocolate blood-agar plates may speed the appearance of obligately aerobic organisms. Commercially available penicillinase can be added to blood cultures from patients who have received penicillin therapy. Penicillinase preparations should be checked for sterility to eliminate them as a potential source of contamination. Resins incorporated in special blood-culture media can neutralize a broad spectrum of antibiotics.

Once a Gram's stain has rendered some information concerning the type of organism involved, special supplementary or differential media should be inoculated. *MacConkey* or *eosin–methylene blue* plates should be streaked if gram-negative rods are present, and prereduced media should be inoculated if obligate anaerobes such as *Bacteroides* or *Fusobacterium* are suspected. Table 36-2 lists a few of the more common organisms that could be isolated from blood, with their colonial appearances on certain specialized media.

The finding of organisms that constitute the normal flora or are frequent inhabitants of the skin (eg, diphtheroids, *Staphylococcus epidermidis*, *Bacillus* sp) usually is viewed with suspicion, unless the frequency of isolation or the clinical setting indicates they did not arrive as contamination during the collection of the blood.

RESPIRATORY TRACT AND MOUTH

Because of the myriad normal resident flora in the upper respiratory tract, the isolation of lower respiratory tract infectious agents can be difficult and confusing. This is complicated further by the occasional presence of small numbers of potential pathogens such as pneumococci, meningococci, streptococci, *Staphylococcus aureus*, *Haemophilus influenzae,* or enteric organisms that are indigenous to the upper respiratory tract.

Specimen Collection From the Respiratory Tract

The microbiologist must be certain that lower respiratory tract specimens represent sputum that has been brought up by a deep cough. However, it may not be possible to obtain a good sputum sample from a young child, a debilitated older person, or someone who is comatose. In such situations, other procedures must be carried out to obtain a specimen from the lower respiratory tract. One technique is transtracheal aspiration, which, as shown diagrammatically in Figure 36-1, uses a needle and tube inserted into the trachea. This technique also overcomes the problem of contamination from the oro-

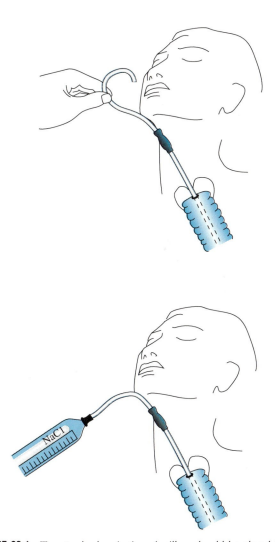

FIGURE 36-1 Transtracheal aspiration. A pillow should be placed beneath the neck to permit maximum extension of the neck. After cleansing the skin, a 14-gauge needle is inserted into the trachea, and a polyethylene tube is passed through the needle into the lung. The needle is withdrawn, and the tube is connected to a syringe containing 3 ml to 4 ml of physiologic saline. The saline is injected into the lung and immediately withdrawn for culture.

coccus neoformans, less frequently cause meningitis. Essentially any organism that gains entrance to the fluid surrounding the brain and spinal cord can grow and cause an inflammation of the meninges. Such infections frequently are severe and, unless promptly and adequately treated, can result in the death of the patient in a matter of hours.

Specimen Collection of Cerebrospinal Fluid

Cerebrospinal fluid (CSF) is obtained by a puncture into the lumbar region of the spine. It is of utmost importance that the puncture site be decontaminated in the manner described previously for venipunctures to ensure that no contaminating organisms are mechanically injected into the CSF. The collected specimen should be placed into a sterile screw-cap tube and delivered immediately to the diagnostic laboratory.

Media Inoculated With Cerebrospinal Fluid

A diagnosis of meningitis usually is based on the microbiologic findings in the CSF, chemical determination of the total protein and glucose present in the fluid, and its cellular content. Because the total specimen frequently is only 1 to 2 mL, the sample must suffice for the hematology, chemistry, and microbiologic findings. Therefore, after the cell count, the CSF is routinely centrifuged for 10 minutes at 1200 times gravity; part of the supernatant is used for the chemical assays, and the sediment is the source for the bacteriologic evaluation.

The sediment from the centrifuged sample is inoculated onto one *blood* and one *chocolate blood-agar* plate. Both plates are incubated aerobically under 5% to 10% CO_2 at 35°C, and disks of hematin and NAD are added to allow the growth of *H influenzae*. Another method of providing these required factors is to make a single streak of *S aureus* across the plate. The staphylococci release these factors by lysis of the red blood cells in the agar, and *H influenzae* will be found growing only as satellite colonies adjacent to the growth of the staphylococci. The chocolate-agar plate is incubated under an atmosphere of 10% CO_2. Both nutrient broth and a special broth for the growth of anaerobes should be inoculated with the CSF sediment. All cultures should be inspected daily and, in the event of growth, broth media should be subcultured onto an appropriate agar medium.

Identification of Isolates From Cerebrospinal Fluid

Because meningitis frequently presents an emergency situation, it is imperative that a tentative diagnosis be made as soon as possible. It is mandatory that the sediment from the centrifuged CSF be subjected to Gram's stain and examined microscopically. Because the number of organisms often is small, it is recommended that at least 30 minutes be spent for such an examination. If organisms are seen, additional procedures sometimes can be used to substantiate immediately a tentative identification. The most common of these are to carry out a coagglutination reaction using latex beads with known specific antiserum or to stain with specific, fluorescence-labeled antiserum. Capsular antigens of certain streptococci, *N meningitidis*, and *H influenzae* can be present even in the absence of bacteria on the Gram's smear, and using latex bead agglutination procedures may speed up the diagnosis of meningitis. Spinal fluid from a possible case of tuberculosis meningitis should be stained for acid-fast organisms, and a possible infection by *C neoformans* can be diagnosed tentatively using wet mounts of spinal fluid sediment mixed with India ink or nigrosin to demonstrate the large capsules surrounding the yeast cells. A latex bead test for cryptococci also is available.

An evaluation of a patient's inflammatory response also aids in the diagnosis of a meningeal infection. In general, polymorphonuclear leukocytes predominate in the CSF in acute bacterial infections, whereas meningitis resulting from fungi, leptospira, or *M tuberculosis* is characterized by the presence of lymphocytes.

WOUNDS AND ABSCESSES

Pus and exudate from an infected wound or open abscess would be expected to contain the etiologic agent of the infection. However, in open wounds, skin and soil contaminants almost invariably are found that, under appropriate growth conditions, could outgrow the true infectious organism, resulting in an erroneous laboratory report.

Collection of Specimens From Wounds and Abscesses

Whenever possible, a sterile syringe and needle should be used to collect specimens from wounds and abscesses. The use of a swab is routinely unsatisfactory because of the limited amount of material collected by this method, making it difficult or impossible to isolate the etiologic agent or agents. It also is important to remember that wounds and abscesses are commonly infected with obligately anaerobic bacteria, which quickly die on a swab that is exposed to the atmosphere. Therefore, all aspirates should be transported to the laboratory in special tubes containing oxygen-free gas. Such containers, which can be obtained commercially, usually contain a few drops of 0.0003% resazurin, an oxidation-reduction indicator that turns pink if air contaminates the bottle. Table 36-4 lists some of the more common types of infections in which the obligate anaerobes are involved.

Burns often are infected with opportunists such as *Pseudomonas aeruginosa*, enteric organisms, staphylo-

TABLE 36-4
Infections in Which Anaerobes Are the Predominant Pathogens or Are Commonly Present

Region	Type of Infection
Head and neck	Brain abscess
	Otogenic meningitis, extradural or subdural empyema
	Chronic otitis media
	Dental infection
Pleuropulmonary	Pneumonia secondary to obstructive process
	Aspiration pneumonia
	Lung abscess
	Bronchiectasis
	Thoracic empyema
Intraabdominal	Liver abscess
	Pylephlebitis
	Peritonitis
	Appendicitis
	Subphrenic abscess
	Other intraabdominal abscess
	Wound infection after bowel surgery or trauma
Female genital	Puerperal sepsis
	Postabortal sepsis
	Endometritis
	Tuboovarian abscess
	Other gynecologic infection
Other	Perirectal abscess
	Gas-forming cellulitis
	Gas gangrene
	Breast abscess

cocci, and yeast, making isolation of the definitive infectious agent extremely difficult. Quantitative cultures may assist in the interpretation of laboratory findings. Specimens of burned tissue and any drainage material should be sent to the laboratory for culture and evaluation.

Media Inoculated With Wound and Abscess Specimens

Because the array of organisms that can infect a wound is so great, the choice of inoculation media can be difficult. In general, obligate anaerobes, such as those in the genera *Clostridium, Bacteroides, Eubacterium, Fusobacterium,* and *Actinomyces,* must be considered. Table 36-5 lists a few of the features that suggest the involvement of one of these anaerobes.

Numerous specialized media can be used successfully for the growth of the obligate anaerobes. Most contain whole or lysed blood from sheep, complex infusions such as brain–heart infusion or chopped meat, vitamin supplements such as yeast extract and additional vitamin K, and, in broths, a reducing agent such as thioglycollate or cysteine with 0.1% agar added to reduce convection currents.

Because most wound infections or abscesses contain multiple organisms, the use of liquid media alone is not satisfactory. In fact, if isolated colonies are obtained on agar plates, little is gained by the examination of broth cultures. However, agar plates must be incubated in an anaerobic jar (a jar from which all oxygen has been removed) or a similar device.

Because most infections are caused by mixtures of aerobic and anaerobic bacteria, blood-agar plates as well as selective and differential media (eg, eosin–methylene blue or MacConkey) also must be inoculated and then incubated aerobically at 36°C.

Identification of Wound Isolates

The multiplicity of genera that can be found in a wound makes it difficult to list firm rules for their identification. A Gram's stain of all specimens should be observed first. The results of microscopic examination may provide information that will aid in a decision regarding which media should be inoculated and under what conditions the culture should be incubated. It is no simple affair to differentiate between the true etiologic agents of wounds and abscess infection and the contaminants that "go along for the ride."

FECES

Gastrointestinal illnesses usually are characterized by diarrhea or the presence of blood, mucus, and, in certain cases, white blood cells in voided stools. Many such disturbances are cases of food poisoning resulting from the ingestion of a preformed toxin. Symptoms of such intoxication rarely last beyond 24 hours, and treatment usually is confined to the intravenous replacement of lost fluids and electrolytes.

A bacteriologic examination of food suspected of causing an illness would be more likely to yield informative data concerning the etiology of an intoxication than would an examination of a fecal specimen. For example, a Gram's stain revealing large numbers of straphylococci, together with a history and the clinical symptoms of staphylococcal food poisoning (see Chap. 24), would provide strong circumstantial evidence that the gastroenteritis was due to the ingestion of food contaminated with staphylococcal enterotoxin. A similar situation would be seen in food poisoning due to *Clostridium perfringens* (see Chap. 29). In both cases, the organisms would be present in large numbers in the contaminated food; however, because the staphylococcal enterotoxin is more stable to heat inactivation than are the staphylococi themselves, it would not be unusual to see large numbers of staphylococci in a Gram's stain (ie, of a heated cream soup) and yet not be able to culture significant numbers of organisms from the suspected food. On the other hand, because the *C perfringens* enterotoxin is produced only dur-

TABLE 36-5
Clinical and Bacteriologic Features Suggesting Possible Infection With Anaerobes

Clinical	Bacteriologic
Foul-smelling discharge	Unique morphology on Gram's stain
Location of infection in proximity to a mucosal surface	Failure to grow aerobically; organisms seen on Gram's stain of orig-
Necrotic tissue, gangrene; pseudomembrane formation	inal exudate (failure to obtain growth in fluid thioglycollate me-
Gas in tissues or discharges	dium is not adequate assurance that anaerobes were not present)
Endocarditis with negative routine blood culture results	Growth in anaerobic zone of fluid media or of agar deeps
Infection associated with malignancy or other process producing	Growth anaerobically on media containing 100 µg/mL of kanamy-
tissue destruction	cin, neomycin, or paromomycin (or medium also containing 7.5
Infection related to the use of aminoglycosides (oral, parenteral, or	µg/mL of vancomycin for gram-negative anaerobic bacilli)
topical)	Gas and foul odor in specimen or culture
Septic thrombophlebitis	Characteristic colonies on agar plates anaerobically
Bacteremic features with jaundice	Young colonies of *Bacteroides melaninogenicus* may fluoresce red
Infection after human or other bites	under ultraviolet light
Black discoloration of blood-containing exudates; these exudates	
may fluoresce red under ultraviolet light (*Bacteroides melanino-*	
genicus infections)	
"Sulfur granules" in discharges (actinomycosis)	
Classic clinical features of gas gangrene	

ing sporulation, large numbers of viable organisms might be found in a similar situation. It is likely that many cases of gastroenteritis are of viral origin, and some of these agents are discussed in Unit Five. With these qualifications as a preface, the laboratory diagnosis of gastrointestinal infections that result from the presence of the etiologic agent in the intestinal contents is discussed.

Specimens From Intestinal Contents

In culturing intestinal contents, the choice of material to be taken from the patient is obvious, although best results are obtained when the fecal specimen is collected during the acutge stage of an episode of diarrhea. If a specimen contains blood or mucus, these should be included in material to be sent to the laboratory. When a sterile swab is used instead of a fecal specimen, the swab must be inserted past the anal sphincter and rotated several times before being withdrawn.

It is a common misconception that the microorganisms found in feces are rather hearty and that special precautions to preserve the viability of suspected pathogens are not required. Nothing could be further from the truth! Unless fecal specimens can be taken directly to the laboratory for culturing, they should be refrigerated or placed in a stool preservative containing a buffer that will maintain the pH near neutrality. One such preservative uses about equal parts of sterile glycerol (containing 0.033 M phosphate buffer, pH 7.4) and feces. A pH indicator also can be included to ensure that a drop in pH does not go unnoticed. Failure to use a preservative will result in the death of many of the enteric pathogens, especially the shigellae and, to a lesser extent, the salmo-

nellae. Fecal specimens of 1 to 2 g are adequate for bacteriologic procedures.

Media Inoculated With Intestinal Specimens

As discussed in Chapter 26, the major intestinal flora consists of obligately anaerobic gram-negative rods, including organisms in the genera *Bacteroides, Fusobacterium, Eubacterium,* and *Clostridium.* All these can cause serious abscesses but, with the exception of the enterotoxins from *C perfringens* and *Clostridium difficile,* none of the obligate anaerobes has been implicated in gastrointestinal disease characterized by diarrhea. Therefore, unlike the processing of blood or abscess specimens, it is not usual to culture fecal specimens under anaerobic conditions.

When species of either *Salmonella* or *Shigella* are the possible pathogens, it is advisable to inoculate an enrichment medium that will selectively permit the growth of these organisms over that of the normal gram-negative flora. Many such media are available, and it is probable that some diagnostic laboratories use various modifications of these media. Two of the more common enrichment media are a *tetrathionate* and a *selenite F* medium, both of which are commercially available. After incubation of the inoculated enrichment medium for 12 to 16 hours at 35°C to 37°C, it should be streaked on standard, differential media such as *MacConkey* or *eosin–methylene blue* and *deoxycholate* agar plates. *Hektoen* enteric or *xylose-lysine-deoxycholate* plates also can be used. Many other differential and selective media are available that can be used for the isolation of the pathogenic Enterobacteriaceae, and it is likely that diagnostic laboratories vary somewhat in their preference of one medium over another.

In cases of suspected cholera, fecal specimens or rectal swabs should be plated directly on nonselective media such as taurocholate gelatin agar and on nutrient agar. In addition, selective agar plates containing thiosulfate citrate bile salts or tellurite taurocholate gelatin should be heavily streaked. Because *Vibrio cholerae* will grow at a more alkaline pH than most enteric organisms, an enrichment peptone broth, pH 8.5, should be inoculated. All enrichment cultures should be streaked on nonselective media after 8 to 18 hours of incubation at 35°C.

Vibrio parahaemolyticus, a major source of food poisoning acquired from eating undercooked seafood, is a halophilic (salt-loving) organism that can be enriched by growth in a medium containing excess NaCl. Thus, the inoculation of a fecal specimen into a 1% peptone broth (pH 7.1) containing 3% NaCl greatly increases the chances of isolation of this organism. The enrichment broth then can be streaked on any of several nonselective agar plates (such as described for *V cholerae*) for final isolation.

In addition to staphylococcal food poisoning resulting from the ingestion of preformed enterotoxin, *S aureus* on rare occasions causes an ulcerative enteritis as a consequence of the actual invasion of the bowel wall. In such cases, blood or mucus present in the stool should be plated on a blood-agar medium and a selective medium such as mannitol salt agar.

Identification of Fecal Isolates

Because of the large numbers of facultative, gram-negative rods that make up the normal intestinal flora, the isolation and identification of the morphologically similar shigellae and salmonellae requires the use of selective and differential media as well as considerable experience in working with these organisms. Table 36-6 lists a few of the enteric organisms for some of the media commonly used to culture these organisms.

As outlined in Chapter 26, numerous kits are available for use in identifying members of the Enterobacteriaceae. One widely used kit, termed the *API 20E,* consists of a plastic strip containing wells of dehydrated media and appropriate indicators. The wells are inoculated with a suspension of the unknown organisms and, after 24 hours, a numerical value is assigned to each positive reaction. Using the sum of these values, a complete identification can be made from tables that accompany the kit.

The identification of staphylococci from a fecal specimen is a moderately easy task if the laboratory has been instructed that the clinical symptoms are compatible with those of a staphylococcal enteritis. Large colonies on selective sheep blood-agar plates showing β-hemolysis and grape-like clusters of gram-positive cocci should be tested

additionally for coagulase production and, if specific antiserum is available, for the production of enterotoxin.

Intestinal infections by yeast, such as species of *Candida,* or any of the many parasitic protozoa or worms are diagnosed by the direct microscopic examination of a fecal specimen. Additional details concerning these agents are discussed in Chapter 35 and in Unit Six.

URINE

Most urinary tract infections are initiated by organisms that gain entrance to the bladder by ascending through the urethra, and they are more common in women than in men. In men, however, a chronic infection of the prostate gland also can be the source of a bladder infection (cystitis) or a kidney infection (pyelonephritis). In both sexes, most urinary tract infections are caused by normal flora enteric organisms, among which can be species of *Escherichia, Klebsiella, Enterobacter, Proteus, Pseudomonas,* and *Enterococcus.*

Collection of Urine Specimens

Urethral catheterization can yield samples with minimal contamination, but the danger of introducing organisms from the urethra into the bladder provides some risk to this procedure. Moreover, microbial flora in the urethra, particularly in men, can contaminate the specimen, leading the microbiologist to an erroneous conclusion. Therefore, catheterization is not performed routinely for the collection of urine samples. Instead, voided samples are obtained after careful cleansing of the external genitalia. However, the following considerations must be adhered to strictly if bacteriologic reports on voided urine samples are to be meaningful.

First, all voided urine samples will contain some bacteria; therefore, a quantitative assay for the number of bacteria present must be carried out. Second, this number will be grossly misleading unless the exterior genitalia are carefully cleaned to remove contaminating bacteria from the female vulva and perineal area and from the male urethral meatus. The patient must be carefully instructed in how to wash these areas with soap and water, then rinse them thoroughly to remove any residual soap. Women must be instructed to keep the labia continuously apart during the washing, rinsing, and voiding of urine. Urine from either sex should be collected in a sterile cup only after the first 20 to 25 mL has been voided, because the flushing action of the initial flow will remove many of the organisms present in the urethra.

On rare occasions, it is necessary to collect the urine directly from the bladder with a needle and syringe. This procedure is done by a puncture of the abdominal wall directly into the bladder. In other cases, a urine sample is required from a patient who has an indwelling catheter in place. In such situations, the urine should be collected with a needle and syringe directly from the catheter tubing

TABLE 36-6
Growth Characteristics on Some Commonly Used Agar Media of Bacteria Frequently Isolated From Feces

Organism	Eosin Methylene Blue Agar	MacConkey Agar	Hektoen Enteric Agar	Salmonella-Shigella Agar	Bismuth Sulfite Agar	Xylose-Lysine-Deoxycholate Agar	Selective Enterococcus Agar
Arizona	Translucent, colorless	Uncolored, transparent; red (LF)	Similar to Salmonella	Black centered, clear periphery	Black; green-brown (LF)	Black-centered red colonies	Inhibited
Citrobacter	Translucent colonies, greenish metallic sheen (LF)	Uncolored, transparent; red (LF)	Usually inhibited; when present, colonies are small and bluish green	Similar to Arizona	Black; green-brown	Opaque, yellow	Inhibited
Enterobacter, Serratia	Metallic sheen, similar to E coli but somewhat larger	Red-pink	Green centers with yellow to brown periphery	White or cream colored, opaque, mucoid	Raised mucoid colonies, silvery sheen	Opaque, yellow	Inhibited
Escherichia coli (rapid lactose fermenters)	Dark center; greenish metallic sheen	Red or pink; may be surrounded by a zone of precipitated bile	Moderately inhibited; orange to salmon-pink	Red to pink; colorless with a pink center	Mostly inhibited; black-brown, greenish surface; no metallic sheen	Opaque, yellow	Inhibited
Klebsiella	Larger than E coli. mucoid, brownish, tend to coalesce, often convex	Pink, mucoid	Yellow centers, periphery orange	Red to pink; colorless with a pink center	Mostly inhibited	Opaque, yellow	Inhibited
Proteus	Translucent, colorless	Uncolored, transparent	Most strains are inhibited; dark centered, greenish (H$_2$S producers), similar to Salmonella	Black centered, clear periphery	Green; black (H$_2$S producers); mostly inhibited	Opaque, yellow (P mirabilis, P vulgaris), red (P rettgeri, P morganii)	Small gray colonies (few)
Pseudomonas	Translucent, colorless amber	Uncolored, transparent	Most strains are inhibited; colonies are small, flat, and green to brown	Mostly inhibited; transparent colorless colonies	Inhibited	Sometimes red colonies	Inhibited
Salmonella	Translucent, amber colonies; colorless	Uncolored, transparent	Blue to blue-green; most colonies have black centers (H$_2$S producers)	Opaque; transparent; uncolored; black centered, clear periphery	S typhi black with sheen or dotted black or greenish-gray; other Salmonella are black or green	Black-centered red (H$_2$S producers); red color (no H$_2$S)	Inhibited
Shigella	Translucent, amber colonies; colorless	Uncolored, transparent	Blue to blue-green; periphery of colonies lighter than center portion	Opaque, transparent	Mostly inhibited; S flexneri and S sonnei are brown, raised and crater-like	Red	Inhibited

LF, lactose fermenter.

504

and never from the drainage bag, because considerable bacterial growth may have occurred in the urine receptacle.

Media Inoculated With Urine Specimens

All voided urine samples, as well as most samples collected by catheterization, contain some bacteria, so the clinical diagnosis of an infection is based on the numbers of bacteria in the urine. Considerable experimental data have resulted in the formulation of the following rules: (1) 10^5 bacteria or more per milliliter from a clean, voided specimen indicates a urinary tract infection; (2) a value of 10^3 to 10^4 bacteria per milliliter in a symptomatic patient requires a second culture; and (3) 10^3 or fewer bacteria per milliliter usually is not considered significant in a voided sample. Single samples cannot be considered to be 100% accurate, and it frequently is advisable that duplicate samples collected at different times be sent to the diagnostic laboratory.

Because of the need to measure the bacteria present in a sample of urine, several different techniques have been devised to accomplish a rapid enumeration.

A standard platinum dilution loop (commercially available) holds about 0.001 mL of liquid. Such a loop can be used to streak a urine specimen directly onto a nutrient-agar plate. If the loop is calibrated monthly and compared with counts obtained by the pour-plate method, the overall accuracy of the calibrated-loop technique is equivalent to that of a pour plate.

A variety of screening kits are commercially available for suspected urinary tract infections. One, called a paddle or dip-slide type, has a selective agar medium coated on one side and a nonselective agar medium on the other side. The paddle is dipped into the urine specimen, reinserted into its sterile container, and incubated at 35°C

for 18 to 24 hours before counting the colonies (Fig. 36-2). The amount of urine adhering to a paddle has been determined experimentally by the manufacturer, and this kit is reported to be about 95% as accurate as the pour-plate procedure. Other kits also are available, and it is likely that each laboratory has its preferred method for enumerating the microorganisms present in a urine specimen.

Identification of Urine Isolates

If a speedy result is required, a Gram's stain of the uncentrifuged urine specimen can be examined, primarily because if one drop is allowed to dry on a slide without spreading, the appearance of one or more bacteria per oil-immersion field (sometimes with leukocytes present) is indicative of a total bacterial count greater than 10^5 organisms per milliliter of urine.

Blood-agar plates, as well as MacConkey and eosin–methylene blue plates, should be streaked with the urine specimen. Because members of the Enterobacteriaceae are, by far, the most frequent causes of urinary tract infections, final identification of the organism is accomplished as outlined in Chapter 26.

Serologic Techniques

The measurement of antibodies arising in response to an infectious agent can aid in the diagnosis of some infections. In the case of syphilis, for example, a diagnosis usually depends on demonstrating the presence of antibodies that were formed in response to the infection. These tests are discussed in detail in Chapter 32.

Examples of other diseases for which the patient's

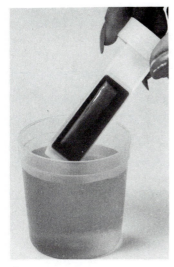

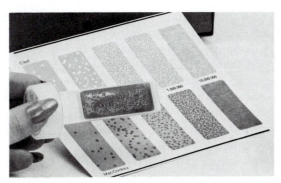

FIGURE 36-2 Uricult provides one method for screening urine samples. **A.** An agar-coated paddle is dipped in the urine sample. **B.** After incubation, the colony count may be quickly (and roughly) determined by comparison of growth on the paddle with a chart for the appropriate type of agar medium.

A

B

antibody response can be used as an aid in making a diagnosis include typhoid fever, brucellosis, and tularemia. In these cases, antibody is measured by determining the agglutination titer of the patient's serum against the known organisms. However, such tests are not a substitute for the isolation and identification of the etiologic agent, and should be used only to support culture techniques or to provide a retrospective diagnosis when attempts to isolate the disease-producing agent have failed. Moreover, the mere presence of specific antibodies cannot be used to support a serologic diagnosis for a disease, because such information does not indicate when the antibody formation occurred. It is necessary to show that a rise in antibody titer occurred during the course of the illness. This is accomplished by using paired sera, an acute-phase serum taken early in the illness and a convalescent-phase serum taken 2 weeks later. The usual rule of thumb is that for data to be significant, there should be at least a four-fold rise in antibody titer in these paired sera.

For some diseases, such as leptospirosis, mycoplasma pneumonia, and rickettsial infections, it sometimes can be arduous to isolate or visualize the causative agent, and an increase in antibody may provide the only information for a diagnosis. Other diseases, such as the late sequelae that can follow a group A streptococcal infection (eg, rheumatic fever or acute glomerulonephritis), occur after recovery from the bacterial infection, and the causative organisms are no longer present. In these cases, the occurrence of a recent streptococcal infection can be established only by showing the presence of antibodies to a group A streptococcal antigen such as streptolysin O (see Laboratory Diagnosis of Group A Streptococcal Infections, Chap. 24).

FLUORESCEIN-LABELED ANTIBODY

Fluorescein-labeled antibodies are used in a procedure for rapidly determining the presence of specific antigens or antibodies to a known antigen. As illustrated in Figure 36-3, the indirect method can be used to detect the presence of antibodies to any bacterium. All that is required is known bacteria, the patient's serum, and some fluorescein-labeled antihuman γ-globulin.

The direct method, also illustrated in Figure 36-3, can be used to confirm a tentative identification of an isolated organism. In this case, however, the microbiologist is limited by the availability of fluorescein-labeled specific antibody to the bacterium in question.

The commercial availability of many different monoclonal antibodies has facilitated the rapid identification of many bacteria and viruses. Such antibodies can be selected to provide a much higher specificity than can be obtained with a heterologous population of antibodies. Monoclonal antibodies can be linked to fluorescent dyes and used to detect microorganisms in tissues and infected cell cultures.

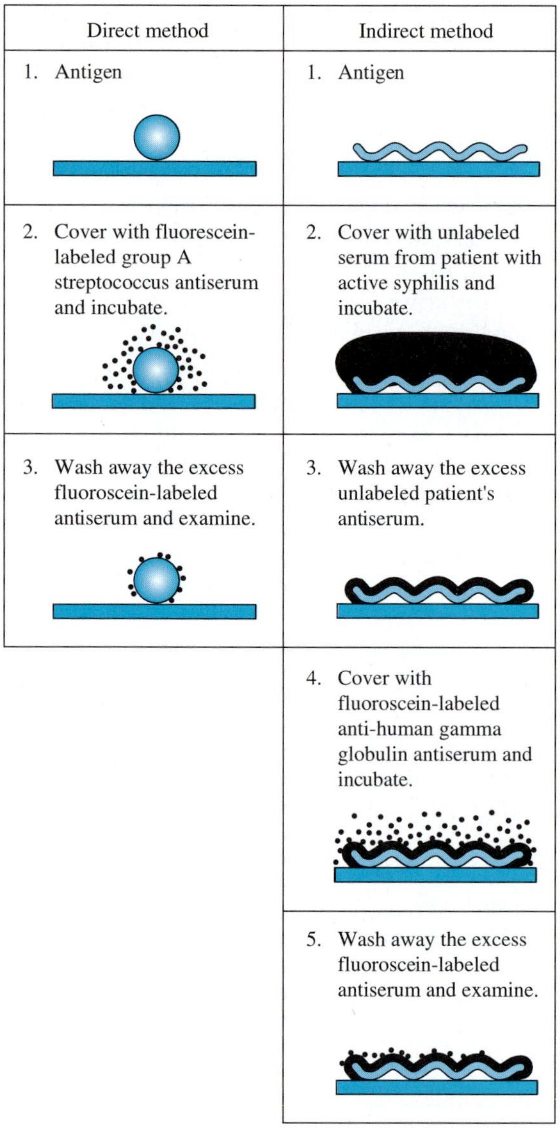

Direct method	Indirect method
1. Antigen	1. Antigen
2. Cover with fluorescein-labeled group A streptococcus antiserum and incubate.	2. Cover with unlabeled serum from patient with active syphilis and incubate.
3. Wash away the excess fluoroscein-labeled antiserum and examine.	3. Wash away the excess unlabeled patient's antiserum.
	4. Cover with fluorescein-labeled anti-human gamma globulin antiserum and incubate.
	5. Wash away the excess fluoroscein-labeled antiserum and examine.

FIGURE 36-3 Fluorescein-labeled antibody test methods. Note that one must have fluorescein-labeled antibody that is specific for the organism in question in order to use the direct method; however, the indirect method can be adapted to any organism using fluorescein-labeled antihuman gamma globulin as the only labeled antiserum.

ENZYME-LINKED IMMUNOSORBENT ASSAY

Enzyme-linked immunosorbent assay (ELISA) methods are techniques in which an enzyme, such as alkaline phosphatase or horseradish peroxidase, is conjugated to an antispecies immunoglobulin such as antihuman IgG. To carry out an ELISA assay, a specific antigen is used to coat a polystyrene well or tube. Dilutions of an unknown serum are added and allowed to react for about 1 hour. Excess serum then is removed by repeated washing.

To determine whether the unknown serum contained the specific antibody in question, the enzyme-linked antihuman immunoglobulin is added and allowed to bind before thoroughly washing the reaction well. At this point, the enzyme-linked immunoglobulin will still be present only if human antibodies bound to the antigen used to coat the polystyrene well. The appropriate substrate for the enzyme then is added and enzyme activity is measured.

ELISA methods are extremely sensitive and are used for detecting antibodies to a wide variety of viruses, bacteria, and parasites.

COUNTERIMMUNOELECTROPHORESIS

Counterimmunoelectrophoresis is designed to detect specific antigens (see Chap. 6). Clinically, it has been used to detect the presence of capsular material in CSF, blood, or urine. It has now been replaced largely by latex bead agglutination.

Latex Bead Agglutination

Latex beads are small, perfect spheres of uniform size and surfaced properties. Their value for serologic diagnosis resides in the ability of proteins to bind firmly to the polystyrene surface of the particles. Thus, they can be coated readily with either antibodies or antigens, and such sensitized particles can be used in slide agglutination reactions.

Latex beads that have been precoated with specific antibodies are commercially available for use in the detection of hundreds of different antigens. Thus, they can be used to detect the presence of many infectious disease agents (fungi, bacteria, viruses, and parasites) as well as hormones, drugs, immunoglobulins, and many more biologic proteins, such as kangaroo meat that has been used to adulterate beef products. To use such beads, the appropriate coated beads are mixed with a drop of urine, serum, CSF, or other substance; if the specific antigen is present, the beads will form large visible clumps. This procedure can be made quantitative by mixing a dilute suspension of sensitized beads with serial dilutions of the material to be tested. Such immunoassays then are read in a spectrophotometer or nephelometer, or directly on cards or glass plates.

DNA PROBES

A DNA probe consists of a radiolabeled or chromogenically labeled, single-stranded piece of DNA that will bind to DNA that is complementary to the probe using hybridization techniques. *Because all organisms contain some unique sequences of DNA, probes can be designed that are totally specific for any given genus or species of microorganism.* For example, probes can be used to identify *Salmonella, Shigella,* or *Legionella,* or to hybridize with genes encoding toxins such as LT, ST, or cholera toxin. Hybridization is accomplished in tubes or by spotting the un-

known organisms onto a filter (ie, nitrocellulose paper), lysing them to release the DNA, and denaturating in mild alkali. The probe then can be added and, after thorough washing to remove any unbound probe, the tube or spot is examined for evidence of hybridization. Formalin-fixed, paraffin-embedded tissues also can be probed, particularly for viral DNA sequences. However, the most specific procedure is to cleave the nucleic acid from the unknown organism with a restriction enzyme, and then to perform electrophoresis of the hydrolyzed DNA in agarose. The separated fragments then are transferred to nitrocellulose and are hybridized with the labeled DNA probe (Southern hybridization).

DNA probes also can be designed that will bind to RNA, and this procedure has been used specifically to locate ribosomal RNA (rRNA). This can be specific, because rRNA has been highly conserved within a species. It also can be a sensitive technique, because a single cell can contain many thousands of molecules of a particular rRNA.

Nucleic acid probes must be labeled in some manner to ascertain whether hybridization has occurred. The most common procedure is to attach radioactive phosphate groups to the probe. Several nonradioactive labels also are available, most of which involve the attachment of an enzyme to the probe either directly or through the use of a ligand, which binds to the probe. Enzymes used are those that form highly colored products, such as alkaline phosphatase or horseradish peroxidase. Chemiluminescent indicators also have been introduced recently to routine diagnostic work.

MOLECULAR EPIDEMIOLOGY

It frequently is necessary for the epidemiologist to determine whether a single strain of microorganism is responsible for an infectious disease outbreak. For many years, such a question was answered using serologic reactions with known antibodies, antibiotic-resistance profiles, or biochemical analyses of metabolic end products or enzymes. However, during the past decade, many newer procedures have been developed using techniques of molecular epidemiology such as plasmid profiles, genomic fingerprinting, and the polymerase chain reaction.

Plasmid Profiles

Bacteria that have arisen from a single clone also contain identical or very similar plasmids. Such plasmids often encode for antibiotic resistance, as well as for virulence factors such as enterotoxins and adhesins. It is a fairly simple procedure to extract plasmid DNA from several different isolates and determine their migration after separation by agarose-gel electrophoresis. Different isolates then can be compared by examination of the gel for the number and size of the plasmids in each lane of the gel.

What properties does *S mutans* possess that endow it with its cariogenic activity? As previously mentioned, it is extremely aciduric, growing well at a pH range of 4.5 to 5, and it produces large amounts of lactic acid from the fermentation of carbohydrates. However, *S mutans* has one other attribute that is especially important for this function. It produces a cell-wall–bound *glucosyltransferase* that splits sucrose to form glucose and fructose, and it then transfers the glucose to a growing polysaccharide chain to form a large extracellular glucan, as shown below:

$$\text{n sucrose} \xrightarrow{\text{glucosyl transferase}} (\text{glucan})_n + \text{n fructose}$$

The glucan adheres tightly to the surface of the tooth and to the bacterium, bringing viable streptococci into intimate association with the tooth enamel. The fructose is fermented to form lactic acid, resulting in decalcification and decay. Most strains of *S mutans* produce two or more hexosyltransferases that catalyze the synthesis of both cell-associated and soluble glucans and fructans. It seems clear, however, that it is the cell-bound form that is responsible for adherence to the tooth surface.

ROLE OF THE PLAQUE. Normal individuals produce more than 1 L of saliva daily. This saliva acts as a buffer to neutralize the acids formed by the oral bacteria. It appears to exert an effect on plaque acids, inasmuch as the removal of the salivary glands of rodents greatly enhanced caries activity. However, the organisms, polysaccharides, and glycoproteins making up the plaque act as a physical barrier to slow down acid neutralization, permitting some acids formed within the plaque to interact with the tooth enamel.

Therefore, it can be seen that the production of dental caries requires two major events: (1) the formation of a plaque, which brings the organisms into close contact with the tooth enamel and inhibits the buffering action of saliva; and (2) the inclusion of an aciduric organism that can ferment dietary carbohydrates to form one or more organic acids.

PREVENTION OF DENTAL CARIES

Methods for the prevention of dental caries can be grouped into three categories: (1) mechanical removal of the plaque by thorough brushing and flossing; (2) limitation of dietary carbohydrate intake, especially sucrose; and (3) treatment of the teeth with fluoride.

There is little to be added concerning plaque removal. If there is no plaque, there will be no decay. Dietary restrictions, however, are receiving considerable attention. Because sucrose is the only substrate for the glucosyltransferase of *S mutans*, its exclusion from the diet will inhibit the inclusion of *S mutans* in the plaque. After the plaque is formed, however, most dietary carbohydrates will be fermented by the plaque inhabitants to form organic acids. Because completely eliminating sucrose from the diet is difficult for most individuals, particularly in developed countries, the best preventive measures are the mechanical removal of plaque and dietary restrictions to prevent plaque formation.

There are two possible mechanisms whereby fluoride inhibits caries formation. The first is well documented and is the result of the incorporation of the fluoride into the tooth enamel, converting the hydroxyapatite into a fluorapatite. The latter material is considerably more resistant to acid demineralization than is non–fluoride-containing enamel. The second mechanism suggests that the dental plaque itself might accumulate a sufficient amount of fluoride to reach inhibitory levels for the growth of the microorganisms making up the plaque. This is supported by one report that demonstrated that plaques rinsed with dilute fluoride produced considerably less lactic acid from sucrose than did control plaques. Many cities add fluoride to their water supplies, and it also is incorporated into various brands of toothpaste. In addition, dentists frequently apply topical applications of concentrated fluoride solutions.

The immunobiology of dental caries has received considerable attention during the past decade, and numerous attempts have been made to induce an immune response to *S mutans* and its glucosyltransferases. Immunization by a systemic route results in the formation of serum antibodies, but these are of no value for inhibiting the formation of *S mutans*–containing dental plaque. The induction of a secretory IgA response in animals, however, has resulted in a marked reduction in dental caries. Such local immunity has been stimulated by direct injection of *S mutans* into the salivary glands and by feeding cultures of *S mutans*. It also has been reported that immunization of monkeys by the application to the gingival crevices of a 3.8-kilodalton antigen from *S mutans* resulted in a significantly lower incidence of dental caries over that seen in control subjects. It is within the realm of possibility that an effective vaccine for humans will be available some day.

Periodontal Disease

Periodontal disease derives its name from the fact that it is a disease that occurs around (*peri-*) the tooth (*dontal*). Thus, it is an infection that involves the *gingiva* (gums) and the *alveolar bone,* which supports the teeth. Periodontal disease is a slow, chronic, painless infection that affects about 80% of teenagers and adults. It is a mostly preventable disease and is the major cause of tooth loss. Before the role of bacteria as etiologic agents of periodontal disease is discussed, the anatomy and histology of tooth attachment will be examined briefly.

ANATOMY OF THE TEETH AND SURROUNDING TISSUE

A somewhat simplistic view of tooth attachment is shown in Figure 37-1. Here it can be seen that the gingiva forms

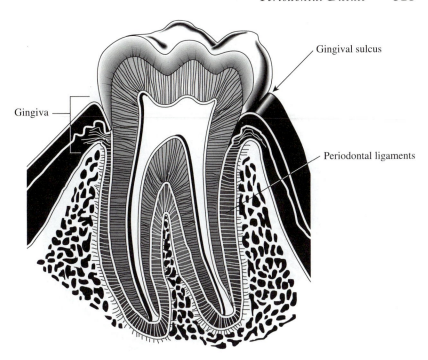

FIGURE 37-1   Normal tooth showing support through linkage of the periodontal ligaments to the alveolar bone.

a tight collar around the neck of the tooth, and that a structure called the *periodontal ligament* attaches the roots of the tooth to the alveolar bone. It also can be seen that there is a shallow furrow, called a *gingival sulcus*, found between the gingival margin and the tooth surface. The depth of a normal, healthy gingival sulcus should not exceed 3 mm. Several other types of epithelial tissue also are involved in tooth attachment, but the structures illustrated in Figure 37-1 provide a sufficient background for a discussion of periodontal disease.

PLAQUE FORMATION IN PERIODONTAL DISEASE

As described for dental caries, the same plaque formation is the initiating event in periodontal disease. In this case, however, the overall process is considerably more complex than simple decalcification by organic acids, and there appear to be many species of bacteria that are directly involved in the pathology of periodontal disease.

Periodontal disease begins when plaque formation occurs at the gingival margin and extends into the gingival sulcus. If this plaque is not removed by brushing or flossing, calcium is deposited on the plaque surface, forming a rough, stony crust, termed *calculus* or *tartar,* which clings tenaciously to the tooth surface. More plaque continues to be laid down on calculus surfaces, eventually forming a thick layer of calcified plaque.

BACTERIOLOGY OF PERIODONTAL DISEASE

The initial plaque is a thin layer that consists primarily of *S sanguis, Streptococcus mitis, A viscosus, Actinomyces naeslundii,* and *Actinomyces israelii.* As this plaque thickens, the absolute number of bacteria increases, as does

the percentage of actinomycetes. There also is an increase in gram-negative rods such as *Haemophilus, Veillonella, Fusobacterium,* and *Campylobacter.* The flora in the plaque at the bottom of the gingival sulcus consists primarily of obligately anaerobic gram-negative rods such as *Porphyromonas, Prevotella, Bacteroides, Fusobacterium, Eikenella,* and the spirochete, *Treponema denticola.*

Capnocytophaga gingivalis is a member of the oral flora that also has been associated with advanced periodontal disease, particularly in persons with juvenile-onset diabetes. These organisms are gram-negative, flexible rods that can be isolated routinely from dental plaques, and the numerous reports that have associated them with colonization of the gingival sulcus undoubtedly indicate that they may play a major role in progressive periodontal disease.

Porphyromonas gingivalis is another important constituent of plaque that has been shown to act as a primary pathogen in experimental periodontal disease in monkeys and rats. It is a gram-negative, obligately anaerobic coccobacillus that produces at least two proteases and a collagenase. Infection of gnotobiotic (germ-free) rats with *P gingivalis* induces alveolar bone loss, but immunization with its 43-kilodalton fimbrial protein protects them from periodontitis after a similar infection. Its repeated isolation from advanced periodontal lesions also indicates that it is a prime contributor to this disease.

T denticola is present in small numbers in the normal healthy mouth, but can account for up to 30% of the flora in cases of progressive periodontitis. It forms at least two proteases as well as several hydrolytic enzymes, and possesses the ability to attach to host tissues and other bacteria.

THERE probably are few cells, eucaryotic or procaryotic, that cannot be infected by a virus. In addition to the bacteriophages described in the bacteriology section of this book, there are viruses that infect other procaryotic cells, such as actinomycetes (actinophages), blue-green algae (cyanophages), and even free-living mycoplasmas. Among the invaders of eucaryotic cells, viruses have been described that infect fungi, protozoa, invertebrates, and probably every higher animal in existence. Some of the most serious infectious diseases of humans are caused by viruses. In addition, viruses, because of their simple structure and limited genetic content, serve as indispensable tools for molecular biologists and cell biologists. Viruses also have been used experimentally as vectors for the delivery of genes for vaccinations and gene therapy. It is likely that viruses will be used extensively for such purposes in the future.

Much scientific speculation has surrounded the origin of viruses. Because viruses require host cells for their replication, they are most likely younger on the evolutionary scale than are their more complex host cells. This suggests two major possibilities: (1) viruses are the result of a retrograde evolution of procaryotic or eucaryotic cells; or (2) viruses originated from genetic material in host cells that mutated in such a manner that it not only could reproduce independently within a host cell, but could exist outside the cell and still maintain its ability to infect other cells. It is not absolutely clear which of these theories of viral origins is correct, but most virologists believe that the latter is the more probable explanation.

Many changes occur in a host cell once it is infected by a virus. Sometimes these changes are subtle, and the virus causes an inapparent infection or benign disease. Other times, virus infection leads to extensive and often profound consequences for the host. This is illustrated dramatically when cells of the nervous system are infected and destroyed by viruses such as polio or rabies; the destruction of the infected nerve cells can result in permanent disability or death of the entire host organism. Another example is human immunodeficiency virus, which infects and destroys cells of the immune system, ultimately resulting in a breakdown of this system and the development of the acquired immunodeficiency syndrome. In many instances, however, viruses do not cause any noticeable damage to either the infected cells or the host. In such cases, viruses appear to have reached the ultimate state of parasitism in which both the virus and the host cell continue to prosper. This delicate balance can be tipped by changes in the metabolic or immune state of the host.

Many viruses exhibit the capacity to stimulate the growth and proliferation of infected cells. This often results in benign, self-limiting manifestations such as the common warts caused by papillomaviruses or infectious mononucleosis caused by Epstein-Barr virus. However, these viruses and many others can contribute to the uncontrolled and malignant growth of cells, eventually leading to the development of life-threatening conditions.

Many factors influence the delicate balance that exists between the host and the virus that seeks to replicate within that host. Of particular importance is the host's ability to mount cellular and humoral immune responses to the virus. In addition, the induction of cellular proteins called interferons plays an important role in limiting virus spread. To understand how viruses cause disease, one must know the essential features of virus replication, the ways in which viruses influence (for better or for worse) the hosts that harbor them, and the ways in which hosts respond to the presence of viruses. It is the purpose of this unit to address these questions, as well as to describe the essential features of those viruses that cause disease in humans.

Bibliography

BOOKS

Evans AS, ed. Viral infections of humans, ed 3. New York, Plenum Publishing, 1989.

Fields BN, Knipe DM, eds. Virology, ed 2. New York, Raven Press, 1990.

Joklik WK, Willett HP, Amos DB, Wilfert CM. Zinsser microbiology, ed 19. Norwalk, CT, Appleton & Lange, 1988.

Mandell GL, Douglas RG Jr, Bennett JE. Principles and practices of infectious diseases, ed 3. New York, Churchill Livingstone, 1990.

White DO, Fenner FJ. Medical virology, ed 3. Orlando, FL, Academic Press, 1986.

Essentials of Medical Microbiology, Fifth Edition, edited by Wesley A. Volk,
Bryan M. Gebhardt, Marie-Louise Hammarskjöld, and Robert J. Kadner.
Lippincott-Raven Publishers, Philadelphia © 1996.

Chapter 38

Structure and Classification of Animal Viruses

All viruses are obligate intracellular parasites and are absolutely dependent on a host cell for their replication. Replication inside a host cell eventually leads to the release of virus particles. These particles (called virions) have no metabolism and no organelles. However, they carry all the genetic information necessary for the generation of more virus particles after infection of a new host cell. Viruses are unique in that the genetic information can be carried as either RNA or DNA. The type of nucleic acid contained in a virion is a determining factor in its replicative pathway and, hence, is a major consideration when classifying viruses. The genetic material in the virion is surrounded by protein that forms a symmetric structure called the capsid. One of the major functions of the capsid is to protect the viral nucleic acid. In some viruses, the capsid is in turn surrounded by a lipid bilayer membrane known as the viral envelope.

Virus replication requires expression of the information carried in the genetic material of the virus through the classic pathways of transcription and translation of this information into proteins. However, because viruses do not contain a machinery for these processes, they must infect new host cells and subvert normal cellular mechanisms for their own replication. The extent to which they rely on host cellular factors for replication depends in large part on the complexity of their own genetic structure. For example, the large and complex viruses, such as herpesviruses, encode many of the proteins required for their replication, whereas genetically less complex viruses, such as papovaviruses, must rely almost totally on host functions for their replication.

Our understanding of the structure and organization of viral genetic information has been facilitated by a complete sequence analysis of many viral genomes, both large and small. This has contributed greatly to our understanding of viral protein structure, virus replication, and viral pathogenesis. In addition, knowledge of virus protein sequences has allowed new approaches to the design of viral vaccines and therapies.

Sizes of Viruses

Viruses vary considerably in size but are in general well below the limit of visibility in the light microscope. The original name for these agents was ultrafilterable viruses (virus being the Greek word for poison), because they were small enough to pass through filters that retained bacteria and other infectious agents.

Virus sizes range from 20 to 250 nm. However, because many viruses are pleomorphic in size and shape, precise measurements can be difficult to attain. Historically, several techniques have been used to determine virus sizes, but direct observation using an electron microscope is now the method of choice.

Chemical Composition and Structure of Viruses

VIRAL CAPSIDS

The capsid of a virus is made up of repeating identical morphologic protein subunits termed *capsomers,* which are held together by noncovalent bonds. Each capsomer consists of one or more polypeptides. The use of small identical subunits allows viruses to build the capsid using only a small amount of genetic material. The viral capsid performs several functions, such as protecting the enclosed nucleic acid from both physical destruction and enzymatic hydrolysis by the extracellular milieu. In non-enveloped viruses, it also provides binding sites that enable the virus to attach to specific receptors on the host cell. Finally, the capsid facilitates the assembly and packaging of the viral genetic information. Electron microscopy has revealed that, with the exception of the relatively complex poxviruses, the capsids of all animal viruses show either icosahedral or helical symmetry. Virtually all DNA-containing animal viruses exhibit icosahedral symmetry, an exception being the more complex, brick-shaped poxviruses; RNA-containing animal viruses show either icosahedral or helical symmetry.

Virus Symmetry

ICOSAHEDRAL SYMMETRY. The capsids of icosahedral viruses appear to be in the shape of a regular icosahedron (*icosa,* meaning 20 in Greek), with each particle showing 20 facets, each of which is an equilateral triangle. These facets come together to form 12 vertices. Icosahedral viruses have their nucleic acid (RNA or DNA) packaged inside the capsid. In some viruses, the capsid is surrounded by a viral envelope (see later); in other viruses, the capsid is naked. Schematic and electron microscopic views of an icosahedral virus are shown in Figure 38-1. As can be seen in this figure, the capsomer at each of the 12 vertices is surrounded by only 5 other capsomers, whereas all other capsomers are adjacent to 6 other capsomers. The

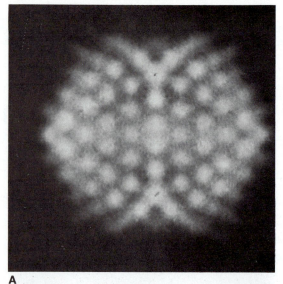

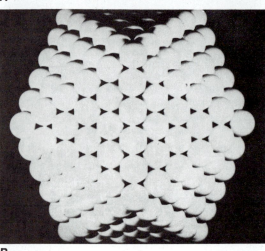

FIGURE 38-1 **A.** Electron micrograph of a negatively stained adenovirus virion. **B.** Model of the same virion showing 252 spheres in icosahedral symmetry.

capsomers at the vertices are called *pentons* and the remaining capsomers are referred to as *hexons.*

A special property of an icosahedral structure is its multiple axes of symmetry. Figure 38-2 shows that it is possible to discern three different types of symmetry as the icosahedron is rotated, through the edges, the faces, and the vertices, resulting in what is referred to as 5:3:2 symmetry.

One means of classifying an icosahedral virus is based on the number of capsomers present in the viral capsid. This number can be calculated for many viruses with icosahedral symmetry by using the formula, $N = 10(n - 1)^2 + 2$, where n is the number of capsomers on one side of each equilateral triangle. Examples that fit this formula include herpesvirus, with 5 capsomers on the side of each triangular surface and a total of 162 capsomers (150 hexons and 12 pentons) making up the

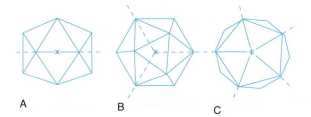

FIGURE 38-2 Features of icosahedral symmetry. Depending on the angle of observation, the icosahedron shows two, three, or five axes of symmetry. **A.** Looking down on the edge between two triangular facets, the same symmetry is observed as the icosahedron is rotated 180 degrees (two axes). **B.** Looking at the center of a triangular facet, an identical symmetry is observed with each 120 degrees of rotation (three axes). **C.** Looking directly down on a penton capsomer, identical axes of symmetry can be observed by rotating the icosahedron in a series of 72-degree steps (five axes).

intact capsid, and adenovirus, with 6 capsomers per side and a total of 252 capsomers per intact virion (240 hexons and 12 pentons).

HELICAL VIRUSES. In many RNA viruses, the viral nucleic acid is closely associated with the protein capsomers, forming a coil-shaped, helical nucleocapsid. The exact nature of the nucleic acid interactions within the capsid is not well understood, but the protein seems to protect the RNA from enzymatic degradation by nucleases after infection of a new host cell, while still allowing the transcription of RNA from the intact nucleoprotein. Helical animal viruses are always surrounded by a viral envelope. Figure 38-3 shows electron micrographs of rhabdovirus virions, in which the striations of nucleic acid can be seen wound in a helical pattern in the interior of the particles. With the exception of the bullet-shaped rhabdoviruses, helical animal viruses exist as spherical virions containing a helical-shaped nucleocapsid surrounded by a more or less spherical membrane envelope.

VIRAL ENVELOPES

In many animal viruses, the capsid is surrounded by a lipid bilayer membrane envelope. This envelope is acquired by the virus during the final stage of replication as the immature particles bud through special areas of the host-cell membrane (Fig. 38-4). These special areas of host-cell membrane are characterized by the presence of virus-specified glycoproteins. In the mature virus particle, the glycoproteins often appear as projections or spikes on the outer surface of the envelope; these protrusions have been given the name *peplomers*. Many of these glycoproteins have special functions and mediate the attachment of the virus to host-cell receptors to initiate the entrance of the virion into a new host cell. Some viral glycoproteins also attach to receptors on red blood cells, causing these cells to agglutinate (hemagglutination). Others possess enzy-

matic activity (neuraminidase) and cleave neuraminic acid from host-cell glycoproteins. In light of these important functions, it is not surprising that antibodies capable of neutralizing viral infectivity frequently are directed against envelope glycoproteins.

In addition to proteins and glycoproteins, the viral envelope contains 20% to 30% lipid, derived totally from the host-cell membrane. Therefore, the infectiousness of

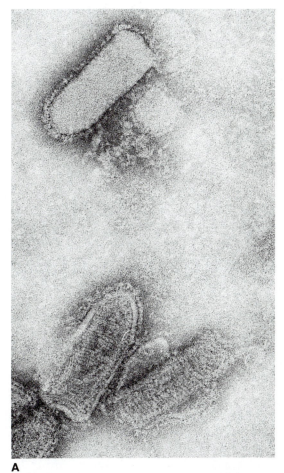

A

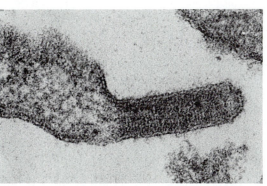

B

FIGURE 38-3 **A.** Virions of vesicular stomatitis virus (VSV); the helical nucleocapsid is visible as cross striations. (Original magnification ×207,000.) **B.** VSV budding from a cell. (Original magnification ×147,000.)

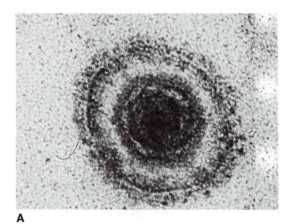

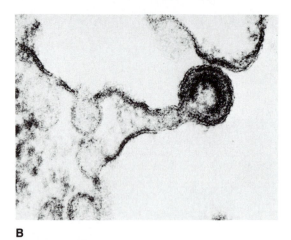

FIGURE 38-4   **A.** Section through a herpesvirus, showing envelope, capsid, and electron-dense internal core. (Original magnification about ×330,000.) **B.** A C-type renovirus particle budding from an infected cell. (Original magnification ×168,000.)

enveloped viruses is inactivated by lipid solvents such as ether and chloroform, whereas viruses existing as naked capsids usually are resistant to such treatments. The sensitivity of viruses to lipid solvents can be used to facilitate the characterization of new or unknown viruses.

VIRAL NUCLEIC ACID

Each family of viruses possesses a nucleic acid characteristic for that group, which, along with the properties of the virion capsid, is used for the classification of the virus. As listed in Tables 38-1 and 38-2, viruses possess single- (SS) or double-stranded (DS) DNA and RNA. In addition, the nucleic acid can exist in a linear or circular form. For most viruses, the genome consists of a single nucleic acid molecule, but some viruses have a genome made up of several different fragments. The genetic complexity of the nucleic acid varies greatly among different virus families. In some cases, the genetic material contains enough information to encode only a few proteins (eg, parvoviruses, picornaviruses). In other cases, it is large enough to encode hundreds of proteins (eg, herpesviruses, poxviruses).

Structure of Viral DNA

Differences in viral DNA structure between viruses have required them to evolve different strategies for replicating their genetic information. As discussed later, the elucidation of these mechanisms by molecular biologists has yielded invaluable insights into the mechanisms of cellular DNA replication.

The genetic material of animal DNA viruses exists as either linear molecules (in the form of SS or DS DNA) or circular forms of DNA. The DS DNA of papovaviruses consists of covalently closed DNA that forms a molecule known as a *supercoil* (Fig. 38-5). Supercoiled DNA results from extra turns in the helical structure of DS DNA, which are introduced by an enzyme called *DNA gyrase*. Supercoiled DNA can be converted into a simple circular structure by enzymatically breaking (nicking) one strand of the DS DNA. This relieves the supercoiled twist, permitting the relaxation of the molecule to form a "relaxed" circular molecule. Supercoiling occurs in all types of covalently closed DS circular DNA (eg, mitochondrial DNA, chloroplast DNA, bacterial plasmid DNA).

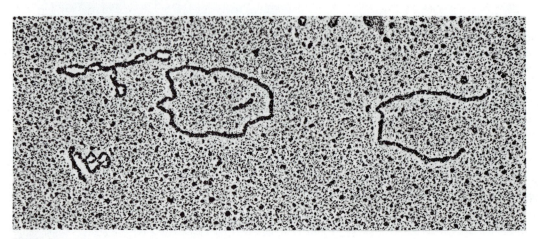

FIGURE 38-5   Electron micrograph of SV40 DNA, showing linear, circular, and supercoiled molecules.

TABLE 38-1
Chemical and Physical Properties of Animal DNA Viruses

Families and Genera of DNA Viruses	Capsid Symmetry (Capsomers)	Envelope	Virion Size (nm)	Genome Size (Kilobases)
ADENOVIRIDAE				
Mastadenovirus	Icosahedral (252)	No	60–90	36 DS, linear
HERPESVIRIDAE				
Herpesvirus				
Varicella-zoster	Icosahedral	Yes	150–200	130–220
Cytomegalovirus	(162)			DS, linear
Epstein-Barr virus				
POXVIRIDAE				
Orthopoxvirus	Complex	Yes (ether-resistant)	240 × 300	130–280 DS, linear
PAPOVAVIRIDAE				
Polyomavirus	Icosahedral	No	40–55	5, 8*
Papillomavirus	(72)			DS, closed circular
PARVOVIRIDAE				
Parvoviruses	Icosahedral	No	22	5
Dependoviruses	(32)			SS, linear
HEPADNAVIRIDAE				
Hepatitis B virus	Icosahedral	Yes	42	3 DS, circular†

DS, double-stranded; SS, single-stranded.

* Five kilobases for polyomaviruses, 8 kilobases for papillomaviruses.

† Genome is partially double-stranded.

Molecular biologists have long appreciated the fact that bacteriophage DNAs frequently have repeated sequences at the ends of their genome that facilitate virus replication. For example, the bacteriophage λ genome contains direct repeats at the termini that make it possible for the DNA to form circular structures during the process of DNA replication (Fig. 38-6A). The termini of the DNA of many animal viruses also have sequences that facilitate the formation of SS or DS circular forms. For example, the DNA of adenoviruses contains inverted repeat sequences in which the end of each strand of DNA can be represented as 5'-ABC–C'B'A' 3' (where ABC is complementary to and can base pair with A'B'C'). This kind of sequence organization can be visualized in the electron microscope if the DS DNA is heated and the separated strands are permitted to reanneal. On reannealing, part of the DNA base pairs to re-form the original DS DNA, but some of the DNA molecules form base pairs between their complementary 3' and 5' ends to create a panhandle or lollipop structure (see Fig. 38-6B) similar to that described for a transposon (see Chap. 21). Herpes simplex virus DNA possesses a more complicated organization of repeated DNA sequences. Here, sequences complementary to the terminally repeated sequences also are found within the viral DNA sequence, providing an internal repetition (see Fig. 38-6C).

The existence of terminal redundancy in viral DNA provides a unique structural feature important for the replication of the virus. Such a terminal redundancy makes it possible for the same protein to recognize both ends of DS linear DNA. In addition, inverted terminal repetitions in SS DNA can provide a DS region necessary for the initiation of replication of the SS DNA.

Structure of Viral RNA

The genomes of animal RNA viruses consist of linear RNA molecules that can be either DS or SS. In addition, the RNA genome within a virion can be made up of several different RNA fragments. For example, reoviruses contain 10 different segments of DS RNA, rotaviruses contain 11 separate segments of DS RNA, and influenza viruses possess 8 different segments of SS RNA. Other RNA viruses containing a segmented genome include the bunyaviruses (3 segments) and the arenaviruses (2 segments). Retroviruses are unique in that they contain

TABLE 38-2
Chemical and Physical Properties of Animal RNA Viruses

Families and Genera of RNA Viruses	Capsid Symmetry (Capsomers/Envelope)	Virion Size (nm)	Genome Size* (Kilobases) Polarity	Virus-associated Transcriptase
PICORNAVIRIDAE				
Enterovirus (enteric)	Icosahedral	27	7–7.5	No
Rhinovirus (respiratory)	(60/no envelope)		SS, positive	
CALICIVIRIDAE				
Calicivirus (Norwalk virus)	Icosahedral	30	8	No
	(32/no envelope)		SS, positive	
CORONAVIRIDAE				
Coronavirus	Helical, enveloped, petal-shaped spikes	120	27	No
			SS, positive	
TOGAVIRIDAE				
Alphavirus	Icosahedral, enveloped	60–70	11–12	No
Rubivirus† (rubella)			SS, positive	
FLAVIVIRIDAE				
Flavivirus	Icosahedral, enveloped	45	11	No
			SS, positive	
BUNYAVIRIDAE				
Bunyavirus	Helical, enveloped	90–120	14	Yes
Phleboviruses			(3 segments)	
Hantaviruses			SS, negative‡	
Nairoviruses				
ORTHOMYXOVIRIDAE				
Influenza virus (influenza)	Helical, enveloped	80–100	14	Yes
			(8 segments)	
			SS, negative	
PARAMYXOVIRIDAE				
Paramyxovirus (Parainfluenza, mumps)	Helical, enveloped	120–250	15	Yes
Morbillivirus (measles)			SS, negative	
Pneumovirus (respiratory syncytial)				
RHABDOVIRIDAE				
Lyssavirus (rabies group)	Helical, enveloped	70 × 170	11	Yes
Vesiculovirus (vesicular stomatitis group)		(bullet-shaped)	SS, negative	
FILOVIRIDAE				
(Marburg/Ebola)	Helical, enveloped	Pleomorphic	13	Yes
			SS, negative	
ARENAVIRIDAE				
Arenavirus (lymphocytic choriomeningitis, Tacaribe complex, Lassa fever)	Helical, enveloped	60–350	11 (2 segments) SS, negative‡	Yes
RETROVIRIDAE				
Oncovirus	Icosahedral, enveloped	65–150	5–9	Yes
Spumavirus			(2 segments)§	(reverse transcriptase)
Lentivirus			SS, positive	
REOVIRIDAE				
(DS RNA viruses)	Icosahedral, no envelope (double capsid)	60–80	23	Yes
Reovirus			(10–11 segments)	
Rotavirus				
Orbivirus			DS	

SS, single-stranded; DS, double-stranded.

* Approximate size of genome in kilobases; the polarity of the genome is designated as positive or negative.

† Has been placed in the family Togaviridae on the basis of its physical and chemical similarities to the other togaviruses.

‡ Some bunyaviruses and arenaviruses contain genome segments with ambisense polarity.

§ Both segments are identical.

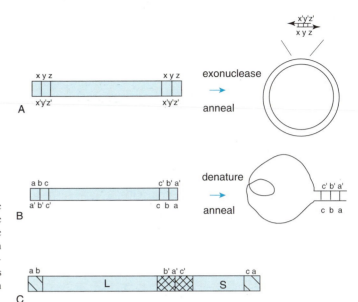

FIGURE 38-6 Viral DNAs have different terminal sequences. **A.** The base pairing between the ends of a DNA molecule with cohesive termini after treatment of the DNA with exonuclease. **B.** The possible base pairing between the ends of a DNA molecule containing an inverted repeated sequence after denaturation of the DNA and annealing of the separated strands. **C.** The distribution of repeated sequences within the DNA genome of herpesvirus. Note the presence of both internal and terminal repeats.

two identical SS genomes and, hence, are diploid in genetic content. The complex organization of genetic information in viruses with segmented genomes requires unique mechanisms to ensure the proper segregation of genetic material. It also provides the viruses with unique opportunities for alteration of the genetic composition of the virus by facilitating the exchange of individual RNA segments if two closely related viruses are infecting the same host cell (eg, strains of influenza A; see Chap. 48).

Positive and Negative Strands of Nucleic Acid

Viruses containing DS nucleic acid usually package only one of the two strands within the virion. Viruses containing SS RNA can be classified based on the polarity (or sense) of the genomic RNA. Viruses that contain SS RNA, which is of the correct polarity to act directly as messenger RNA (mRNA), have been designated as positive-strand viruses, whereas those that first must transcribe their RNA to form a complementary strand (which then acts as the mRNA) are designated as negative-strand viruses. As might be expected, the naked RNA of positive-strand viruses, such as poliovirus, can infect an animal cell, directing replication and the synthesis of complete new virus particles. This is possible because the viral genome contains all the genetic information of the virus and can act directly as mRNA to be translated into protein by the host ribosome translation machinery. The naked RNA from negative-strand viruses, however, is not infectious, because it first must be transcribed to form the complementary RNA that serves as mRNA. During natural infection, this transcription is always catalyzed by a virus-specified, RNA-dependent RNA polymerase carried within the virion (see later). A unique situation has been

noted for arenaviruses and some bunyaviruses, where one of the RNA segments exhibits both a positive and a negative polarity. These viruses have been termed *ambisense* because part of the RNA strand can function directly as mRNA, whereas the remainder of the RNA must be transcribed to yield mRNA. Classification of a virus as either a positive- or negative-strand virus is extremely useful, because it immediately reveals certain features of the strategy of virus replication.

DNA viruses also can exist as positive- or negative-strand viruses, but the DNA from SS DNA viruses is converted to DS DNA before being transcribed into mRNA.

NONSTRUCTURAL VIRAL PROTEINS

Viruses often carry within their capsids enzymes that are liberated after the virus is uncoated in the host cell. By far the most common enzymes are viral-encoded polymerases. As mentioned earlier, all negative-strand RNA viruses carry within the virion an RNA-dependent RNA polymerase that is responsible for initiating the early steps in virus replication. All retroviruses carry a unique enzyme in their virions called reverse transcriptase. This enzyme is an RNA-dependent DNA polymerase that catalyzes the formation of a DS DNA molecule from the SS RNA molecules present in the virion. Retroviruses also carry an integrase, which enables this DS DNA to integrate into the host-cell DNA.

The positive-strand RNA viruses encode their own RNA polymerase, which is synthesized by host-cell translation of the viral mRNA. This RNA polymerase catalyzes the formation of negative-strand RNA, which then serves as a template for the formation of more positive-strand RNA. Many DNA viruses encode virus-specific, DNA-dependent DNA polymerases and other enzymes that facilitate replication of their DNA. However, these are not necessary to initiate the infection process and, thus, are not usually found in the virus particles.

Classification of Animal Viruses

As our knowledge of viruses has increased, the properties used to classify them into families, groups, or genera have shifted from the symptomatology or pathology of the infections they cause to the physical characteristics of the viruses themselves. To standardize the naming of new viruses, the International Committee on Nomenclature of Viruses was established at the Ninth International Congress for Microbiology in 1966. In the decades since, this committee has adopted the following criteria for the classification of viruses: (1) the chemical nature of the nucleic acid (ie, DNA or RNA, SS or DS, single or segmented genome, approximate molecular weight of nucleic acid, and whether the virion contains a positive or negative strand of nucleic acid); (2) the symmetry of the nucleocapsid (ie, icosahedral or helical); (3) the presence or absence of an envelope; and (4) the number of capso-

mers for icosahedral virions, or the diameter of the nucleocapsids for helical viruses.

Based on these criteria, most of the viruses infecting mammalian hosts have been assigned to one of several virus families (Fig. 38-7). Within these families, viruses have been subdivided into one or more genera based on serologic, morphologic, and other important differences. Table 38-1 lists the current classification for DNA viruses that are discussed in this text, along with some of their chemical and physical properties. Table 38-2 provides similar information for RNA viruses.

It should be emphasized to readers new to the field of medical virology that, although a generic-type classification of viruses is essential to provide a systematic handle, some of the generic names rarely are used by medical virologists, who are more likely to refer to many of the viruses by the name of the disease for which they are responsible. This text introduces the generic terminology, but discussion of individual viruses, for the most part, uses those virus names that are more commonly used.

FAMILIES OF DNA VIRUSES

Adenoviridae

Adenoviruses are nonenveloped icosahedral viruses that contain linear DS DNA and replicate in the nucleus of

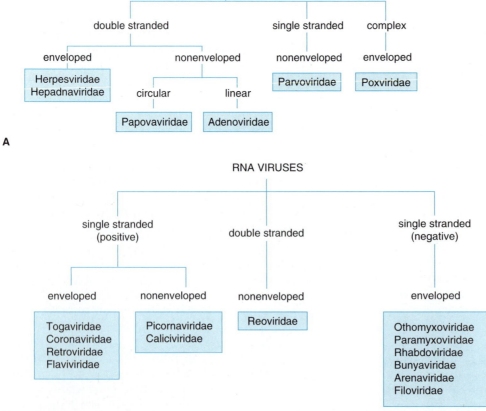

FIGURE 38-7 Summary of the classification of DNA viruses **A.** and RNA viruses **B.**

infected cells. There are at least 47 serologically distinct human adenoviruses, many of which cause infection of the respiratory tract. Others cause eye and gastrointestinal tract infections. Adenoviruses are characterized by their ability to persist in tissues for long periods. Their name derives from the fact that they originally were isolated from seemingly normal human adenoids.

Parvoviridae

Parvoviruses are small, nonenveloped icosahedral DNA viruses. Parvoviruses are the only animal viruses that contain SS DNA. The genus *Parvovirus* includes viruses that infect mice, rats, and swine, as well as a single virus that infects humans.

A second genus, termed *Dependovirus,* includes five types of "adeno-associated" viruses. These viruses are unable to replicate within susceptible cells without coinfection of the cell with a "helper" adenovirus or herpesvirus. Thus, they are found in association with adenoviruses or herpesviruses, but are not known to be the direct cause of any disease in humans.

Papovaviridae

Papovaviruses (*pa* for papilloma, *po* for polyoma, *va* for vacuolating) are small, DS, icosahedral, nonenveloped DNA viruses that replicate in the nucleus of infected cells and often have the ability to transform cells and induce tumors. The DS DNA consists of a covalently closed circular supercoiled molecule. Viruses included in this family include *Papillomavirus, Polyomavirus,* and simian virus 40. There are two genera, *Papillomavirus* and *Polyomavirus.* The papillomaviruses cause warts on the skin or on mucous membranes in humans, and some types show a strong association with the development of cervical carcinoma. Human polyomaviruses commonly produce inapparent infections in humans, generally early in life. These viruses often are reactivated in immunosuppressed individuals. One of these viruses is the cause of a progressive neurologic disease. Two polyomaviruses (mouse polyomavirus and simian virus 40) and bovine papillomavirus have served as important model systems for the study of virus replication and structure as well as tumor transformation.

Herpesviridae

Herpesviruses are large, enveloped icosahedral viruses that contain linear DS DNA. Herpesviruses replicate in the nucleus of their host cells and mature by budding through the inner part of the nuclear membrane, thus acquiring their lipid envelope. Herpesviruses generally are characterized by their ability to establish latent infections in the host and by their propensity to be reactivated months to many years after a primary infection. Human herpesviruses have been classified into three genera: (1)

Alphaherpesvirinae, which includes herpes simplex types 1 and 2, viruses that are responsible for oral and genital infections, as well as varicella-zoster virus, the agent that causes chickenpox and herpes zoster (also known as shingles); (2) Betaherpesvirinae, which includes the cytomegaloviruses, such as the human cytomegalovirus that can cause congenital infections as well as serious infections in immunocompromised individuals; and (3) Gammaherpesvirinae, which includes Epstein-Barr virus, the etiologic agent of infectious mononucleosis. Epstein-Barr virus also shows a strong association with human cancers such as Burkitt's lymphoma and nasopharyngeal carcinoma.

Poxviridae

The poxviruses are a group of complex viruses that contain linear DS DNA surrounded by a complex array of virus-encoded structures. Poxviruses are unique among DNA viruses in that they replicate solely in the cytoplasm of infected cells. The human poxviruses (*Orthopoxvirus*) include the etiologic agent of smallpox, as well as vaccinia (the virus used in smallpox vaccination) and related viruses.

Hepadnaviridae

Hepadnaviruses are small, spherical viruses. The virion contains an icosahedral core with a partially DS, partially SS circular DNA genome surrounded by an envelope containing a virus-encoded surface antigen. Hepadnaviruses replicate in the nucleus of infected cells. Hepadnaviruses of humans and other animal species are characterized by their unique retrovirus-like replication cycle and the ability to induce chronic infection of the liver. In humans, infection with the hepadnavirus hepatitis B virus can result in a hepatitis that can progress to a chronic, persistent disease. The virus shows a strong association with the development of primary hepatocellular carcinoma.

FAMILIES OF RNA VIRUSES

Picornaviridae

The Picornaviridae (*pico* for small, *rna* for RNA) consist of small, nonenveloped icosahedral viruses that contain a single molecule of positive-strand SS RNA. These viruses replicate solely in the cytoplasm of infected cells. The family Picornaviridae contains two genera that cause human disease. The members of the genus *Enterovirus* are transmitted to humans primarily by a fecal–oral route and usually cause inapparent enteric infections. Some of these viruses can invade the bloodstream and infect the central nervous system, where they can cause serious disease. Other manifestations of enterovirus infections include rashes, myocarditis, myositis, respiratory tract infections, and hepatitis. Common human enteroviruses include the polioviruses, coxsackieviruses, echoviruses (*enteric cytopathic human orphan viruses*), and the etiologic agent of one form of human viral hepatitis (hepatitis A virus) .

The second genus of Picornaviridae, *Rhinovirus,* causes a great deal of misery in humans because it encompasses some of the major etiologic agents of the common cold. There are more than 100 different serotypes of rhinoviruses, which undoubtedly helps to account for the "commonness" of the common cold.

Caliciviridae

Formerly classified as a genus of Picornaviridae, the Caliciviridae differ enough in their morphology and mode of replication to warrant classification as a distinct family. The major human viruses of this family include the caliciviruses and the Norwalk and Norwalk-like viruses. Some of these viruses are important causes of gastroenteritis. Hepatitis E, an agent responsible for large outbreaks of human hepatitis spread by the fecal–oral route, has been shown to be a Norwalk-like virus.

Togaviridae

Togaviridae are a family of positive-strand SS RNA viruses possessing icosahedral symmetry and a lipoprotein envelope, hence the prefix *toga-,* meaning coat or mantle. These viruses replicate in the cytoplasm and acquire their lipid envelope by budding from the plasma membrane of the infected cell. Included in this family are many of the insect-borne arboviruses (*ar*thropod-*bo*rne viruses). Two genera (*Alphavirus* and *Rubivirus*) contain virus species that cause disease in humans. *Alphavirus* includes viruses that cause the arboviral diseases eastern equine encephalitis, western equine encephalitis, and Venezuelan equine encephalitis. These viruses infect humans through mosquito bites. *Rubivirus* is not transmitted by an arthropod vector, but is classified with the togaviruses, because rubella virus, the sole member of this genus, shares several properties with the other togaviruses. Rubella virus is the causative agent of German measles, a common childhood disease.

Flaviviridae

The flavivirus family has been separated from the Togaviridae based on differences in replication strategy. Structurally, flaviviruses resemble togaviruses in that they are small icosahedral viruses containing SS, positive-strand RNA with a cell-derived lipid envelope. The genus, *Flavivirus,* includes viruses that cause yellow and dengue fever, and several forms of encephalitis (St. Louis, Japanese, Murray Valley, and Russian tick-borne encephalitis).

These flaviviruses all are transmitted by arthropod vectors. *Hepatitis C Virus,* a major cause of transfusion-associated hepatitis, has been classified as a separate genus within the flavivirus family.

Coronaviridae

Coronaviruses are enveloped positive-strand RNA viruses that are so named because of the large, petal-like peplomers on their envelopes (*corona* means crown). Virus particles contain a single molecule of positive-strand RNA in a helical nucleocapsid. Coronaviruses have been isolated from humans and other animals with upper respiratory tract infections and are frequent causes of such infections. Coronaviruses have the largest genome of all RNA viruses (about 30,000 nucleotides).

Orthomyxoviridae

Orthomyxoviruses are segmented, negative-strand RNA viruses whose enveloped virions contain a nucleocapsid with helical symmetry. The virion contains an RNA-dependent RNA polymerase. Projecting from the viral envelope are two different kinds of peplomers. One is designated a *hemagglutinin,* because it reacts with a glycoprotein present on the surface of red blood cells, causing them to agglutinate. The other is an enzyme, *neuraminidase,* which can liberate neuraminic acid from the red blood cell glycoprotein, causing the spontaneous elution of the virus from the agglutinated red blood cells. Virus particles contain seven or eight SS RNA segments. Virus RNA transcription and replication takes place in the nucleus, but virus particles assemble in the cytoplasm and mature by budding from the plasma membrane of the host cell. The orthomyxovirus family includes three serologically distinct species: influenza virus A, strains of which infect humans as well as birds, horses, and swine; influenza virus B, a human pathogen; and influenza C, an uncommon human pathogen.

Paramyxoviridae

Paramyxoviruses are enveloped viruses that contain a single molecule of negative-strand RNA. The nucleocapsid shows a helical symmetry. Virus particles carry a virion-associated, RNA-dependent RNA polymerase and replicate in the cytoplasm of their host cells. The envelope glycoproteins exhibit hemagglutinin and, often, a neuraminidase activity. The Paramyxoviridae consist of three genera: *Paramyxovirus, Morbillivirus,* and *Pneumovirus.* The genera *Paramyxovirus* and *Pneumovirus* cause respiratory tract infections (parainfluenza and respiratory syncytial viruses) or generalized infections with parotid gland involvement (mumps virus), whereas the genus *Morbillivirus* contains the virus that causes measles.

Rhabdoviridae

Rhabdoviruses are enveloped helical viruses that are characteristically bullet shaped. The genome is made up of a single molecule of negative-strand RNA. The two best-studied members of this family are rabies virus and vesicular stomatitis virus (a pathogen for cattle). However, there are many other rhabdoviruses, including several fish pathogens. Because rhabdoviruses contain the negative strand of the RNA, the virus particles carry their own RNA polymerase.

Filoviridae

Members of the family Filoviridae previously were classified in the family Rhabdoviridae. However, the unique morphology of these viruses prompted a new designation. The Marburg and Ebola viruses in this family are among the most lethal of human viruses but infect humans only rarely. Monkeys probably are the natural host, although human antibody levels to both viruses are high in areas of endemic infection.

Bunyaviridae

Bunyaviruses have been known for many years as the Bunyamwera supergroup. This group includes many (more than 100) of the arthropod-borne viruses. Unlike the togaviruses and flaviviruses, however, the bunyaviruses are helical viruses containing SS RNA that exists in three segments with negative or ambisense polarity. Bunyaviruses replicate in the cytoplasm and bud into Golgi vesicles. Many of the virus species are transmitted by arthropod vectors. The genus, *Bunyavirus,* includes the mosquito-transmitted, California-group arboviruses, which cause encephalitis in humans. The genus, *Phlebovirus,* includes sandfly fever and Rift Valley fever. The genus, *Nairovirus,* includes the virus of Congo-Crimean hemorrhagic fever, and the genus, *Hantavirus,* includes rodent-borne viruses that cause hemorrhagic fever.

Arenaviridae

Arenaviruses originally were grouped together because of their morphologic similarities and acquired their name because the cellular ribosomes present in the pleomorphic, enveloped virions look like grains of sand in the electron microscope. Arenaviruses contain two segments of negative or ambisense SS RNA, each maintained in a circular configuration, as well as a virion-associated RNA polymerase. The best-studied arenavirus is lymphocytic choriomeningitis virus, which characteristically produces an asymptomatic infection in mice and occasionally causes meningitis in humans. Much more serious diseases produced by this group of viruses are the hemorrhagic fevers found in South America and Lassa fever, a disease found principally in Africa.

Retroviridae

Retroviridae is the family name given to a ubiquitous group of RNA viruses that replicate through DNA intermediates. All retroviruses contain two identical molecules of SS, positive-sense RNA. The replication of retroviruses begins by copying (or reverse transcribing) of the SS RNA into DS linear DNA. The DNA copy of the RNA genome subsequently is integrated into the host chromosomes (this form of the viral genome is called the "provirus"), where it is both inherited by daughter cells and transcribed by host RNA polymerase to yield new progeny viral RNA molecules. Retroviruses produce a variety of neoplasms, including leukemias and solid tumors in birds and rodents. In humans, retroviruses are etiologic agents in adult T-cell leukemias (human T-cell leukemia virus [HTLV]) and the acquired immunodeficiency syndrome (human immunodeficiency virus 1 and 2). HTLV-I also is associated with a demyelinating neurologic disease known as tropical spastic paraparesis, or HTLV-associated myelopathy. Retroviruses have been studied for many years as model systems for cellular transformation.

Reoviridae

Reoviridae (*r*espiratory, *e*nteric, *o*rphan) is a family of viruses that contains a genome consisting of 10 to 12 segments of DS RNA. Human reoviruses possess a double icosahedral capsid and replicate solely in the cytoplasm of host cells. Reoviruses are involved in mild respiratory tract infections in humans and also are found in the human intestinal tract.

Orbivirus, a genus of Reoviridae, includes viruses that are primarily animal pathogens, although Colorado tick fever virus (an arbovirus) infects humans.

The genus, *Rotavirus,* so named because of the wheel-like morphology of the viral particles (*rota* means wheel), includes five serologically distinct viruses that cause severe human diarrhea, particularly in infants. Rotavirus infections are common causes of severe dehydration and death in children in undeveloped countries.

UNCONVENTIONAL AGENTS

Several slowly progressing, usually fatal neurologic diseases are known to be associated with the transmission of an infectious agent. These diseases include kuru and Creutzfeldt-Jakob diseases in humans, scrapie in sheep, and transmissible mink encephalopathy in mink. Model studies on the scrapie agent of sheep have led to the suggestion that the infectious agent may represent unique proteinaceous materials termed *prions.*

cases, obtaining immunologic evidence of a virus infection is as important as knowing precisely the level of virus particles in an individual. A variety of different serologic methods, as well as enzyme-linked immunosorbent assays and radioimmunoassays, can be used to determine the level of antibody response to a specific virus. These methodologies were discussed previously (see Chap. 9).

NUCLEIC ACID HYBRIDIZATION

The advent of molecular cloning of viral genomes has given rise to a new repertoire of DNA "probes" for individual viruses. Using techniques based on the principles of RNA—DNA and DNA—DNA hybridization, new approaches to the *detection* and *characterization* of viruses are rapidly becoming a part of viral diagnostics. The use of either radioactively labeled or nonisotopically labeled DNA probes provides sensitive methods for the detection of viruses in infected cells, tissues, and extracellular fluids (see Fig. 39-4). The use of DNA probes combined with cleavage of viral DNA with restriction endonucleases also allows the identification and molecular "fingerprinting" of individual viral isolates. This has become of special importance for certain DNA viruses, such as herpesviruses.

POLYMERASE CHAIN REACTION TECHNIQUES

Polymerase chain reaction (PCR) techniques have been developed for the detection of many different viruses. These techniques are capable of detecting minute amounts of viral genetic material in a tissue or cells. PCR techniques involve the selective amplification of specific DNA sequences using small synthetic oligonucleotide primers (usually around 20 nucleotides) that hybridize to opposing strands of the DNA several hundred nucleotides or more apart. The DNA first is denatured, allowing the primers to hybridize. A heat-stable DNA polymerase then is used to copy the DNA segment between the primers. After heating to separate the newly synthesized DNA, the cycle can be repeated. After 30 polymerization cycles, up to 1 billion copies of the DNA are obtained. This DNA can be visualized directly on a gel or detected by hybridization to a specific radiolabeled DNA probe. The method is sensitive enough to detect the presence of one virus particle in several million cells. For the detection of mRNA or the RNA of RNA viruses, reverse transcriptase can be used to convert the RNA into complementary DNA before DNA amplification by PCR. In situ PCR techniques, capable of detecting viral DNA directly in tissue without extraction, also have been developed. PCR techniques have become invaluable for the detection and characterization of many viruses that cause human disease.

Purification of Viruses

The ability to grow most viruses in cell cultures has made it possible to obtain large amounts of pure virions of many different viruses. The methods by which viruses are purified from the culture medium of infected cells vary from one virus to another, but generally rely on ultracentrifugation.

Purification using centrifugation can be done with either rate zonal or isopyknic (equilibrium density) centrifugation. Rate zonal centrifugation is achieved by carefully filling a centrifuge tube with a solution of sucrose or glycerol with a linearly decreasing concentration. When filled, the solution will increase in density from the top to the bottom of the tube. A virus suspension then is layered carefully over the top of the gradient, and the tube is subjected to high-speed centrifugation in an ultracentrifuge. The rate at which the virus moves through the gradient is a function of its size and weight. The centrifuge is stopped when the virus particles have moved part way through the gradient, and a hole is punched in the bottom or side of the centrifuge tube to collect the contents in a series of fractions. Isopyknic centrifugation is initiated by suspending the virus preparation in a solution of an alkali metal chloride, such as cesium chloride. When such a solution is subjected to high-speed centrifugation, a salt gradient is automatically established during the time of centrifugation, and the virus will form a narrow band in the centrifuge tube at that depth where its buoyant density exactly equals the density of the salt solution. The band of concentrated virus, free of host-cell proteins and nucleic acids, then can be collected as described earlier.

Consequences of Virus Infection

In the introduction to Unit Five, different reactions of the host cell to viral infection were described; these are summarized in Table 39-1. The same virus can produce various effects, depending on the type of host cell infected. Different manifestations of a virus infection (lytic infection and cell death, latent and persistent infections, cell transformation) and cell immunity to virus infection are discussed later.

LYTIC INFECTION

In general, those viruses that kill their host cells do so by inhibiting cellular macromolecular synthesis in favor of virus production. Details of how this occurs are in many cases unknown, but it is clear that infection by cytolytic viruses (those causing death and lysis of the host cell) results in the cessation of many of the processes of cellular macromolecular synthesis. For example, 2 to 3 hours after

TABLE 39-1
Reaction of Host Cell to Viral Infection

Reaction	Representative Viruses Causing These Effects
Death of host cell	Most viruses
Proliferation of host cells	Poxvirus
	Papovaviruses
	Papillomavirus
Fusion of membranes of adjacent cells to form multinucleate cells	Respiratory syncytial virus
	Measles virus
	Sendai virus
	Herpesvirus
	Human immunodeficiency virus (HIV)
Transformation of normal cells into malignant cells	Polyomaviruses
	Herpesvirus
	Adenovirus
	Retroviruses
No histologic change in host-cell appearance for several weeks	Rubella virus
	Some adenoviruses

infection of HeLa cells with poliovirus, the rate of cellular protein synthesis is only about 10% to 20% of that of uninfected cells. For many viruses, cellular RNA and DNA synthesis also is rapidly inhibited. In some cases, these effects may be due to an excess of viral mRNA competing for host-cell ribosomes and enzymes. In other cases, such as reported for poliovirus infections, the virus appears to synthesize products that selectively inhibit the synthesis of host-cell proteins. Regardless of the mechanism involved, the effect is a channeling of the cellular biosynthetic abilities of the cell toward the production of virus, ultimately resulting in the death of the cell.

Evidence of virus infection often is revealed by the presence of intracellular inclusions in the infected host cell. These *inclusion bodies* frequently, but not always, are areas of assembly of new virus particles, and their intracellular location and appearance are characteristic of a particular virus. Accordingly, many inclusion bodies have been given specific names, and their appearance within a cell often can be used as a diagnostic criterion. Figure 39-6 shows one such body, designated a *Negri body*, which is characteristically formed during the replication of rabies virus.

Insertion of viral-coded proteins into the plasma membrane of infected cells often induces profound changes in the interaction of the infected cells with its neighbors. For example, paramyxoviruses, herpesviruses, and some retroviruses (most notably HIV) can cause cell fusion between infected cells and adjacent noninfected cells, thereby producing distinctive polykaryotic giant cells known as syncytia. This facilitates the transmission of virus to neighboring cells.

LATENT AND PERSISTENT INFECTIONS

In view of the fact that a virus needs to multiply and survive within an infected host organism, it is not surprising that many viruses have evolved mechanisms that allow them to persist even in the face of a strong host immune response. For the virologist, understanding the mechanisms of latency and viral persistence is a particular challenge, because, in most cases, apparent evidence of virus multiplication within the host disappears after the initial primary infection, leaving the investigator little to study. Nonetheless, careful manipulation of virus-infected cell cultures, the use of animal model systems, and molecular detective work looking for traces of virus replication have begun to shed light on this complicated process. Three of the better studied examples of latent and persistent infections are discussed here.

Latent Infection

Members of the herpesvirus family provide clinically important examples of viruses that seemingly disappear after a primary infection, often early in life, only to be reactivated months or years later. Although the factors leading to reactivation of these viruses remain largely uncharacterized, with the exception of the involvement of immune suppression, information about the events leading to the establishment of latency is rapidly accumulating. In the case of herpes simplex types 1 and 2 and varicella-zoster viruses, the virus, after primary infection of the skin or mucous membranes, travels up peripheral nerves to the sensory ganglia. There, the virus remains, probably as unintegrated, episomal DNA with no evidence of virus replication. However, if such ganglion cells are cocultivated in vitro with susceptible cells, the viral DNA can be triggered to replicate, with ensuing virus production. In the case of many latent herpes simplex virus infections, periodic virus replication occurs. During this reactivation, the virus migrates down the peripheral nerves and establishes recurrent lesions at or near the site of the primary infection. This usually gives rise to cold sores in the case of HSV1 and genital sores in the case of HSV2. In the case of varicella-zoster virus, a similar reactivation of virus that has remained dormant after a primary chickenpox can cause herpes zoster (shingles), usually in the abdominal area. The site of reactivation depends on the innervation area of the ganglia in which the latent infection originally was established.

Two other members of the herpesvirus family, cytomegalovirus and Epstein-Barr virus, also are known to establish latent lifelong infections once a primary infection has occurred. In these instances, the viruses reside in a latent state in monocytes and macrophages (cytomegalovirus) or in B lymphocytes (Epstein-Barr virus). Reactivation of these infections often is seen in immunosuppressed

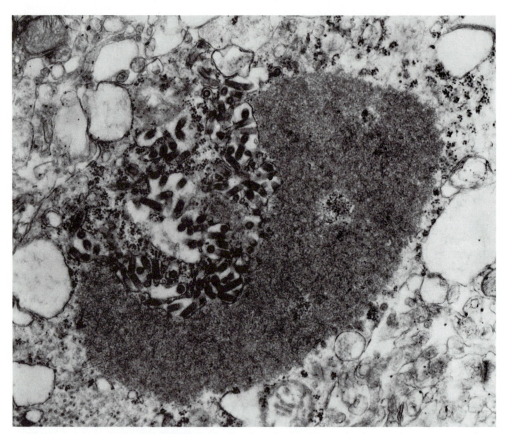

FIGURE 39-6   Rabies virus inclusion body in fox brain tissue. Note the individual virions close to the inclusion. (Original magnification ×50,000.)

individuals (eg, transplant recipients and persons with the acquired immunodeficiency syndrome).

Chronic Infections

The continued production of virus over months and even years is a hallmark of a chronic virus infection, the prime example being hepatitis B virus. Such infections can continue in the absence of overt clinical disease, and affected persons can transmit the virus to a naive recipient (ie, through blood transfusions). In the case of hepatitis B infection, the carrier state is established by the persistent infection of a population of hepatocytes and is characterized by the presence of viral antigens and infectious virus in the bloodstream. Chronic infections, although usually clinically inapparent for many years, can lead to more serious consequences, such as cirrhosis or hepatocellular carcinoma in the case of hepatitis B.

Slow Progressive Infection

A prime example of slow progressive infection is subacute sclerosing panencephalitis, a disease that occurs between 1 and 10 years after recovery from a primary measles virus infection. Although rare (1 in 1 million cases of measles), this is a feared complication because it is invariably lethal. The disease is characterized by high antibody levels in the cerebrospinal fluid to some of the measles virus proteins. Evidence suggests that in the final stages of subacute sclerosing panencephalitis, most infected cells in the central nervous system synthesize readily detectable levels of viral positive- and negative-strand RNA. In addition, the infected cells contain measles nucleocapsids but lack a specific viral protein, the matrix protein. The apparent constraint of virus expression thus appears to result from the lack of a viral protein (the matrix protein) required for virus maturation. This impaired virus assembly seems to permit the persistence of the virus in the face of the host's immune response, allowing slow virus spread, most likely by cell–cell fusion.

Other examples of slow progressive diseases caused by viruses are progressive multifocal leukoencephalopathy, a rare complication of a human polyomavirus infection, and a variety of diseases caused by the lentivirus subfamily of retroviruses. Of major importance in recent years have been persistent infections caused by HIV. HIV infections produce severe immune deficiency 1 to 10 years or longer after the initial infection. More is said about these viruses later, in the discussion of the Retroviridae.

CELL TRANSFORMATION

Infection of cells with certain RNA or DNA viruses does not result in lytic infection and cell death, but instead leads to an alteration in the growth properties of these cells. Such alterations in growth properties frequently are manifested by the formation of a tumor if the virus is used to infect an animal. In infected cell cultures, alterations in morphology, growth properties, and cellular metabolism are observed. Collectively, these changes are referred to as *cellular transformation*. Transformation is a direct result of the expression of one or more viral genes.

Because these differences arise from the expression of viral genetic information within the transformed cell, the changes are passed on to the infected cell's progeny when the cell divides. Some of the biologic and biochemical consequences of viral transformation are summarized later. In subsequent chapters, the role of individual viruses in this process is discussed.

Persistence of Viral DNA

The persistence of all or part of the viral genome in the host cell is required to initiate the events leading to transformation. In most cases, such persistence also is required for maintenance of the transformed state. This usually is achieved by a process of genetic recombination, resulting in the integration of viral genes into the host chromosome. For some viruses (eg, many DNA tumor viruses), this occurs as a chance event at a low frequency (1 in 10^4 to 10^5 cells) and relies on host cellular processes. In other cases (retroviruses), the process of viral DNA integration is a regular part of the virus replication and is catalyzed by specific viral enzymes. This leads to a high frequency of cellular transformation. In the case of some viruses (Epstein-Barr virus and papillomaviruses), the viral genome can persist in a free episomal state in transformed cells.

The extent of expression of viral information varies widely from cell to cell, depending on the virus and the host cell. However, for most transformed cells, the prerequisite intervention of the virus is revealed by the presence of viral DNA, viral mRNA, and viral-encoded proteins. It has been speculated that certain viruses (eg, herpesviruses) can actively initiate events leading to transformation and, having triggered the process, silently leave the doomed cell. Such hit-and-run mechanisms may be common in the etiology of virus-associated human cancers.

Morphology and Altered Growth Properties

Transformation of cells results in pronounced and varied changes in cell morphology. Whereas normal cells grow in consistently oriented patterns, transformed cells orient themselves randomly and are more rounded and refractile.

In cell culture, normal cells grow only to a certain density. For example, adherent cells growing in a tissue culture flask or plate continue to divide only until they form a confluent single cell layer (a monolayer). Confluency serves as a signal to the normal cell to cease cell division. Density-dependent inhibition reflects mechanisms needed to ensure orderly growth in the host. Transformed cells exhibit loss of such density-dependent inhibition (ie, transformed cells continue to divide and pile up on each other after reaching confluency). This process leads to the overt overgrowth of transformed cells.

All cells require factors present in serum for growth in culture. However, transformed cells usually need much lower levels of serum to sustain growth compared to their normal counterparts. This reduced dependence of transformed cells on growth factors present in serum often is due to the fact that transformed cells produce their own growth factors, providing autocrine growth stimulation.

ANCHORAGE-INDEPENDENT GROWTH AND TUMORIGENICITY. In contrast to normal cells, many transformed cells form colonies of cells in semisolid agar. This property of *anchorage independence* goes hand in hand with other alterations of growth properties. Such transformed cells generally form tumors when inoculated into syngeneic or immunologically deficient animals, such as athymic nude mice. Transformed cells exhibit a broad spectrum of growth properties in animals, particularly variations in invasiveness and the ability to form metastases.

Biochemical and Genetic Changes in Transformed Cells

Transformed cells exhibit wide and variable alterations in biochemical properties. The changes can include alterations in membrane transport, acquisition of new surface components, alterations in plasma membrane components, alterations in cyclic nucleotide levels, increased secretion of certain proteases, and alterations in cytoskeletal matrix components. Transformed cells also typically show alterations in their karyotype; these include deletions, duplication, and amplification of portions of their chromosomes. Translocations and duplications of entire chromosomes often are observed.

In summary, transformation gives rise to profound alterations of growth properties, cellular metabolism, and genetic content. How viruses mediate these many and diverse effects is one of the most basic and important questions in cell biology.

HOST RESPONSE TO VIRUS INFECTION

Interferon-Type Interference

Virus infection of cells often leads to the production and secretion of substances (termed *interferons*) that protect uninfected cells from a broad spectrum of viruses. Interferon-mediated resistance is the result of the production of a family of proteins encoded in the genome of the infected animal cell. This type of interference originally was described when it was discovered that allantoic fluid obtained from a chicken embryo infected with influenza virus could prevent the subsequent infection of uninfected chicken embryos. Interferons later were shown to be soluble proteins produced by cells infected with a variety of animal and human viruses.

An important property of interferon is that it is not virus specific; rather, it is host-species specific. This means that interferon produced by chicken embryo cells infected with influenza virus is effective in preventing the infection of other chicken embryo cells with almost any virus. On the other hand, interferon produced in a mouse is effective in protecting other mice from a virus infection, but is of little value when used with chicken or human cells. In fact, interferons from different host cells vary in their molecular weight as well as in other physical properties. Thus, the generalization can be made that interferon inhibits viral replication most effectively in the species in which it was produced, but that it is nonspecific with respect to the types of viruses it can inhibit.

TYPES OF INTERFERON. Interferons originally were named according to the cell type from which they were produced (ie, leukocyte interferon, fibroblast interferon, and immune interferon [also called *T-cell interferon*]). The current classification is based on antigenic differences among the interferons, as shown in Table 39-2.

Molecular cloning and DNA sequencing of the human interferon genes revealed that the interferons are encoded by a structurally related multigene complex. Fourteen distinct human α-interferon genes have been identified, as well as single genes for β-interferon and γ-interferon. DNA sequence analysis has shown that the α-interferon subtypes are structurally related, sharing 80% to 95% sequence homology. In contrast, β-interferon and γ-interferon are more distantly related, sharing only about 30% to 40% sequence homology with α-interferon. Most of the mature human α-interferon subtypes and β-interferon are 166 amino acids in length and contain a 20– to 23–amino acid signal peptide, which is cleaved after translation.

INDUCTION OF INTERFERON. The synthesis of α- and β-interferon occurs when a cell becomes infected with a virus. Essentially any virus is effective, although the amount of interferon induced varies, depending on both the cell line and the individual virus used. The properties shared by the wide array of interferon-inducing viruses are not understood; however, double-stranded RNA alone can act as an efficient inducer of interferon synthesis. Moreover, an excellent inducer of interferon is a synthetic polynucleotide called *poly-rI: poly-rC (poly-IC)*. This is a small, double-stranded RNA molecule consisting of paired homopolymer strands of polyriboinosinic acid (poly-rI) and its complementary base, polyribocytidylic acid (poly-rC). It generally is believed that double-stranded RNA plays a role, perhaps being the actual inducer of interferon synthesis during a viral infection.

γ-Interferon can be differentiated from type I interferons serologically and by the observation that it is destroyed rapidly at a pH level of 2, whereas α- and β-interferon are stable at that level. Induction of γ-interferon follows the addition of an antigen to which the cells have been sensitized, such as the addition of tuberculin to T cells from a tuberculin-positive individual. γ-Interferon also can be induced by the addition of a

TABLE 39-2
Physiochemical Properties of Human Interferons (IFNs)

Property	Interferon		
	α	β	γ
Previous designations	Le-IFN	F-IFN	Immune IFN
Subtypes	14	1	1
Principal source	Epithelium, leukocytes	Fibroblasts	Lymphocyte
Molecular weight*			
Major subtypes	16,000–23,000	23,000	20,000–25,000
Glycosylation	No†	Yes	Yes
pH 2 stability	Stable†	Stable	Labile
Induction	Viruses	Viruses	Mitogens
Introns in gene	No	No	Yes
Homology with Hu-IFN-α	80%–95%	30%–50%	<10%

* Molecular weight of monomeric form. Interferons often occur as polymers.

† Most subtypes, but not all.

mitogen (which causes the cells to divide) such as endotoxin or phytohemagglutinin to normal, unprimed T cells.

The overall importance of γ-interferon is not clear, but it has been shown to regulate natural killer cell activity and to enhance macrophage activation. Moreover, individuals with autoimmune diseases, such as systemic lupus erythematosus and rheumatic fever, have been shown to have γ-interferon in their serum. Thus, γ-interferon can be considered to be a lymphokine that exerts a protective effect by regulation of nonspecific host immunity.

MECHANISM OF ANTIVIRAL EFFECT. Interferon is secreted in minute amounts by the virus-infected cell. It is inactive against viruses in cell-free extracts, and only after it enters or reacts with a cell can it exert its antiviral activity. It is now known that interferon induces the formation of at least three enzymes: (1) a 2′, 5′-oligoadenylate synthetase; (2) ribonuclease L; and (3) a protein kinase. These enzymes are detected in cells within 2 to 6 hours after treatment with interferon, and they reach peak activity within 15 to 30 hours. A fourth protein, induced by α- and β-interferon treatment of mouse cells, appears to reside in the nucleus and inhibit influenza virus mRNA synthesis.

INTERFERON-INDUCED 2′, 5′-OLIGOADENYLATE SYNTHESIS AND ACTIVATION OF RIBONUCLEASE L. This unusual nucleotide synthesized by interferon-induced 2′, 5′-oligoadenylate synthetase contains 2′, 5′-phosphodiester bonds and is designated as pppA(2′p5′A)n, where n can be three or more. The synthetase is active only when bound to double-stranded RNA. After the oligoadenylate is synthesized, it acts as a positive effector to activate an inactive endonuclease, ribonuclease L. The activated endonuclease then catalyzes the degradation of viral and host-cell mRNA. It should be noted that double-stranded RNA is both an inducer of interferon and a necessary factor for the activation of two different enzymes involved in virus inactivation.

INTERFERON-INDUCED PROTEIN KINASE. Interferon-induced protein kinase catalyzes the phosphorylation of one protein initiation factor known as eIF-2. The protein kinase is active only in the presence of double-stranded RNA; however, after phosphorylation of this protein, translation of viral mRNA is greatly reduced. Much work remains before the mechanisms of interferon action can be delineated, although evidence has shown that interferon activity is pleiotropic in nature and likely exerts its activity on several molecular pathways.

CLINICAL USES OF INTERFERON. Human interferons have been purified to homogeneity from human cells and from bacteria and yeasts expressing genetically engineered human interferon genes. Although each method of production has advantages and disadvantages, the net result is that significantly large amounts of interferon are available for clinical trials. Interferon normally is administered intramuscularly or intravenously. Unfortunately, the half-life of both α- and β-interferon is short after intravenous injection. Toxic side effects are observed regularly, even when low doses of highly purified interferon are administered. Fever is a common side effect, but it lasts only a day or so. Severe fatigue also is common and can be accompanied by malaise, anorexia, myalgia, headache, nausea, vomiting, weight loss, erythema, reversible partial alopecia, dry mouth, reversible peripheral sensory neuropathy, or central nervous system signs. Interferon administration often leads to an antiinterferon response. It is now apparent that this is a common development in patients receiving human α- and β-interferon, although the short- or long-term clinical significance of such antibodies remains to be established.

The clinical efficacy of interferon treatment is the subject of much discussion. Some of the clinical conditions against which interferon appears to show some promise of success are summarized here.

Reports have indicated that interferon delivered by intranasal aerosol spray confers protection against rhinovirus-induced colds. Other studies using human α-interferon produced in *Escherichia coli* confirmed that colds can be prevented by intranasal installation of interferon in high dosage at frequent intervals before exposure to the virus. In spite of such encouraging news, this approach to chemoprophylaxis may be impractical for routine prevention of the common cold.

Interferon may play an important role in the treatment of specific viral diseases. Certain herpesvirus infections, chronic hepatitis B, and asymptomatic hepatitis appear amenable to prolonged therapy with high doses of α- or β-interferon. Interferon also has proved extremely useful in the treatment of juvenile laryngeal papilloma, a severe recurrent viral condition that normally requires repeated surgical therapy. However, these benign tumors tend to recur after withdrawal of interferon treatment. Interferon also has been used successfully to treat other types of human papillomavirus, including common warts and genital warts. In addition, rabies virus infections appear to be amenable to treatment with interferon. Animal studies clearly show that interferon is effective in protecting animals after challenge with rabies virus. Many lethal viral diseases of humans may prove to be vulnerable to interferon treatment. The increased availability of natural and genetically engineered interferon should greatly hasten our understanding of the role of interferon in the treatment of viral diseases.

The value of interferon in the treatment of cancer remains to be firmly established. Several groups have reported promising results using interferon to treat osteosarcoma, multiple myeloma, Hodgkin's disease, and acute leukemia. Partial regression of metastatic breast carcinoma, multiple myeloma, and malignant (non-

Hodgkin's) lymphoma was reported in an uncontrolled pilot study using leukocyte interferon. However, several other carefully conducted trials have yielded less encouraging results. It is too soon to declare definitively the importance of interferon in the treatment of viral infections and cancer, although evidence does indicate that interferon treatment alters the course of several viral diseases and has demonstrable effects on certain types of cancers. In addition, it has been shown that treatment with β-interferon slows the progression of multiple sclerosis in some patients. Continual research and clinical trials undoubtedly will establish the efficacy of interferon as a modern chemotherapeutic agent.

Immune Response to Viral Infection

VIRAL VACCINES

Because viral capsids are made of protein, and because viral envelopes contain both viral proteins and glycoproteins, it is not surprising that most viral infections induce immunologic responses. These responses usually include the production of specific antibodies directed against various virus components, as well as the induction of cytotoxic T cells capable of recognizing and killing virus-infected cells. The specific responses that are generated in the case of different viruses are discussed in more detail in the following chapters. The capacity of the host to generate these specific responses against viral antigens can be used to protect against viral disease using different kinds of vaccines. These vaccines usually contain either inactivated virus particles or live, attenuated (mutant) viruses, which still possess the same antigenic properties as the virulent virus, but have lost the ability to produce disease. Many novel approaches to vaccine development have been introduced. No longer do we have a simple choice between live or killed vaccine—modern molecular biology has revolutionized our thinking about vaccine development. Recombinant DNA technology has provided a means of synthesizing large amounts of individual viral gene products, an advance that provides readily available viral components for immunization. Such approaches to modern vaccine technology are discussed in later chapters.

Bibliography

JOURNALS

Ho H. Interferon for the treatment of infections. Annu Rev Med 1987;38:51.

Tyrrell DAJ. Interferons and their clinical value. Rev Infect Dis 1987;9:243.

BOOK

White DO. Antiviral chemotherapy, interferons and vaccines. Basel, Karger, 1984.

Essentials of Medical Microbiology, Fifth Edition, edited by Wesley A. Volk,
Bryan M. Gebhardt, Marie-Louise Hammarskjöld, and Robert J. Kadner.
Lippincott-Raven Publishers, Philadelphia © 1996.

Chapter 40

Herpesviridae

The Herpesviridae are a large group of viruses found widely throughout the animal kingdom. The property that most herpesviruses share is their ability to induce latent infections. Such infections can be reactivated after months or years, producing identical symptoms for each sporadic recurrence, or producing a disease totally unlike the original infection.

Classification

Seven different human herpesviruses have been identified. There also are several additional members of the herpesvirus family that infect different species of animals. Herpesviruses generally show a strict species specificity (ie, human viruses do not infect animals). The nomenclature of the human herpesviruses has evolved haphazardly; varicella-zoster virus (VZV) is named after the disease it causes, Epstein-Barr virus (EBV) is named for its codiscoverers, and cytomegalovirus (CMV) is named to describe the pathology of the infection. The four other human herpesviruses are referred to as herpes simplex viruses type 1 (HSV1) and type 2 (HSV2), and human herpesviruses 6 (HHV6) and 7 (HHV7).

In an attempt to classify the herpesviruses on the basis of their biologic properties and host ranges, the International Committee on Taxonomy of Viruses has established three subfamilies; Table 40-1 shows how the common human herpesviruses fit into this classification. In general, alpha herpesviruses have a variable host range and a short replicative cycle, and are cytopathic on host cells. Beta herpesviruses show a more narrow host range and a longer replicative cycle, resulting in less of a cytopathic effect, whereas gamma herpesviruses have a narrow host range and infect lymphocytes, often inducing a self-limiting transformation.

In humans, herpesvirus infections can cause several different diseases. Among the more common manifestations are fever blisters or cold sores (which can involve the eye) caused by HSV, and varicella (chickenpox) and zoster (shingles) caused by VZV. CMV can cause congenital defects in newborns and severe disease in immunosuppressed individuals. EBV causes infectious mononucleosis

TABLE 40-1
Members of the Family Herpesviridae

Virus	Subfamily	Primary Infections	Recurrent Infections
Herpes simplex virus 1	Alpha	Gingivostomatitis	Herpes labialis
		Keratoconjunctivitis	Keratoconjunctivitis
		Eczema herpeticum	Cutaneous herpes
		Meningoencephalitis	Encephalitis
Herpes simplex virus 2	Alpha	Genital infections	Genital infections
		Neonatal infections	—
Varicella-zoster virus	Alpha	Varicella	Zoster
Cytomegalovirus	Beta	Congenital cytomegalic inclusion disease	—
		Mononucleosis	
Epstein-Barr virus	Gamma	Mononucleosis	
		Hepatitis	—
Human herpesvirus 6	—	Exanthem subitum	—
Human herpesvirus 7	—	?	?

(IM), a disease seen mainly in adolescents and young adults. HHV6, which was identified only recently, has been shown to be the cause of exanthem subitum, a usually mild childhood disease. In recent years, genital herpes, a sexually transmitted disease caused by HSV2, has become a worldwide problem. There also is evidence that EBV plays an etiologic role in the induction of some human cancers (ie, Burkitt's lymphoma, Hodgkin's lymphoma, nasopharyngeal carcinoma). In addition, EBV has been shown to be linked to many cases of lymphoma in immunosuppressed individuals (eg, transplant recipients, patients with the acquired immunodeficiency syndrome [AIDS]).

Structure

Herpesviruses contain linear double-stranded DNA. The icosahedral virus particle is surrounded by an envelope acquired as the virion buds from the nuclear membrane of the host cell (Fig. 40-1). The diameter of the enveloped virion is 150 to 200 nm, whereas that of the naked capsid is about 100 nm. The capsids of all herpesviruses are made up of 162 capsomers. The molecular weight of the DNA from different herpesviruses varies from 130 to 220 kilobases. The DNA sequences of several human herpesviruses have been completely determined.

Herpes Simplex Virus

DNA STRUCTURE

The DNA of HSV possesses unique structural features not found in the DNA of other viruses. If the 3′ ends of the double-stranded DNA are partially digested with DNA exonuclease III, subsequent annealing will result in the formation of double-stranded circles, indicating the

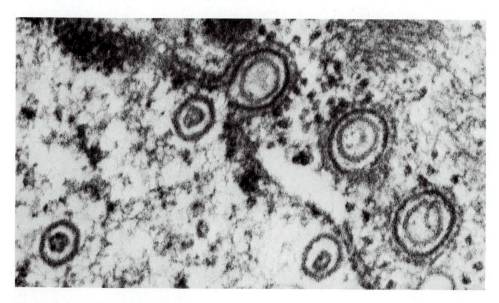

FIGURE 40-1 Virions of herpesvirus acquire an envelope as they bud through a nuclear envelope. To the left in the nucleus are icosahedral capsids containing DNA; viruses in the cytoplasm to the right are enveloped after budding. In this section, one bud has not yet pinched off from the nuclear envelope. (Original magnification ×100,000.)

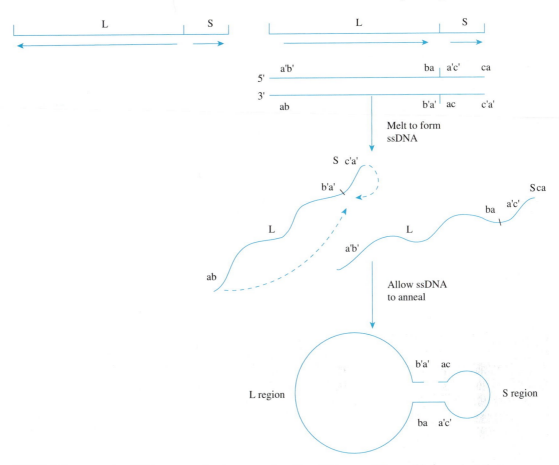

FIGURE 40-2 Herpesvirus DNA structure showing two regions (*L* and *S*) in two of the possible four orientations. The internal inverted repeats are detected by denaturing the DNA and allowing the single-stranded DNA to reanneal. Base pairing between the terminal bases and the internal repeats leads to the formation of a double circle that can be visualized in the electron microscope.

presence of terminally redundant sequences. However, if HSV DNA is denatured and the single strands are allowed to reanneal, some of the DNA will form circles stabilized by the formation of a short stretch of double-stranded DNA. Such forms result from the presence of internal sequences complementary to the terminally redundant sequences (Fig. 40-2). The biologic significance of the internal reiterated sequences is unclear, because mutants of HSV lacking such sequences replicate efficiently. The HSV genome is made up of two separate regions of DNA, which can exist in different orientation relative to one another. Each of these regions possesses unique sequences as well as terminally and internally repeated sequences. The longer of the two regions has been designated L and constitutes 82% of the DNA, and the shorter region has been designated S and contains the remainder of the molecule (see Fig. 40-2). Because of the capacity of the L and S segments to invert during replication, the DNA extracted from a single virus plaque consists of four populations, each exhibiting a different orientation of the L and S regions relative to one another.

REPLICATION

Attachment of a herpesvirus particle to a host cell will occur at 4°C; however, subsequent penetration of the virion requires energy and results in a virus-induced fusion of the viral envelope with the cell membrane. This event releases the naked capsid into the cytoplasm. The exact nature of the cellular receptor is not known.

Relatively little is known about the uncoating or initial processing of the herpesvirus capsid, but the transcription of viral DNA and the final assembly of new nucleocapsids occur in the nucleus of the host cell. The time course of virus replication varies depending on the nature of the host cell and the multiplicity of virus infection. The initial transcription of the viral DNA is catalyzed by cellular DNA-dependent RNA polymerase II that transcribes mRNAs from a limited set of viral genes known as alpha genes (Fig. 40-3). The initial transcription is directed to the regions containing alpha genes with the help of a virally encoded protein known as VP16 that is present in the virion. VP16 associates with cellular transcription factors, and the complex specifically binds to

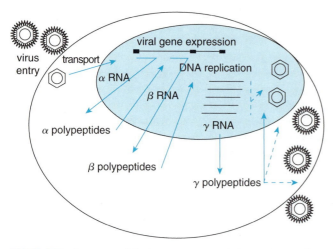

FIGURE 40-3   Summary of the important events in herpesvirus replication. See text for details.

DNA sequences upstream of the alpha promoters, leading to the induction of transcription. The alpha genes are distributed throughout the genome, including the repeated regions. The alpha mRNAs encode a set of proteins referred to as immediate early, or alpha, proteins. The alpha proteins all appear to play a role in the regulation of viral gene expression. The synthesis of alpha proteins is required for the transcription of a second set of genes, beta genes, which encode a class of mRNAs that are translated into early, or beta, proteins. Alpha genes can be transcribed in the absence of protein synthesis, but the transcription of beta genes requires the synthesis of alpha-gene products. Many of the beta proteins are involved in and necessary for viral DNA replication. The beta proteins identified thus far include a DNA polymerase, a thymidine kinase, and a DNA-binding protein. Most of the genes encoding alpha and beta proteins have been mapped within the HSV genome, and the mecha-

nisms that regulate the viral expression cascade are under intense investigation.

The final steps in HSV replication depend on viral DNA synthesis. The synthesis and translation of late viral mRNAs results in the formation of the gamma proteins, which consist mainly of structural proteins. The structural proteins are transported back into the nucleus, where they self-assemble to form empty capsids. Head-to-tail concatemeric DNA, the product of viral DNA replication, then is cleaved into genome-size DNA and inserted into the capsid shells, and maturation proceeds through budding of the viral nucleocapsid at the nuclear membrane of the cell. Several virally encoded glycoproteins present in the virion are inserted into both the nuclear and the plasma membrane of the host cell.

Curiously, even though the plasma membrane of an infected cell contains viral glycoprotein, the nucleocapsid derives its envelope as it buds through the inner lamina of the cell's nuclear membrane. The virus particles then are enclosed within a vacuole that traverses the Golgi and finally fuses with the plasma membrane to release the virus particles. A single cell can produce as many as 10,000 infectious particles. The production of virus results in the eventual death of the host cell. Herpesvirus replication is shown schematically in Figure 40-3.

Herpes Simplex Virus Infections in Humans

Herpes simplex virus infections in humans are caused by two antigenically distinct viruses. HSV1 is characteristically responsible for oral infections (Fig. 40-4), whereas HSV2 normally is associated with genital tract infections. Less than 1% of all primary HSV infections are clinically overt. However, a latent infection is regularly established even when the primary infection is asymptomatic. About 25% of all individuals with latent HSV infections eventu-

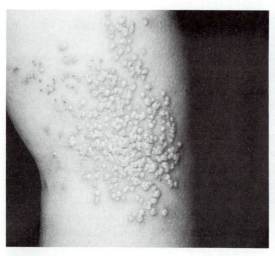 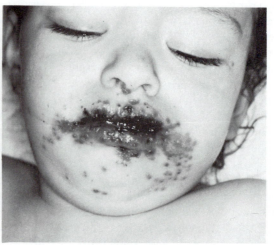

FIGURE 40-4   Herpes fever blisters on the left (*left*), and on the lips and face (*right*).

ally exhibit symptoms of recurrent infections. Infection with HSV1 frequently occurs early in life, with antibodies prevalent in 30% to 100% of adults, depending largely on socioeconomic status. HSV2 infections occur coincident with increased sexual activity and their incidence has risen dramatically in recent years. The major clinical syndromes associated with HSV infections are summarized.

HERPES SIMPLEX VIRUS TYPE 1

Gingivostomatitis

The primary infection often causes no symptoms and usually is undiagnosed; however, about 15% of primary infections are manifested by an acute gingivostomatitis in which the gums become red and swollen, and multiple ulcerated lesions occur on the membranes of the mouth. The lesions also can involve the tonsils, pharynx, or nose. Infectious virus can be isolated from the lesions. The disease generally is self-limiting, and lesions disappear in 2 to 3 weeks.

Eczema Herpeticum and Traumatic Herpes

More serious primary infections can occur if the virus infects multiple sites on the skin of a person with eczema. This can cause the loss of large areas of epithelium, resulting in the subsequent loss of body fluids and the development of secondary bacterial infections. Traumatic (wound) herpes can result from infection of an open injury. Such infections occur most frequently on the fingers and are an occupational hazard for dentists, physicians, and nurses.

Meningoencephalitis

Herpetic encephalitis in adults is probably the most devastating disease produced by HSV1 and represents the most common cause of fatal, sporadic encephalitis in the United States (one case per million population per year). The virus produces necrotic lesions (areas of dead cells) in localized areas of the brain, frequently causing death or residual neurologic abnormalities such as partial paralysis, mental retardation, or abnormal behavior patterns. Herpetic encephalitis can occur after a primary infection; however, most patients have a previous history of HSV1 infections, indicating that the encephalitis is a result of the reactivation of a latent infection.

Keratoconjunctivitis

Infection of the eye by HSV1 causes an extremely painful ulceration of the cornea. It is estimated that this virus infects the eyes of 275,000 Americans each year. In most cases, the primary lesions heal within 2 to 3 weeks. However, recurrent keratitis can result in severe corneal ulcers

and is a frequent cause of corneal blindness in the United States.

Latent and Recurrent Infections

Recovery from a primary infection by HSV frequently is followed by an asymptomatic latent infection. During latency, the virus appears to be harbored in the nervous system within the sensory ganglion cells (Fig. 40-5). In animals infected with virus, or in seropositive cadavers, the virus cannot be detected in ganglia at the time of autopsy; however, virus subsequently can be rescued when the ganglia are cocultivated in cell culture with susceptible cells. Such results, as well as molecular biologic studies of infected ganglia, support the concept that the herpesvirus DNA exists in a sequestered (episomal) form within the infected ganglion.

Even after latency has been established, it is likely that small amounts of infectious virus are produced sporadically, because the virus occasionally can be isolated from oral secretions, and humoral antibody levels remain high. In some individuals, the latent virus never manifests itself clinically. Other patients experience more or less frequent bouts of recurrent herpes lesions (cold sores). The molecular events that trigger secondary recurrent disease are unknown. It is well established that reactivation frequently follows fever, menstruation, emotional stress, or exposure to sunlight. The most common signs of reactivation are clusters of vesicles at the mucocutaneous junction of the lips. These vesicles contain infectious virus. Recurrent herpes also can occur in the nose or eyes, or on areas of the skin that have experienced a primary infection.

Patients with defects in cellular immune functions or those who are immunosuppressed as a consequence of organ transplants or immunosuppressive diseases (eg, AIDS) are much more likely to have chronic herpetic ulcers or severe disseminated herpetic infections, particularly of the skin or respiratory tract.

HERPES SIMPLEX VIRUS TYPE 2

Herpes simplex virus type 2 causes one of the most prevalent forms of sexually transmitted disease. Primary infections can be asymptomatic but frequently are associated with fever, malaise, and tender, swollen regional lymph nodes. In women, lesions can occur on the perineum, vagina, cervix, or vulva, producing symptoms of burning, itching, and severe pain during urination. In men, lesions can occur on the glans, prepuce, or shaft of the penis. Although 70% to 90% of genital herpes is caused by HSV2, an increasing number of HSV1 infections are being reported. HSV2 also can be involved in oral infections. In addition, HSV2 establishes latent infections in neuronal ganglia and frequently reactivates to cause recurrent genital sores.

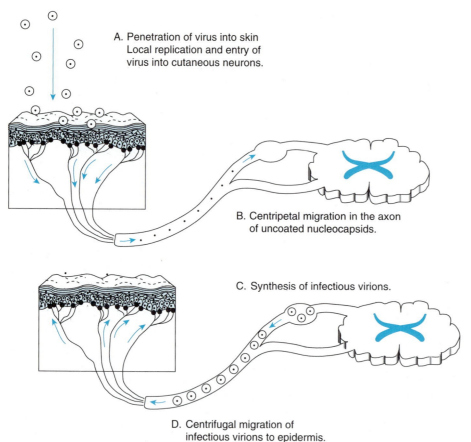

A. Penetration of virus into skin
Local replication and entry of
virus into cutaneous neurons.

B. Centripetal migration in the axon
of uncoated nucleocapsids.

C. Synthesis of infectious virions.

D. Centrifugal migration of
infectious virions to epidermis.

FIGURE 40-5   Diagram of the pathogenesis of primary and recurrent herpes simplex virus infection.

Neonatal Herpesvirus Infections

Childbirth during a primary or recurrent HSV2 infection can result in an unusually severe infection in the newborn during the first month of life. Such infections frequently are fatal; those who survive can have residual damage of the central nervous system or the eyes, although current evidence also indicates that HSV2 infections of the newborn sometimes cause no symptoms. In addition, HSV2 infections during pregnancy can result in spontaneous abortions or congenital defects.

Herpes Simplex Virus Type 2 Infections and Cervical Cancer

Herpes simplex virus type 2 infections have been linked to cervical cancer, one of the most common malignancies of the female reproductive organs. Antibodies to HSV2 have been found in a much higher percentage of women with cervical carcinoma than in appropriate control groups. However, conflicting data are accumulating, casting doubt on the significance of the link between HSV2 infection and cervical carcinoma. It has been established that other sexually transmitted viruses, namely papillomaviruses, play a much more important role in the etiology of this malignancy.

LABORATORY DIAGNOSIS OF HERPES SIMPLEX VIRUS INFECTIONS

Herpes simplex virus can be readily isolated from the herpetic lesions and from the saliva during a primary infection. Small amounts of virus also can be excreted during asymptomatic periods. The virus can be grown in several different cell lines, but it is propagated routinely in primary human embryonic kidney or human amnion cells. Cytopathic effects include the presence of intranuclear inclusion bodies and the formation of multinucleated giant cells. Skin scrapings from herpetic lesions reveal similar giant cells and inclusion bodies.

New approaches to the identification of herpesvirus infections have used virus-specific monoclonal antibodies and virus-specific DNA probes. Biopsy material can reveal herpesviruses when it is stained with fluorescence labeled antibodies or analyzed with labeled DNA probes. Such techniques are particularly important when a rapid diagnosis is essential, as in herpesvirus meningoencephalitis. Primary infections lead to a marked increase in antibody titer. In contrast, a recurrent infection may not result in an increase in antibody levels, making traditional serology difficult.

TREATMENT OF HERPES SIMPLEX VIRUS INFECTIONS

Several drugs, including 5-iodo-2′-deoxyuridine and adenine arabinoside (ara-A), have been used with some success in the treatment of herpes keratitis, although drug-resistant mutants can arise. However, these drugs have been disappointingly unsuccessful in the treatment of skin and mucous membrane lesions. Ara-A has been licensed by the US Food and Drug Administration for the treatment of herpes meningoencephalitis. Such treatment appears to be moderately successful, particularly if it is started early in the infection. It also has been used for neonatal disseminated HSV infections and for progressive infections in immunosuppressed patients. The successful use of acyclovir to treat herpesvirus infection has diminished the use of ara-A (see later).

The most recent drug to be licensed for use in treating HSV infections is acyclovir (9-[[2 hydroxyethoxy] methyl]guanine). Acyclovir is phosphorylated by a herpesvirus thymidine kinase, and its triphosphate analogue inhibits herpesvirus DNA polymerase without blocking the function of the host-cell DNA polymerases. Acyclovir has been licensed in the United States for the treatment of primary genital herpes infections and mucocutaneous infections in immunosuppressed patients. Intravenous acyclovir has been used to treat herpes encephalitis. Acyclovir is not effective against latent HSV infections, but will suppress recurrences in patients with frequent episodes of infection. Unfortunately, cases of acyclovir-resistant HSV have been reported, and it is likely that widespread use of acyclovir will make such strains more common.

Varicella-Zoster Virus

Varicella (chickenpox) is principally a disease of childhood, characterized by pock-type lesions (raised skin lesions containing fluid) occurring over essentially the entire body surface. Zoster (shingles) is a disease of adults characterized by similar pock-type lesions. However, these are restricted to an area of the skin supplied by the sensory nerves of a single dorsal root ganglion or a small group of ganglia in which the virus previously established a latent infection. Both diseases are caused by the same virus, and zoster has been shown to represent a reactivation of a latent chickenpox infection in an immune individual.

REPLICATION

Varicella-zoster virus is morphologically similar to HSV1 and HSV2. It can be propagated in human diploid fibroblast cells. Varicella occurs worldwide, usually in children and frequently in epidemics during the winter and spring. The virus probably is acquired by the respiratory route and, during an incubation period of 14 to 16 days, it multiplies in the respiratory tract and the regional lymph nodes. It then is released into the bloodstream and disseminated throughout the body. Fever, headache, and malaise are the usual symptoms that precede a maculopapular rash (one that contains flat discolorations and spots elevated above the level of the skin in the same area). The rash develops into vesicles that eventually form scabs, which, in the absence of secondary bacterial infection, heal without leaving a scar. A prominent characteristic of the lesions of chickenpox is that they occur in crops (ie, new lesions begin to develop in the same areas where older lesions are crusting over and healing). Neutralizing antibodies to the virus can be detected about 1 week after the rash, and recovery usually is complete 2 weeks after the onset of initial symptoms.

Although varicella generally is a mild disease of childhood, it can be severe in adults or in persons with a defective or suppressed immune response. Meningoencephalitis is a rare complication, with a high fatality rate in all age groups. Varicella pneumonia is encountered frequently as an adult complication.

Zoster is the result of the reactivation of a latent VZV infection and can be seen in patients of all ages. Individuals who have recovered from chickenpox often carry the latent VZV in their ganglionic nerve cells. Activation of the latent virus can occur after physical trauma, tuberculosis, or cancer, but in most cases, the factors that lead to reactivation are unknown. Zoster is relatively common in patients with leukemia or Hodgkin's disease, and in those receiving immunosuppressive drug therapy, suggesting that immune mechanisms play an important role in the prevention of symptomatic reactivation. After activation, the virus travels along a nerve (or nerves) to the skin, where it produces lesions over the area of the skin supplied by the affected nerves. Paralysis can result from infection of the spinal cord, but the more usual prognosis is recovery in 2 to 4 weeks. Children who are exposed to an adult with zoster can develop a typical case of chickenpox, because the zoster lesions contain infectious virus.

DIAGNOSIS OF CHICKENPOX AND ZOSTER

The diagnosis of VZV infections almost always is made on the basis of the characteristic clinical picture. Varicella lesions contain giant cells and cells with typical intranuclear inclusion bodies. In addition, the virus can be grown in cell culture, permitting a positive identification using serologic techniques with known antiserum.

PREVENTION OF VARICELLA-ZOSTER VIRUS INFECTIONS

Live attenuated vaccines have been tested in clinical trials. However, because of the mildness of chickenpox in normal children, these vaccines are more likely to be of value for high-risk or immunocompromised individuals.

Zoster immune globulin, prepared from the serum of patients recovering from zoster, has been shown to be protective if it is administered within 2 to 3 days after exposure to the VZV. Such a procedure is particularly important for children with leukemia or immunodeficiency syndromes, or for patients who are taking immunosuppressive drugs. However, exposure often is not recognized, because an infected individual can spread the virus before clinical symptoms appear. Because the source of infectious virus in zoster is reactivated latent virus, there is no known way to prevent this secondary disease.

Cytomegalovirus

Cytomegaloviruses are typical herpesviruses, both in their structure and in their mode of replication. CMV-infected cells become distinctly enlarged (ie, exhibit cytomegaly) and possess both intranuclear and cytoplasmic inclusion bodies (Fig. 40-6). CMV can be propagated in several human embryonic fibroblast cell lines.

CMV infection is the cause of the most common congenital virus infections and also is the etiologic agent for a serious disease in immunocompromised patients. There is a single serotype of human CMV, although different strains can be identified using restriction endonuclease mapping techniques. Worldwide surveys show that about 80% of adults older than 35 years of age have circulating antibody to the virus. Most infections in immunocompetent individuals appear to be asymptomatic.

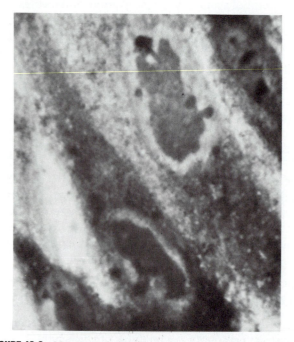

FIGURE 40-6 Numerous dark cytomegalovirus inclusion bodies are evident in these Giemsa-stained human fibroblast cells 3 days after infection. (Original magnification ×3000.)

Evidence indicates that after a primary infection, CMV is excreted in the urine and saliva for long periods, and perhaps for life. Virus can be isolated from over 90% of patients who are receiving immunosuppressive therapy as a consequence of organ transplantation. If the primary infection occurs during pregnancy, the virus is capable of crossing the placenta and infecting the fetus. This can cause either the death of the fetus or a wide variety of congenital defects. Alternatively, it can cause a persistent infection without any immediately obvious defects in the newborn.

Although the congenital effects of CMV are extremely varied, it appears to be the most common viral cause of mental retardation. Estimates indicate that about 1% of all newborn infants are infected with CMV. Most infants do not show obvious abnormalities, but about 10% of those infected in utero develop congenital abnormalities, such as microcephaly (an abnormally small head), central nervous system damage resulting in seizures and deafness, mental retardation, psychomotor retardation, ocular abnormalities, chronic gastroenteritis, jaundice, pneumonia, or thrombocytopenia (lack of thrombocytes). These newborns often show no signs of CMV infection, but have extensive abnormalities that become evident only later in life.

Because the disease in the mother is asymptomatic, it usually is not possible to determine the age at which the fetus became infected. Like other herpesviruses, CMV is believed to produce infections that can persist in a latent state and flare up periodically, resulting in the excretion of infectious virus. Therefore, fetal infection can result from a flare up of CMV during pregnancy, and it appears that endogenous CMV is the most frequent source of intrauterine transmission in immune women. Primary CMV infections of pregnant women also can result in a high incidence of congenital infections, but more babies with intrauterine infections are born to mothers with recurrent CMV infections than to mothers with primary infections. However, primary infections lead to a higher incidence of symptomatic infections, perhaps because maternal antibody present during recurrent infections may modify cell damage in the fetus.

CMV also causes a type of IM in young adults and recipients of blood transfusions. This disease has been named *CMV mononucleosis*. It resembles the classic IM caused by EBV (see later), but apparently does not cause the severe sore throat or the rise in heterophile antibodies usually seen in EBV IM.

Organ transplant recipients who are receiving immunosuppressive drugs to prevent rejection are susceptible to various CMV-induced complications. Numerous studies have reported the isolation of CMV from such patients. In many cases, the problems are caused by a reactivation of a latent infection. Alternatively, patients can acquire primary CMV infections from the transplanted organs or from blood transfusions. Infections can be asymptomatic, or they can cause pneumonia, disseminated infection, and, sometimes, death. Patients with leukemia or lymphoma, particularly children, also are susceptible to CMV disease. In addition, CMV infections are a problem in patients with AIDS.

DIAGNOSIS OF CYTOMEGALOVIRUS INFECTIONS

Cytomegalovirus usually is excreted in the urine of infected patients, and virus isolated from urine or saliva can be grown on human fibroblasts. Infected cells exhibit cytopathic effects, appearing as swollen, rounded cells possessing large intranuclear inclusion bodies. CMV infections also can be diagnosed by measuring the presence of complement-fixing antibodies formed in response to the virus. However, these tests often are not sensitive enough for reliable diagnosis of perinatal infections. Sensitive radioimmunoassay or enzyme-linked immunosorbent assay techniques, as well as nucleic acid hybridization and polymerase chain reaction techniques, frequently are used to confirm a diagnosis. Infected infants often produce IgM antibodies against the virus; such antibodies can be detected using immunologic techniques.

CONTROL OF CYTOMEGALOVIRUS INFECTIONS

Because adult infections usually are asymptomatic, controlling the spread of this virus is difficult. The virus is excreted primarily in the urine and, in some instances, can be sexually transmitted. In addition, blood transfusions containing infected lymphocytes are a frequent source of infection. Therefore, it is important to screen blood for the presence of CMV before giving a transfusion to a seronegative immunosuppressed patient.

Epstein-Barr Virus

Epstein-Barr virus originally was isolated during a search for an etiologic agent for Burkitt's lymphoma, a malignancy originating in the cells of the lymph nodes. In this disease, the lower jaw is the most common site of the tumor, although tumors can occur in the kidneys, liver, ovaries, thyroid, adrenals, or upper jaw.

Burkitt's lymphoma first received worldwide attention in 1958 when Dennis Burkitt reported a large number of cases of lymphoma in children, primarily in certain parts of East Africa. The rarity of the disease elsewhere prompted a search for an infectious agent as the cause of Burkitt's lymphoma. Although no virus was observed in fresh Burkitt's lymphoma tumor cells, continued cultivation of the tumor cells revealed that some cells contained herpes-like virus particles that on subsequent isolation

and characterization proved to be a previously undescribed herpesvirus.

PROPERTIES OF EPSTEIN-BARR VIRUS

Epstein-Barr virus is morphologically and structurally similar to other human herpesviruses. It exhibits a distinctive tropism for human B lymphocytes and certain epithelial cells. This tropism is due to the presence of a specific receptor for the virus on these cells. This receptor is the CD21 or CR2 molecule, which is the receptor for the C3d complement factor. Infection usually is initiated by virus in saliva that infects epithelial cells in the oropharynx. These epithelial cells become productively infected and are killed by the virus. Virus produced in these cells then goes on to infect normal B lymphocytes. Infection of B lymphocytes usually results in a nonproductive viral infection that leads to the transformation and expansion of the infected B-cell population (Fig. 40-7). Unlike normal lymphocytes, which are unable to divide in cell culture without the addition of specific growth factors, cells transformed by EBV can proliferate continuously in regular culture medium. Only a small percentage of the transformed cells ever go on to produce EBV. The isolation and cultivation of a single transformed clone, however, can give rise to a population of cells, some of which are activated to produce EBV. This observation indicates that the transformed cells carry the complete viral genome, but that virus production is restricted in these cells (ie, the virus has established a latent infection). The fact that all EBV-transformed cells actually carry the complete EBV genome has been confirmed by hybridization with labeled DNA probes. In most transformed cells, the EBV genome exists as covalently closed, circular, nonintegrated (episomal) DNA present at 2 to 200 copies per cell. These cells express only a small subset of the viral gene products. The proteins expressed in many latently infected cells include several nuclear proteins (Epstein-Barr nuclear antigens) as well as proteins that are inserted into the membrane of the transformed cells (latent membrane proteins). However, it has been shown that in other cells, only a single gene product (Epstein-Barr nuclear antigen 1) is expressed. This gene product is essential for maintenance of the viral episome. A few transformed cells containing latent viral genomes are activated spontaneously to produce virus. This process can be enhanced by treatment with bromodeoxyuridine or 5-azacytidine.

INFECTIOUS MONONUCLEOSIS

Epstein-Barr virus is the etiologic agent of IM, a benign lymphoproliferative disease. IM is primarily a disease of young adults, in which the usual clinical symptoms are high fever, headache, chills and sweats, fatigue, hepatomegaly and splenomegaly, and a severe sore throat. The

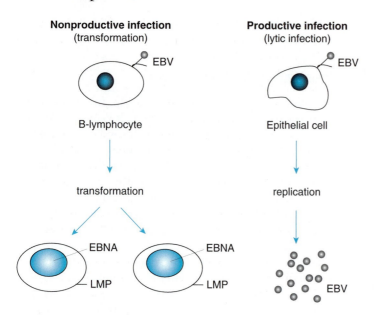

FIGURE 40-7 Pathways of Epstein-Barr virus infection in humans. See text for details.

duration of the illness can vary from several days to several weeks, and the disease occasionally is accompanied by mild hepatitis or signs of meningitis. EBV infections occur frequently in very young children, particularly among the lower socioeconomic groups. In such cases, infections usually are asymptomatic or associated with only mild, flu-like symptoms.

Clinically, IM is diagnosed based on the characteristic symptoms and on the presence of abnormal, large lymphocytes in the blood (Table 40-2). In addition, most

TABLE 40-2
Some Differential Diagnostic Problems in Infectious Mononucleosis

Signs and Symptoms	Anatomic Lesions	Analogous Disorders
Sore throat	Ulcerative or membranous pharyngitis	Diptheria
Painful and stiff ncek; occasionally convulsions and coma	Rapidly enlarged retrocervical lymph nodes; acute hyperplastic lymphadenitis; pleocytosis in cerebrospinal fluid can be present	Meningitis (serous meningitis can be present)
Generalized lymphadenopathy	Acute hyperplastic lymphadenitis	Leukemia
Abdominal pain and tenderness	Rapidly enlarged abdominal lymph nodes	
Right lower quadrant		Acute appendicitis
Left upper quadrant	Acute splenomegaly; acute diffuse hyperplasia	Acute pleuritis; perinephritic abscess
Acute tenderness and pain in right upper quadrant	Acute diffuse hepatitis; periportal infiltrations; enlarged lymph nodes around common bile duct	Acute hepatitis, especially if jaundice is present
Acute general abdominal pain, followed by shock	Ruptured spleen	Acute abdominal emergency
Cough (resembling whooping cough)	Enlarged mediastinal lymph nodes	Pertussis; Hodgkin's disease; tuberculosis
Cutaneous rashes		Exanthematous disease (measles); scarlet fever, especially if angina is present; secondary syphilis, especially if enlarged inguinal lymph nodes and positive test for syphilis are present
Puffiness around eyes	Swelling of retrobulbar tissues	Trichinosis
Toothache	Acutely swollen submandibular lymph nodes	Pulpitis
Hematuria	Specific infiltration of renal parenchyma or purpuric renal hemorrhage	Acute glomerulonephritis

TABLE 40-3
Relation of Epstein-Barr Virus (EBV) and EBV Antibodies to Infectious Mononucleosis

EBV	EBV Antibody
Regularly present in cultured lymphocytes from infectious mononucleosis patients	Absent before illness
	Appears during illness
Persists in lymphocytes after infectious mononucleosis	Persists for years after illness
Is necessary for lymphocyte proliferation in vitro	Shows no such relation to any other illness
Produces infectious mononucleosis in susceptible recipients through blood transfusion	When present, indicates immunity to infectious mononucleosis
Has produced infectious mononucleosis in one transmission experiment	When absent, indicates susceptibility to infectious mononucleosis

patients have high titers of so-called heterophile antibodies, which are characterized by their ability to agglutinate red blood cells from sheep. The first indication that EBV might be the causal agent of IM occurred when a laboratory technician developed IM while working with EBV (Table 40-3). After recovery, it was found that she had developed antibodies to EBV. Furthermore, her B lymphocytes could be cultivated as a continuous cell line that, after several months in tissue culture, yielded infectious EBV. IM appears to be an excellent example of a self-limiting malignancy. Initially, infected lymphocytes are transformed by the infecting virus, resulting in the polyclonal expansion of the B-cell population. Although these cells have many characteristics of malignant cells, the subsequent disappearance of most of the EBV-transformed B lymphocytes after recovery from IM probably results from the host's immune response to EBV infection. This response undoubtedly requires the active participation of both cell-mediated and humoral response mechanisms.

IM frequently is referred to as the "kissing disease," a term arising from the fact that it often is transmitted through close oral contact. This is due to the production and release of infectious virus in the oropharynx. Studies have shown that virus is shed not only during the primary infection, but also periodically throughout the life of an infected individual.

EPSTEIN-BARR VIRUS INFECTIONS IN IMMUNODEFICIENT INDIVIDUALS

Epstein-Barr virus infections in individuals with hereditary X-linked recessive immunodeficiency syndrome result in an often fatal polyclonal B-cell proliferation, leading to aplastic anemia, hypogammaglobulinemia, fatal IM, or malignant lymphoma. Affected individuals exhibit normal measurable parameters of cellular and humoral immunity before EBV infection, but have an aberrant immune response to the infection. Progressive lymphoproliferative diseases also are observed in children with primary immunodeficiencies, in transplant recipients, and in immunosuppressed patients. Such diseases appear to result from the activation and unrestricted proliferation of latently infected B cells. In addition, the incidence of EBV-associated lymphomas has risen dramatically in recent years concomitant with an increase in the number of patients who have AIDS or who receive immunosuppressive drug therapy after organ transplantation. As many as 5% to 10% of individuals infected with the human immunodeficiency virus eventually develop some kind of lymphoma, often associated with EBV. Most of the EBV-associated lymphomas in these patients are non-Hodgkin's lymphomas, but several cases of Hodgkin's lymphoma also have been reported. The presence of EBV has been noted in Reed-Sternberg cells, which are characteristic for Hodgkin's disease.

CHRONIC FATIGUE SYNDROME

Recently, considerable interest and speculation arose regarding the possible involvement of EBV in *chronic fatigue syndrome*. Typically, patients with this syndrome complain of chronic fatigue, myalgias, headache, fevers, and cognitive problems after the resolution of an acute infectious-type illness. However, controlled studies have clearly shown that EBV is not involved in most cases of this syndrome.

EPSTEIN-BARR VIRUS AND HUMAN CANCER

Epstein-Barr virus is associated with several human malignancies, including Burkitt's lymphoma and nasopharyngeal carcinoma (a condition characterized by the proliferation of epithelial cells in the upper pharynx). Both these cancers exhibit a limited geographic distribution (Burkitt's lymphoma occurs mainly in central Africa and nasopharyngeal carcinoma is found in Asia and Northern Africa). In addition, several studies have shown the association of EBV with other types of human lymphomas.

The etiologic role of EBV in Burkitt's lymphoma is unclear, particularly in light of the fact that EBV is found worldwide and that most cases of Burkitt's lymphoma outside the endemic area in Africa are not associated with EBV. However, several facts point to the likely role of EBV as a facilitating agent or cocarcinogen in Burkitt's lymphoma. The unique geographic distribution of Burkitt's lymphoma suggests that another agent may be a cofactor in producing a high incidence of malignancy. Areas in which Burkitt's lymphoma is most prevalent also have high incidences of malaria. Malaria is known to suppress the immune system, thereby enhancing the opportunity for EBV infection and subsequent B-cell prolifera-tion. Virtually all Burkitt's lymphoma cells carry unique and characteristic chromosomal abnormalities. These chromosomal alterations involve reciprocal translocation of the long arm of chromosome 8 with chromosome 14, 2, or 22. The regions of chromosomes 14, 2, and 22 that are involved in these translocations are actively transcribed in B cells, because they contain immunoglobulin genes. It is now clear that the translocations activate the expres-sion of a cellular oncogene, c-*myc,* which is located on chromosome 8. As discussed in Chapter 44, activation of c-*myc* is thought to be a critical event in the establishment of human B-cell lymphomas. It is possible that EBV infec-tion of B lymphocytes enhances the level of B-cell prolifer-ation and, thereby, the frequency of translocation events.

New Human Herpesviruses

Two new human herpesviruses have been identified. Both these viruses initially were isolated from stimulated human peripheral blood mononuclear cells. The viruses have been given the names HHV6 and HHV7. HHV6 first was observed in 1986 in cells from patients with lympho-proliferative disorders and later was isolated from many patients with AIDS. It soon became clear that HHV6 is a ubiquitous virus that is the cause of a childhood rash disease known as exanthem subitum or roseola infantum. Antibodies to HHV6 are found in the serum of 10% to 40% of normal American adults. HHV6 differs from EBV in that infection of B lymphocytes leads to cell lysis rather than immortalization.

HHV7 is yet another lymphotropic herpesvirus that first was isolated from CD4-positive lymphocytes of a healthy adult in 1990. No disease has been associated with this virus.

Bibliography

JOURNAL

Masucci MG, Ernberg J. Trends. Microbiol 1994;2:125.

BOOKS

Miller G. Epstein-Barr virus: biology, pathogenesis and medical aspects. In: Fields VN, Knipe DM, eds. Virology, ed 2. New York, Raven Press, 1990:1921.

Roizman B, Sears AE. Herpes simplex viruses and their replication. In: Fields BN, Knipe DM, eds. Virology, ed 2. New York, Raven Press, 1990:1795.

Stinski MF. Cytomegalovirus and its replication. In: Fields BN, Knipe DM, eds. Virology, ed 2. New York, Raven Press, 1990:1959.

Essentials of Medical Microbiology, Fifth Edition, edited by Wesley A. Volk,
Bryan M. Gebhardt, Marie-Louise Hammarskjöld, and Robert J. Kadner.
Lippincott-Raven Publishers, Philadelphia © 1996.

Chapter 41

Papovaviridae, Adenoviridae, and Parvoviridae

PAPOVAVIRIDAE

The family Papovaviridae consists of a group of DNA viruses that induce both lytic infections and either benign or malignant tumors. The name *papovavirus* was coined by using the first two letters of the original three viruses included in this family: (1) human and animal *pa*pillomaviruses, (2) mouse *po*lyomavirus, and (3) simian *vac*uolating virus (now named SV40). The family now includes human polyomaviruses, two of which, BK and JC, are discussed later in this chapter. All papovaviruses have a similar structure, being icosahedral virions with 72 capsomers (Fig. 41-1), and contain double-stranded circular DNA. All papovaviruses have the capacity to replicate efficiently in appropriate cell types, causing death and lysis of the host cell. Papovaviruses also are capable of inducing a nonproductive infection in certain cells, resulting in cell transformation.

Polyomavirus and Simian Vacuolating Virus

Polyomavirus can be isolated routinely from secretions of wild and laboratory mice. Under natural conditions, the infection does not cause symptoms, even though the mice can excrete the virus for long periods. Inoculation of polyomavirus into mouse embryo cells yields a productive infection in which virions are produced and infected host cells are destroyed. However, if the virus is injected into newborn mice, hamsters, or rats, the animals develop multiple malignant tumors in essentially every organ of the body. Thus, this virus appears to be essentially harmless when acquired naturally by adult mice but causes highly fatal malignancies if injected into newborn animals. The in vitro infection of hamster or rat cells in culture by polyomavirus does not yield infectious virus (ie, the cells are nonpermissive for complete virus replication). However, the infection can result in the transformation of some of the cells in the culture, because the early genes that are required for transformation are expressed in these cells.

557

in young adults. These viruses generally are transmitted by sexual contact. Genital warts may regress spontaneously, but can recur and result in extensive lesions.

Laryngeal papillomas, another group of HPV-induced lesions, occur in both young children and adults. These benign tumors often show frequent and rapid recurrence, even after surgical removal, but rarely develop into malignant tumors. HPV types 6, 11, and 30 are recovered most often from these warts.

PAPILLOMAVIRUS INFECTIONS AND CANCER

The relationship between papillomaviruses and the progression to malignant disease is supported by several observations. Studies in animals have shown that infection with papillomaviruses consistently is associated with specific malignant lesions. For example, a high percentage (over 70%) of the papillomas induced in the cottontail rabbit with Shope papillomavirus progress to a malignant carcinoma within 1 year. In humans, cutaneous lesions in patients with epidermodysplasia verruciformis consistently are observed to progress to carcinomas. In addition, progression to cancer has been recognized in cervical dysplasias associated with infection with specific HPVs (particularly types 16 and 18; see Table 41-1). The evidence suggests that HPV plays an etiologic role in the development of many cases of cervical cancer. However, cervical cancer usually requires a long latency period to develop (20 to 40 years after primary infections). This, and the fact that only a few infected individuals ever develop cervical cancer, clearly indicate that virus infection alone is not sufficient for cancer development.

ADENOVIRIDAE

In 1953, the first of the viruses that constitute the large group of adenoviruses was isolated from cultures of normal adenoids. To date, 47 different serologic types of adenoviruses producing a variety of human respiratory tract, conjunctival, and gastrointestinal tract infections have been identified and placed in the genus *Mastadenovirus*. These viruses frequently have been isolated from normal (or at least apparently normal) adenoids and tonsils, as well as from both respiratory tract and ocular secretions. This has been shown to be due to a high frequency of chronic adenovirus infections. The mechanism of this persistence remains obscure. Most individuals harboring adenoviruses do not shed virus, possibly because of the presence of specific cellular and humoral immune responses.

Structure and Replication of Adenoviruses

Adenoviruses are icosahedral virions containing double-stranded linear DNA. They are 60 to 90 nm in diameter, and each capsid is made up of 252 capsomers. Twelve penton capsomers reside at the 12 vertices of the icosahedral capsids, with hexons occupying all the other positions in this structure. Extending from each penton is a long fiber projection that binds specifically to receptor sites on the host cell. Nine proteins constitute the outer capsid and inner core structures, and their organization is depicted in Figure 41-4. The linear adenovirus DNA genome contains about 36,000 base pairs. The termini of adenovirus DNA are covalently linked to a specific viral protein that serves an important function in DNA replication within the host cell. After adsorption, the virus is taken rapidly into the cell, either by phagocytosis or by direct penetration of the membrane. The virus then is partially uncoated, and the viral DNA is transported to the host-cell nucleus.

The replication cycle of adenoviruses extends over a period of 36 to 48 hours and is characterized by an early and a late stage, as in the case of the papovaviruses. Using restriction endonucleases and DNA cloning and sequencing, investigators have been able both to map the position of the different viral genes within the adenovirus genome and to examine the expression of these individual genes during the replication cycle. Early in the replication cycle (8 to 12 hours after infection), before DNA replication, four distinct regions of the adenovirus genome are expressed (Fig. 41-5). These regions, designated E1, E2, E3, and E4, contain the early genes encoding proteins necessary for DNA replication and the expression of late genes. Some of the early gene products help the virus escape host immune responses. Synthesis and accumulation of the early proteins trigger DNA replication and the subsequent expression of late genes. Transcription of late genes starts at a single point on the adenovirus genome, designated the *major late promoter*. Many different mRNAs are generated from transcripts initiating from this promoter through differential polyadenylation and splicing. This creates individual mRNAs for the different late proteins. These RNAs then are transported to the cytoplasm, where they are translated into all the proteins required for virus particle assembly and maturation. The complex nature of adenovirus transcription and RNA processing reflects the requirement for the virus to use a limited amount of coding information in the most advantageous manner, analogous to the situation observed for polyomaviruses.

Adenovirus DNA replication depends on the synthesis of early viral proteins, one of which is a virus-encoded DNA polymerase. Replication begins at the ends of the adenovirus DNA molecule and proceeds in a 5′-to-3′ direction, yielding a double-stranded duplex and a free single-stranded molecule (Fig. 41-6). Initiation of DNA replication requires another virus-specific protein, the terminal protein. A newly made copy of this protein binds to the end of the parental DNA molecule. The protein also binds a single nucleotide triphosphate that serves as a primer for DNA replication. The free single-stranded

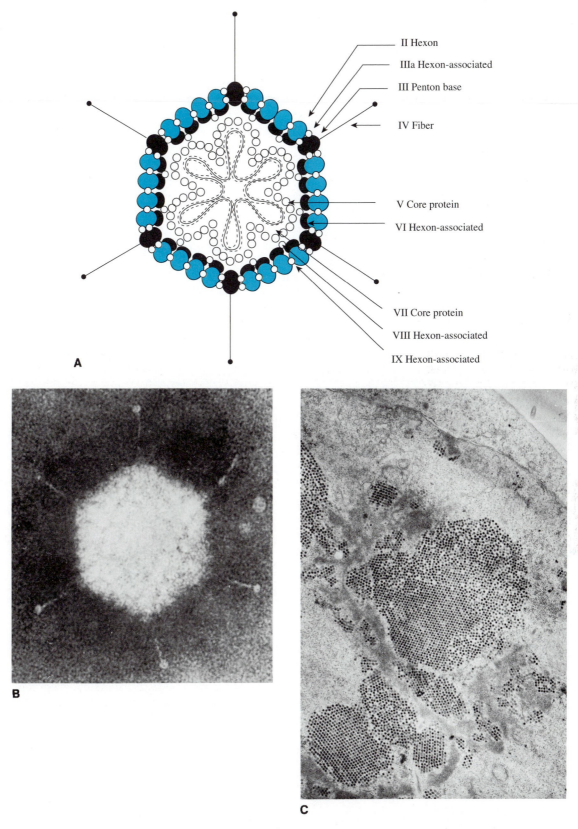

FIGURE 41-4 **A.** Model of adenovirus. The location of each of the major capsid proteins is designated. **B.** Negatively stained virion of adenovirus; note fibers extending from the vertices. (Original magnification about ×500,000.) **C.** Crystalline aggregates of adenovirus in the nucleus of a HeLa cell 24 hours after infection. (Original magnification ×8870.)

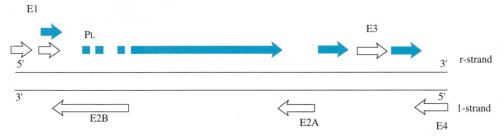

FIGURE 41-5 A transcriptional map of the adenovirus genome. Open arrows denote early messenger RNA transcripts; closed arrows denote late messenger RNA transcripts. P_L marks the position of the major late promoter for transcription.

DNA molecule that is generated is believed to circularize by virtue of the inverted terminally repeated sequences, so then the small region of double-stranded DNA can serve as the initial point for copying the single-stranded DNA into a complete double-stranded progeny molecule. The newly synthesized DNA then is packaged into preformed capsids. Mature particles, as well as empty capsids and excess viral structural protein, accumulate in the cell nucleus, forming crystalline inclusion bodies (see Fig. 41-4C).

Host-Cell Response to Infection

Adenoviruses can be grown in continuous human cell lines such as HeLa cells, or they can be grown in primary

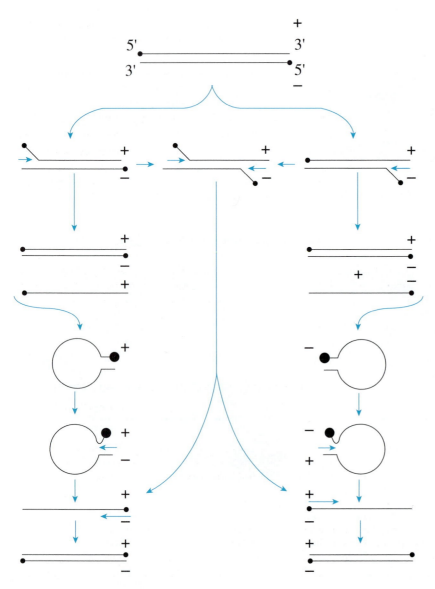

FIGURE 41-6 A model for the replication of adenovirus DNA. Replication can begin at either end, resulting in the displacement of the viral negative (−) or positive (+) strand. The single strands generated in step one circularize and are transcribed again, yielding double-stranded DNA. The ● symbol denotes a terminal protein linked covalently to the 5′ end of both DNA strands.

cell cultures such as human embryo kidney cells. They are cytopathic for such permissive cells, and plaque assays can be carried out in cell monolayers. Cell death is manifested by a "rounding up" of the infected cell; however, because lysis is not a normal event, only a small amount of virus is released into the culture medium. To obtain large yields of adenovirus, infected cells must be disrupted (by sonication, mechanical grinding, or the use of mild detergents) to release the virions from the cell nucleus. Many of the cytopathic effects appear to result from the toxicity of the penton subunit, because the addition of purified pentons to a growing cell culture will cause the cells to round up and detach from the substrate on which the cells are growing.

At least 12 of the human adenoviruses have the capacity to produce malignant carcinomas if injected into newborn hamsters, mice, or rats. Infection of cultured rat or hamster cells in vitro also results in transformation. These cells are nonpermissive for complete adenovirus replication (ie, infectious virus is not produced). However, early genes are expressed after infection of these cells. Molecular analysis of transformed cells has shown that they possess both viral DNA and viral mRNA. The DNA is found integrated into the chromosome of transformed cells. It has been demonstrated that transformation does not require the complete viral genome. In fact, cells can be transformed by DNA transfection using only the E1 region (the leftmost 11% of the adenovirus genome).

The E1 region encodes several proteins required for stable transformation. Two such proteins, designated the E1A proteins, are known to activate the expression of viral and cellular genes in "trans." It is likely that the ability of the E1A proteins to stimulate expression of new host-cell proteins contributes directly to the process of cellular transformation. One of the E1A proteins binds to the cellular Rb protein, whereas one of the E1B gene products binds to the p53 protein. Thus, the ability to bind to these two cellular gene products is common to all the transforming viruses described in this chapter,

showing that these associations are likely to play a crucial role in the ability of these viruses to cause transformation.

The oncogenicity of adenoviruses in rodents and rodent cells in culture originally gave rise to a concern that human adenoviruses may cause cancer in humans. However, several careful studies using DNA hybridization techniques capable of detecting less than one copy of the adenovirus genome per cell have failed to detect adenovirus DNA in any human tumors.

Classification of Adenoviruses

All adenoviruses except avian adenoviruses contain a common group-specific antigen associated with the hexon capsomers and a second group-specific determinant in the penton subunit. In addition, hexons possess an additional antigenic determinant used to subdivide these viruses into specific serotypes. The fiber contains a hemagglutinin that can bind to receptors on the surface of certain red blood cells. The antigenic determinants on the hemagglutinin are distinct for each serotype. As a result, type specificity can be determined using a hemagglutinin-inhibition test, which depends on the ability of a specific antihemagglutinin to prevent hemagglutination. However, because there occasionally are cross-reactions with this antigen, hemagglutination inhibition does not provide as reliable a test for type specificity as do antibody reactions (eg, neutralizing infectivity) directed toward the type-specific hexon antigen. To date, 47 serotypes of human adenoviruses have been identified. These can be divided into seven subgroups based on their biologic, biochemical, and immunologic properties (Table 41-2).

Adenovirus Infections in Humans

In adults, the incidence of overt respiratory tract infection caused by adenoviruses appears to be low. As shown in Table 41-2, different serologic types can cause various

TABLE 41-2
Properties of the Human Adenovirus Subgroups

Subgroup	Type	Pathogenicity	Oncogenicity
A	12, 18, 31	Not defined	Rapidly form tumors in most animals
B	3, 7, 11, 14, 16, 21, 34, 35	Acute respiratory tract infections, conjunctivitis, pharyngitis, gastroenteritis, hemorrhagic cystitis	Slowly induce tumors in some animals
C	1, 2, 5, 6	Respiratory tract infections in infants	None
D	8–10, 13, 15, 17, 19, 20, 22–30, 32, 33, 36, 37, 38, 39	8, 19, and 37 keratoconjunctivitis	None
E	4	Acute respiratory tract infections	None
F	40	Diarrhea in children	None
G	41	Diarrhea in children	None

manifestations of respiratory tract and conjunctival infections. Major epidemics seem to occur primarily in new army recruits in the form of an acute respiratory tract disease caused by types 3, 4, and 7. For unknown reasons, these types occur much less frequently in civilian populations.

Little doubt exists, however, that adenoviruses are responsible for a significant percentage of both upper and lower respiratory tract infections in children. A Swedish study estimated that adenoviruses are responsible for up to 19% of febrile upper respiratory tract infections in children, and another study involving 18,000 infants and children concluded that 10% of all childhood respiratory tract infections are caused by adenoviruses. Lower respiratory tract infections can result in a syndrome similar to the primary atypical pneumonia caused by *Mycoplasma pneumoniae*. Adenoviruses also cause epidemic keratoconjunctivitis, primarily in an environment in which the eyes are subjected to mild trauma by the presence of dust. Adenovirus types 11 and 21 have been shown to be associated with a hemorrhagic cystitis, particularly in young boys. The pathogenesis of this syndrome and the reason for its prevalence in boys are not known.

Adenoviruses 40 and 41 have been associated with gastroenteritis, especially in young children. However, the adenoviruses involved in this malady have been difficult to study because they do not replicate well in tissue culture. Adenoviruses also can cause fatal disseminated disease in immunosuppressed transplant recipients and in patients with immunodeficiency syndromes.

CONTROL OF ADENOVIRUS INFECTIONS IN HUMANS

Because humans seem to be the only reservoir for the human adenoviruses, the spread from person to person appears to occur directly through respiratory tract or conjunctival discharges. Recovery from adenovirus infections results in a long-lasting, type-specific immunity, and it seems possible that the extended duration of immunity might result from subsequent subclinical infections. It seems likely that vaccines would be effective for the prevention of adenovirus infections, and the United States Army has shown this to be the case using inactivated viral vaccines. In addition, live vaccines of nonattenuated viruses incorporated into a capsule that dissolves in the intestine have produced solid immunity (probably by stimulating the synthesis of specific IgA antibodies) without causing overt disease. However, the general absence of epidemics of acute respiratory tract disease in the adult civilian population and the multiplicity of serologic types of adenoviruses discourages the widespread use of adenovirus vaccines.

DIAGNOSIS OF ADENOVIRUS INFECTIONS IN HUMANS

Diagnosis of adenovirus infections can be accomplished either by isolating and identifying the virus or by demonstrating a rise in specific antibody titer during a patient's convalescent period. Isolation is accomplished by placing respiratory tract or conjunctival secretions on monolayers of cell cultures and observing the cultures for cytopathic effect. General identification of an adenovirus is accomplished using known complement-fixing antibody that reacts with all adenoviruses; neutralizing or hemagglutination-inhibition antibodies are required to determine type specificity. More recently, radioimmunoassay and enzyme-linked immunosorbent assay and DNA hybridization techniques have been used for virus identification. These techniques are of particular importance in the diagnosis of enteric adenoviruses, where conventional cell-culture techniques fail.

PARVOVIRIDAE

Parvoviruses are among the smallest icosahedral viruses found in vertebrates. They contain single-stranded linear DNA about 5 kilobases in size and have been divided into two genera on the basis of whether they are nondefective (parvoviruses) or defective (dependoviruses) for replication. In general, the parvoviruses are resistant to physical destruction. They survive heating at 56°C for hours and are resistant to treatment with either chloroform or ether. They often remain viable after years of storage.

Parvoviruses

The genus *Parvovirus* contains nondefective viruses that infect rats, mice, hamsters, cats, dogs, pigs, and humans. In some of these animals, such as rats, they produce a variety of congenital defects in the fetus. In 1983, a parvovirus designated B19 was isolated and identified as a highly infectious human virus.

HUMAN INFECTIONS BY PARVOVIRUS B19

Erythema infectiosum (also known as fifth disease) is a mild childhood disease that is characterized by a facial rash resembling a slapped cheek. Many children experience asymptomatic infections, and by 5 years of age, 15% to 60% are seropositive for the virus. However, it is not healthy children that are the source of concern for this virus, but patients with hemolytic anemia and pregnant women.

Parvovirus B19 has a propensity to infect and promote the lysis of erythroid precursor cells, thus interrupting normal red blood cell production. Although this usually is clinically inapparent in normal persons, individuals with chronic hemolytic anemias who require increased hematopoiesis to maintain stable red blood cell counts are at risk for a transient aplastic crisis. In addition, immunodeficient persons can become persistently infected with B19, resulting in a chronic anemia.

Studies of B19 infections during pregnancy have indicated that the fetus is not adversely affected in most cases. However, some spontaneously aborted fetuses have tested positive for B19 infection, and it is likely that these abortions were attributable to B19 infection. However, unlike some animal parvoviruses, there is no evidence that B19 causes congenital anomalies.

Dependoviruses

The dependoviruses are unable to grow unless the host cell is coinfected with a helper virus, either adenovirus or herpesvirus. As a result, dependoviruses also are referred to as adeno-associated viruses. The nature of the functions provided by the helper virus is not fully understood, although adenovirus temperature-sensitive mutants unable to replicate their DNA at a nonpermissive temperature in a host cell are still capable of providing the helper function, showing that expression of the early adenovirus genes is sufficient. Data suggest that proteins from the E1, E2, and E4 regions are required for helper function.

All dependoviruses contain single-stranded DNA. However, the virus particles are unusual in that some virions contain a positive strand of DNA, whereas others contain the complementary negative strand. All five human serotypes appear to be widespread, based on the observation that most children acquire antibodies to the human types before reaching their teenage years. However, none of the serotypes have been associated with any disease. In the infected cell, the dependovirus genome is maintained in the form of double-stranded DNA integrated into the host-cell chromosome. The process of viral DNA integration does not require helper virus, but virus replication does. Therefore, the ability of a dependovirus to establish a long-lasting latent infection in the absence of a helper virus essentially allows the virus to bide its time waiting for the encounter with a cytopathic adenovirus. There has been a growing interest in the development of adeno-associated viruses as a vector for human gene therapy and intracellular immunization.

Bibliography

JOURNAL

Pipas JM. Common and unique features of T antigens encoded by the polyomavirus group. J Virol 1992;66:3979.

BOOKS

Berns KI. Parvoviridae and their replication. In: Fields BN, Knipe DM, eds. Virology, ed 2. New York, Raven Press, 1990:1743.

Eckhart W. Polyomavirinae and their replication. In: Fields BN, Knipe DM, eds. Virology, ed 2. New York, Raven Press, 1990:1593.

Horwitz MS. Adenoviridae and their replication. In: Fields BN, Knipe DM, eds. Virology, ed 2. New York, Raven Press, 1990:1679.

Howley PM. Papillomavirinae and their replication. In: Fields BN, Knipe DM, eds. Virology, ed 2. New York, Raven Press, 1990:1625.

zurHauzen H. Papillomaviruses as carcinomaviruses. In: Klein G, ed. Tumorigenic DNA viruses, vol 8. New York, Raven Press, 1989:1.

Essentials of Medical Microbiology, Fifth Edition, edited by Wesley A. Volk, Bryan M. Gebhardt, Marie-Louise Hammarskjöld, and Robert J. Kadner. Lippincott-Raven Publishers, Philadelphia © 1996.

Chapter 42

Poxviridae

Poxviruses are large, complex, brick-shaped viruses classified into genera on the basis of their ability to replicate in different natural hosts, their morphologic differences, and their distinguishing group-specific antigens. All poxviruses induce cell proliferation to some degree in a susceptible host. The most common manifestation of this proliferation is pox lesions, the external sign of such diseases as smallpox, cowpox, rabbitpox, sheep-pox, and fowlpox.

Structure and Replication

Poxviruses are structurally the most complex of any of the animal viruses. Their double-stranded DNA, capable of coding for several hundred proteins, is enclosed in a dense, dumbbell-shaped core, along with several enzymes necessary for viral replication. The core is surrounded by a tubular-shaped lipoprotein membrane, and fitting into the concave portions of the dumbbell-shaped core are dense structures that have been named *lateral bodies*. This entire structure is enclosed in a second membrane envelope, which is acquired when the virus is naturally released from the cell (Fig. 42-1). A better concept of poxvirus structure can be gained by examining the events that occur during the replication of vaccinia virus, the avirulent virus used to vaccinate against smallpox.

REPLICATION OF VACCINIA VIRUS

The replication of vaccinia virus in cell culture is in all likelihood similar to that occurring in human smallpox infection, and probably is similar to that of most other poxviruses (Fig. 42-2).

After the infection of cells in culture, the virus is rapidly adsorbed to receptors on the surface of the host cell. The nature and specificity of these cellular receptors is not known. Penetration occurs as a result of fusion of viral and cellular membranes or endocytosis of the intact virion into host-cell lysosomal vesicles. At this stage, the

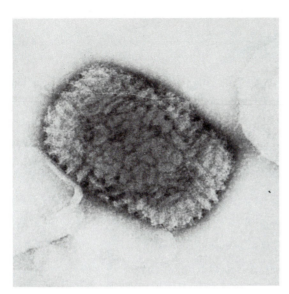

FIGURE 42-1 Smallpox (variola) virus. Note the "brick" shape and the globular subunits on the surface. (Original magnification ×147,000.)

first uncoating step occurs through the degradation of the outer viral membrane by host-cell enzymes. The viral core, without the lateral bodies, then leaves the lysosomal vesicle and enters the cytoplasm of the host cell.

Transcription of the viral genome begins at this point. A virus-encoded, DNA-dependent RNA polymerase within the virus core transcribes early mRNAs corresponding to about 14% of the viral DNA genome. These early mRNAs exit the viral core and are translated on host-cell ribosomes, producing several proteins. One of these early proteins is an uncoating enzyme that degrades the viral core, releasing the naked DNA. After release of the DNA, additional early transcription occurs (before DNA replication begins), producing several structural proteins and several enzymes, including a DNA polymerase. The appearance of the DNA polymerase is followed by the replication of the viral DNA. At the same time, the synthesis and translation of late mRNA begins, resulting in the formation of more viral enzymes and most of the structural proteins of the virus. At this time, host-cell protein synthesis is inhibited, and transport of host-cell mRNA from the nucleus is blocked. The molecular mechanism by which the virus prevents these cellular events is not known.

Two aspects of poxvirus replication are different from that of other DNA viruses such as adenoviruses and herpesviruses. First, the entire replication occurs in the cytoplasm of the host cell, and second, viral assembly does not begin until viral DNA replication is essentially complete. The assembly of the viral DNA and viral enzymes into the complex virion is far from understood. Maturation of the virus is complex and appears to involve several important steps. Immature particles first are enclosed in a lipid bilayer membrane. This membrane encloses the lateral bodies and core to form the complete virion. The

release of completed virions from the host cell by the Golgi results in the acquisition of a second lipid envelope. However, this is an inefficient process, and at least 90% of the virions remain inside the cell. Those virions that leave the cell can exit through the microvilli or by fusion with portions of the plasma membrane of the host cell. Both extracellular, enveloped and intracellular, nonenveloped virus particles are infectious.

Poxvirus Infections in Humans

SMALLPOX

Smallpox is an ancient disease that has caused the deaths of untold millions of people during its 3000-year recorded history. As recently as 65 years ago, thousands of cases of smallpox occurred annually in the United States. However, because of an intensive vaccination and surveillance program carried out by the World Health Organization, there have been no reported cases of smallpox since 1977, and it is now believed that smallpox has been successfully eradicated from the world. This section, therefore, is primarily of historic interest; however, it would seem inappropriate to omit a discussion of a disease that has been so important in the history of mankind.

Two variants of the smallpox virus are pathogenic for humans. The first variant, variola major, causes a severe illness, with a mortality rate of 25% to 50%. The second variant, variola minor (frequently called alastrim), produces a much milder disease, with a mortality rate of less than 1%. Although there is no doubt that these two variants actually exist as separate entities, they are morphologically and serologically identical. Both viruses show similar pathogenesis, although the skin lesions of variola minor are more superficial.

Pathogenicity

The usual site of entry for the smallpox virus was the respiratory tract. An incubation period of 12 to 16 days followed, during which the virus multiplied, probably in the regional lymph nodes. Symptoms, characterized by chills, fever, headache, back pains, and prostration, began when the virus entered the bloodstream. Viremia (virus in the bloodstream) resulted in spread of the virus throughout the body, infecting internal organs, mucous membranes, and skin. Several days later, pox lesions appeared on the face and then spread to the forearms, hands, and lower extremities. Lesions occurred over the entire body, but usually were more abundant on the shoulders and chest than on the abdomen. Unlike those of chickenpox, the lesions of smallpox typically were at the same stage of development in any given body area (ie, they occurred as a single crop that progressed from macules [unraised discolorations] to papules [raised lesions] to

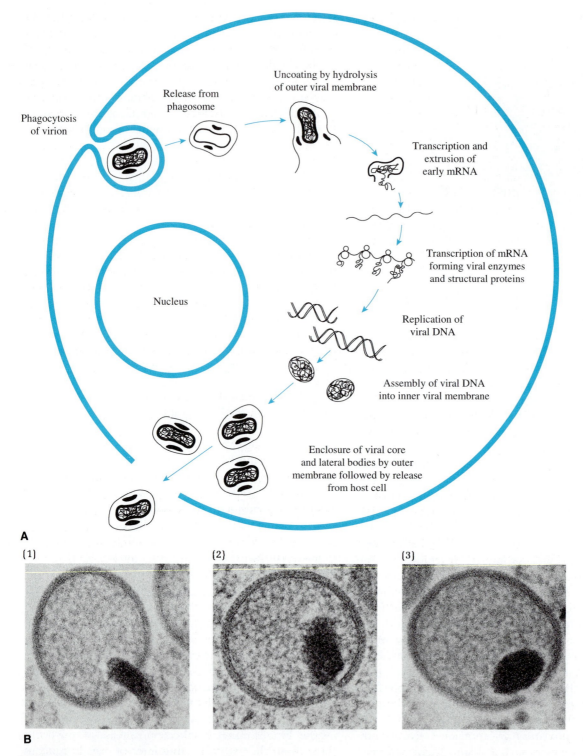

A

(1)   (2)   (3)

B

FIGURE 42-2 **A.** Replication of vaccinia. Note that replication takes place entirely within the cytoplasm of the host cell. **B.** Insertion of nucleoprotein into viral membranes to form immature vaccinia proviruses. The first frame shows deoxyribonucleoprotein at mid-stage of condensation and insertion; the second frame shows insertion nearly completed, with some material still extending into the host cell's cytoplasm; and the third frame shows a fully developed nucleoid, or provirus, with a small orifice remaining to close. (Original magnification ×102,900.)

vesicles [containing fluid]). Finally, rupture occurred, followed by crusting over and healing.

Spread of the virus most often was from direct or indirect contact with the pox lesions of an infected person. However, because mucous membranes also can be infected, any contact with secretions or discharges of an infected patient could spread the disease.

Diagnosis

The diagnosis of smallpox was made on the basis of appearance and clinical symptoms, but a positive confirmation required one or more laboratory procedures for identification of the virus. Such methods included the direct inoculation of vesicle fluid onto the chorioallantoic membrane of chicken embryos.

Control

The complete eradication of smallpox was possible for the following reasons: (1) a successful vaccination strategy was developed with a vaccine that provided solid immunity to smallpox; (2) the virus infects only humans, meaning that there is no animal reservoir; and (3) there were no asymptomatic or undiagnosed cases.

The long road to smallpox eradication began when Edward Jenner pointed out in 1798 (long before anyone had any concept of a virus) that the milkmaids in England rarely came down with smallpox, although the incidence was high in the general population. Jenner postulated that their immunity stemmed from an earlier infection with cowpox that they had acquired from milking infected cows. In spite of much ridicule and opposition for proposing such an unorthodox concept, a primitive vaccination program (termed *variolation*) using ground scabs obtained from the lesions of infected cows was started in both Europe and the United States. These early methods provided the basis for modern vaccine strategies, the efficacy of which is now readily apparent.

Several viral strains called *vaccinia virus* have been used for vaccination against smallpox. Although the origins of these viruses are somewhat vague, their properties resemble in many aspects those of cowpox virus.

Although the smallpox vaccine is no longer administered, there has been considerable research in recent years on the possible use of vaccinia virus as a delivery vector for "foreign genes." It is possible that, using hybrid vaccinia viruses, new and potentially more efficacious strategies will be devised to administer vaccines for serious diseases (eg, acquired immunodeficiency syndrome). For this reason, a brief discussion of vaccine delivery is in order.

In modern vaccination practice, the vaccinia virus was introduced into the skin of a susceptible person, using a specially designed instrument to prick the skin in a small area. About a week later, a local pox lesion developed in the area, in which the vaccinia virus was actively replicat-

ing. This lesion usually healed about 2 weeks later, leaving a small scar. This series of events was called a *primary take*. In a previously vaccinated person, the severity of the vaccination reaction varied according to the degree of residual immunity. In comparison with a primary take, the lesion progressed through its stages more rapidly and healed considerably sooner in a partially immune person. The completely immune person acquired only a small red papule, which appeared 2 or 3 days after vaccination and healed in a few more days, leaving no scar.

Several complications could follow vaccination with vaccinia virus. Progressive vaccinia, or vaccinia necrosum, occurred when the primary lesion failed to heal and continued to enlarge and spread. This was extremely rare and seemed to occur only in persons who were unable to raise a cellular immune response against the virus. A condition known as *generalized vaccinia* was sometimes observed in persons with eczema. It was characterized by the presence of vaccinia lesions all over the eczematous area, resulting from transplantation of the virus (usually by the fingers) from the original vaccination site. This was an extremely severe and sometimes fatal complication.

Postvaccinal encephalitis was another rare complication that followed smallpox vaccination. The incidence seemed to vary, but it probably occurred in about 1 of every 50,000 persons vaccinated. The symptoms of encephalitis usually began about 10 to 12 days after vaccination, and the mortality rate was as high as 50%.

RECOMBINANT VACCINIA VIRUSES. Using recombinant DNA technology, it is possible to insert 22 to 25 kilobases of foreign DNA into vaccinia virus without diminishing its ability to replicate. Various recombinant vaccinia virus strains have been made that encode for the surface antigens of hepatitis B virus, influenza viruses, and herpesviruses. Experimental infection of animals with such strains has shown the formation of antibodies against the proteins that are expressed from the inserted virus genes. In many cases, these have been shown to be protective, making it probable that recombinant vaccinia viruses of this kind will enable the development of effective vaccines for several important diseases that will be widely used in the future. Because so much foreign DNA can be inserted, recombinant viruses might be engineered that will give rise to immunity to several different viruses using a single vaccine. It is hoped that vaccine complications with the recombinant vaccinia virus strains will be rare, because of reduced virulence of these strains compared to the wild-type virus.

COWPOX

Cowpox occurs in cows as a mild infection transmitted to humans by direct contact. Thus, human infections usually occur on the hands and fingers, causing lesions not unlike a primary take from vaccinia virus. The disease is self-limiting and, after healing of the lesions, infected humans possess immunity to the much more virulent smallpox virus.

MOLLUSCUM CONTAGIOSUM

Molluscum contagiosum involves a lesion that proliferates on the skin, most frequently on the face, arms, buttocks, genitals, and legs. The lesions appear as small, white nodules about 2 mm in diameter that result from the proliferation of epithelial cells. Infected cells contain large cytoplasmic inclusion bodies containing poxvirus, which have been given the name *molluscum bodies*.

The nodules usually disappear after several months, probably after the development of a cellular immune response. The virus has not been studied extensively, and the mechanism by which it stimulates cell proliferation is unknown.

YABA MONKEY POXVIRUS

Yaba monkey poxvirus causes a benign tumor in Asian and African monkeys, which regresses after 5 to 6 weeks. Laboratory workers occasionally can be infected by handling infected animals.

Bibliography

JOURNAL

Mackett M, Smith GL. Vaccinia virus expression vectors. J Gen Virol 1986;67:2067.

BOOKS

Fenner F, Henderson DA, Arita I, Jezek Z, Ladnyi ID. Smallpox and its eradication. Geneva, World Health Organization, 1988.

Fenner F, Wittek R, Dumbell KR. The orthopoxviruses. New York, Academic Press, 1989.

Essentials of Medical Microbiology, Fifth Edition, edited by Wesley A. Volk,
Bryan M. Gebhardt, Marie-Louise Hammarskjöld, and Robert J. Kadner.
Lippincott-Raven Publishers, Philadelphia © 1996.

Chapter 43

Retroviridae

The retroviruses are a large group of RNA viruses, many of which readily induce neoplastic disease in their natural host. The first of these viruses was described in the early 1900s when it was shown that leukemias and sarcomas of chickens could be transmitted to newborn healthy chickens using cell-free extracts of the tumors. At that time, the phenomenon was considered an intellectual curiosity, and few scientists realized the implications of this discovery in relation to the role of viruses in cancer.

It is now known that retroviruses are widespread in nature. These viruses have been isolated from a variety of vertebrate species, including birds, mice, rats, cats, hamsters, cattle, horses, and, recently, humans. Many of these RNA-containing viruses cause leukemia (a malignancy of primitive blood cells such as lymphoblasts, myeloblasts, or erythroblasts) carcinomas, or sarcomas (solid tumors). Several other members of the retrovirus family have been shown to cause severe immunodeficiency or neurologic disease in their respective hosts.

Structure of Retroviruses

Retroviruses generally are spherical, with an overall diameter varying from 65 to 150 nm. The mature virion has three morphologic components (Fig. 43-1): (1) an outer envelope made up of a lipid bilayer membrane containing virus-specific glycoprotein spikes; (2) an internal protein capsid; and (3) within the capsid, a nucleocapsid and two virally encoded enzymes (reverse transcriptase and integrase). The retrovirus genome is a dimeric structure consisting of two identical single-stranded RNA segments (7 to 10 kilobases in length). In addition, unique cellular tRNAs are associated with each segment of the viral genome. These tRNAs play an essential role in viral replication by providing a primer for the RNA-dependent DNA polymerase (reverse transcriptase) that replicates the viral genome (see later).

The retrovirus family is divided into three subfamilies; Oncovirinae, Lentivirinae, and Spumavirinae. The On-

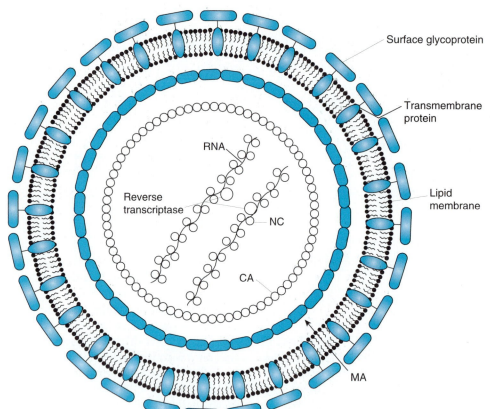

FIGURE 43-1 Structure of the retrovirus particle. See text for details.

covirinae, or RNA tumor virus subfamily, includes all the transforming retroviruses. Electron micrographs of different types of RNA tumor viruses reveal several morphologic types of particles. The most common is a spherical, enveloped virus with a centrally located dense core. This structure has been designated as a C-type virion (Fig. 43-2A), and it is differentiated from morphologically similar B-type virions (see Fig. 43-2B), whose spherical, dense nucleocapsid is located eccentrically within the particle. A-type particles are observed only within the cytoplasm of a host cell and do not possess an envelope. A-type particles (see Fig. 43-2C), which are often seen within the cisternae of the endoplasmic reticulum, may represent defective retroviruses. A fourth type of retrovirus, designated D-type virus, has been isolated from several nonhuman primates. These viruses resemble B-type particles in that they have an eccentric core. However, they differ in structure, having less prominent surface glycoprotein spikes.

The Lentivirinae subfamily (to which human immunodeficiency virus [HIV] belongs) is characterized by a distinctive nucleocapsid core, viewed in the electron microscope as a bar or truncated, cone-shaped nucleocapsid.

The spumaviruses (from the Greek *spuma,* meaning foam) derive their name from the foam-like vacuoles they cause in infected cells.

Replication of Retroviruses

Retrovirus replication begins with the interaction of the viral envelope glycoprotein spikes with cellular receptor proteins of the host-cell membrane. The cellular receptors are different for different retroviruses. The interaction between the viral glycoprotein and the receptor activates a hydrophobic fusion protein that is part of the viral spike. After fusion of the viral envelope with the host-cell membrane, the viral core is released into the cell. At this point, the replication of the retroviruses differs from that of all other viruses, because the first step is the copying of the viral RNA into complementary double-stranded DNA. This reaction is catalyzed by a virus-encoded *RNA-dependent DNA polymerase* that is present in the virus particle. This enzyme is commonly called reverse transcriptase, because the "transcription" it catalyzes is opposite to the normal pathway of information flow (DNA to RNA).

Viral DNA synthesis occurs initially within the cytoplasm of the host cell. A model for viral DNA synthesis consistent with experimental data is shown in Figure 43-3.

DNA synthesis is initiated on a cellular tRNA primer that base pairs with the viral RNA 100 to 300 nucleotides from the 5′ end of the RNA at a location known as the primer binding site. Synthesis proceeds in a 5′-to-

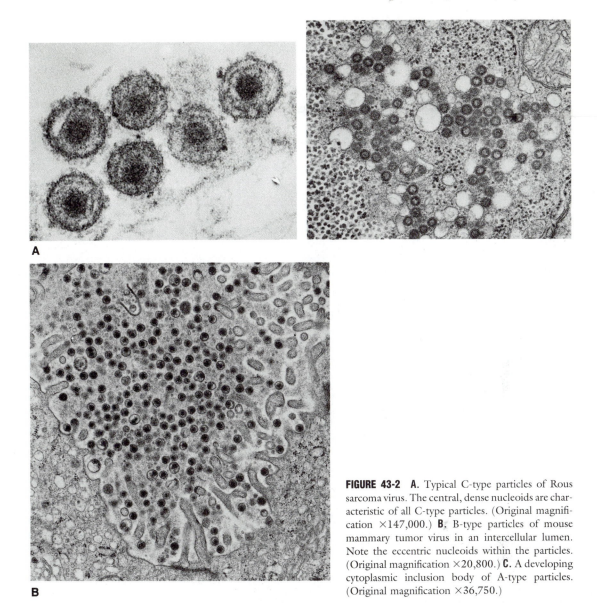

FIGURE 43-2 **A.** Typical C-type particles of Rous sarcoma virus. The central, dense nucleoids are characteristic of all C-type particles. (Original magnification ×147,000.) **B.** B-type particles of mouse mammary tumor virus in an intercellular lumen. Note the eccentric nucleoids within the particles. (Original magnification ×20,800.) **C.** A developing cytoplasmic inclusion body of A-type particles. (Original magnification ×36,750.)

3′ direction, stopping after traversing a short sequence designated R (repeated). The R sequence is present at both ends of the retroviral RNA genome; hence, the newly synthesized DNA can base pair either with the sequence present at the 5′ end or with the R sequence present at the 3′ end of the RNA genome. This terminal redundancy allows a first "jump" to take place, in which the newly synthesized DNA "jumps" to base pair with RNA sequences at the 3′ end of either the same RNA molecule (an intrastrand jump) or the second RNA molecule in the core (an interstrand jump; see Fig. 43-3). After the jump has taken place, DNA synthesis can continue, resulting in the formation of a minus-strand DNA molecule. Plus-strand DNA synthesis then is initiated at a unique site in the 3′ end of the RNA and proceeds from

5′ to 3′ using the newly synthesized minus-strand DNA as a template. The process of plus-strand synthesis again generates intermediates with complementary terminal sequences, enabling a second jump to take place. A complete double-stranded DNA molecule then can be made, probably through a circular intermediate similar to that depicted in Figure 43-3. The final DNA product has a longer terminally repeated sequence than the original RNA molecule because, during the process of reverse transcription, some sequences are copied twice. This long terminal repeat (LTR) is made up of U_3 (a unique 3′ sequence in the RNA), R, and U_5 (a unique 5′ sequence in the RNA) sequences. The LTR sequences vary in length between different retroviruses (300 to 600 base pairs).

Linear duplex DNA synthesis takes place in the cyto-

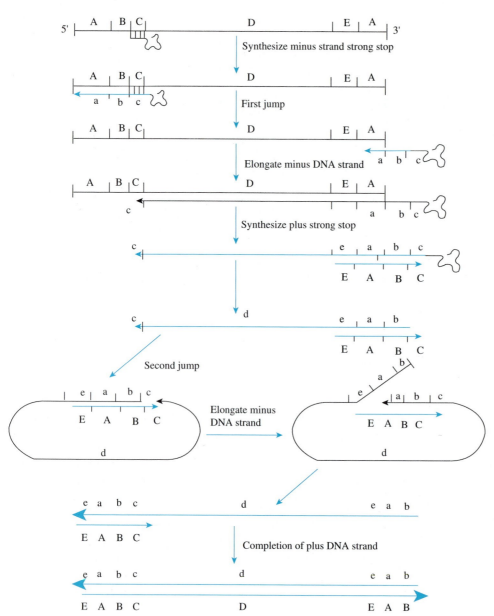

FIGURE 43-3 Schematic diagram of retroviral DNA synthesis. A, B, C, D, and E denote viral RNA sequences important for reverse transcription and are not drawn to scale. The sequence A represents the terminally repeated sequence R; the sequences B and E represent the U_5 and U_3 regions of the viral RNA, respectively; and the sequence C denotes the primer binding site. The various steps in replication are discussed in the text.

plasm of infected cells, generally within the first 8 to 24 hours of infection. At later periods, circular forms of viral DNA are observed in the nucleus (Fig. 43-4). These DNAs contain either one or two copies of the LTR sequence. These DNA molecules integrate into the cellular chromosomes with the help of the viral enzyme *integrase*. The integration of retroviral DNA shows striking similarities with the insertion of bacterial transposable elements. Integrated proviral DNA is identical to the linear DNA precursor except that it always lacks two base pairs present at each end of the linear precursor. In addition, a four–base-pair repeat is generated in the host-cell target sequence. The process of viral DNA integration requires the presence of specific sequences near the ends of the viral LTR sequences; these sequences are considered analogues of bacteriophage attachment (*att*) sites.

Integration of viral DNA generally occurs at a single site in the host chromosome, but the site of integration varies from cell to cell. After integration, transcription of viral DNA is controlled by viral transcriptional elements (promoter and enhancer sequences) located within the U_3 sequence of the LTR (see Fig. 43-4). Synthesis of viral RNA, carried out by the host cell's RNA polymerase II, starts at the 5′ end of R in the 5′ LTR and terminates at the 3′ end of R in the 3′ LTR. The primary RNA product is polyadenylated using the cellular machinery. This "full-length" RNA is used to translate the viral gag and pol proteins (see later) and also is the viral genome that gets packaged into new virus particles. Some of the viral RNA molecules are spliced to generate smaller subgenomic mRNAs that are used to translate env proteins (and regulatory proteins in the case of complex retrovi-

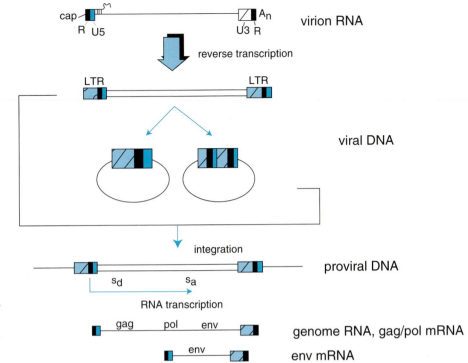

FIGURE 43-4 Summary of retrovirus DNA synthesis, integration, and expression during the life cycle. *Cap,* capped nucleotide at the 5' end of the viral RNA; A_n, polyadenylic acid at the 3' end of the RNA; *R,* repeated sequence at the ends of the RNA; *U3* and *U5,* unique sequences at the ends of the RNA duplicated during DNA synthesis; *LTR,* long terminal repeat; S_d and S_a, RNA splice donor and acceptor sites, respectively.

ruses such as HIV). After processing, the viral mRNA molecules are transported to the cytoplasm and viral proteins are synthesized on cytoplasmic polyribosomes. The env proteins are modified by glycosylation in the Golgi apparatus of the host cells and then are incorporated into the host-cell plasma membrane. The assembly of viral RNA and viral gag and gag/pol proteins occurs at the cell membrane in regions where the env proteins have been incorporated, after which the virus is released by budding from the membrane. Unlike most other viral infections, infections with many retroviruses do not kill the host cell, and both host-cell division and virus production can continue indefinitely. Figure 43-5 summarizes these steps in retrovirus replication.

RETROVIRUS GENE STRUCTURE

Many of the oncoviruses are *defective* (ie, they lack one or more genes necessary for replication). These viruses can replicate only in the presence of a second helper virus.

Oncoviruses that can replicate independently within a host cell are termed *nondefective.*

Based on the biologic properties of an oncovirus in cell culture, and on the pathology of the disease induced in an animal, the oncoviruses can be subdivided further into two classes: acute transforming viruses and nonacute transforming viruses. The former induce a rapid formation of leukemia or sarcoma in the host, usually within a period of weeks, and cause a malignant transformation of cells in culture. Viruses belonging to the latter class cause disease in the host only after a long latent period of several months (or even years) and do not induce malignant transformation of cells in culture, although they replicate in such cells. Biochemical and genetic analysis of these two classes of retroviruses has shown that the nonacute viruses contain only the genes required for viral replication: the *gag* gene, encoding the structural proteins of the viral capsid and core; the *pol* gene, encoding the virion-associated RNA-dependent DNA polymerase and integrase; and the *env* gene, encoding the env glycoproteins of the virus (Fig. 43-6). The nonacute viruses contain all the information required for efficient virus replication and, therefore, are nondefective viruses.

Acute transforming viruses, on the other hand, lack all or parts of the genes required for replication and in their place have acquired unique cellular sequences termed *oncogene sequences.* It is the virus-mediated expression of these oncogene sequences that gives rise to the rapid onset of malignant disease in the animal host and to the transformation of cells in culture (see Fig. 43-6). However, because the oncogene sequences have replaced (either totally or in part) the genes required for virus replication, acute transforming viruses are "defective" for replication and, therefore, require the concomitant replication of a helper virus, a nonacute virus, to provide the viral proteins necessary for virus replication and integration. The one exception to this rule is Rous sarcoma virus (RSV), an avian retrovirus. Interestingly, in RSV, the resident oncogene sequence (*src*) lies outside the boundaries of the genes required for replication (see Fig. 43-6). Hence, RSV is the only known example of a nondefective,

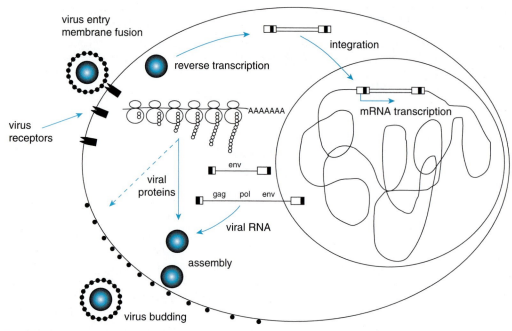

FIGURE 43-5   Summary of the steps required for retrovirus replication. See text for details.

acute sarcoma virus. For this reason, RSV has been one of the most intensely studied retroviruses.

The lentiviruses and spumaviruses show a more complex gene structure and are characterized by the presence in the genome of one or more regulatory genes in addition to *gag, pol,* and *env.* These genes play important roles in the replication of these viruses (see later).

SYNTHESIS OF RETROVIRUS PROTEINS

The retrovirus core is made up of the genomic RNA and several nucleocapsid proteins. The multiple core proteins (known as gag [group antigen] proteins) are encoded in a single gene, the *gag* gene. They are synthesized as a polyprotein precursor, termed Prgag, that subsequently is cleaved into the component *gag* proteins by a protease usually encoded within gag. In the case of some viruses, the protease is encoded within pol. A standardized nomenclature for the gag proteins that are common to all retroviruses has been established. The individual proteins have been designated capsid protein, matrix protein, nucleocapsid protein, and protease. The organization of the proteins within the virus is shown in Figure 43-1. The products of the *pol* gene, reverse transcriptase and integrase, also are cleaved from a precursor protein, which is known as Prgag/pol because it contains the *gag* as well as the *pol* protein sequences. This precursor protein is cleaved by the viral protease during the assembly process to yield the different gag proteins as well as the two *pol* gene products.

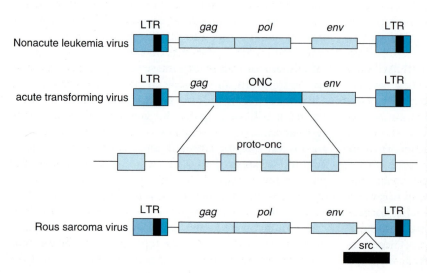

FIGURE 43-6   Organization of the genomes of various transforming and nontransforming retroviruses. The three viral genes required for virus replication are denoted by the terms *gag, pol,* and *env* (see text). The sequences acquired by transforming retroviruses by recombination with cellular sequences (here, denoted proto-onc) are indicated by the term *onc.* Insertion of *onc* sequences into the viral genome results in the partial or complete deletion of *gag, pol,* and *env* sequences. Such viruses are replication defective. Rous sarcoma virus contains the *onc* gene denoted *src* inserted 3' to the *env* gene and, therefore, is replication competent.

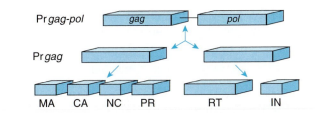

A

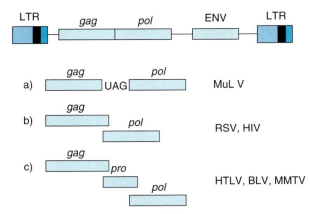

B

FIGURE 43-7 Processing of retrovirus structural proteins. **A.** The events leading to the proteolytic cleavage of the *gag* and *pol* gene products. Prgag is the precursor to the viral structural proteins MA, CA, NC, and PR (see text for further description of these proteins). Prgag-pol is the precursor to reverse transcriptase (*RT*) and integrase (*IN*). **B.** The arrangement of *gag* and *pol* coding sequences within the genomes of various retroviruses. (**a**) The genes *gag* and *pol* are in the same reading frame and are separated by a UAG termination codon. (**b**) The genes *gag* and *pol* are in different reading frames. (**c**) The genes *gag*, *pro*, and *pol* are in three different reading frames.

All retroviruses, including those of human origin, share a similar organization of genetic information (Fig. 43-7). A novel and interesting feature of retrovirus translation is that *gag* and *pol* genes always are expressed as gag—pol fusion proteins, in spite of the fact that these genes are either interrupted by translational stop codons or present in different translational reading frames. This paradox is explained by the ability of eucaryotic ribosomes to occasionally insert amino acids in response to nonsense codons or, alternatively, to shift reading frames at defined sites and frequencies when translating viral RNAs. Such mechanisms provide clear advantages to the retroviruses: structural *gag* proteins can be made in large amounts, whereas catalytic proteins (*pol* and *int*) are made in relatively small amounts. In addition, this process allows *pol* proteins to be packaged into virions attached to their *gag* counterparts.

The envelope gene encodes two glycoproteins that make up the envelope spikes: a larger protein forming the "knob" of the spike (also referred to as SU, *su*rface protein), and a smaller protein forming the base (also referred to as TM, *trans*membrane protein). These two proteins are like the other viral gene products synthesized

as a precursor protein. They then are cleaved specifically by a cellular protease to yield the SU and TM proteins. The surface protein binds to the receptor on the host cell, whereas the transmembrane protein serves as a fusion protein that enables fusion of the viral and host-cell membranes once binding has occurred (see earlier).

Exogenous Retroviruses

DEFECTIVE, ACUTE TRANSFORMING VIRUSES

In 1911, Peyton Rous demonstrated that chicken sarcomas could be transmitted from one chicken to another using cell-free filtrates of the original tumors, thus establishing the viral etiology of this malignancy. The RSV has been the subject of intense investigation for many years; these studies have revealed that the oncogenic properties of this virus can be attributed to a single viral gene, termed *src*. Other avian retroviruses since have been isolated that induce a wide variety of sarcomas and other malignant diseases in chickens, including erythroblastosis, myelocytomatosis, and myeloblastosis. In addition, many retroviruses isolated from other species, such as cats, mice, and monkeys, induce malignant sarcomas and lymphomas.

Nonacute, nondefective mouse retroviruses can give rise to acute, defective transforming viruses if passed multiple times in a susceptible host (eg, a mouse or rat). This will give rise to an occasional malignant tumor that often yields a new, highly oncogenic (and defective) virus. These new viruses exhibit the properties of the acute transforming viruses, readily inducing disease in the natural host and causing transformation of cells in culture. From a wide variety of experimental results, it is now known that each of these acute transforming viruses has acquired a novel gene from the host cell that is responsible for the malignant properties. Such genes are collectively termed *oncogenes* and, for each virus, the oncogene is designated by a three-letter acronym denoting its origin. The properties of individual oncogenes are discussed in Chapter 44. The reader is referred to Table 44-2, which summarizes some of the acute transforming viruses isolated and the oncogenes they have acquired. Examination of this table reveals several interesting facts. For example, the same oncogene sequence has been acquired by two different retroviruses from different species. The *fes* oncogene of feline sarcoma virus is structurally identical to the *fps* oncogene of the avian retrovirus Fujinami sarcoma virus. Therefore, it can be concluded that the oncogenic potential of these genes can be manifested equally well in different species. In addition, some viruses have acquired two oncogenes (eg, the *erb* A and *erb* B oncogenes of avian erythroblastosis virus). A growing body of evidence suggests that the two oncogenes provide a synergistic effect in the animal for the rapid and efficient outgrowth of tumor cells.

ORIGIN OF VIRAL ONCOGENES

Two major questions arose immediately on identification of the first retroviral oncogenes: (1) Where do such transforming genes come from? (2) How have retroviruses acquired them? The first question was answered when investigators prepared highly radioactive DNA probes complementary to the viral oncogene sequence. When these probes were hybridized to normal-cell DNA, it was observed that all normal DNA from birds, rodents, and humans contained one or two copies of a gene virtually identical to the oncogene under investigation. Such experiments, coupled with more sophisticated molecular cloning and DNA sequencing experiments, have now shown that viral oncogenes have normal cell counterparts (termed *proto-oncogenes*) in the DNA of all vertebrate species. Hence, it is generally accepted that proto-oncogenes encode normal cellular proteins that perform some essential function during the lifetime of a specific cell.

If proto-oncogenes encode normal cellular proteins, how are these genes acquired by the retrovirus genome, and what alterations in the structure of the gene convert it to an oncogenic element? First, although definitive data regarding the mechanism of oncogene "capture" do not exist, an educated guess can be made as to how this process might take place. Because nonacute retroviruses are ubiquitous in nature, it is postulated that, rarely, a nondefective virus may integrate adjacent to a proto-oncogene sequence. A deletion of chromosomal DNA then could result in the joining of part of the retrovirus genome with the coding sequences of the proto-oncogene. Transcription of the fused genes could readily produce a hybrid RNA containing both retrovirus sequences and proto-oncogene sequences. Such an RNA molecule can undergo recombination with an existing nonacute leukemia virus transcript, thereby yielding an RNA species similar in structure to the known acute transforming virus genome. A comparative analysis of the DNA sequences of viral oncogenes and their cellular homologues has revealed interesting structural modifications in viral oncogene sequences. In general, when the proto-oncogene is captured by the retrovirus, only a portion of the proto-oncogene is found in the virus. In those instances in which the entire proto-oncogene is captured, there often are multiple mutations within the captured viral gene. Therefore, it has been suggested that the oncogenic potential exhibited by the viral oncogene often is due to the fact that only a portion of the gene is present in the virus, or to the fact that the whole gene that is present is mutated in a specific manner that alters its functional activity.

It is clear from many studies that proto-oncogene activation is a complex event (or set of events), and considerable investigation is required before the details of such processes can be understood. It also is clear that the biochemical events mediated by viral oncogene products can differ, perhaps substantially, from the biochemical events mediated by their normal cellular counterparts.

NONDEFECTIVE, NONACUTE RNA TUMOR VIRUSES

Nonacute viruses contain the three essential genes (gag, pol, and env) required for replication (see Fig. 43-6) and, when used to infect cells in culture, these viruses replicate efficiently. However, they do not induce distinguishable morphologic changes in the cells. Introduction of these viruses into a susceptible host (either in a laboratory setting or by transmission in nature) results in a widespread viremia. After several months, perhaps a year, a variety of neoplastic diseases (eg, lymphocytic or myeloid tumors, erythroblastic leukemias, osteopetrosis, nephroblastoma, thymic sarcomas, or lymphosarcomas) often can be observed. Examination of the cells of these tumors shows that, in most cases, the tumors are monoclonal in origin (ie, originating from a single transformed cell). In the case of induction of leukemia by avian leukosis virus (ALV), the mechanism of the oncogenic event is understood. Analyses of ALV lymphomas have shown that each tumor contains a portion of the ALV proviral genome integrated adjacent to the cellular proto-oncogene, c-*myc*. The integration of ALV sequences activates the expression of the c-*myc* proto-oncogene considerably above the levels observed in normal lymphocytes. Such an "insertional" activation is a critical step in the establishment of the neoplastic lymphoma, and insertional activation of different oncogenes can occur in different tumors.

Endogenous Retroviruses

Endogenous retroviruses can be found in virtually all vertebrate species (including man). For the most part, expression of these sequences is tightly regulated, and viral genes are expressed only at defined times during cellular differentiation or during the lifetime of the animal. However, in the case of chickens and mice, the extensive experimentation with these species has led to the development of highly inbred strains. Individual strains often show a unique and definable pattern of endogenous virus expression and subsequent development of malignant disease. For example, in some strains of mice, such as AKR mice, the endogenous mouse leukemia virus is activated soon after birth. These animals develop acute viremia, and within 6 to 12 months, a high percentage develop leukemia. Other strains of mice (low-incidence strains) may fail to acquire leukemia until late in life, if at all. High-incidence strains of mice contain two dominant loci (AKV-1 and AKV-2) that code for the *ecotropic* viruses AKV-1 and AKV-2. Expression of either locus results in expression of the leukemia virus and the induction of neoplastic disease. In low-incidence strains of mice, resistance to leukemia results from the host's resistance to infection by his own endogenous virus. Some mouse strains do not develop leukemia; these mice lack the endogenous leukemia virus loci.

In addition to endogenous viruses that are induced naturally and will replicate (hence the designation, *ecotropic viruses*) in the host, most animal cells contain endogenous retroviruses that can be induced to replicate only in cells different from the natural host. For example, treatment of mouse cells in culture with inhibitors of protein synthesis, such as halogenated deoxyribonucleosides, or inhibitors of nucleic acid synthesis induces viruses that do not grow on mouse cells but that replicate on cells of a different species. These viruses are termed *xenotropic viruses,* and their host range (ie, the cells in which they will replicate) is determined by the ability of the *env* glycoprotein to bind specifically to the appropriate cellular receptors.

Considerable interest has centered on the role of the readily inducible ecotropic mouse virus in the development of thymic lymphomas. It has become increasingly clear that the ecotropic virus itself is not responsible for the induction of malignant disease. However, isolation of virus from late preleukemic or leukemic AKR mice has revealed several new viruses that have the properties of both ecotropic and xenotropic endogenous viruses. These viruses can multiply in both mouse cells and mink cells, and have been termed *dual tropic,* or *MCF (mink cell focus-forming)* viruses. These viruses are not endogenous viruses in the sense that their composite genomes are not present in the germline DNA of the host. However, these novel recombinant viruses appear to exhibit a unique tissue-cell tropism, and they are important elements in establishing malignant disease. The precise mechanism by which these viruses mediate cellular transformation most certainly involves the insertional activation of cellular oncogene sequences by the integrated viruses.

Murine Mammary Tumor Viruses

In 1936, the first murine mammary tumor viruses (MMTVs) were discovered in the milk of a strain of mice showing a high incidence of mammary carcinomas. MMTVs are generally similar to the other RNA tumor viruses, but their dense nucleocapsid is slightly off-center in the spherical virion; hence, they are called *B-type particles* (Fig. 43-8).

MMTV represents a class of mouse endogenous viruses that are expressed in different inbred strains of mice in varying degrees. In C3H mice, MMTV is highly oncogenic and is expressed at high levels in most tissues of the mouse. The virus also is found in large amounts in lactating mammary tissue and in milk. Transfer of the virus to the offspring through the milk results in a high incidence of mammary carcinomas within 6 to 12 months. If newborn mice of a high-incidence strain are nursed by

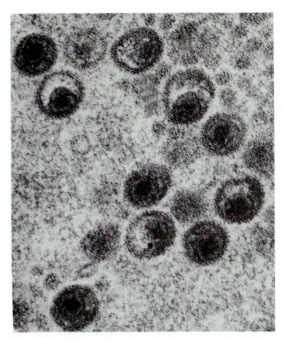

FIGURE 43-8 B-type particles of mouse mammary tumor virus at high magnification, clearly showing the off-center nucleoids. (Original magnification ×136,000.)

a foster mother of a low-incidence strain, few tumors develop. Conversely, if newborn mice of a low-incidence strain are nursed by a foster mother producing MMTV, those low-incidence mice will acquire mammary tumors within the 6- to 12-month period.

MMTV is a nondefective virus and, therefore, has the usual complement of viral genes: *gag, pol,* and *env.* However, expression of the MMTV provirus is regulated by both genetic and hormonal factors. Glucocorticoids greatly enhance the level of expression of MMTV RNA through binding of the glucocorticoid receptor complex to a unique glucocorticoid response element in the MMTV LTR. The mechanism of tumor induction is thought to resemble that of other nondefective, nonacute leukemia viruses, in that tumor cells contain integrated MMTV provirus at two distinct loci in the DNA of mouse mammary tumors. These loci, termed *int*-1 and *int*-2, encode products that appear to be related to cellular growth factors.

Human Retroviruses

HUMAN T-CELL LEUKEMIA VIRUSES

There was an extensive search for human leukemia viruses during the 1970s that was fraught with skepticism. Virus-like particles were observed frequently in human leukemia cells, but several early isolates subsequently were shown to be laboratory contaminants of nonhuman origin. However, in 1981, investigators in both the United States and

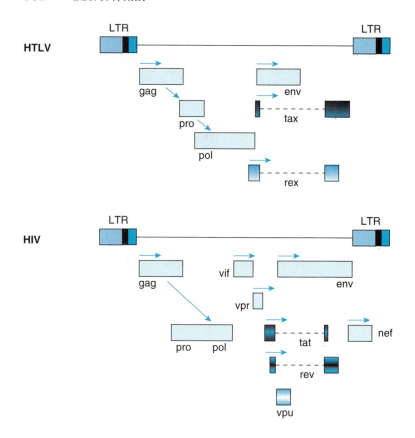

FIGURE 43-9 Genome structure of the human retroviruses human T-cell leukemia/lymphoma virus (HTLV–I, HTLV-II), and human immunodeficiency virus (HIV). See text for details.

Japan reported that a virus could be isolated from patients with certain T-cell malignancies. This virus was isolated from several cultivated cell lines derived from malignant tissue as well as from fresh blood obtained from patients with adult T-cell leukemia (ATL).

The virus, designated human T-cell leukemia virus I (HTLV-I), has now been clearly shown to be associated with T-cell malignancies in humans. HTLV-I–related T-cell leukemias are endemic to parts of Japan, the Caribbean, South America, and Africa. About 10% of the population in southwest Japan has antibodies to HTLV-I, whereas seropositive individuals are rare in parts of the world where ATL is not endemic. HTLV-I also shows an association with a neurologic disease that is common in the endemic areas. Known as tropical spastic paraparesis (TSP) or HTLV-associated myelopathy (HAM), this is a demyelinating disease characterized by the development of a progressive weakness of the leg and lower body muscles. The link between HAM/TSP and HTLV-I infection was first established by the serologic analysis of patients with TSP on the Caribbean islands of Martinique and Jamaica. Continued seroepidemiologic testing has shown that patients with HAM/TSP in Columbia, Trinidad, and Seychelles, as well as in Japan, also exhibit high incidences of HTLV-I infections. Thus, the link between this disease and HTLV-I has been clearly established. Although some HTLV-I infections eventually lead to overt clinical disease in the form of ATL or HAM/TSP, most remain subclinical throughout the life of the infected individual. The lifetime risk of developing disease has been estimated at only a few percent or less.

A second related virus, designated HTLV-II, originally was isolated from a patient with T-cell variant hairy-cell leukemia. HTLV-II has been shown to be endemic in Native American populations, but has not been clearly linked to any human disease. HTLV-I and HTLV-II can be transmitted in three different ways: through sexual contact, through contaminated blood, and from an infected mother to her child during the perinatal period. The last mode of transmission occurs mainly through infected cells in breast milk. Therefore, it is recommended that infected mothers do not breastfeed their children.

Because HTLV can be spread by blood, and thus by transfusions, blood banks routinely test their blood supply for the presence of HTLV. Intravenous drug abusers in the United States are showing an increasing prevalence of HTLV infection (mainly HTLV-II). Many of these individuals also are infected with HIV. It is unclear whether such patients progress more rapidly to the acquired immunodeficiency syndrome (AIDS), and whether they have a higher incidence of ATL or HAM/TSP.

Structure and Replication of Human T-Cell Leukemia Viruses I and II

The genome of HTLV closely resembles that of other vertebrate retroviruses in that it encodes the three essential gene products (gag, pol, and env) required for virus replication (Fig. 43-9). However, the HTLV genome contains additional genes that contribute to the ability of HTLV to autoregulate its replication in infected cells. This distinguishes the replication cycle of this virus from that of more conventional retroviruses. The best characterized of these genes, designated *tax* and *rex,* reside downstream of the *env* gene. Together, the *tax* and *rex* gene products regulate the production of HTLV RNA. The *tax* protein is a strong "transactivator" of cellular and viral gene expression. The tax protein binds to host-cell transcription factors that, in turn, actively promote efficient transcription of virus RNA. The tax protein also promotes or enhances (transactivates) the expression of certain cellular genes (eg, the interleukin-2 receptor). The *rex* protein acts specifically to promote the expression of the viral structural proteins gag, pol, and env. The rex protein binds to an element present in the 5' end of the mRNAs for these proteins, known as the rex response element, and promotes the transport of the RNAs from the nucleus to the cytoplasm of infected cells. The function of the rex protein appears to be similar to that of the HIV rev protein discussed later. The tax and rex genes both are situated at the 3' end of the viral genome. This region, previously known as the pX region, also encodes other gene products. The exact functions of these in viral replication are unknown.

The relationship between HTLV replication and the appearance of ATL is unclear. Analysis of cell lines derived from patients with ATL has shown that each individual ATL cell line has HTLV sequences integrated at a different site in the chromosomal DNA. No evidence for "insertional" activation of a cellular oncogene has been obtained. What, then, is the mechanism for HTLV-induced disease? One model suggests that the HTLV-encoded *tax* gene product may act to transactivate cellular genes that, in turn, stimulate T-cell proliferation. The rapid proliferation of a population of T cells then could give rise to the activation of cellular oncogenes through additional mutational mechanisms (see Chap. 44). Evidence for this model comes from the observation that *tax* expression in T lymphocytes increases the level of expression of interleukin-2 and interleukin-2 receptors, cellular components that are required for T-cell proliferation.

Much remains to be done to elucidate the role of HTLV in human malignancies and other diseases. However, insights into the role of virus replication and the contributions of novel viral gene products will help to paint a clearer picture of virus-induced cellular changes, both malignant and otherwise.

HUMAN IMMUNODEFICIENCY VIRUSES

In 1981, a novel, epidemic form of immunodeficiency, termed *AIDS,* was recognized. Between 1981 and 1991, there was a virtual explosion in the number of AIDS cases in the United States, and this disease is now one of the leading causes of death in young individuals. In 1981, there were 310 cases of AIDS reported in this country and 135 deaths attributed to the disease. In 1991 alone, more than 40,000 new AIDS cases were reported and more than 30,000 people died of the disease. AIDS is now known to be caused by a human retrovirus, designated HIV. The disease is characterized by opportunistic infections and malignant diseases in patients without a recognized cause for immunodeficiency. Numerous opportunistic infections have been observed, predominantly caused by *Pneumocystis carinii,* cytomegalovirus, atypical mycobacteria, *Toxoplasma gondii, Candida,* herpes simplex virus, *Cryptococcus neoformans,* and *Cryptosporidium.* Active tuberculosis also is seen at an increasing frequency. Other highly distinctive features of AIDS are the occurrence of Kaposi's sarcoma (particularly in gay men) and dementing neurologic disorders. As many as 5% to 10% of infected individuals develop lymphomas that frequently are positive for Epstein-Barr virus. In addition, the incidence of cervical carcinoma is significantly increased in HIV-infected women. AIDS is a disease of the immune system, and a hallmark of the disease is an abnormally low number of CD4-positive cells.

Like HTLV, HIV is transmitted by sexual contact, through infected blood, and from mother to child. HIV can be transmitted during both pregnancy and the neonatal period, and recent studies suggest that vertical transmission can be reduced significantly by azidothymidine (AZT) treatment of the mother during pregnancy. Without treatment, about 25% of children born to infected mothers acquire the virus. Many of these go on to rapidly develop AIDS. The blood supply is now routinely tested for HIV, but before tests were developed, many individuals became infected as a result of blood transfusions. Blood-derived products used in the treatment of hemophilia also were contaminated frequently with HIV, and a large percentage of patients with severe hemophilia were infected early on in the epidemic. Many of these have now died of AIDS.

In the United States and Europe, HIV infection and, subsequently, AIDS still occurs mostly in certain high-risk groups. These include gay and bisexual men, intravenous drug abusers, heterosexual partners of members of these groups, and infants born to HIV-positive mothers. AIDS is still mainly a male disease in these countries. However, the number of cases in women is increasing rapidly. In the United States, most infected women belong to minority groups (74%), and many women infected in recent years have reported heterosexual activity as their only risk factor. This indicates that heterosexual transmission is becoming more common in this country. In many other areas of the world, the disease already is spread primarily by heterosexual transmission and affects men and women in equal proportions. In Africa, where the epidemic is thought to have originated, as many as 10 million people

A Closer Look

In the spring of 1981, the first cases of the disease that soon became known as AIDS (*A*quired *I*mmune *D*eficiency *S*yndrome) started to appear at hospitals in New York City, San Francisco, and Los Angeles. The patients all presented with severe opportunistic infections, and several of them had a form of pneumonia caused by *Pneumocystic carinii* that had previously been extremely rare in the United States. Almost all of the patients were gay men. At the same time, several young gay men were diagnosed with a strange skin condition. The lesions were soon recognized to be consistent with Kaposi's sarcoma, a rare form of cancer that causes characteristic skin lesions. What was particularly puzzling was that this disease had previously been diagnosed almost exclusively in elderly Jewish and Italian men. In addition, the skin cancer in the young men seemed much more aggressive than the usual cases of Kaposi's sarcoma.

The underlying cause of all these problems was soon recognized to be a severe defect in the patients' immune systems. The low numbers of CD4 helper T cells in their blood were particularly striking. Up to this time, severe immunodeficiencies had been relatively rare and were usually associated with genetic defects or aggressive immunosuppressive treatments.

As the number of cases started to increase, it became clear that an epidemic was emerging among gay men. Soon, similar cases were reported from several countries in Europe. Although an infectious agent was suspected almost from the beginning, it was also possible that the disease could be caused by an environmental agent. Potential candidates were some of the drugs that were commonly used in the gay community. However, many virologists started to suspect that the disease might be caused by a virus, and by 1982, the hunt for the potential culprit was on.

Tissues and blood from patients with the disease were examined for every possible virus, and for a while, the disease was believed to be caused by a herpesvirus or an adenovirus. In the spring of 1983, however, a group at the French Pasteur Institute led by Dr. Luc Montagnier, reported that they had isolated what seemed to be a novel retrovirus from several patients with AIDS. Their findings were later confirmed by isolations of similar viruses by Dr. Robert Gallo's group at the National Institutes of Health (NIH) and by Dr. Jay Levy's group in San Francisco.

By the time the novel retrovirus was discovered, it had become obvious that AIDS was transmitted in three different ways: by sexual transmission, through contaminated blood, and from an infected mother to her child. Indications of these routes of transmission included the findings that an increasing number of cases involved intravenous drug users and children born to mothers who were intravenous drug users. Several cases of the disease had already been reported in recipients of blood transfusions, in hemophiliacs who had received blood concentrates, and in children of each of these two groups. It thus became imperative to quickly develop a blood test for the virus. Through collaborative efforts between the groups that had first isolated the virus (originally named LAV by the French group, ARV by the California group, and HTLV-III by the NIH group), such a test soon became available. It thus became possible to test every batch of blood and blood concentrate for the presence of the virus, which was now called *human immunodeficiency virus,* or *HIV*. Testing of blood supply and blood products soon became mandatory in most countries of the world.

As soon as the blood test became available, researchers saw that the picture of AIDS was even more chilling than originally suspected. It was soon established that the virus was present not only in the United States and Europe, but also in several other areas of the world. The picture was especially grim in Africa, which is now believed to be where the virus originated. Random testing showed that the epidemic was rampant in several different African countries, with some cities showing overall seroprevalence levels of approximately 10% to 15%. This testing also showed that AIDS was already a major killer in Africa—a fact that had been largely unrecognized because of the multitude of other medical problems and deaths caused by malnutrition and a low standard of living.

The blood test also showed that 30% to 40% of hemophiliacs were infected and that many more recipients of blood transfusions were infected than had originally been suspected. Many of these individuals showed little or no symptoms of AIDS. Because the exact date on which these patients had been infected was usually possible to pinpoint, researchers realized that many of these patients had already lived several years with the virus. We now know that the latency period between HIV infection and the development of AIDS can be 10 or more years. Some long-term survivors have shown little or no signs of a declining immune system 10 to 15 years after they were infected. About 5% of patients seem to belong in this group.

were infected with HIV by mid-1994. It is unclear how many already have died of AIDS, because most cases are not reported, but the estimated figure is 2.5 million (50% women). Latin America also has a serious problem, with millions of infected individuals. HIV infection also is spreading rapidly in parts of Asia, especially in Thailand and India, and it is clear that AIDS soon will be a serious problem in these countries. It has been estimated that about 1 million individuals in the United States are infected with HIV. Many of these have no symptoms, and many do not know that they are infected. By mid-1994, the total number of reported AIDS cases in the United States alone had reached almost 400,000, and about 60% of these patients already had died from the disease.

The initial isolation of HIV from the cells of patients with AIDS was reported by a group of French scientists in 1983. This was followed by the isolation and continuous propagation of other isolates by scientists in both France and the United States in 1984, clearly documenting the link between the virus and AIDS. Several lines of evidence have now established HIV as the main etiologic agent for AIDS. Infected individuals often remain free of symptoms for many years. Recent estimates indicate that 80% to 90% of those infected go on to develop AIDS within 10 to 12 years of infection. The time for progression to AIDS varies greatly. Long-term survivors (ie, infected patients who have been observed for 7 years or more) include individuals with normal levels of CD4-positive cells. Some of these may never go on to develop AIDS. In other patients, levels of CD4-positive cells drop dramatically within years after infection, leading to rapid development of the disease and death. The factors that determine these different outcomes are still largely unknown.

Human Immunodeficiency Virus Genome Structure

Human immunodeficiency virus belongs to the Lentivirus subfamily. Lentiviruses are characterized by a complex genome structure with several more genes in addition to *gag, pol,* and *env.* They also are characterized by their efficient replication and their ability to cause a lytic infection (ie, an infection that kills the host cell). It is now recognized that there are two different types of HIV (HIV-1 and HIV-2). HIV-2 is most prevalent in parts of West Africa, and only a few cases of HIV-2 infection have been reported in the United States.

The HIV genome has been shown to contain at least six extra genes. Three of these genes (*tat, rev,* and *nef*) encode regulatory proteins that are likely to play important roles in viral pathogenesis (see Fig. 43-9). The HIV-1 genome contains three additional accessory genes (*vpu, vif,* and *vpr*) that are dispensable for replication in some tissue-culture cells. The HIV-2 genome differs from HIV-1 in that the *vpu* gene is missing. However, the

HIV-2 genome contains a gene (*vpx*) that is not present in HIV-1. The exact role of the accessory gene products in virus replication is unclear.

The *tat* gene plays a major role in the regulation of viral gene expression, and its expression is essential for virus growth. The tat protein is an 82–amino acid protein found in the nucleus of infected cells. The *tat* gene contains two coding exons interrupted by an intron, and the virus RNA has to be multiply spliced to generate the mRNA for this protein. The *tat* gene product (like the HTLV-*tax* gene product) is a powerful transactivator of viral transcription. *Tat* functions to enhance virus RNA transcription by specifically interacting with sequences at the 5′ end of the viral genome, the TAR (*tat* response) sequences. The TAR sequences are the first sequences to be transcribed from the viral promoter. The newly transcribed TAR RNA forms a stem-loop structure that specifically binds the tat protein. This promotes elongation of the RNA chain and probably also initiation of new RNA synthesis. Thus, TAR acts as an enhancer at the RNA level. In the presence of tat, the amounts of full-length viral transcripts are increased several hundredfold. Hence, in an infected cell, the presence or absence of the tat protein has marked effects on the efficiency of virus transcription.

The *rev* protein also is made from a multiply spliced mRNA. This protein functions similarly to the HTLV-*rex* protein. *Rev* (a 116–amino acid protein in HIV-1) promotes the transport from the host-cell nucleus to the cytoplasm of the mRNAs encoding the structural proteins gag, gag/pol, and env, as well as the mRNAs for vif, vpr, and vpu. In the absence of rev, only the nef, rev, and tat mRNAs reach the cytoplasm. The rev-regulated mRNAs all are incompletely spliced and contain complete introns.

The nef protein is dispensable for virus replication in most tissue-culture cells. However, nef is likely to play an important role in pathogenesis. The nef protein downregulates the CD4 receptor and also may affect cellular signal transduction pathways.

Human Immunodeficiency Virus Replication and Pathogenesis

The basis for the immunopathogenesis of HIV infection is a severe depletion of the helper/inducer subset of T lymphocytes expressing the CD4 marker. This depletion causes a severe combined immunodeficiency, because the T4 lymphocytes play a central role in the immune response to foreign antigens.

HIV's tropism for T4 lymphocytes reflects the utilization of the CD4 molecule as a high-affinity receptor for the virus. Other cells that express the CD4 molecule, such as macrophages and monocytes, also are targets for HIV infection. After binding of the HIV SU protein gp120 to the CD4 molecule, fusion of viral and cellular membranes enables the virus to enter the host cell. The fusion is mediated by the transmembrane portion of the env protein (gp41). After the core is internalized, the HIV genome is transcribed to DNA, and proviral DNA is integrated into the host chromosome. After integration of the provirus, the infection can become latent or virus replication can be initiated. The frequency at which a latent infection rather than a productive infection is established is unclear. However, it is known that a large number of cells are actively replicating virus even during the clinical latency period. The precise relationship between cell activation and virus replication has not been delineated, but the extent of antigenic stimulation of the immune system may play a role in determining the period between virus infection and severe T4-cell depletion.

Several mechanisms have been proposed to explain the depletion of the CD4 cells. In addition to cells being killed directly by HIV replication, cells expressing viral envelope protein on the cell surface may interact with uninfected CD4-bearing cells, thereby promoting the fusion of infected and uninfected T4 lymphocytes. This might lead to the death of noninfected cells. In addition, cell–cell fusion could promote efficient spread of virus from cell to cell. Immune mechanisms also may play an important role in T4-cell depletion. For example, infected T4 cells expressing envelope protein on their surface may be recognized as nonself and efficiently cleared from the system. In addition, binding of circulating gp120 to the surface of uninfected T4 cells also may designate these cells as nonself, leading to their destruction.

The importance of macrophages and monocytes in the course of HIV infection and disease is becoming more evident. Monocytes can be infected with HIV in vitro, and virus can be isolated from monocytes obtained from the blood and organs of HIV-infected individuals, indicating that monocytes serve as a major reservoir for HIV in the body. The infected monocyte may transport the virus to various organs of the body. Macrophages also may contribute to the unique neurologic symptoms associated with AIDS, because they are the major cell type harboring HIV in the brain, giving rise to the speculation that these cells contribute to the spread of virus within the central nervous system.

It has been postulated that antigenic stimulation of an infected individual's immune system might stimulate T-cell proliferation, thereby promoting virus spread. In addition, it is possible that concomitant virus infections (ie, Epstein-Barr virus, cytomegalovirus, hepatitis B, or herpes simplex virus) can induce HIV expression, leading to more rapid disease progression.

Acquired Immunodeficiency Syndrome Treatment and Prevention

Strategies for the treatment and prevention of HIV infection have focused in large part on inhibiting different stages of the HIV replication cycle. The most successful treatment modality makes use of the drug AZT, 3'-azido-3'-deoxythymidine, also known as zidovudine or Retrovir. AZT, first synthesized in 1964, is a potent inhibitor of HIV replication in vitro and specifically inhibits reverse transcription. The antiretroviral activity of AZT is a result of a preferential interaction of the 5'-triphosphate of AZT with the viral reverse transcriptase, inhibiting viral reverse transcriptase activity about 100 times more efficiently than do cellular DNA polymerases. After clinical trials in 1986, AZT was licensed in the United States during 1987 for the treatment of patients with symptomatic HIV infections. AZT is not without sometimes serious side effects, the major ones being macrocytic anemia and granulocytopenia. However, the most severe problem is that HIV variants resistant to AZT invariably arise in treated patients. Thus, although the initial effects of treatment often are dramatic, with diminishing viral replication and sometimes increasing T4-cell levels, the effects are transient. Several other reverse transcriptase inhibitors have been developed, but resistance is a problem with these drugs as well. Most recently, novel drugs have been developed that specifically inhibit another enzyme, the viral protease. Some of these compounds are undergoing clinical trials, but it already has been documented that the rapid development of resistant virus variants is going to limit the usefulness of these drugs.

In spite of global efforts, an effective vaccine for HIV has not been developed. Most of the potential vaccines that have been tested have consisted of different forms of the HIV envelope protein. It has been shown in both human vaccine trials and animal experiments that these vaccines are capable of inducing good immune responses, including the induction of neutralizing antibodies. However, these antibodies are only able to protect against an infection with a virus that contains the same or a similar envelope protein. This presents a serious problem, because many different virus variants with vastly different envelope proteins are circulating in the human population. In fact, it has been shown that many different viruses may exist simultaneously within the same patient, and that the predominant variant changes from time to time. This is likely due to the selection of viruses that are not neutralized by the prevalent neutralizing antibodies, which helps to explain why the virus can continue to replicate in infected individuals in spite of a generally good initial immune response. Vaccines based on other viral components are under development, and preparations containing a mixture of several different envelope proteins also are under consideration.

Bibliography

JOURNALS

AIDS: the unanswered questions. Science 1993;260:1253.
Bishop JM. Viral oncogenes. Cell 1985;42:23.
Varmus H. Retroviruses. Science 1988;240:1427.

BOOKS

Coffin JM. Structure and classification of retroviruses. In: Levy JA, ed. The Retroviridae, vol 1. New York, Plenum Press, 1992:19.

Green PL, Chen ISY. Molecular features of the human T-cell leukemia virus. In: Levy JA, ed. The Retroviridae, vol 3. New York, Plenum Press, 1994:277.

Loh PC. Spumaviruses. In: Levy JA, ed. The Retroviridae, vol 2. New York, Plenum Press, 1993:362.

Luciw PA, Leung NJ. Mechanisms of retrovirus replication. In: Levy JA, ed. The Retroviridae, vol 1. New York, Plenum Press, 1992:159.

Mann J, Tarantola DJM, Netter TW, eds. AIDS in the world: a global report. Cambridge, MA, Harvard University Press, 1992.

Sugamura K, Hinuma Y. Human retroviruses: HTLV-I and HTLV-II. In: Levy JA, ed. The Retroviridae, vol 2. New York, Plenum Press, 1993:399.

Temin HM. Origin and general nature of retroviruses. In: Levy JA, ed. The Retroviridae, vol 1. New York, Plenum Press, 1992:1.

Essentials of Medical Microbiology, Fifth Edition, edited by Wesley A. Volk, Bryan M. Gebhardt, Marie-Louise Hammarskjöld, and Robert J. Kadner. Lippincott-Raven Publishers, Philadelphia © 1996.

Chapter 44

Oncogenes and Cancer

Studies on the structure and replication of RNA and DNA tumor viruses have provided a unique perspective on the molecular basis of cancer. The identification of genes (oncogenes) that can confer the malignant phenotype to normal cells has provided the molecular biologist with the key to understanding some of the underlying steps leading to the establishment of the cancer cell. In the past decade, there has been a veritable explosion in our understanding of the role of oncogenes in neoplasia. In the brief space available here, it is not possible to consider all the experimental data that have brought us to our current knowledge of the role of oncogenes in the development of malignancies. Therefore, only a short summary of some of the major concepts linking oncogenes and cancer is presented.

Viral Oncogenes and Cellular Transformation

The realization that acute transforming retroviruses contain oncogenes that are both necessary and sufficient for the transformation of cells in culture and for the induction of animal tumors led investigators to initiate an analysis of the proteins encoded by these oncogenes. Between 25 and 30 viral oncogenes have been identified and are designated by three-letter acronyms. In most cases, the viral oncogene products have been identified. Table 44-1 summarizes our knowledge of representative members of the different oncogene families. The discovery that viral oncogenes were acquired from normal host genes (proto-oncogenes) supported the notion that viral oncoproteins would likely be related structurally and functionally to important cellular host proteins and enzymes. In many cases, DNA and protein sequence analysis has permitted the identification of the cellular homologue of the viral oncogene, verifying this notion. For example, the oncoprotein encoded by the simian sarcoma virus, v-*sis,* is structurally identical to a growth factor secreted by platelets, platelet-derived growth factor (PDGF), whereas the oncoprotein encoded by the avian erythroblastosis virus *erb*-B gene is structurally identical to a portion of the receptor for epidermal growth factor (EGF). These and other examples are summarized in Table 44-1.

TABLE 44-1
Viral Oncogenes and Cellular Homologues of Known Function

Oncogene	Activity	Cellular Homologue
src	Tyrosine protein kinase	Membrane-associated tyrosine kinase
erb B	Tyrosine protein kinase	Epidermal growth factor receptor
fms	Tyrosine protein kinase	Colony-stimulating factor I receptor
sis	Growth stimulation	Platelet-derived growth factor-B chain
raf	Serine/threonine kinase	Cytoplasmic-receptor linked kinase
ras	GTP/GDP binding	Receptor-coupling factors
jun	DNA binding	Transcription factor (AP-1 related)
erb A	DNA binding	Thyroxin receptor

GTP, guanosine triphosphate; GDP, guanosine diphosphate.

Understanding of the biochemical functions mediated by oncoproteins has provided important insights into the types of cellular perturbations that lead to cellular transformation. The properties of some of these proteins are summarized here.

Oncogene Families

Viral oncoproteins can function in either the nucleus or the cytoplasm. Sequence analysis and intracellular location, as well as functional activity, have permitted the general classification of these proteins into families (Table 44-2). The largest family is made up of the tyrosine kinase oncogenes (representative members being *src, abl, fps, yes, fgr, fms, ros,* and *erb* B). The proteins encoded by these oncogenes are found associated with cellular membranes and exhibit protein tyrosine kinase activity (ie, the transfer of phosphate from adenosine triphosphate to tyrosine residues in the acceptor protein). The members of this family can be subdivided further into membrane-spanning

TABLE 44-2
Viral Oncogenes and Their Products

Oncogene	Virus	Animal of Origin	Virus Disease	Protein Product	Activity
src	RSV	Chicken	Sarcoma	$pp60^{src}$	Tyrosine kinase
fps/fes	Fujinami ASV/ST FeSV	Chicken	Sarcoma	$pp140^{gag-fps}$	Tyrosine kinase
		Cat	Sarcoma	$p85^{gag-fes}$	Tyrosine kinase
yes	Y73 ASV	Chicken	Sarcoma	$p90^{gag-yes}$	Tyrosine kinase
ros	UR-2 ASV	Chicken	Sarcoma	$p68^{gag-ros}$	Tyrosine kinase
fgr	GR FeSV	Cat	Sarcoma	$p70^{gag-fgr}$	Tyrosine kinase
abl	Abelson MLV	Mouse	Pre–B-cell leukemia	$p160^{gag-abl}$	Tyrosine kinase
fms	SM FeSV	Cat	Sarcoma	$p180^{gag-fms}$	Tyrosine kinase
erb B	AEV-H, AEV-ES4	Chicken	Erythroblastosis	$p68^{erbB}$	Tyrosine kinase
erb A	AEV-ES4	Chicken	Erythroblastosis	$p75^{gag-erbA}$	Nuclear, DNA binding
myc	MC29	Chicken	Myelocytomatosis	$p110^{gag-myc}$	Nuclear, DNA binding
myb	AMV	Chicken	Myeloblastosis	$p45^{myb}$	Nuclear, DNA binding
fos	FBR MSV	Mouse	Osteosarcoma	$p75^{gag-fos}$	Nuclear, DNA binding
jun	ASV-17	Chicken	Osteosarcoma	$p65^{gag-jun}$	Nuclear, DNA binding
H-ras	Harvey MSV	Rat	Sarcoma and erythroleukemia	$p21^{Hras}$	GTP/GDP-binding protein
K-ras	Kirsten MSV	Rat	Sarcoma and erythroleukemia	$p21^{Kras}$	GTP/GDP-binding protein
N-ras	Neuroblastoma*	Human	†	$p21^{Nras}$	GTP/GDP-binding protein
raf/mil	3611 MSV	Mouse	Sarcoma	$p75^{gag-raf}$	Serine kinase
	MH-2	Chicken	Sarcoma	$p100^{gag-mil}$	Serine kinase
mos	Moloney MSV	Mouse	Sarcoma	$p37^{mos}$	Serine kinase
sis	SSV	Monkey	Sarcoma	$p28^{sis}$	PDGF-B chain
	P1 FeSV	Cat	Sarcoma	$p76^{gag-sis}$	PDGF-B chain
rel	REV*	Chicken	Reticuloendotheliosis	$p59^{v-rel}$	‡
ets	E26	Chicken	Erythroblastosis	$p135^{gag-myb-ets}$	‡

AVS, avian sarcoma virus; FeSV, feline sarcoma virus; MLV, mouse leukemia virus; AEV, avian erythroblastosis virus; SSV simian sarcoma virus; AMV, avian myeloblastosis virus; REV, reticuloendotheliosis virus; MSV, mouse sarcoma virus; RSV, Rous sarcoma virus; ST, Synder-Theilin; GR, Gardner-Rasheed; SM, Susan McDonough; FBR, Finkel-Biskis-Reilly; GTP, guanosine triphosphate; GDP, guanosine diphosphate; PDGF, platelet-derived growth factor.

* Identified by DNA transfection of mouse cells.

† Not found in a retrovirus.
‡ Function unknown.

tyrosine kinases that resemble growth factor receptors (v-*fms*, v-*erb* B) and tyrosine kinases that associate with the inner side of the plasma membrane (v-*src*, v-*yes*, v-*fps*). The significance of this distinction is discussed later. A closely related family of oncogenes (*mos, raf, mil,* and *rel*) has been shown to have partial sequence similarity with the tyrosine kinase family of oncogenes. Several members of this family exhibit protein serine/threonine kinase activity. Also in the cytoplasm is the *ras* family of oncogenes (Ha-*ras*, K-*ras*, and N-*ras*). Members of this highly conserved family of oncoproteins are characterized by their ability to bind guanine nucleotides and hydrolyze guanosine triphosphate (GTP) (guanosine diphosphate [GDP]/GTP-binding/GTPase activity). The nuclear oncogene family includes *erb* A, *jun, fos, myc, myb, ski,* and two DNA tumor virus gene products, adenovirus E1A and SV40/polyoma T antigen. Nuclear oncogenes function in a variety of ways to alter the pattern of gene expression. For example, DNA sequence analysis has shown that *erb* A is an altered form of the thyroxine receptor and appears to interact with a unique receptor-binding site. Similarly, *jun* and *fos* appear to function as "transcription" factors by binding directly to DNA and promoting gene expression.

THE TYROSINE KINASE FAMILY

Perhaps the best studied of all the viral oncoproteins is the *src* protein of the acute transforming virus, Rous sarcoma virus (RSV). RSV induces sarcomas in chickens at the site of injection and transforms a variety of avian and rodent cells in cell culture. All cells transformed by RSV produce a 60-kilodalton protein that can be identified in whole cell extracts by immunoprecipitation with antisera from rabbits or mice bearing RSV-induced tumors. The most striking feature of the *src* protein, designated pp60^{src}, is that it is a protein tyrosine kinase capable of phosphorylation of either itself (autophosphorylation) or certain other proteins on tyrosine residues. This unusual kinase activity of pp60^{src} is particularly interesting in light of the observation that in normal cells, only about 0.01% of all phosphoamino acids in proteins are phosphotyrosine, most being phosphoserine (99%) and phosphothreonine (0.09%). In cells transformed with RSV, the level of tyrosine phosphorylation in cellular proteins is elevated tenfold, clearly showing the biochemical consequences of expression of the *src* tyrosine protein kinase. Members of the tyrosine kinase family of oncogenes (see Table 44-2) all encode proteins that exhibit tyrosine protein kinase activity. Sequence analysis has revealed the functional relatedness of this family of oncoproteins, in that they all contain a conserved tyrosine kinase domain flanked by divergent domains presumably required to define the "targets" of the kinase activity and regulate enzyme activity.

Oncogene-encoded proteins belonging to the tyrosine kinase family that span the plasma membrane are related to specific receptor molecules, such as the EGF receptor, the PDGF receptor, and the insulin receptor (Fig. 44-1A). The functional relationship between these proteins and growth factor/mitogen receptors has been confirmed by the demonstration that the amino acid sequence of the *erb*-B gene product is virtually identical to a portion of the EGF receptor and represents a truncated version of the EGF receptor. It is likely that the membrane-spanning tyrosine kinase oncoproteins induce cellular transformation by interrupting or altering in some way signal transduction across the plasma membrane. The exact mechanism by which the *src* protein and its close relatives induce transformation is less clear. However, their presence on the inner face of the plasma membrane suggests that these proteins may be "coupled" to other "receptor-like" molecules and may play a role in transmitting cellular signals in response to extracellular stimuli. Several cellular proteins that interact directly or indirectly with the src protein have been identified.

The proteins encoded by the oncogenes *mos, raf, mil,* and *rel* exhibit distant, but clearly identifiable, homology to the tyrosine kinase family of proteins. At least two members of this family, the *raf* and *mos* proteins, possess an associated serine/threonine kinase activity. The proteins in this family also are likely to exert their oncogenic effects by altering the pattern of serine/threonine phosphorylation in transformed cells.

THE *RAS* FAMILY

The third family of cytoplasmic oncoproteins is made up of three highly conserved proteins encoded by three distinct *ras* genes in humans (see Table 44-2). The human Ha-*ras* gene is the homologue of the oncogene of Harvey murine sarcoma virus, whereas the human K-*ras* gene is the homologue of the oncogene of the Kirsten murine sarcoma virus. N-*ras*, the third member of this gene family, was identified in human tumor cells using DNA transfection techniques (see later). Each *ras* gene encodes a protein of 21 kilodaltons, p21, which is associated with the inner face of the plasma membrane. The *ras* proteins are not protein kinases but instead bind guanine nucleotides, both GDP and GTP. Studies have shown that the *ras* proteins have the capacity to hydrolyze GTP to GDP, a property shared with several other known GTP-binding proteins that function as coupling factors in hormone-mediated signaling. Interestingly, the transforming *ras* proteins encoded by either the Ha-*ras* or K-*ras* genes (or by activated cellular *ras* genes; see Fig. 44-1B) have an impaired ability to hydrolyze GTP compared with the *ras* protein encoded by a normal cellular *ras* gene. This is the result of a single nucleotide change in the normal cellular *ras* gene. The structural and functional similarities between *ras* proteins and coupling factors prompt conjec-

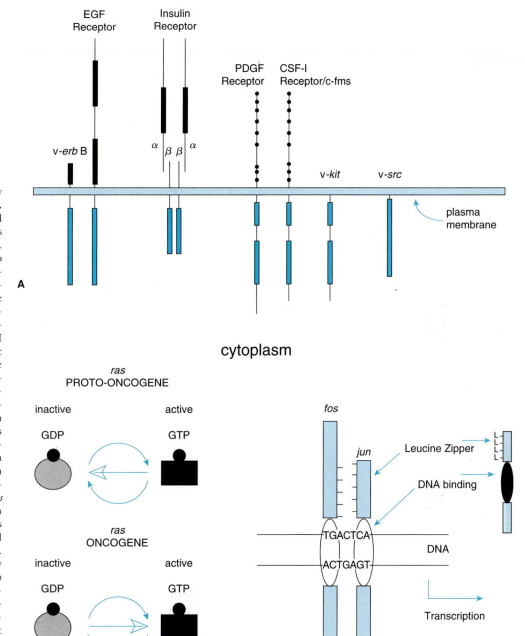

FIGURE 44-1 Proteins encoded by oncogenes and proto-oncogenes. **A.** Structural organization of several receptor tyrosine protein kinases and their oncogenic counterparts. The proteins depicted from left to right are: the epidermal growth factor (EGF) receptor and the oncogene-encoded protein v-*erb* B; the insulin receptor; the platelet-derived growth factor (PDGF) receptor; the colony-stimulating factor-I (CSF-I) receptor and its oncogenic derivative v-*fms*; the oncogene product, v-*kit*; and the viral oncogene product v-*src*. Open boxes denote the location of the highly conserved "kinase" domains for each protein; filled boxes and filled circles denote highly conserved extracellular structural motifs involved in growth factor binding. **B.** Activation of the *ras* protein. Inactive GDP–*ras* complexes and active GTP–*ras* complexes are shown. The open arrows denote the relative amounts of the two forms found in normal (*top*) and transformed (*bottom*) cells. **C.** Regulation of gene expression by *fos* and *jun*. The binding of *fos–jun* protein complexes to the transcriptional regulatory sequence, TGAC-TCA, is depicted. The "leucine zipper" denotes sequences important for the formation of *fos–jun* complexes.

ture that normal cellular p21^{ras} has a receptor-coupling factor function, and that the activated oncogenic version may transmit a continuous signal rather than a highly regulated one.

NUCLEAR ONCOGENES

Several oncoproteins appear to mediate cellular transformation by altering events taking place in the nucleus. The role of these gene products in the regulation of gene transcription has been suggested by several experimental results. Among the most provocative are experiments in which the treatment of quiescent cells with mitogens or growth factors results in the rapid induction of *fos* and *myc* gene expression. In addition, it is clear that enhanced expression of the *myc* gene in certain mouse and human tumors results in sustained growth of the tumor in the animal. These results suggest that alterations in the expression of gene products that normally control or regulate gene expression (nuclear proto-oncogenes) can provoke stable cellular transformation.

The continued characterization of nuclear oncoproteins, particularly *fos* and *jun* (the so-called *fos–jun* connection) has provided unique insights into how gene transcription is altered in transformed cells. The *fos* oncogene was first identified as the oncogenic component of a retrovirus that caused osteosarcomas in mice. The *jun* oncogene was initially found within the genome of the avian retrovirus, ASV-17, a virus that causes fibrosarcomas in chickens. The first clue regarding the function of the *jun* oncogene came from the observation that the amino acid sequence of v-*jun* was strikingly similar to that of a cellular transcription factor called AP-1. AP-1 stimulates the transcription of genes that carry an AP-1–binding site upstream from the cellular transcriptional promoter. Hence, it was concluded that v-*jun* triggers transformation by promoting the unregulated expression of certain cellular genes. The role of the *fos* protein in the control of gene expression became apparent when it was recognized that the *fos* protein formed stable complexes with a cellular protein. This protein is the cellular homologue of *jun*. Therefore, v-*fos* appears to induce transformation by binding to c-jun (a cellular transcription factor) and presumably altering gene expression (see Fig. 44-1C). The recurring theme in all aspects of oncogene study is that cellular signaling pathways that result in altered gene expression are well paved with oncogene products.

Proto-Oncogenes and Oncogenes: Mechanisms of Activation

As discussed in Chapter 43, acute transforming retroviruses induce transformation because they express a "cap-tured" cellular oncogene sequence. In addition, it is well documented that nonacute retroviruses can transcriptionally activate cellular proto-oncogenes by insertional mutagenesis (see Chap. 43), thereby inducing cellular transformation. Proto-oncogenes also can be activated by mechanisms other than retrovirus integration. Three such mechanisms have been described: somatic mutations, chromosomal translocations, and proto-oncogene amplification.

PROTO-ONCOGENE MUTATIONS

The first clues indicating that cells transformed by agents other than viruses contained activated oncogenes came from experiments using the techniques of DNA transfection. In these experiments, investigators prepared DNA from several human tumor cell lines and applied this DNA to normal mouse cell lines in culture (NIH-3T3 cells). It was observed that DNA from certain tumors induced the formation of foci or patches of transformed NIH-3T3 cells at a frequency much greater than that generated by DNA from normal cells (Fig. 44-2). If DNA was prepared from transformed recipient cells and used in a second experiment to artificially infect normal NIH-3T3 cells, an elevated frequency of transformed foci again was observed. Finally, if cells derived from such transformed foci were injected into mice, tumors were observed (see Fig. 44-2). The ability to detect and transfer genes capable of inducing transformation of NIH-3T3 cells led rapidly to the molecular cloning and characterization of the genes responsible for such transformation. DNA sequence analysis of the first gene that was cloned in this way showed that it was identical to the *ras* gene of the Harvey sarcoma virus (Ha-*ras;* see earlier). In addition, the activated human *ras* gene differed from its normal cellular homologue

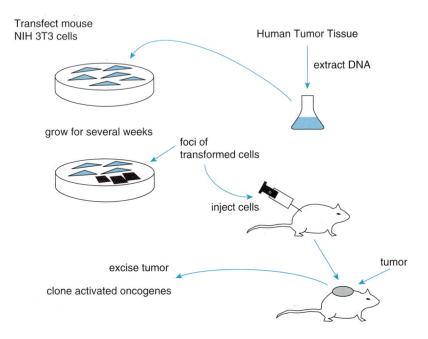

Transfect mouse NIH 3T3 cells

Human Tumor Tissue

extract DNA

grow for several weeks

foci of transformed cells

inject cells

excise tumor

clone activated oncogenes

tumor

FIGURE 44-2 Schematic diagram of the steps required for the molecular cloning of oncogenes from human tumor-cell DNA. See text for details.

at a single position, the codon for amino acid 12, the precise position at which the Ha-*ras* gene was altered.

These data, as well as other evidence, corroborate the conclusion that a single codon mutation in the sequence of the human Ha-*ras* gene is sufficient to activate this proto-oncogene. Many other human tumor cells have now been examined for activated oncogenes, using the DNA transfection method. Soon after the isolation of Ha-*ras*, such experiments identified two other oncogenes present in human tumor cells: the K-*ras* gene (structurally identical to the K-*ras* gene of Kirsten sarcoma virus) and the N-*ras* gene (structurally similar to Ha-*ras* and K-*ras*). Both the activated human K-*ras* and N-*ras* oncogenes encode proteins containing a single amino acid change compared with their normal cellular homologues. Although it is difficult to ascertain directly the role of the activated *ras* gene in the etiology of the human tumor in which it is found, the presence of a specific mutation suggests that such a change is likely to be an important step in the genesis of the tumor.

The search for additional human oncogenes using the NIH-3T3-DNA transfection assay has led to the identification of several other putative oncogenes (see Table 44-2).

CHROMOSOMAL TRANSLOCATIONS, NEOPLASIA, AND ONCOGENE ACTIVATION

The association between specific chromosomal translocations and certain human neoplasms has been recognized for many years. Consistent chromosomal aberrations are found primarily in hematologic malignancies, as well as in tumors of embryonic origin. Specific translocations are a prominent feature of many types of leukemia and lymphoma. Translocations are principally of two types: (1) constitutional (ie, carried by all cells of the affected individual); and (2) somatic (ie, alterations that occur in a particular cell and are carried only by its neoplastic progeny). Constitutional translocations (and other chromosomal abnormalities) are thought to predispose an organism to the development of a malignancy, but this requires additional mutations to fix the malignant transformation. An example of this is hereditary renal cell carcinoma, in which a constitutional translocation involving chromosomes 3 and 8 is associated with the development of renal cell carcinoma during the fourth decade of life.

Somatic translocations, on the other hand, arise in a single cell and contribute in some way to the malignant transformation of that initial cell and its progeny. Although it is difficult to assess the precise role of the translocation in the neoplastic process, the close association between particular malignancies and specific translocations (Table 44-3) makes a strong, yet somewhat circumstantial, argument that these translocations are causally related to the development of the neoplasm.

The localization of proto-oncogene sequences on

TABLE 44-3
Neoplasms With Consistent Chromosomal Defects

Disease	Chromosomal Defect
(UNIQUE CHROMOSOMAL DEFECTS)	
Acute lymphocytic leukemia, L2	t(4;11)(q21;q23)
Acute myelogenous leukemia, M2	t(8;21)(q22.1;q22.3)
Acute promyelocytic leukemia, M3	t(15;17)(q22;q11.2)
Acute myelomonocytic leukemia, M4	inv(16)(p13.2;q22)
(CONSISTENTLY SHARED CHROMOSOMAL DEFECTS)	
Acute nonlymphocytic leukemias, subtypes M1, M2, M4, M5, M6	del(5)(q22;q23) mde 17(q33;q36) +8
Burkitt's lymphoma	t(8;14)(q24.1;q32.3)
Acute lymphocytic leukemia, L3	
Small noncleaved non-Burkitt's lymphoma	
Immunoblastic lymphoma*	
Acute monocytic leukemia	t(9;11)(p22;q23)
Acute myelomonocytic leukemia	
Chronic myelogenous leukemia	t(9;22)(q34.1;q11.2)
Acute myelogenous leukemia, M1	
Acute lymphocytic leukemia, L1, L2	
Chronic lymphocytic leukemia	t(11;14)(q13;32)*
Small cell lymphocytic lymphoma (transformed to diffuse large cell lymphoma)	
Chronic lymphocytic lymphoma	+12
Small cell lymphocytic lymphoma	
Follicular small cleaved cell lymphoma	t(14;18)(q32.3;q21.3)
Follicular mixed cell lymphoma	
Follicular large cell lymphoma	

* Few cases reported.

various chromosomes of humans and mice led to the recognition that somatic translocations associated with certain neoplasms involved chromosomal segments containing proto-oncogene sequences. Such discoveries suggested the possibility that translocations of a proto-oncogene sequence may transcriptionally activate proto-oncogene expression or perhaps alter its gene structure.

One of the better understood examples of tumor-associated chromosomal translocation is that of Burkitt's lymphoma (BL). Three characteristic somatic translocations are associated with BL; 90% of the tumors have a reciprocal translocation involving the long arms of chromosomes 8 and 14 (t8;t14). The remaining tumors contain translocations involving chromosome 8 and either chromosome 2 (t2;t8) or chromosome 22 (t8;t22). Molecular cloning and DNA sequence analysis have demonstrated that in BL, the chromosomal translocations result in the juxtaposition of the c-*myc* proto-oncogene to a portion of the immunoglobulin heavy-chain gene

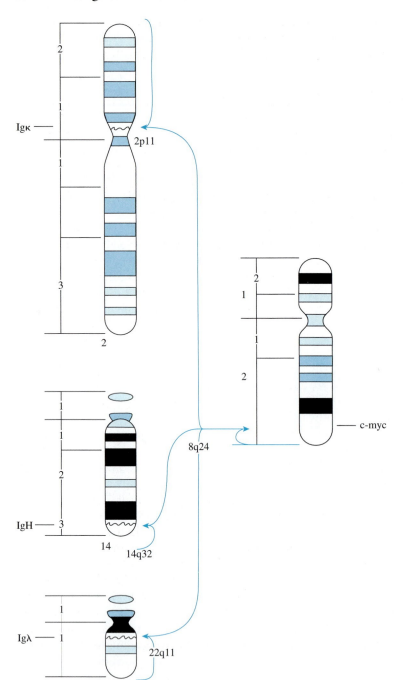

FIGURE 44-3 Chromosomal rearrangements involved in Burkitt's lymphoma. The human chromosomes 2, 14, and 22 are depicted with the positions of the Igκ, IgH, and Igλ genes. Chromosome 8 also is shown with the position of the c-*myc* gene. The arrows denote the positions of the various breakpoints observed in reciprocal translocations involving chromosome 8 and chromosome 14, 2, or 22.

(t8;t14) or to the κ (t2;t8) or λ light-chain (t8;t22) genes (Fig. 44-3). In the case of t8;t14 translocations, the c-*myc* gene resides adjacent to the break point and is transcribed in the direction opposite from that of the heavy-chain gene. In most cases, the break point occurs in the switch region of the heavy-chain gene locus, although some variability is observed. DNA sequences from the variable region of the immunoglobulin heavy-chain gene also are found on chromosome 8, indicating that the chromosomal exchange is reciprocal.

The translocation of the c-*myc* gene to chromosome 14 can result in an enhancement of transcription of the translocated c-*myc* gene. Because the absolute level of c-*myc* expression is different in individual cases of BL, it is not clear what mechanisms modulate *myc* expression. However, the consistent association of c-*myc* translocation and BL leaves little doubt that the transcriptional activation of the *myc* gene is an important prerequisite step in the development of BL.

Several other observations suggest that proto-oncogene expression may be activated by specific chromosomal translocations. The proto-oncogene c-*mos* is located on chromosome 8 near the break point observed in the translocation (t8;t21) associated with myeloblastic leukemia. In chronic myelogenous leukemia, the c-*abl* proto-oncogene, normally present on chromosome 9, is translocated to chromosome 22, resulting in an aberrant chromosome designated the Philadelphia (22q−) chromosome. Chronic myelogenous leukemia cells express an aberrant form of the c-*abl* protein, suggesting that the t9;t22 translocation gives rise to the expression of an altered oncogene product. Finally, in follicular lymphoma cells (a B-cell neoplasm), the characteristic translocation involving chromosomes 14 and 18 has been examined. In these cells, a portion of chromosome 18 is translocated to the immunoglobulin heavy-chain gene in a manner similar to the translocations observed in BL. The translocated gene locus on chromosome 18 is unrelated to any known oncogene and may represent a novel oncogene important for the pathogenesis of B-cell neoplasms.

In summary, it is clear that oncogene activation and somatic translocations go hand in hand with the process of neoplastic transformation. In addition, continued study of the gene sequences involved in unique translocations should provide a new dimension to our understanding of neoplastic development.

CHROMOSOMAL AMPLIFICATION

Solid tumors often contain chromosomes with homogeneous staining regions and acentric chromosomal fragments termed *double minutes*. This chromosomal material has been shown to be the result of gene amplification. Of special interest is the gene amplification observed in a particular subset of small cell lung carcinoma (SCLC), termed *variant SCLC* (SCLC-V). Patients with SCLC-V have an inferior response to chemotherapy and radiotherapy and a much shorter survival than do other patients with SCLC. SCLC-V cell lines often have double minutes and homogeneous staining regions, and an analysis of proto-oncogene levels in these cells has revealed a 20- to 40-fold amplification of c-*myc* and L-*myc* (a closely related *myc* gene) DNA sequences. The increased copy number of *myc* genes is accompanied by a commensurate increase in the level of *myc* RNA and protein expression. These observations suggest that *myc*-gene amplification plays a role in the development of this type of tumor.

An analogous amplification of a second gene structurally related to c-*myc*, termed the N-*myc* gene, has been observed in many human neuroblastoma cell lines and in some SCLC-V tumor lines. The amplification of these genes indicates that they play an important role in the malignant progression of certain types of neuroblastomas and carcinomas.

AUTOCRINE GROWTH FACTORS

Evolving knowledge about the role of growth factors, mitogens, receptors, and oncogenes has focused intense interest on the possible role of these factors in the establishment of the neoplastic phenotype. The relatively autonomous nature of malignant cells has been known for many years. For example, tumor cells require fewer exogenous growth factors for optimal growth and multiplication than do their normal counterparts. To help explain this phenomenon, it has been suggested that transformed cells produce polypeptide growth factors, which, in turn, act on their own functional external receptors, thereby exerting the effect of the polypeptide growth factor on the same cell that produces it. Such a process has been designated *autocrine stimulation*.

Many types of tumor cells release polypeptide growth factors into the medium when grown in cell culture. These tumor cells usually possess receptors for the released factor. Several peptide growth factors have been demonstrated to function through the autocrine stimulation mechanism. These include transforming growth factor-α, peptides related to PDGF, bombesin, and transforming growth factor-β. The activity of each of these four growth factors, and likely many others, is mediated by a different cell-surface receptor. Activation of the receptor triggers a signaling mechanism that eventually leads to a mitogenic response. Support for the autocrine hypothesis derives in large part from experiments establishing the structural relationship between the oncogene of simian sarcoma virus v-*sis* and PDGF. The amino-terminal 109 amino acids of the β chain of PDGF are almost identical to the amino acid sequence of the v-*sis* gene product, p28$^{\text{v-sis}}$. Therefore, the oncogenicity of simian sarcoma virus is related directly to the ability of this virus to express a PDGF-like growth factor.

These observations lend further support to the concept that proteins encoded by oncogenes (or inappropriately expressed or mutated proto-oncogenes) can function at several points in the cellular signaling cascade. Some oncoproteins confer growth-factor autonomy, some appear to activate postreceptor signaling pathways, and some lead to an alteration in synthesis and the release of a specific growth factor. Therefore, a cancer cell is likely to generally be a product of one or more genetic events that lead to profound changes in growth control.

Recessive Oncogenes: Antioncogenes

As long ago as the middle of the last century, it was observed that certain forms of cancer can cluster in families. In such cases, the genetic predisposition to cancer often behaves as an autosomal dominant trait. The childhood cancer retinoblastoma, a tumor of the eye, occurs in two forms: heritable, characterized by its autosomal inheritance within families, and sporadic, arising in children with no family history of disease or apparent risks. Epidemiologic studies led to the hypothesis that heritable retinoblastoma results from the inheritance of a predisposing mutation from the affected parent, and that, under normal circumstances (ie, in most cells), the mutation itself was not sufficient to induce the cancer (ie, it behaved

Nonhereditary
retinoblastoma

Hereditary
retinoblastoma

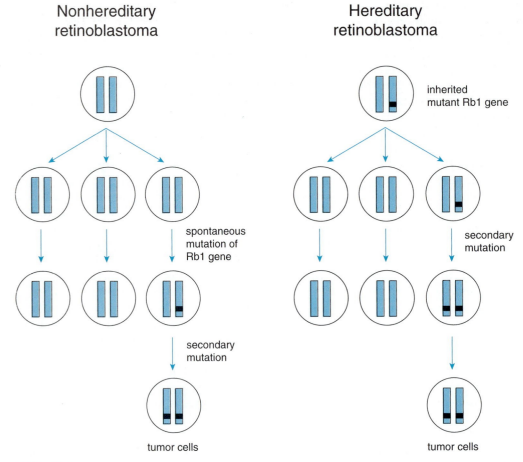

inherited
mutant Rb1 gene

spontaneous
mutation of
Rb1 gene

secondary
mutation

secondary
mutation

secondary
mutation

tumor cells

tumor cells

FIGURE 44-4 Diagram of the genetic events leading to retinoblastoma. Filled boxes denote deletions of the Rb 1 locus. See text for details.

like a recessive mutation). Genetic studies at the molecular level have now shown that the original hypothesis was correct. Retinoblastoma tumor cells have a characteristic genetic abnormality in that chromosome 13 always contains a deletion of band 14, designated the Rb1 locus. On the other hand, normal cells from the same individual are heterozygous for this locus, containing one unaltered chromosome 13 and one copy of chromosome 13 with a deleted Rb1 locus (Fig. 44-4). One hypothesis to explain the appearance of the tumor is that the wild-type Rb1 allele serves to suppress the tumor phenotype, and that the rare genetic events that give rise to the loss of that allele result in the formation of tumor cells. This would occur by chance much more frequently in an individual who was genetically heterozygous for this allele than in a homozygous person. Hence, heritable retinoblastoma is much more common than is the rare sporadic form, in which both alleles must be lost. The concept that certain genes, such as the Rb gene, can suppress tumor formation has led investigators to coin the term *antioncogenes,* or *tumor suppressor genes,* to designate genes that act in a positive way to promote the normal growth of cells. The observation that the introduction of a cloned Rb gene into retinoblastoma or osteosarcoma

cell cultures suppresses the neoplastic phenotype strongly supports its role as an antioncogene.

The cellular gene known as p53 is another example of a tumor suppressor gene that is capable of counteracting transformation. It has been shown that p53 mutations are common in certain human cancers (eg, certain forms of colon cancer). Evidence suggests that both the p53 protein and the Rb gene product play important roles in cell-cycle regulation.

Several lines of evidence indicate that the protein products of antioncogenes and oncogenes may interact functionally to promote changes in cell growth leading to transformation. For example, in cells transformed by the DNA virus, SV40, the protein encoded by the transforming oncogene of this virus, large T antigen, is found to be tightly associated with the product of the normal Rb gene. Mutations in the SV40 oncogene that block the transformation of cells by SV40 also change the structure of the T-antigen protein such that it no longer binds to the normal Rb protein. Large T antigen also binds to the p53 protein, and this interaction is important for transformation as well. As described in Chapter 41, the oncogene products of adenoviruses as well as oncogenic papillomaviruses also bind to the same two cellular proteins. Thus, it is likely that these viruses transform cells at least partially by preventing (or inhibiting) the action of these tumor suppressor proteins.

Bibliography

JOURNALS

Bishop JM. Cellular oncogenes and retroviruses. Annu Rev Biochem 1983;52:301.

Bishop JM. Viral oncogenes. Cell 1985;42:23.

Bishop JM. The molecular genetics of cancer. Science 1987;235:305.

Curran T, Franza BR. Fos and jun: the AP-1 connection. Cell 1988;55:395.

Hansen MF, Cavenee WK. Tumor suppressors: recessive mutations that lead to cancer. Cell 1988;53:172.

Nowell PC, Croce CM. Chromosomal approaches to oncogenes and oncogenesis. FASEB J 1988;2:3054.

Varmus HE. Oncogenes and transcriptional control. Science 1987;238:1337.

Weinberg WA. Finding the anti-oncogene. Sci Am 1988;259:44.

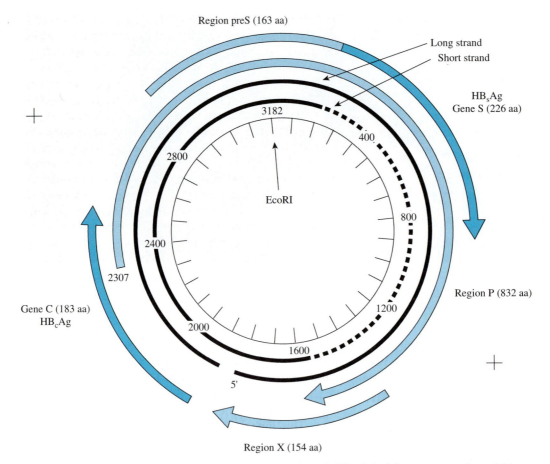

FIGURE 45-3 Organization of the genes in hepatitis B virus (HBV). The dashed line represents the variable single-stranded region. The EcoRI site denotes the point of origin for the physical map. The broad arrows define the four large open reading frames of the L strand transcript. The four coding regions are designated S (made up of pre-S and S genes), P (polymerase), X (regulatory gene), and C. The two regions encoding the S (surface antigen) and C (core antigen) proteins are represented by stippling.

REPLICATION OF HEPATITIS B VIRUS

Studies on the replication of HBV and HBV-related viruses (ie, woodchuck, ground squirrel, and duck hepatitis viruses) have suggested a unique mode of replication for HBV. This replication involves reverse transcription, indicating that HBV is phylogenetically related to the retrovirus family. The viral genome of HBV is about 3000 to 3300 nucleotides in length, and molecular cloning and DNA sequencing experiments have established the relative organization of the genes for the various structural proteins (Fig. 45-3). In addition, an open reading frame encoding a putative DNA polymerase has been identified.

Although the viral DNA is circular, both strands of the duplex are linear, and the circular conformation is maintained solely by extensive base pairing between the two gapped DNA strands (Fig. 45-4). Within the virus particle, the negative strand appears to be uniform in length, about 3200 nucleotides. In contrast, the positive strand is shorter and varies in length between different virions, due to single-stranded gaps of variable size. On infection, the DNA polymerase in the nucleocapsid core

is activated and completes the synthesis of the positive strand, using the negative strand as a template.

The important steps of this model of HBV replication are summarized in Figure 45-5. After the conversion of gapped double-stranded viral DNA to fully double-stranded DNA, a full-length positive-strand RNA (a "pre-genome") is transcribed from the HBV DNA template. This RNA serves as the mRNA for the translation of the HB_cAg. Evidence suggests that this form of RNA also is packaged with viral core proteins and the viral DNA polymerase within the cell to form an "immature core." A DNA strand of negative polarity then is synthesized through reverse transcription. This step is followed by the synthesis of a partial positive strand and the full maturation of the virus particle containing a gapped DNA genome.

EPIDEMIOLOGY OF HEPATITIS B VIRUS INFECTIONS

Early volunteer studies failed to show a normal portal of exit for HBV and, for years, it was believed that a person

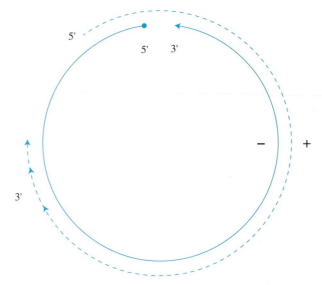

FIGURE 45-4 Structure of hepatitis B DNA. The long, dashed arrow denotes the incomplete minus strand. The short arrows denote the relative position of new DNA synthesis. The ● symbol represents covalently bound terminal protein.

by a long incubation period, ranging from 50 to 180 days. Symptoms such as fever, rash, and arthritis begin insidiously, and the severity of the infection varies widely. Mild cases that do not result in jaundice are termed *anicteric*. In more severe cases, characterized by headache, mild fever, nausea, and loss of appetite, icterus (jaundice) occurs 3 to 5 days after the initial symptoms. The duration and severity of the disease vary from clinically inapparent to fatal fulminating hepatitis. The overall fatality rate is estimated to be 1% to 2%, with most deaths occurring in adults older than 30 years of age. The duration of uncomplicated hepatitis rarely is more than 8 to 10 weeks, but mild symptoms can persist for more than 1 year. The mechanism of hepatic damage of HBV is not established, but considerable data support the notion that most of the liver damage that occurs during acute or chronic

could become infected only by the injection of blood or serum from an infected person or by the use of contaminated needles or syringes. As a result, the older name for this disease was serum hepatitis. It has now been shown that this supposition is not true. Using serologic techniques, HB_sAg has been found in feces, urine, saliva, vaginal secretions, semen, and breast milk. Undoubtedly, the mechanical transmission of infected blood or blood products is one of the most efficient methods of viral transmission, and infections have been traced to tattooing, ear piercing, acupuncture, and drug abuse. About 5% to 10% of intravenous drug abusers are HBV carriers, and as many as 60% show evidence of previous HBV infections. Neonatal transmission also appears to occur during childbirth. The incidence is increased significantly if the mother's blood contains HB_eAg. For example, in a study from Taiwan, a 32% transmission rate was observed, and the transmission could be correlated with HB_eAg-positive cord blood. The presence of HB_sAg in breast milk also suggests an additional vehicle for the transmission of HBV to the newborn. The demonstration of infectious virus in semen presents the possibility that virus can be sexually transmitted. In hospitals, HBV infections are a risk for both hospital personnel and patients because of constant exposure to blood and blood products.

PATHOGENESIS OF HEPATITIS B VIRUS INFECTIONS

Acute hepatitis caused by HBV cannot be clinically distinguished from hepatitis caused by HAV. However, several characteristics differentiate the infections caused by these viruses (see Table 45-2). HBV infections are characterized

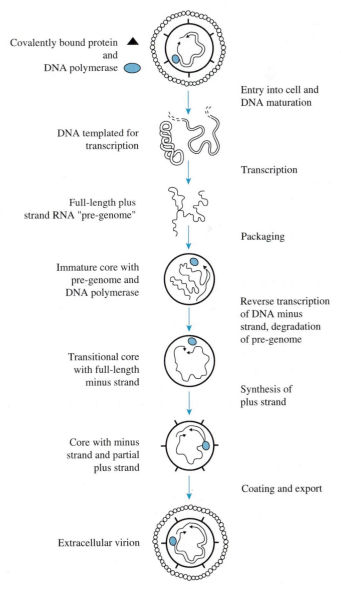

Covalently bound protein ▲
and
DNA polymerase ⬭

Entry into cell and
DNA maturation

DNA templated for
transcription

Transcription

Full-length plus
strand RNA "pre-genome"

Packaging

Immature core with
pre-genome and
DNA polymerase

Reverse transcription
of DNA minus
strand, degradation
of pre-genome

Transitional core
with full-length
minus strand

Synthesis of
plus strand

Core with minus
strand and partial
plus strand

Coating and export

Extracellular virion

FIGURE 45-5 A model for the replication of hepatitis B–like viruses. See text for details.

hepatitis is mediated by a cellular immune response directed toward the new antigens deposited in the cell membrane of the infected cell.

Based on the ultimate pattern of the disease, this disease can be divided into two categories: self-limiting acute infections and chronic infections.

Self-Limiting Hepatitis B Virus Infections

Self-limiting infections can be inapparent or can result in a clinical hepatitis with jaundice lasting 4 to 5 weeks. HB$_s$Ag may or may not be present in the blood, but, if present, it usually disappears as the symptoms of hepatitis subside and the jaundice clears. Antibodies to HB$_c$Ag, HB$_e$Ag, and HB$_s$Ag arise at different periods during the infection and can remain detectable for years after recovery. There seems to be a good immune response to group-specific determinants, because recovery appears to provide immunity to different subtypes of the virus.

Chronic Hepatitis B Virus Infections

Between 6% and 10% of clinically diagnosed patients with hepatitis B become chronically infected and continue to have HB$_s$Ag in their blood for at least 6 months, and sometimes for life. Chronic infections can be subdivided into two general categories: chronic persistent hepatitis and chronic active hepatitis. The latter is the most severe and often eventually leads to cirrhosis or the development of primary hepatocellular carcinoma. Worldwide, it has been estimated that there are more than 200 million permanently infected carriers of HBV, of which about 1 million reside in the United States. The prevalence of chronic carriers varies widely in different parts of the world, from 0.1% to 0.5% in the United States to up to 20% in China, Southeast Asia, and some African countries. The perinatal infection of newborn infants born to chronically infected mothers results in a high incidence of chronic infection (90%), which often is lifelong. This is particularly disquieting in the developing countries of Asia and Africa, where carrier rates are high. It has been estimated that HBV is the most common single cause of liver disease in the world.

All carriers have antibodies to HB$_c$Ag, and some have antibodies to HB$_e$Ag. Those who do not possess anti-HB$_e$ may have circulating HB$_e$Ag. Carriers with high concentrations of Dane particles and circulating HB$_e$Ag appear to be more likely to suffer liver damage than those in whom only HB$_s$Ag can be detected, but the validity of this proposal is yet to be established. However, such persons are much more likely to be transmitters of the disease than are those who have solely HB$_s$Ag in their blood. Several cases of membranous glomerulonephritis have been described in HB$_s$Ag-positive children, and it has been reported that the glomerulonephritis results from the deposition of immune complexes consisting of anti-HBe IgG and HB$_e$Ag.

The mechanism by which carriers can remain persistently infected and yet be asymptomatic is unknown. However, prolonged carrier status is seen in association with chronic hepatitis in patients with lowered immunity and in those infected during the neonatal period or early childhood.

Primary Hepatocellular Carcinoma

A considerable amount of evidence has documented the close association between HBV infection and the development of primary hepatocellular carcinoma. Hepatocellular carcinoma is the most common cancer in the world, with at least 250,000 new cases reported annually. Patients with hepatocellular carcinoma often have high levels of HB$_s$Ag, and the carcinoma cells often contain integrated HBV DNA. Further evidence for the link between persistent HBV infections and hepatocellular carcinoma comes from epidemiologic data showing that the risk of developing primary hepatocellular carcinoma is more than 200 times higher in HBV carriers than in noncarriers. Within some populations, the risk of developing primary hepatocellular carcinoma is as high as 50% in male chronic carriers. However, HBV infection is not solely responsible for tumor development, because the carrier state often exists for a lengthy period (often 40 years or more) before the onset of liver cancer. In addition, the predominance of hepatocellular carcinoma in men indicates that other factors, including sex-related factors, contribute to the development of this cancer. Nonetheless, an important component of chronic liver disease is the continual regeneration of damaged or destroyed hepatocytes, which, coupled with HBV replication and exposure to environmental carcinogens, likely contributes in a significant fashion to tumor development and progression. The relationships between oncogene activation, loss of tumor suppressor genes, and the HBV are under active investigation.

Because of the close epidemiologic link between chronic HBV infection and hepatocellular carcinoma, it is hoped that mass vaccination of susceptible individuals in such countries as China and Taiwan will reduce the overall incidence of HBV infection, and that this eventually will reduce dramatically the incidence of hepatocarcinoma.

DIAGNOSIS OF HEPATITIS B VIRUS INFECTIONS

As in all cases of viral hepatitis, abnormal liver function is indicated by increased levels of liver enzymes such as serum glutamic-oxaloacetic transaminase and alanine aminotransferase (ALT). The presence of HB$_s$Ag confirms a diagnosis of hepatitis B, and its serologic detection is routinely carried out in diagnostic laboratories and blood banks using radioimmunoassays or enzyme-linked immunosorbent assays.

CONTROL OF HEPATITIS B VIRUS INFECTIONS

The examination of all donor blood for the presence of HB$_s$Ag is now routine, and this practice has done much to control the occurrence of posttransfusion hepatitis B infections.

Passive immunization of human volunteers with hepatitis B immune globulin (HBIG) has been shown to prevent disease when the volunteers were challenged with infectious material, but the use of immune globulin is not effective for the treatment of active disease. One important and effective use for HBIG, however, is the prevention of active hepatitis B infections in neonates born to mothers who are chronic carriers of HB$_s$Ag. HBIG also can be given to nonimmune individuals known to have been exposed to HBV.

Active immunization with HB$_s$Ag promises to provide a vehicle for the control of hepatitis B. Clinical trials in high-risk populations have shown that the incidence of hepatitis B in persons actively immunized with HB$_s$Ag is decreased by about 95%. Moreover, immunization even during the long incubation period may be efficacious in preventing HBV infections. Because HBV has not been grown in cell cultures, the first vaccine consisted of highly purified, formalin-inactivated HB$_s$Ag particles obtained from the plasma of persistently infected carriers. This vaccine has now been superseded by a recombinant vaccine, in which the gene for HB$_s$Ag has been cloned in yeast, enabling the production of polypeptides carrying the antigenic determinants of HB$_s$Ag in large amounts. The yeast-produced vaccine has been licensed for use and has been given to more than 2 million people in the United States. The vaccine is considered safe and provides effective protection. Administration of the HBV vaccine worldwide has the potential to reduce drastically the incidence of HBV infection. Early studies have shown that its use in HBV-positive pregnant women reduces the percentage of infants who become carriers from 90% to 23%. In addition, if HBIG is used in conjunction with the vaccine, the newborn carrier incidence can be reduced to less than 5%. Taking note of the fact that many chronic HBV carriers eventually die of liver disease, this vaccine represents the first prophylactic measure to substantially reduce or prevent cirrhosis and human cancer.

Non-A, Non-B Hepatitis

About 20 years ago, as diagnostic assays to detect HAV and HBV became readily available, it was demonstrated that most cases of transfusion-associated infection were caused by neither HAV nor HBV. Thus, it seemed clear that other hepatitis viruses remained to be isolated. The disease caused by these unknown agents became known as *non-A, non-B (NANB) hepatitis*. It has now been shown that most cases of transfusion-associated hepatitis are caused by an RNA virus that has been named HCV. Two other RNA viruses responsible for some cases of NANB hepatitis also have been identified. One of these viruses (HDV) requires HBV to replicate and, therefore, is seen only in individuals who are infected with HBV. A third RNA agent of NANB hepatitis, which is called HEV and is spread by a fecal–oral route, has been shown to be the cause of large outbreaks of hepatitis in developing countries.

HEPATITIS C VIRUS

When it became clear that most cases of transfusion-associated hepatitis probably were caused by a hitherto unknown virus, molecular genetic and recombinant DNA techniques were used to identify, clone, and sequence putative agents. This led to the isolation of a new RNA virus, HCV. Sequence analysis has revealed that HCV is organized in a manner similar to the flaviviruses and that it shares biologic characteristics with this family. This has led to a classification of HCV as a genus within the flavivirus family. About 80% of patients with chronic, posttransfusion NANB hepatitis in Italy and Japan have been shown to have antibodies to HCV, and 58% of patients with NANB hepatitis in the United States, with no known parenteral exposure to the virus, have HCV antibodies. Based on these data, it seems likely that HCV is a major contributor to NANB hepatitis throughout the world. Most infected individuals become chronic carriers of the virus, and many develop chronic hepatitis. Studies in several urban areas have shown that as many as 80% of intravenous drug abusers have been infected with HCV. The development of commercial antibody tests to detect HCV infection has markedly reduced the number of cases of NANB hepatitis acquired from transfusions and blood products.

HEPATITIS DELTA VIRUS

Hepatitis delta virus was first described in 1977 as a novel antigen–antibody complex detected by immunofluorescence in hepatocyte nuclei of patients with chronic HBV infection and chronic hepatitis. Although HDV antigen was initially observed in Italy, it has been detected worldwide, primarily in HBV carriers who have had multiple exposures to blood and blood products (Table 45-3). Transmission experiments in chimpanzees and other studies have shown that HDV is a transmissible and pathogenic agent that requires concomitant replication of HBV to provide certain helper functions. The HDV virion is a spherical, 36-nm enveloped particle with a chimeric structure; the genome consists of a 1.7-kilobase RNA molecule specific for HDV, whereas the envelope contains

Group	Number of Groups Studied	Delta Prevalence (%)
HBV carriers (blood donors)	15	1.4–8.0
Acute hepatitis	6	1.5–7.2
Fulminant hepatitis	2	16–34
Chronic hepatitis	4	13–41
Cirrhosis	1	25
Primary hepatocellular carcinoma	3	0–3

From Maynard JE, Hadler, SC, Fields HA: Delta hepatitis in the Americas. Prog Clin Biol Res 1987;234:493.

HBV-encoded HB$_s$Ag. The HDV genomic RNA is a circular, single-stranded RNA similar in structure to certain pathogenic RNAs of plants (viroids), and its replication requires the concomitant expression of HBV gene products.

Two principal modes of HDV infection have been described: (1) coinfection (the simultaneous introduction of both HBV and HDV into a susceptible host); and (2) superinfection (the infection of an HBV carrier with HDV). Simultaneous exposure to HBV and HDV leads to a typical pattern of HBV disease, with the duration of HBV infection being the limiting factor to the expression of HDV. The outcome of such HBV/HDV coinfections usually is similar to that of infection with HBV alone, and chronic infections seem to be established with the same frequency.

The clinical outcome from HDV superinfection of an HBV carrier is markedly different. In this case, the persistent HBV infection promotes the efficient replication of the defective HDV and leads to a fulminant HB$_s$Ag-positive hepatitis with a significant mortality rate (5% to 15%). In addition, the chronic infection with HBV potentiates the continued replication of HDV, establishing a chronic HDV infection. There are few data to support a role for HDV in the development of primary hepatocellular carcinoma.

HDV transmission is linked closely to that of its helper, HBV. Parenteral inoculation accounts for the worldwide distribution of HDV among drug addicts. In parts of the world with a low incidence of HBV, HDV infections are found mostly in drug addicts and other individuals at risk for being HBV carriers. HDV infection of newborns occurs only in babies born to HB$_s$Ag-positive, HDV-infected mothers. Although HDV is found worldwide, an interesting anomaly exists in that

HDV infection is endemic in South America, resulting in severe outbreaks of fulminant hepatitis. In contrast, HDV infections are rare in Asia, although the prevalence of HB$_s$Ag carriers is similar to that in South America. Overall, it has been estimated that about 5% of chronic HBV carriers also are infected with HDV.

Because no HDV vaccine is available, controlling the transmission of HBV is the only approach to controlling the spread of HDV. Unfortunately for the estimated 200 million HB$_s$Ag carriers in the world, there is no effective measure to prevent HDV infection per se.

HEPATITIS E VIRUS

Many cases of acute viral hepatitis in Asia and Africa are caused by a virus that is transmitted through the fecal–oral route but is unrelated to HAV. Outbreaks of this disease also have been confirmed in other parts of the world, including the Middle East and Mexico. The disease usually is caused by the ingestion of fecally contaminated water. The virus causing this kind of hepatitis has been named HEV. The first verified hepatitis E outbreak was documented in New Delhi, India, in 1955. In this epidemic, 29,000 cases of icteric hepatitis were reported after fecal contamination of the city's drinking water. Several other outbreaks have been linked to HEV since then. HEV is a small, nonenveloped RNA virus. Recent information about the genomic organization and other properties of the virus strongly suggests that it is a calicivirus and should be placed in a new genus within this family.

Bibliography

JOURNALS

Beasley RP. Hepatitis B virus. The major etiology of hepatocellular carcinoma. Cancer 1988;61:1942.

Lemon SM. Hepatitis A virus: current concepts of the molecular virology, immunobiology and approaches to vaccine development. Rev Med Virol 1992;2:73.

Reyes GR, Baroudy BM. Molecular biology of non-A, non-B hepatitis agents: hepatitis C and hepatitis E viruses. Adv Virus Res 1991;40:57.

BOOKS

Gerin JL, Purcell RH, Rizetto M, eds. The hepatitis delta virus. New York, Raven Press, 1991.

Gust ID, Feinstone SM. Hepatitis A. Boca Raton, FL, CRC Press, 1988.

Robinson WS. Biology of human hepatitis viruses. In: Zakim D, Boyer T, eds. Hepatology: a textbook of liver disease. Philadelphia, WB Saunders, 1990.

Robinson WS. Hepadnaviridae and their replication. In: Fields BN, Knipe DM, eds. Virology, ed 2. New York, Raven Press, 1990.

Mason WS, Seeger C. Hepadnaviruses. In: Current topics in microbiology and immunology, vol 168. Berlin: Springer-Verlag, 1991.

McLachlan A. Molecular biology of hepatitis B viruses. Boca Raton, FL, CRC Press, 1991.

Essentials of Medical Microbiology, Fifth Edition, edited by Wesley A. Volk,
Bryan M. Gebhardt, Marie-Louise Hammarskjöld, and Robert J. Kadner.
Lippincott-Raven Publishers, Philadelphia © 1996.

Chapter 46

Picornaviridae, Caliciviridae (Norwalk Viruses), and Coronaviridae

The viruses discussed in this chapter are all RNA viruses that infect humans through an oral or respiratory route. Many of these viruses are spread through fecal–oral transmission. Others are strict respiratory tract pathogens that are transmitted mainly through a respiratory route.

PICORNAVIRIDAE

Human pathogens in the family Picornaviridae (*pico* means small) have been subdivided into three different genera: enteroviruses, rhinoviruses, and hepatitis A virus (discussed in Chap. 45). The enteroviruses include five major subgroups: (1) poliovirus (3 serotypes); (2) echoviruses (31 serotypes); (3) coxsackievirus A (23 serotypes); (4) coxsackievirus B (6 serotypes); and (5) new enteroviruses (4 serotypes, designated 68 through 71). The rhinoviruses comprise about 100 different serotypes.

In addition, several important groups of nonhuman pathogens belong to the picornavirus group, including the cardioviruses and foot-and-mouth disease virus. This discussion is restricted to the human pathogens.

Structure and Replication of Picornaviruses

In spite of the diversity of human diseases caused by the picornaviruses, there do not appear to be major differences in their modes of replication or general structures. Minor differences in structure do exist, as revealed by the observation that the enteroviruses can maintain their structural stability and infectivity at a pH level of 3, whereas the rhinoviruses are inactivated at this level of acidity. Thus, the enteroviruses can pass through the enteric system without inactivation and frequently are spread through the fecal–oral route.

Picornaviruses contain a single molecule of linear single-stranded RNA (about 7400 nucleotides for poliovirus RNA) enclosed in a naked icosahedral capsid (Fig. 46-1) made up of 60 protomers. All picornavirus particles con-

of the virus from throat swabs, feces, or, in rare cases, spinal fluid, or on the demonstration of an increase in neutralizing antibody to one of the three serotypes of poliovirus during convalescence.

CONTROL OF POLIOVIRUS INFECTIONS

Paradoxically, a dramatic increase in paralytic poliomyelitis was seen in several geographic areas during the early part of the 20th century as a result of increasing living standards. Because poliovirus is transmitted primarily by a fecal–oral route, the better sanitation became, the older an average person would be before becoming infected with the virus. Because the incidence of paralysis increases markedly with age, this led to epidemics of much more serious disease. Therefore, paralytic poliomyelitis has been called a *civilization* disease.

Because of the devastating crippling effects of paralytic poliomyelitis, it became one of the most feared diseases of the 20th century. As recently as 1958, almost 6000 cases of paralytic polio were reported annually in the United States. However, during 1974, after the introduction of a comprehensive vaccination program, the incidence of paralytic poliomyelitis dropped dramatically. Nonetheless, it is estimated that 250,000 to 2 million cases of paralytic poliomyelitis occur each year in developing countries.

Paralytic polio has become an extremely rare disease in the United States because of the development of two effective vaccines. The original vaccine, developed by Jonas Salk in the mid-1950s, contained formalin-killed viruses of each of the three serotypes. The injection of this vaccine stimulates the production of IgG antibodies in the serum. After infection, a virulent virus is neutralized as it enters the viremic stage (bloodstream), thus preventing involvement of the central nervous system.

A live vaccine, the Sabin vaccine, has now largely replaced the Salk vaccine in the United States. The Sabin vaccine is made up of attenuated live polioviruses of each of the three types. The vaccine is administered orally, and current practice is to administer all three types together in three successive doses. The live virus present in the vaccine multiplies in the cells of the gastrointestinal tract and oropharynx, stimulating both IgG and IgA antibodies, and providing the same solid immunity that the natural infection would provide.

The efficacy of the Salk and Sabin vaccines in preventing paralytic polio is well established, but the safety of the live Sabin vaccine remains a matter of discussion. The vaccine virus can revert to neurovirulence in vaccinated individuals, although this occurs rarely. Today in the United States, virtually all cases of poliomyelitis are vaccine associated, based on both epidemiologic and laboratory classifications. Vaccine-associated poliomyelitis is rare, but predictable, within this country (about 4 to 5 cases per year). Because vaccinated individuals shed virus in their feces, nonvaccinated contacts can become infected with the vaccine virus. Between 1972 and 1983, 278.8 million doses of the oral vaccine were distributed. During this period, 87 vaccine-associated cases of paralytic polio were reported, 32 among vaccinees and 55 among their household and nonhousehold contacts. Many of these cases occurred in immunodeficient individuals. Because the number of susceptible vaccine recipients or subsequent susceptible contacts is not known, the actual risk of vaccine-associated poliomyelitis is impossible to determine. The Sabin vaccine should not be given to known immunodeficient individuals or their close contacts. These individuals should be immunized with a killed vaccine.

Although the polio vaccine has essentially eliminated the paralytic aspects of this disease, the virus (largely replaced by the vaccine strain) is still widespread in countries that use primarily the live vaccine. Thus, public complacency could easily result in a large population lacking immunity and the resultant spread of neurovirulent virus.

Other Enteroviruses

The enterovirus group, in addition to poliovirus, includes numerous viruses that cause many different respiratory tract, central nervous system, and febrile diseases. These viruses cause a variety of clinical symptoms, with significant overlap among the different serologically defined viruses. The following sections summarize the major properties and diseases associated with the enteroviruses.

Enteroviruses are classified based on their reactivity with specific antisera, their ability to replicate in cultured cells, and their pathogenesis in animals. Their classification is complicated in that some enteroviruses are named for their initial origin of isolation (eg, coxsackieviruses were first isolated in Coxsackie, NY) and some for their apparent lack of disease specificity (echoviruses). More recently isolated enteroviruses simply have been given the name enterovirus (enterovirus types 68 through 72).

COXSACKIEVIRUSES

Coxsackieviruses were named for Coxsackie, NY, where the first virus in this group was isolated from stools of a patient in 1948. Coxsackievirus originally was believed to be a new type of poliovirus. Although its structure and replication appeared to be that of a typical poliovirus, the high virulence of the newly discovered virus for newborn mice led to its assignment into a new group of picornaviruses. Since the initial discovery, numerous other coxsackieviruses have been isolated and characterized.

The coxsackieviruses are placed into one of two groups based on the pathology observed after the infection of newborn mice. Group A viruses, serologically divided into 23 types by virtue of type-specific neutralizing and complement-fixing antigens, produce a fulminating, lethal infection resulting in total flaccid paralysis and death of the mouse. Pathologically, group A virus lesions are restricted to the necrosis and degeneration of skeletal muscle. Group B viruses, divided into six serotypes, cause a less severe infection in mice; however, these viruses can produce localized lesions in the liver, pancreas, myocardium, brain, and brown fat pads, as well as in the skeletal muscle. Some types of group B coxsackievirus produce a diabetes-like syndrome in mice, and this has fueled speculation concerning the possible viral etiology of human juvenile diabetes. In addition, all group B coxsackieviruses share a common group antigen, whereas no common antigen has been observed with group A coxsackieviruses.

Climate plays a major role in the epidemiologic pattern of coxsackieviruses. In temperate climates, their circulation culminates in summer and autumn, whereas in tropical areas, these viruses occur endemically throughout the year.

ECHOVIRUSES

The echoviruses illustrate the dilemma virologists faced as they discovered many new viruses in the feces of persons who had no clinical illness. At one time, these viruses often were referred to facetiously as "viruses in search of disease." Later, they were given the rather long name of enteric cytopathogenic human orphan viruses, indicating that they were isolated from human feces and caused a cytopathic effect in cell cultures, but could not be associated with any specific disease. From this name came the acronym *echovirus.* Echoviruses have been subdivided into 31 types based on the presence of a type-specific neutralizing antigen in their capsid. Echoviruses originally were differentiated from the coxsackieviruses by their lack of pathogenicity for suckling mice. However, a few variant types have now been shown to produce lesions in newborn mice. Most echovirus infections are asymptomatic or associated with minor respiratory tract symptoms. However, these viruses also have been associated with more serious diseases, such as aseptic meningitis, encephalitis, paralysis, myocarditis, Reye's syndrome, and Guillain-Barré syndrome. They also can cause gastrointestinal disorders.

ENTEROVIRUS

Since 1970, new, serologically distinct enteroviruses have been designated by assigning them new serotype numbers (types 68 through 72).

Epidemiology and Pathogenesis of Enterovirus Infections

Enteroviruses occur worldwide, and humans appear to be their only natural host. They also seem to be transmitted easily, and most infections are asymptomatic or mild (and

TABLE 46-1
Clinical Symptoms Associated With Enteroviruses

Syndrome	Coxsackievirus A	Coxsackievirus B	Echoviruses/Enteroviruses
Asymptomatic infections	+	+	+
Aseptic meningitis	+	+	+
Herpangina	+	−	−
Pleurodynia	−	+	−
Respiratory tract disease	+	+	+
Myocarditis	−	+	−
Pericarditis	−	+	+
Congenital anomalies	+	+	−
Rash diseases	+	+	+
Hepatitis	−	−	+

hence, undiagnosed). Enteroviruses grow in the pharynx and intestines, and virus spread occurs through oral secretions or a fecal–oral route. In addition to poliomyelitis, human enterovirus diseases vary considerably from one virus type to another. Table 46-1 lists the more common clinical syndromes, along with the virus usually involved.

ASEPTIC MENINGITIS. Nonpolio enteroviruses are a major cause of acute central nervous system infections worldwide, with aseptic meningitis being the most common. In general, enterovirus meningitis occurs more frequently in young patients, especially those under 1 year of age. Clinical symptoms of enterovirus central nervous system disease in young children are largely nonspecific and mimic symptoms of bacterial sepsis or meningitis. Symptoms can include fever, headache, nausea, stiffness in the neck, gastrointestinal or respiratory tract symptoms, and rash. Recovery usually is complete; however, some evidence suggests that children with enterovirus meningitis, especially at young ages, exhibit long-term neurologic abnormalities, including smaller head size, deficits in speech and language development, and lower intelligence.

HERPANGINA. Herpangina is predominantly a childhood ailment and can be caused by several of the group A coxsackieviruses. This disease is an acute illness characterized by fever and lesions on the tonsils, soft palate, and pharynx. Difficulty in swallowing (dysphagia), loss of appetite (anorexia), vomiting, and abdominal pain also can occur. The disease is benign, with a usual duration of 1 to 4 days.

PLEURODYNIA AND RESPIRATORY TRACT DISEASE. Pleurodynia (also called Bornholm disease or devil's grip) is caused primarily by group B coxsackieviruses and is characterized by fever, headache, severe pleuritic pain, and malaise. Symptoms can last several days to several weeks. Enteroviruses also cause upper respiratory tract infections. Such infections are of short duration and are characterized by fever, sore throat, headache, malaise, and vague pains. Many cases are considered to be "common colds."

MYOCARDITIS AND PERICARDITIS. Carditis caused by group B coxsackieviruses (and, less often, by other enteroviruses) can occur in both adults and children, causing permanent cardiac abnormalities. Myocarditis in newborns frequently is fatal. Furthermore, if a pregnant woman becomes infected, it appears that the virus can pass the placental wall and cause congenital heart defects in the fetus.

RASH DISEASES. Enterovirus infections often cause febrile illnesses and rashes. These diseases generally are transient and most always inconsequential for the patient. It often is difficult to distinguish enterovirus-caused rashes from those caused by other viruses, particularly rubella virus.

CONJUNCTIVITIS. Enterovirus 70 and a variant of coxsackievirus A24 were associated with severe outbreaks of acute hemorrhagic conjunctivitis in West Africa, Asia, and Japan in 1969. In 1981, the disease was seen again in Central and South America, the Caribbean, and the southeastern United States. The conjunctivitis occurred mainly in adults, and infections resolved in 1 to 2 weeks, usually without complication.

Diagnosis and Control of Enterovirus Infections

Nonpolio enteroviruses can be isolated from throat washings, spinal fluid, or feces. The injection of virus into newborn mice, or the use of monkey and human cell cultures that show cytopathic effects, allows recovery of the virus. Identification requires the use of specific neutralizing antiserum. A retrospective diagnosis also can be made by showing a rise in neutralizing antibodies between the acute and convalescent phases of the disease. There are no effective control measures for nonpolio enterovirus infections. Although vaccines would likely be effective, the multiplicity of virus types makes their development and production impractical.

Rhinoviruses

The very "commonness" of the common cold was a stumbling block for many years to understanding the etiology of this disease. Although initially a single viral agent was sought, it is now known that many different viruses can cause the mild respiratory tract infections we refer to as the common cold. The largest number of these viruses have been classified into a group known as the rhinoviruses.

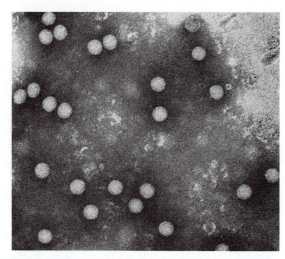

FIGURE 46-3 Virions of human rhinovirus type 14. (Original magnification ×120,000.)

CLASSIFICATION

Only a few of the rhinoviruses have been studied extensively; however, these small RNA viruses are morphologically and biochemically similar to other members of the picornavirus family (Fig. 46-3). They can be differentiated from the enteroviruses on the basis of their acid lability, buoyant density, and temperature sensitivity. Rhinoviruses are inactivated if maintained at a pH level of 3 at 37°C for 1 hour. This same treatment has little or no effect on the enteroviruses. Immunologically, the rhinoviruses have been subdivided into more than 100 serotypes based on a type-specific antigen in their capsid.

EPIDEMIOLOGY AND PATHOGENESIS OF RHINOVIRUS INFECTIONS

Infections in humans appear to be restricted to the cells of the upper respiratory tract and, during the first 5 to 10 days of an illness, the virus can be isolated from nasopharyngeal secretions. Therefore, it follows that a person acquires the virus by coming into contact with virus shed from the respiratory tract. Although transmission studies have shown that the virus can be spread by aerosols under intimate conditions, a more efficient mode of transmission appears to involve hand contact and self-inoculation of mucous membranes of the eye and nasal mucosa. Because viral contamination of objects in the environment is commonplace, hand contact followed by self-inoculation is the most likely and important mode of infection. Studies have shown that experimental transmission of the virus can be inhibited by local application of aqueous iodine solutions to the hands.

Although rhinovirus infections are observed throughout the year, there appears to be an increased incidence from April to October. Infections are caused routinely by several different serotypes; however, occasional "epidemics" caused by a single serotype have been noted.

Repeated infections with different serotypes occur throughout life, giving rise to a general increase in antibody titer with age. Immunity to rhinovirus infections is type-specific, and it probably is effective for at least 2 years. As might be expected, immunity can be correlated better with the amount of IgA present in the nasal mucous secretions than with the serum IgG.

DIAGNOSIS AND CONTROL OF RHINOVIRUS INFECTIONS

The clinical symptoms of the common cold hardly require description to anyone old enough to read this text. The virus can be grown in HeLa cells, human embryo kidney cells, human embryonic nasal or tracheal epithelium, and human diploid cell lines. Some strains grow in both monkey and human cell lines; these are designated M strains to differentiate them from H strains, which grow only in human cells. Identification of isolated viruses is accomplished using standard known neutralizing antiserum.

An unusual and unexpected property of rhinoviruses is that on initial isolation, their growth and cytopathic effects occur maximally at 33°C (a condition similar to that of the nasal mucosa) and hardly at all at normal cell-culture temperatures of 36°C or 37°C.

The impracticality of a rhinovirus vaccine can easily be understood, given the following reasons: (1) immunity is type-specific for more than 100 serotypes; (2) immunity appears to result from IgA antibody, and experimental vaccines must be administered through the nose; and (3) 2 years is probably the longest period of immunity that could be expected from even the best vaccine. Therefore, the control of rhinovirus infections continues to rely on avoidance of infected persons.

NORWALK AND NORWALK-LIKE VIRUSES (CALICIVIRIDAE)

The association of a specific virus-like agent with acute infectious nonbacterial gastroenteritis was first suggested in 1968 after an outbreak of gastroenteritis in an elementary school in Norwalk, Ohio. After more than 50% of the student population was stricken, the highly contagious nature of the etiologic agent was demonstrated by infecting human volunteers. The disease caused by the Norwalk virus is characterized by diarrhea and often severe vomiting, which occur 24 to 48 hours after exposure. Studies have been hampered by the fact that the virus cannot be propagated in tissue culture. Immune electron microscopy is the method of choice to diagnose infection with this virus and other viruses causing gastroenteritis. Norwalk virus is a small, nonenveloped virus that has been classified within the Caliciviridae family.

Since the original description of the Norwalk agent, additional agents with similar properties have been described in England and the United States. Thus, the term *Norwalk-like viruses* is now used to designate these viruses.

Structure and Replication of Norwalk Viruses

Norwalk and Norwalk-like viruses observed in the electron microscope are 27 to 30 nm in diameter and resemble picornaviruses and parvoviruses. Norwalk viruses have not been cultivated in cell culture, so characterization of their structure and replication is limited to analysis of virus purified from diarrheal stools of infected patients and analysis of viral genes using recombinant DNA technology. Norwalk virions lack a lipid envelope and appear to contain a single structural protein of about 59,000 daltons molecular weight. The positive-polarity RNA genome consists of a single molecule of RNA, about 8000 nucleotides in length.

Epidemiology and Pathogenesis of Norwalk Viruses

Norwalk and Norwalk-like viruses have been responsible for many outbreaks of acute infectious gastroenteritis occurring in grade schools, colleges, families, cruise ships at sea, and hotels and restaurants. Epidemiologic studies have shown that infections have resulted from virus contamination of municipal water supplies, recreational swimming pools, seafood, and food handlers. Antibodies to Norwalk viruses are present in healthy blood donors worldwide, and five distinct serotypes have been identified. The incubation period for the onset of clinical symptoms is 24 to 48 hours, and the disease is characterized by a sudden onset of nausea and vomiting, often severe. Other symptoms include fever and diarrhea. The epidemiologic and clinical features of gastroenteritis caused by Norwalk and Norwalk-like viruses are similar. Although these agents are antigenically distinct, it is likely that Norwalk and Norwalk-like viruses comprise a common family of viruses.

Diagnosis and Control of Norwalk Virus Infections

Laboratory diagnosis of Norwalk and Norwalk-like virus infections has been hindered by the inability to grow these viruses in cell culture. Routine laboratory diagnosis is not carried out, especially because most patients do not require hospitalization. However, virus can be visualized in the stools of infected patients using immune electron microscopy techniques. Vaccine development is unlikely because the sporadic and brief nature of the disease is not particularly life threatening. The best prevention is good personal hygiene and sound water and sewage treatment policies.

CORONAVIRIDAE

Coronaviruses cause gastroenteritis in swine and calves, and hepatitis in mice; however, it seems that human strains of these viruses are associated predominantly with upper respiratory tract infections indistinguishable from the common colds caused by the rhinoviruses.

Structure and Replication of Coronaviruses

Coronaviruses derive their name from a series of club-like projections covering the surface of their envelopes that resemble a solar corona (Fig. 46-4). The genome consists of a single strand of RNA with positive polarity. Coronaviruses replicate in the cytoplasm of infected cells and mature by budding into the cisternae of the endoplasmic reticulum and Golgi apparatus, from which they are transported in vesicles to the plasma membrane. The human coronaviruses are difficult to propagate in cell culture, and some isolates replicate only in human ciliated embryonic tracheal or nasal organ culture, whereas others can be cultivated only in the brains of newborn mice. As a result, research on these agents has been difficult.

Epidemiology and Pathogenesis of Coronavirus Infections

Coronavirus infections occur mainly in the winter and spring, and undoubtedly are spread through respiratory tract secretions. It is estimated that coronaviruses cause about 15% of adult common colds. Surprisingly, based on surveys of antibody titers, they seem to infect young adults more frequently than children. However, this observation may be an erroneous conclusion, because complement-fixing antibodies may not reach measurable or lasting titers until after multiple infections. Human coronaviruses appear to belong to one of two serotypes, distinguished by virus neutralization or hemagglutination inhibition.

Because of the limited range of cells in which coronaviruses can be propagated, it seems probable that during a human infection, the virus grows only in the cells of the respiratory tract. Studies of volunteers have shown an average incubation period of 3 days and an illness lasting about 1 week. Symptoms include a sore throat plus other effects normally associated with an acute upper respiratory tract infection. Enteric coronaviruses have been identified using electron microscopic examination of stools of patients with acute nonbacterial gastroenteritis. However, virus particles also have been found in stools of healthy individuals, bringing into question the role of coronaviruses in human gastroenteritis.

Diagnosis and Control of Coronavirus Infections

Virus isolation is difficult and is not done routinely. The most common laboratory diagnostic procedure is the demonstration of complement-fixing antibodies against the human prototype strain 229E. Red blood cells also can be coated with the coronavirus antigen and the serum tested for hemagglutination.

Bibliography

JOURNALS

Christensen ML. Human viral gastroenteritis. Clin Microbiol Rev 1989;2:51.

Greenberg HB, Matsul SM. Astroviruses and caliciviruses: emerging enteric pathogens. Infect Agents Dis 1992;1:71.

Melnick JL. Vaccination against poliomyelitis: present possibilities and future prospects. Am J Public Health 1988;78:304.

BOOKS

Brinton MA, Heinz FX, eds. New aspects of positive-strand RNA viruses. Washington, DC, American Society for Microbiology, 1990.

Crouch RB. Rhinoviruses. In: Fields BN, Knipe DM, eds. Virology, ed 2. New York, Raven Press, 1990:607.

Holmes KV. Coronaviridae and their replication. In: Fields BN, Knipe DM, eds. Virology, ed 2. New York, Raven Press, 1990:841.

Melnick JL. Enteroviruses: poliovirus, coxsackieviruses, echoviruses, and newer enteroviruses. In: Fields BN, Knipe DM, eds. Virology, ed 2. New York, Raven Press, 1990:549.

Rueckert RR. Picornaviruses and their replication. In: Fields BN, Knipe DM, eds. Virology, ed 2. New York, Raven Press, 1990:507.

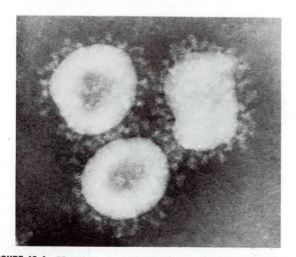

FIGURE 46-4 Human coronavirus. Surface projections create a corona effect around each virion. (Original magnification ×230,000.)

Essentials of Medical Microbiology, Fifth Edition, edited by Wesley A. Volk,
Bryan M. Gebhardt, Marie-Louise Hammarskjöld, and Robert J. Kadner.
Lippincott-Raven Publishers, Philadelphia © 1996.

Chapter 47

Togaviridae, Flaviviridae, and Bunyaviridae

The viruses comprising the families Togaviridae, Flaviviridae, and Bunyaviridae previously were referred to collectively as arboviruses, for *ar*thropod-*bo*rne viruses. This name reflects the ability of most members of these families to multiply both in arthropod vectors (most frequently mosquitoes and ticks) and in a wide variety of vertebrates, including humans. As a consequence, the infections produced by such viruses share a common epidemiology in that the virus is ingested by a blood-sucking arthropod from an infected animal and, after multiplication within the arthropod, is injected into an uninfected animal during a subsequent blood meal.

As more became known about the arboviruses, it became clear that they showed differences in structure and replication that warranted their division into three separate families. It also became clear that some of these viruses are related to other viruses that are non–arthropod-borne, which are now included in these families.

Members of the Togaviridae, Flaviviridae, and Bunyaviridae often derive their names from the geographic regions in which the viruses first were isolated or from the areas of the world where the viruses are endemic (Table 47-1). In general, humans play little or no part in the natural replication cycle of arboviruses (Fig. 47-1). However, as a result of human encroachment into the natural ecosystem of the different arboviruses, these viruses often are transmitted to humans, in whom they can cause severe disease, including encephalitis and hemorrhagic fevers. Rodents, cattle, sheep, and monkeys have been identified as reservoirs for the tick-borne encephalitis viruses, whereas wild birds, rodents, cattle, and horses constitute the major reservoir for many of the mosquito-borne arboviruses. Under circumstances in which the virus-carrying vector is found in proximity to humans, such as urban yellow fever virus or dengue virus, humans serve as an efficient reservoir.

The arthropod–vertebrate cycle is a continuous one in tropical areas of the world. However, where colder climates contribute to the temporary disappearance of the

TABLE 47-1
Classification and Description of Togaviruses, Flaviviruses, and Bunyaviruses

Family	Group (Genus)	Viral Species	Vector	Clinical Diseases in Humans	Geographic Distribution
Togaviridae	*Alphavirus*	Eastern equine encephalitis (EEE)	Mosquito	Encephalitis	Eastern U.S., Canada, Brazil, Cuba, Panama, Philippines, Dominican Republic, Trinidad
		Venezuelan equine encephalitis (VEE)	Mosquito	Encephalitis	Brazil, Columbia, Ecuador, Trinidad, Venezuela, Mexico, U.S. (Florida and Texas)
		Western equine encephalitis (WEE)	Mosquito	Encephalitis	Western U.S., Canada, Mexico, Argentina, Brazil, British Guiana
		Sindbis	Mosquito	Subclinical	Egypt, India, South Africa, Australia
		Chikungunya	Mosquito	Headache, fever, rash, joint and muscle pains	East Africa, South Africa, Southeast Asia
		Semliki Forest	Mosquito	Fever or none	East Africa, West Africa
		Majora	Mosquito	Headache, fever, joint and muscle pains	Bolivia, Brazil, Colombia, Trinidad
	Rubivirus	Rubella	None	Rubella	Worldwide
Flaviviridae	*Flavivirus*	St. Louis encephalitis	Mosquito	Encephalitis	U.S., Trinidad, Panama
		Japanese B encephalitis	Mosquito	Encephalitis	Japan, Guam, Eastern Asian mainland, Malaya, India
		Murray Valley encephalitis	Mosquito	Encephalitis	Australia, New Guinea
		West Nile	Mosquito	Headache, fever, myalgia, rash, lymphadenopathy	Egypt, Israel, India, Uganda, South Africa
		Dengue (4 types)	Mosquito	Headache, fever, myalgia, prostration, rash (sometimes hemorrhagic)	Pacific Islands, South and Southeast Asia, northern Australia, New Guinea, Greece, Caribbean Islands, Nigeria, Central and South America
		Yellow fever	Mosquito	Fever, prostration, hepatitis, nephritis	Central and South America, Africa, Trinidad
		Tick-borne group (Russian spring-summer encephalitis group)	Tick	Encephalitis; meningoencephalitis, hemorrhagic fever	Russian spring-summer encephalitis: Russia; Powassan: Canada, U.S.; Others: Japan, Siberia, Central Europe, Russia, India, Malaya, Great Britain (Louping iLL)
Bunyaviridae	*Bunyamwera*	*Bunyamwera* and 13 others	Mosquito	Headache, fever, myalgia; just fever; or none	Uganda, South Africa, India, Malaya, Colombia, Brazil, Trinidad, West Africa, Finland, U.S.
	California group	California encephalitis La Crosse	Mosquito	Encephalitis, or none	U.S., Trinidad, Brazil, Canada, Czech The Republic, Slovakia, Mozambique
	Phlebovirus	Rift Valley fever	*Phlebotomus* Sandfly	Headache, fever, myalgia	Italy, Egypt, Russia, India, Central and South America
	Nairovirus	Congo-Crimean hemorrhagic fever	Tick	Hepatitis, hemorrhagic fever	Russia, Middle East, Africa
	Hantavirus	Hantavirus	Rodents	Acute interstitial nephritis, respiratory disease	Asia, Europe, US

vector, the diseases are seasonal. It is not known for certain where arboviruses are harbored during the winter months, but they may remain in the vector, being transferred from one generation to the next (transovarial transmission). Alternatively, viruses may remain in the primary or secondary reservoir, being reintroduced into the area by migratory birds, or they may remain in secondary hosts such as rodents. Thus, arboviruses have evolved several useful strategies to adapt to the many different environmental challenges.

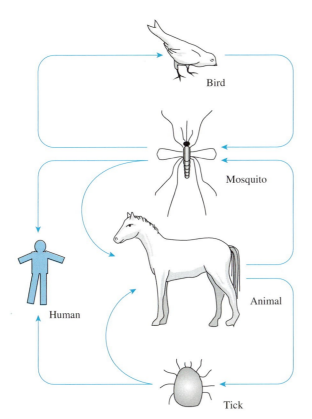

FIGURE 47-1 Epidemiology of arbovirus infections. Although the bird–mosquito cycle probably is most important for the maintenance of these viruses, lower animals and ticks also participate in the epidemiology of the arboviruses. Humans come into contact with one of these cycles when they become infected by either mosquitoes or ticks (varying among the different arboviruses).

TOGAVIRIDAE AND FLAVIVIRIDAE

Togaviruses are icosahedral, contain single-stranded RNA (about 11,500 nucleotides), and are surrounded by a membrane envelope (*toga* means mantle). Based on similarities in their RNA genomes, capsid structures, lipoprotein envelopes, and multiplication cycles, four genera of viruses are included in the Togaviridae family. Members of the genus *Alphavirus* are spread to vertebrates through an arthropod vector and, hence, are arboviruses. Non–arthropod-borne members of this family are placed either in the genus *Rubivirus,* which contains the etiologic agent of rubella (German measles), or in the genera *Pestivirus* or *Arterivirus,* which contain numerous viruses that cause animal diseases.

Until recently, *Flavivirus* was classified as a genus in the family Togaviridae. However, evidence now indicates that the flaviviruses differ from the togaviruses with respect to size, structure, gene sequence, and replication strategy. Accordingly, the International Committee on Taxonomy of Viruses has designated Flaviviridae a new family.

Structure and Replication of Togaviruses

Togavirus virions, as exemplified by Semliki Forest virus, the best studied of these viruses, consist of an icosahedral nucleocapsid comprising a single capsid protein, the C protein. The capsid is surrounded by a lipid envelope containing virus-specified glycoproteins (Fig. 47-2). Three viral glycoproteins form the spike; these are designated E1, E2, and E3. Interestingly, the glycoproteins E1 and E2 not only are glycosylated but also are acylated, containing covalently bound fatty acid. These modifications appear important for the association of the glycoprotein with the lipid bilayer of the host cell. Both neutralizing antibodies and hemagglutination-inhibition antibodies are directed against one or more of these glycosylated envelope proteins.

Togaviruses obtain their envelopes as they bud through areas of the host-cell membrane that have been modified by the incorporation of viral glycoproteins. Thus, release of the virions does not elicit lysis of the host cell, but generally does cause the eventual death of vertebrate cells. In contrast, in vitro infection of cultured arthropod cells results in a chronic infection in which small amounts of virus continue to be produced over a long period without causing destruction of the infected cell. This corresponds to the in vivo situation, in which the virus multiplies without apparent damage to its arthropod vector.

Togavirus reproduction occurs entirely within the cytoplasm of the infected cell. After adsorption, penetration, and uncoating, the virion RNA acts as its own mRNA to code for the synthesis of an RNA polymerase and the structural proteins that form the nucleocapsid and are incorporated into the envelope of the completed virion.

Although the virions contain only one molecule of 49S RNA, two different molecules of RNA are involved in virus replication (Fig. 47-3). The 5′ terminal two thirds of the virion 49S RNA encodes four nonstructural polypeptides. These polypeptides catalyze the transcription of the positive-strand RNA, generating a negative strand that subsequently is used as a template for the production of more virion RNA. A smaller 26S RNA, which is made by partial transcription of the virion RNA, serves as mRNA for the synthesis of viral structural proteins. Proteins translated from this 26S mRNA are synthesized as a single polypeptide precursor molecule, which then is cleaved into the proteins found in the virion capsid (C protein) and envelope (E1, E2, and E3).

Structure and Replication of Flaviviruses

Flaviviruses are uniformly spherical particles about 45 nm in diameter with a lipid envelope that surrounds a densely staining core measuring about 30 nm in diameter. Spikes

decline in incidence has been noted in Asia and reflects changes in agricultural practices, increased spraying to eliminate the mosquito vector, and increased immunization of susceptible individuals. At the same time, a dramatic increase in the incidence of Japanese B encephalitis has occurred in northern parts of the Indian subcontinent and Southeast Asia. Apparently, the reservoir is birds, and spread of the virus occurs through mosquitoes. An inactivated vaccine has been administered in Taiwan and Japan, and a live vaccine is being evaluated in the United States.

Russian spring-summer encephalitis virus is one of the flaviviruses for which the vector is the wood tick. Wild animals appear to serve as the reservoir, but because the virus can be passed transovarially (from mother to egg) in the tick, an additional reservoir is not necessary for the maintenance of this disease. In humans, the disease is characterized by headache, fever, nausea, and, occasionally, coma. The virus is found in both the blood and the spinal fluid, and can cause paralysis early in the infection. The mortality rate can be as high as 30%, although the use of a vaccine grown in mouse brains has been beneficial in reducing the incidence and severity of the disease. At least nine other tick-borne flaviviruses infect animals, including occasional infections of humans causing mild to severe symptoms. Several of the best-studied flaviviruses include louping ill (primarily a disease of sheep), Omsk hemorrhagic fever (from Russia), and Kyasanur Forest disease (from India). The last two can cause severe hemorrhagic diseases in humans.

YELLOW FEVER

Yellow fever virus causes an acute infectious disease characterized by severe liver damage. Symptoms include headache, backache, fever, prostration, nausea, and vomiting. As a result of liver damage, jaundice can be evident as early as the fourth or fifth day of the illness. The incubation period is 3 to 6 days, and recovery from the disease results in lifelong immunity.

One of the first major insights into the control of viral diseases in general occurred when Dr. Walter Reed and associates described the epidemiology of yellow fever. Their research resulted in the elimination of this disease from many urban areas of the world, including Panama (which, at least indirectly, made it possible to complete the construction of the canal). The disease is transmitted by one or more species of mosquito from person to person, monkey to human, or monkey to monkey. Humans are the reservoir of infection in urban areas, and the mosquito *Aedes aegypti* is the vector for urban yellow fever. Monkeys, marmosets, and, perhaps, marsupial animals serve as reservoirs in the jungle. Jungle yellow fever differs from urban yellow fever only in the fact that different genera of mosquitoes are the vectors for its transmission.

There is only one antigenic strain of yellow fever virus, so a single vaccine is effective.

Clinical observations usually are sufficient for diagnosis of yellow fever during epidemics, but mild cases can be difficult to diagnose. Diagnosis can be accomplished by the microscopic examination of liver biopsy samples for necrotic lesions and for intranuclear inclusion bodies characteristic of yellow fever, by isolation of the virus from mice after intracerebral inoculation with a patient's serum, or by demonstration of a rise in the level of neutralizing antibodies during convalescence.

The eradication of *A. aegypti* mosquitoes in urban areas is an effective control measure. This sort of attack on the vector has virtually eliminated the disease from the urban populations of Central and South America, as well as the southern cities of the United States.

An attenuated vaccine for yellow fever, the 17D strain of the virus, is grown in chick embryos and has proved to be effective in stimulating active immunity to the disease.

DENGUE FEVER

Dengue fever occurs throughout the tropics, including the Caribbean area, where the disease is endemic in Puerto Rico and the Virgin Islands. Dengue fever virus is transmitted from person to person by several species of mosquitoes of the genus *Aedes*.

The disease, dengue fever, is an acute infection usually manifested by headache, backache, fatigue, stiffness, loss of appetite, chilliness, and, occasionally, a rash. Probably the most characteristic symptom is emphasized by the other name for this disease, break-bone fever. Many of the symptoms precede the first rise in temperature. In some cases, the onset is sudden, with a sharp temperature rise, severe headache, backache, pain behind the eyes, and muscle and joint pains. The virus is found in the blood of the infected person shortly before the onset of fever.

There are four serologically distinct types of dengue fever virus. However, considerable antigenic cross-reactivity is observed among the different serotypes, and recovery from an infection by one type does not provide complete immunity against infection by other types. The normal incubation period is 5 to 6 days, but this seems to be influenced by the amount of infecting virus and can vary from 3 to 15 days. Humans and the *Aedes* mosquito are the recognized reservoir and vector, respectively; however, as in yellow fever, monkeys also can serve as a major reservoir.

Dengue hemorrhagic fever (DHF) and dengue shock syndrome (DSS) appear to be relatively new manifestations of dengue virus infection that have become more and more prevalent since the early 1950s. Before that time, the disease had a low fatality rate and was particularly mild in children. However, in the Philippines and in Southeast Asia, the disease appears to have become much more severe, especially in children, with symptoms of shock and hemorrhage and a mortality rate that approaches 10%. The appearance of DHF/DSS relates directly to the introduction of two or more different dengue virus serotypes into the general population (a result of better transportation facilities) and increased movement of persons between the various endemic areas of dengue fever. DHF/DSS appears to result from the antibody-dependent enhancement of dengue virus infection of cells of the mononuclear phagocyte lineage. Patients with DHF/DSS show acute physiologic derangements brought about by increased vascular permeability, abnormal hemostasis, and inflammation, consistent with mononuclear phagocytes being a major target for virus infection. DHF/DSS occurs primarily in infants, less than 1 year of age, who are born to dengue-immune mothers, and in children 1 year or older who are immune to one of the dengue virus serotypes and are undergoing an infection by a second serotype. The replication of dengue virus in mononuclear phagocytes is enhanced by the presence of subneutralizing amounts of cross-reacting antibody to the dengue virus (provided by an earlier encounter with a particular serotype or by the transmission of maternal antibodies). These antibodies are not sufficient to neutralize the newly acquired virus but instead bind to the virus particle and concomitantly to the Fc receptors on the mononuclear phagocytes. In this fashion, the antibody promotes the efficient binding and entry of virus into the cell, thus accelerating the infection process.

Serologic tests useful in the diagnosis of dengue fever include tests for complement-fixing, neutralizing, and hemagglutination-inhibition antibodies. The major types of the virus are adapted for growth in mice, and mice are used for the preparation of specific antigen for the diagnostic serologic test.

Control measures are directed toward the elimination of *Aedes* mosquitoes. Vaccines against dengue virus are not available for general use. The possibility of provoking or enhancing DHF/DSS in vaccinated persons has engendered considerable discussion regarding the potential effectiveness of dengue vaccines. It would appear that potential vaccines must effectively prevent infection by all four serotypes of virus.

Rubivirus Infections in Humans

The agent that causes rubella is spread from person to person through respiratory tract secretions. This virus is a typical togavirus and is classified in the genus *Rubivirus* within this family. The virus can be grown in a variety of human and primate cell cultures; cytopathic effects occur only in some cells.

Rubella is a mild disease spread through respiratory tract secretions. After replication in the cervical lymph nodes, the virus is disseminated throughout the body through the bloodstream, with the first overt signs of disease being moderate catarrhal symptoms and mild fever; the extent of the rash tends to be irregular. The incubation period varies from 2 to 3 weeks, but virus can be isolated from nasopharyngeal secretions for as long as a week before there are recognizable symptoms. The illness is of short duration, and recovery usually is complete within 3 to 4 days after the appearance of the rash. Transient arthritis is a fairly frequent symptom in adult women, but other complications are rare.

The tragic aspect of rubella can become evident if infection occurs during pregnancy. The virus can cross the placental wall, particularly early in pregnancy, and infect the fetus, where it disseminates and grows in every fetal organ. Infection can result in a large variety of congenital defects or death of the fetus. Defects can include hearing loss, mental retardation, cerebral palsy, cataracts, microcephaly, and heart abnormalities, as well as other congenital anomalies. Collectively, these are referred to as the congenital rubella syndrome. A fetus that survives initial infection can continue to shed rubella virus for 1 to 2 years after birth, in spite of the presence of circulating antibody to the virus. It is estimated that 10% to 20% of such babies die during the first year after birth.

The prognosis of an infected fetus born with rubella syndrome depends largely on its stage of development at the time of infection. Congenital defects can occur in as many as 80% of the fetuses of mothers infected during the first month of pregnancy; however, the incidence drops to about 15% by the third month, and by the end of the first trimester, the percentage of fetuses with congenital defects is small. The most serious congenital abnormalities appear to occur when the fetus is infected during the period of maximum cell differentiation. The observation that rubella-infected human embryo cells show significant chromosomal breakage and inhibition of normal mitosis sheds some light on the reasons for the congenital defects. Infection of the fetus during cell differentiation could easily interfere with development, causing a variety of defects.

Laboratory diagnosis of rubella requires isolation of the virus, usually from nasopharyngeal secretions. The lack of cytopathic effects in some types of cell cultures can be overcome by using the knowledge that rubella-infected cells, although outwardly normal, are resistant to infection by many picornaviruses that ordinarily cause cytopathic effects. In addition, because rubella virus possesses a hemagglutinin, infected areas can be located by hemadsorption. Other methods of diagnosis measure a rise in antibody titer using hemagglutination inhibition, complement fixation, neutralization tests, or enzyme-linked immunosorbent assays.

There is only one antigenic strain of rubella virus, and infection induces immunity that appears to be lifelong, although second infections occur occasionally as inapparent disease. Rash does not occur in some cases of rubella, even though such persons are excreting virus. Thus, there are three major reasons for virus spread: (1) inapparent infections, (2) an asymptomatic period of about 1 week before apparent symptoms, and (3) congenitally infected babies who can appear normal even though they are excreting virus. Therefore, control through isolation of patients with the disease is impossible.

The live attenuated rubella vaccine (RA 27/3) induces effective immunity in about 95% of recipients. However, the vaccine can cause fever, mild rash, and, in adult women, transient arthritis. Although it appears that vaccinated persons subsequently can experience mild to inapparent rubella virus infections, the frequency of fetal infections in partially immune vaccinated women is unknown.

Inadvertent administration of the vaccine to pregnant women can result in infection of the fetus. However, there is no evidence that the vaccine causes congenital abnormalities. Nonetheless, use of the vaccine in pregnant women is not recommended. In the United States, the vaccine is administered to all prepubertal children of both sexes in an attempt to provide herd immunity and maximum protection to at-risk women. In European countries, 10- to 14-year-old girls are administered the vaccine in an attempt to establish immunity among women of childbearing age.

BUNYAVIRIDAE

The bunyaviruses at one time were placed together with other groups in the large taxonomic group known as the arboviruses. However, sufficient information about this group has since been obtained to give it the status of a family, called the Bunyaviridae. This family contains more than 250 viruses and is divided into five genera: *Bunyavirus, Hantavirus, Phlebovirus, Uukuvirus,* and *Nairovirus.* Viruses of this family, with the exception of hantaviruses, are transmitted by arthropod vectors, including mosquitoes, ticks, biting midges, and sandflies. Hantaviruses are transmitted by rodents. Viruses of the Bunyaviridae are important human and veterinary pathogens throughout the world (see Table 46-1).

Structure and Replication of Bunyaviruses

Structurally, bunyaviruses differ from togaviruses in that they possess a helical nucleocapsid (Fig. 47-4) and three single-stranded, negative-sense RNAs. The viruses are lipid-enveloped spherical structures, 90 to 120 nm in diameter, that contain 5- to 10-nm surface projections (spikes). The virion spikes are made up of two surface glycoproteins (G1 and G2), and the virion core contains a single nucleocapsid protein, termed N. The virus also encodes a virion-associated polymerase that can be detected in purified virus preparations. The G1 or G2 proteins likely serve as hemagglutinin and targets for neutralizing antibody.

The three negative-strand RNA genomic segments are termed large (L), medium (M), and small (S). The viral nucleocapsids are circular in configuration because of the presence of complementary 3' and 5' sequences at the termini of each RNA segment. The M RNA segment has been shown to encode a polyprotein that is processed in infected cells to form the G1 and G2 glycoproteins as well as a nonstructural protein, designated NS_M. The S RNA segment has been shown to encode the N protein and a nonstructural protein NS_s. The L RNA segment likely encodes the virion-associated RNA polymerase.

The replication strategy of bunyaviruses resembles that of other negative-strand viruses. After attachment, penetration, and entry of the virus into the cytoplasm of the cell, each segment is transcribed by the virion-

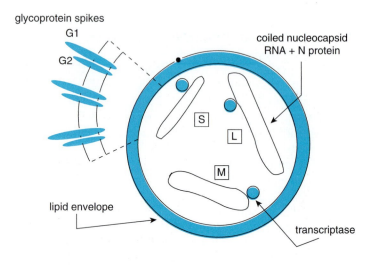

FIGURE 47-4 Diagram of a bunyavirus particle. Glycoprotein spikes present in the virus envelope are denoted by the filled ellipses. The hatched circles represent virion-encoded transcriptase present in virus particles. S, M, and L denote the three RNA segments that make up the bunyavirus genome. See text for additional details.

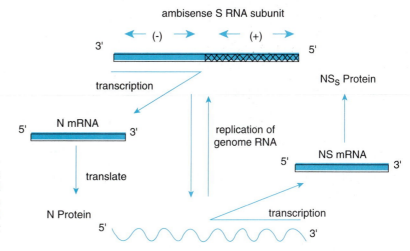

FIGURE 47-5 Ambisense expression of the S RNA segment of a phlebovirus. The diagram depicts the steps leading to expression of the N protein form (−) strand sequences present in the S RNA segment. The NS protein is encoded by an mRNA transcribed from the (+) strand sequences present in the S RNA segment. See text for further details.

associated polymerase, giving rise to positive-strand mRNAs that are translated on host ribosomes. Like influenza virus mRNAs, bunyavirus mRNAs contain 5″ sequences derived from the host, presumably through mechanisms similar to those used by influenza viruses (see Chap. 48). The phleboviruses exhibit a remarkable variation on this theme in that the S segment contains both negative- and positive-sense information (Fig. 47-5). After infection, the negative-sense, 3′ half of this virion RNA segment is transcribed into positive-sense mRNA, which in turn encodes the N protein. The positive-sense portion (5′ half) of the viral genome is not translated directly. However, after transcription (replication) of the entire S segment to form a complementary strand, selective transcription occurs to provide an mRNA encoding the nonstructural protein NS$_s$. This unique arrangement of genetic information is termed *ambisense*.

The segmented nature of bunyaviruses renders the clear possibility of genetic exchange among two or more viruses. Indeed, high-frequency reassortment of genome segments has been observed among viruses of several genera.

Bunyaviridae Diseases in Humans

Most of the Bunyaviridae are carried by arthropod vectors and only a few cause severe infections in humans. Among the most important of these diseases are California encephalitis, Rift Valley fever, sandfly fever, and hemorrhagic fevers.

BUNYAVIRUSES: CALIFORNIA ENCEPHALITIS GROUP

The California encephalitis serogroup contains at least 15 serologically related viruses (of the genus *Bunyavirus*), all of which are found in the United States and Western Europe. LaCrosse virus is one of the better-studied members of this group and is among the most important agents of California encephalitis in the United States. LaCrosse virus is transmitted by the bite of the mosquito *Aedes triseriatus* and causes disease in children and forest workers in heavily wooded areas of the Midwest and West.

The virus is transmitted transovarially in infected mosquitoes and is maintained by overwintering in the infected mosquito eggs. Mosquitoes also transmit the virus to several animals that serve as a reservoir for the infection of more mosquitoes. The disease occurs most frequently in children and can cause a mild, undiagnosed febrile illness or severe central nervous system involvement, which can lead to convulsions. Other symptoms include headache, stiff neck, nausea, and vomiting. Mortality is low, even in severe cases, although there have been reports of residual personality changes and learning disorders.

A specific diagnosis of California encephalitis usually is based on a four-fold rise in antibody to the virus after recovery from the infection. Prevention depends on mosquito control.

PHLEBOVIRUSES: RIFT VALLEY FEVER, SANDFLY FEVER

Rift Valley fever virus is characterized by its pathogenicity for domestic animals and its ability to cause serious and often fatal infections in humans. The virus originally was isolated in the Rift Valley of Kenya, but has been distributed over the entire sub-Saharan African continent for centuries. Repeated infections of sheep, cattle, and goats have been reported, with mortality rates of 10% to 30%. As for other bunyaviruses, virus transmission is mediated by the mosquito.

The viruses causing sandfly fever are spread to humans through the bite of the female sandfly, *Phlebotomus papatasii*. The disease, found primarily in the areas of the Mediterranean Sea, Russia, India, and Central and South

A Closer Look

The death of a young Navajo woman from the Four Corners area in the Southwestern United States, which occurred after a brief illness in May 1993, originally did not cause much attention. Her major symptom had been difficulty breathing, and she had a history of asthma. However, when her previously healthy fiancé died only 5 days later at the Indian Medical Center in Gallup, New Mexico, the chief of internal medicine became quite alarmed. The 20-year-old Navajo man was a physically fit person who suddenly started gasping for air on the way to his fiancée's funeral. Autopsies showed that both victims had died of severe pneumonia and that their lungs were filled with fluid. At this time, the doctor recalled that he had three other patients that had died of a similar disease within the preceding half-year period. They had all been young Navajos without known medical problems. Considering all these facts, the doctor first suspected a possible outbreak of bubonic plague. Sporadic occurrence of this flea-borne disease is seen in this part of the United States from time to time. The tests came back negative, however, as did several other tests for common causes of pneumonia. Finding himself with a potential unknown infectious agent, the physician decided to notify the state health department.

About 2 weeks later, a team from the Centers for Disease Control (CDC) in Atlanta, Georgia, arrived to investigate the possible cause of these pneumonia cases. By this time, several other cases of the disease had been reported, causing a nationwide concern and media attention. The disease had already been named the "Navajo flu" by the newspapers, increasing the prejudice against Native Americans in the area. Initially, there were many possibilities for the cause of the "epidemic." Among them were several infectious agents (eg, organisms of the genera *Legionella, Mycoplasma, Chlamydia, Rickettsia;* adenovirus; herpesvirus), but it was also possible that the disease was caused by an environmental problem (eg, heavy metals or a pesticide).

The team from CDC carefully investigated all the case histories and started to limit the number of possible causes. The fact that high fever was a common symptom made an infectious agent appear more likely. Also, some of the characteristics seemed to indicate that the disease might be a form of hemorrhagic fever. Because hemorrhagic fever outbreaks caused by viruses have been seen in several different parts of the world, the CDC team started to look for a virus that could explain this new epidemic. Because the victims were rural people who might have had exposure to rodents, a rodent-borne hantavirus or an arenavirus soon became prime suspects. Also, when antibodies from the patients were tested against a panel of infectious agents, they consistently reacted with only three hantaviruses. These results indicated that the patients had been exposed to a hantavirus.

Previous outbreaks in other parts of the world have made clear that hantaviruses are frequently spread through rodent droppings. Cleaning out of such droppings can create an aerosol that is then inhaled, causing the disease. It took the CDC team less than 1 week to determine that the probable cause of the epidemic was a hantavirus. In the meantime, however, several other cases of the disease had been reported in the Four Corners area. As soon as a hantavirus became the prime suspect for the outbreak, the CDC "rat trapping" team was called in. They trapped mice in the homes of the patients and sent blood and tissue back to CDC in Atlanta. By using the polymerase chain reaction (PCR) technique on DNA extracted from this material, they were able to confirm the presence of a hantavirus in several deer mice that had been trapped in and around the homes of some of the victims.

To prove that the hantavirus was the cause of the mysterious disease, PCR also had to be performed on samples taken from the victims. These tests showed the presence of genetic material from the same hantavirus, making it clear that the virus was the cause of the disease outbreak. Interestingly, the virus was shown to represent a novel hantavirus that had never been isolated before. The final identification was made only 1 month after the first death had been reported. The people living in the Four Corners area were cautioned to avoid contact with mouse droppings, to protect their food and dishes from the mice, and to eliminate mice with mouse traps or rat poison. These and other precautions to avoid direct contact with mice and mice droppings soon curbed the epidemic.

About 1 year after the first outbreak, a total of 74 cases of hantavirus infections in the United States had been reported to the CDC, and 42 people had died. Interestingly, several of the cases were not from the Four Corners area. In fact, 18 different states reported hantavirus cases, showing that hantaviruses are present in several different areas. Random trapping and testing of deer mice have shown that up to 15% of deer mice nationwide are infected with these viruses, indicating that hantaviruses have been present in the United States for many years.

America, causes headache, nausea, fever, photophobia, and abdominal pain. Complete recovery is usual.

HANTAVIRUSES: HEMORRHAGIC FEVER, RODENT-BORNE NEPHROPATHY

Hantaviruses are unusual among the bunyaviruses in that they are spread by rodents. These viruses were responsible for sizable outbreaks of hemorrhagic fever or hemorrhagic fever associated with renal syndrome during the Korean War. In addition, hantaviruses have been identified as the cause of a similar related condition, termed *nephropathia epidemica,* which has been recognized in Scandinavia for many years. Rodent-borne hantaviruses have been identified worldwide. An outbreak of disease among Native Americans living in an area of the southwestern United States in 1993 was shown to be caused by a hantavirus. The disease caused by this virus was characterized by fever, general malaise, and sometimes severe respiratory problems, and it had a significant mortality rate. The vector was shown to be a deer mouse, and those infected had been in contact with mouse droppings. Hantaviruses since have been found in deer mouse populations in many states, and isolated cases of disease with a few deaths have been reported in several different areas.

NAIROVIRUSES: CONGO-CRIMEAN HEMORRHAGIC FEVER

Tick-borne nairoviruses are responsible for an exceptionally severe hemorrhagic fever that occurs throughout Central Asia, the Middle East, and Africa. The virus is maintained in ticks by transovarial transmission, and vertebrate species comprise an important host. Transmission of the virus to humans results in a disease characterized by abrupt fever, severe headache, and back and abdominal pain, followed by extensive hemorrhages from many sites. Internal bleeding can lead to shock, edema, and death in 5% to 50% of cases. Preventive measures center on the elimination or control of ticks in endemic areas.

Bibliography

JOURNALS

Bouloy M. Bunyaviridae: genome organization and replication strategies. Adv Virol Res 1991;40:235.

Elliott RM. Molecular biology of the Bunyaviridae. J Gen Virol 1990;71:501.

Freij BJ, South MA, Sever JL. Maternal rubella and the congenital rubella syndrome. Clin Perinatol 1988;15:247.

Halstead SB. Pathogenesis of dengue: challenges to molecular biology. Science 1988;239:476.

Westaway EG. Flavivirus replication strategy. Adv Virus Res 1987;33:45.

BOOKS

Brinton MA, Heinz FX, eds. New aspects of positive-strand RNA viruses. Washington, DC, American Society for Microbiology, 1990.

Monath TP. Flaviviruses. In: Fields BN, Knipe DM, eds. Virology, ed 2. New York, Raven Press, 1990:763.

Schlesinger S, Schlesinger MJ. Replication of Togaviridae and Flaviviridae. In: Fields BN, Knipe DM, eds. Virology, ed 2. New York, Raven Press, 1990:697.

FIGU
ativel
spike
tion
enza

The HA plays a central role in virus replication and pathogenicity. It directs the binding of virus particles to host-cell receptors (sialic acid). It is a major target of the host cell's immune response, and it catalyzes an important step in virus entry into the host cell. The HA activity of influenza viruses results from the ability of the HA spike present on the surface of the viruses to attach to the sialic acid present on glycoproteins on the surface of erythrocytes, causing them to agglutinate. Numerous studies have shown that each HA spike is made up of three identical polypeptide chains, which are cleaved after translation to form two subunits, HA1 and HA2. These subunits are arranged to form a stalk embedded in the lipid bilayer and a globular head (see Fig. 48-1). Antibodies that neutralize virus infectivity bind to epitopes present on the surface of the globular head of the HA. In addition, there is a small depression in each of the HA heads. The amino acid residues making up the depression or pocket are highly conserved among different influenza viruses and, together, these residues form a pocket for binding to the host-cell receptor molecule. Antibodies that block or neutralize infectivity of the virus do not bind to sites within the depression but to amino acid residues that surround the receptor-binding pocket. Thus, neutralization is accomplished by antibody sterically inhibiting the binding of virus to a cellular receptor.

The viral NA activity was first recognized when it was observed that virus particles would catalyze the cleavage of terminal neuraminic acid from erythrocyte virus receptors. During the course of virus infection, the NA appears important in allowing the virus to penetrate mucin within the respiratory tract, enhancing access of the virus to epithelial cells. In addition, NA plays an important role in mediating the release of virus from infected cells and promoting the spread of the virus within the infected host. The NA also is the target for neutralizing antibodies, although these antibodies appear to be more important in blocking the spread of virus than in blocking initial infection. The NA spike is made up of four polypeptide chains arranged to form a membrane-anchored stalk attached to a roughly box-like head (see Fig. 48-1). The head of the NA contains the biologically important sites, the catalytic site for enzymatic cleavage and the major antigenic determinants involved in virus neutralization.

Virus particles contain several important proteins necessary for virus structure and replication. The M1 protein lies beneath the lipid bilayer, forming a shell surrounding the nucleocapsid (see Fig. 48-1). It is postulated that the M1 protein serves as an anchor for the envelope-associated HA and NA glycoproteins, as well as functions as a binding site for ribonuclear protein segments during virus maturation. The NP binds to the negative strands of viral RNA and appears to be important in the organization of the viral RNA segments. Three proteins encoded by the virus, PB1, PB2, and PA, catalyze viral transcription and are discussed in more detail later in this chapter.

Adsorption of virus to cellular receptors requires the specific reaction between the HA spike and a sialic acid residue present on glycoproteins on the host-cell surface. Antibodies directed specifically against the viral HA will neutralize infection by preventing adsorption of the virus. In addition, treatment of potential host cells with NA to remove terminal sialic acid residues from the specific glycoprotein receptor will prevent adsorption of the virus.

There is a growing body of evidence concerning the actual mechanism of penetration and uncoating of the infecting virion. The HA appears to play an important role in the fusion of the viral envelope with the host-cell membrane. The amino terminus of the HA2 subunit is created by posttranslational cleavage of the HA precursor polypeptide. This portion of HA2 is hydrophobic and exhibits sequence similarity with the amino-terminal region of fusion proteins of paramyxoviruses (see later). After attachment, the virus is internalized into an intracellular endosome. The acid pH of this vesicle promotes a conformational alteration in the HA, leading to an interaction between the hydrophobic N terminus of the HA2 polypeptide and the endosome membrane. As a result, this membrane is fused with the viral envelope and the viral nucleocapsid is released into the cytoplasm of the infected cell. Influenza virus grown in cells that do not cleave HA to HA1 and HA2 exhibits reduced virus infectivity. Infectivity can be restored by in vitro incubation of virus with known proteases, which restore the cleavage of HA to HA1 and HA2.

After the release of viral ribonucleoprotein into the cytoplasm, the viral RNA segments are transported to the cell nucleus, where the virus-encoded polymerase transcribes each individual segment of viral RNA into complementary RNA (cRNA). Detailed studies on the replication of influenza virus RNA have shown that in the infected cell, virion RNAs are transcribed into two different types of transcripts (Fig. 48-2). The first type of viral transcript is complete cRNA copies of the virion RNAs. These full-length RNAs function as templates for the synthesis of new progeny virion RNAs. The second type of transcript is viral messenger RNAs (mRNAs). These molecules contain a 5'-capped terminus consisting of 10 to 13 nucleotides derived from host-cell mRNAs (see later). They lack the 3' 15 to 16 nucleotides of the cRNA, having instead a poly A tail. Viral mRNAs are transported to the cytoplasm, where they direct the synthesis of viral proteins. An unusual aspect of influenza virus replication is the fact that it can be blocked by actinomycin D, an inhibitor of DNA-dependent RNA synthesis. An explanation for the paradoxical requirement for DNA-dependent RNA synthesis was provided when it was observed that host-cell mRNAs could stimulate the in vitro transcription of influenza virus RNA. It is now known that the synthesis of viral mRNAs is dependent on the presence of cellular "capped" primers (see Fig. 48-2). A viral-specified endonuclease, a part of the viral transcription complex, cleaves host mRNAs, generating 5'-capped oligonucleotides 10 to 13 nucleo-

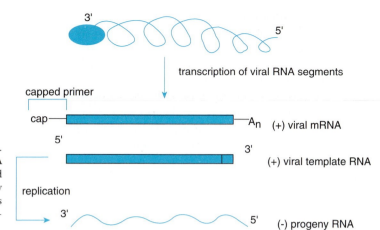

FIGURE 48-2 Transcription of influenza virus RNA segments. The diagram depicts the steps in the synthesis of viral mRNA and virus progeny RNA. The (+) viral RNA contains a 5′ "capped primer" sequence derived from host cell RNA and a 3′ poly A sequence (A_n). Virion template RNA contains 3′ sequences (*hatched box*) not present in viral mRNA. The filled ellipse denotes the virus-encoded polymerase complex.

tides in length. These primers bind to the polymerase complex (made up of PB1, PB2, and PA) and initiate transcription of the mRNA from virion RNA. The viral protein PB2 seems to be involved in recognition and cleavage of the capped oligonucleotides from host-cell mRNAs, and the viral protein PB1 is required to initiate transcription and carry out chain elongation. The third member of the polymerase complex, PA, may play a role in virion RNA replication. About 3 hours after infection, progeny RNA synthesis commences using template RNAs sequestered in the nucleus. The molecular mechanisms that direct the change from synthesis of viral mRNAs to synthesis of viral progeny are unknown.

Ten viral proteins are encoded by the eight segments of the influenza virus genome. At least one protein is encoded by each segment, and alternative RNA splicing appears to be responsible for the generation of mRNAs for the remaining viral proteins. There also appears to be a mechanism for regulating the synthesis of individual viral proteins, because not all viral polypeptides are synthesized in equimolar amounts. This control appears to operate at the level of mRNA transcription, but its precise nature remains unclear.

Maturation of the influenza virus is initiated as HA and NA proteins are incorporated into areas of the plasma membrane. The viral ribonuclear protein (RNP) complex formed in the nucleus is transported out of the nucleus, probably with the help of the M1 protein. The complex then associates with the morphologically altered areas of the host-cell membrane containing the viral envelope proteins, and virus particles are formed by budding. Because of the segmentation of the viral genome, simultaneous infection of a cell by two genetically distinct influenza viruses leads to a high level of genetic exchange. The consequent reassortment of viral genes can result in the formation of novel strains with new antigenic properties, changed virulence, and different host-cell dependence (see later).

Influenza viruses can be subdivided into three types based on the serologic cross-reactivity of the internal NP.

Type A has been isolated from humans, animals, and birds; types B and C appear to infect only humans. In addition, type A and B influenza viruses are subdivided into strains based on antigenic differences in their HA and NA. There is a single strain of type C influenza virus.

Influenza in Humans

Influenza virus infections in humans are characterized by respiratory symptoms, fever, chills, headache, generalized muscle aches, and loss of appetite. The virus is restricted to the upper respiratory tract, where spread is facilitated by the ability of the viral NA to hydrolyze the mucoproteins lining the respiratory tract. The death and sloughing of ciliated epithelial cells may be responsible for many of the respiratory symptoms.

Although a patient can be very ill during the acute infection, an uneventful recovery after 3 to 7 days is the usual prognosis. However, the disease can take a more severe course, especially in persons older than 65 years of age and in individuals with other health problems, such as heart and lung disease or immunodeficiency. Deaths resulting from influenza are caused most frequently by pneumonia. Although cases occur in which the influenza virus is the sole etiologic agent of the pneumonia, secondary bacterial pneumonia is a much more frequent cause of death. As a result, it is difficult to obtain accurate statistics regarding the number of deaths directly attributable to an influenza epidemic. The most common bacterial invaders are staphylococci (causing toxic shock syndrome), followed by pneumococci, *Haemophilus influenzae,* and, somewhat less frequently, β-hemolytic streptococci.

REYE'S SYNDROME

Reye's syndrome is characterized by a severe encephalomyelitis and serious liver damage resulting in elevated blood ammonia values. It occurs exclusively in children (2 to 6 years of age) and has a mortality rate of 10% to

40%. The etiology of this syndrome is unknown, but it has been reported after infection by many different viruses. Clustered cases of Reye's syndrome have been seen frequently during influenza epidemics. The syndrome often has been associated with type B influenza virus infections, but, during the winter of 1978 to 1979, 85 cases were reported after infection by type A influenza virus. Studies have shown that the use of aspirin greatly enhances the incidence of Reye's syndrome, and the number of cases has declined with reduced use of these compounds in children.

EPIDEMIOLOGY

Epidemics of type A influenza occur every 2 or 3 years, whereas those caused by type B influenza virus usually are seen at 4- to 6-year intervals. In addition, type A influenza epidemics are more widespread, and the illnesses are more severe than those caused by type B influenza virus. Type C influenza virus produces a mild illness and has not been associated with epidemics.

Four major types of influenza virus HA have been defined using serologic methods: H0, H1, H2, and H3. Similarly, three major types of NA have been observed: N1, N2, and N8. Individuals having antibodies to one HA (ie, H1) are susceptible to infection by a virus bearing a different HA (ie, H2).

Recovery from influenza results in solid immunity to the infecting virus. Antibodies to the HA molecule neutralize viral infectivity and protect from infection, whereas antibodies to NA do not prevent infection, but help to limit the spread of virus. Major epidemics of influenza still arise because each succeeding epidemic is caused by a virus that is antigenically different from those that caused the earlier epidemics. Two different mechanisms contribute to the variability of the HA and NA that permit new epidemics to occur.

The first, termed *antigenic drift,* is caused by minor antigenic changes in the HA, the NA, or both (Fig. 48-3). Such changes result from mutations in the HA or the NA and enable the mutated virus to survive in a population that is immune to the original strain. Furthermore, there seems to be a finite possible number of such changes, so that with each succeeding influenza epidemic, the adult population acquires a greater immunity. This results in either a mild disease, inapparent infection, or complete resistance to the virus. Epidemics resulting from antigenic drift of the virus, therefore, are more likely to cause disease in children and young adults.

The second mechanism, termed *antigenic shift,* results in a major change in the antigenic nature of either the HA, the NA, or both. This type of major alteration occurs only in type A influenza virus, and it is viruses of this serotype that can cause devastating pandemics.

Seroarcheologic studies (ie, studies using serum from individuals who lived during the major pandemics of the

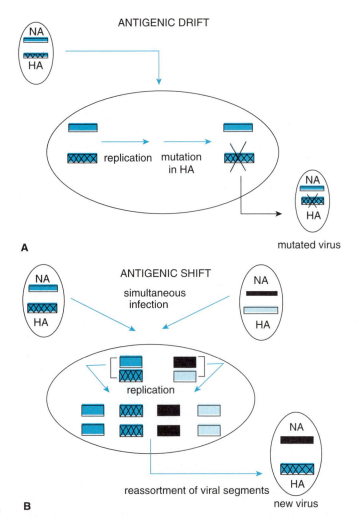

FIGURE 48-3 Antigenic drift and antigenic shift in influenza virus infections. **A.** Antigenic drift due to mutations in the HA gene. Open boxes denote the RNA segments encoding the NA protein; hatched boxes denote the RNA segments encoding the HA protein. The "X" denotes a mutation in the HA coding sequence that gives rise to an amino acid alteration in the HA protein. **B.** Antigenic shift due to the simultaneous replication of two genetically distinct influenza viruses. The individual virus segments encoding HA and NA from two different influenza viruses are denoted by the open, filled, and hatched boxes, respectively. The formation of a "new" influenza virus is depicted by the presence of a new complement of HA and NA genes, neither of which was present in the original infecting viruses.

late 1800s and early 1900s) have revealed an interesting ebb and flow of influenza viruses (Fig. 48-4). The epidemic of 1889 to 1890 was caused by a virus bearing an H2 HA subtype and an N8 NA subtype. A new virus (H3N8) appeared around 1900, and was supplanted in 1918 by a particularly virulent virus that was different from the previous viruses (H1N1, known as the Spanish strain). Interestingly, in 1957, a virus containing the H2 HA reappeared (H2N2, known as the Asian strain), followed in 1968 by yet another virus (H3N2, known as Hong Kong). In 1977, an H1N1 virus reappeared.

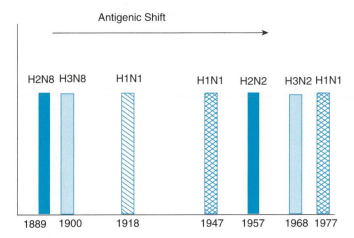

Antigenic Shift →

H2N8 H3N8   H1N1   H1N1 H2N2 H3N2 H1N1

1889 1900   1918   1947 1957 1968 1977

FIGURE 48-4 Appearance of new influenza viruses. The individual bars denote the antigenic composition of viruses that appeared in the designated years. Note the recent reappearance of antigenically distinct viruses.

The major changes in HA and NA result from reassortment of genetic information among avian, animal, and human strains of type A influenza viruses (see Fig. 48-3). Two major factors contribute to the exchange of genetic information. First, type A influenza viruses are found naturally in birds, animals, and humans. Second, the segmented nature of the influenza virus genome contributes to the observed high recombination frequency. Antigenic hybrids can readily be produced between avian and animal influenza viruses by the multiple infection of cell cultures with different viruses (see Fig. 48-3). Phylogenetic evidence suggests that new pandemic strains most commonly arise when human viruses acquire gene segments from avian viruses. Most major pandemics begin in China. Pigs in some areas of China have been shown to be infected with both avian and human viruses, and they may be the source of most of the new strains.

DIAGNOSIS

Although a presumptive diagnosis of influenza can be made on the basis of clinical evidence, especially during documented outbreaks, other viruses (respiratory syncytial virus [RSV], adenovirus, and parainfluenza) often produce similar clinical symptoms. Therefore, a positive diagnosis requires either isolation of the virus or demonstration of a rise in antibody titers after the acute illness. Rapid diagnosis of influenza virus infection can be accomplished using fluorescence-tagged antibodies to stain cells recovered from the nasopharynx. Alternatively, throat washings can be used to infect either Madin-Darby canine kidney cells or primate cell culture lines. Growth of the virus in these cells is detected by hemadsorption or reactivity with type-specific, fluorescence-labeled antibody to the virus. Inoculation of the amniotic membranes of 11- to 12-day-old fertilized chicken eggs is still used for the growth of suspected influenza virus strains and for the large-scale production of virus for laboratory studies and vaccines.

HA-inhibition assays using dilutions of patients' acute- and convalescent-phase sera with a known influenza virus are the easiest way to detect an antibody increase. However, sera first must be treated with trypsin or NA to destroy any glycoproteins that may nonspecifically inhibit hemagglutination. Complement-fixing antibodies also increase after an influenza infection. Those directed against the nucleocapsid have broad specificity, whereas those directed against the HA spike are type-specific. In general, these diagnostic strategies have more epidemiologic than clinical value.

CONTROL

The parenteral injection of formalin-inactivated influenza virus grown from chick embryos remains the major mechanism for controlling influenza. The efficacy of such vaccines has been the subject of much debate, and a general consensus is that even though such immunization does not always provide absolute protection, it at least modifies the disease. Maximum protection requires annual immunization with vaccines to the current and projected influenza strains; in the event of an antigenic shift and appearance of a new virus, these vaccines become ineffective. The development of protection against such influenza strains requires that each new virus be isolated, adapted to give high yields in chick embryos, and then grown in large amounts and dispensed for use in vaccines.

Current influenza vaccines are made from highly purified, egg-grown viruses that have been inactivated. Most vaccines administered in the United States have been chemically treated (so-called split-virus preparations) to reduce the incidence of febrile side effects in children. These vaccines usually contain three virus strains, two type A and one type B, representing viruses either circulating in the population or anticipated to be prevalent during the coming influenza season.

Forewarning of the appearance of new variants is essential, and World Health Organization surveillance teams are continually isolating and identifying current strains throughout the world. Present terminology of type A influenza virus strains designates the geographic area where the strain was first isolated, the year it was isolated, and the antigenic composition of its HA and NA. Thus, an HD3N2 strain isolated in Georgia in 1974 would be designated as $A/Georgia/74H_3N_2$, whereas a similar strain isolated in Texas in 1977 would be listed as $A/Texas/77H_3N_2$. As might be suspected, the isolation of a strain with a new antigenic makeup sets in motion the rapid production of a vaccine against the new strain.

A particularly dramatic example of this process occurred during the spring of 1976, when a swine-like strain of type A influenza virus (so-called "swine" flu) was isolated from a case of human influenza. Such a finding normally might not evoke much excitement among the medical community, but all available data indicated that it was similar to the influenza strain that caused the devastating influenza pandemic of 1918. The magnitude of this pandemic can be appreciated by examining some mortality statistics from 1918. The United States' death toll over a period of a few weeks is listed as 548,452 persons, more than 10 times the number killed during World War I (53,513). India put its toll at 12.5 million, and the Dutch East Indies at 800,000. Many villages throughout the world were virtually wiped out by this virus, and the final worldwide mortality was estimated to be 20 million people. It is likely that the severity of this pandemic was enhanced by the fact that it occurred right at the end of World War I. In addition, no antibiotics were available at that time, and many of the fatalities were caused by bacterial superinfections rather than by the virus itself. In spite of this, it was not surprising that the isolation of a similar influenza virus in 1976 evoked concern.

In April 1976, the United States government appropriated $135 million to produce sufficient vaccine to immunize all Americans against the swine flu virus, in spite of the fact that there was no evidence of the threat of a serious human epidemic caused by this virus. Immunization of the American population was begun by late September of 1976, and by mid-December, more than 35 million persons had received the swine flu vaccine. At that point, however, a disturbing problem came to light—some vaccinees experienced an ascending paralysis (known as Guillain-Barré syndrome) that began a few days after they received the swine influenza vaccine. Even though the incidence of the syndrome was low (about 1 in 100,000 recipients of the swine flu vaccine), the mass immunization program was halted because there was a possibility that factors present in the swine flu vaccine may have precipitated this disease. Fortunately, no recurrence of Guillain-Barré syndrome has been observed during the administration of subsequent influenza vaccines. It since has been shown that transmission of swine viruses to humans occurs frequently in the United States, but has never resulted in a human epidemic. Thus, it is unlikely that the swine flu was ever a serious threat.

The research aimed at future control of influenza epidemics involves several different approaches. Attenuated influenza virus strains, or so-called cold-adapted strains, have been isolated that retain their antigenicity but no longer cause overt disease. Such vaccines are used experimentally and are administered intranasally, resulting in the production of high levels of IgA and IgG antibodies. A concern regarding this approach is that vaccines for newly isolated strains might be difficult to produce in time to efficiently prevent new epidemics.

A second approach is based on the belief that even antigenic shifts are limited to a finite number of variations. This is supported, in part, by the observation that the pandemic from 1889 to 1890 was caused by a virus

thought to have the same HA (H2) as the Asian influenza pandemic of 1957; at that time, only persons 67 years or older possessed neutralizing antibody to the new H2 virus. Consequently, some laboratories are attempting to make new influenza strains by genetic reassortment. In this way, a high-yield laboratory strain would be immediately available for vaccine preparation as soon as a new variant appeared in nature.

In spite of the inadequacies of current vaccines, annual immunization is recommended for high-risk groups such as persons with diabetes and chronic heart or lung disorders, persons older than 65 years of age, and persons with suppressed immune systems. Vaccination also is recommended for health care workers and vital community personnel.

Chemical prophylaxis by 1-adamantan-amine hydrochloride (amantadine), a drug that inhibits viral uncoating, appears to be effective in preventing influenza. However, most individuals are reluctant to obtain a prescription, purchase the drug, and take it daily during the period of an epidemic. This factor, coupled with reports of the side effects of the drug, has hindered its extensive use. Nonetheless, amantadine is recommended for at-risk persons, unvaccinated high-risk persons, immunodeficient persons, and persons for whom the influenza vaccine is contraindicated.

PARAMYXOVIRIDAE

Classification

The family Paramyxoviridae is made up of three genera: *Paramyxovirus, Morbillivirus,* and *Pneumovirus.* Members of the genus *Paramyxovirus* include five human parainfluenza viruses and mumps virus. *Morbillivirus* includes measles virus and two important animal pathogens: canine distemper and rinderpest virus of cattle. *Pneumovirus* includes RSV, a human respiratory virus.

Most of the paramyxoviruses possess properties that outwardly resemble the more obvious characteristics of the orthomyxoviruses (see Table 48-1), the most notable of which are the ability to adsorb to neuraminic acid–containing glycoproteins (causing hemagglutination), the presence of NA activity associated with the glycoproteins present in their lipid envelopes, and a unique fusion protein that enables the viruses to fuse cells to form large syncytia. However, their structure, mode of replication, and even the types of infections they cause differ markedly from those of the influenza viruses (Table 48-2).

Structure and Replication

Paramyxoviruses contain a single piece of single-stranded negative-sense RNA (about 15,000 nucleotides), and they exhibit helical symmetry within the RNP core. The

TABLE 48-2
Properties of Human Paramyxoviruses

Virus	Serotypes	Fusion Protein	Hemagglutinin	Neuraminidase	Clinical Features (Complications)
Mumps	1	+	+	+	Parotitis (orchitis, meningitis, encephalitis)
Measles	1	+	+	−	Rash (encephalitis)
Parainfluenza	5*	+	+	+	Croup, pneumonia, bronchiolitis†
Respiratory syncytial	2	+	−	−	Bronchiolitis, pneumonia, croup†

* Four serotypes found predominantly in humans, type 5 in monkeys.

† Listed in order of relative frequency of occurrence.

RNP is enclosed in a protein coat, and this entire structure is surrounded by a lipid bilayer membrane containing numerous spikes (Fig. 48-5). Thus, the overall structure is similar to that of the influenza viruses but differs in the following properties: (1) the nucleic acid exists as a single piece of RNA; (2) the diameter of the enveloped virions is about twice that of the orthomyxoviruses, and there tends to be greater pleomorphism (more varied forms), with the frequent formation of filamentous forms; (3) HA and NA activity both reside on the same glycoprotein (hemagglutinin-neuraminidase [HN]), whereas the fusion protein (F) is a separate second envelope protein; and (4) replication takes place in the cytoplasm of the host cell. It is important to note that morbilliviruses (eg, measles) and pneumoviruses (eg, RSV) do not possess an NA.

Adsorption, penetration, and uncoating of paramyxoviruses are not completely understood; however, those possessing an HA and an NA appear to bind to neuraminic acid–containing glycoprotein receptor sites on the cell surface in a manner similar to that described for the influenza virus. Penetration requires the action of the virion-associated fusion protein. The virus nucleocapsid is released into the cytoplasm after a direct fusion at the plasma membrane. As with the influenza virus HA, the fusion protein must be activated during virus maturation through specific cleavage by a host-cell protease. Cells lacking such proteases produce only noninfectious virus.

Transcription of the negative-strand viral genome into mRNA occurs in the cytoplasm and is catalyzed by a viral polymerase present in the virus particle. Thus, like the influenza viruses, the paramyxoviruses carry their genetic information on negative strands of single-stranded RNA, which must be transcribed into mRNA before viral protein synthesis begins. However, unlike influenza viruses, there is no requirement for host-cell RNA primers. Although the viral RNA exists as a single molecule, multiple mRNAs are found in the cytoplasm

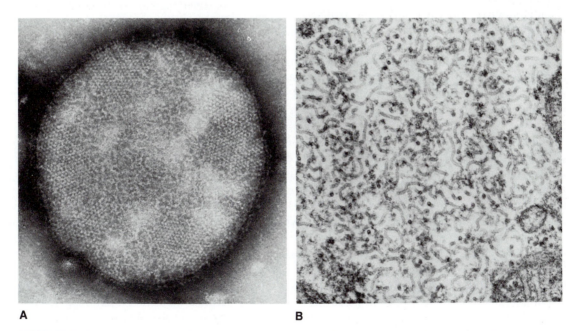

A　　　**B**

FIGURE 48-5 **A.** Electron micrograph of parainfluenza virus type 4A. (Original magnification ×116,800.)
B. Portions of a paramyxovirus inclusion body consisting of nucleocapsids. (Original magnification ×58,400.)

of infected cells. Each of these mRNAs encodes a single viral protein (an exception has been noted for the mRNA encoding the P protein of Sendai virus; this mRNA contains a second gene sequence embedded within the P coding sequence). All paramyxovirus mRNAs are capped at the 5′ terminus and polyadenylated at the 3′ end, just like cellular mRNAs. Evidence suggests that transcription of viral mRNA commences at a unique site at the 3′ end of the template viral genome, at which point individual mRNAs are generated by a stop–start mechanism that allows for the capping and addition of poly A at specific sites along the transcript.

Replication of viral RNA is catalyzed by the virus-encoded polymerase (L protein) and requires first the synthesis of complete positive-strand copies of the virion RNA. These copies then are used as templates for the production of viral progeny RNAs. NPs are synthesized in large excess, and most are assembled into empty capsids that give rise to cytoplasmic inclusion bodies. The NPs bind to newly synthesized viral RNA, after which the resulting RNP complexes migrate to areas of the host-cell membrane where viral envelope proteins have replaced cell proteins. The arrival of the nucleoprotein at the cell membrane is followed quickly by the appearance of the glycoprotein spikes in the lipid bilayer of the host cell. The nucleocapsid then is enclosed by a lipid membrane containing the glycoprotein spikes, and the virion is released by budding from the host cell.

The fate of the host cell varies considerably, depending on both the particular virus involved and the type of cell infected. However, two general properties of paramyxovirus infections deserve emphasis. First, many paramyxoviruses cause adjacent host cells to fuse into multinucleate giant cells. This fusion is mediated by interactions between the viral glycoproteins and receptors in the membrane of the cells. Thus, infected cells can fuse with all the surrounding uninfected cells. This process eventually results in the death of the cell. Paramyxovirus glycoproteins have been used extensively as a laboratory tool to cause the fusion of cells of different origin for genetic studies of the resulting hybrid cells. Second, essentially all the paramyxoviruses have been shown to establish persistent infections in cultured cells. These infections can result in the production of small amounts of virus, or they can be manifested only by the intracellular presence of viral antigens. Still, the fact that such persistently infected cells can continue to survive indefinitely has broad implications in human and animal infections. Measles virus is the only human paramyxovirus for which it has been shown that a persistent infection can cause severe disease. This disease is a deadly neurologic condition known as subacute sclerosing panencephalitis (SSPE) that occurs rarely after measles. However, indirect evidence has suggested the possible role of paramyxoviruses in other chronic diseases, such as multiple sclerosis, lupus erythematosus, and polymyositis.

Paramyxovirus Infections in Humans

PARAINFLUENZA VIRUS

Although there are five serologic types of parainfluenza viruses, type 5 usually is referred to as simian virus 5 (SV5) because it originally was isolated from monkey kidney cells.

All parainfluenza viruses produce upper respiratory tract infections in adults, although illnesses caused by type 4 parainfluenza virus usually cause no symptoms. Types 1 and 2 parainfluenza virus, and, to a lesser extent, type 3 parainfluenza virus, cause infections in adults that would be diagnosed clinically as common colds. In infants and children, these viruses can invade the lower respiratory tract, causing pneumonia. Types 1 and 2 parainfluenza virus seem to be particularly frequent invaders of the larynx in infants, causing a sometimes deadly syndrome called laryngotracheobronchitis, or croup (see Table 48-2).

All parainfluenza virus types can be grown in human or monkey cell cultures, but they usually produce few cytopathic changes. Infected areas can be recognized by hemadsorption or by the use of specific immunofluorescent antibody. Antibody levels can be determined by hemagglutination inhibition or by complement fixation, but the mere presence of antibody is not diagnostic because of the widespread occurrence of these viruses.

Inactivated vaccines have been used against parainfluenza viruses, but the stimulated IgG response is not protective. Living attenuated vaccines to be administered intranasally are being developed and, if successful, may be of value in preventing the serious lower respiratory tract disease caused by these viruses in infants and young children. Because immunity to reinfection is not solid, attenuated vaccines do not seem practical for adult use.

MUMPS

The familiar clinical picture of mumps hardly needs description. Infection of the parotid glands produces inflammation, with marked swelling behind the ears and difficulty in swallowing.

The mumps virus is transmitted through respiratory tract secretions; it multiplies in the upper respiratory tract and in the local lymph nodes. The virus then enters the bloodstream, and viremia results in spread of the virus throughout the body. Most commonly, the major manifestation is the painful swelling of one or both parotid glands, occurring 18 to 21 days after exposure. In addition, infection can develop in the meninges, pancreas, ovaries, testes, or heart. Of these, the most feared complication is infection of the testes (orchitis), which occurs in 20% of 30% of infected boys who have reached puberty. This complication is extremely painful, primarily because the lining surrounding the testes does not allow the inflamed organs to swell. As a result, the disease occasionally causes sterility. Infection of the ovaries also can occur, but because swelling is not prevented, it is not as painful. In addition, aseptic meningitis is a frequent, although usually not severe, complication. Postinfection encephalitis or encephalomyelitis is a more severe, but less common, manifestation of central nervous system infection, occurring in 1 to 2 per 1000 cases of mumps infection. This disease is caused by damage resulting from immune responses to the virus.

A diagnosis of mumps is made most frequently by observing the characteristic clinical picture. Virus can be detected in cell cultures using either immunofluorescent antibodies or hemadsorption of chicken or guinea pig erythrocytes. In either case, a positive identification can be completed by demonstrating hemagglutination inhibition with a known antiserum to the virus.

Mumps is not nearly as contagious as many of the other childhood diseases, and it is common for persons to reach adulthood and still be completely susceptible to infection by mumps virus.

After recovery, a patient develops antibodies to both the NP and the HA surface antigen. Antibodies induced by the HA are protective, but, even though immunity is lifelong, detection of these antibodies several years after recovery may not be possible.

Because there is only one antigenic type of mumps virus, a live attenuated vaccine grown in chick embryos has been widely used since 1967, and the incidence of mumps has declined steadily since then, with the fewest cases being reported in 1985 (2982 cases). It appears that at least 95% of susceptible persons develop adequate antibody titers as a result of vaccine administration. Although the duration of the vaccine-induced immunity is not known, it appears to be long term. From 1967 to 1987, more than 82.3 million doses of live mumps virus vaccine were administered in the United States. The major objective of the current vaccine strategy is to achieve and maintain high immunization levels among infants and young children. The vaccine is given as a part of the trivalent measles-mumps-rubella vaccine. Recent increases in the number of mumps cases (7790 in 1986, 12,848 in 1987, and 12,299 in 1988) do not appear to be caused by waning immunity in persons previously vaccinated, but likely reflect an underimmunized group of children born between 1967 and 1977. Enforcement of comprehensive mumps immunization school entry laws appears to reduce the number of children in this underimmunized group.

MORBILLIVIRUS: MEASLES

Measles virus is morphologically similar to other paramyxoviruses and possesses an HA that causes weak agglutination of monkey erythrocytes. In contrast to members of the genus *Paramyxovirus,* measles virus does not contain an NA (see Table 48-2).

Although measles, a previously common childhood disease, is now rare in the United States (2900 cases in 1988) due to a comprehensive vaccination program, measles virus is responsible for about 2 million deaths worldwide. Most of these deaths occur in undeveloped countries where immunization is unavailable and malnutrition is rampant.

Measles (rubeola, or morbilli) is a sometimes severe, acute, highly contagious disease spread by respiratory secretions that can occur in epidemics every 2 to 3 years in unimmunized populations. Humans are the only normal reservoir of the virus, although exposed monkeys readily develop the disease.

The virus multiplies in the upper respiratory tract and conjunctiva during the early phase of the incubation period. Late in the incubation period, the virus enters the bloodstream (viremia) and is transported to all parts of the body. The disease frequently is severe, with high fever (often leading to convulsions), delirium, cough, and photophobia. It usually is accompanied by severe conjunctivitis and a rash over the entire body. In immunosuppressed individuals and in children with congenital defects in cell-mediated immunity, measles takes an especially serious, often fatal, course.

As a result of the spread of the virus throughout the cells of the body, complications are common. As in influenza, secondary infections causing pneumonia and ear infections frequently are the result of bacterial invaders. By far the most feared complication is encephalitis, which can cause permanent neurologic injury and even death. Although encephalitis is relatively rare, it does follow about 1 of 1000 cases of measles. In such cases, symptoms of encephalitis appear about 3 to 5 days after recovery from the acute illness and include seizures, confusion, and coma. The observed demyelination seems to be due to an autoimmune reaction triggered by the virus. The mortality rate in such cases approaches 25%. SSPE is a late and extremely rare, but always fatal, complication of measles. It is a slowly progressing neurologic disease that starts an average of 6 to 8 years after a primary infection. In most cases, the primary infection occurred before 2 years of age. SSPE usually leads to death within 1 to 2 years.

The incubation period of measles is uniform, with the first symptoms of fever, cough, headache, sore throat, and conjunctivitis beginning 11 days after exposure; the rash appears 3 days later. Infected persons secrete virus from their respiratory tracts and conjunctiva and in their urine from about 3 days before to about 5 days after the appearance of the rash. Measles is one of the most contagious of all infectious diseases.

A diagnosis of measles almost always is made on clinical grounds. An early diagnosis frequently can be made by observing Koplik spots (small bluish yellow spots), which occur in the mouth on the buccal mucosa 2 or 3 days before the rash appears. In addition, the virus can

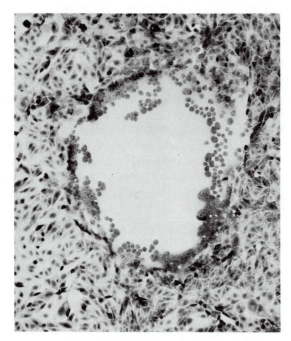

FIGURE 48-6 Giant cell formed of fused Vero cells in culture 48 hours after infection with measles virus. (Original magnification ×70.)

be obtained from specimens taken from respiratory tract secretions and grown in tissue cultures of many primary or continuous cell lines. Virus can be detected by the hemadsorption of infected cells with chicken erythrocytes or by immunofluorescence with labeled antibodies.

The presence of giant cells in nasal secretions, resulting from the ability of measles virus to cause cell fusion of infected cells, also is characteristic of measles (Fig. 48-6). Serologic tests can be carried out for neutralizing and complement-fixing antibodies.

There is only one antigenic type of measles virus, and recovery from the disease imparts lifelong immunity.

Isolation of persons who have measles has not been an effective control measure because these individuals are infective several days before the appearance of the rash and usually are unaware of their infection. Antibodies to measles virus pass through the placenta and protect infants for about the first 6 months of life.

Because measles can be a severe disease with grave complications, much effort has been expended in developing an effective vaccine. The first attenuated vaccines were developed in 1962 by John Enders after passage of the virus through human kidney cells, human amnion cells, and, finally, chick embryo tissue culture. Newer attenuated vaccines produce few side effects and induce immunity in over 95% of recipients. The vaccine usually is given at 9 to 15 months of age. Mass immunization has reduced the incidence of measles in the United States by about 90%. In 1983, a record low of 1497 measles cases was reported. Recent increases in the incidence of measles have occurred in unimmunized, indigent, inner

city children, often from families of immigrants or illegal aliens. In addition, a smaller, but significant, number of cases have appeared in populations of well-immunized individuals, mainly high school and college students. The appearance of measles within this latter group has prompted concern regarding the possibility of vaccine failure among a small (5%) group of vaccine recipients. Such outbreaks on college campuses are of particular concern, because measles is a more serious disease among adults than among schoolchildren.

RESPIRATORY SYNCYTIAL VIRUS

Respiratory syncytial virus is structurally similar to other members of the Paramyxoviridae family. The name for this virus derives from the fact that RSV causes serious respiratory tract infections in young children and induces a characteristic fusion of infected cells leading to the appearance of giant multinucleated cells. The two serotypes of RSV resemble other members of the paramyxovirus family in that the envelope contains a membrane fusion (F) protein responsible for the fusigenic properties of the virus (see Table 48-2). However, RSV lacks both HA and NA activity, prompting its assignment to a separate genus, *Pneumovirus*. RSV contains a second envelope protein (G) that binds to host cell receptors but lacks hemagglutinating activity.

RSV is the single most frequent cause of serious respiratory disease in very young children. RSV infecting infants younger than 6 months of age frequently results in lower respiratory tract infections, causing pneumonia or bronchiolitis. The virus has been proposed to be a frequent cause of sudden infant death syndrome. RSV is widespread, as evidenced by the fact that 95% of children possess antibodies to it by the age of 5 years. Outbreaks occur annually, usually in the winter and spring, accounting for a rise in the number of young children with lower respiratory tract infections. It is common for both serotypes of RSV to circulate within a population simultaneously. RSV infections are highly contagious, and nosocomial infections of both hospital personnel and hospitalized children are common. The virus is believed to be spread throughout the hospital in large part by infected hospital staff. RSV infection is a particular hazard for premature infants, infants with congenital heart or lung disease, and immunodeficient infants and children.

Infection does not result in lasting immunity, and older children and adults can be reinfected. However, unlike primary infections, reinfections usually do not involve the lower respiratory tract. Instead, such infections are manifested as upper respiratory tract disease and normally are diagnosed as bad colds.

The relationship between the severity of an RSV infection and the age of the patient seems paradoxic, because severe disease is seen in infants, who often possess circulating maternal antibodies to RSV. Furthermore, in a clinical trial in which inactivated virus was injected into infants in an attempt to immunize them to RSV, infants who received the vaccine had more serious infections during a subsequent RSV epidemic than did nonimmunized control subjects.

These early observations led to speculation that serum antibodies may play a direct role in the severity of RSV disease. It is now clear from several studies that although there may be an immunologic component to the pathogenesis of RSV bronchiolitis and pneumonia, the predominant cause of pathology is the severe cytopathic effect of the virus infection. The role of virus-induced antibody in the prevention of and recovery from infection remains controversial. Immunity is only partially effective, as evidenced by infection of small infants having circulating maternal antibodies and reinfection of older infants, sometimes within weeks of recovery from a primary infection. Both serum and secretory antibodies appear to play a major, albeit incomplete, role in protection. Local immunity (presence of IgA) appears to be one of the most important aspects of protection from upper respiratory tract infection, whereas serum antibodies play a major role in resistance to infection in the lower respiratory tract. Impaired IgA and IgG immune responses to RSV infection seem to be common manifestations of RSV infection in early infancy. Although the exact reasons for this unresponsiveness are not known, it has been speculated that immunologic immaturity and immunologic suppression may be contributing factors.

As mentioned earlier, previous attempts to use formalin-inactivated virus vaccine met with failure. These preparations failed to provide protective immunity, and actually enhanced disease during subsequent infection by RSV. Experiments since have shown that the enhanced immunopathogenicity elicited by the formalin-inactivated vaccine was caused by the selective action of formalin on certain neutralizing epitopes present on the G and F proteins of the virus. Neither live virus nor heat-inactivated virus produces a similar effect. Immunization with formalin-inactivated virus preparations results in an unbalanced immune response and the production of antibodies to a large number of nonneutralizing epitopes. On subsequent infection with RSV, these antibodies fail to halt virus spread, and in the face of continued virus production, the formation of immune complexes results in complement fixation, tissue destruction, and inflammation.

The development of vaccines for RSV poses several challenging problems, foremost of which is the task of inducing an effective immune response in young infants with immature immunologic systems. Nonetheless, new approaches using recombinant DNA techniques to produce viral protein components such as purified F and G proteins hold out the possibility that new and innovative strategies for immunization will be available soon.

Laboratory diagnosis of RSV infections can be made by direct isolation of the virus after inoculation of human cell cultures with nasal and pharyngeal secretions. Alternately, viral antigens can be detected in nasopharyngeal washings by enzyme-linked immunosorbent assay techniques, by indirect immunofluorescence in exfoliated cells, or by demonstration of a rise in serum antibodies during recovery from infection.

Bibliography

JOURNALS

Barrett T. The molecular biology of the Morbillivirus (measles) group. Biochem Soc Symp 1988;53:25.

Klenk H-D, Rott R. The molecular biology of influenza virus pathogenicity. Adv Virus Res 1988;34:247.

Welliver RC. Detection, pathogenesis, and therapy of respiratory syncytial virus infections. Clin Microbiol Rev 1988;1:27.

Welliver RC, Ogra PL. Immunology of respiratory viral infection. Annu Rev Med 1988;39:147.

BOOKS

Chanock RM, McIntosh K. Parainfluenza viruses. In: Fields BN, Knipe DM, eds. Virology, ed 2. New York, Raven Press, 1990:963.

Kingsbury DW. Orthomyxoviridae and their replication. In: Fields BN, Knipe DM, eds. Virology, ed 2. New York, Raven Press, 1990:1075.

Kingsbury DW, ed. The paramyxoviruses. New York, Plenum Press, 1991.

Murphy BR, Webster RG. Orthomyxoviruses. In: Fields BN, Knipe DM, eds. Virology, ed 2. New York, Raven Press, 1990:1091.

Norrby E, Oxman MN. Measles virus. In: Fields BN, Knipe DM, eds. Virology, ed 2. New York, Raven Press, 1990:1013.

Wolinsky JS, Waxham MN. Mumps virus. In: Fields BN, Knipe DM, eds. Virology, ed 2. New York, Raven Press, 1990:989.

Essentials of Medical Microbiology, Fifth Edition, edited by Wesley A. Volk, Bryan M. Gebhardt, Marie-Louise Hammarskjöld, and Robert J. Kadner. Lippincott-Raven Publishers, Philadelphia © 1996.

Chapter 49

Rhabdoviridae, Filoviridae, Arenaviridae, Reoviridae, and Slow Virus Diseases

RHABDOVIRIDAE

Rhabdoviruses form a large family of agents that infect both animals and plants. The assignment of a virus to this family has in the past been based primarily on the structure of the virion: all rhabdoviruses are rod shaped or bullet shaped (Fig. 49-1). Biochemical studies have supported this classification by demonstrating the extensive similarities of these viruses in spite of the diversity of the hosts they infect. Rabies virus is the only agent of this group that normally infects humans, although laboratory infections with vesicular stomatitis virus (VSV), a pathogen of cattle, have occasionally occurred. This section deals only with rabies virus infections, but as far as is known, the general structure and mode of replication for all rhabdoviruses are similar.

Structure and Replication

The rhabdoviruses differ in shape from the paramyxoviruses, but they are similar in the helical symmetry of their virion RNA and in their mode of replication. Infection is initiated when the envelope glycoproteins of the virion attach to specific host-cell receptors. Removal of the viral glycoprotein with trypsin causes a marked decrease in infectivity, presumably because the virus can no longer attach to the host cell. Fusion of the viral envelope with the host-cell membrane results in the liberation of the nucleocapsid into the host-cell cytoplasm. The nucleocapsid contains one molecule of single-stranded RNA of a negative-strand polarity. The initial events in replication involve two steps: (1) the synthesis of positive-strand RNAs to serve as mRNAs for viral protein synthesis; and (2) the synthesis of a genome-length RNA to serve as a template for progeny RNA synthesis. Both of these processes are carried out in the cytoplasm by a viral-

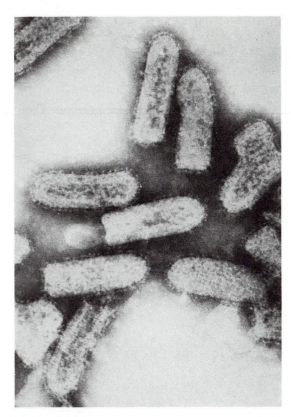

FIGURE 49-1 Virions of vesicular stomatitis virus, a typical rhabdovirus that infects animals. Notice the external spikes protruding from virion membranes and striations within the core resulting from spirally wound RNA within the nucleoprotein.

encoded transcriptase, which is a component of the infectious virus particle. VSV has proved to be an excellent model for the study of rhabdovirus replication. The basic steps of VSV replication are summarized in Figure 49-2.

Assembly of virions occurs at specific sites on the host-cell membrane where viral glycoproteins have been inserted into the membrane, replacing host-cell membrane proteins. Release of virus occurs as the completed virion buds from the cell membrane.

Rabies virus replication differs from that of most other rhabdoviruses in that infected cells develop characteristic cytoplasmic inclusion bodies, which have been given the name *Negri bodies* (Fig. 49-3). Some disagreement concerning the origin or function of the Negri bodies exists, but it seems likely that they are the site of virus replication or accumulation of viral antigens.

Rabies

Few diseases can induce the psychologic terror caused by the bite of a "mad" dog. The scope of this fear is indicated by the fact that each year in the United States about 35,000 persons receive treatment for potential rabies after dog bites. Fortunately, the development of the disease is unlikely in any single case, because effective postexposure immunization procedures are available and vaccination programs have virtually eliminated rabies in domestic dogs and cats in the United States. However, wildlife rabies continues to be a major reservoir for the virus and constitutes a source of exposure for humans and nonimmune dogs and cats.

PATHOGENESIS AND EPIDEMIOLOGY

Rabies infections are almost always acquired from the bite of a rabid animal, although reports show that animals and humans frequenting caves inhabited by rabid bats have contracted rabies by the respiratory route. The most unusual feature of rabies is the long and variable incubation period after infection, before the appearance of overt symptoms. These periods vary from 13 days to 9 months, but the average incubation period is about 30 days. Several factors influence the incubation period, the route by which the virus reaches the brain, and the mechanism by which the virus infects the salivary glands of the rabid animal. Experimental observations reveal that the length of the incubation period is determined by the severity of the lacerations from the bite, the amount of virus introduced at the site of the wound, and the distance the virus must travel in the body to reach the brain. Thus, head and face wounds usually result in a shorter incubation period than wounds on the extremities, feet, and hands.

After introduction into a wound, the virus may remain at the site of injection for 1 to 4 days, after which it seems to progress along nerve paths to the central nervous system (CNS). Once in the CNS, it produces an encephalitis that is usually fatal. Experimental evidence supports the possibility of virus dissemination by way of both the bloodstream and nerve paths. The exact mechanism whereby the salivary glands become infected also is unknown, but such infections likely occur from the centrifugal spread of the virus by way of nerve paths or as a result of viremia.

Initial symptoms of headache, nausea, sore throat, and sensitivity around the original wound site are followed by a period of excitation and nervousness. During this stage, the person has great difficulty in swallowing, and even the sight of liquid may induce painful contractions of the throat muscles. This stage is followed by convulsions, coma, and death.

Rabies virus is capable of infecting all warm-blooded animals, and wild mammals are a major reservoir for the virus worldwide. Interestingly, the type of animal most frequently involved varies from one part of the world to another. This may represent a strain-dependent tropism of the virus for different animal species. Skunks, foxes, coyotes, and raccoons are common sources in North America. Dogs and cats, which may become infected by a wild animal, particularly in rural areas, constitute a dan-

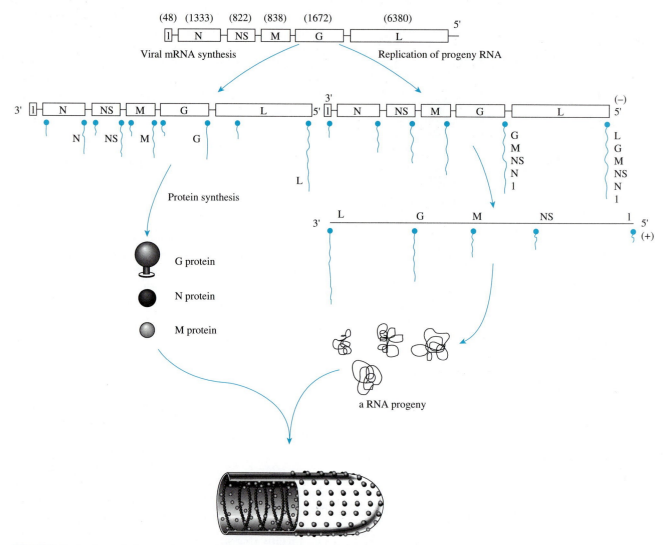

FIGURE 49-2   A schematic diagram depicting the replication of vesicular stomatitis virus (VSV). The VSV genome encodes five viral proteins: N, the major nucleocapsid protein; NS, a nonstructural protein of unknown function; M, the matrix protein; G, the envelope glycoprotein; and L, the viral transcriptase. Two pathways of synthesis are shown, one indicating the synthesis of viral proteins and a second indicating the pathway of viral RNA replication. Virus maturation takes place in the cytoplasm, resulting in the assembly of mature virus particles.

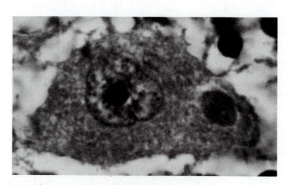

FIGURE 49-3   An oval Negri body is seen to the right of the nucleus in a brain cell from a case of rabies in a human.

gerous source of infection for humans. Over 4500 cases of animal rabies per year were reported to the Centers for Disease Control in 1988, with most cases occurring in wild animals (skunks, raccoons, and bats), and only a small proportion occurring in domestic animals. Human rabies is rare: only one case has been reported since 1985.

Both vampire and insectivorous bats make up an exceedingly dangerous reservoir for rabies virus, inasmuch as it seems that these animals may be asymptomatic carriers of the virus for many months. In Latin America, more than 150 cases of human rabies have been attributed to bat bites over the last few years, and it is estimated that vampire bats cause the death of 500,000 to 1 million head of cattle each year.

DIAGNOSIS AND CONTROL

The major criterion for a laboratory diagnosis of rabies is the presence of the characteristic Negri bodies in the cytoplasm of infected brain cells (see Fig. 49-3). In addition, a suspension of infected brain or salivary gland cells can be injected intracerebrally into mice; after paralysis of the mice, their brains can be examined for the presence of Negri bodies. Detection of virus with fluorescent-labeled antibody to rabies virus also is an effective means of identifying Negri bodies in infected cells. This technique is much more sensitive than the older method of staining for Negri bodies and is preferred in most laboratories. Diagnosis can sometimes be made using fluorescent antibodies to detect Negri bodies in skin biopsy specimens, usually from the buccal mucosa or nape of the neck.

Rabies control in the United States is primarily directed toward the prevention of rabies in domestic dogs and cats. This is accomplished by mandatory vaccination of all dogs, using a living attenuated virus (Flury LEP) that has been adapted to grow in chick embryos. Vaccinated animals can become mildly ill, but the resulting immunity is effective for about 3 years. Control in wild animals is more difficult; however, limited trials are underway in Switzerland and Germany using live oral vaccines contained in animal bait. The number of rabies cases in animals reported annually in the United States undoubtedly represents only a small fraction of actual infections present in the animal population, and control of rabies infections in humans requires constant surveillance and immunization of domestic animals against infection.

TREATMENT

Although there is one documented case of recovery from overt rabies in humans, the disease still can be considered essentially 100% fatal. Thus, treatment is designed to induce an effective immune response in a potentially infected person during the long incubation period of the disease. This approach was employed by Pasteur in 1885 when he injected a young boy, bitten by a rabid dog, with ground-up spinal cords of rabies-infected rabbits. The infected spinal cords had been dried for various lengths of time to partially inactivate the virus. This somewhat altered rabies virus was called "fixed" virus to differentiate it from the wild-type strain, which Pasteur referred to as "street" virus. The viral vaccines used today are somewhat different from that used in 1885, but the principle is the same. Vaccines used during the last decades have consisted of either a phenol-inactivated virus grown in rabbit brain or a β-propiolactone-inactivated virus grown in duck embryos. The vaccine grown in rabbit brains induced a better immunologic response, but because of the presence of brain tissue in the vaccine, a small percentage of treated persons developed a severe and often fatal encephalitis. The rabies vaccine licensed for

use in the United States consists of killed rabies virus that has been grown in human diploid cells. This vaccine provides complete protection after only five injections, and because the vaccine contains essentially no extraneous foreign proteins, allergic reactions seldom occur. Another promising experimental rabies vaccine consists of only the glycoprotein isolated from rabies virus grown in human diploid cells.

An unprovoked bite by a wild animal, bat, or dog must be considered a potential exposure to rabies. If the animal can be apprehended, it should be confined for observation. If no symptoms develop in the animal during the subsequent 10 days, there is no danger of rabies from the bite. If the animal is destroyed immediately after the bite, the rabies virus should be assayed either by examining the brain for the presence of Negri bodies or by injecting brain suspensions intracerebrally into mice.

FILOVIRIDAE

MARBURG-EBOLA VIRUS

Marburg and Ebola viruses represent two agents that at first seemed to be similar to rhabdoviruses. However, these viruses are considered unique based on their structure, antigenic composition, and disease spectrum. Marburg virus was first identified in 1967 in Marburg, Germany, where 25 primary and 6 secondary cases of hemorrhagic fever were reported, resulting in seven deaths. All of the primary cases were laboratory workers who had contact with monkeys shipped from Uganda. In 1976, an antigenically distinct but morphologically similar virus was isolated from patients experiencing a hemorrhagic fever outbreak in southern Sudan and northeastern Zaire. This virus, designated Ebola virus (for the region in Zaire), was seen again in Zaire in 1977 to 1978. The epidemiology of virus infection is not well understood, although transmission within outbreaks seems to come from close personal contact. Clinically, Marburg-Ebola virus infections begin with fever, headaches, nausea, vomiting, and diarrhea. Five to 7 days later, severe bleeding begins, mostly within the gastrointestinal tract, with shock and death often following. In locations lacking adequate medical facilities, these viruses cause a disease with virtually a 100% fatality. The availability of modern treatment facilities, however, reduces the fatality rate to about 20%.

ARENAVIRIDAE

The establishment of the Arenaviridae as a taxonomic group was based primarily on the morphologic features and the grainy appearance of the virions when viewed in

A Closer Look

The level of sophistication at which we have arrived in molecular biology could lull us into a state of complacency insofar as new diseases or infections are concerned. But, we would soon find out that this is a mistake. For example, it is only a little over a decade ago since the virus causing AIDS was isolated, and even more recently, did the "flesh-eating" *streptococci* come to the fore.

In 1995 another emerging human disease brought panic to parts of Africa. This disease, caused by Ebola virus, was known to infect monkeys, but human infections were rare and occurred primarily in rural areas where human to human spread did not readily happen. Not so for the 1995 epidemic which was first reported in Kikwit, Zaire, a city of about 600,000 people.

What do we know about this infection and why is it so feared? The infection, known as hemorrhagic fever, has about a 90% mortality rate. Its symptoms include fever, vomiting, destruction of internal organs, and bleeding from the eyes, nose, and other orifices. Fortunately, Ebola virus is not spread as a respiratory disease. Thus, person to person spread occurs through an exchange of body fluids and many of the cases in Zaire took place in hospitals among patients and health care workers. Medical personnel are most likely to become infected from exposure to blood occurring during bleeding in the late stages of the disease.

What can be done to halt the epidemic that has infected hundreds of individuals in Zaire? There is no vaccine nor is there any cure. Better sanitary conditions will undoubtedly help to halt its spread. The major fear, however, is that the virus will spread to other large cities in Africa or even to other parts of the world. To this end, the entire city of Kikwit was quarantined by Zairian solders who prevented anyone from entering or leaving the city. In spite of these measures, the disease was reported to be present in several additional villages.

Where do we go from here? Scientists are searching for the natural reservoir of Ebola virus as well as a closely related hemorrhagic fever virus known as Marburg virus. But, until more is learned about these viruses, preventive measures are difficult to carry out.

---

thin sections with the electron microscope (*arenosus* is Latin for sandy; Fig. 49-4).

Arenaviruses comprise a group of 14 serologically distinct viruses, of which four cause severe disease in humans. These viruses are characterized by their lifelong persistence in rodent populations and their occasional transmission to humans. One member of this family, Lassa fever virus, gained notoriety after causing severe and fatal infections of nurses and, subsequently, laboratory workers after an outbreak of Lassa fever in northeastern Nigeria in 1969.

Structure and Replication

The arenavirus particles are pleomorphic, varying in diameter from 60 to 350 nm. The replication cycle of arenaviruses resembles that of bunyaviruses. Virus particles contain four to five species of RNA, two of which, designated large (L) and small (S), represent the viral genome and are of negative polarity. The other RNAs seem to be derived from ribosomes that become encapsulated within the virus on maturation from the infected cell (giving the sandy appearance), but there is no evidence that these ribosomes are necessary for virus replication. Like the viral segments of bunyaviruses, the L and S RNAs of arenaviruses are circular. The L segment encodes at least the viral polymerase, whereas the S segment encodes both the nucleocapsid (N) protein and the envelope glycoprotein (G). In the latter case, the N and G proteins are transcribed from different regions of the S segment, each of which exhibits a different translational polarity. Hence, the S segment of arenaviruses, like the S segment of bunyaviruses, is *ambisense*. Replication of arenaviruses takes place in the cytoplasm of the host cell, and mature virus particles seem to bud from the plasma membranes of infected cells.

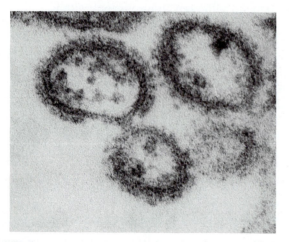

FIGURE 49-4   Lassa fever virus present in a Vero cell culture. Ribosomes incorporated from the host cell can be seen within the virus particles. (Original magnification ×173,000.)

Based on shared complement-fixing antigens, the arenaviruses have been subdivided as follows into three groups: (1) lymphocytic choriomeningitis virus (LCM), (2) the Tacaribe complex of viruses (which include the two human pathogens, Junin and Machupo viruses), and (3) Lassa fever virus.

Lymphocytic Choriomeningitis Virus

Lymphocytic choriomeningitis virus causes a unique congenital infection in mice that leads to an essentially asymptomatic condition in which the adult animal continues to excrete the virus. The ability of most congenitally infected mice to become permanent virus carriers results from the development of an immunologic tolerance to the virus and from the fact that replication of the virus does not result in the cytopathic destruction of the infected host cell. Tolerance is not always complete, and virus may be present in the bloodstream as a virus–immunoglobulin complex. This complex does not, however, neutralize the virus, and such complexes are infectious.

Injection of LCM virus into adult mice, in contrast, causes acute disease and death. Interestingly, LCM virus does not seem to cause a cytopathic effect in tissues of these mice. Instead, as the virus replicates, new virally coded antigens are inserted into the infected host-cell membranes. The adult mouse reacts with a cell-mediated immune response directed against the LCM-infected cells, which results in the destruction of the host cells in a manner analogous to a graft-versus-host reaction.

Although it was formerly believed that LCM virus was a major cause of aseptic meningitis in humans, careful studies have shown that meningitis is a fairly rare manifestation of this virus. When infections do arise, they are influenza-like, with symptoms of fever, headache, malaise, and nausea. When CNS invasion does occur, the symptoms ordinarily are mild, and recovery usually is complete in 1 to 3 weeks.

Tacaribe Virus Complex: Junin and Machupo Viruses

As shown in Figure 49-5, eight serotypes of the Tacaribe virus complex have been isolated from Florida and South America. Only two of the Tacaribe viruses have been shown to infect humans: Junin and Machupo viruses, which cause Argentine and Bolivian hemorrhagic fever, respectively. Both of these diseases are characterized by bleeding from the mouth, stomach, intestine, and nose, and occasionally from the vagina. Although blood loss is not great, patients may go into shock and die. The overall mortality rate varies from 10% to 50%. Both Junin and Machupo viruses seem to reside in a rodent reservoir and, like LCM, cause a silent chronic infection in their rodent

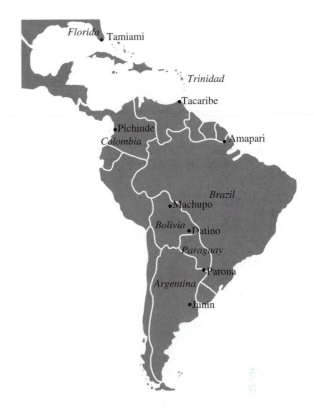

FIGURE 49-5 Partial map of the Western Hemisphere showing the geographic localities in which viruses of the Tacaribe complex have been recognized.

host. This infection is characterized by a persistent viremia in the absence of detectable circulating antibodies. These diseases were once believed to be arthropod borne; however, no evidence supports this concept. Human infection probably results from contact with infected rodent secretions, from dust contaminated with excretions, or by ingestion of contaminated food and drink.

Lassa Fever Virus

Lassa fever was first described in Nigeria in 1969, and several epidemics have since been reported in other areas of Africa. The virus produces a chronic infection in its host, usually rodents, and humans become infected through contact with infected rodents or rodent urine and feces. Person-to-person spread also may occur, particularly as a hospital-acquired nosocomial infection.

Although Lassa fever may occur as a mild or inapparent infection, the more severe infections seen in hospitalized patients have had a high mortality rate. Early symptoms include most of the influenza-like complaints. Later, subcutaneous hemorrhages may occur on the arms and legs as a result of diffuse capillary leakage. Death usually is attributed to cardiac failure. Case fatality rates can be as high as 20% in hospitalized individuals but are only 2% overall.

REOVIRIDAE

The family Reoviridae was established to include those icosahedral viruses (60 to 80 nm in diameter) whose genome consists of 10 or 11 segments of double-stranded RNA. The name was coined because original isolates obtained from the respiratory and intestinal tracts did not seem to cause disease. As a result, the family name Reoviridae arose from the first letter of each word in the designation *r*espiratory *e*nteric *o*rphan. The three morphologically similar but entirely unrelated groups of viruses that infect humans and animals are (1) reoviruses (genus *Orthoreovirus*) isolated from humans, other mammals, and birds; (2) rotaviruses (genus *Rotavirus*), which cause acute diarrhea in humans; and (3) orbiviruses (genus *Orbivirus*), which cause arthropod-borne diseases of humans and animals.

Structure and Replication

Reoviruses are unusual because they contain 10 separate segments of double-stranded RNA, and also because this complex genome is enclosed in a double-walled icosahedral capsid (Fig. 49-6).

After adsorption to cellular receptors, the virion enters the cell by phagocytosis, and the phagocytic vacuole fuses with a lysosome. Hydrolytic enzymes from the lysosome partially degrade the outer capsid wall, producing subviral particles that are released into the cytoplasm. This process activates the RNA transcriptase present in the inner capsid, and mRNA molecules are extruded from holes at the 12-pentomer vertices (Fig. 49-7). Transcription occurs semiconservatively, because only one strand

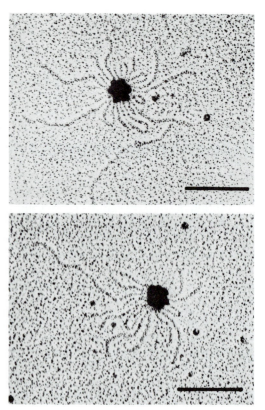

FIGURE 49-7 Reovirus reaction cores with RNA extruded from the vertices. Notice the loops in some strands of RNA. (Bar = 0.2 μm)

of the double-stranded RNA is copied, and only positive-strand mRNAs are released from the virion. All 10 strands are transcribed, yielding 10 mRNAs that are translated individually on host-cell polyribosomes.

The 10 segments of the genome are divided into three molecular sizes: large (segments L1, L2, and L3), medium (M1, M2, and M3), and small (S1, S2, S3, and S4). Each segment encodes a unique mRNA that is translated into a polypeptide. Like the genome segments that encode them, viral proteins are grouped into large, medium, and small classes.

Replication of new viral RNA progeny begins with replication of the mRNA to form double-stranded RNA. This occurs within a polypeptide structure, which eventually becomes the virion core. These "cytoplasmic factories" form crystalline aggregates of virions and empty capsids. The mechanisms that regulate the assembly of virus particles, so that each virion receives its total complement of 10 double-stranded RNA molecules, are not well understood. The completed virions are released from the cell without budding. Simultaneous replication of two different reoviruses within the same cell results in the mixing or reassortment of viral RNA segments from each of the viruses. Such a mechanism of "recombination" can rapidly lead to the generation of new viruses with altered phenotypes.

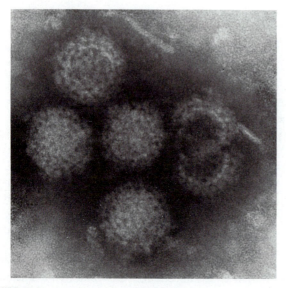

FIGURE 49-6 Reovirus capsids. (Original magnification ×272,000.)

Epidemiology and Pathogenesis

Reoviruses are extremely widespread in nature, and essentially all mammals possess antibodies to these agents. Only three serologic types infect humans and, because the antigenic differences reside in their surface hemagglutinin, they can be typed either by hemagglutination-inhibition or by neutralization tests. By 16 years of age, 50% to 80% of the general population have antibodies to reovirus.

Reoviruses have been isolated from persons with mild respiratory disease or diarrhea and from many completely healthy persons. Experimental infections frequently have been unsuccessful in the production of symptoms, and, when illness is occasionally produced, it is a mild respiratory disease. Hence, the acronym *reovirus* seems to be appropriate.

Reovirus can be isolated from throat washings or feces and can be grown on a number of human or monkey tissue cultures. All human strains possess a common complement-fixing antigen that allows a single screening test for human reoviruses.

Reoviruses are likely spread from person to person by both a respiratory and a fecal–oral route. Attempts at control seem unwarranted in view of the mildness of the diseases for which they may be responsible.

Rotaviruses

Human rotaviruses were first detected in 1973 by electron microscopic examination of duodenal biopsy specimens obtained from children with acute diarrhea. The virus is 75 nm in size, contains 11 double-stranded RNA segments, and has an inner and outer capsid. Neutralizing antibodies to two outer capsid proteins define the five serotypes of human rotaviruses.

Rotaviruses are the principal cause of acute infectious diarrhea, a major cause of death in the young. It has been estimated that more than one million rotavirus-associated deaths occur annually, with most of these in underdeveloped countries. These agents have been given the official generic name *Rotavirus,* stemming from the morphologic similarity of their double-walled capsid to a wheel (Fig. 49-8).

EPIDEMIOLOGY AND PATHOGENESIS

The ubiquity of rotaviruses throughout the animal kingdom is supported by the observation that piglets and calves deprived of colostrum (the first milk, containing high concentrations of the mother's antibodies) invariably develop a severe diarrhea caused by a virus related to human rotavirus. About 75% of newborn humans possess maternally acquired antibodies to rotavirus. The antibody titer declines during the first 6 months of life, but, by 5 or 6 years of age, about three fourths of all children have normally acquired an active immunity to rotavirus infections.

The incubation period of the gastroenteritis is 1 to 3 days; in infants, infection may result in death from dehydration and loss of electrolytes from the diarrhea and vomiting. In one study involving 21 fatal cases of rotavirus gastroenteritis, the children's ages varied from 4 to 30 months. Death occurred within 1 to 3 days after the onset of symptoms.

Only cholera leads to dehydration with a frequency equal to or greater than rotaviral gastroenteritis. Early hospitalization with fluid and electrolyte replacement all

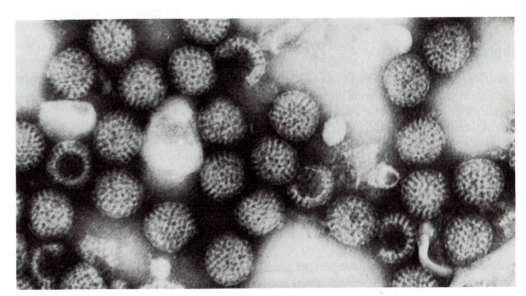

FIGURE 49-8 Rotavirus particles; each is about 75 nm in diameter. Notice the resemblance of some capsids to a wheel with spokes.

obligate parasites in animals and can produce chronic to acute diseases in humans.

NUTRITION

Unlike bacteria, which obtain nutrients by the transport of dissolved substances into the cell, most protozoa are *holozoic,* that is, they ingest solid particles of food through a mouth opening, or *cytostome.* The ingested food usually consists of bacteria, algae, or other protozoa. After ingestion, the food becomes enclosed in a food vacuole, and enzymes are secreted into the vacuole to catalyze the degradation of complex materials into soluble substances. Once dissolved, the nutrients can enter the cytoplasm to be used for the synthesis of cellular material or to be metabolized further to provide energy for the cell. Ingested material not dissolved in the vacuole either is expelled from the cell body through an *anal pore* or is moved to the surface, where the vacuole breaks open to free the undigested material from the cell.

Many members of one class of protozoa, the *Sporozoa,* are unable to engulf solid particles of food; these organisms obtain their nutrients by the transport of soluble nutrients into the cell in the same manner as bacteria.

REPRODUCTION

Many protozoa are able to reproduce both sexually and asexually. Asexually, most divide by splitting into two cells of equal size after nuclear division. Some protozoa divide by simple transverse fission (crosswise), whereas other classes divide longitudinally (lengthwise). Unequal fission, budding, or multiple fission is found in some species.

Sexual reproduction occurs when two morphologically different cells fuse (conjugate), resulting in the exchange of nuclear material and subsequent segregation into daughter cells. Some protozoa have complex reproductive cycles in which part of the life cycle must occur in humans or other vertebrates and another stage of the cycle must occur in a different host. In such cases, the host in which sexual reproduction occurs is termed the *definitive* host, whereas the host in which only asexual multiplication takes place is known as the *intermediate* host.

ENCYSTMENT

Under certain adverse environmental conditions, some protozoa can become *encysted,* that is, the cell can assume a fairly round or oval shape and secrete a protective coating around itself. At this stage, the cell can survive a lack of food or moisture, adverse temperature changes, or contact with toxic chemical agents. The *cyst* is particularly valuable in permitting parasitic forms to survive outside the host until they can enter a new host. With a return

to favorable conditions, water is absorbed into the cyst, and the organism emerges and resumes its growth.

In addition to the parasitic species, free-living forms are found in most classes of protozoa. In rare cases, the protozoan exists in its host in a mutualistic relationship, one in which the host benefits from the presence of the guest and the guest benefits from the host. One notable example of mutualism is the termite, which could not live if its gut were not inhabited by a protozoan capable of digesting wood ingested by the termite. On the other hand, these protozoa are unable to live if they are removed from the intestine of the termite.

Many animals infected by protozoa are not this fortunate, however, and the resulting infections vary from chronic to acute diseases. Such dire infections are most common in tropical areas, where conditions seem to be most favorable for the growth and spread of parasites.

Classification

Of the approximately 40,000 species of protozoa that have been described, only a few cause disease in humans. These pathogenic species are distributed in various phyla, subphyla, and classes of protozoa, and, thus, a study of the medically important species requires a general knowledge of each of these groups.

Amoebae form the subphylum *Sarcodina* and are characterized by their ability to send out finger-like projections called *pseudopodia* (false feet), which serve both for motility and for the engulfment of food particles (Fig. 50-1*A*). The cells do not contain complex organelles, and these organisms do not have a sexual mechanism of reproduction. Actively growing cells reproduce by binary fission, but, under adverse conditions, many species form dormant cysts. When environmental conditions are favorable, the amoeba can emerge to become an active feeding cell, called a *trophozoite.* Most amoebic infections of humans are confined to the intestine, but they sometimes are carried by the blood to other organs of the body, causing abscess formation in the liver, lungs, brain, pericardium, and spleen.

The phylum *Ciliophora* encompasses the ciliates. Most ciliates are free-living, and *Balantidium coli* is the single species causing disease in humans. The organisms in this class are characterized by the possession of *cilia* responsible for rapid movement through an aqueous environment (see Fig. 50-1*B*). Most divide by transverse fission, and many possess two nuclei, one a larger, less dense structure termed a *macronucleus* and the other a small, dense nucleus called a *micronucleus.* Sexual conjugation also occurs in many ciliates.

Organisms known as flagellates form the *Mastigophora* and differ grossly from the ciliates by possessing long, filamentous flagella. Although the fine structure is much the same, flagella are readily distinguishable from

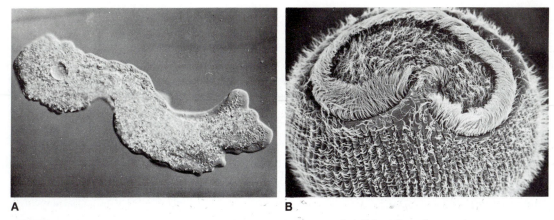

FIGURE 50-1 **A.** *Amoeba proteus.* (Original magnification ×154.) Normarski differential interference microscopy. **B.** Scanning electron micrograph of the ciliate *Stentor coeruleus.* (Original magnification ×336.)

cilia in that a flagellate usually possesses only one or several of these long, whip-like appendages; ciliates, on the other hand, are covered with hundreds of cilia. Numerous protozoan flagellates infect humans, causing intestinal, genital, and systemic diseases. All divide by longitudinal fission, and some also possess a sexual cycle of reproduction.

All members of the class *Sporozoa* (in the phylum, *Apicomplexa*) are parasitic for one or more animal species; they are unable to engulf solid food particles and must obtain their nutrients by the transport of soluble substances into the cytoplasm or, as in the case of *Plasmodium*, by *endocytosis*. Furthermore, these organisms normally lack obvious organs of locomotion, but all are probably motile at one stage of the life cycle. Both an amoeboid-type motility and gliding along the substrate using surface ridges or folds are seen. The most unusual aspect of their reproductive cycles is their frequent requirement for two different animal hosts for the completion of asexual and sexual cycles. Malaria and toxoplasmosis are the major human diseases caused by the Sporozoa.

Table 50-1 summarizes the major human diseases caused by some of the protozoa discussed in this chapter.

Sarcodina

ENTAMOEBA HISTOLYTICA

Entamoeba is the most prevalent genus of the Sarcodina found associated with humans. Most species of *Entamoeba* appear to exist in the human intestines as commensals much like other normal flora, but one species, *Entamoeba histolytica*, is potentially a human intestinal pathogen.

Human infections with *E histolytica* are referred to as *amoebiasis* and overt intestinal disease is termed *amoebic dysentery*. The active amoebae, called trophozoites, move by extruding *pseudopodia*, with the remaining cytoplasm flowing into the pseudopodium. In cases of amoebic dys-

entery, the trophozoites invade the intestinal mucosa, and examination of stool specimens can reveal ingested red blood cells in the amoebae. Because *E histolytica* is essentially the only parasitic amoeba to engulf red blood cells, their presence within the amoeba provides strong evidence for its identification.

Trophozoites of *E histolytica* reproduce by binary fission. In a specimen stained with hematoxylin, the nucleus appears as a granular structure containing a small, dense mass of chromatin (called a *karyosome*) in its center (Fig. 50-2).

The cyst stage of the life cycle of *E histolytica* occurs as trophozoites are scraped from the intestinal wall and carried down the colon with the fecal mass. During cyst formation, the amoebae usually excrete their ingested food particles, shrink to form rounded, nonmotile cells,

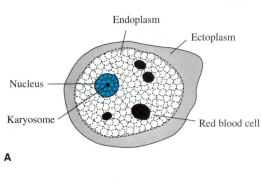

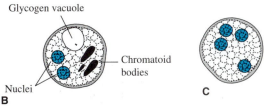

FIGURE 50-2 *Entamoeba histolytica.* **A.** Trophozoite containing red blood cells. **B.** Binucleated cyst containing chromatoid bars. **C.** Mature tetranucleated cyst.

TABLE 50-1
Major Protozoa Causing Specific Human Diseases

Parasites (Diseases)	Definitive Hosts	Intermediate Hosts	Important Reservoir Hosts	Transmission to Humans
Entamoeba histolytica (amoebiasis)	Humans	None	Humans	By ingestion (mature cyst)
Balantidium coli (balantidiasis)	Hogs, humans	None	Hogs, humans	By ingestion (mature cyst)
Giardia lamblia (giardiasis)	Humans	None	Humans	By ingestion (mature cyst)
Trichomonas vaginalis (trichomonad vaginitis)	Humans	None	Humans	By contact (flagellate)
Trypanosoma gambiense *Trypanosoma rhodesiense* (African sleeping sickness)	Humans, animals	Tsetse flies (*Glossina* species)	Humans, animals	By inoculation (bite of fly)
Trypanosoma cruzi (Chagas' disease)	Animals, humans	Reduviid bugs	Armadillos, opossums, humans	By contamination (infective feces of bug)
Leishmania donovani (kala-azar)	Humans, dogs	Sandflies (*Phlebotomus* species)	Dogs, humans	By inoculation (bite of fly; direct transmission possible)
Leishmania tropica (oriental sore) *Leishmania braziliensis** (espundia)				
Plasmodium vivax *Plasmodium falciparum* *Plasmodium malariae* *Plasmodium ovale* (malaria)	Anopheline mosquitoes	Humans	Humans	By inoculation (bite of mosquito; also by transfer of infected blood)

* Dogs and other animals have been implicated in the life cycles of *L donovani* and *L tropica*, but the part played by hosts other than humans in the case of *L braziliensis* is yet questionable. Naturally infected dogs have been found in South America.

and begin to secrete a thin, refractile covering. As this structure, known as a *precyst*, moves down the intestine, the nucleus undergoes two divisions, resulting in the formation of a mature cyst containing four small, identical nuclei. Ribosomes, which aggregate in the form of bars that stain with Gomori's trichrome stain or iron hematoxylin, normally are seen in the one- or two-nucleated precysts, but most of the mature four-nucleated cysts do not possess them. Because of their staining properties, these bars are referred to as *chromatoidal bars*. Thus, trophozoites of *E histolytica* can be identified by observing the granular appearance of the nuclear chromatin and, in some cases, the presence of ingested red blood cells. Mature cysts are characterized by the presence of four identical nuclei (all containing karyosomes) and by the occasional presence of chromatoidal bars within the cytoplasm.

Symptomatology and Pathogenesis of Amoebic Dysentery

For many years, it has been said that *E histolytica* infects about 10% of the world's population. However, about 90% of all such infections are asymptomatic, and it recently has been established that these individuals are infected with a nonpathogenic *Entamoeba* that is morphologically identical to the pathogenic species. These distinct species can be differentiated from each other by isoenzyme analysis, ribosomal RNA sequence analysis, restriction fragment length polymorphism analysis, and typing with specific monoclonal antibodies. Therefore, it has been proposed that the nonpathogenic variety be named *Entamoeba dispar* and the name of *E histolytica* be retained for the pathogenic strain. As a result, we can now state that about 1% of the world's population is infected with *E histolytica*, and that these infections cause between 40,000 and 100,000 deaths annually.

In a typical case of amoebic dysentery, the organisms first penetrate the intestinal mucosa. The resulting lesions can be minor and the symptoms confined to a few daily loose stools containing flecks of blood and mucus. In acute cases, there can be numerous intestinal ulcers, and these can coalesce and become secondarily infected with bacteria. When this happens, a person can have severe diarrhea characterized by the presence of considerable blood and mucus.

In 2% to 20% of such cases, the intestinal ulcers erode into adjoining blood vessels, causing intraluminal bleeding and permitting the spread of the amoebae to the liver. Painful hepatic abscesses can develop and erode through the diaphragm into the lung, causing bronchial abscesses. Individuals over the age of 40 years who use corticosteroids appear to be predisposed to systemic complications.

Other organs also can be infected, but such sequelae are extremely rare.

Epidemiology of Amoebic Dysentery

The presence and frequency of amoebic dysentery can be correlated with the sanitary conditions prevailing within a given area. The disease is considerably more prevalent in tropical and subtropical areas than in temperate latitudes. It has been estimated that 0.1% to 0.5% of persons in the United States are infected with *E histolytica,* contrasted with an infection rate of 5% to 8% in some tropical regions. Infections also have been reported to occur in as many as 32% of homosexual men, but almost all these have now been shown to be the nonpathogenic species, *E dispar.*

Paradoxically, the normal spread of *E histolytica* usually is not caused by persons with acute cases of amoebic dysentery, but by asymptomatic chronic carriers of the organisms. This is because persons with the acute disease pass actively growing trophozoites in their stools, and this form of the organism has a short survival time outside the host. Chronic carriers, however, excrete primarily the cyst form of the organism, and cysts are much more resistant to external conditions. In addition, it is extremely unlikely that the fragile trophozoites would withstand normal gastric acidity long enough to pass through the stomach into the intestinal area, so it probably is the ingestion of the cyst form of *E histolytica* that causes

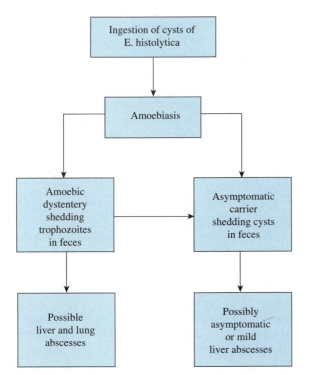

FIGURE 50-3 Possible courses of infection occurring during amebiasis.

disease. Figure 50-3 schematically summarizes the various courses that can occur in amoebiasis.

Diagnosis of Amoebic Dysentery

A definitive diagnosis of amoebic dysentery requires that the parasite be identified in feces or infected tissues. Feces must be examined soon after voiding, because the trophozoites have a short survival time outside the host. Trophozoites containing ingested red blood cells, showing invasion of the intestinal mucosa, are indicative of active disease. Stained cysts greater than 10 μm in diameter that possess four nuclei also indicate an *E histolytica* infection. Because it is not necessary to treat patients infected with the nonpathogenic *E dispar,* it is important to differentiate between these two organisms. To that end, Dr. William Petri, Jr. at the University of Virginia has developed an enzyme-linked immunosorbent assay using monoclonal antibodies to a galactose-specific adhesin on the parasites that can be used to differentiate the pathogenic and nonpathogenic amoebae.

Control and Treatment of Amoebic Dysentery

Control of amoebic dysentery is essentially synonymous with adequate sanitation. Most sporadic cases in the Western Hemisphere occur in rural areas and in lower socioeconomic groups. Breaks in the normal sanitation chain resulting in fecally contaminated drinking water or food bring about occasional epidemics. Normal chlorination procedures used for the treatment of municipal water sources are generally effective in eliminating the cysts of *E histolytica.* Control in tropical and developing countries will require increased health education to bring about improved methods of fecal disposal.

The most recent advance in the control of amoebic dysentery is the potential development of an effective vaccine. Dr. William Petri Jr. and his collaborators have identified a galactose-specific lectin that attaches the amoebae to the intestinal epithelium. They have reported that antibodies to this galactose lectin elicit a partial protective response in a gerbil model of amoebic liver abscesses and they are studying its role in the cytotoxicity of the amoebae.

Many effective drugs are available for the treatment of amoebic dysentery. Most of these drugs, such as dehydroemetine, diiodohydroxyquin, chloroquine (Aralen), or metronidazole, exhibit varying degrees of toxicity and should be taken only under the supervision of an experienced physician.

NONPATHOGENIC *ENTAMOEBA*

Several species of the genus *Entamoeba* have a worldwide distribution but do not appear to cause disease. A knowledge of these species is of value in differentiating the harmless commensals from the potentially pathogenic *E histolytica*. One amoeba usually considered to be non-pathogenic is *Entamoeba hartmanni*. This organism is differentiated from *E histolytica* primarily on the basis that both its trophozoites and its cysts are smaller than those of *E histolytica*. The lack of ingested red blood cells in *E hartmanni* also can be of value in distinguishing between these two species.

Entamoeba coli is a widely dispersed nonpathogenic amoeba that is difficult to differentiate from *E histolytica*. The trophozoites are described as sluggish organisms exhibiting a nondirectional motility, and, like other nonpathogenic amoebae, they do not contain ingested red blood cells. The nucleus of *E coli* contains peripheral chromatin irregularly distributed on the nuclear envelope. Cysts of *E coli* are somewhat easier to identify, because they routinely possess eight nuclei within a granular cytoplasm.

Other nonpathogenic amoebae, such as *Entamoeba polecki* and *Entamoeba gingivalis*, also can be confused with *E histolytica*. *E polecki* is an intestinal parasite, and *E gingivalis* can be found in pyorrheal pockets between the teeth and gums, and in the crypts of the tonsils. *E gingivalis* does not form cysts, and the trophozoites in all likelihood are transmitted from human to human through close oral contact or contaminated drinking utensils. The organism can be found in the gingival tissues around the teeth and its widespread occurrence is attested to by the fact that it can be found in the mouths of about 50% of seemingly normal persons. Its incidence approaches 75% to 90% in individuals with gingival lesions, but there is no proof that *E gingivalis* is the etiologic agent of such lesions. Treatment and prevention of infections are achieved by good oral hygiene.

Dientamoeba fragilis is a small parasite that formerly was considered to be an amoeba. However, it has been reclassified as an amoeba-like flagellate, which does not possess a flagellum and is related to the Trichomonas group. It is found as an intestinal parasite. This organism does not form cysts and can be recognized only by staining the trophozoites occurring in fresh stool specimens. The trophozoites of *D fragilis* usually are differentiated from other intestinal amoebae by their possession of two nuclei within the cell. Infections with *D fragilis* generally are asymptomatic, but some persons experience a mild, persistent diarrhea, along with gastrointestinal distress.

The mode of transmission of *D fragilis* is unknown. The oral ingestion of cultured trophozoites by human volunteers fails to produce infection, and there is considerable evidence that this organism may be carried inside the eggs of the nematode, *Enterobius vermicularis*, the common pinworm. This would explain how the delicate trophozoites could withstand the acids of the stomach to reach the intestine.

PRIMARY AMOEBIC MENINGOENCEPHALITIS

In recent years, strains of the free-living amoebo-flagellates *Naegleria fowleri* and *Acanthamoeba* species have been isolated from patients with meningoencephalitis. *Naegleria* is characterized by a life cycle in which the amoeboid phase alternates with organisms possessing two or four flagella, but *Acanthamoeba* has no flagellate form.

Both are widespread in fresh water and also are found in moist soils, decaying vegetables, and fecal wastes. Cases of human meningoencephalitis occur during the summer months (most often caused by *Naegleria*) and usually are manifested within a week after swimming in contaminated water; however, because both lakes and swimming pools are apparent sources of infection, the use of the phrase "contaminated water" does not necessarily imply foul or brackish waters.

The dramatic clinical course of the disease is characteristic of a typical fulminating meningoencephalitis and almost invariably ends with the death of the patient within 3 to 6 days after the initial symptoms.

Little is known about the pathogenesis of this infection, but it is believed that the nasal mucosa may provide the portal of entry. Diagnosis is based on the observation of the motile amoebae in unstained preparations of spinal fluid and on the finding of stained amoebae in sections of the brain at autopsy.

Acanthamoeba also is known to cause a severe keratitis, which can lead to blindness. Infection frequently follows ocular trauma or exposure to contaminated water, but more and more cases are occurring in persons wearing contact lenses. One survey of such infected persons indicated that they were significantly more likely than control subjects not to disinfect their lenses as frequently or as thoroughly as recommended by lens manufacturers.

Results of treatment have been exceedingly disappointing, and none of the usual amoebicidal drugs appear to be particularly effective. However, initial reports suggest that amphotericin B has clinical potential for the treatment of amoebic meningoencephalitis.

Ciliophora

BALANTIDIUM COLI

Ciliophora, an extremely large class of ciliated protozoa, is made up largely of free-living organisms, and *B coli* is the only species that causes disease in humans.

B coli can attain a length of 200 μm and is the largest of the parasitic protozoa that can be found in the human intestine. The organisms reside primarily in the lumen of the intestine and obtain food by the ingestion of bacteria. Occasionally, however, *B coli* causes a bloody diarrhea not unlike the acute episodes of amoebic dysentery.

Trophozoites of the organism are oval structures covered with cilia (Fig. 50-4). Like other ciliates, *B coli* possesses two nuclei, a *macronucleus* and a *micronucleus*. The

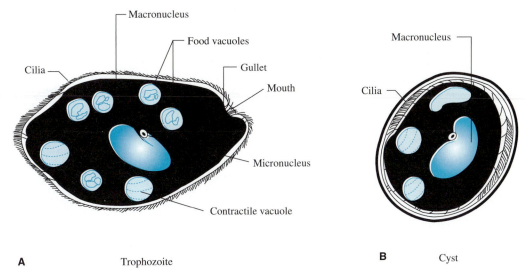

FIGURE 50-4 *Balantidium coli.* **A.** Trophozoite. **B.** Cyst.

micronucleus functions in sexual reproduction of the cell, and the macronucleus controls the metabolic activities within the organism. *B coli* forms a cyst about 60 to 70 μm long. The cyst is covered with a thin, refractile covering, and in newly formed cysts, the ciliated organisms can be seen within the cyst wall.

B coli appears to be routinely present in swine, and it seems possible that humans become infected by the ingestion of water or food contaminated with cysts present in swine feces. Overt disease is rare, however, and it appears that most infections produce no demonstrable symptoms. Spread of the organisms to the liver, lymph nodes, and lungs has been reported, but such complications are exceedingly rare. Treatment with oxytetracycline, carbarsone, or diiodohydroxyquin appears to be effective for the elimination of this potential parasite.

Mastigophora

The parasitic flagellated protozoa fall into two categories with respect to the type of disease produced in humans. One group, commonly called the intestinal flagellates, is found only in the digestive or genital tracts; these organisms can produce infections varying from asymptomatic to severe disease. Members of the second group, the hemoflagellates, are transmitted by blood-sucking insects to humans, in whom they produce severe and frequently fatal infections.

Intestinal Flagellates

GIARDIA LAMBLIA

Giardia lamblia is the only flagellated protozoan that produces frank intestinal disease. It is easy to recognize because the trophozoites are bilaterally symmetric; each organelle and structure is paired, as shown in Figure 50-5*A*. *Giardia* possess two nuclei, each containing a central karyosome, and four pairs of flagella, which impart an erratic motility and result in a slow osscillation around its long axis. Cysts of *G lamblia* are ovoid structures about 8 by 12 μm in size, containing four nuclei and numerous refractile threads in the cytoplasm.

Infections in adults can be asymptomatic, and for many years, the organism was considered a nonpathogen. It has been amply demonstrated, however, that this organism does cause an intestinal disease (particularly in children) that varies in severity. It is likely that most overt cases of intestinal infections by *Giardia* are manifested by diarrhea and abdominal cramps, but severe cases also can be accompanied by malabsorption deficiencies in the small intestine.

G lamblia is a worldwide distribution, and its spectrum of occurrence in the United States is similar to that of *E histolytica*, in that it is seen most frequently in rural and lower socioeconomic areas. (An outbreak in Aspen, Colorado, during the 1966 ski season hardly fits this geographic definition, but this epidemic occurred when sewage from defective pipes leaked into a well supplying drinking water.) Estimates indicate that *G lamblia* is carried by 4% to 7% of adults, making it the most frequent cause of water-borne diarrhea in the United States, as well as being the most frequently identified intestinal parasite found in stool specimens submitted to the US public health laboratories. Outbreaks occurring among campers are thought to result from various animal species of *Giardia* that are harbored by many domestic animals, as well as beavers and other rodents. In addition, there have been outbreaks of giardiasis attributed to municipal water supplies, and it is possible that the cysts can survive some forms of water treatment. Contact with diaper-age

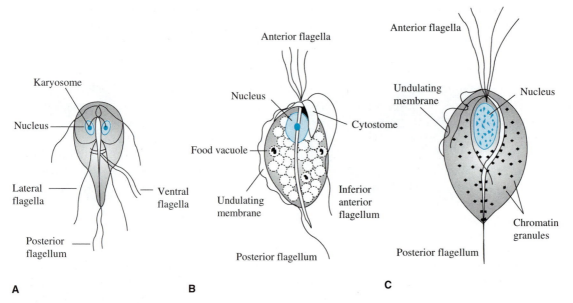

FIGURE 50-5 Flagellates infecting the human genital and intestinal tracts. **A.** *Giardia lamblia* trophozoite. **B.** *Trichomonas hominis* trophozoite. **C.** *Trichomonas vaginalis* trophozoite.

children also serves as a frequent source of infection. The prevalence of *Giardia* infections among male homosexuals also is considerably higher than that of control subjects.

Commercial immunoassay kits are available that can detect a specific *Giardia* antigen in aqueous extracts of stool specimens. Stool specimens also can be examined for ova and parasites, but this is more laborious and less sensitive than the available enzyme immunoassay procedures. Infections can be treated effectively with quinacrine hydrochloride (Atabrine). In addition, metronidazole, mebendazole, and tinidazole are highly effective for the treatment of giardiasis.

CHILOMASTIX MESNILI

Chilomastix mesnili is not known to cause symptomatic disease in humans, but because it is found throughout the world as an intestinal parasite, it must be differentiated from organisms such as *Giardia*. The organism possesses several anterior flagella and a single large anterior nucleus. (Note that *Giardia* has two nuclei and four pairs of flagella.) Cysts of *C mesnili* are lemon-shaped and contain a single large nucleus.

TRICHOMONAS HOMINIS

Trichomonas hominis appears to exist only as a commensal in the intestinal tract of humans and, along with *Trichomonas vaginalis*, possesses the dubious honor of being the only flagellate parasitizing humans that does not form cysts. Morphologically, it is characterized by four anterior flagella plus a posterior flagellum that forms the outer edge of an undulating membrane (see Fig. 50-5*B*). The

organism appears to be an obligate parasite of the intestinal tract; therefore, its presence elsewhere is a result of recent fecal contamination.

TRICHOMONAS VAGINALIS

T vaginalis, the etiologic agent of *trichomoniasis,* is morphologically similar to *T hominis,* but is larger, with a shorter undulating membrane (see Fig. 50-5*C*). However, *T vaginalis* is found only in vaginal secretions, whereas *T hominis* is never observed in this area of the body.

Trichomoniasis is a common sexually transmitted disease, infecting both men and women and causing an estimated 2 to 3 million symptomatic infections per year among sexually active women in the United States. In one survey of 177 women attending a sexually transmitted disease clinic, 49% were found to be infected with *T vaginalis.* The infection in women can be asymptomatic, or it can cause a thin, watery, vaginal discharge accompanied by burning and itching. One study of infected women demonstrated that strains of *T vaginalis* isolated from symptomatic infections were β-hemolytic on human red blood cells, whereas strains from asymptomatic infections were not, suggesting that the β-hemolysin may be a virulence factor. Infection in men usually is asymptomatic, except in cases involving the prostate and seminal vesicles.

Before the introduction of metronidazole, many women remained infected throughout their reproductive lifetime. Now, most cases respond to treatment, although cases of refractory vaginal trichomoniasis caused by strains that are relatively resistant to metronidazole have been reported. Because the infection is sexually transmitted and frequently asymptomatic in men, both male and female sexual partners should receive treatment.

Hemoflagellates

Flagellated protozoa transmitted to humans by the bites of infected, blood-sucking insects are referred to as the *hemoflagellates*. These organisms can be found in the blood, lymph, and cerebrospinal fluid, and as intracellular parasites in various organs of the body.

Hemoflagellates that infect humans are classified in two genera, *Trypanosoma* and *Leishmania*, and it is believed that they originally were parasites of insects that later acquired the ability to propagate in humans and other animals. This is supported by the observation that some genera still are exclusively insect parasites, and even those species that infect higher animals undergo part of their development in the insect.

Cells of *Leishmania* and *Trypanosoma* pass through similar morphologic states during their life cycles in vertebrate and invertebrate hosts (Fig. 50-6). The *trypomastigote* form characteristically possesses an undulating membrane composed of a thin protoplasmic extension along the entire length of the organism. A single flagellum forms the outer edge of this membrane and, in usual circumstances, extends anterior to the cell, where it functions as an organ of locomotion. The undulating membrane of the *epimastigote* stage originates in the central part of the cell anterior to the nucleus, whereas the *promastigote* form lacks an undulating membrane but is motile through a single flagellum inserted in the anterior end of the cell. *Amastigote* forms appear as rounded, nonmotile organisms. Of the major pathogens discussed here, *Trypanosoma gambiense* grows as a trypomastigote form in the vertebrate host but is seen in both the trypomastigote and epimastigote forms in the invertebrate host. On the other hand, all four stages are seen when *Trypanosoma cruzi* grows in the vertebrate host, but only the trypomastigote and epimastigote forms are found in the invertebrate host. All species of *Leishmania* grow only in the amastigote form in the vertebrate host and the promastigote form in the invertebrate host. It is obvious, therefore, that no sharp anatomic dividing line exists between the genera *Trypanosoma* and *Leishmania*.

TRYPANOSOMA

Trypanosomes are the etiologic agents for African sleeping sickness, a disease that affects about 1 million people in Central and East Africa and that causes about 20,000 new cases annually. The disease occurs in a 4.5 million square mile area that is sometimes referred to as the *tsetse fly belt*.

T gambiense causes *West African sleeping sickness*, which is sometimes referred to as *Gambian trypanosomiasis*. A more virulent form of this disease is seen in Central and Eastern Africa, where it is called *East African sleeping sickness* or *Rhodesian trypanosomiasis*. The etiologic agent of this latter form has been named *Trypanosoma rhodesiense*. Although there is no dispute concerning the difference in the severity of these two diseases, the two trypanosomes are indistinguishable morphologically. A third hemoflagellate, *Trypanosoma brucei*, produces a severe infection in domestic animals but is not known to affect humans. Oddly, this species also is indistinguishable from *T gambiense* and *T rhodesiense*, and many parasitologists considered these to be subspecies of *T brucei* (ie, *T brucei* subspecies gambiense and *T brucei* subspecies rhodesiense). For simplicity, however, the three species names are used in this section.

West African Sleeping Sickness (Gambian Trypanosomiasis)

After the bite of an infected tsetse fly, there usually is a period of 2 to 3 weeks before the occurrence of overt symptoms of West African sleeping sickness. In some cases, an ulcer develops at the site of the bite, but this normally heals after 1 to 3 weeks. During the incubation period, trypanosomes can be seen in small numbers in blood smears, but the attacks of fever do not begin until the organisms invade the lymph nodes. At this time, the number of trypanosomes in the bloodstream and lymph nodes increases dramatically. After several days to a week, the fever subsides, and the patient has no symptoms for several weeks before the occurrence of a subsequent similar episode. These intermittent attacks can continue over a period of several months, normally causing the face to swell and often leading to heart damage. As the disease

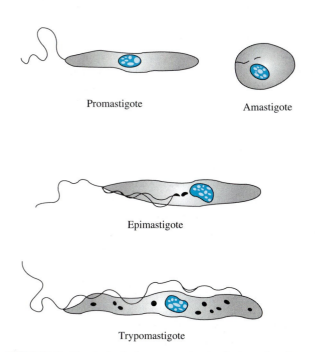

FIGURE 50-6   Morphologic forms occurring in the hemoflagellates.

Promastigote

Amastigote

Epimastigote

Trypomastigote

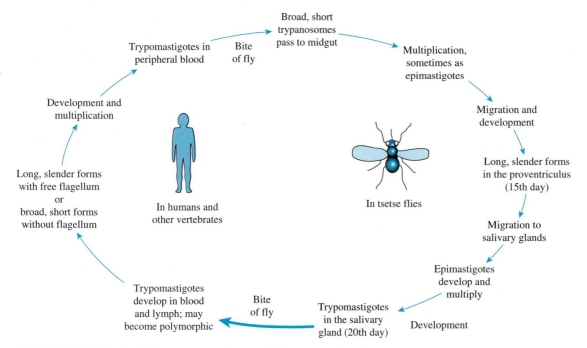

FIGURES 50-7   Life cycle of *Trypanosoma gambiense* and *Trypanosoma rhodesiense*.

progresses, the trypanosomes invade the central nervous system, causing a meningoencephalitis frequently manifested by slurred speech and difficulty in walking. Later stages are characterized by convulsions, paralysis, mental deterioration, and increasing sleepiness. The central nervous system symptoms can last for many months before the person finally becomes comatose and dies.

T gambiense has been shown to infect some game animals of Africa, as well as many domestic animals, particularly cattle, pigs, and goats, which can be infected for long periods without symptoms. However, most human infections probably result from transmission from a human to a tsetse fly and back to a human (Fig. 50-7).

For many years, the most puzzling aspects of this disease were the unexplained, recurrent febrile attacks and the apparent lack of an effective immune response to the trypanosomes, in spite of the presence of high titers of IgM antibodies to trypanosomal antigens. Experimental infection of animals with *T brucei* yielded an explanation for this paradox. These experiments showed conclusively that during an infection, trypanosomes undergo surface changes with the formation of a new surface antigen. This surface antigen consists of about 10 million molecules of a single glycoprotein, which is termed the *variable surface glycoprotein (VSG)*. Using recombinant DNA techniques, it has been shown that a single trypanosome can possess several thousand different VSG genes, of which only one is transcribed at any one time. Interestingly, there are 12 to 14 of these VSGs that always are expressed first when a tsetse fly bites a mammalian host. These particular genes, called *metacyclic genes,* all are expressed at the time of the initial infection; thus, one trypanosome expresses one

metacyclic gene, another a different metacyclic gene, and so on for the expression of all the metacyclic genes. About 5 days after infection, all the surface antigens expressed by the metacyclic genes disappear, and the infection progresses with the expression of one VSG gene after another.

It is not known how an organism can express only one VSG at a time, or why the first VSG to appear after the disappearance of the metacyclic VSGs is the one that was being expressed at the time the fly became infected. It is known that there are multiple expression sites existing on different chromosomes, and that any VSG gene that is being expressed is located near the telomere of its chromosome. Thus, VSG genes that normally occupy sites in the interior of the chromosome must be duplicated and translocated to a site near the telomere to be expressed. On the other hand, many VSG genes that normally are situated near the telomere can be expressed without duplication and translocation.

A model with multiple expression sites must have an exquisite form of regulation so that only one is active at any given time, but the mechanism of such regulation is presently unknown.

The diagnosis of trypanosomiasis depends on observation of the parasites in blood, lymph nodes, or spinal fluid, or on demonstration of IgM antibody directed toward the basic antigen of the trypanosome. The presence of this antibody in spinal fluid provides a definitive diagnosis of trypanosomal meningoencephalitis. The organisms can be grown on a concentrated blood agar, but continuous cultivation is too difficult to be of practical value as a diagnostic technique. However, good growth does occur on the chorioallantoic membrane of the chick embryo.

An immunologic control of Gambian trypanosomiasis seems exceedingly unlikely, particularly because there is no antigenic cross-reactivity among the myriad of potential VSGs as they exist on the surface of the trypanosome. A vaccine consisting of metacyclic VSGs could be effective, but it seems possible that other VSG genes could take over and serve as metacyclic genes.

Control of Gambian trypanosomiasis is directed toward elimination of the vectors, *Glossina palpalis* and *Glossina tachinoides*. These species of tsetse flies normally inhabit the banks of shaded streams near human habitations, and the use of insecticides plus the clearing of streamside brush provides effective control.

A variety of drugs can be used for the successful treatment of trypanosomiasis, although the more effective ones exhibit some toxicity to the host. Pentamidine isethionate, suramin, and melarsoprol are the usual therapeutic agents for the treatment of Gambian trypanosomiasis.

East African Sleeping Sickness (Rhodesian Trypanosomiasis)

T rhodesiense, the etiologic agent of Rhodesian trypanosomiasis, is morphologically indistinguishable from *T gambiense*, but the corresponding disease is more severe than its West African counterpart. The pathogenesis is similar to that of Gambian trypanosomiasis, but the disease progresses more rapidly, and death frequently occurs before the development of meningoencephalitis. Myocarditis occurs commonly and is a major cause of mortality. When encephalitis does occur, central nervous system involvement takes place earlier than in Gambian trypanosomiasis.

The vector of Rhodesian sleeping sickness also is a tsetse fly (*Glossina morsitans*), but this vector usually becomes infected from feeding on wild animals. Thus, *T gambiense*, the etiologic agent of Rhodesian trypanosomiasis, is found more commonly in several wild animals; although the disease tends to occur sporadically, control is more difficult than in the West African variety.

The treatment of choice is a drug called suramin; however, because of the high toxicity of this drug for the host, administration of drugs normally used in the treatment of Gambian trypanosomiasis may be preferable.

American Trypanosomiasis (Chagas' Disease)

Chagas' disease also is caused by a trypanosome, *T cruzi*, but its epidemiology and pathogenesis are different from those of African trypanosomiasis, as shown in Figure 50-8.

The disease occurs in the southern United States, Central America, and as far south as Argentina. The reservoir for the trypanosomes includes a wide variety of wild animals, particularly rodents, opossums, and armadillos. The vector can be any one of several species of infected *reduviid bugs* (also called *triatomids*). These vectors characteristically inhabit houses; trypanosomes grow in the gut of the bug and are passed in its feces. Humans become

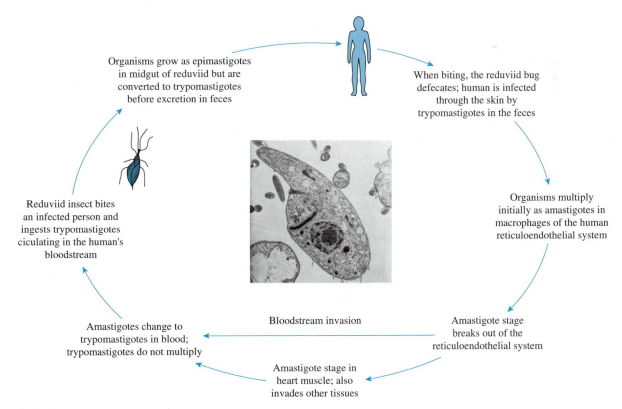

Organisms grow as epimastigotes in midgut of reduviid but are converted to trypomastigotes before excretion in feces

When biting, the reduviid bug defecates; human is infected through the skin by trypomastigotes in the feces

Reduviid insect bites an infected person and ingests trypomastigotes ciculating in the human's bloodstream

Organisms multiply initially as amastigotes in macrophages of the human reticuloendothelial system

Amastigotes change to trypomastigotes in blood; trypomastigotes do not multiply

Bloodstream invasion

Amastigote stage breaks out of the reticuloendothelial system

Amastigote stage in heart muscle; also invades other tissues

FIGURE 50-8 Life cycle of *Trypanosoma cruzi*. The electron micrograph shows a thin section through the epimastigote form. (Original magnification ×3740.)

infected because the bug habitually defecates while feeding, and the trypanosomes are introduced into the site of the bite from the fecal contamination of the infected vector. The parasites also can be acquired congenitally from an infected mother or through a blood transfusion from an infected asymptomatic person.

T cruzi differs from the other trypanosomes discussed in that it is unable to multiply outside the cell in a vertebrate host. Instead, after entering the bloodstream, the organisms undergo a morphologic change in which they round up and lose their undulating membrane and flagellum. This morphologic stage, depicted in Figure 50-6, is called an *amastigote* form, and it is this form of *T cruzi* that multiplies within the cell in essentially every organ of the body. After infected cells rupture, the trypomastigote form can be found in the blood, but the parasites do not multiply in the mammalian host while in this stage.

Ordinarily, an erythematous lesion (termed a *chagoma*) develops at the site of infection. The organisms infect the regional lymph nodes and from there are spread through the bloodstream to other organs of the body. The liver and macrophages in the spleen are commonly infected, but the organ most characteristically affected is the heart. Growth of the amastigote forms within the heart induces an inflammatory response and an enlarged heart with electrocardiographic changes typical of Chagas' disease.

Central nervous system involvement resulting in a fatal meningoencephalitis is not unusual in infants infected with *T cruzi*. However, older children and adults can show few or no signs of encephalitis, and these infections are characterized most often by myocarditis (an inflammation of the muscular tissue of the heart). Interestingly, the myocarditis, which can lead to congestive heart failure, appears to be caused by an autoimmune reaction. However, the organ-specific autoantigen for chronic Chagas' disease myocarditis remains unknown.

The initial illness resolves spontaneously over a period of 4 to 6 months in most patients, but this usually is followed by a chronic, indeterminate phase in which there are no symptoms but a lifelong low-grade parasitemia persists. It is in this phase that the organisms are transmitted through blood transfusions. In 10% to 30% of such individuals, a symptomatic chronic infection occurs years after the initial infection accompanied by major pathologic changes in the heart. Death usually results from disturbances of rhythm or congestive heart failure.

Chagas' disease can be diagnosed early in the infection by observing the trypanosomes in blood smears. During later stages of the disease, the organisms can be grown from blood cultures. A fluorescence-labeled antibody also is used successfully in diagnosis. An unusual technique, called *xenodiagnosis,* occasionally is used for the diagnosis of this disease; this method involves the use of uninfected reduviid bugs that are allowed to feed on a suspected case. The bugs are examined at a later date for the presence of trypanosomes. This procedure actually is an enrichment technique designed to overcome the paucity of trypanosomes present in the blood during the later stages of the disease.

The drugs used to treat African trypanosomiasis are of no value against the American variety. Nifurtimox and benznidazole reduce the severity of acute Chagas' disease but do not eliminate the parasites. Moreover, both must be taken for extended periods, frequently causing severe side effects. As a result, no successful therapy is available for Chagas' disease.

LEISHMANIA

Taxonomic classification of the genus *Leishmania* seems to be an almost insurmountable problem. The situation is confusing because there are no obvious morphologic differences between any of the *Leishmania* and, apparently, a myriad of serologic types produce essentially identical infections. However, restriction digests of kinetoplast DNA (*schizodeme analysis*) and isoenzyme patterns (*zymodeme analysis*) have been used to suggest taxonomic groups.

All species of *Leishmania* are transmitted from one animal to another (including humans) by the bite of infected sandflies belonging to the genus *Phlebotomus.* Each species of parasite has an extreme host specificity for a particular species of sandfly, and if more than one serologic species of *Leishmania* exists in a given area, each will be transmitted by a different species of *Phlebotomus.* In addition, each *Leishmania* exists in two different morphologic forms. The organisms introduced by the bite of the sandfly exist as flagellated promastigote forms (see Fig. 50-6). The parasites then transform into a nonmotile, ovoid cell (amastigote form), and this stage proliferates within the host's macrophages and endothelial cells. When a sandfly acquires the parasites from an infected host, the organisms proliferate in the insect's gut as motile promastigotes, which eventually accumulate in the pharynx and buccal cavity in a position to infect a new host.

The diseases caused by members of the genus *Leishmania* occur as two major types: *cutaneous leishmaniasis* and *visceral leishmaniasis.* However, the cutaneous variety can be manifested by different species of *Leishmania* as a dermatrophic form producing skin lesions and as a mucocutaneous variety producing ulcers on the oral or nasal mucosa. All forms of leishmaniasis are intracellular infections of the reticuloendothelial system (fixed phagocytic cells scattered throughout the body, especially in the liver, spleen, bone marrow, and lymph nodes), and the different types of this disease really are manifestations of the invasive properties of the parasite. Therefore, it would seem that the cutaneous infections are caused by a species of low invasive power in which the parasites are confined to the reticuloendothelial cells in the skin and subcutaneous area of the body. On the other hand, the organisms causing visceral leishmaniasis are able to invade the reticuloendothelial system throughout the body, particularly the reticuloendothelial cells of the spleen and liver.

Cutaneous Leishmaniasis

Numerous serologic variants of *Leishmania* serve as the etiologic agents of cutaneous leishmaniasis. Because of the similarity of these parasites, they usually are classified as *Leishmania tropica* or are referred to by some parasitologists as the *L tropica* species complex.

The prototype of the cutaneous ulcer is called an *Oriental sore* (Fig. 50-9); the disease occurs primarily in the Near East, the Mediterranean region, Africa, southern Russia, and southern Asia. As in all cases of leishmaniasis, the parasites are transmitted to the host by the bite of an infected sandfly. After an incubation period varying from several weeks to several months, a papule eventually evolves into an ulcer at the site of the bite. Routinely, the ulcer also is the site of a secondary bacterial infection. The lesion usually heals in about 1 year, leaving a disfiguring and depigmented scar. Immunity is solid, and because an endemic area usually is infested with only one serologic type of *L tropica,* it is not unusual for parents to infect their children intentionally in a part of the body where the resulting scar normally will not be visible.

Dermal leishmaniasis also occurs in Central and South America, and some investigators have given new species names to these variants of American leishmaniasis. A mild cutaneous infection occurring in the mountainous areas of Peru is called *uta,* and the causative agent frequently is referred to as *Leishmania peruviana.* A similar infection prevalent in the Brazilian forest region is called *chiclero's ulcer,* and many persons have used the name of *Leishmania mexicana* for the etiologic agent of this disease.

The normal reservoir for *L tropica* varies from one endemic area to another. For example, in India, both humans and dogs appear to be the reservoirs of infection. Elsewhere, rodents play this role, and in some regions, gerbils and ground squirrels provide the source of parasites from which the sandflies become infected.

Diagnosis of cutaneous leishmaniasis usually is based on observation of the parasites in stained scrapings from infected areas; however, the intradermal injection of a killed suspension of promastigotes (called the Montenegro test) gives a delayed-type skin reaction in a large percentage of infected persons.

Treatment with arsenical compounds usually is effective. The most effective therapeutic agent is pentavalent antimony available as sodium stibogluconate, although the antibiotic amphotericin B also is reported to yield good results.

Mucocutaneous Leishmaniasis

Mucocutaneous leishmaniasis is a variant of the cutaneous disease, but it is considered by most investigators suffi-

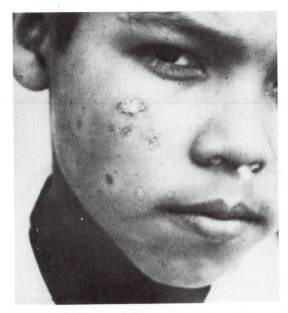

FIGURE 50-9 Oriental sores resulting from cutaneous leishmaniasis.

ciently distinct to warrant the naming of a new species, *Leishmania braziliensis,* as its causative agent. Particularly prevalent in Brazil, the disease frequently is fatal.

The infection normally begins as a dermal lesion similar to that described for cutaneous leishmaniasis. The lesion heals and, after an interval of months to years, the organisms reappear, causing lesions in the mucous membranes of the nasopharyngeal area. If the lesions are untreated, the nasal septum, the lips, and the soft palate can be destroyed. Death can occur by asphyxiation due to airway collapse or as a result of secondary bacterial infections. This form of leishmaniasis may represent a hypersensitivity phenomenon.

The major reservoir of infection for American leishmaniasis seems to be a large number of rodents inhabiting the forest regions of South America although, on occasion, animals such as dogs and opossums have been implicated. As with other leishmanial infections, the sandfly appears to be the vector in the spread of these organisms from animals to humans.

The diagnosis and treatment of mucocutaneous leishmaniasis are essentially the same as described for the cutaneous variety. However, the mucocutaneous type is somewhat unresponsive to therapy, and treatment with γ-interferon (γ-IFN) along with pentavalent antimony has been reported to increase success rates.

Visceral Leishmaniasis

Visceral leishmaniasis, caused by *Leishmania donovani,* is more commonly known by its Indian name of *kala-azar.* It is seen in the Near and Far East, southern Russia, the Mediterranean area, parts of Africa, and Central and South America.

Humans acquire the parasites from the bite of an

adult humans become infected with *Toxoplasma* either by ingesting undercooked meat that contains trophozoites or cysts of *T gondii,* or by ingesting sporulated oocysts in cat feces. It also is noteworthy that oocysts excreted by cats require 2 to 3 days to form spores and become infectious. Thus, transmission can be minimized by disposing of cat litter daily.

Diagnosis and Treatment

The inoculation of infected tissue into mice usually results in the intraperitoneal occurrence of intracellular proliferative trophozoites. This is rarely done, however; the usual diagnosis is based on serologic tests. One such test, the Sabin-Feldman dye exclusion test, requires living organisms of the genus *Toxoplasma* and is carried out by staining the parasites with alkaline methylene blue in the presence of the patient's serum. In the absence of specific antibodies, the organisms are stained by the dye. If antibodies are present, the dye is excluded from the organisms. Routinely, complement fixation and fluorescently-labeled antibodies are used as additional diagnostic aids. Both radioimmunoassays and enzyme-linked immunosorbent assays also are being developed for the serologic diagnosis of toxoplasmosis.

Experimental vaccines using *T gondii* strains of low human and animal pathogenicity have been used successfully to immunize cats, a procedure that would reduce infection of pregnant women and children. Such vaccines also could be used for livestock that transmit the parasite in their meat.

Treatment of toxoplasmosis with pyrimethamine in combination with trisulfapyrimidines or sulfadiazine is the best effective chemotherapy. However, these drugs do not eradicate the tissue cysts and, as a result, patients with AIDS must continue on lifelong suppressive therapy.

ISOSPOROSIS

Isospora belli causes an intestinal infection in humans that is characterized primarily by fever and diarrhea. The disease can be chronic, lasting for several decades, or it can be acute, particularly in immunosuppressed individuals and patients with AIDS.

The parasite is acquired by the ingestion of fecally contaminated food. Both asexual and sexual cycles take place within the human intestinal epithelial cells. During the sexual cycle, the male gamete fertilizes the female gamete, and the resulting zygote becomes enclosed within a wall, converting it to an oocyst. The oocyst is excreted in the feces and serves as the source of additional infections. It is thought that during chronic infections, the oocyst may form spores in the intestine, allowing additional cycles of sexual and asexual reproduction to continue.

A diagnosis usually is based on finding characteristic oocysts in the feces or observing the parasite in biopsy samples.

Numerous drugs are effective for the treatment of isosporosis, the most commonly used ones including sulfamethoxazole/trimethoprim and pyrimethamine plus sulfadiazine.

SARCOCYSTICOSIS

Members of the genus *Sarcocystis* require two separate hosts to complete their asexual and sexual reproductive cycles. For two species, humans are the final host and, hence, the source of continued infections. The intermediate hosts for these parasites are cattle (*Sarcocystis hominis*) and pigs (*Sarcocystis suihominis*).

Cattle and pigs acquire the infection by the ingestion of food contaminated with human feces that contain the oocysts of these parasites. Within the animal, the sporozoites are released and, after penetrating the intestinal epithelium, they enter the endothelial cells of blood vessels throughout the body. It is in these cells that the asexual reproduction involving schizonts and merozoites continues for several weeks. At that time, the parasite enters the muscles and becomes encysted.

Humans become infected by eating raw or undercooked beef or pork containing the encysted parasite. Within the human intestinal cells, the organisms differentiate into male and female gametes, which, after fertilization, mature into oocysts. The oocysts are passed in the feces and serve as a source of infection for cattle and pigs.

The disease in humans normally is mild or asymptomatic but can cause acute abdominal symptoms. The disease usually is self-limiting and can be prevented by properly disposing of human feces and by not eating undercooked pork or beef.

CRYPTOSPORIDIOSIS

Until the last decade, *Cryptosporidium* was thought to cause infections in animals or humans only rarely. It has now been established, however, that cryptosporidiosis is common in several newly born animals. It is particularly prevalent in calves aged 1 to 4 weeks, in which it causes a mild to severe diarrhea lasting an average of 7 days before spontaneous recovery. The disease also occurs in lambs and goats, as well as in many birds and wild animals.

The organism is a protozoan parasite, which is included in the class Sporozoa. Both the asexual and sexual reproductive cycles occur within a single host, and the sexually produced oocyst is passed in the feces to produce additional infections when ingested by a susceptible animal. Although there appears to be some host specificity, many isolates are able to infect and to cause diarrhea in a wide range of hosts.

It is becoming evident that human infections resulting in diarrhea and abdominal cramps may not be as rare as previously thought. In fact, cases of typical traveler's diarrhea in persons returning from Mexico have been ascribed to *Cryptosporidium*. Nosocomial infections also have occurred and, in 1987, a large community outbreak of cryptosporidiosis, involving an estimated 13,000 persons, was shown to be due to the contamination of a filtered public water supply. In 1993, the city of Milwaukee, Wisconsin had its water supply contaminated with *Cryptosporidium,* and it is estimated that 370,000 city residents experienced severe diarrhea, nausea, and stomach cramps. The source of this contamination is unproven, but may have resulted from a spring water runoff carrying contaminated animal feces into an overstressed treatment facility.

Many infections appear to be asymptomatic or are self-limiting, resulting in recovery within 1 to 10 days after the onset of symptoms. In immunocompromised patients, however, *Cryptosporidium* produces a severe, persistent diarrhea in which the patient can pass 3 to 17 L of watery stool per day. This manifestation is becoming more and more frequent in persons with AIDS and, in such patients, therapy has proved unsuccessful in preventing death. The source of most such infections in an urban setting is unknown, but rodents, kittens, and puppies are easily infected with human isolates of *Cryptosporidium* and may serve as a natural reservoir for this parasite. Human-to-human transmission also is probable, occurring through either direct or indirect contact with contaminated feces.

PNEUMOCYSTIS CARINII PNEUMONIA

Pneumocystis carinii appears to occupy a taxonomic niche in which it shares certain properties of both protozoa and fungi. Its protozoan classification was based on the amoeboid appearance of a small developmental form, the structure of its mitochondria, its insensitivity to amphotericin B, and the absence of growth in fungal media. The fungal classification considered the similarity of *Pneumocystis* spores to ascospores and its lack of invasive organelles as being more fungal than protozoan. Based on sequence data of its ribosomal RNA, the latter concept appears to be correct, but there is not yet agreement as to exactly where *Pneumocystis* belongs in the fungal taxonomic tree, although several reports show a close association with the Ascomycetes. For this edition, however, we shall leave it with the protozoa, confident that in the next revision, it will move to a definitive place in the chapter on mycology.

This parasite is found in a wide variety of animals, and it is responsible for a common infection in humans. Until recently, however, few people had even heard of *P carinii*, because the infection usually is mild or asymptomatic. As judged by their IgM–IgG levels, between 75% and 90% of healthy children experience a respiratory infection with *P carinii* by the age of 4 years. On rare occasions, though, this parasite is responsible for a severe and often fatal pneumonia in premature, malnourished infants.

These types of infections, however, are not responsible for the notoriety that *P carinii* has acquired during the past decade. Rather, it is the frequently fatal interstitial pneumonia it produces in immunosuppressed patients. Such infections are seen in persons with neoplastic disease or other disorders of the immune system, as well as in those undergoing immunosuppressive therapy after organ transplants. However, by far the most common victims of *P carinii* pneumonia are patients with AIDS; this infection has been documented in three fourths of these patients. Such cases are believed to result from the reactivation of a latent infection.

Diagnosis of *P carinii* pneumonia usually is accomplished by observation of the organism in lung biopsy samples. Examination of induced sputum with an indirect immunofluorescent stain using monoclonal antibodies also is effective in establishing a diagnosis. Patients are treated with either intravenous sulfamethoxazole/trimethoprim or intramuscular pentamidine; in spite of treatment, however, this infection carries about a 50% mortality rate in immunoincompetent patients.

Bibliography

JOURNALS

Adam RD. The biology of *Giardia* spp. Microbiol Rev 1991;55:706.

Bartlett MS, Smith JW. *Pneumocystis carinii,* an opportunist in immunocompromised patients. Clin Microbiol Rev 1991;4:137.

Bruckner DA. Amebiasis. Clin Microbiol Rev 1992;5:356.

Current WL, Garcia LS. Cryptosporidiosis. Clin Microbiol Rev 1991;4:325.

Edwards DD. Troubled waters in Milwaukee. ASM News 1993;59:342.

Grimaldi G Jr, Tesh RB. Leishmaniases of the new world: current concepts and implications for future research. Clin Microbiol Rev 1993;6:230.

Guerrant RL, Bobak DA. Medical progress: bacterial and protozoal gastroenteritis. N Engl J Med 1991;325:327.

Marciano-Cabral F. Biology of *Naegleria* spp. Microbiol Rev 1988;52:114.

Pomeroy C, Filice GA. Pulmonary toxoplasmosis: a review. Clin Infect Dis 1992;14:863.

Reed SL. Amebiasis: an update. Clin Infect Dis 1992;14:385.

Tanowitz HB, et al. Chagas' disease. Clin Microbiol Rev 1992;5:400.

Wolfe MS. Giardiasis. Clin Microbiol Rev 1992;5:93.

Wyler DJ. Malaria: overview and update. Clin Infect Dis 1993;16:449.

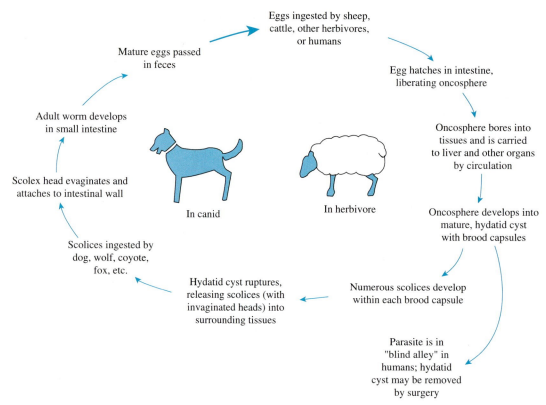

FIGURE 51-5   Life cycle of *Echinococcus granulosus.*

Hymenolepis nana

The definitive hosts for *Hymenolepis nana* are humans, mice, and rats, and no intermediate host is required. Humans are the major reservoir for this cestode, also known as the *dwarf tapeworm.* Infection with *H nana* is the most common tapeworm infection in the United States. Infection occurs under conditions of poor sanitation, usually by the direct transfer of fertilized eggs from hand to mouth. *H nana* also can develop in the grain beetle, and the ingestion of uncooked grain also provides a means of infection by this cestode. After reaching the intestine, the embryos hatch from the eggs, enter the mucosa, and develop into a larval stage, the cysticercoid. These larvae subsequently enter the intestinal lumen and develop into adult worms.

Symptoms routinely are limited to mild abdominal discomfort, unless the infection is heavy, in which case they can include abdominal pain, nausea, diarrhea, and headaches. The diagnosis is made by observing typical eggs in the feces. Niclosamide is used for chemotherapy.

EXTRAINTESTINAL INFECTIONS OF HUMANS BY CESTODES

Echinococcus granulosus

As described for *T solium,* a tapeworm infection in which the larvae are distributed throughout the body of the intermediate host causes symptoms different from those that occur in the definitive host when the adult worm is confined to the intestinal tract.

Humans can serve as hosts for several other larval cestodes in addition to *T solium,* but our discussion includes only one common species, *Echinococcus granulosus.* The usual intermediate hosts of this worm are sheep, cattle, and other herbivores. Humans almost always acquire the infection from dogs, although wolves, coyotes, and foxes also serve as definitive hosts.

After the ingested eggs hatch, the liberated larvae (oncospheres) penetrate the intestinal wall and are disseminated throughout the body through the lymphatics and the bloodstream. The liver is the organ most frequently infected, but the larvae also can settle in the lungs, kidneys, bone, or brain. Each larva forms a fluid-filled bladder—a *hydatid cyst*—that continues to increase in size and to form secondary interior cysts known as *brood capsules.* The primary and secondary cysts contain countless scoleces, and each scolex can develop into an adult worm when ingested by a dog. Rupture of the hydatid cyst can release thousands of scoleces into the surrounding tissues. Because of the highly allergenic nature of the cyst fluid, rupture of the cyst can result in a fatal anaphylactic reaction. The life cycle is summarized in Figure 51-5.

In humans, a single cyst usually develops, and it frequently impairs organ function by pressure on the surrounding tissues. An inflammation develops, mediated, in part, by a hypersensitivity response to the scoleces, and adjacent tissues either atrophy or undergo pressure necrosis.

The diagnosis of hydatid disease is commonly based on finding a tumor mass, usually in the liver, and a history of association with dogs in an endemic area. Radiographs may reveal a calcified cyst wall. The diagnosis can be confirmed by demonstrating brood capsules and scoleces in the fluid of the surgically removed cyst.

Most human cases of hydatid disease occur in grazing countries where an intimate association between humans and dogs is common, and the disease occasionally is seen in the United States, particularly in California. Infections follow a hand-to-mouth transfer of the eggs from contaminated soil or dog fur. Most drugs are ineffective as chemotherapy for hydatid disease, and treatment usually relies on surgical removal of the hydatid cyst. However, mebendazole has been used successfully to treat early disease. Control is directed at prevention of the infection in dogs; dogs should not be fed uncooked viscera from slaughtered animals. Dogs in endemic areas should be treated periodically with quinacrine (Atabrine) or niclosamide.

Trematodes

Trematodes also are referred to as *flukes*. Adult worms can vary in size from 1 mm to several centimeters, and all exhibit suckers used for attachment to host tissue.

Trematodes are of worldwide distribution, and each species is found in association with the specific species of snail required as its intermediate host. Most human infections, however, occur in the Far and Near East (particularly in areas with rice paddies), Africa, Latin America, and other tropical areas.

Comprehension of the epidemiology of trematode infections requires a general knowledge of the complex events that occur between the excretion of the egg of the definitive host and the formation of the final larval stage. During this period, five different larval forms occur (except in the blood flukes, which have only three):

1. The hatching of the egg usually occurs only in fresh water. Within the egg is formed a *miracidium,* a small, ciliated larva. The miracidium escapes from the egg and swims about until it finds a snail of the right species for its first intermediate host.
2. After finding the snail, the miracidium bores into the snail's tissues.
3. The larva then loses its cilia and undergoes a metamorphosis to form a long, tubular larva called a *sporocyst.*
4. The sporocyst migrates to the hepatic tissue of the snail, where it continues to form masses of germ cells within a sac-like structure. With the exception of certain flukes, such as schistosomes, the sporocyst then undergoes another morphologic change to become a more differentiated larva possessing a mouth and a rudimentary digestive tract. This stage is called a *redia.*
5. Within each redia, germ cells develop into more rediae, but eventually a final larval change occurs when *cercariae* begin to develop within the rediae. A cercaria resembles the adult worm, possessing suckers and a rudimentary digestive and excretory system. It also possesses a tail for locomotion after leaving the snail. The cercaria can infect a new intermediate host, which may be a freshwater fish, a crab, another snail, or aquatic vegetation. In many cases, after infection, the cercaria loses its tail and secretes a cyst wall around the larva. This cyst form is called a *metacercaria* and, except for the schistosomes, humans are infected *only* by the ingestion of metacercariae. These stages are reviewed in Figure 51-6.

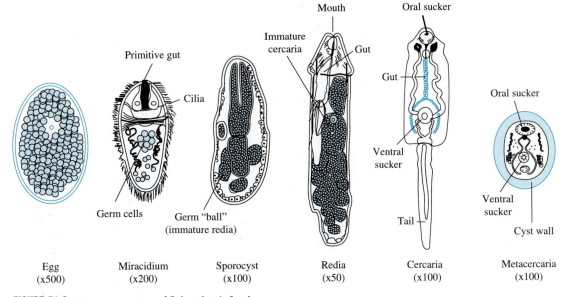

FIGURE 51-6 Immature stages of flukes that infect humans.

Egg (x500)   Miracidium (x200)   Sporocyst (x100)   Redia (x50)   Cercaria (x100)   Metacercaria (x100)

The life cycle of the schistosomes differs from that of most other trematodes in that they do not form rediae; the results of asexual reproduction within the sporocysts are motile cercariae. The cercariae of schistosomes do not encyst, but rather infect by burrowing directly through the unbroken skin of the definitive host.

We are now ready to consider the trematodes that infect humans. These parasites usually are divided into the intestinal flukes, the liver flukes, the lung flukes, and the blood flukes.

INTESTINAL FLUKES

Intestinal flukes are basically parasites of other animals, and humans become accidental hosts during the development of these flatworms.

Fasciolopsis buski

Fasciolopsis buski normally infects pigs in Southeast Asia, although the incidence of infection in humans can reach 100% in some areas. After leaving the snail, the cercariae attach themselves to various types of vegetation, where they develop into metacercariae. Humans become infected by eating contaminated plants such as water chestnuts, bamboo, and water hyacinths (Fig. 51-7).

The metacercariae evolve into adult worms that attach to the mucosa of the small intestine. Symptoms vary according to the degree of infection. In small children, heavy infections can be particularly severe, occasionally resulting in death. Diagnosis is confirmed by the presence of characteristic eggs in the feces. Praziquantel is effective for treatment.

Metagonimus yokogawai and Heterophyes heterophyes

The metacercariae of both *Metagonimus yokogawai* and *Heterophyes heterophyes* are formed under the scales of freshwater fish. Dogs and cats usually serve as the definitive hosts in Asia, and humans become infected by eating raw fish.

The adult worms attach to the mucosa of the small intestine, and symptoms usually are mild. Eggs occasionally are carried by the lymphatics to the heart or central nervous system, which can cause severe reactions. Praziquantel is the drug of choice for the treatment of these infections.

LIVER FLUKES

Flatworms that mature into adults in the bile ducts of the definitive host are commonly referred to as *liver flukes.* The World Health Organization estimates that as many as 20 million people are infected with these flukes.

Fasciola hepatica

Sheep and, to a lesser extent, cattle constitute the usual hosts for *Fasciola hepatica.* Human infections occur in many parts of the world, and cases have been reported from southern France, Algeria, Cuba, and the Latin American countries.

Fertilized eggs pass through the common bile duct into the intestinal tract. If they reach water that contains the appropriate snails, the miracidia will infect this intermediate host, and motile cercariae will be released at the end of larval development. The cercariae encyst on local

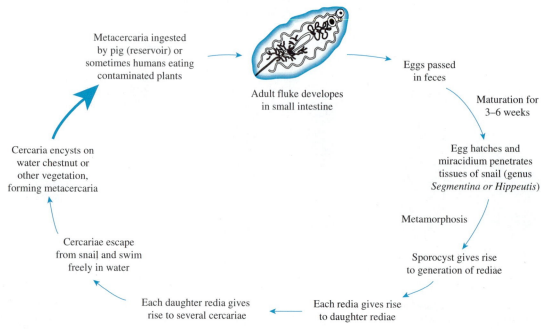

FIGURE 51-7   Life cycle of the intestinal fluke, *Fasciolopsis buski.*

vegetation (eg, grass or watercress) to form metacercariae. Sheep, cattle, and, occasionally, humans become the definitive hosts after the ingestion of metaceracariae on contaminated vegetation.

In the definitive host, the metacercariae penetrate the intestine and migrate from the peritoneal cavity to infect the liver parenchyma and, eventually, the bile ducts. There, they produce mechanical and toxic injuries, which, in severe infections, terminate with cirrhosis. Eggs entering the intestines from the common bile duct are passed and reinitiate the larval cycle.

Bithionol is the drug of choice for the treatment of infections caused by these liver flukes.

Clonorchis sinensis

Clonorchis sinensis, also known as *Chinese liver fluke,* exists primarily in the Far East. The intermediary larval stages in the snail are as described for trematodes in general; the definitive hosts (usually dogs and cats, but also humans) become infected from eating raw fish infected with the metacercariae (Fig. 51-8). The encysted metacercariae can survive for extended periods in dried, salted, or pickled freshwater fish.

Symptoms vary considerably, depending on the degree of infection. Light infections can be asymptomatic, whereas heavy and repeated ingestion of the larvae can cause abscesses and liver impairment.

Two other liver flukes that occasionally infect humans are *Opisthorchis felineus* and *Opisthorchis viverrini.* Cats and, to a lesser extent, dogs are the primary definitive hosts for the adult stage of these parasites.

Praziquantel is effective and widely used for the treatment of infections by *Clonorchis* and *Opisthorchis* species.

LUNG FLUKES

Paragonimus westermani

Paragonimus westermani causes a major disease, *Paragonimiasis,* in which the adult worm parasitizes the lungs. It is restricted to the Far East. Other species of *Paragonimus* are responsible for human infections in Africa and South America.

After leaving the snail, the cercariae infect crabs or crayfish (in which they become encysted) as second intermediate hosts. Humans are infected by eating raw or improperly cooked crabs or crayfish containing metacercariae (Fig. 51-9).

After ingestion, the cercariae leave the small intestine and migrate from the peritoneal cavity through the diaphragm into the bronchioles, where a fibrous capsule forms around the larva. After the development of the adult worm, the capsule ruptures into the bronchioles, releasing eggs, which are coughed up and expectorated or swallowed. In fresh water, the eggs hatch into miracidia, and infection of the appropriate snails starts the cycle over again.

Symptoms of paragonimiasis are lacking or restricted to occasional coughing up of rusty sputum, depending on the number of parasites in the lungs. The disease responds to the oral administration of bithionol. However, this drug can cause side effects such as rashes, nausea, diarrhea, headaches, and dizziness. It also can induce a contact dermatitis, and, because bithionol was at one time

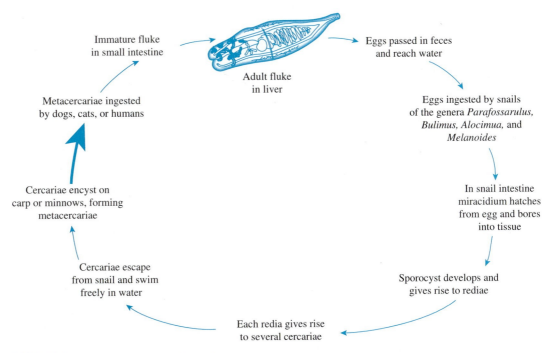

FIGURE 51-8 Life cycle of the liver fluke, *Clonorchis sinensis.*

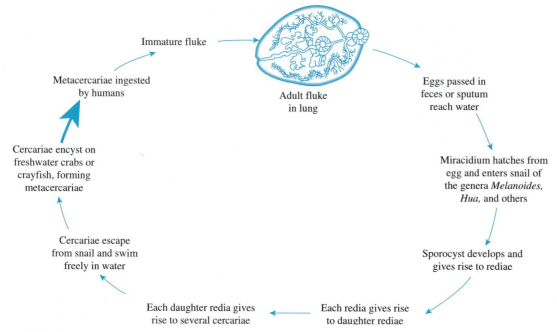

FIGURE 51-9   Life cycle of the lung fluke, *Paragonimus westermani.*

incorporated into several medicated soaps and shampoos, patients should be checked for hypersensitivity reactions before using this drug. Therapy for 2 days with oral praziquantel also appears to be effective and, at least in most situations, does not result in serious adverse reactions to the medication.

BLOOD FLUKES

The human *blood flukes* belonging to the genus *Schistosoma* infect 5% to 10% of the world's population. The life cycles of these parasites differ from those of the trematodes previously described in the following ways:

1. The adult worms are not hermaphroditic and exist as two separate sexes. The sexes can easily be differentiated, because the male worm is much larger than the female (Fig. 51-10).
2. Schistosomes do not require a secondary intermediate host and, hence, do not form metacercariae; animals, including humans, become infected by the *direct penetration of the cercariae through the skin.*

In general, after penetrating the skin, the cercariae migrate through the heart and the lungs, eventually reaching the intrahepatic part of the portal system. There, they mature and mate, after which (depending on the species) they migrate together to the mesenteric venules, where the fertilized eggs are deposited.

It is estimated that more than 200 million persons worldwide are infected with schistosomes, and perhaps as many as 400,000 cases of schistosomiasis exist in immigrants to the United States. However, the disease cannot be spread in the United States because of a lack of the specific snail intermediate host.

Human schistosomiasis occurs in three fairly distinct stages:

1. The invasion stage, unless overwhelming, usually is asymptomatic. This stage also includes the migration of the cercariae to the hepatic veins. (The cercariae are referred to as *schistosomula* after losing their tails following penetration.)
2. The acute stage occurs with the start of egg laying after the mature worms have migrated to the mesenteric veins. This stage is characterized by diarrhea, fe-

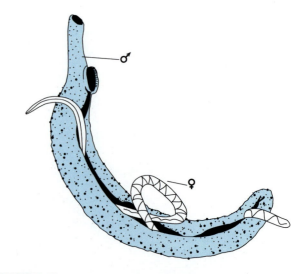

FIGURE 51-10   Adult schistosomes. The larger male is coupled with the slender female worm.

ver, malaise, and general discomfort. Most of the symptoms of this second stage appear to be due to a hypersensitivity reaction to the eggs.

3. The final stage is chronic and occurs as a tissue reaction to the eggs. Eggs are passed in the urine or feces, but they also are deposited in various organs of the body, particularly the liver. In these cases of deposition, a tissue reaction is manifested by walling off of the foreign material to form granulomas similar to the tubercles that occur in tuberculosis.

Three species of *Schistosoma* constitute the major causes of human schistosomiasis, namely, *Schistosoma mansoni*, *Schistosoma japonicum*, and *Schistosoma haematobium*. Each of these is tightly restricted to the genus of snail that it can use for its intermediate host. In addition, during the adult stage (a period that can last as long as 30 years), each species is located in a different area of the human body.

Schistosoma mansoni

S mansoni is found in Africa, as well as in South America, the West Indies, and Puerto Rico. In human infections, the parasites characteristically leave the liver, and the adult worms take up permanent residence in the inferior mesenteric veins of the large intestine. In this environment, they deposit eggs in the wall of the intestine; the eggs eventually break through the mucosa into the lumen and are passed with feces. After reaching fresh water, the eggs hatch, and, if the appropriate species of snail is present, the miracidia enter the intermediate host to become cercariae that will initiate a new cycle of human infection (Fig. 51-11).

Schistosoma japonicum

S japonicum occurs exclusively in the Far East, and its definitive hosts include horses, cattle, pigs, dogs, cats, rodents, and water buffalo, in addition to humans.

The life cycle and pathogenesis of *S japonicum* are as described for *S mansoni*. The final residence for the adult worms is found in the superior mesenteric veins of the small intestine. The eggs break through the wall into the lumen and are passed with the feces. *S japonicum* is the most prolific egg layer of the parasites causing human schistosomiasis, and it is common for the eggs to be carried to the liver and other organs of the body, including the central nervous system. As a result, both cirrhosis and brain lesions are more commonly associated with this species than with the other schistosomes.

Schistosoma haematobium

Large areas of Africa, the Nile River Valley, and the Near East are endemic for *S haematobium,* a predominantly human parasite. The adult worms characteristically migrate into the rectal vessels and eventually reach veins surrounding the bladder. Unlike the other schistosomes, the eggs of *S haematobium* penetrate the bladder mucosa and are passed in the urine. Ulceration of the bladder causes numerous small hemorrhages, and the passage of blood in the urine is common. In Egypt, this infection dates back to at least the year 2000 BC, and it is interesting that the hieroglyphic symbol for schistosomiasis is a penis dripping blood, a characteristic symptom of this disease.

Schistosoma Dermatitis

Individuals exposed to species of *Schistosoma* that infect humans usually experience itching within 1 hour after

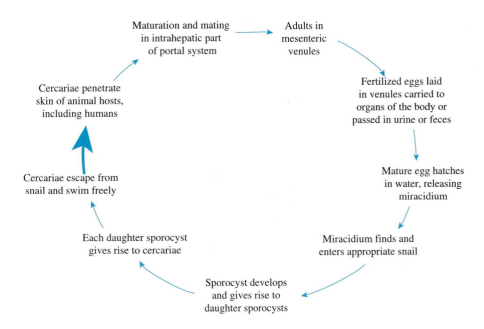

FIGURE 51-11 Life cycle of the blood flukes in the genus *Schistosoma*. Refer to the text for minor differences among species.

contact. This can persist as a rash and papular eruption that can take days to disappear. In the United States, however, a cercarial dermatitis called *swimmers' itch* is most often caused by nonhuman schistosomes. This is particularly true for lakes in the American Midwest, where duck schistosomes can cause a severe dermatitis, particularly in reinfected individuals. After penetration, the cercariae of duck schistosomes die in the skin, but their antigens induce a sensitization that is responsible for the dermatitis.

DIAGNOSIS, TREATMENT, AND CONTROL OF SCHISTOSOMAL INFECTIONS. The diagnosis of all schistosomal infections is based on a history of exposure to an endemic area and on the finding of eggs in the urine or stools of the infected person.

Praziquantel has supplanted all other drugs for the treatment of schistosomiasis, because it is effective in a single day when administered orally. Side effects are frequent, but mild and transient. In endemic areas, however, reinfection is an almost inevitable event.

Efforts to control schistosomal infections (estimated by the World Health Organization to be second only to malaria as a cause of morbidity and mortality in the tropics) are directed toward the elimination of the snails that act as intermediate hosts and the protection of water from human fecal contamination. Several chemicals, such as copper sulfate, can be used to kill snails, but the migration of snails from untreated areas frequently neutralizes this method of control. In the Far East, the task is complicated further by the common use of human feces as a primary source of fertilizer. It would seem that a major hope for controlling schistosomiasis lies in a program of education designed to teach methods for the sanitary disposal of feces and urine; however, such programs alone have not been effective.

It is noteworthy that the immune system appears to be inefficient in combating an active schistosomal infection. A ready explanation for this immunologic impotence is obscure, but there are reports that the worms coat themselves with blood group and histocompatibility antigens to prevent recognition by the immune system. This does not seem to be the whole story, however, and other investigators have reported that the schistosomes secrete one or more small peptides that inhibit T-cell activation. In spite of these observations, human volunteer studies indicate that some individuals do appear to acquire some immunity to reinfection, and considerable research has been directed toward the identification and isolation of specific antigens from the worms that could serve as a vaccine. Toward this end, various *Schistosoma* genes have been cloned into *Escherichia coli* and the recombinant proteins used as experimental vaccines in animals. Initial results indicate that several cell types and different antibody classes may be involved in a multifactorial immunity to this parasite. For example, Andre Capion and his colleagues at Lille, France, successfully immunized rats and hamsters with a 25-kilodalton recombinant schistosomal protein. In this case, immunity appeared to be caused primarily by IgE antibodies and eosinophils. Others, using purified surface antigens isolated from adult schistosomes, also have demonstrated some induced immunity in experimental animals. Thus, although an effective vaccine probably is some years away, there is some hope for its eventual use.

ASCHELMINTHES

Nematodes

Nematodes are round, elongated worms; the sexes are separate and, unlike the flatworms, adult nematodes possess complete digestive systems that include both a mouth and an anus (Fig. 51-12). Human infections caused by these roundworms usually are divided into two large categories: the *intestinal roundworms* and the *blood and tissue roundworms*.

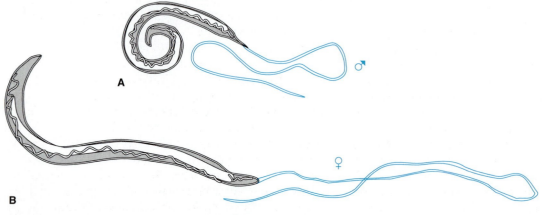

FIGURE 51-12   The nematode *Trichuris trichiura*. **A.** Male. **B.** Female.

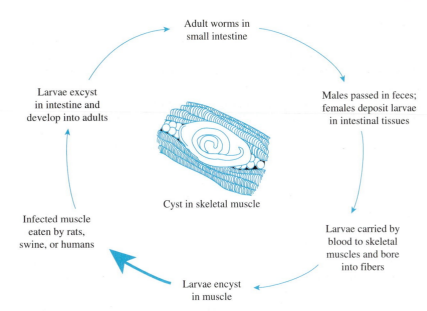

FIGURE 51-13 Life cycle of *Trichinella spiralis*.

INTESTINAL NEMATODE INFECTIONS IN HUMANS

Roundworms that exist in the intestine during their adult stage generally are categorized as intestinal nematodes. However, the larval stages of some intestinal species can be widely distributed throughout the body of an infected person.

Trichinella spiralis

Trichinella spiralis is the etiologic agent of *trichinosis* (also called *trichinellosis*), a disease disseminated in carnivorous animals. Human infections occur worldwide, and as recently as the 1930s, the incidence of the disease in the United States was estimated to include 20% of the population (control measures have now reduced this to about 4%). Most human infections result from the ingestion of improperly cooked pork containing the *encysted larvae;* however, bears, walruses, and other wild game also are responsible for many infections. After ingestion, the cysts reach the intestine, where larvae are liberated and develop into adult worms. After copulation, the male worms are passed in the feces, and the females penetrate the intestinal mucosa, where they produce as many as 1500 larvae over a period of 1 to 3 months. The larvae enter the bloodstream, primarily through the lymphatics, after which they penetrate the skeletal muscles and become encysted (Fig. 51-13).

As with many helminthic infections, the symptoms depend in large part on the magnitude of the initial infection. Light infections normally are asymptomatic, but the ingestion of large numbers of encysted larvae can cause a severe disease culminating in the death of the patient. Initial symptoms, occurring within 4 to 14 days after infection and resulting from the intestinal activities of the adult worms, characteristically include diarrhea, malaise, and fever. This stage can be mild to severe but persists for only about 1 week, and it frequently is attributed to the "flu." The second stage of the infection, involving the migration of the larvae into skeletal muscle, begins about 1 week after the initial infection, and in cases of moderate to heavy infection, muscle pain throughout the body can be significant. Moreover, although encystment occurs only in muscle, the larvae can infect other organs of the body, including the lungs, heart, eyelids, meninges, and brain. Myocarditis is the most common cardiac lesion, leading to arrhythmias and congestive heart failure. Massive invasion of any of these organs can result in death during the early weeks of the infection. The usual pathogenic effects, however, result from the destruction of striated muscle fibers and occur during the encystment and subsequent calcification of the larval cysts.

Barring reinfection, major symptoms subside in several months, but weakness, rheumatic pain, and loss of dexterity can persist for long periods.

Several laboratory tests are available for the diagnosis of trichinosis, but the only definitive one is observation of the larvae or larval cysts in biopsy samples of infected muscles. Complement fixation and a skin reaction using an antigen prepared from *Trichinella* are used to support a tentative diagnosis.

Thiabendazole appears to be effective against the intestinal phase of this parasite, but its efficacy against larvae in muscles is not clearly established. In addition, this drug is associated with a high incidence of allergic reactions. Mebendazole has a lethal effect in experimentally infected animals and has been reported to be effective for the treatment of human trichinosis. In severe cases, steroids are given to lessen the extent of inflammation and to provide symptomatic relief. Because the ingestion of undercooked infected meat is the only mechanism of infection, it would seem possible to eliminate this disease from domestic animals. However, an important reservoir for *T spiralis* occurs in cannibalistic brown and black rats, and it is essentially impossible to control completely this source of infection for pigs. Laws requiring the sterilization of garbage used for feeding hogs are in force throughout the United States, and such measures, coupled with the thorough cooking of pork (or freezing, which also destroys the encysted larvae), have done much to decrease the incidence of trichinosis.

In many countries of Western Europe, each slaughtered pig is checked individually for the presence of *Trichinella*. This requires a microscopic examination of the pork muscle, and the expense involved undoubtedly has been an influence in the lack of such inspection in the United States. More recently, a serologic test has been described in which pig serum is added to ELISA wells that have been coated with *Trichinella* antigens. This simple assay is reported to be 100% accurate in detecting *Trichinella*-infected pigs, and it is hoped that its adoption will lead to certified *Trichinella*-free pork in the United States. Such a procedure would remove the ban on the sale of American pork to many European countries.

Trichuris trichiura

Trichuriasis, also known as *whipworm disease* because of its resemblance to a buggy whip, is caused by the nematode *Trichuris trichiura*. This disease occurs extensively in the tropics and occasionally in lower socioeconomic areas in the southern United States. It is a disease associated with filth and is seen primarily in children. Its prevalence is indicated by the estimate that between 500 and 800 million persons are infected with this nematode.

The adult worm lives mainly in the human cecum attached to the intestinal mucosa, where it produces 1000 or more eggs per day for 6 to 8 years. The eggs are passed in the feces, and in a moist, warm environment, infective larvae develop within the eggs in 3 to 6 weeks. Ingestion of the *mature eggs,* either directly from the soil or through contaminated food and water, initiates a new cycle during which the larvae develop into mature adults in the cecum (Fig. 51-14).

Heavy infections usually are accompanied by chronic diarrhea. Abdominal pain, vomiting, constipation, headache, and anemia also can accompany whipworm infections.

Observation of the barrel-shaped eggs in the feces provides a definitive diagnosis for trichuriasis. Adult worms rarely are seen in the feces, because they normally remain attached to the intestinal mucosa. By proctoscopy, heavy infections of worms can be observed attached to the rectal mucosa.

The drug mebendazole is an effective treatment when given orally for several days. Enemas containing hexylresorcinol previously were used to treat heavy infections. The major effective control measures are those directed toward the sanitary disposal of human feces. Secondary measures involve thorough sanitary procedures such as the washing of hands before meals and the complete cleansing of uncooked vegetables before consumption.

Ascaris lumbricoides

Ascaris lumbricoides can attain a length of 20 to 30 cm and is the largest nematode that infects humans. It occurs most frequently in young children in the tropics and, to a lesser extent, in certain areas of the southern United States. It is estimated that more than 900 million persons are infected, and that about 1 million of these live in

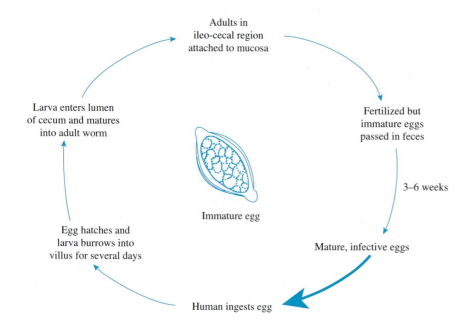

Adults in
ileo-cecal region
attached to mucosa

Larva enters lumen
of cecum and matures
into adult worm

Fertilized but
immature eggs
passed in feces

Immature egg

3–6 weeks

Egg hatches and
larva burrows into
villus for several days

Mature, infective eggs

Human ingests egg

FIGURE 51-14   Life cycle of *Trichuris trichiura.*

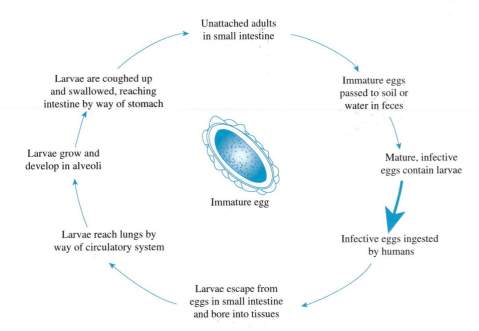

Unattached adults
in small intestine

Larvae are coughed up
and swallowed, reaching
intestine by way of stomach

Immature eggs
passed to soil or
water in feces

Larvae grow and
develop in alveoli

Immature egg

Mature, infective
eggs contain larvae

Larvae reach lungs by
way of circulatory system

Infective eggs ingested
by humans

FIGURE 51-15 Life cycle of *Ascaris lumbricoides.*

Larvae escape from
eggs in small intestine
and bore into tissues

the mountainous regions of the southern United States. Moreover, *Ascaris,* along with *Trichuris,* is the most common intestinal parasite found in immigrants to the United States from Southeast Asia.

Second-stage larvae develop within the eggs while in the soil, and humans are infected through the ingestion of the infective eggs (Fig. 51-15). After reaching the intestine, the larvae hatch, penetrate the intestinal mucosa, and (after being picked up in the portal circulation and passed through the heart and liver) eventually reach the lungs. There, they undergo additional differentiation and are coughed up, swallowed, and returned to the intestine.

Adult worms remain unattached in the small intestine, and, in the absence of a heavy infection, symptoms are mild or absent. Heavier infections cause abdominal pain, and complications occasionally occur as a result of invasion of the liver, bile ducts, gallbladder, and appendix by adult worms. Hypersensitivity reactions occurring during the pulmonary migration of larvae in subsequent infections can result in an asthma-like condition known as *Loeffler's syndrome.*

Because the adult female is capable of producing more than 20 million eggs at the rate of 200,000 per day, not many females are needed to cause the excretion of large numbers of *Ascaris* eggs. The primary technique used in the diagnosis of ascariasis is visualization and identification of the eggs voided in the feces.

Mebendazole is the treatment of choice; however, piperazine citrate also is effective, as well as inexpensive and relatively nontoxic to the host. In addition, cyclobendazole appears to be effective for the treatment of *Ascaris* infections. As with parasitic infections in which humans

are the major reservoir, control depends on the sanitary disposal of human feces.

Enterobius vermicularis

Humans are the only known host of *Enterobius vermicularis* or, as the organisms are frequently called, *pinworms.* Contrary to popular belief, dogs and cats do not carry this human parasite.

Humans, often children, become infected by the ingestion of the fertilized *eggs.* The adult worms live and copulate in the cecum. When gravid, the female migrates to the anus, where she deposits her eggs in the perianal area, usually at night. On rare occasions, such eggs gain reentry into the intestine, but infections ordinarily result from the ingestion of fertilized eggs. Their presence in the anal area causes an intense itching; the subsequent scratching contaminates the hands, leading to reinfection through hand-to-mouth contact or through the contamination of materials such as food, drink, bed linen, and towels, where the eggs can survive for weeks. Most infections are asymptomatic and, barring reinfection, a cure is spontaneous after all the females have died. There have been moderately rare instances in which the worms have migrated up the vagina and become encapsulated in the fallopian tubes. Such infections can result in a chronic salpingitis and sterility. A schematic cycle is shown in Figure 51-16.

Because eggs are not deposited in the feces, a diagnosis is made by recovering eggs from the perianal skin. If a piece of adhesive tape looped over a microscope slide is pressed firmly into the anal area, the eggs will attach and be visible when the tape is examined under the micro-

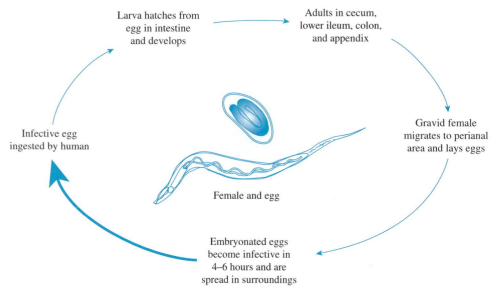

Larva hatches from
egg in intestine
and develops

Adults in cecum,
lower ileum, colon,
and appendix

Infective egg
ingested by human

Gravid female
migrates to perianal
area and lays eggs

Female and egg

Embryonated eggs
become infective in
4–6 hours and are
spread in surroundings

FIGURE 51-16   Life cycle of the pinworm, *Enterobius vermicularis.*

scope. In addition, examination of the anus during periods of intense itching—usually occurring shortly after retiring for the night—frequently reveals the presence of adult female worms.

Several therapeutic drugs can be used to treat pinworm infections. A single dose of pyrantel pamoate (Antiminth) or mebendazole ordinarily is effective. Treatment should be repeated after 2 weeks. If scratching and subsequent reinfection can be prevented, spontaneous recovery normally occurs after several months.

Strongyloides stercoralis

Strongyloides stercoralis is unique among nematodes in that it is capable of having a free-living generation and a parasitic generation, as shown in Figure 51-17. The parasites exist worldwide but are most commonly found in tropical climates that provide a warm, damp environment for the free-living stage of the parasite.

In most cases, the infective larvae in the soil enter humans by penetration of the skin (direct cycle). They then pass through the heart by way of the venous circulation, eventually reaching the lungs. After penetration of the alveoli, the larvae are coughed up, are swallowed, and gain entrance to the mucosa of the small intestine, where they develop into adult parthenogenetic females. The progeny of these worms pass in the feces as first-stage larvae (*rhabditiform*), which then develop into infective *filariform* larvae.

In other cases, it appears that larvae in the soil can develop into adult males and females that copulate and produce fertilized eggs (indirect cycle). Larvae infective for humans can develop in the soil from these eggs. This cycle requires a suitably warm, moist environment.

In still a third life cycle, called *internal autoinfection,*

the larvae undergo partial development to form filariform larvae in the intestine. The filariform larvae then penetrate the intestinal mucosa to enter the venous circulation, complete the entire developmental cycle in the lungs, and are coughed up and swallowed again, reaching the intestine without leaving the host. The extent of this autoinfection generally is thought to be controlled by the host's cell-mediated immunity. Infected persons who are taking corticosteroids frequently experience increasing numbers of autoinfective larvae, which can result in a fatal *disseminated strongyloidiasis.* Because other causes of immunosuppression do not appear to result in a disseminated strongyloidiasis, however, Dr. Robert Genta of Baylor College of Medicine has proposed that it is the corticosteroids themselves that induce the hyperinfection and the dissemination of the larvae.

Most infections are light and asymptomatic, but vomiting and diarrhea can occur. Heavy infections can cause anemia, weight loss, and chronic diarrhea. Fatal cases seem to follow extensive dissemination of the larvae throughout the body as a result of massive autoinfection. Persistent infections lasting more than 40 years have been reported in previous prisoners of war who worked on the Burma–Thailand railroad during World War II. Interestingly, many such persons had only minor gastrointestinal symptoms, but some experienced a creeping skin eruption or recurrent urticaria that varied in frequency from once a year to almost daily eruptions. The mechanism of the cutaneous symptoms is unknown.

Observation of the larvae in freshly passed stools provides the most definite diagnosis. Because the larvae can exist in extremely small numbers, special techniques (eg, examination of duodenal fluid) often are necessary for detection. Even then, it is difficult to diagnose chronic strongyloidiasis. A serologic procedure using filariform

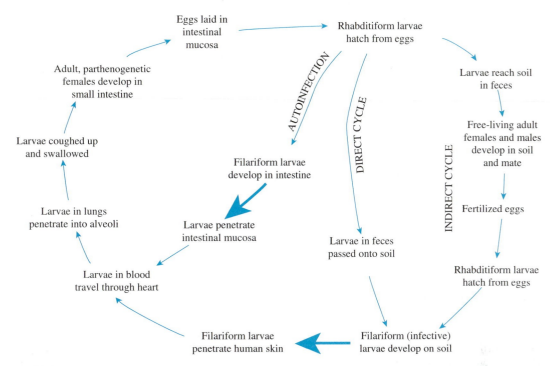

FIGURE 51-17 Life cycle of *Strongyloides stercoralis*, and some ways in which humans can become infected.

larvae as an antigen in an ELISA also has been used to verify a diagnosis. Thiabendazole is the treatment of choice. Because contaminated human feces are the major source of infection, the only effective control is the sanitary disposal of human sewage.

Necator americanus and Ancylostoma duodenale

Necator americanus and *Ancylostoma duodenale* are the major etiologic agents of *human hookworm disease*. Their life cycles differ only in that a pulmonary migration and development in the lungs is an obligatory requirement for *N americanus*, whereas some species of *Ancylostoma* can bypass this stage in their life cycle. However, neither the larval stages nor the eggs can be differentiated, and, because treatment and control are similar, it usually is not necessary to complete a diagnosis beyond determining that a hookworm infection exists.

Both species are widespread in tropical areas, but *A duodenale* also occurs extensively in Europe. On the other hand, *N americanus* was brought from Africa by slaves, and it is now the major hookworm species in the United States. As a result, infections by *A duodenale* sometimes are referred to as Old World hookworm, whereas those caused by *N americanus* are called New World hookworm.

As shown in Figure 51-18, the eggs of both species are passed in the feces and hatch into first-stage larvae (rhabditiform) that feed on bacteria and vegetation in the soil. After 5 days, they become longer, more slender forms called filariform larvae. The filariform larvae gain access

to the host by penetrating the skin, usually on the foot or between the toes. The larvae migrate through the blood to the lungs, where they break through the alveoli and are coughed up and swallowed. The adults reside in the small intestine attached to the mucosa. Unlike *N americanus, A duodenale* can infect the host orally as well as by skin penetration.

Symptoms of hookworm disease can be mild, although the simultaneous passage of many larvae through the lungs can cause headaches, fever, and nausea, and can result in the production of sputum containing blood. The primary intestinal symptoms are diarrhea, vomiting, and fever. Heavy infection causes significant anemia through the loss of blood from the intestine because of the feeding activities of the worms. There also is a clear correlation between hookworm infection and impairments in growth and physical fitness in children.

Another manifestation of hookworm disease is known as *creeping eruption* or *cutaneous larva migrans*. This cutaneous infection can be caused by the larva of several different hookworms, but the most common cause in the United States is *Ancylostoma braziliense*, a hookworm of dogs and cats. This infection can become extensive, involving large areas of the skin, but dog and cat larvae do not mature to adult nematodes in humans.

Recovery and identification of eggs from voided feces provides the only definitive diagnosis. Because anemia is a prominent feature of heavy infections, treatment with iron, vitamins, and a high-protein diet frequently alleviates the symptoms. Pyrantel pamoate and mebendazole are the drugs of choice, although tetrachlorethylene is an

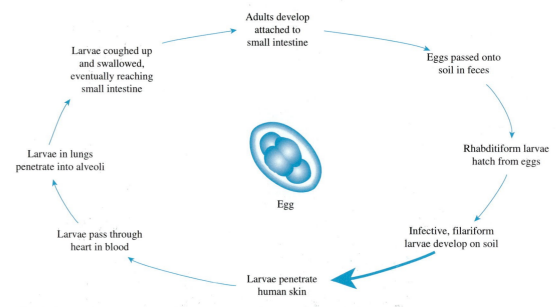

Egg

FIGURE 51-18 Life cycle of the hookworms, *Necator americanus* and *Ancylostoma duodenale*.

effective drug for *Necator* and has been used for many years. Control requires the sanitary disposal of human feces, plus protection from infection by means such as wearing shoes in endemic areas.

BLOOD AND TISSUE NEMATODE INFECTIONS IN HUMANS

Unlike intestinal roundworm infections, nematodes infecting blood and tissue are not spread through fecal contamination. Most of the latter parasites are carried from human to human by the bite of an arthropod vector.

With one exception, the worms discussed in this section belong to the superfamily *Filarioidea,* and a resulting human infection is called *filariasis.* Adult worms generally range from 2 to 30 cm in length, with the female being about twice the size of the male. One property distinguishing the filariae from other nematodes is that the female does not lay eggs, but instead gives birth to prelarval forms called *microfilariae.* The ingestion of the microfilariae by blood-sucking insect vectors provides for the transmission of filariae from one person to another.

Based on the habitat of the adult worms, these parasites can be divided into two major groups: (1) the lymphatic group, which includes *Wuchereria bancrofti* and *Brugia malayi;* and (2) the cutaneous group, which includes *Loa loa* and *Onchocerca volvulus. Dracunculus medinensis* does not belong to the family Filarioidea, but is included here because of its morphologic similarity to the filariae.

Wuchereria bancrofti

Bancroft's filariasis (a cause of *elephantiasis*) is seen extensively in the Pacific islands, as well as in much of Africa. Sporadic cases occur in European countries bordering the Mediterranean Sea, and the disease also is found scattered throughout the Near and Far East and in Central and South America.

W bancrofti is transmitted to humans through the bite of an infected mosquito—a species of *Culex, Aedes,* or *Anopheles* (Fig. 51-19). However, the mosquito provides more than a mere mechanical vector for transmission; the ingested microfilariae must undergo transformation within the mosquito to form larvae infective for the definitive host, that is, humans. This development requires about 10 days, after which time infective larvae enter the proboscis of the mosquito and are transmitted to a human during the next blood meal.

Within humans, the larvae enter the lymphatic vessels and nodes, where they develop into adult worms during the ensuing 6 months. The worms appear to infect preferentially the lymphatics of the lower extremities, and pathologic changes occur most frequently in the groin and genital areas. Once the worms are ensconced, mating occurs, and the resulting microfilariae migrate through the walls of the lymphatics into the adjacent blood vessels.

Symptoms result from the presence of the adult worms in the lymphatics, but light infections often go unnoticed, with the only physical signs being slightly enlarged lymph nodes, particularly in the groin. However, in endemic areas where frequent exposure occurs, attacks are characterized by fever, chills, vomiting, malaise, and tender, swollen lymph nodes. Such attacks last several days and can result in the formation of draining ulcers in the lymph nodes or along the lymphatic vessels. Surprisingly, the major symptoms seem to be the result of a hypersensitivity reaction directed against antigens present in the adult worms. In rare cases, multiple exposure to the filariae results in the proliferation of fibrous tissue around the dead worms, leading to an obstruction of

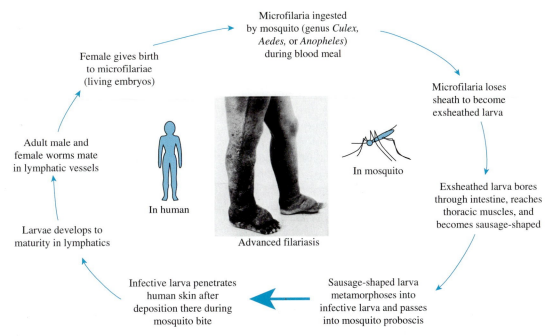

Female gives birth to microfilariae (living embryos)

Microfilaria ingested by mosquito (genus *Culex, Aedes,* or *Anopheles*) during blood meal

Microfilaria loses sheath to become exsheathed larva

Adult male and female worms mate in lymphatic vessels

In mosquito

Exsheathed larva bores through intestine, reaches thoracic muscles, and becomes sausage-shaped

In human

Advanced filariasis

Larvae develops to maturity in lymphatics

Infective larva penetrates human skin after deposition there during mosquito bite

Sausage-shaped larva metamorphoses into infective larva and passes into mosquito proboscis

FIGURE 51-19 Life cycle of *Wuchereria bancrofti*. The photograph demonstrates an advanced case of filariasis caused by blockage of the lymphatics in both legs of a child by this parasite.

lymphatic flow and causing extensive edema (swelling due to the accumulation of fluid) in the legs, scrotum, female genitalia, or breasts. This obstructive filariasis, more commonly called elephantiasis (see Fig. 51-19), is rare, even in endemic areas, and occurs only after repeated infections and many years of chronic filariasis.

The physical signs of inflamed lymph vessels (lymphangitis), swollen, tender lymph nodes (lymphadenitis), and edema of the extremities, genitalia, or breasts (elephantiasis) occurring in an endemic area are sufficient to make a tentative diagnosis of chronic filariasis. However, an unequivocal diagnosis requires observation of the microfilariae in the blood. This can prove difficult for two reasons: (1) few microfilariae are present during the chronic stage, and (2) with the exception of the South Pacific strain, the microfilariae show a definite periodicity in which few are present in the blood during daylight hours while the patient is active, but large numbers can be found during the night. This nocturnal periodicity is not fully understood, but it could be influenced by an increased partial pressure of oxygen in the lungs during normal activity. This phenomenon necessitates collection of blood samples between 10:00 PM and 2:00 AM. A monoclonal antibody-based enzyme immunoassay for detecting soluble parasite antigen in the sera of infected persons has been reported to be a sensitive, specific, and practical test for detecting active *W bancrofti* infections. Diethylcarbamazine (Hetrazan) kills the microfilariae of *W bancrofti* but is not always effective in eliminating adult worms. Antihistamines and corticosteroids are used to decrease hypersensitivity reactions. Advanced cases of ele-

phantiasis, however, usually require surgery to control lymphatic obstructions. This may require removal of an enlarged scrotum or anastomosis (joining together) of the deep and superficial lymphatics in the legs.

Efforts to control *W bancrofti* can be directed toward two vulnerable stages in the life cycle of filariae: (1) the elimination of the mosquito, as was achieved against yellow fever; and (2) the mass administration of diethylcarbamazine to all persons within an endemic region. The latter procedure destroys the microfilariae and has proved successful in several isolated island areas, such as the Virgin Islands and Tahiti.

Brugia malayi

B malayi, the etiologic agent of *Malayan filariasis,* differs slightly in morphology from *W bancrofti* but shares many life cycle characteristics. In addition, the clinical and pathologic features of Malayan filariasis are similar to those described for the bancroftian variety. The Malay Peninsula is one of the major endemic areas of this disease, although the parasites also are seen in India, Vietnam, Indonesia, Thailand, and Ceylon. The microfilariae can develop in the same mosquito species as *W bancrofti,* but the principal mosquito vector for *B malayi* is a mosquito belonging to the genus *Mansonia.* Unlike *W bancrofti,* for which humans are the only known reservoir, *B malayi* has been found in monkeys, dogs, and cats, and it is assumed that many mammalian hosts can serve as reservoirs for this nematode.

Laboratory diagnosis requires visualization of the microfilariae in a blood smear. As described for *W bancrofti*, microfilariae from most strains also exhibit a nocturnal periodicity, but some strains have been reported to lack this feature.

Treatment and control of this parasite involve essentially the same procedures as for the bancroftian variety. The major vectors, mosquitoes of the genus *Mansonia*, breed in ponds heavily populated with the water plant *Pistia stratiotes*, an essential component of the life cycle of these mosquitoes. As a result, herbicides such as sodium methyl chlorphenoxyacetate provide effective control.

Brugia timori causes a similar lymphatic filariasis, but this parasite is restricted to parts of Indonesia.

Loa loa

The scientific designation of *L loa* for this species of nematode is derived from its African name. It is found only in Africa, and a common name is the *African eye worm*.

The transmission of *loiasis*, the disease resulting from an infection of *L loa*, is much the same as with diseases from other filarial parasites, except that in this case, the vector is one of several species of mango or deer flies (genus *Chrysops*). The microfilariae undergo development within the fly and are transmitted to humans through the bite of an infected fly. Monkeys and humans appear to be the only definitive hosts.

After infection, the larvae develop into adult worms, which migrate throughout the subcutaneous tissues of the definitive host. The infection generally is asymptomatic, although occasional inflammatory reactions known as *Calabar swellings* occur at irregular intervals. These swellings are thought to result from hypersensitivity reactions and normally disappear within a week. The disquieting and somewhat painful manifestation of a *Loa* infection occurs when adult worms migrate into the facial area. There, they frequently can be seen (and removed) as they pass over the bridge of the nose or migrate through the subconjunctival tissue of the eye. Untreated, the infection can last for many years without major apparent damage to the host. Chronic loiasis sometimes results in an allergic dermatitis in which abscesses can form after secondary bacterial infections.

The occurrence of Calabar swellings in an endemic zone suggests an *L loa* infection; however, a definitive diagnosis of loiasis is based on finding the microfilariae in the blood or observing the adult worms beneath the conjunctiva. The oral administration of diethylcarbamazine is effective in eliminating adult worms and microfilariae. The worms also can be removed surgically, but because chemotherapy is effectual, this procedure probably is unwarranted.

Prevention of infection is directed at eliminating the carriers by mass treatment with diethylcarbamazine in endemic regions; nets, screens, and repellents also are used to ward off infected flies.

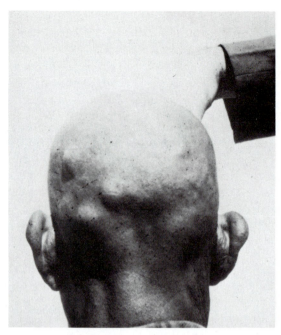

FIGURE 51-20   Skin nodules containing the filarial parasite *Onchocerca volvulus*.

Onchocerca volvulus

Most infections by *O volvulus* are found in Central Africa, but they also occur in restricted areas of Central America and northern South America. Larvae are transmitted to humans through the bites of infected black flies (genus *Simulium*). The adult worms occur in the subcutaneous tissue of the definitive host. There, the male and female worms routinely become enclosed in fibrous capsules that can be seen grossly as small nodules under the skin (Fig. 51-20).

Microfilariae migrate from the capsules and move throughout the dermis and connective tissue; these microfilariae induce the major pathologic lesions of *onchocerciasis*. The most serious lesions occur after migration of the microfilariae into the eyes. Ocular lesions can be caused, in part, by toxic products, but it generally is thought that the chief destructive changes are the effect of allergic reactions to the invading microfilariae. The severity of the damage can be emphasized by statistics obtained from some endemic regions of Africa, which reveal that about 20 million people in the developing world are infected, and 500,000 of these become permanently blinded each year as a result of onchocerciasis. The prevalence of infection in some hyperendemic areas is virtually 100%, and by the age of 50 years, about 40% of such individuals are blinded. Because rivers and streams provide the breeding areas for the black fly vectors of onchocerciasis, the disease frequently is referred to as *river blindness*.

Skin inflammation also is a frequent manifestation of this disease. *Onchocerca* dermatitis, which is the result of an allergic reaction to the microfilariae in the skin, can be seen (after long-established, chronic disease) as thick, wrinkled, hyperpigmented skin. In extreme cases, a sac of pelvic tissue hangs down to the knees because of loss of elasticity in the skin. However, this elephantiasis is not the result of lymphatic obstruction, as described for bancroftian elephantiasis.

The appearance of characteristic skin nodules in endemic areas is highly suggestive of onchocerciasis, but a definitive laboratory diagnosis requires detection of the microfilariae. Because they do not occur in the blood, skin biopsy samples or superficial snips of the skin can be examined for the presence of microfilariae. More recently, a serologic diagnosis has become available using a cloned antigen designated OV-16.

It now appears possible to rid the world of this disease. Merck and Company has developed a drug termed *mectizan*, a derivative of another drug called *ivermectin*. Two doses per year provide protection with minimal side effects. Mectizan kills the microfilariae in the body and prevents the adults worms from producing new microfilariae. Thus, if an entire population can be treated for a period of about 10 years, all adult worms should have died and the disease eliminated from the world.

To make this possible, Merck and Company has offered the drug free to developing countries. The World Health Organization, along with a review committee set up by Merck, will establish distribution and reporting systems. It now seems possible that, if appropriate antiparasitic drugs can be developed, all the filarial diseases in which humans comprise the sole definitive host can be eliminated.

Prevention of infection is directed toward elimination of the disease in humans (the only definitive host from which the vector, the intermediate host, becomes infected with the microfilariae) and eradication of the vector itself. The latter procedure involves the addition of insecticides to local waters to destroy the aquatic developmental stages of the black flies.

Dracunculus medinensis

D medinensis, known as the *guinea worm,* is believed to be the "fiery serpent" that, according to the Old Testament, infected the Israelites during one of their earlier ventures into the Sinai Peninsula. This nematode is found in Africa and large areas of Asia, and it is estimated that about 48 million persons are infected. In the past, these worms have been observed in the West Indian islands and in Brazil, but they are no longer believed to cause human disease in the Western Hemisphere.

Unlike other nematode infections of blood and tissue, guinea worm infections are acquired by drinking water that contains the intermediate host for this parasite, *infected copepods* (minute freshwater and marine crustaceans). When a person digests the copepods, the ingested larvae penetrate the intestinal wall and move through the

A Closer Look

Inasmuch as there are no known animal reservoirs, a global eradication plan for dracunculiasis (guinea worm disease) was proposed in 1980. Like the eradication of smallpox, however, such a campaign requires incredible effort to locate each village in India, Pakistan, and the 17 African countries where dracunculiasis occurs. This is particularly challenging because most infections occur in remote rural villages where travel is exceedingly difficult.

The key to surveillance is to identify each new case of dracunculiasis as soon as possible to prevent further transmission associated with that case. The goal is to detect each new case within 24 hours after the emergence of the worm and to report it to the next-level supervisor. To this end, Pakistan and India have offered cash rewards to any villager, health worker, or patient who reports cases of dracunculiasis.

The magnitude of such a village-by-village search can be appreciated by noting that persons are at risk for this disease in more than 20,000 villages in India, Pakistan, and Africa. Such searches require the mobilization of thousands of public health and other workers for several weeks for each periodic search so that all villages can be visited quickly. Once cases are located, villagers are trained to boil all drinking water or they are provided with fine cloth filters to remove infected copepods from drinking water.

Although dracunculiasis remains prevalent, such methods are beginning to show promise. For example, from June 1991 to June 1992, 201,453 cases of dracunculiasis were reported in 4576 villages in Nigeria—a decrease of 68.5% since 1988 to 1989. Moreover, in almost one fourth of infected villages, this parasite was eradicated completely. The goal in Nigeria is to eradicate dracunculiasis entirely by the end of 1995.

So, there is a light at the end of the tunnel, and it is only a matter of time before other parasitic diseases (eg, schistosomiasis) suffer a similar fate.

lymphatics to the deep subcutaneous tissues. There, they develop into adult worms. It is believed that the male worm dies after mating. About 1 year after the initial infection, the female (which can exceed a length of 100 cm) migrates to a position just beneath the skin. A local ulcer develops, exposing a loop of the worm's uterus that, on contact with water, will discharge huge numbers of motile larvae. When ingested by an appropriate copepod, these larvae undergo metamorphosis and are able to initiate a new cycle of human infection within about 3 weeks.

Systemic symptoms of vomiting, diarrhea, hives, and shortness of breath seem to result from an allergic reaction rather than from direct toxicity of the parasite. Symptoms can last for several weeks, while the female discharges her larvae, after which the worm may be expelled or may penetrate again to deeper tissues before dying. Local healing occurs at this time, and subsequent radiographs reveal calcified lesions surrounding the remains of the dead worms.

Intracutaneous injection of an extract of the worms will induce a delayed-type skin reaction, but the appearance of the worm just under the skin provides the most common means of diagnosis.

Diethylcarbamazine is an effective treatment if used early, before the larvae develop into mature worms; however, niridazole is the drug of choice for the adult parasite. This latter drug is toxic and can cause several severe reactions.

The most common technique for removing the adult guinea worm is to insert a stick into the ulcer beneath the worm and slowly turn it to wind the worm around the stick. This must be done carefully to avoid rupturing the parasite and causing secondary infections. Because only a few centimeters of the worm can be wound about the stick each day, considerable time is necessary to extract a worm 100 cm long.

The life cycle of *D medinensis* could be interrupted easily by using protected springs or wells as sources of drinking water. Water supplies can be rendered noninfectious by boiling or by filtering through cloth filters to remove infected copepods. This latter technique has resulted in a substantial decline in dracunculiasis in Africa since the international eradication campaign began in the early 1980s.

Bibliography

JOURNALS

Boros DL. Immunopathology of *Schistosoma mansoni* infection. Clin Microbiol Rev 1989;2:250.

Cherfas J. New hope for vaccine against schistosomiasis. Science 1991;251:630.

Genta RM. Dysregulation of strongyloidiasis: a new hypothesis. Clin Microbiol Rev 1992;5:345.Gottstein B. Molecular and immunological diagnosis of echinococcosis. Clin Microbiol Rev 1992;5:248.

Greene BM. Modern medicine versus an ancient scourge: progress toward control of onchocerciasis. J Infect Dis 1992;166:15.

Harms G, et al. Trichinosis: a prospective controlled study of patients ten years after acute infection. Clin Infect Dis 1993;17:637.

Maizels RM, et al. Immunological modulation and evasion by helminth parasites in human populations. Nature 1993;365:797.

Nanduri J, Kazura JW. Clinical and laboratory aspects of filariasis. Clin Microbiol Rev 1989;2:39.

Schantz PM, et al. Neurocysticercosis in an orthodox Jewish community in New York city. N Engl J Med 1992;327:692.

Steel C, et al. Immunologic responses to repeated ivermectin treatment in patients with onchocerciasis. J Infect Dis 1991;164:581.

FIGURE AND TABLE CREDITS

Unit-Opening Photos

FRONTISPIECE. A computer-generated model of an equine herpes nucleocapsid superimposed on an electron micrograph of frozen, hydrated equine herpes nucleocapsids. Magnification × 167,000. Courtesy of Tim Baker, Purdue University, William W. Newcomb and Jay Brown, University of Virginia, and Frank Booy and Alisdair Steven, National Institutes of Health.

UNIT ONE. Electron micrograph showing a plasmid released from a lysed cell of *Escherichia coli.* The plasmid is a recombinant molecule in which the *trp* operon carrying the genes for tryptophan biosynthesis has been cloned into the plasmid vecor pBR322. The plasmid, on the left, is a circular molecule of double-stranded DNA. A large number of RNA products can be seen transcribing the *trp* operon. Courtesy of S. French and O. L. Miller, Jr., University of Virginia.

UNIT TWO. Murine myeloma cell, an example of the cell type used in preparation of hybridoma cell lines for monoclonal antibodies (× 9000). Generously provided by Dr. John Herr and Mr. Donald Spell, Department of Anatomy, University of Virginia.

UNIT THREE. Bacteriophase λ. Negative stain at × 195,000. Courtesy of William W. Newcomb, University of Virginia.

UNIT FOUR. Scanning electron micrograph of *Clostridium tetani.* Magnification × 12,600.

UNIT FIVE. A mixture of herpesvirus, adenoviruses, lambda phage, and nucleocapsids of vesicular stomatitis virus. Magnification × 100,000. Courtesy of William W. Newcomb and Jay Brown, University of Virginia.

UNIT SIX. Electron micrograph of *Leishmania donovani* (× 7,700), the etiologic agent of kalaazar. Courtesy of the Central Electron Microscope Facility, University of Virginia School of Medicine.

Figures

1-1A. Bausch and Lomb, Rochester, NY

1-2A, 1-5, 3-2, 6-2, 20-1, 31-1, 31-4B. S.C. Holt, Dept. of Microbiology, University of Massachusetts, Amherst

2-3. Champe PC and Harvey RA. Biochemistry, 2nd ed. Philadelphia: JB Lippincott, 1994.

2-11. Janet Dunn-Coleman and Oscar Miller, Jr., Department of Biology, University of Virginia

4-1. Austrian R. J Exp Med 98:21, 1953

4-2, 4-3. Bainton DF. J Cell Biol 28:277-301, 1966

4-4. D.F. Bainton, Department of Pathology, University of California, San Francisco

4-6. I. Carr, Department of Pathology, University of Saskatchewan

4-8. Root RK, Rosenthal AS, Balestra DJ. J Clin Invest 51:649-665, 1972

5-3B. N.M. Green, National Institute for Medical Research, London, UK

5-6B, 5-6C. A. Feinstein, Institute for Animal Physiology, Agricultural Research Council, Cambridge, U.K.

6-4, 6-5A, 6-6. D.E. Normansell, University of Virginia School of Medicine

6-5. M.R. Greaves, Department of Zoology, University College London, U.K.

8-2. Adapted from Williams AF, Nature 314:579, 1985

12-2. Adapted from Reid KBM, Porter RR, Biochem J 155:19, 1976

13-5. Reproduced with permission. Yanelli JR et al. J Immunol

15-1A, 15-1B, 15-1D, 24-1. Z. Skobe, Forsyth Dental Center, Boston, Massachusetts

15-1C (top). L.M. Pope, Department of Microbiology, The University of Texas at Austin

15-1C (bottom), 17-1. T.J. Beveridge, Department of Bacteriology and Immunology, The University of Western Ontario

17-4. Singer DJ, Nicolson GL. Science 175:720–731, 1972 (Copyright 1972 by the American Association for the Advancement of Science)

17-9A. Rietschel ET, Ernst TH et al. Structure and conformation of the lipid: a component of lipopolysaccharides. In

Rietschel ET (ed), Handbook of Endotoxin, Vol 1: Chemistry of Endotoxin. New York: Elsevier Science Publishers, 1984

17-11E. W.L. Dentler, Department of Physiology and Cell Biology, University of Kansas, Lawrence

17-12. DePamphilis ML, Adler J. J Bacteriol 105:384–395, 1971

18-6. M. R. Greaves, Department of Zoology, University College London, U.K.

18-8. Lorian V. Time 115(16):77, 1980

21-2. C.C. Brinton, Jr., and J. Chapman, Department of Life Sciences, University of Pittsburgh

24-2, 24-3A. Krause RM. Fed Proc 29:59–65, 1970

24-3B and C. P.P. Cleary, Department of Microbiology, University of Minnesota Medical School

24-4. R.R. Facklam, Centers for Disease Control, Atlanta

24-5, 24-6B. C.A. Schnaitman, University of Virginia School of Medicine

24-6A, 25-2, 28-6, 29-5. L.J. LeBeau, Department of Pathology and Department of Microbiology, University of Illinois Hospital at the Medical Center, Chicago

24-7, 31-2. American Society for Microbiology, Washington, D.C.

25-1A, 25-4, 26-5, 29-2, 30-2, 31-2A, 34-3, 34-4, 35-3A, 35-6C (bottom), 35-10, 35-11, 35-12, 35-13B, 35-14, 35-15, 35-17 (top), 35-18, 50-9, 50-13, 51-19 (center), 51-20. Photo-Art Resource Library, Instructional Media Division, Centers for Disease Control, Atlanta

25-1B, 25-5. J.S. Hook and D. Leith, Department of Microbiology and Immunology, University of Oregon Health Sciences Center

25-3. DeVoe IW, Gilchrist JE. Infect Immun 10:872–876, 1974

26-3. I. Snyder, Department of Microbiology, West Virginia University Medical Center

26-4. D.G. Evans, Program in Infectious Diseases and Clinical Microbiology, The University of Texas Medical School

26-6. E.T. Nelson, Department of Biological Sciences, Southeastern Louisiana University

26-8. R.L. Guerrant, Department of Internal Medicine, University of Virginia School of Medicine

27-2. M.J. Tufte, Department of Biology, University of Wisconsin, Platteville

27-4. Bibel DJ, Chen TH. Bacteriol Rev 40:633–651, 1976

27-5. U.S. Army Medical Research Institute of Infectious Diseases, Fort Detrick, Frederick, MD

28-1. F.L.A. Buckmire, Department of Microbiology, The Medical College of Wisconsin

28-2. J. Mayhew, Milwaukee, WI

28-4. Flesher AR, Ito S, Mansheim BJ, Kasper DL. Ann Intern Med 90:628–630, 1979

29-1. Heckley RJ, Goldwasser E. J Infect Dis 84:92–97, 1949

29-4. V.R. Dowell, Centers for Disease Control, Atlanta

30-1. S.M. Gibson, General Bacteriology Lab., Texas Department of Health Resources, Austin

30-4. Collier RJ, Bacteriol Rev 39:54–85, 1975

31-1. R.W. Smithwick, Centers for Disease Control, Atlanta

31-4B. E.H. Runyon, Salt Lake City, UT

32-4A. Burgdorfer W. Infect Immun 2:256–259, 1970

32-5A. D. Bromley, Department of Microbiology, West Virginia University Medical Center

33-1A. Boatman ES, Kenny GE. J Bacteriol 106:1005, 1971

33-1B, 33-2. M.G. Gabridge, Department of Microbiology, University of Illinois, Urbana

33-3. Shepard MC, Howard DR. Ann NY Acad Sci 1wa74:809–819, 1970

33-4. S. Madoff (Dienes Collection), Department of Bacteriology, Massachusetts General Hospital, Boston

34-1, 34-2. W. Burdorfer, Rocky Mountain Lab., Hamilton, MT

34-5. McCaul TF, Williams JC. J Bacteriol 147:1063, 1981

34-6, 34-7. L.A. Page, National Animal Disease Center, Ames, IA

35-1. Duda J, Slack JM. J Gen Microbiol 71:63–68, 1972

35-2, 35-3B. Slack JM, Gerencser MA, Actinomyces, Filamentous Bacteria: Biology and Pathogenicity. Minneapolis: Burgess Publishing Co, 1975

35-4, 35-9. Sinski JR. Dermatophytes in Human Skin, Hair and Nails. Springfield, IL: Charles C. Thomas, 1974

35-5A, 35-6A, 35-6C (top), 35-7, 35-8. Copyright Carroll H. Weiss, RBP, 1978

35-13A. Dolan CT et al. Atlases of Clinical Mycology II: Systemic Mycosis—Deep Seated. Chicago: American Society of Clinical Pathologist, 1975

35-16. Dolan CT et al. Atlases of Clinical Mycology I: Systemic Mycosis—Yeasts. Chicago: American Society of Clinical Pathologists, 1975

35-17 (bottom). F. Marsik, Department of Clinical Pathology, University of Virginia School of Medicine

36-2. Uricult, Medical Technology Corp, Hackensack, NJ

36-3. Blundell GP. In Stefanini M (ed). Progress in Clinical Pathology, Vol 3. New York: Grune & Stratton, 1970

38-1. Horne RW et al. J Mol Biol 1:84–86, 1959

38-3A. G. Wertz, Department of Bacteriology and Immunology, School of Medicine, The University of North Carolina at Chapel Hill

38-3B. J.W. Heine, Department of Medical Viral Oncology, Roswell Park Memorial Institute, Buffalo, NY

38-6A, 40-1, 40-4. B. Roizman, Committee on Virology, The University of Chicago

38-6B. J.J. Cardamone, Jr. and J.S. Youngner, Department of Microbiology, University of Pittsburgh School of Medicine

39-3. J.S. Lazuick and W.S. Archibald, Vector-Borne Diseases Division, Center for Disease Control, Ft. Collins, CO

39-5. D.J. Muth and W.S. Archibald, Vector-Borne Diseases Division, Center for Disease Control, Ft. Collins, CO

39-6, 42-1. 46-4, 48-5A, 48-6, 49-3. F.A. Murphy, Centers for Disease Control, Atlanta

41-1. R.C. Williams, Virus Laboratory, University of California, Berkeley

41-4B. Valentine RC, Pereira HG. J Mol Biol 13:13–20, 1965

41-6. Adapted from Lechner RL, Kelly TJ. Cell 12:1007, 1977

42-2B. Morgan C. Science 193:591–592, 1976 (Copyright 1976 by The American Association for the Advancement of Science)

43-2A, 43-2B. G.H. Smith, Lab Molecular Biology, National Cancer Institute, Bethesda, MD

43-2C. N. Salomonsky and J.T. Parsons, University of Virginia School of Medicine

43-3. Adapted from Gilboa E et al. Cell 18:93–100, 1979

44-2. J. Griffith, Department of Biochemistry, Stanford University School of Medicine

45-4, 45-5. Adapted from Summers J, Mason WS. Cell 29:403, 1982

46-1B. B.A. Phillips, Department of Microbiology, University of Pittsburgh School of Medicine

47-2. Compans RW, Dimmock NJ. Virology 39:499–515, 1969

48-5B. Compans RW et al. Virology 30:411–426, 1966

49-1. N. Salomonsky, Department of Microbiology, University of Virginia School of Medicine

49-4. Murphy FA, Whitfield SG. Bull WHO 52:409–419, 1975

49-5. Johnson KM, Webb PA, Justines G. In Lehmann-Grube F (ed): Lymphocytic Choriomeningitis: Virus and Other Arena Viruses. New York: Springer-Verlag, 1973

50-1A. D.L. Taylor, Department of Biology, Harvard University

50-1B. J.J. Paulin and A. Steiner, Department of Zoology, University of Georgia

50-8 (center). J.J. Paulin, Department of Zoology, University of Georgia

Tables

9-1. Adapted from Heidelberger M, Kendall FE. J Exp Med 62:697–720, 1935

20-1. Benveniste R, Davies J. Ann Rev Biochem 42:471–506, 1973

24-5. MMWR Oct 11, 1975

26-4. World Health Organization International, Reference Centre for Salmonella, Pasteur Institute, Paris

26-5, 26-6. Pavlovskis OR, Callahan LT III, Pollack M. In Schlessinger D (ed), Microbiology 1975. Washington DC, American Society for Microbiology, 1975

26-7. Iglewski BH, Kabat D. Proc Nat Acad Sci USA 72:2284–2288, 1975

26-8. Bennett JV. J Infect Dis 130(suppl):S4–S7, 1974

27-2. MMWR September 24, 1976

29-2. MMWR June 22, 1974

29-3. Davis BD et al. Microbiology, 2nd ed. Hagerstown: Harper & Row, 1973

30-2. Data from Centers for Disease Control, Atlanta

31-2. After Arnold HL Jr, Fasal P. Leprosy: Diagnosis and Management, 2nd ed. Springfield IL: Charles C. Thomas, 1973

34-1. Ormsbee RA. In Lennette EH, Spaulding EH, Truant JP (eds), Manual of Clinical Microbiology, 2nd ed. Washington DC: American Society for Microbiology, 1974

35-3. Adapted from Saito M, Enomoto M, Tatsuno T. In Ciegler A, Kadis S, Ajl SJ (eds), Microbial Toxins, Vol 6. New York: Academic Press, 1971

36-1. Isenberg HD, Berkman JI. In Stefanini M (ed), Progress in Clinical Pathology, Vol 1. New York: Grune & Stratton, 1966

36-2, 36-6. Isenberg HD, Washington JA II, Balows A, Sonnenwirth AC. In Lennette EH, Spaulding EH, Truant JP (eds), Manual of Clinical Microbiology, 2nd ed. Washington DC: American Society for Microbiology, 1974

36-4, 36-5. Sutter VL, Finegold SM. In Stefanini M (ed), Progress in Clinical Pathology, Vol 5. New York: Grune & Stratton, 1973

40-1. Herpesvirus Study Group, International Committee

for the Nomenclature of Viruses. J Gen Virol 20:417–419, 1973

40-2. Davidson I, Henry JB. Clinical Diagnosis by Laboratory Methods, 14th ed. Philadelphia: WB Saunders, 1969

42-2. MMWR November 1984

45-2. MMWR December 23, 1972

50-1. Medical Protozoology and Helminthology. Bethesda, US Naval Medical School, National Naval Medical Center, 1962

Cover Art

Computer drawn figure of herpes simplex virus. Courtesy of Professor Jay Brown, Department of Microbiology, University of Virginia

INDEX

Page numbers followed by f *indicate figures; page numbers followed by* t *indicate tabular material.*

Nalidixic acid, mechanism of action, 267

Nannizzia, 480

Nasopharyngeal carcinoma, 527, 546, 555–556

Nasopharyngeal cultures, 499

Natural killer (NK) cells, 170, 176
  properties of, 171*t*
  in tumor immunity, 189

Natural selection theory, of antibody formation, 43

Necator americanus, 687–688, 688*f*

nef gene, in HIV, 585

Negri body, 539, 540*f*, 639, 641*f*

Neisseria
  growth characteristics of, 498*t*
  morphology of, 348, 349*f*
  in normal flora, 496*t*
  nutrition of, 348–349
  oxidase test for, 349, 349*f*
  protease, 349

Neisseriaceae, 348–358

Neisseria flavescens, growth characteristics of, 352*t*

Neisseria gonorrhoeae, 206*t*, 348, 352–357, 399
  antibiotic sensitivity, 244
  antigenic classification of, 353–355
  colony types of, 353, 353*f*
  fimbriae, 324
  fimbrial phase variation, 311
  growth characteristics of, 352*t*, 498*t*
  immune evasion, 283–284, 311
  outer membrane proteins, 354–355
  penicillin resistance in, 356–357
  pili, 353*f*, 353–354, 355
  protein II, 283, 311
  virulence factors, 355

Neisseria meningitidis, 206*t*, 316, 348, 349–352, 399
  antigenic classification of, 350, 350*t*
  growth characteristics of, 351–352, 352*t*, 498*t*
  identification of, 499, 499*t*, 500
  infections
    epidemiology of, 350
    laboratory diagnosis of, 351–352, 352*t*
    pathogenesis of, 350–351, 351*f*
    prevention of, 352
    spectrum of, 351
    treatment of, 352
  meningitis, 328, 499
  oxidase test for, 349, 349*f*
  serotyping of, 350, 350*t*
  vaccine, 352

Neisseria sicca, 357
  growth characteristics of, 352*t*

Neisseria subflava, 357

Nematoda, 672

Nematodes, 682–692
  blood and tissue, 688–692
  intestinal, 682–688

Neomycin
  mechanism of action, 271
  structure of, 270*f*

Neoplasia
  autocrine growth factors in, 595
  chromosomal amplification in, 595
  chromosomal defects in, 593, 593*t*
  chromosomal translocations in, 593–595, 594*f*

Nephritis, complex, 186

Nephropathia epidemica, 625

Netilmicin, mechanism of action, 271

Neuraminidase, 521, 528
  influenza virus, 630*f*, 630–631
  orthomyxovirus, 626, 628
  paramyxovirus, 632–633, 633*t*

Neuroblastoma, chromosomal amplification in, 595

Neurotoxin(s), 326

Neutrophil(s), 49
  impaired intracellular killing in, 54–56

Niclosamide, 673, 675, 676, 677

Nifurtimox, 662

NIH-3T3-DNA transfection assay, 592*f*, 592–593

Nitric oxide, 228, 335

Nitrofurans, mechanism of action, 272

Nitrofurantoin, mechanism of action, 272

N-linked glycosylation, 12

Nocardia, 476–477
  of medical importance, 206*t*

Nocardia asteroides, 206*t*, 476, 477*f*

Nocardia brasiliensis, 476, 477

Nocardia caviae, 476

Nocardioses, human
  control of, 477
  diagnosis of, 476–477
  epidemiology of, 476
  pathogenesis of, 476
  treatment of, 477

Non-A, non-B hepatitis, 605–606

Nonactivator surface, 163, 164*f*

Nongonococcal urethritis
  chlamydial, 468, 469, 471
  Ureaplasma urealyticum, 455–456

Nonphotochromogens, mycobacterial, 436–437

Nonsense mutations, 18

Normal flora, 315–317, 319*t*
  of digestive tract, 318
  of eye, 317, 319*t*
  of genitourinary tract, 318, 319*t*
  of respiratory tract, 317–318, 319*t*
  of skin, 317, 319*t*
  spirochetes in, 440
  of vagina, 318, 319*t*

North American blastomycosis. *See* Blastomycosis

Norwalk-like virus, 528, 613–614

Norwalk virus, 528, 613–614
  infection
    control of, 613–614
    diagnosis of, 613–614
    epidemiology of, 613
    pathogenesis of, 613
  properties of, 524*t*
  replication, 613
  structure of, 613

Nosocomial infection(s), 314

Novobiocin, mechanism of action, 267

N-*ras* gene, 589*t*, 590
  activation of, 593

N-Region addition, in B cells, 109–110

Nuclear oncogenes, 589*t*, 591–592

Nucleic acid hybridization techniques, 20, 22*f*, 205–207
  for viral assay, 536*f*, 538

Nucleic acid probes, 209–210

Nucleic acids
  structure of, 14–16, 15*f*
    antibiotics acting on, 266–267
  synthesis of, 266–268
    antibiotics acting on, 266–268

Nucleoprotein hypothesis, of prions, 648

Nucleosomes, 25, 26*f*

Nucleotide bases, 14–16, 15*f*

Nucleus, eucaryotic cell, 8, 10*f*

Nutrition, protozoan, 652

Nystatin, 484
  mechanism of action, 262

O

O antigen, 361. *See also* Lipopolysaccharide, O-specific polysaccharide side chains (O antigen)
  Salmonella, 370, 370*t*

Ochratoxins, 493

Okazaki fragments, 26

Old tuberculin, 168

2′,5′-Oligoadenylate synthetase, interferon-induced, 543

OmpA protein, 242

Omsk hemorrhagic fever, 620

onc genes, in oncoviruses, 577, 578*f*

Onchocerca dermatitis, 690–691

Onchocerca volvulus, 688, 690*f*, 690–691

Onchocerciasis, 690–691

Oncofetal antigens, 187–188

Oncogene(s). *See also specific gene*
  acquisition by defective, acute transforming retroviruses (oncogene capture), 579, 592
  activation of, 592–595
    chromosomal translocations and neoplasia and, 593–595
  and cancer, 588–597
  cellular, 187
  c-*myc*
    activation, 556
    in lymphoma, 556
  families of, 589–592
  insertional activation of, 580, 592
  molecular cloning of, 592, 592*f*
  nuclear, 589*t*, 591–592
  ras family, 589*t*, 590–591
  recessive, 595–597
  retroviral, origin of, 580
  tyrosine kinase family, 589, 589*t*, 590
  viral
    cellular homolgues of, 588–589, 589*t*